DICTIONARY OF
MEDICINE

third edition

Titles in the series

Workbooks

Visit our web site for full details of all our books

http://www.petercollin.com

DICTIONARY OF
MEDICINE

third edition

P.H. Collin

PP

PETER COLLIN PUBLISHING

First published in Great Britain 1987
as *English Medical Dictionary*
Second edition published 1993
Third edition published 2000

Published by Peter Collin Publishing Ltd
1 Cambridge Road, Teddington, Middlesex, TW11 8DT

British Library Cataloguing-in-Publication Data

A catalogue record for this book is available from the British Library

ISBN 1-901659-45-3

Text computer typeset by PCP
Printed and bound by Creative Print and Design
Cover artwork by Gary Weston

PREFACE TO THE FIRST EDITION

This dictionary provides the user with the basic vocabulary used in British and American medical practice. The subject matter covers terms used in surgery, general practice, hospitals, nursing, pharmacy, dentistry and other specializations. The level of language varies from the very technical to informal usage as between professionals or between professionals and patients.

Each of the 12,000 headwords is defined in simple English, using a limited vocabulary of 500 words over and above those words which actually appear in the dictionary as main words. Very many examples are given to show how the words and phrases are used in context, and many of the more difficult phrases are also explained in simple and clear English. Words which pose particular grammatical problems have short grammar notes attached, giving irregular forms, and notes on constructions, together with differences between British and American English where appropriate. Comments are also given for many words with notes on symptoms and treatment, as well as more encyclopaedic information. Some of the anatomical features are illustrated by line drawings. Also included in the text are quotations from medical journals and magazines from various parts of the world to show how the language is used in practice.

At the back of the book are a series of supplements which give useful information in tabular form: these refer to vitamins, incubation periods, SI equivalents, diets, and notes on eponymous words.

Very many people have helped or advised on the compilation and checking of this dictionary: in particular we would like to thank G. H. Hooton (who provided most of the supplementary material), Erica Ison, Dr. G. Lewis and Dr. D. W. Macintosh. Illustrations are by SM Design.

PREFACE TO THE SECOND EDITION

The text of the original edition has been entirely revised and updated, with the addition of many new entries. We are grateful again to G. H. Hooton for his contributions, and to Hazel Curties who provided much new material.

PREFACE TO THE THIRD EDITION

Again the text of the previous edition has been revised and updated, with the addition of many new items. We are particularly grateful to Dr Ruth Maxwell for her contributions to the new text, as well as new material for the supplement.

Because the pronunciation of some specialized words can cause problems, we have added the phonetic transcription of all the main words, using the International Phonetic Alphabet.

Phonetics

The following symbols have been used to show the pronunciation of the main words in the dictionary.

Stress has been indicated by a main stress mark ('), but these are only guides as the stress of the word may change according to its position in the sentence.

Vowels			*Consonants*	
æ	back		b	buck
ɑː	harm		d	dead
ɒ	stop		ð	other
aɪ	type		dʒ	jump
aʊ	how		f	fare
aɪə	hire		g	gold
aʊə	hour		h	head
ɔː	course		j	yellow
ɔɪ	loyalty		k	cab
e	head		l	leave
eə	fair		m	mix
eɪ	make		n	nil
ə	abroad		ŋ	bring
əʊ	float		p	post
əʊə	lower		r	rule
ɜː	word		s	save
iː	keep		ʃ	shop
ɪ	fit		t	take
ɪə	near		tʃ	change
u	supreme		χ	loch
uː	pool		θ	theft
ʊ	book		v	value
ʌ	shut		w	work
			z	zone
			ʒ	measure

Aa

AA = ALCOHOLICS ANONYMOUS

A & E ['eɪ ənd 'iː] = ACCIDENT AND EMERGENCY; *A & E department*; *an A & E ward*; *A & E nurses*

Vitamin A ['vɪtəmɪn 'eɪ] *noun* retinol, a vitamin which is soluble in fat and can be formed in the body from precursors but is mainly found in food, such as liver, vegetables, eggs and cod liver oil.

> COMMENT: Lack of Vitamin A affects the body's growth and resistance to disease and can cause night blindness or xerophthalmia. Carotene (the yellow substance in carrots) is a precursor of Vitamin A, which accounts for the saying that eating carrots helps you to see in the dark

A band ['eɪ 'bænd] *noun* part of the pattern in muscle tissue, seen through a microscope as a dark band

ABC ['eɪ 'biː 'siː] *abbreviation for* Airway, Breathing and Circulation: the basic initial checks of a casualty's condition

ab- [æb] *prefix meaning* away from

abdomen ['æbdəmən] *noun* space in front of the body below the diaphragm and above the pelvis, containing the stomach, intestines, liver and other vital organs; *pain in the abdomen*; **acute abdomen** = any serious condition of the abdomen which requires surgery

> COMMENT: the abdomen is divided for medical purposes into nine regions: at the top, the right and left hypochondriac regions with the epigastrium between them; in the centre, the right and left lumbar regions with the umbilical between them; and at the bottom, the right and left iliac regions with the hypogastrium between them

abdomin(o)- [æb'dɒmɪn(ə)] *prefix* referring to the abdomen

abdominal [æb'dɒmɪnəl] *adjective* referring to the abdomen; **abdominal aorta** = *see* AORTA; **abdominal cavity** = space in the body below the chest; **abdominal distension** = condition where the abdomen is stretched (because of gas or fluid); **abdominal pain** = pain in the abdomen caused by indigestion or more serious disorders; **abdominal viscera** = organs contained in the abdomen (such as the stomach, liver, etc.); **abdominal wall** = muscular tissue which surrounds the abdomen

abdominoperineal excision [æb'dɒmɪnəuperɪ'niːəl ɪk'sɪʒn] *noun* cutting out of tissue in both the abdomen and the perineum

abdominoscopy [æbdɒmɪ'nɒskəpi] *noun* internal examination of the abdomen, usually with an endoscope

abdominothoracic [æbdɒmɪnəuθɔː'ræsɪk] *adjective* referring to the abdomen and thorax (NOTE: for other terms referring to the abdomen, see words beginning with **coeli-**)

abducens *or* **abducent nerve** [æb'djuːsens *or* æb'djuːsənt 'nɜːv] *noun* sixth cranial nerve, which controls the muscle which makes the eyeball turn outwards

abduct [æb'dʌkt] *verb* to pull away from the centre line of the body; **vocal folds abducted** = normal condition of the vocal cords in quiet breathing (NOTE: the opposite is **adduct**)

abduction [æb'dʌkʃn] *noun* movement of part of the body away from the midline or away from a neighbouring part (NOTE: the opposite is **adduction**)

> Mary was nursed in a position of not more than 90° upright with her legs in abduction
> *British Journal of Nursing*

abductor (muscle) [æb'dʌktə 'mʌsl] *noun* muscle which pulls a part of the body away from the midline of the body or from a neighbouring part (NOTE: the opposite is **adductor**)

aberrant [æ'berənt] *adjective* not normal

aberration [æbə'reɪʃn] *noun* action or growth which is not normal; **chromosome** *or* **chromosomal aberration** = abnormality in the number, arrangement, etc. of chromosomes; **mental aberration** = slight forgetfulness, slightly abnormal mental process

ability [ə'bɪləti] *noun* being able to do something

ablation [æ'bleɪʃn] *noun* removal of an organ or of part of the body by surgery; **segmental ablation** = surgical removal of part of a nail, as treatment for an ingrowing toenail

able ['eɪbl] *adjective* **after the injection he was able to breathe more easily** = he could breathe more easily (NOTE: the opposite is **unable**. Note also that **able** is used with **to** and a verb)

abnormal [æb'nɔːməl] *adjective* not normal; **abnormal behaviour** = conduct which is different from the way normal people behave; **abnormal motion** *or* **abnormal stool** = faeces which are different in colour, which are very liquid

> the synovium produces an excess of synovial fluid, which is abnormal and becomes thickened. This causes pain, swelling and immobility of the affected joint
>
> *Nursing Times*

abnormality [æbnɔː'mæləti] *noun* form or action which is not normal

> Even children with the milder forms of sickle-cell disease have an increased frequency of pneumococcal infection. The reason for this susceptibility is a profound abnormality of the immune system in children with SCD
>
> *Lancet*

abnormally [æb'nɔːməli] *adverb* in a way which is not normal; *he had an abnormally fast pulse*; *her periods were abnormally frequent* (NOTE: for other terms referring to abnormality, see words beginning with **terat-**)

abocclusion [æbɒ'kluːʒn] *noun (dentistry)* condition where the teeth in the top and bottom jaws do not touch

abort [ə'bɔːt] *verb* (i) to eject the embryo or fetus and so end a pregnancy before the fetus is fully developed; (ii) to have an abortion; *the doctors decided to abort the fetus*; *the tissue will be aborted spontaneously*

abortifacient [əbɔːtɪ'feɪʃnt] *noun* drug which provokes an abortion

abortion [ə'bɔːʃn] *noun* situation where an unborn baby leaves the uterus before the end of pregnancy, especially during the first twenty-eight weeks of pregnancy when it is not likely to survive birth; **to have an abortion** = to have an operation to make a fetus leave the uterus during the first period of pregnancy; *the girl asked the clinic if she could have an abortion*; *she had two abortions before her first child was born*; **complete abortion** = abortion where the whole contents of the uterus are expelled; **criminal abortion** *or* **illegal abortion** = abortion which is carried out illegally; **habitual abortion** *or* **recurrent abortion** = condition where a woman has several miscarriages with successive pregnancies; **incomplete abortion** = abortion where part of the contents of the uterus is not expelled; **induced abortion** = abortion which is produced by drugs or by surgery; **legal abortion** = abortion which is carried out legally; **spontaneous abortion** = MISCARRIAGE; **therapeutic abortion** = abortion which is carried out because the health of the mother is in danger; **threatened abortion** = possible abortion in the early stages of pregnancy, indicated by bleeding

> COMMENT: in the UK an abortion can be carried out legally if two doctors agree that the mother's life is in danger, that she risks grave permanent injury to the physical or mental health of herself or her children, or that the fetus is likely to be born with severe handicaps

abortionist [ə'bɔːʃənɪst] *noun* person who makes a woman abort, usually a person who performs an illegal abortion

abortive [ə'bɔːtɪv] *adjective* which does not succeed; **abortive poliomyelitis** = mild form of polio which only affects the throat and intestines

abortus fever [ə'bɔːtəs 'fiːvə] *noun* brucellosis, a disease which can be caught from cattle, or from drinking infected milk, spread by a species of the bacterium Brucella

COMMENT: symptoms include tiredness, arthritis, headaches, sweating and swelling of the spleen

ABO system [ˈeɪ ˈbiː ˈəʊ ˈsɪstəm] *noun* system of classifying blood groups; *see note at* BLOOD GROUP

above [əˈbʌv] *preposition & adverb* higher than; *his temperature was above 100 degrees*; *her pulse rate was far above normal*; *babies aged six months and above*

abrasion [əˈbreɪʒn] *noun* condition where the surface of the skin has been rubbed off by a rough surface and bleeds

COMMENT: as the intact skin is an efficient barrier to bacteria, even minor abrasions can allow infection to enter the body and thus should be cleaned and treated with an antiseptic

abreaction [æbriˈækʃn] *noun* (*in psychology*) treatment of a neurotic patient by making him think again about past bad experiences

abscess [ˈæbses] *noun* painful swollen area where pus forms, often accompanied by high temperature; *he had an abscess under a tooth*; *the doctor decided to lance the abscess*; **acute abscess** = abscess which develops rapidly; **chronic abscess** = abscess which develops slowly over a period of time (NOTE: the plural is **abscesses**)

COMMENT: an acute abscess can be dealt with by opening and draining when it has reached the stage where sufficient pus has been formed; a chronic abscess is usually treated with drugs

absence [ˈæbsəns] *noun* not being here or there; **in the absence of any other symptoms** = because no other symptoms are present

absent [ˈæbsənt] *adjective* not here, not there; *normal symptoms of malaria are absent in this form of the disease*; *three children are absent because they are ill*

absolutely [ˈæbsəluːtli] *adverb* really, completely; *he's still not absolutely fit after his operation*; *the patient must remain absolutely still while the scan is taking place*

absorb [əbˈzɔːb] *verb* to take in (a liquid); *cotton wads are used to absorb the discharge from the wound*

absorbable suture [əbˈzɔːbəbl ˈsuːtʃə] *noun* suture which will eventually be absorbed into the body, and does not need to be removed

absorbent [əbˈzɔːbənt] *adjective* which absorbs; **absorbent cotton** = soft white stuff used as a dressing to put on wounds

absorption [əbˈzɔːpʃn] *noun* (i) action of taking a liquid into a solid; (ii) taking substances into the body, such as proteins or fats which have been digested from food and are taken into the bloodstream from the stomach and intestines; **absorption rate** = rate at which a liquid is absorbed by a solid; **percutaneous absorption** = absorbing a substance through the skin (NOTE: the spellings: **absorb** but **absorption**)

abstain [əbˈsteɪn] *verb* not to do something voluntarily; *he abstained from taking any drugs for two months*; *they decided to abstain from sexual intercourse*

abstainer [əbˈsteɪnə] *noun* person who does not drink alcohol

abstinence [ˈæbstɪnəns] *noun* not doing something voluntarily; *the clinic recommended total abstinence from alcohol or from drugs*

abulia [əˈbuːliə] *noun* lack of willpower

abuse 1 [əˈbjuːs] *noun* (**a**) using something wrongly; **alcohol abuse** *or* **amphetamine abuse** *or* **drug abuse** *or* **solvent abuse** = being mentally and physically dependent on regularly taking alcohol, amphetamines, drugs or on inhaling solvents (**b**) bad treatment of a person; *child abuse or sexual abuse of children* (NOTE: no plural) **2** [əˈbjuːz] *verb* (**a**) to use something wrongly; *heroin and cocaine are commonly abused drugs*; **to abuse one's authority** = to use one's powers in an illegal or harmful way (**b**) to treat someone badly; *he had sexually abused small children*

a.c. [ˈeɪ siː] *abbreviation of* 'ante cibum': meaning 'before food' (used on prescriptions)

acanthosis [əkənˈθəʊsɪs] *noun* disease of the prickle cell layer of the skin, where warts appear on the skin or inside the mouth

acaricide [əˈkærɪsaɪd] *noun* substance which kills mites

acatalasia [ækætəˈleɪziə] *noun* inherited condition which results in a defect of catalase in all tissue

accelerate [əkˈseləreɪt] *verb* to go faster, make something go faster

acceleration [əkselə'reɪʃn] *noun* going faster, making something go faster; *the nurse noticed an acceleration in the patient's pulse rate*

accentuate [ək'sentjueɪt] *verb* to make stronger; *to accentuate pain*

accessory [ək'sesəri] *adjective* (thing) which helps, without being most important; **accessory nerve** = eleventh cranial nerve which supplies the muscles in the neck and shoulders; **accessory organ** = organ which has a function which is controlled by another organ

accident ['æksɪdənt] *noun* (a) something which happens by chance; *I met her by accident at the bus stop* (b) unpleasant event which happens suddenly and harms someone's health; *she had an accident in the kitchen and had to go to hospital*; *three people were killed in the accident on the motorway*; **accident and emergency department (A & E)** = department of a hospital which deals with accidents and emergency cases; **accident prevention** = taking steps to prevent accidents from happening; **accident ward** = ward in a hospital for victims of accidents

accidentally [æksɪ'dentəli] *adverb* (a) by chance; *I found the missing watch accidentally* (b) in an accident; *he was killed accidentally*

accident-prone ['æksɪdənt'prəun] *adjective* (person) who has awkward movements and frequently has or causes minor accidents

accommodation (reflex) [əkɒmə'deɪʃn] *noun (of the lens of the eye)* ability to focus on objects at different distances, using the ciliary muscle

accommodative squint [əkɒmə'deɪtɪv 'skwɪnt] *noun* squint when the eye is trying to focus on an object which is very close

accompany [ə'kʌmpni] *verb* to go with; *he accompanied his wife to hospital*; *the pain was accompanied by high temperature*

according to [ə'kɔːdɪŋ 'tʊ] *preposition* as someone says or writes; *according to the dosage on the bottle, the medicine can be given to very young children*

accretion [ə'kriːʃn] *noun* growth of a substance which sticks to an object; *an accretion of calcium round the joint*

accumulate [ə'kjuːmjəleɪt] *verb* to grow together in a group; *large quantities of fat accumulated in the arteries*

accumulation [əkjuːmjə'leɪʃn] *noun* (i) act of accumulating; (ii) material which has accumulated; *the drug aims at clearing the accumulation of fatty deposits in the arteries*

accurate ['ækjərət] *adjective* very correct; *the sphygmomanometer does not seem to be giving an accurate reading*; *the scan helped to give an accurate location for the operation site*; *the results of the lab tests should help the consultant make an accurate diagnosis*

accurately ['ækjərətli] *adverb* very correctly; *the GP accurately diagnosed a brain tumour*

ACE inhibitor = ANGIOTENSIN-CONVERTING ENZYME INHIBITOR

acephalus ['eɪsefələs] *noun* fetus born without a head

acetabuloplasty [æsɪ'tæbjʊləuplæsti] *noun* surgical operation to repair or rebuild the acetabulum

acetabulum [æsɪ'tæbjʊləm] *noun* the cotyloid cavity, the part of the pelvic bone, shaped like a cup, into which the head of the femur fits to form the hip joint (NOTE: the plural is **acetabula**)

acetic acid [ə'siːtɪk 'æsɪd] *noun* acid which turns wine into vinegar

> COMMENT: a weak solution of acetic acid can be used to cool the body in hot weather; a strong solution can be used to burn away warts

acetonaemia [əsiːtəʊ'niːmiə] = KETONAEMIA

acetone ['æsɪtəʊn] *noun* colourless, volatile substance, used in nail varnish, also formed in the body after vomiting or during diabetes; *see also* KETONE

acetonuria [əsiːtəʊ'njuːriə] *noun* presence of acetone in the urine, giving off a sweet smell

acetylcholine [æsɪtaɪl'kəʊliːn] *noun* substance released from nerve endings, which allows nerve impulses to move from one nerve to another or from a nerve to the organ it controls. Found in nerves of the sympathetic and parasympathetic divisions of the autonomic nervous system

acetylsalicylic acid [æsɪtaɪlsæləˈsɪlɪk ˈæsɪd] *noun see* ASPIRIN

achalasia [ækəˈleɪzɪə] *noun* being unable to relax the muscles; **cardiac achalasia** *or* **achalasia of the cardia** = being unable to relax the cardia (the muscle at the entrance to the stomach), with the result that food cannot enter the stomach; *see also* CARDIOMYOTOMY

ache [eɪk] **1** *noun* pain which goes on for a time, but is not very acute; *he complained of various aches and pains*; *used with other words to show where the pain is situated: see* BACKACHE, HEADACHE, STOMACH ACHE, TOOTHACHE **2** *verb* to have a pain in part of the body; *his tooth ached so much he went to the dentist*

Achilles tendon [əˈkɪliːz ˈtendən] *noun* tendon at the back of the ankle which connects the calf muscles to the heel and which acts to pull up the heel when the calf muscle is contracted

achillorrhaphy [əkɪˈlɔːrəfi] *noun* surgical operation to stitch a torn Achilles tendon

achillotomy [əkɪˈlɒtəmi] *noun* act of dividing the Achilles tendon

aching [ˈeɪkɪŋ] *adjective* with a continuous pain

achlorhydria [eɪklɔːˈhaɪdrɪə] *noun* condition where the gastric juices do not contain hydrochloric acid, a symptom of stomach cancer or pernicious anaemia

acholia [eɪˈkəʊlɪə] *noun* absence of bile

acholuria [eɪkɒˈluːrɪə] *noun* absence of bile colouring in the urine

acholuric jaundice [ækəˈluːrɪk ˈdʒɔːndɪs] *noun* hereditary spherocytosis, a disease where abnormally round red blood cells form, leading to anaemia, enlarged spleen and the formation of gallstones

achondroplasia [eɪkɒndrəˈpleɪzɪə] *noun* hereditary condition where the long bones in the arms and legs do not grow fully, while the rest of the bones in the body do so, producing dwarfism

acid [ˈæsɪd] *noun* **(a)** chemical compound containing hydrogen, which reacts with an alkali to form a salt and water; *hydrochloric acid is secreted in the stomach and forms part of the gastric juices*; **bile acids** = acids (such as cholic acid) found in the bile; **inorganic acids** = acids which come from minerals, used in dilute form to help indigestion; **organic acids** = acids which

come from plants, taken to stimulate the production of urine **(b)** any bitter juice

acidity [əˈsɪdəti] *noun* **(a)** level of acid in a liquid; *the alkaline solution may help to reduce acidity* **(b)** acid stomach, a form of indigestion where the patient has a burning feeling in his stomach caused by too much acid forming there

acidosis [æsɪˈdəʊsɪs] *noun* **(a)** condition when there are more acid waste products (such as urea) than normal in the blood because of a lack of alkali; **metabolic acidosis** = acidosis caused by a defect in the body's metabolism **(b)** = ACIDITY

acid stomach [ˈæsɪd ˈstʌmək] = ACIDITY

acinus [ˈæsɪnəs] *noun* (i) tiny alveolus which forms part of a gland; (ii) part of a lobule in the lung (NOTE: the plural is **acini**)

acne *or* **acne vulgaris** [ˈækni] *noun* inflammation of the sebaceous glands during puberty, which makes blackheads appear on the skin, usually on the face, neck and shoulders, and these then become infected; *he suffers from acne*; *she is using a cream to clear up her acne*

acoustic [eˈkuːstɪk] *adjective* referring to sound or hearing; **acoustic nerve** = *see* NERVE; **acoustic neurofibroma** *or* **acoustic neuroma** = tumour in the sheath of the auditory nerve, causing deafness

acquired [əˈkwaɪəd] *adjective* (condition) which is neither congenital nor hereditary and which a person develops after birth in reaction to his environment; **acquired immunity** = immunity which a body acquires and which is not congenital; **acquired immunodeficiency syndrome** *or* **acquired immune deficiency syndrome** = AIDS; *see also* CONGENITAL, HEREDITARY

acro- [ˈækrəʊ] *prefix* referring to a point or tip

acrocyanosis [ækrəʊsaɪəˈnəʊsɪs] *noun* blue colour of the extremities (fingers, toes, ears and nose) due to bad circulation

acrodynia [ækrəʊˈdɪnɪə] *noun* pink disease, a children's disease where the child's hands, feet and face swell and become pink, with a fever and loss of appetite, caused by allergy to mercury

acromegaly [ækrəʊˈmegəli] *noun* disease caused by excessive quantities of growth hormone produced by the pituitary gland, causing a slow enlargement of the hands, feet and jaws in adults

acromial [ə'krəʊmiəl] *adjective* referring to the acromion; **coraco-acromial** = referring to both the coracoid process and the acromion

acromion [ə'krəʊmiən] *noun* pointed top of the scapula, which forms the tip of the shoulder; *see illustrations at* SHOULDER, SKELETON

acronyx ['ækrɒnɪks or 'eɪkrɒnɪks] *noun (of a nail)* growing into the flesh

acroparaesthesia [ækrəʊpærɪs'θiːziə] *noun* condition where the patient suffers sharp pains in the arms and numbness in the fingers after sleep

acrophobia [ækrə'fəʊbiə] *noun* fear of heights

acrosclerosis [ækrəʊskle'rəʊsɪs] *noun* sclerosis which affects the extremities

act [ækt] *verb* to do something, to have the effect of; *the connecting tissue acts as a supporting framework*; *he had to act quickly to save his sister*

ACTH = ADRENOCORTICOTROPHIC HORMONE

actin ['æktɪn] *noun* protein which, with myosin, forms the contractile tissue of muscle

actinomycosis [æktɪnəmaɪ'kəʊsɪs] *noun* disease transmitted by cattle, where the patient is infected with fungus which forms abscesses in the mouth and lungs (pulmonary actinomycosis) or in the ileum (intestinal actinomycosis)

action ['ækʃn] *noun* something which is done, effect; *the injection will speed up the action of the antibiotic*

activate ['æktɪveɪt] *verb* to make something start to work; *the muscle activates the heart*; *hormones from the pituitary gland activate other glands*

active ['æktɪv] *adjective* **(a)** *(of person)* lively, energetic; *although he is over eighty he is still very active*; **active movement** = movement made by a patient using his own willpower and muscles **(b)** *(of disease)* which affects a patient, which is not dormant; *after two years of active rheumatoid disease* **(c)** which acts, does something; **active ingredient** = main medicinal ingredient of an ointment or lotion (as opposed to the base); **active principle** = main medicinal ingredient of a drug which makes it have the required effect on a patient

activity [æk'tɪvəti] *noun* what something does; *the drug's activity did not last more than a few hours*; **antibacterial activity** = effective action against bacteria; **activities of daily living** = scale used by geriatricians and occupational therapists to assess the capacity of elderly or disabled patients to live independently

actomyosin [æktəʊ'maɪəsɪn] *noun* combination of actin and myosin, which forms the contractile tissue of muscle

act on *or* **upon** ['ækt or ɑ'pɒn] *verb* **(a)** to do something as the result of something which has been said; *he acted upon your suggestion* **(b)** to have an effect on; *the antibiotic acted quickly on the infection*

actual ['æktʃuəl] *adjective* real; *what are the actual figures for the number of children in school?*

actually ['æktʃəli] *adverb* really; *is he actually going to discharge himself from the hospital?*

acuity [ə'kjuːəti] *noun* sharpness; **auditory acuity** = being able to hear sounds clearly; **visual acuity** = being able to see objects clearly

acupressure [ækju'preʃə] *noun* treatment which is based on the same principle as acupuncture but where, instead of needles, fingers are used on some specific points on the body, called pressure points

acupuncture ['ækjupʌŋktʃə] *noun* treatment originating in China, where needles are inserted through the skin into nerve centres in order to relieve pain, to treat a disorder, etc.

acupuncturist ['ækjupʌŋktʃərɪst] *noun* person who practises acupuncture

acute [ə'kjuːt] *adjective* (i) (disease) which comes on rapidly and can be dangerous; (ii) (pain) which is sharp and intense; *she had an acute attack of shingles*; *he felt acute chest pains*; *after the acute stage of the illness had passed he felt very weak*; **acute abdomen** = any serious condition of the abdomen which may require surgery; **acute bed** = hospital bed reserved for acute cases (NOTE: the opposite is **chronic**)

twenty-seven adult patients admitted to hospital with acute abdominal pains were referred for study

Lancet

the survey shows a reduction in acute beds in the last six years. The bed losses forced one hospital to send acutely ill patients to hospitals up to sixteen miles away

Nursing Times

acute yellow atrophy   [əˈkjuːt   ˈjeləʊ ˈætrəfi] *see* YELLOW

acystia [əˈsɪstiə] *noun* congenital defect, where a baby is born without a bladder

Adam's apple [ˈædəmz ˈæpl] *noun* piece of the thyroid cartilage surrounding the voice box, which projects from the neck below the chin in a man and moves up and down when he speaks or swallows

adapt [əˈdæpt] *verb* to change to fit a new situation; *she has adapted very well to her new job in the children's hospital*; *the brace has to be adapted to fit the patient*

adaptation [ædæpˈteɪʃn] *noun* (i) changing something so that it fits a new situation; (ii) process by which sensory receptors become accustomed to a sensation which is repeated; **dark adaptation** *or* **light adaptation** = changes in the eye in response to changes in light conditions

addict [ˈædɪkt] *noun* **drug addict** = person who is physically and mentally dependent on taking drugs regularly; *a heroin addict*; *a morphine addict*

addicted [əˈdɪktɪd] *adjective* **addicted to alcohol** *or* **drugs** = being unable to live without taking alcohol or drugs regularly

addiction [əˈdɪkʃn] *noun* **drug addiction** *or* **drug dependence** = being mentally and physically dependent on taking a drug regularly

three quarters of patients aged 35–64 on GPs' lists have at least one major risk factor: high cholesterol, high blood pressure or addiction to tobacco

Health Services Journal

addictive [əˈdɪktɪv] *adjective* (drug) which is habit-forming, which people can become addicted to; *certain narcotic drugs are addictive*

Addison's anaemia [ˈædɪsənz əˈniːmiə] = PERNICIOUS ANAEMIA

Addison's disease [ˈædɪsənz dɪˈziːz] *noun* disease of the adrenal glands, resulting in general weakness, anaemia, low blood pressure and wasting away

COMMENT: the most noticeable symptom of the disease is the change in skin colour to yellow and then to dark brown. Treatment consists of corticosteroid injections

additive [ˈædɪtɪv] *noun* chemical substance which is added, especially one which is added to food to improve its appearance or to prevent it going bad; *the tin of beans contains a number of additives*; *asthmatic and allergic reactions to additives are frequently found in workers in food processing factories*

adducted [əˈdʌktɪd] *adjective* brought towards the middle of the body; **vocal folds adducted** = position of the vocal cords for speaking (NOTE: the opposite is **abducted**)

adduction [əˈdʌkʃn] *noun* movement of part of the body towards the midline or towards a neighbouring part (NOTE: the opposite is **abduction**)

adductor (muscle) [əˈdʌktə (ˈmʌsl)] *noun* muscle which pulls a part of the body towards the midline of the body (NOTE: the opposite is **abductor**)

aden- *or* **adeno-** [ædɪn or ædɪnəʊ] *prefix* referring to glands

adenectomy [ædɪˈnektəmi] *noun* surgical removal of a gland

adenine [ˈædəniːn] *noun* one of the four basic elements in DNA

adenitis [ædəˈnaɪtɪs] *noun* inflammation of a lymph gland; *see also* LYMPHOADENITIS

adenocarcinoma [ædɪnəʊkɑːsɪˈnəʊmə] *noun* malignant tumour of a gland

adenohypophysis [ædɪnəʊhaɪˈpɒfɪsɪs] *noun* front lobe of the pituitary gland which secretes several hormones which themselves stimulate the adrenal and thyroid glands, or which stimulate the production of sex hormones, melanin and milk

adenoid [ˈædɪnɔɪd] *adjective* like a gland

adenoidal [ædɪˈnɔɪdl] *adjective* referring to adenoids; **adenoidal expression** = common symptom of child suffering from adenoids, where his mouth is always open, the nose is narrow and the top teeth appear to project forward; **adenoidal tissue** = the pharyngeal tonsils, glands at the back of the throat where the passages from the nose join the throat

adenoidectomy [ædɪnɔɪˈdektəmi] *noun* surgical removal of the adenoids

adenoidism [ˈædɪnɔɪdɪzm] *noun* condition of a person with adenoids; *the little boy suffers from adenoidism*

adenoids [ˈædɪnɔɪdz] *plural noun* condition where growths form on the glands at the back of the throat where the passages from the nose join the throat, which prevent the patient breathing through the nose; **enlargement of the adenoids** *or* **adenoid vegetation** = condition in children where the adenoidal tissue is covered with growths and can block the nasal passages or the Eustachian tubes; *removal of the adenoids is sometimes indicated*

adenoma [ædɪˈnəʊmə] *noun* benign tumour of a gland

adenomyoma [ædɪnəʊmaɪˈəʊmə] *noun* benign tumour made up of glands and muscle

adenopathy [ædɪˈnɒpəθi] *noun* disease of a gland

adenosclerosis [ædɪnəʊskləˈrəʊsɪs] *noun* hardening of a gland

adenosine triphosphate (ATP) [əˈdenəʊsiːn traɪˈfɒsfeɪt] *noun* chemical which occurs in all cells, but mainly in muscle, where it forms the energy reserve

adenosis [ædɪˈnəʊsɪs] *noun* any disease or disorder of the glands

adenovirus [ædɪnəʊˈvaɪrəs] *noun* virus which produces upper respiratory infections and sore throats and can cause fatal pneumonia in infants

adequate [ˈædɪkwət] *adjective* enough; *the brain must have an adequate supply of blood*; *does the children's diet provide them with an adequate quantity of iron?*

ADH = ANTIDIURETIC HORMONE

ADHD = ATTENTION DEFICIT HYPERACTIVITY DISORDER; *see* HYPERACTIVITY

adhesion [ədˈhiːʒn] *noun* abnormal connection between two surfaces in the body which should not be connected

adhesive [ədˈhiːzɪv] *adjective* which sticks; **adhesive dressing** *or* **adhesive plaster** *or* **adhesive tape** = dressing with a sticky substance on the back so that it can stick to the skin; **adhesive strapping** = overlapping strips of adhesive plaster used to protect a lesion

adipo- [ˈædɪpəʊ] *prefix meaning* fat

adipose [ˈædɪpəʊz] *adjective* containing fat, made of fat; **adipose tissue** = body fat, tissue where the cells contain fat; **adipose degeneration** = *see* DEGENERATION

> COMMENT: normal fibrous tissue is replaced by adipose tissue when more food is eaten than is necessary

adiposis dolorosa [ædɪˈpəʊsɪs dɒləˈrəʊsə] *noun* Dercum's disease, a disease of middle-aged women where painful lumps of fatty substance form in the body

adiposogenitalis [ædɪpsəʊdʒenɪˈteɪlɪs] = DYSTROPHIA ADIPOSOGENITALIS; *see* FRÖHLICH'S SYNDROME

adiposuria [ædɪpəʊˈsjuːriə] *noun* fat in the urine

adiposus [ædɪˈpəʊsəs] *see* PANNICULUS

aditus [ˈædɪtəs] *noun* opening or entrance to a passage

adjuvant [ˈædʒuːvənt] **1** *adjective* (treatment) which uses drugs, radiation therapy, etc. following surgery for cancer **2** *noun* substance added to a drug to enhance the effect of the main ingredient

administer [ədˈmɪnɪstə] *verb* to give (a medicine) to a patient; **to administer orally** = to give a medicine by mouth

administration [ədmɪnɪsˈtreɪʃn] *noun* **(a)** giving of a medicine; *administration of drugs must be supervised by a qualified doctor or nurse* **(b)** management, running of a hospital, service, etc.; **medical administration** = running of hospitals and other health services; *she started her career in medical administration*

administrative [ədˈmɪnɪstrətɪv] *adjective* referring to administration; *most of the GP's spare time is taken up with administrative work*

administrator [ədˈmɪnɪstreɪtə] *noun* person who runs (a hospital, district health authority, etc.)

admission [ədˈmɪʃn] *noun* being allowed into a place; **admission to the hospital** = official registering of a patient in a hospital; **admission form** = form which has to be filled for each patient who is admitted to a hospital

admit [ədˈmɪt] *verb* to allow (someone) to go in; to register a patient in a hospital; *children are admitted free*; *he was admitted (to hospital) this morning*

> 80% of elderly patients admitted to geriatric units are on medication
>
> *Nursing Times*

> ten patients were admitted to the ICU before operation, the main indications being the need for evaluation of patients with a history of severe heart disease
>
> *Southern Medical Journal*

adnexa [æd'neksə] *plural noun* structures attached to an organ

adolescence [ædə'lesns] *noun* period of life when a child is developing into an adult

adolescent [ædə'lesnt] *noun & adjective* (person) who is at the stage of life when he is developing into an adult

adopt [ə'dɒpt] *verb* to become the legal parent of a child who was born to other parents; **adopted child** *or* **son** *or* **daughter** = child, son or daughter who has been adopted

adoption [ə'dɒpʃn] *noun* act of becoming the legal parent of a child who was born to other parents; **adoption order** = order by a court which legally transfers the rights of the natural parents to the adoptive parents; **adoption proceedings** = court action to adopt someone

> COMMENT: if a child's parents are divorced or if one parent dies, the child may be adopted by a step-father or step-mother

adoptive [ə'dɒptɪv] *adjective* **adoptive child** *or* **son** *or* **daughter** = child, son or daughter who has been adopted; **adoptive parent** = person who has adopted a child

adoptive immunotherapy [ə'dɒptɪv ɪmjunə'θerəpi] *noun* treatment for cancer in which the patient's own white blood cells are used to attack cancer cells

> COMMENT: this technique was discovered in 1980 and can halt the growth of cancer cells in the body. Much of the more recent research has examined ways of minimizing the distressing toxic side-effects of the substances used

adrenal [ə'driːnl] *adjective* situated near the kidney; **adrenal body** = an adrenal gland; **adrenal cortex** = firm outside layer of an adrenal gland, which secretes a series of hormones affecting the metabolism of carbohydrates and water; **adrenal glands** *or*

suprarenal glands, *US* **the adrenals** = two endocrine glands at the top of the kidneys, which secrete cortisone, adrenaline and other hormones; **adrenal medulla** = soft inner part of the adrenal gland which secretes adrenaline and noradrenaline; *see illustration at* KIDNEY

adrenalectomy [ədriːnə'lektəmi] *noun* surgical removal of one of the adrenal glands; **bilateral adrenalectomy** = surgical removal of both adrenal glands

adrenaline [ə'drenəlɪn] *noun* hormone secreted by the medulla of the adrenal glands which has an effect similar to stimulation of the sympathetic nervous system (NOTE: American English is **epinephrine**)

> COMMENT: adrenaline is produced when a person experiences surprise, shock, fear, excitement: it speeds up the heartbeat and raises blood pressure; it is administered as emergency treatment of acute anaphylaxis and in cardiopulmonary resuscitation

adrenergic [ædrə'nɜːdʒɪk] *adjective* (neurones or receptors) stimulated by adrenaline

> COMMENT: three types of adrenergic receptor act in different ways when stimulated by adrenaline. Alpha receptors constrict the bronchi, beta 1 receptors speed up the heartbeat and beta 2 receptors dilate the bronchi. See also ALPHA BLOCKER, BETA BLOCKER

adrenoceptor [ədrenəʊ'septə] *noun* cell or neurone which is stimulated by adrenaline; *see also* ADRENERGIC

adrenocortical [ədriːnəʊ'kɔːtɪkl] *adjective* referring to the cortex of the adrenal glands

adrenocorticotrophic hormone (ACTH) [ədriːnəʊkɔːtəkəʊ'trɒfɪk 'hɔːməʊn] *noun* corticotrophin, a hormone secreted by the pituitary gland, which makes the cortex of the adrenal glands produce corticosteroids

adrenocorticotrophin [ədriːnəʊkɔːtəkəʊ'trəʊfɪn] *noun* adrenaline extracted from animals' adrenal glands and used to prevent haemorrhages or to help asthmatic conditions

adrenogenital syndrome [ədriːnəʊ'dʒenɪtəl 'sɪndrəʊm] *noun* condition caused by overproduction of male sex hormones, where boys show rapid sexual development and females show virilization

adrenolytic [ədriːnəʊ'lɪtɪk] *adjective* acting against the secretion of adrenaline

adrenoreceptor [ədrenəʊrɪ'septə] see ADRENOCEPTOR

adsorbent [æd'sɔːbənt] *adjective* capable of adsorption

adsorption [æd'sɔːpʃn] *noun* bonding of a solid with a gas or vapour which touches its surface

adult ['ædʌlt or ə'dʌlt] *noun & adjective* grown-up (person, animal); *adolescents reach the adult stage about the age of eighteen or twenty*

advanced [əd'vɑːnst] *adjective* which has developed; *the advanced stages of a disease*; *he is suffering from advanced syphilis*

adventitia [ædven'tɪʃə] *noun;* **(tunica) adventitia** = outer layer of the wall of an artery or vein

adventitious [ædvən'tɪʃəs] *adjective* which is on the outside or in an unusual place; **adventitious bursa;** *see* BURSA

adverse ['ædvɜːs] *adjective* harmful, unfavourable; **the treatment had an adverse effect on his dermatitis** = it made it worse; **adverse occurrence** = harmful event which occurs during treatment; **adverse reaction from a drug** = situation where a patient suffers harmful effects from the application of a drug

advice [əd'vaɪs] *noun* suggestion about what should be done; *he went to the psychiatrist for advice on how to cope with his problem*; *she would not listen to my advice*; *the doctor's advice was that he should take a long holiday*; *the doctor's advice was to stay in bed*; *he took the doctor's advice and went to bed* (NOTE: no plural: **some advice** or **a piece of advice**)

advise [əd'vaɪz] *verb* to suggest what should be done; *the doctor advised him to stay in bed*; *she advised me to have a checkup*; *I would advise you not to drink alcohol*

advise against [əd'vaɪz ə'genst] *verb* to suggest that something should not be done; *he wanted to leave hospital but the consultant advised against it*; *the doctor advised against going to bed late*

adynamic ileus [ædɪ'næmɪk 'ɪliəs] *noun* obstruction in the ileum caused by paralysis of the muscles of the intestine

aegophony [iː'gɒfəni] *noun* high sound of the voice heard through a stethoscope, where there is fluid in the pleural cavity

aer- *or* **aero-** [eə or 'eərəʊ] *prefix meaning* air

aeroba *or* **aerobe** [eə'rəʊbə or 'eərəʊb] *noun* tiny organism which needs oxygen to survive

aerobic [eə'rəʊbɪk] *adjective* needing oxygen to live; **aerobic respiration** = process where the oxygen which is breathed in is used to conserve energy as ATP

aerobics [eə'rəʊbɪks] *plural noun* exercises which aim to increase the amount of oxygen taken into the body

aerogenous [eə'rɒdʒənəs] *adjective* (bacterium) which produces gas

aerophagy *or* **aerophagia** [eə'rɒfədʒi or eərə'feɪdʒə] *noun* habit of swallowing air when suffering from indigestion, so making the stomach pains worse

aerosol ['eərəsɒl] *noun* **(a)** tiny particles of liquid suspended in a gas under pressure, sprayed from a container and used as a medicine, sterilizing agent, etc. **(b) aerosol** *or* **aerosol dispenser** = container, device from which liquid can be sprayed in tiny particles

aetiological agent [iːtiə'lɒdʒikl 'eɪdʒnt] *noun* agent which causes a disease

aetiology *US* **etiology** [iːti'ɒlədʒi] *noun* (study of) the cause or origin of a disease

> a wide variety of organs or tissues may be infected by the Salmonella group of organisms, presenting symptoms which are not immediately recognized as being of Salmonella aetiology
> *Indian Journal of Medical Sciences*

afebrile [æ'fiːbraɪl] *adjective* with no fever

affect [ə'fekt] *verb* to make something change; *some organs are rapidly affected if the patient lacks oxygen for even a short time*

affection *or* **affect** [ə'fekʃn or ə'fekt] *noun* type of feeling; general state of a person's emotions

> Depression has degrees of severity, ranging from sadness, through flatness of affection or feeling, to suicide and psychosis
> *British Journal of Nursing*

affective disorder [ə'fektɪv dɪs'ɔːdə] *noun* condition which changes the mood of a patient, making him or her depressed or excited

afferent ['æfrənt] *adjective* which conducts liquid or electrical impulses towards the inside (NOTE: the opposite is **efferent**)

affinity [ə'finəti] *noun* attraction between two substances

afford [ə'fɔ:d] *verb* to have enough money to pay for something; *I can't afford to go to hospital*; *how can you afford this expensive treatment?*

after- ['ɑ:ftə] *prefix* which comes later, which take place later

afterbirth ['ɑ:ftəbɜ:θ] *noun* tissues (including the placenta and umbilical cord) which are present in the uterus during pregnancy and are expelled after the birth of the baby; *see also* PLACENTA

aftercare ['ɑ:ftəkeə] *noun* care of a person who has had an operation; care of a mother who has just given birth; *aftercare treatment involves changing dressings and helping the patient to look after himself again*

after-effects ['ɑ:ftəri'fekts] *plural noun* changes which appear only some time after the cause; *the operation had some unpleasant after-effects*

after-image ['ɑ:ftər'imidʒ] *noun* image of an object which remains in a person's sight after the object itself has gone

afterpains ['ɑ:ftəpeinz] *plural noun* regular pains in the uterus which are sometimes experienced after childbirth

aftertaste ['ɑ:ftəteist] *noun* taste which remains in the mouth after the substance which caused it has been removed; *the linctus leaves an unpleasant aftertaste*

Ag *chemical symbol for* silver

agalactia [ægə'lækʃiə] *noun (of mother after childbirth)* being unable to produce milk

agammaglobulinaemia
[ægæməglɒbjuli'ni:miə] *noun* deficiency or absence of gamma globulin in the blood, which results in a reduced ability to provide immune responses

agar *or* **agar agar** ['eigə *or* 'eigər'eigə] *noun* jelly made from seaweed, used to cultivate bacterial cultures in laboratories and also as a laxative

age [eidʒ] **1** *noun* number of years which a person has lived; *what's your age on your next birthday?*; *he was sixty years of age*; *she looks younger than her age*; *the size varies according to age*; **mental age** = age of a person's mental state, measured by intelligence tests (usually compared to that of a normal person of the same chronological age); **old age** = period when a person is old (usually taken to be after the age of sixty-five) **2** *verb* to grow old

aged *adjective* **(a)** [eidʒd] with a certain age; *a boy aged twelve*; *he died last year, aged 64* **(b)** ['eidʒid] very old; *an aged man*

ageing *US* **aging** ['eidʒiŋ] *noun* growing old; **the ageing process** = the physical changes which take place in a person as he grows older

COMMENT: changes take place in almost every part of the body as the person ages. Bones become more brittle, skin is less elastic. The most important changes affect the blood vessels which are less elastic, making thrombosis more likely. This also reduces the supply of blood to the brain, which in turn reduces the mental faculties

agency ['eidʒənsi] *noun* **(a)** action of causing something to happen; *the disease develops through the agency of certain bacteria present in the bloodstream* **(b)** office, organization which provides nurses for temporary work in hospitals, clinics, in private houses

the cost of employing agency nurses should be no higher than the equivalent full-time staff
Nursing Times

growing numbers of nurses are choosing agency careers, which pay more and provide more flexible schedules than hospitals
American Journal of Nursing

agent ['eidʒənt] *noun* **(a)** person who acts for another, often in another country; *he is the agent for an American pharmaceutical firm* **(b)** chemical substance which makes another substance react **(c)** substance or organism which causes a disease or condition

agglutinate [ə'glu:tineit] *verb* to form into groups or clusters

agglutination [əglu:ti'neiʃn] *noun* action of grouping together of cells (as of bacteria cells in the presence of serum or blood cells when blood of different types is mixed); **agglutination test** = (i) test to identify bacteria; (ii) test to identify if a woman is pregnant

agglutinin [əˈgluːtɪnɪn] *noun* factor in a serum which makes cells group together

agglutinogen [æglʊˈtɪnədʒən] *noun* factor in red blood cells which reacts with a specific agglutinin in serum; *see also* PAUL-BUNNELL, WEIL-FELIX, WIDAL

aggravate [ˈægrəveɪt] *verb* to make worse; *playing football only aggravates his knee injury; the treatment seems to aggravate the disease*

aggression [əˈgreʃn] *noun* state of feeling violently angry towards someone, something

aggressive [əˈgresɪv] *adjective* (treatment) involving frequent high doses of medication

agitans [ˈædʒɪtəns] *see* PARALYSIS

agitated [ˈædʒɪteɪtɪd] *adjective* moving about or twitching nervously (because of worry or other psychological state); *the patient became agitated and had to be given a sedative*

agnosia [ægˈnəʊziə] *noun* brain disorder where the patient cannot understand what his senses tell him and so fails to recognize places, people, tastes, or smells which he used to know well

agonist [ˈægənɪst] *noun* substance which produces an observable physiological effect by acting through specific receptors; *see also* ANTAGONIST

agony [ˈægənɪ] *noun* very severe pain; *he lay in agony on the floor; she suffered agonies until her condition was diagnosed*

agoraphobia [ægərəˈfəʊbiə] *noun* fear of being in open spaces

agoraphobic [ægərəˈfəʊbɪk] *noun & adjective* (person) suffering from agoraphobia (NOTE: the opposite is **claustrophobia**)

agranulocytosis [əgrænjʊləʊsaɪˈtəʊsɪs] *noun* usually fatal disease where the number of granulocytes (white blood cells) falls sharply because of a defect in the bone marrow

agraphia [eɪˈgræfiə] *noun* being unable to put ideas in writing

agreement [əˈgriːmənt] *noun* action of agreeing; **they are in agreement with our plan** = they agree with it

agree with [əˈgriː ˈwɪð] *verb* (a) to say that you think the same way as someone; to say yes; *the consultant agreed with the GP's diagnosis* (b) to be easily digested by

someone; *this rich food does not agree with me*

aid [eɪd] **1** *noun* **(a)** help; **medical aid** = treatment of someone who is ill or injured, given by a doctor; *see also* FIRST **(b)** machine or tool or drug which helps someone do something; *he uses a walking frame as an aid to exercising his legs* **2** *verb* to help; *the reason for the procedure is to aid repair of tissues after surgery*

AID [ˈeɪ ˈaɪ ˈdiː] = ARTIFICIAL INSEMINATION BY DONOR

aider [ˈeɪdə] *noun* person who helps; **first-aider** = person who gives first aid to someone who is suddenly ill or injured

AIDS *or* **Aids** [eɪdz] *noun* (= ACQUIRED IMMUNODEFICIENCY SYNDROME *or* ACQUIRED IMMUNE DEFICIENCY SYNDROME) viral infection which breaks down the body's immune system; **there are two patients with AIDS** *or* **two AIDS patients in the clinic**; **AIDS-related condition** *or* **complex (ARC)** = early symptom or illness, such as loss of weight, fever, herpes zoster, etc., exhibited by a patient infected with the HIV virus

COMMENT: AIDS is a disease, spread by the human immunodeficiency virus (HIV). It is spread mostly by sexual intercourse and although at first associated with male homosexuals, it is now known to affect anyone. It is also transmitted through infected blood and plasma transfusions, through using unsterilized needles for injections, and can be passed from a mother to a fetus. The disease takes a long time, even years, to show symptoms, so there are many carriers. It causes a breakdown of the body's immune system, making the patient susceptible to any infection and often results in the development of rare skin cancers. It is not curable

AIH [ˈeɪ ˈaɪ ˈeɪtʃ] = ARTIFICIAL INSEMINATION BY HUSBAND

ailing [ˈeɪlɪŋ] *adjective* not well for a period of time; *he stayed at home to look after his ailing parents*

ailment [ˈeɪlmənt] *noun* illness, though not generally a very serious one; *chickenpox is one of the common childhood ailments*

ailurophobia [aɪlʊərəˈfəʊbiə] *noun* fear of cats

aim [eɪm] *verb* **(a)** to point at; *the X-ray beam is aimed at the patient's jaw* **(b)** to intend to do something; *we aim to eradicate tuberculosis by the end of the century*

air [eə] *noun* mixture of gases (mainly oxygen and nitrogen) which cannot be seen, but which exists all around us and which is breathed; *the air in the mountains felt cold*; *he breathed the polluted air into his lungs*; **air bed** = mattress which is filled with air, used to prevent the formation of bedsores; *see also* CONDUCTION; **air embolism** = interference with blood flow caused by air bubbles; **air hunger** = condition where the patient needs air because of lack of oxygen in the tissues; **air passages** = tubes, formed of the nose, pharynx, larynx, trachea and bronchi, which take air to the lungs; **air sac** = alveolus, a small sac in the lungs which contains air

airsick ['eəsɪk] *adjective* feeling sick because of the movement of an aircraft

airsickness ['eəsɪknəs] *noun* sickness caused by the movement of an aircraft

airway ['eəweɪ] *noun* passage through which air passes, especially the trachea; **airway clearing** = making sure that the airways in a newborn baby or an unconscious person are free of any obstruction; **airway obstruction** = something which blocks the air passages

akathisia [eɪkə'θɪsiə] *noun* restlessness

akinesia [ækɪ'niːziə] *noun* lack of voluntary movement (as in Parkinson's disease)

akinetic [ækɪ'netik] *adjective* without movement

AI = ALUMINIUM

alactasia [ælæk'teɪziə] *noun* condition where there is a deficiency of lactase in the intestine, making the patient incapable of digesting milk sugar (lactose)

alanine ['æləniːn] *noun* amino acid in protein

alar cartilage ['eɪlə 'kɑːtəlɪdʒ] *noun* cartilage in the outer wings of the nose

alba ['ælbə] *see* LINEA

Albee's operation ['ɔːlbiːz ɒpə'reɪʃn] *noun* (i) surgical operation to fuse two or more vertebrae; (ii) surgical operation to fuse the femur to the pelvis

albicans ['ælbɪkænz] *see* CANDIDA ALBICANS, CORPUS ALBICANS

albinism ['ælbɪnɪzm] *noun* condition where the patient lacks melanin and so has pink

skin and eyes and white hair; *see also* VITILIGO

COMMENT: albinism is hereditary and cannot be treated

albino [æl'biːnəʊ] *noun* person who is deficient in melanin, with little or no pigmentation in skin, hair or eyes

albuginea [ælbjuˈdʒɪniə] *noun* layer of white tissue covering a part of the body; **albuginea oculi** = sclera, the white outer covering of the eyeball; *see also* TUNICA

albumin ['ælbjumɪn] *noun* common protein, soluble in water and found in plant and animal tissue and digested in the intestine; **serum albumin** = major protein in blood plasma

albuminometer [ælbjuːmɪ'nɒmɪtə] *noun* instrument for measuring the level of albumin in the urine

albuminuria [ælbjuːmɪ'njʊəriə] *noun* condition where albumin is found in the urine, usually a sign of kidney disease, but also sometimes of heart failure

albumose ['ælbjuməʊz] *noun* intermediate product in the digestion of protein

alcohol ['ælkəhɒl] *noun* pure colourless liquid, which forms part of drinks such as wine and whisky, and which is formed by the action of yeast on sugar solutions; **alcohol abuse** *or* **alcohol addiction** = condition where a patient is addicted to drinking alcohol and cannot stop; **alcohol poisoning** = poisoning and disease caused by excessive drinking of alcohol; **alcohol rub** = rubbing a bedridden patient with alcohol to help protect against bedsores and as a tonic; **absolute alcohol** *or* **anhydrous alcohol** = alcohol which contains no water; **denatured alcohol** = ethyl alcohol (such as methylated spirit, rubbing alcohol, surgical spirit) with an additive (usually methyl alcohol) to make it unpleasant to drink; **methyl alcohol** = wood alcohol (poisonous alcohol used for heating); **pure alcohol** *or* **ethyl alcohol** *or* **ethanol** = colourless liquid, which is the basis of drinking alcohols (whisky, gin, vodka, etc.) and which is also used in medicines and as a disinfectant;

COMMENT: alcohol is used medicinally to dry wounds or harden the skin. When drunk, alcohol is rapidly absorbed into the bloodstream. It is a source of energy, so any carbohydrates taken at the same time are not used by the body and are stored as fat.

Alcohol is a depressant, not a stimulant, and affects the mental faculties

alcohol-fast ['ælkəhɒl'fɑːst] *adjective* (organ stained for testing) which is not discoloured by alcohol

alcoholic [ælkə'hɒlɪk] **1** *adjective* (i) containing alcohol; (ii) caused by alcoholism; *children should not be encouraged to take alcoholic drinks*; *alcoholic poisoning*; *alcoholic cirrhosis* = cirrhosis of the liver caused by alcoholism **2** *noun* person who is addicted to drinking alcohol and shows changes in behaviour and personality

Alcoholics Anonymous (AA) [ælkə'hɒlɪks ə'nɒnɪməs] *noun* organization of former alcoholics which helps sufferers from alcoholism to overcome their dependence on alcohol by encouraging them to talk about their problems in group therapy

alcoholicum [ælkə'hɒlɪkəm] *see* DELIRIUM

alcoholism ['ælkəhɒlɪzm] *noun* excessive drinking of alcohol which becomes addictive

alcoholuria [ælkəhɒ'ljuəriə] *noun* condition where alcohol is present in the urine (the level of alcohol in the urine is used as a test for drunken drivers)

aldosterone [æl'dɒstərəun] *noun* hormone secreted by the cortex of the adrenal gland and which regulates the balance of sodium and potassium in the body and the amount of body fluid

alert [ə'lɜːt] *adjective* (person) who takes an intelligent interest in his surroundings; *the patient is still alert, though in great pain*

aleukaemic [ælu'kiːmɪk] *adjective* (i) (state) where leukaemia is not present; (ii) (state) where leucocytes are not normal

alexia [ə'leksiə] *noun* word blindness, a condition where the patient cannot understand printed words

algae ['ældʒiː] *plural noun* class of lower plants, many of which are seaweeds

algesimeter [ældʒɪ'sɪmɪtə] *noun* instrument to measure the sensitivity of the skin to pain

-algia ['ældʒiə] *suffix meaning* pain

algid ['ældʒɪd] *adjective* cold, (stage in an attack of cholera or malaria) where the body becomes cold

alimentary canal [ælɪ'mentri kə'næl] *noun* tube in the body going from the mouth to the anus and including the throat, stomach, intestine, etc., through which food passes and is digested

alimentary system [ælɪ'mentri 'sɪstəm] *noun* arrangement of tubes and organs, including the alimentary canal, salivary glands, liver, etc., through which food passes and is digested

alimentation [ælɪmen'teɪʃn] *noun* feeding, taking in food

alive [ə'laɪv] *adjective* living, not dead; *the patient was still alive, even though he had been in the sea for two days* (NOTE: **alive** cannot be used in front of a noun: **the patient is alive** but **a living patient** Note also that **live** can be used in front of a noun: **the patient was injected with live vaccine**)

alkalaemia [ælkə'liːmiə] *noun* excess of alkali in the blood

alkali ['ælkəlaɪ] *noun* one of many substances which neutralize acids and form salts (NOTE: British English plural is **alkalis,** but American English is **alkalies**)

alkaline ['ælkəlaɪn] *adjective* containing more alkali than acid

alkalinity [ælkə'lɪnəti] *noun* level of alkali in a body; *hyperventilation causes fluctuating carbon dioxide levels in the blood, resulting in an increase of blood alkalinity*

COMMENT: alkalinity and acidity are measured according to the pH scale. pH7 is neutral, and pH8 and upwards are alkaline. Alkaline solutions are used to counteract the effects of acid poisoning and also of bee stings. If strong alkali (such as ammonia) is swallowed, the patient should drink water and an acid such as orange juice. Alkalosis can be caused by vomiting.

alkaloid ['ælkəlɔɪd] *noun* one of many poisonous substances (such as atropine, morphine or quinine) found in plants and used as medicines

alkalosis [ælkə'ləusɪs] *noun* condition where the alkali level in the body tissue is high, producing cramps; **metabolic alkalosis** = alkalosis caused by a defect in the body's metabolism

alkaptonuria [ælkæptə'njuəriə] *noun* hereditary condition where dark pigment is present in the urine

allantoin [ə'læntəʊɪn] *noun* powder from the herb comfrey, used to treat skin disorders

allantois [ə'læntəʊɪs] *noun* one of the membranes in the embryo, shaped like a sac, which grows out of the embryonic hindgut

allele [ə'li:l] *noun* one of two or more alternative forms of a gene, which can imitate each other's form: they are situated in the same area of a pair of chromosomes and produce different characteristics

allergen ['ælədʒen] *noun* substance which produces hypersensitivity; **food allergen =** substance in food which produces an allergy

COMMENT: allergens are usually proteins, and include foods, dust, hair of animals, as well as pollen from flowers. Allergic reaction to serum is known as anaphylaxis. Treatment of allergies depends on correctly identifying the allergen to which the patient is sensitive. This is done by patch tests in which drops of different allergens are placed on scratches in the skin. Food allergens discovered in this way can be avoided, but other allergens (such as dust and pollen) can hardly be avoided and have to be treated by a course of desensitizing injections

allergenic [ælə'dʒenɪk] *adjective* which produces an allergy; **the allergenic *properties of fungal spores*; **allergenic agent =** substance which produces an allergy; *see also* NON

allergic [ə'lɜ:dʒɪk] *adjective* suffering from an allergy; *she is allergic to cats*; *I'm allergic to penicillin*; *he showed an allergic reaction to chocolate*; **allergic agent =** substance which produces an allergic reaction; **allergic person =** person who has an allergy to something; **allergic reaction =** effect (such as a skin rash or sneezing) produced by a substance to which a person has an allergy; **allergic rhinitis =** inflammation in the nasal passages and eyes caused by an allergic reaction to plant pollen (hayfever), mould spores, dust mites or animal hair

allergist ['ælədʒɪst] *noun* doctor who specializes in the treatment of allergies

allergy ['ælədʒɪ] *noun* sensitivity to certain substances such as pollen or dust, which cause a physical reaction; *she has an allergy to household dust*; *he has a penicillin allergy*; **drug allergy =** reaction to a certain drug; **respiratory allergy =** allergy caused by a substance which is inhaled; *see also*

ALVEOLITIS, FOOD (NOTE: you have an allergy or you are allergic **to** something)

alleviate [ə'li:vɪeɪt] *verb* to make (a pain) less, to relieve (a pain); *he was given injections to alleviate the pain*; *the nurses tried to alleviate the suffering of the injured*

allo- ['æləʊ] *prefix* different

allograft ['æləʊgrɑːft] *noun* homograft, the graft of an organ or tissue from a donor to a recipient of the same species (as from one person to another); *compare* AUTOGRAFT

allopathy [ə'lɒpəθi] *noun* treatment of a condition using drugs which produce opposite symptoms to those of the condition; *compare* HOMEOPATHY

all or none law ['ɔːl ɔː 'nʌn 'lɔː] *noun* rule that the heart muscle either contracts fully or does not contract at all

all over ['ɔːl 'əʊvə] *preposition* **(a)** everywhere; *there were red marks all over the child's body*; *she poured water all over the patient's head* **(b)** finished; *when it was all over we went home*

allow [ə'laʊ] *verb* to say that someone can do something; *the consultant allowed him to watch the operation*; *patients are not allowed to go outside the hospital*; *he is allowed to eat certain types of food*

allowance [ə'laʊəns] *noun* money paid regularly; *she gets a weekly allowance from her father*

all right ['ɔːl 'raɪt] *adjective* fine, well, not ill; *he's feeling very sick at the moment, but he will be all right in a few hours*; *my mother had flu but she is all right now*; *his hearing is all right, but his sight is failing*

almoner ['ɑːmənə or 'ælmənə] *noun* formerly a person working in a hospital, looking after the welfare of patients and the families of patients (now called medical social worker)

alopecia [ælə'piːʃə] *noun* baldness; **alopecia areata =** condition where the hair falls out in patches

COMMENT: baldness in men is hereditary; it can also occur in men and women as a reaction to an illness or to a drug

alpha ['ælfə] *noun* first letter of the Greek alphabet; **alpha blocker =** drug (such as alfuzosin hydrochloride) which blocks the alpha adrenoceptors in the nervous system; **alpha cell =** one of the types of cells in glands (such as the pancreas) which have more than one type of cell

alpha-adrenoceptor antagonist (alpha-blocker) ['ælfəædri:nəʊrı'septə æntægənıst] *noun* alpha blocker, a drug (such as alfuzosin hydrochloride) used to relax smooth muscle, used in urinary retention and hypertension

alpha-fetoprotein ['ælfəfi:təʊ'prəʊti:n] *noun* protein found in the amniotic fluid when the fetus has an open neurological deficiency such as meningomyelocele

ALS ['eı 'el 'es] = AMYOTROPHIC LATERAL SCLEROSIS, ANTILYMPHOCYTIC SERUM

altitude sickness ['æltıtju:d 'sıknəs] = MOUNTAIN SICKNESS

aluminium *US* **aluminum** [ælju:'mınıəm *US* ə'lu:mınəm] *noun* metallic element extracted from the ore bauxite (NOTE: the chemical symbol is **Al**; the atomic number is **13**)

aluminium hydroxide *US* **aluminum hydroxide (Al(OH)₃)** [ælə'mınıəm haı'drɒksaıd or ə'lu:mınəm] *noun* chemical substance used as an antacid to treat indigestion

alveolar [ælvı'əʊlə or æl'vi:ələ] *adjective* referring to alveoli; **alveolar bone** = part of the jawbone to which the teeth are attached; **alveolar duct** = duct in the lung which leads from the respiratory bronchioles to the alveoli; **alveolar walls** = walls which separate the alveoli in the lungs

alveolitis [ælvıə'laıtıs] *noun* inflammation of an alveolus in the lungs or the socket of a tooth; **extrinsic allergic alveolitis** = condition where the lungs are allergic to fungus and other allergens

alveolus [ælvı'əʊləs or æl'vi:ələs] *noun* small cavity, such as one of the air sacs in the lungs or the socket into which a tooth fits (NOTE: the plural is **alveoli**); *see illustration at* LUNGS

Alzheimer's disease ['æltshaıməz dı'zi:z] *noun* disease where the patient suffers from progressive dementia due to nerve cell loss in specific brain areas, resulting in loss of mental faculties including memory; **Alzheimer plaques** = disc-shaped plaques of amyloid found in the brain in Alzheimer's disease

COMMENT: no single cause has been identified, although an early onset type occurs more frequently in some families,

due to a mutation in a gene on chromosome 21. Risk factors include age, genes, head injury, lifestyle and environment

amalgam [ə'mælgəm] *noun* mixture of metals (based on mercury and tin) used by dentists to fill holes in teeth

amaurosis [æmɔ:'rəʊsıs] *noun* blindness where there is no visible defect in the eye, caused by a defect in the optic nerves; **amaurosis fugax** = temporary blindness on one eye, caused by problems of circulation

amaurotic familial idiocy [æmɔ:'rɒtık fə'mılıəl 'ıdıəsı] = TAY-SACHS DISEASE

amb(i)- ['æmbi] *prefix* meaning both

ambidextrous [æmbi'dekstrəs] *adjective* (person) who can use both hands equally well and who is not right- or left-handed

ambisexual [æmbi'sekʃuəl] *adjective* bisexual, (person) who is sexually attracted to both males and females

amblyopia [æmbli'əʊpiə] *noun* partial blindness, leading to blindness, for which no cause seems to exist, although it may be caused by the cyanide in tobacco smoke or by drinking methylated spirits (toxic amblyopia)

amblyopic [æmbli'ɒpık] *adjective* suffering from amblyopia

amblyoscope ['æmbliəʊskəʊp] *noun* surgical instrument for checking and training an amblyopic eye

ambulance ['æmbjələns] *noun* van for taking sick or injured people to hospital; *the injured man was taken away in an ambulance*; *the telephone number of the local ambulance service is in the telephone book*; *see also* ST JOHN

ambulanceman ['æmbjələnsmæn] *noun* man who drives or assists in an ambulance (NOTE: the plural is **ambulancemen**)

ambulant ['æmbjələnt] *adjective* (patient) who can walk

ambulation [æmbju'leıʃn] *noun* walking; **early ambulation is recommended** = patients should try to get out of bed and walk about as soon as possible after the operation

ambulatory ['æmbjulətəri] *adjective* (patient) who is not confined to bed but is able to walk; **ambulatory fever** = mild fever (such as the early stages of typhoid fever) where the patient can walk about and can therefore act as a carrier

ambulatory patients with
essential hypertension were
evaluated and followed up at
the hypertension clinic
British Medical Journal

ameba [ə'miːbə] *US* = AMOEBA

amelia [ə'miːliə] *noun* congenital absence of a limb, condition where a limb is congenitally short

amelioration [əmiːliə'reɪʃn] *noun* improvement, getting better

ameloblastoma [əmeləublæ'stəumə] *noun* tumour in the jaw, usually in the lower jaw

amenity bed [ə'miːnəti 'bed] *noun* bed (usually in a separate room) in an NHS hospital, for which the patient pays extra

amenorrhoea [eɪmenə'riːə] *noun* absence of one or more menstrual periods, normal during pregnancy and after the menopause, but otherwise abnormal in adult women; **primary amenorrhoea** = condition where a woman has never had menstrual periods; **secondary amenorrhoea** = situation where a woman's menstrual periods have stopped

amentia [eɪ'menʃə] *noun* being mentally subnormal

ametropia [æmɪ'trəupiə] *noun* condition where the eye cannot focus light correctly onto the retina, as in astigmatism, hypermetropia and myopia; *compare* EMMETROPIA

amino acid [ə'miːnəu 'æsɪd] *noun* chemical compound which is broken down from proteins in the digestive system and then used by the body to form its own protein; *proteins are first broken down into amino acids*; **essential amino acids** = eight amino acids which are essential for growth, but which cannot be synthesized and so must be obtained from food or medicinal substances

COMMENT: amino acids all contain carbon, hydrogen, nitrogen and oxygen, as well as other elements. Some amino acids are produced in the body itself, but others have to be absorbed from food. The eight essential amino acids are: isoleucine, leucine, lysine, methionine, phenylalanine, threonine, tryptophan and valine

aminobutyric acid [əmiːnəubju'tɪrɪk 'æsɪd] *see* GAMMA

aminoglycoside [əmiːnəu'glaɪkəsaɪd] *noun* drug used to treat many Gram-negative and some Gram-positive bacterial infections, such as in septicaemia (NOTE: includes drugs ending in **-cin: gentamicin**)

amitosis [æmɪ'təusɪs] *noun* multiplication of a cell by splitting the nucleus

ammonia (NH₃) [ə'məuniə] *noun* gas with a strong smell, a compound of nitrogen and hydrogen, which is a normal product of human metabolism

ammonium [ə'məuniəm] *noun* ion formed from ammonia

amnesia [æm'niːziə] *noun* loss of memory; **general amnesia** = loss of all memory, a state where a person does not even remember who he is; **partial amnesia** = being unable to remember certain facts, such as names of people

amniocentesis [æmniəusen'tiːsɪs] *noun* taking a test sample of the amniotic fluid during pregnancy using a hollow needle and syringe

COMMENT: amniocentesis and amnioscopy are the examination and testing of the amniotic fluid, giving information about possible congenital abnormalities in the fetus and also the sex of the unborn baby

amnion ['æmniən] *noun* thin sac (containing the amniotic fluid) which covers an unborn baby in the uterus

amnioscopy [æmni'ɒskəpi] *noun* examination of the amniotic fluid during pregnancy

amniotic [æmni'ɒtɪk] *adjective* referring to the amnion; **amniotic cavity** = space formed by the amnion, full of amniotic fluid; **amniotic fluid** = fluid contained in the amnion, which surrounds an unborn baby; **amniotic sac** = AMNION

amniotomy [æmni'ɒtəmi] *noun* puncture of the amnion to help induce labour

amoeba [ə'miːbə] *noun* form of animal life, made up of a single cell (NOTE: the plural is **amoebae**. Note also the American spelling **ameba, amebiasis, amebic, etc**)

amoebiasis [æmɪ'baɪəsɪs] *noun* infection caused by amoeba, which can result in amoebic dysentery in the large intestine (intestinal amoebiasis) and can sometimes infect the lungs (pulmonary amoebiasis)

amoebic [ə'mi:bɪk] *adjective* referring to an amoeba; **amoebic dysentery** = mainly tropical form of dysentery which is caused by *Entamoeba histolytica* which enters the body through contaminated water or unwashed food

amoebicide [ə'mi:bɪsaɪd] *noun* substance which kills amoebae

amorphous [ə'mɔ:fəs] *adjective* with no regular shape

amount [ə'maʊnt] **1** *noun* quantity; *he is not allowed to drink a large amount of water*; *she should not eat large amounts of fried food* **2** *verb* to be equal (to); *the bill for surgery amounted to £1,000*

amphetamine [æm'fetəmi:n] *noun* addictive drug, similar to adrenaline, used to give a feeling of wellbeing and wakefulness; **amphetamine abuse** = repeated addictive use of amphetamines which in the end affects the mental faculties

amphiarthrosis [æmfɑ:'θrəʊsɪs] *noun* joint which only has limited movement (such as the joints in the spine)

amphotericin [æmfəʊ'terɪsɪn] *noun* antifungal agent, used against *Candida*

ampicillin [æmpɪ'sɪlɪn] *noun* type of penicillin, used as an antibiotic

ampoule *or* **ampule** ['æmpu:l *or* 'æmpju:l] *noun* small glass container, closed at the neck, used to contain sterile drugs for use in injections

ampulla [æm'pʊlə] *noun* swelling of a canal or duct, shaped like a bottle (NOTE: the plural is **ampullae**)

amputate [æmpjʊteɪt] *verb* to remove a limb or part of a limb in a surgical operation; *a patient whose leg needs to be amputated below the knee*; *after gangrene set in, surgeons had to amputate her toes*

amputation [æmpjʊ'teɪʃn] *noun* surgical removal of a limb or part of a limb

amputee [æmpjʊ'ti:] *noun* patient who has had a limb or part of a limb removed in a surgical operation

amuse [ə'mju:z] *verb* to make someone happy; *the nurses amused the children at Christmas*

amusement [ə'mju:zmənt] *noun* being made happy; *Father Christmas gave out presents to the great amusement of the children in the ward*

amusing [ə'mju:zɪŋ] *adjective* which makes you happy

amygdala *or* **amygdaloid body** [ə'mɪgdələ *or* ə'mɪgdəlɔɪd 'bɒdi] *noun* almond-shaped body in the brain, at the end of the caudate nucleus of the thalamus

amyl- ['æməl] *prefix* meaning starch

amylase ['æmɪleɪz] *noun* enzyme which converts starch into maltose

amyloid ['æmɪlɔɪd] *noun* wax-like protein, associated with various diseases

amyloid disease *or* **amyloidosis** ['æmɪlɔɪd dɪ'zi:z *or* æmɪlɔɪ'dəʊsɪs] *noun* disease of the kidneys and liver, where the tissues are filled with amyloid

COMMENT: amyloid is also found in disc shaped plaques in the brain in Alzheimer's disease

amyloid precursor protein (APP) ['æmɪlɔɪd prɪ'kɜ:sə 'prəʊti:n] *noun* compound found in cell membranes from which beta amyloid is derived, a mutation of the gene causes early-onset Alzheimer's disease in a few rare families

amylopsin [æmɪ'lɒpsi:n] *noun* enzyme which converts starch into maltose

amylose ['æmɪləʊz] *noun* carbohydrate of starch

amyotonia [eɪmaɪə'təʊniə] *noun* lack of muscle tone; **amyotonia congenita** *or* **floppy baby syndrome** = congenital disease of children, where the muscles lack tone

amyotrophia [eɪmaɪə'trəʊfiə] *noun* wasting away of a muscle

amyotrophic lateral sclerosis (ALS) [eɪmaɪə'trɒfɪk 'lætərl sklə'rəʊsɪs] *noun* Gehrig's disease, a motor neurone disease, similar to muscular sclerosis, where the limbs twitch and the muscles gradually waste away

amyotrophy [eɪmaɪə'trəʊfi] = AMYOTROPHIA

an(a)- [æn] *prefix* meaning without or lacking

anabolic [ænə'bɒlɪk] *adjective* (substance) which synthesizes protein; **anabolic steroid** = drug which encourages the synthesis of new living tissue (especially muscle) from nutrients

insulin, secreted by the islets of Langerhans, is the body's major anabolic hormone,

regulating the metabolism of
all body fuels and substrates

Nursing Times

anabolism [æ'næbəlɪzm] *noun* process of
building up complex chemical substances on
the basis of simpler ones

anae- [ə'niː or 'ænɪ] (NOTE: words beginning
with anae- are spelt ane- in American English)

anaemia *US* **anemia** [ə'niːmiə] *noun*
condition where the level of red blood cells
is less than normal or where the haemoglobin
is less, making it more difficult for the blood
to carry oxygen; **haemolytic anaemia** =
anaemia caused by the destruction of red
blood cells; **iron-deficiency anaemia** =
anaemia caused by lack of iron in red blood
cells; **megaloblastic anaemia** = anaemia
caused by vitamin B_{12} deficiency;
pernicious anaemia *or* **Addison's anaemia**
= disease where an inability to absorb
vitamin B_{12} prevents the production of red
blood cells and damages the spinal cord;
splenic anaemia = type of anaemia where
the patient has portal hypertension, an
enlarged spleen and haemorrhages, caused
by cirrhosis of the liver; *see also*
APLASTIC, SICKLE-CELL

COMMENT: symptoms of anaemia are
tiredness and pale colour, especially pale
lips, nails and the inside of the eyelids. The
condition can be fatal if not treated

anaemic *US* **anemic** [ə'niːmɪk] *adjective*
suffering from anaemia

anaerobe [æn'eərəʊb] *noun*
microorganism (such as the tetanus bacillus)
which lives without oxygen

anaerobic respiration [ænə'rəʊbɪk
respə'reɪʃn] *noun* biochemical processes
which lead to the formation of ATP without
oxygen

anaesthesia *US* **anesthesia**
[ænəs'θiːziə] *noun* loss of the feeling of pain;
epidural anaesthesia = local anaesthesia
(used in childbirth) in which anaesthetic is
injected into the space between the vertebral
canal and the dura mater; **general
anaesthesia** = loss of feeling and loss of
consciousness; **local anaesthesia** = loss of
feeling in a certain part of the body; **spinal
anaesthesia** = local anaesthesia in which an
anaesthetic is injected into the cerebrospinal
fluid; *see also* NERVE BLOCK

anaesthesiologist [ænəsθiːziˈɒlədʒɪst]
noun specialist in the study of anaesthetics

anaesthesiology [ænəsθiːziˈɒlədʒi] *noun*
study of anaesthetics

anaesthetic [ænəs'θetɪk] **1** *adjective* which
produces loss of feeling; **anaesthetic
induction** = methods of inducing anaesthesia
in a patient; **anaesthetic risk** = risk that an
anaesthetic may cause serious unwanted side
effects **2** *noun* substance given to a patient to
remove feeling, so that he can undergo an
operation without feeling pain; **caudal
anaesthetic** = anaesthetic often used in
childbirth, where the drug is injected into the
base of the spine to remove feeling in the
lower part of the trunk; **general anaesthetic** =
substance (such as nitrous oxide) given to
make a patient lose consciousness so that a
major surgical operation can be carried out;
local anaesthetic = substance (such as
lignocaine hydrochloride) which removes the
feeling in a certain part of the body only;
spinal anaesthetic = anaesthetic given by
injection into the spine, which results in large
parts of the body losing the sense of feeling

Spinal and epidural
anaesthetics can also cause
gross vasodilation, leading to
heat loss

British Journal of Nursing

anaesthetist [ə'niːsθətɪst] *noun* specialist
who administers anaesthetics

anaesthetize [ə'niːsθətaɪz] *verb* to produce
a loss of feeling in a patient or in part of the
body; *the patient was anaesthetized before
the operation*

anal ['eɪnəl] *adjective* referring to the anus;
anal canal = passage leading from the rectum
to the anus; **anal fissure** = crack in the
mucous membrane of the wall of the anal
canal; **anal fistula** *or* **fistula in ano** = fistula
which develops between the rectum and the
outside of the body after an abscess near the
anus; **anal sphincter** = strong ring of muscle
which closes the anus; **anal triangle** *or* **rectal
triangle** = posterior part of the perineum

analeptic [ænə'leptɪk] *noun* drug used to
make someone regain consciousness or to
stimulate a patient

analgesia [ænəl'dʒiːziə] *noun* reduction of
the feeling of pain without loss of
consciousness; **caudal analgesia** = technique
often used in childbirth, where an analgesic is
injected into the extradural space at the base
of the spine to remove feeling in the lower
part of the trunk

analgesic [ænəl'dʒiːzɪk] **1** *adjective* referring to analgesia **2** *noun* painkilling drug which produces analgesia and reduces pyrexia

COMMENT: there are two types: non-opioid, such as paracetamol and aspirin (acetylsalicyclic acid), and opioid such as codeine phosphate. Opioid analgesics are used for severe pain relief such as in terminal care, as cough suppressants and to reduce gut motility in cases of diarrhoea; analgesics are commonly used as local anaesthetics, for example in dentistry.

anally ['eɪnəli] *adverb* through the anus; *the patient is not able to pass faeces anally*

analyse *US* **analyze** ['ænəlaɪz] *verb* to examine something in detail; *the laboratory is analysing the blood samples*; *when the food was analysed it was found to contain traces of bacteria*

analyser *US* **analyzer** ['ænəlaɪzə] *noun* machine which analyses blood or tissue samples automatically

analysis [ə'næləsɪs] *noun* examination of a substance to find out what it is made of (NOTE: the plural is **analyses**)

analyst ['ænəlɪst] *noun* **(a)** person who examines samples of substances or tissue, to find out what they are made of **(b)** = PSYCHOANALYST

anaphase ['ænəfeɪz] *noun* stage in cell division, after the metaphase and before the telophase

anaphylactic shock [ænəfɪ'læktɪk 'ʃɒk] *noun* sudden allergic reaction to an allergen such as an injection, which can be fatal

anaphylaxis [ænəfɪ'læksɪs] *noun* reaction, similar to an allergic reaction, to an injection or to a bee sting

anaplasia [ænə'pleɪsɪə] *noun* loss of a cell's characteristics, caused by cancer

anaplastic [ænə'plæstɪk] *adjective* referring to anaplasia; **anaplastic neoplasm** = cancer where the cells are not similar to those of the tissue from which they come

anasarca [ænə'sɑːkə] *noun* dropsy, presence of fluid in the body tissues

anastomose [ə'næstəməʊz] *verb* to attach two arteries or tubes together

anastomosis [ənæstə'məʊsɪs] *noun* connection made between two vessels or two tubes, either naturally or by surgery

anatomical [ænə'tɒmɪkl] *adjective* referring to anatomy; *the anatomical features of a fetus*

anatomist [ə'nætəmɪst] *noun* scientist who specializes in the study of anatomy

anatomy [ə'nætəmi] *noun* (i) structure of the body; (ii) study of the structure of the body; *he is studying anatomy*; *she failed her anatomy examination*; **human anatomy** = structure, shape and functions of the human body; **the anatomy of a bone** = description of the structure and shape of a bone

ancestor ['ænsestə] *noun* person from whom someone is descended, usually a person who lived a long time ago

ancillary staff [æn'sɪləri 'stɑːf] *noun* staff in a hospital who are not administrators, doctors or nurses (such as cleaners, porters, kitchen staff, etc.)

anconeus [æŋ'kəʊniəs] *noun* small triangular muscle at the back of the elbow

Ancylostoma *or* **Ankylostoma** [ænsɪ'lɒstəmə *or* æŋkɪ'lɒstəmə] *noun* *Ancylostoma duodenale*, the hookworm, a parasitic worm in the intestine, that holds onto the wall of the intestine with its teeth and lives on the blood and protein of the carrier

ancylostomiasis [ænsɪlɒstə'maɪəsɪs] *noun* hookworm disease, a disease of which the symptoms are weakness and anaemia, caused by a hookworm which lives on the blood of the host. In severe cases the patient may die; *see also* NECATOR

androgen ['ændrədʒn] *noun* male sex hormone (testosterone and androsterone), the hormone which increases the male characteristics of the body

androgenic [ændrə'dʒenɪk] *adjective* which produces male characteristics

androsterone [æn'drɒstərəʊn] *noun* one of the male sex hormones

anemia [ə'niːmiə] *US* = ANAEMIA

anencephalous [ænen'sefələs] *adjective* having no brain

anencephaly [ænen'sefəli] *noun* absence of a brain, which causes a fetus to die a few hours after birth

anergy ['ænədʒi] *noun* (i) being weak, lacking energy; (ii) lack of immunity

anesthesia [ænəs'θiːziə] *US* = ANAESTHESIA

aneurine [ə'njuərɪn] *noun* thiamine, vitamin B₁

aneurysm *or* **aneurism** ['ænjərɪzm] *noun* swelling caused by the weakening of a wall of a blood vessel; **congenital aneurysm =** weakening of the arteries at the base of the brain, occurring in a baby from birth

> COMMENT: aneurysm usually occurs in the wall of the aorta, (aortic aneurysm) and is often due to atherosclerosis, and sometimes to syphilis

angiectasis [ænd͡ʒi'ektəsɪs] *noun* swelling of the blood vessels

angiitis [ænd͡ʒi'aɪtɪs] *noun* inflammation of a blood vessel

angina (pectoris) [æn'd͡ʒaɪnə 'pektərɪs] *noun* pain in the chest caused by inadequate supply of blood to the heart muscles, following exercise or eating, because of narrowing of the arteries; **stable angina =** angina which has not changed for a long time; **unstable angina =** angina which has suddenly become worse

> COMMENT: angina is commonly treated with nitrates or calcium channel blocker drugs

anginal [æn'd͡ʒaɪnəl] *adjective* referring to angina; *he suffered anginal pains*

angi(o)- ['ænd͡ʒi(əu)] *prefix* referring to a blood vessel

angiocardiography [ænd͡ʒiəukɑː'dɪɒɡrəfi] *noun* X-ray examination of the cardiac system after injection with an opaque dye so that the organs show up clearly on the film

angiocardiogram [ænd͡ʒiəu'kɑːdiəgræm] *noun* series of pictures resulting from angiocardiography

angiogram ['ænd͡ʒiəugræm] *noun* X-ray picture of blood vessels

angiography [ænd͡ʒi'ɒgrəfi] *noun* X-ray examination of blood vessels after injection with an opaque dye so that they show up clearly on the film

angioma [ænd͡ʒi'əumə] *noun* benign tumour (such as a naevus) formed of blood vessels

angioneurotic oedema [ænd͡ʒiəunju'rɒtɪk ɪ'diːmə] *noun* sudden accumulation of liquid under the skin, similar to nettle rash

angiopathy [ænd͡ʒi'ɒpəθi] *noun* general term for disease of vessels, such as blood and lymphatic vessels

angioplasty ['ænd͡ʒiəplæsti] *noun* plastic surgery to repair a blood vessel, such as a narrowed coronary artery; **percutaneous angioplasty** *or* **balloon angioplasty =** repair of a narrowed artery by passing a balloon into the artery through a catheter and then inflating it

angiosarcoma [ænd͡ʒiəusɑː'kəumə] *noun* malignant tumour in a blood vessel

angiospasm ['ænd͡ʒiəspæzm] *noun* spasm which constricts blood vessels

angiotensin ['ænd͡ʒiətensiːn] *noun* polypeptide which affects blood pressure by causing vasoconstriction and increasing extracellular volume

> COMMENT: the precursor protein, alpha-2-globulin is converted to angiotensin I, which is inactive. A converting enzyme changes angiotensin I into the active form, angiotensin II. Drugs which block the conversion to the active form, ACE inhibitors, are used in the treatment of hypertension and heart failure

angiotensin-converting enzyme inhibitor (ACE inhibitor) ['ænd͡ʒiətensiːnkʌn'vɜːtɪŋ 'enzaɪm ɪn'hɪbɪtə] *noun* drug which inhibits the conversion of angiotensin I to angiotensin II (a potent vasopressor), used in the treatment of hypertension and heart failure (NOTE: ACE inhibitors have names ending in **-pril: Captopril**)

> COMMENT: contra-indications include use with diuretics, when hypotension can occur and should be avoided in patients with renovascular disease

angle ['æŋgl] *noun* bend, corner; *see also* STERNOCLAVICULAR

angular vein ['æŋgjulə 'veɪn] *noun* vein which continues the facial vein at the side of the nose

anhidrosis [ænhɪ'drəusɪs] *noun* condition where the amount of sweat is reduced or there is no sweat at all

anhidrotic [ænhɪ'drɒtɪk] *adjective* drug which reduces sweating

anhydraemia [ænhaɪ'driːmiə] *noun* lack of sufficient fluid in the blood

anidrosis [ænɪ'drəusɪs] *noun* = ANHIDROSIS

animal ['æniml] *noun* living organism which can feel sensation and move voluntarily; *dogs and cats are animals and man is also an animal*; **animal bite =** bite from an animal

COMMENT: bites from animals should be cleaned immediately. The main danger from animal bites is the possibility of catching rabies

aniridia [ænɪˈrɪdiə] *noun* congenital absence of the iris

anisometropia [ænaɪsəʊməˈtrəʊpiə] *noun* state where the refraction in the two eyes is different

ankle [ˈæŋkl] *noun* part of the body where the foot is connected to the leg; **he twisted his ankle** *or* **he sprained his ankle** = he hurt it by stretching it or bending it; **anklebone** = talus, a bone which is part of the tarsus and links the bones of the lower leg to the calcaneus; **ankle fracture** = break in any of the bones in the ankle; **ankle jerk** = sudden jerk as a reflex action of the foot when the back of the ankle is tapped; **ankle joint** = joint which connects the bones of the lower leg (the tibia and fibula) to the talus

ankyloblepharon [æŋkɪləʊˈblefərɒn] *noun* state where the edges of the eyelids are stuck together

ankylose [ˈæŋkɪləʊz] *verb (of bones)* to fuse together; *see also* SPONDYLITIS

ankylosis [æŋkɪˈləʊsɪs] *noun* condition where the bones of a joint fuse together

Ankylostoma *or* **ankylostomiasis** [æŋkɪˈlɒstəmə *or* æŋkɪlɒstəˈmaɪəsɪs] *see* ANCYLOSTOMA, ANCYLOSTOMIASIS

annular [ˈænjʊlə] *adjective* shaped like a ring

annulus [ˈænjʊləs] *noun* ring, structure shaped like a ring

anococcygeal [ænəkɒksɪˈdʒiːəl] *adjective* referring to both the anus and coccyx

anomalous [əˈnɒmələs] *adjective* different from what is usual; **anomalous pulmonary venous drainage** = condition where oxygenated blood from the lungs drains into the right atrium instead of the left

anomaly [əˈnɒməlɪ] *noun* something which is different from the usual

anonychia [ænəˈnɪkiə] *noun* congenital absence of one or more nails

anopheles [əˈnɒfəliːz] *noun* mosquito which carries the malaria parasite

anorchism [ænˈɔːkɪzm] *noun* congenital absence of testicles

anorectal [eɪnəʊˈrektl] *adjective* referring to both the anus and rectum

anorexia [ænəˈreksiə] *noun* loss of appetite; **anorexia nervosa** = psychological condition (usually found in girls) where the patient refuses to eat because of a fear of becoming fat

anorexic [ænəˈreksɪk] *adjective* referring to anorexia; (person) suffering from anorexia; *the school has developed a programme of counselling for anorexic students*

anosmia [ænˈɒzmiə] *noun* lack of the sense of smell

anovular bleeding [ænˈɒvjʊlə ˈbliːdɪŋ] *noun* bleeding from the uterus when ovulation has not taken place

anovulation [ænɒvjuːˈleɪʃn] *noun* condition where a women does not ovulate and is therefore infertile

anoxaemia [ænɒkˈsiːmiə] *noun* reduction of the amount of oxygen in the blood

anoxia [ænˈɒksiə] *noun* lack of oxygen in body tissue

anoxic [ænˈɒksɪk] *noun* referring to anoxia; lacking oxygen

anserina [ˈænseraɪnə] *see* CUTIS

answer [ˈɑːnsə] **1** *noun* reply, words spoken or written when someone has spoken to you or asked you a question; *he phoned the laboratory but there was no answer*; *have the tests provided an answer to the problem?* **2** *verb* to reply or speak or write words when someone has spoken to you or asked you a question; *when asked if the patient would survive, the consultant did not answer*; **to answer an emergency call** = to go to the place where the call came from to bring help

antacid [æntˈæsɪd] *adjective & noun* (substance, such as calcium carbonate or magnesium trisilicate) that stops too much acid forming in the stomach or alters the amount of acid in the stomach; used in the treatment of gastro-intestinal disease such as ulcers

antagonist [ænˈtægənɪst] **1** *adjective* (muscle) which opposes another muscle in a movement; (substance) which opposes another substance **2** *noun* substance which acts through specific receptors to block the action of another substance, but which has no observable physiological effect itself; *atropine is a cholinergic antagonist and blocks the effects of acetylcholine*

ante- [ˈænti] *prefix* meaning before

ante cibum ['ænti 'tʃɪbʌm or 'siːbʌm] *Latin phrase meaning* 'before food' (used in prescriptions)

anteflexion [ænti'flekʃn] *noun* abnormal bending forward, especially of the uterus

antemortem [ænti'mɔːtəm] *noun* period before death

antenatal [ænti'neɪtəl] *adjective* during the period between conception and childbirth; **antenatal diagnosis** *or* **prenatal diagnosis** = medical examination of a pregnant woman to see if the fetus is developing normally; *see also* CLINIC

antepartum [ænti'pɑːtəm] *noun & adjective* period of three months before childbirth

anterior [æn'tɪərɪə] *adjective* in front; **anterior aspect** = view of the front of the body, of part of the body; **anterior superior iliac spine** = projection at the front end of the iliac crest of the pelvis; **anterior jugular** = small jugular vein in the neck; **anterior synechia** = condition of the eye, where the iris sticks to the cornea (NOTE: the opposite is **posterior**)

anteversion [ænti'vɜːʃn] *noun* leaning forward of an organ, especially of the uterus

anthelmintic [ænθel'mɪntɪk] *noun & adjective* (substance) which removes worms from the intestine

anthracosis [ænθrə'kəʊsɪs] *noun* lung disease caused by breathing coal dust

anthrax ['ænθræks] *noun* disease of cattle and sheep which can be transmitted to humans

COMMENT: caused by *Bacillus anthracis*, anthrax can be transmitted by touching infected skin, meat or other parts of an animal (including bone meal used as a fertilizer). It causes pustules on the skin or in the lungs (woolsorter's disease)

anti- ['ænti] *prefix* meaning against

antiallergenic [æntiælə'dʒenɪk] *adjective* (cosmetic, etc.) which will not aggravate an allergy

anti-arrhythmic ['æntiæ'rɪθmɪk] *adjective* (drug) which corrects an irregular heartbeat

antibacterial [æntibæk'tɪərɪəl] *adjective* which destroys bacteria

antibiogram [ænti'baɪəgræm] *noun* laboratory technique which establishes to what degree an organism is sensitive to an antibiotic

antibiotic [æntibaɪ'ɒtɪk] **1** *adjective* which stops the spread of bacteria **2** *noun* drug (such as penicillin) which is developed from living substances and which stops the spread of microorganisms; *he was given a course of antibiotics*; *antibiotics have no use against virus diseases*; **broad-spectrum antibiotic** = antibiotic used to control many types of bacteria

COMMENT: penicillin is one of the commonest antibiotics, together with streptomycin, tetracycline, erythromycin and many others. Although antibiotics are widely and successfully used, new forms of bacteria have developed which are resistant to them

antibody ['æntibɒdi] *noun* substance which is naturally present in the body and which attacks foreign substances (such as bacteria); *tests showed that he was antibody-positive*

anti-cancer drug [ænti'kænsə 'drʌg] *noun* drug which can control or destroy cancer cells

anticoagulant [æntikəʊ'ægjʊlənt] *noun & adjective* (drug) which slows down or stops the clotting of blood, used to prevent the formation of a thrombus (NOTE: anticoagulants have names ending in **-parin: heparin**)

anticonvulsant [æntikən'vʌlsənt] *noun & adjective* (drug, such as carbamazepine) used to control convulsions, as in the treatment of epilepsy

antidepressant [æntidɪ'presənt] *noun & adjective* (drug) used to treat depression by increasing the amount of sympathetic neurotransmitters in the brain

COMMENT: examples are tricyclic antidepressant, selective serotonin reuptake inhibitor, monoamine oxidase inhibitor

antidiabetic [æntidaɪə'betɪk] *noun & adjective* (drug) which is used in the treatment of diabetes

antidiarrhoeal *US* **antidiarrheal** [æntidaɪə'riːəl] *noun & adjective* (drug, etc.) which is used in the treatment of diarrhoea

anti D immunoglobulin ['ænti 'diː ɪmjʊnəʊ'glɒbjulɪn] *noun* immunoglobulin administered to Rh-negative mothers after the birth of a Rh-positive baby, to prevent haemolytic disease of the newborn in the next pregnancy

antidiuretic [æntidaɪjuˈretɪk] *adjective & noun* (substance) which stops the production of excessive amounts of urine; *hormones* *which have an antidiuretic effect on the kidneys*; **antidiuretic hormone (ADH)** = vasopressin, a hormone secreted by the posterior lobe of the pituitary gland which acts on the kidneys to regulate the quantity of salt in body fluids and the amount of urine excreted by the kidneys

antidote ['æntɪdəʊt] *noun* substance which counteracts the effect of a poison; *there is no satisfactory antidote to cyanide*

antiemetic [æntɪɪ'metɪk] *noun & adjective* (drug, such as domperidone) which prevents sickness, vomiting

antiepileptic drug [æntiepɪ'leptɪk 'drʌg] *noun* drug (such as carbamazepine) used in the treatment of epilepsy and convulsions

antifungal [ænti'fʌŋgəl] *adjective* (substance) which kills or controls fungal and yeast infections such as candida and ringworm (NOTE: antifungal drugs have names ending in **-conazole: fluconazole)**

antigen ['æntɪdʒən] *noun* substance (such as a virus or germ) in the body which makes the body produce antibodies to attack it

antigenic [ænti'dʒenɪk] *adjective* (substance) which stimulates the formation of antibodies

antihaemophilic factor [æntihiːmə'fɪlɪk 'fæktə] *noun* factor VIII (used to encourage clotting in haemophiliacs)

antihelmintic [æntihel'mɪntɪk] *noun* drug (such as mebendazole) used in the treatment of worm infection such as threadworm, hookworm, round worm

antihistamine (drug) [ænti'hɪstəmiːn 'drʌg] *noun* drug used to control the effects of an allergy which releases histamine, or reduces gastric acid in the stomach for the treatment of gastric ulcers (NOTE: antihistamines have names ending in **-tidine: loratidine** (allergy), **cimetidine** (gastric ulcer))

anti-HIV antibodies ['æntieɪtʃaɪ'viː 'æntibɒdiz] *noun* antibodies which attack HIV

antihypertensive [æntihaɪpə'tensɪv] *adjective & noun* (drug, such as hydralazine hydrochloride) used to reduce high blood pressure

anti-inflammatory [æntiɪn'flæmətri] *adjective* (drug, such as ibuprofen) which reduces inflammation, as in a joint, etc.

antilymphocytic serum (ALS) [æntilɪmfəʊ'sɪtɪk 'sɪərəm] *noun* serum used to produce immunosuppression in transplants

antimalarial [æntimə'leəriəl] *adjective & noun* (drug) used to treat malaria and in malarial prophylaxis (NOTE: antimalarial drugs have names ending in **-oquine: chloroquine)**

antimetabolite [æntimə'tæbəlaɪt] *noun* substance which can replace a cell metabolism but which is not active

antimigraine [ænti'maɪgreɪn] *noun* drug (such as sumatriptan) used in the treatment of migraine for its properties as a 5-hydroxy tryptamine 1 agonist

antimitotic [æntimaɪ'tɒtɪk] *adjective* which prevents the division of a cell by mitosis

antimuscarinic [æntiməskə'rɪnɪk] *adjective* (drug) which blocks acetylcholine receptors found on smooth muscle in the gut and eye

antimycotic [æntimaɪ'kɒtɪk] *adjective* which destroys fungi

antiperistalsis [æntiperɪ'stælsɪs] *noun* movement in the oesophagus or intestine where the contents are moved in the opposite direction to normal peristalsis, so leading to vomiting

antiperspirant [ænti'pɜːsprənt] *noun & adjective* (substance) which prevents sweating

antipruritic [æntipru'rɪtɪk] *noun & adjective* (substance) which prevents itching

antipsychotic [æntisaɪ'kɒtɪk] *noun* neuroleptic or major tranquilizer drug (such as chlorpromazine hydrochloride) which calms disturbed patients without causing sedation or confusion by blocking dopamine receptors in the brain, used in the treatment of schizophrenia, psychoses, mania

COMMENT: extrapyramidal side effects can occur, including Parkinsonian symptoms and restlessness

antipyretic [æntipaɪ'retɪk] *noun & adjective* (drug, such as aspirin) which helps to reduce a fever

anti Rh body ['ænti 'ɑːr 'eɪtʃ 'bɒdi] *noun* antibody formed in the mother's blood in reaction to a Rhesus antigen in the blood of the fetus

antisepsis [ænti'sepsɪs] *noun* preventing sepsis

antiseptic [ænti'septɪk] **1** *adjective* which prevents germs spreading; *she gargled with an antiseptic mouthwash* **2** *noun* substance which prevents germs growing or spreading; *the nurse painted the wound with antiseptic*

antiserum [ænti'sɪərəm] *noun* serum taken from an animal which has developed antibodies to bacteria and used to give temporary immunity to a disease (NOTE: the plural is **antisera**)

antisocial [ænti'səʊʃəl] *adjective* (behaviour) which is harmful to other people; **antisocial hours** = hours of work (such as night duty) which can disrupt the worker's family life

antispasmodic [æntispæz'mɒdɪk] *noun* drug (such as mebeverine hydrochloride) used to prevent spasms

antitetanus serum (ATS) [ænti'tetənəs 'sɪərəm] *noun* serum which protects a patient against tetanus

antithrombin [ænti'θrɒmbɪn] *noun* substance present in the blood which prevents clotting

antitoxic serum [ænti'tɒksɪk 'sɪərəm] *noun* immunizing agent, formed of serum taken from an animal which has developed antibodies to a disease, used to protect a person from that disease

antitoxin [ænti'tɒksɪn] *noun* antibody produced by the body to counteract a poison in the body

antitragus [ænti'treɪgəs] *noun* small projection on the outer ear opposite the tragus

antituberculous drug [æntitju'bɜːkjʊləs 'drʌg] *noun* drug (such as Isoniazid or rifampicin) used to treat tuberculosis

antitussive [ænti'tʌsɪv] *noun* drug (such as codeine phosphate) used to reduce coughing

antivenene *or* **antivenom (serum)** [æntɪvə'niːn or ænti'venəm 'sɪərəm] *noun* serum which is used to counteract the poison from snake or insect bites

antiviral drug [ænti'vaɪrəl 'drʌg] *noun* drug which is effective against a virus, such as herpes simplex (NOTE: antiviral drugs have names ending in **-ciclovir: aciclovir**)

antral ['æntrəl] *adjective* referring to an antrum; **antral puncture** = making a hole in the wall of the maxillary sinus to remove fluid

antrectomy [æn'trektəmi] *noun* surgical removal of an antrum in the stomach to prevent gastrin being formed

antrostomy [æn'trɒstəmi] *noun* surgical operation to make an opening in the maxillary sinus to drain an antrum

antrum ['æntrəm] *noun* any cavity inside the body, especially one in bone; **mastoid antrum** = cavity linking the air cells of the mastoid process with the middle ear; **maxillary antrum** *or* **antrum of Highmore** = one of two sinuses behind the cheekbones in the upper jaw; **pyloric antrum** = space at the bottom of the stomach, before the pyloric sphincter

anuria [æn'jʊəriə] *noun* condition where the patient does not make urine, either because of a deficiency in the kidneys or because the urinary tract is blocked

anus ['eɪnəs] *noun* opening at the end of the rectum between the buttocks, leading outside the body and through which faeces are passed; *see illustrations at* DIGESTIVE SYSTEM, UROGENITAL SYSTEM (NOTE: for terms referring to the anus, see also **anal** and words beginning with **ano-**)

anvil ['ænvɪl] *noun* incus, one of the three ossicles in the middle ear; *see illustration at* EAR

anxiety [æŋ'zaɪəti] *noun* state of being very worried and afraid; **anxiety disorder** = mental disorder (such as a phobia) where the patient is very worried and afraid

anxiolytic [æŋksiə'lɪtɪk] *noun & adjective* type of drug used in the treatment of anxiety

anxious ['æŋkʃəs] *adjective* **(a)** very worried and afraid; *my sister is ill - I am anxious about her* **(b)** eager; *she was anxious to get home*; *I was anxious to see the doctor*

aorta [eɪ'ɔːtə] *noun* large artery which takes blood away from the left side of the heart and carries it to other arteries; *see illustration at* HEART; **abdominal aorta** = part of the aorta between the diaphragm and the point where it divides into the iliac arteries; *see illustration at* KIDNEY; **ascending aorta** *or* **descending aorta** = first two sections of the aorta as it leaves the heart, first rising and then turning downwards; **thoracic aorta** = part of the aorta which crosses the thorax

COMMENT: the aorta is about 45 centimetres long. It leaves the left ventricle, rises (where the carotid arteries branch off), then goes downwards through the abdomen and divides into the two iliac arteries. The aorta is the blood vessel which carries all arterial blood from the heart

aortic [eɪˈɔːtɪk] *adjective* referring to the aorta; **aortic arch** = bend in the aorta which links the ascending aorta to the descending; **aortic aneurysm** = serious aneurysm of the aorta, associated with atherosclerosis; **aortic hiatus** = opening in the diaphragm through which the aorta passes; **aortic incompetence** = defective aortic valve, causing regurgitation; **aortic regurgitation** = backwards flow of blood caused by a defective aortic valve; **aortic sinuses** = swellings in the aorta from which the coronary arteries lead back into the heart itself; **aortic stenosis** = condition where the aortic valve is narrow, caused by rheumatic fever; **aortic valve** = valve with three flaps, situated at the opening into the aorta

aortitis [eɪɔːˈtaɪtɪs] *noun* inflammation of the aorta

aortography [eɪɔːˈtɒɡrəfi] *noun* X-ray examination of the aorta after an opaque substance has been injected into it

apathetic [æpəˈθetɪk] *adjective* (patient) who takes no interest in anything

aperient [əˈpɪəriənt] *noun & adjective* (substance, such as a laxative or purgative) which causes a bowel movement

aperistalsis [æperɪˈstælsɪs] *noun* lack of the peristaltic movement in the bowel

aperture [ˈæpətʃə] *noun* hole

apex [ˈeɪpeks] *noun* top of the heart or lung; end of the root of a tooth; **apex beat** = heartbeat which can be felt if the hand is placed on the heart

Apgar score [ˈæpɡɑː ˈskɔː] *noun* method of judging the condition of a newborn baby

COMMENT: the baby is given a maximum of two points on each of five criteria: colour of the skin, heartbeat, breathing, muscle tone and reaction to stimuli

in this study, babies having an Apgar score of four or less had 100% mortality. The lower the Apgar score, the poorer the chance of survival
Indian Journal of Medical Sciences

aphagia [əˈfeɪdʒiə] *noun* being unable to swallow

aphakia [əˈfeɪkiə] *noun* absence of the crystalline lens in the eye

aphakic [əˈfeɪkɪk] *adjective* referring to aphakia

aphasia [əˈfeɪziə] *noun* being unable to speak or write or understand speech or writing because of damage to the brain centres controlling speech

aphonia [eɪˈfəʊniə] *noun* being unable to make sounds

aphrodisiac [æfrəˈdɪziæk] *noun & adjective* (substance) which increases sexual urges

aphthae *or* **aphthous ulcers** [ˈæfθiː or ˈæfθəs ˈʌlsəz] *plural noun* ulcers in the mouth

apical abscess [ˈæpɪkəl ˈæbses] *noun* abscess in the socket around the root of a tooth

apicectomy [æpɪˈsektəmi] *noun* surgical removal of the root of a tooth

aplasia [əˈpleɪziə] *noun* lack of growth of tissue

aplastic anaemia [eɪˈplæstɪk əˈniːmiə] *noun* anaemia caused by bone marrow failure which stops the formation of red blood cells

apnoea *US* **apnea** [æpˈniːə] *noun* stopping of breathing; **sleep apnoea** = condition related to heavy snoring, with prolonged respiratory pauses leading to cerebral hypoxia and subsequent daytime drowsiness

apnoeic *US* **apneic** [æpˈniːɪk] *adjective* where breathing has stopped

apocrine gland [ˈæpəkraɪn ˈɡlænd] *noun* gland, such as a sweat gland producing body odour, where part of the gland's cells breaks off with the secretions

ApoE = APOLIPOPROTEIN E

apolipoprotein E (ApoE) [əpɒlɪpəˈprəʊtiːn] *noun* compound found in three varieties which transport lipids within the cell and across cell membranes, the genes for two of which are linked with increased risk of Alzheimer's disease

aponeurosis [æpəʊnjuˈrəʊsɪs] *noun* band of tissue which attaches muscles to each other

apophyseal [æpəˈfɪziəl] *adjective* referring to apophysis

apophysis [əˈpɒfəsɪs] *noun* process, growth of bone

apophysitis [æpəfɪ'saɪtɪs] *noun* type of osteochondritis, inflammation of an apophysis

apoplectic [æpə'plektɪk] *adjective* (person) suffering from apoplexy, likely to have a stroke

apoplexy ['æpəpleksi] *noun* stroke, the sudden loss of consciousness caused by a cerebral haemorrhage or blood clot in the brain

APP = AMYLOID PRECURSOR PROTEIN

apparatus [æpə'reɪtəs] *noun* equipment used in a laboratory or hospital; *the hospital has installed new apparatus in the physiotherapy department; the blood sample was tested in a special piece of apparatus* (NOTE: no plural: **a piece of apparatus; some new apparatus**)

appear [ə'pɪə] *verb* (a) to start being seen; *a rash suddenly appeared on the upper part of the body* (b) to seem; *he appears to be seriously ill*

appearance [ə'pɪərəns] *noun* how a person or thing looks; *you could tell from her appearance that she was suffering from anaemia*

appendage [ə'pendɪdʒ] *noun* part of the body or piece of tissue which hangs down from another part

appendectomy [æpən'dektəmi] *noun US* = APPENDICECTOMY

appendiceal [æpən'dɪsiəl] *adjective* referring to the appendix; *there is a risk of appendiceal infection;* **appendiceal colic** = colic caused by a grumbling appendix

appendicectomy [əpendɪ'sektəmi] *noun* surgical removal of an appendix

appendicitis [əpendə'saɪtɪs] *noun* inflammation of the vermiform appendix

COMMENT: appendicitis takes several forms, the main ones being: acute appendicitis, which is a sudden attack of violent pain in the right lower part of the abdomen, accompanied by a fever. Acute appendicitis normally requires urgent surgery. A second form is chronic appendicitis, where the appendix is continually slightly inflamed, giving a permanent dull pain or a feeling of indigestion

appendicular skeleton [æpən'dɪkjulə 'skelətən] *noun* part of the skeleton, formed of the pelvic girdle, pectoral girdle and the bones of the arms and legs; *compare* AXIAL SKELETON

appendix [ə'pendɪks] *noun* (a) any small tube or sac hanging from an organ (b) **(vermiform) appendix** = small tube shaped like a worm, attached to the caecum, which serves no function but can become infected, causing appendicitis; *she had her appendix removed; an operation to remove the appendix;* **grumbling appendix** = chronic appendicitis (NOTE: the plural is **appendices**); *see illustration at* DIGESTIVE SYSTEM

appetite ['æpɪtaɪt] *noun* wanting food; **good appetite** = interest in eating food; **loss of appetite** = becoming uninterested in eating food; **poor appetite** = lack of interest in eating food

appliance [ə'plaɪəns] *noun* piece of apparatus used on the body; *he was wearing a surgical appliance to support his neck*

application [æplɪ'keɪʃn] *noun* (a) asking for a job (usually in writing); *if you are applying for the job, you must fill in an application form* (b) putting a substance on; *two applications of the lotion should be made each day*

applicator ['æplɪkeɪtə] *noun* device for applying a substance

apply [ə'plaɪ] *verb* (a) to ask for a job; *she applied for a job in a teaching hospital* (b) to refer to; *this order applies to all medical staff; the rule applies to visitors only* (c) to put (a substance) on; *to apply a dressing to a wound; the ointment should not be applied to the face* (d) to carry out a treatment; *to apply traction*

appoint [ə'pɔɪnt] *verb* to give someone a job; *she was appointed night sister*

appointment [ə'pɔɪntmənt] *noun* (a) giving someone a job; **on his appointment as head of the clinical department** = when he was made head of the clinical department (b) arrangement to see someone at a particular time; *I have an appointment with the doctor or to see the doctor on Tuesday or I have a doctor's appointment on Tuesday; can I make an appointment to see Dr Jones?; I'm very busy - I've got appointments all day*

appreciate [ə'priːʃieɪt] *verb* to notice how good something is; *the patients always appreciate a talk with the ward sister*

approach [ə'prəʊtʃ] **1** *noun* (a) way of dealing with a problem; *the authority has adopted a radical approach to the problem of patient waiting lists* (b) *(in surgery)* path used by a surgeon when carrying out an operation; **posterior approach** = (operation) carried out from the back; **transdiaphragmatic approach** = (operation) carried out through the diaphragm **2** *verb* to go, come nearer; *as the consultant approached, all the patients looked at him*

approve [ə'pruːv] *verb;* **to approve of something** = to think that something is good; *I don't approve of patients staying in bed; the Medical Council does not approve of this new treatment; the drug has been approved by the Department of Health*

apraxia [eɪ'præksɪə] *noun* being unable to make proper movements

apron ['eɪprən] *noun* cloth or plastic cover which you wear in front of your clothes to stop them getting dirty; *the surgeon was wearing a green apron*

apyrexia [æpaɪ'reksɪə] *noun* absence of fever

apyrexial [æpaɪ'reksɪəl] *adjective* no longer having any fever

aqua ['ækwə] *noun* water

aqueduct ['ækwɪdʌkt] *noun* canal, tube which carries fluid from one part of the body to another; **cerebral aqueduct** *or* **aqueduct of Sylvius** = canal connecting the third and fourth ventricles in the brain

aqueous ['eɪkwɪəs or 'ækwɪəs] *adjective* (solution) made with water

aqueous (humour) ['eɪkwɪəs 'hjuːmə] *noun* fluid in the eye between the lens and the cornea (NOTE: usually referred to as 'the aqueous')

aquiline nose ['ækwɪlaɪn 'nəʊz] *noun* nose which is large and strongly curved

AR = ATTRIBUTABLE RISK

arachidonic acid [ærəkə'dɒnɪk 'æsɪd] *noun* essential fatty acid

arachnidism [ə'ræknɪdɪzm] *noun* poisoning by the bite of a spider

arachnodactyly [ərækno'dæktɪli] *noun* one of the conditions of Marfan's syndrome, a congenital condition where the fingers and toes are long and thin

arachnoiditis [æræknɔɪ'daɪtɪs] *noun* inflammation of the arachnoid membrane

arachnoid mater *or* **arachnoid membrane** [ə'ræknɔɪd 'meɪtə or ə'ræknɔɪd 'membreɪn] *noun* middle membrane covering the brain

arborization [ɑːbəraɪ'zeɪʃn] *noun* (i) branching ends of some nerve fibres or of a motor nerve in muscle fibre; (ii) normal tree-like appearance of venules, capillaries and arterioles; (iii) branching of capillaries when inflamed

arbor vitae ['ɑːbə 'vaɪtiː] *noun* structure of the cerebellum or of the uterus which looks like a tree

arbovirus [ɑːbəʊ'vaɪərəs] *noun* virus transmitted by blood-sucking insects

arc [ɑːk] *noun* (i) nerve pathway; (ii) part of a curved structure in the body; **arc eye** = temporary painful blindness caused by ultraviolet rays, especially in arc welding; **reflex arc** = nerve pathway of a reflex action

ARC = AIDS-RELATED CONDITION *or* COMPLEX

arch [ɑːtʃ] *noun* curved part of the body, especially under the foot; **aortic arch** = bend in the aorta which links the ascending aorta to the descending; **deep plantar arch** = curved artery crossing the sole of the foot; **palmar arch** = one of two arches in the palm of the hand, formed by two arteries which link together; **longitudinal arch** *or* **plantar arch** = curved part of the sole of the foot running along the length of the foot; **metatarsal arch** *or* **transverse arch** = arched part of the sole of the foot, running across the sole of the foot from side to side; **zygomatic arch** = ridge of bone across the temporal bone, running between the ear and the bottom of the eye socket; **fallen arches** = condition where the arches in the sole of the foot are not high

arcuate ['ɑːkjuɪt] *adjective* arched; **internal** *or* **external arcuate ligament** *or* **medial arcuate ligament** = fibrous arch to which the diaphragm is attached; *see also* ARTERY

arcus ['ɑːkəs] *noun* arch; **arcus senilis** = grey ring round the cornea, found in old people

area ['eərɪə] *noun* **(a)** measurement of the space occupied by something; *to measure the area of a room you must multiply the length by the width; the area of the ward is 250 square metres* **(b)** space occupied by something; *there is a small area of affected tissue in the right lung; treat the infected area with antiseptic;* **bare area of the liver** = large triangular part of the liver, not covered with peritoneum; **visual area** = part of the cerebral cortex which is concerned with sight

areata [æri'eɪtə] *see* ALOPECIA

areola [əˈriːələ] *noun* (i) coloured part round the nipple; (ii) part of the iris closest to the pupil

areolar tissue [əˈriːələ ˈtɪʃuː] *noun* type of connective tissue

arginine [ˈɑːdʒiniːn] *noun* amino acid which helps the liver form urea

Argyll Robertson pupil [ɑːˈgaɪl ˈrɒbətsən ˈpjuːpəl] *noun* condition of the eye, where the lens is able to focus but the pupil does not react to light

COMMENT: a symptom of tertiary syphilis or of locomotor ataxia

arise [əˈraɪz] *verb* (i) to begin in, come from (a place); (ii) to start to happen; *a muscle arising in the scapula*; *two problems have arisen concerning the removal of the geriatric patients to the other hospital* (NOTE: **arising - arose - has arisen**)

the target cells for adult myeloid leukaemia are located in the bone marrow, and there is now evidence that a substantial proportion of childhood leukaemias also arise in bone marrow
British Medical Journal

one issue has consistently arisen - the amount of time and effort which nurses need to put into the writing of detailed care plans
Nursing Times

arm [ɑːm] *noun* one of the limbs, the part of the body which goes from the shoulder to the hand, formed of the upper arm, the elbow and the forearm; *she broke her arm skiing*; *lift your arms up above your head*; **arm bones** = the humerus, the ulna and the radius; **arm sling** = bandage attached round the neck, used to support an injured arm and prevent it from moving; *he had his arm in a sling*

armpit [ˈɑːmpɪt] *noun* the axilla, the hollow under the shoulder, between the upper arm and the body, where the upper arm joins the shoulder (NOTE: for other terms referring to the arm see words beginning with **brachi-**)

Arnold-Chiari malformation
[ˈɑːnɒldkiˈeəri mælfɔːˈmeɪʃn] *noun* congenital condition where the base of the skull is malformed, allowing parts of the cerebellum into the spinal canal

aromatherapist [ərəʊməˈθerəpɪst] *noun* person specializing in aromatherapy

aromatherapy [ərəʊməˈθerəpi] *noun* treatment to relieve tension, etc., in which fragrant oils and creams containing plant extracts are massaged into the skin

arrange [əˈreɪnʒ] *verb* **(a)** to put in order; *the beds are arranged in rows*; *the patients' records are arranged in alphabetical order* **(b)** to organize; *he arranged the appointment for 6 o'clock*

arrangement [əˈreɪnʒmənt] *noun* way in which something is put in order; way in which something is organized

arrector pili muscle [əˈrektə ˈpaɪlaɪ ˈmʌsl] *noun; see* ERECTOR; *see illustration at* SKIN & SENSORY RECEPTORS

arrest [əˈrest] *noun* stopping of a bodily function; *see also* CARDIAC

arrhythmia [əˈrɪðmiə] *noun* variation in the rhythm of the heartbeat; *see also* ANTI-ARRHYTHMIC

Cardiovascular effects may include atrial arrhythmias but at 30°C there is the possibility of spontaneous ventricular fibrillation
British Journal of Nursing

arsenic [ˈɑːsnɪk] *noun* chemical element which forms poisonous compounds, such as arsenic trioxide, and which was once used in some medicines (NOTE: chemical symbol is **As**)

artefact [ˈɑːtɪfækt] *noun* something which is made or introduced artificially; *see also* DERMATITIS

arterial [ɑːˈtɪəriəl] *adjective* referring to arteries; **arterial bleeding** = bleeding from an artery; **arterial block** = blocking of an artery by a blood clot; **arterial blood** = oxygenated blood, bright red blood in an artery which has received oxygen in the lungs and is being taken to the tissues; **arterial supply to the brain** = supply of blood to the brain by the internal carotid arteries and the vertebral arteries

arteriectomy [ɑːtɪəriˈektəmi] *noun* surgical removal of an artery or part of an artery

arterio- [ɑːˈtɪəriəʊ] *prefix* referring to arteries

arteriogram [ɑːˈtɪəriəʊgræm] *noun* X-ray photograph of an artery, taken after injection with an opaque dye

arteriography [ɑːtɪəri'ɒgrəfi] *noun* taking of X-ray photographs of arteries after injection with an opaque dye

arteriole [ɑː'tɪəriəul] *noun* very small artery

arteriopathy [ɑːtɪəri'ɒpəθi] *noun* disease of an artery

arterioplasty [ɑː'tɪəriəuplæsti] *noun* plastic surgery to make good a damaged or blocked artery

arteriorrhaphy [ɑːtɪəri'ɔːrəfi] *noun* stitching of an artery

arteriosclerosis [ɑːtɪəriəusklə'rəusɪs] *noun* hardening of the arteries, condition (mainly found in old people) where the walls of arteries become thicker and more rigid because of deposits of fats and minerals, making it more difficult for the blood to pass and so causing high blood pressure, strokes and coronary thrombosis

arteriosus [ɑːtɪəri'əusəs] *see* DUCTUS

arteriotomy [ɑːtɪəri'ɒtəmi] *noun* puncture made in the wall of an artery

arteriovenous [ɑːtɪəriəu'viːnəs] *adjective* referring to both an artery and a vein

arteritis [ɑːtə'raɪtɪs] *noun* inflammation of the walls of an artery; **giant-cell arteritis** = disease of old people, which often affects the arteries in the scalp

artery ['ɑːtri] *noun* blood vessel taking blood from the heart to the tissues of the body; **arcuate artery** = curved artery in the foot or kidney; **axillary artery** = artery leading from the subclavian artery in the armpit; **basilar artery** = artery which lies at the base of the brain; **brachial artery** = artery running down the arm from the axillary artery to the elbow, where it divides into the radial and ulnar arteries; **brachiocephalic artery** = INNOMINATE ARTERY; **cerebral arteries** = main arteries which take blood into the brain; **common carotid artery** = main artery running up each side of the lower part of the neck; **common iliac artery** = one of two arteries which branch from the aorta in the abdomen and in turn divide into the internal iliac artery (leading to the pelvis) and the external iliac artery (leading to the leg); **communicating arteries** = arteries which connect the blood supply from each side of the brain, forming part of the circle of Willis; **coronary arteries** = arteries which supply blood to the heart muscles; **external iliac artery** = artery which branches from the aorta in the abdomen and leads to the leg; **facial artery** = artery which branches off the

external carotid into the face and mouth; **femoral artery** = continuation of the external iliac artery, which runs down the front of the thigh and then crosses to the back; **gastric artery** = artery leading from the coeliac trunk to the stomach; **hardened arteries** *or* **hardening of the arteries** = arteriosclerosis, a condition (mainly found in old people) where the walls of arteries become thicker and more rigid because of deposits of fats and minerals, making it more difficult for the blood to pass and so causing high blood pressure, strokes and coronary thrombosis; **hepatic artery** = artery which takes the blood to the liver; **ileocolic artery** = branch of the superior mesenteric artery; **inferior and superior gluteal arteries** = arteries supplying the buttocks; **innominate artery** = largest branch of the arch of the aorta, which continues as the right common carotid and right subclavian arteries; **interlobar artery** = artery running towards the cortex on each side of a renal pyramid; **interlobular arteries** = arteries running to the glomeruli of the kidneys; **internal iliac artery** = artery which branches from the aorta in the abdomen and leads to the pelvis; **lingual artery** = artery which supplies blood to the tongue; **lumbar artery** = one of four arteries which supply blood to the back muscles and skin; **internal** *or* **external maxillary arteries** = branches of the external carotid artery, in the face; **mesenteric artery** = one of two arteries ('superior and inferior mesenteric arteries') which supply the small intestine or the transverse colon and rectum; **popliteal artery** = artery which branches from the femoral artery behind the knee and leads into the tibial arteries; **pulmonary arteries** = arteries which take deoxygenated blood from the heart to the lungs for oxygenation; **radial artery** = artery which branches from the brachial artery, running near the radius, from the elbow to the palm of the hand; **renal arteries** = pair of arteries running from the abdominal aorta to the kidneys; **retinal artery** = sole artery of the retina (it accompanies the optic nerve); **spermatic artery** *or* **testicular artery** = artery which leads into the testes; **subclavian artery** = one of two arteries branching from the aorta on the left and from the innominate artery on the right, continuing into the brachial arteries and supplying blood to each arm; **tibial arteries** = two arteries which run down the front and back of the lower leg; **ulnar artery** = artery which branches from the brachial artery at the elbow and runs down the inside of the forearm to join the radial artery in the palm of the hand; **vertebral arteries** = two arteries which go up the back of the neck into the brain; *compare* VEIN

> COMMENT: In most arteries the blood has been oxygenated in the lungs and is bright red in colour. In the pulmonary artery, the blood is deoxygenated and so is darker. The arterial system begins with the aorta which leaves the heart and from which all the arteries branch

arthr(o)- [ˈɑːθrəʊ] *prefix* referring to a joint

arthralgia [ɑːˈθrældʒə] *noun* pain in a joint

arthrectomy [ɑːˈθrektəmi] *noun* surgical removal of a joint

arthritic [ɑːˈθrɪtɪk] **1** *adjective* referring to arthritis; *he has an arthritic hip* **2** *noun* person suffering from arthritis

arthritis [ɑːˈθraɪtɪs] *noun* painful inflammation of a joint; **reactive arthritis** = arthritis caused by a reaction to something; **rheumatoid arthritis** = general painful disabling collagen disease affecting any joint, but especially the hands, feet, and hips, making them swollen and inflamed; *see also* OSTEOARTHRITIS

arthroclasia [ɑːθrəʊˈkleɪʒə] *noun* removal of ankylosis in a joint

arthrodesis [ɑːθrəʊˈdiːsɪs] *noun* surgical operation where a joint is fused in a certain position so preventing pain from movement

arthrodynia [ɑːθrəˈdɪniə] *noun* pain in a joint

arthrography [ɑːˈθrɒgrəfi] *noun* X-ray photography of a joint

arthropathy [ɑːˈθrɒpəθi] *noun* disease in a joint

arthroplasty [ˈɑːθrəʊplæsti] *noun* surgical operation to repair a joint, to replace a joint; **total hip arthroplasty** = replacing both the head of the femur and the acetabulum with an artificial joint

arthroscope [ˈɑːθrəʊskəʊp] *noun* instrument which is inserted into the cavity of a joint to inspect it

arthroscopy [ɑːˈθrɒskəpi] *noun* examining the inside of a joint by means of an arthroscope

arthrosis [ɑːˈθrəʊsɪs] *noun* degeneration of a joint

arthrotomy [ɑːˈθrɒtəmi] *noun* cutting into a joint to drain pus

articular [ɑːˈtɪkjʊlə] *adjective* referring to joints; **articular cartilage** = layer of cartilage at the end of a bone where it forms a joint with another bone; *see illustration at* BONE STRUCTURE; **articular facet of a rib** = point at which a rib articulates with the spine; **articular process** = piece of bone which sticks out of the neural arch in a vertebra and links with the next vertebra

articulate [ɑːˈtɪkjuleɪt] *verb* to be linked with another bone in a joint; **articulating bones** = bones which form a joint; **articulating process** = ARTICULAR PROCESS

articulation [ɑːtɪkjʊˈleɪʃn] *noun* joint or series of joints

artificial [ɑːtɪˈfɪʃl] *adjective* which is made by man, which is not a natural part of the body; **artificial cartilage**; **artificial kidney**; **artificial lung**; **artificial leg**; **artificial insemination** = introduction of semen into a woman's uterus by artificial means; *see also* INSEMINATION; **artificial respiration** = way of reviving someone who has stopped breathing (as by mouth-to-mouth resuscitation); **artificial ventilation** = breathing which is assisted or controlled by a machine

artificially [ɑːtɪˈfɪʃəli] *adverb* in an artificial way

arytenoid [ærɪˈtiːnɔɪd] *adjective* (cartilage) at the back of the larynx

As *chemical symbol for* arsenic

asbestosis [æsbeˈstəʊsɪs] *noun* disease of the lungs caused by inhaling asbestos dust

> COMMENT: asbestos was formerly widely used in cement and cladding and other types of fireproof construction materials; it is now recognized that asbestos dust can cause many lung diseases, leading in some cases to forms of cancer

ascariasis [æskəˈraɪəsɪs] *noun* disease of the intestine and sometimes the lungs, caused by infestation with *Ascaris lumbricoides*

Ascaris lumbricoides [ˈæskərɪs lʌmbrɪˈkɔɪdiːz] *noun* type of large roundworm which is a parasite in the human intestine

ascending [əˈsendɪŋ] *adjective* going upwards; **ascending aorta** = first part of the aorta which goes up from the heart until it turns at the aortic arch; **ascending colon** =

first part of the colon which goes up the right side of the body from the caecum; *see illustration at* DIGESTIVE SYSTEM

Aschoff nodules ['æʃɒf 'nɒdju:lz] *plural noun* nodules which are formed mainly in or near the heart in rheumatic fever

ascites [ə'saɪtiːz] *noun* abnormal accumulation of liquid from the blood in the peritoneal cavity, occurring in heart and kidney failure

ascorbic acid [ə'skɔːbɪk 'æsɪd] *noun* vitamin C

> COMMENT: ascorbic acid is found in fresh fruit (especially oranges and lemons) and in vegetables. Lack of Vitamin C can cause anaemia and scurvy

-ase [eɪz or eɪs] *suffix meaning* an enzyme

asepsis [eɪ'sepsɪs] *noun* state of being sterilized, having no infection

aseptic [eɪ'septɪk] *adjective* referring to asepsis; *it is important that aseptic techniques should be used in microbiological experiments*; **aseptic meningitis** = relatively mild viral form of meningitis; **aseptic surgery** = surgery using sterilized equipment, rather than relying on killing germs with antiseptic drugs; *compare* ANTISEPTIC

asexual [eɪ'sekʃuəl] *adjective* not sexual, not involving sexual intercourse; **asexual reproduction** = reproduction of a cell by cloning

Asian flu US also **Asiatic flu** ['eɪʒn 'fluː or 'eɪzi'ætik 'fluː] *see* FLU

-asis *see* -IASIS

asleep [ə'sliːp] *adjective* sleeping; *the patient is asleep and must not be disturbed*; **she fell asleep** = she began to sleep; **fast asleep** = sleeping deeply; *the babies are all fast asleep* (NOTE: **asleep** cannot be used in front of a noun **the patient is asleep** but **a sleeping patient**)

asparagine [ə'spærədʒiːn] *noun* amino acid found in protein

aspartic acid [ə'spɑːtɪk 'æsɪd] *noun* amino acid found in sugar

aspect ['æspekt] *noun* way of looking at a patient; **anterior aspect** = view of the front of the body, or of the front of part of the body; **posterior aspect** = view of the back of the body, or of the back of part of the body

Asperger's Syndrome ['æspɜːdʒəz 'sɪndrəʊm] *noun* developmental disorder in children, with difficulty in social interaction and a restricted range of interests, more common in boys than girls

aspergillosis [æspɜːdʒɪ'ləʊsɪs] *noun* infection of the lungs with *Aspergillus*, a type of fungus

aspermia [ə'spɜːmiə] *noun* absence of sperm in semen

asphyxia [æs'fɪksiə] *noun* suffocation, condition where someone is prevented from breathing and therefore cannot take oxygen into the bloodstream; **asphyxia neonatorum** = failure to breathe in a newborn baby

> COMMENT: asphyxia can be caused by strangulation or by breathing poisonous gas or by having the head in a plastic bag, etc.

asphyxiate [æs'fɪksieɪt] *verb* to prevent someone from breathing or to be prevented from breathing; *the baby caught his head in a plastic bag and was asphyxiated*; *an unconscious patient may become asphyxiated or may asphyxiate if left lying on his back*

asphyxiation [æsfɪksi'eɪʃn] *noun* being prevented from breathing

aspiration [æspə'reɪʃn] *noun* removing fluid from a cavity in the body (often using a hollow needle); **aspiration pneumonia** = form of pneumonia where infected matter is inhaled from the bronchi or oesophagus

aspirator ['æspəreɪtə] *noun* instrument to suck fluid out of a cavity, out of the mouth in dentistry, from an operation site

aspirin ['æsprɪn] *noun* (i) common pain-killing drug (acetylsalicylic acid); (ii) tablet of this drug; *he took two aspirin tablets or two aspirins before going to bed*; *see* DRUGS TABLE IN SUPPLEMENT

assay [ə'seɪ] *noun* testing of a substance; *see also* BIOASSAY, IMMUNOASSAY

assimilate [ə'sɪməleɪt] *verb* to take into the body's tissues substances which have been absorbed into the blood from digested food

assimilation [əsɪmə'leɪʃn] *noun* action of assimilating food substances

assist [ə'sɪst] *verb* to help; **assisted respiration** = breathing with the help of a machine

assistance [ə'sɪstns] *noun* help; **medical assistance** = help provided by a nurse, by an ambulanceman or by a member of the Red Cross, etc., to a person who is ill or injured

assistant [ə'sɪstnt] *noun* person who helps; *six assistants helped the consultant*

associate [ə'səʊʃieɪt] *verb* to be related to or to be connected with; *the condition is often associated with diabetes*; *side effects which may be associated with the drug*

association [əsəʊsi'eɪʃn] *noun* **(a)** relating one thing to another in the mind; **association area** = area of the cortex of the brain which is concerned with relating stimuli coming from different sources; **association neurone** = neurone which links an association area to the main parts of the cortex; **association tracts** = tracts which link areas of the cortex in the same cerebral hemisphere **(b)** group of people in the same profession, with similar interests; *see also* BRITISH MEDICAL ASSOCIATION

aster ['æstə] *noun* structure shaped like a star, seen around the centrosome during cell division

asthenia [æs'θi:niə] *noun* being weak, not having any strength

asthenic [æs'θenɪk] *adjective* (general condition) where the patient has no strength and no interest in things

asthenopia [æsθɪ'nəʊpiə] *noun* = EYESTRAIN

asthma ['æsmə] *noun* narrowing of the bronchial tubes, where the muscles go into spasm and the patient has difficulty breathing; **cardiac asthma** = difficulty in breathing caused by heart failure; **occupational asthma** = asthma caused by materials with which one comes into contact at work (such as asthma in farmworkers, caused by hay)

asthmatic [æs'mætɪk] **1** *adjective* referring to asthma; *he has an asthmatic attack every spring*; **acute asthmatic attack** = sudden attack of asthma; **asthmatic bronchitis** = asthma associated with bronchitis **2** *noun* person suffering from asthma

asthmaticus [æs'mætɪkəs] *see* STATUS

astigmatic [æstɪg'mætɪk] *adjective* referring to astigmatism; **he is astigmatic** = he suffers from astigmatism

astigmatism [əs'tɪgmətɪzm] *noun* defect in the eye, which prevents the eye from focusing correctly

COMMENT: in astigmatism, horizontal and vertical objects are not both in correct focus

astonish [ə'stɒnɪʃ] *verb* to surprise; *I was astonished to hear that she had recovered*

astonishing [ə'stɒnɪʃɪŋ] *adjective* which surprises; *it's astonishing how many people catch flu in the winter*

astonishment [ə'stɒnɪʃmənt] *noun* great surprise; *to the doctor's great astonishment, she suddenly started to walk*

astragalus [ə'strægələs] *noun* old name for the talus, anklebone

astringent [ə'strɪnʒnt] *noun* & *adjective* (substance) which stops bleeding and makes the skin tissues contract and harden

astrocyte ['æstrəsaɪt] *noun* star-shaped supporting brain cell

astrocytoma [æstrəsaɪ'təʊmə] *noun* type of brain tumour, consisting of star-shaped cells which develop slowly in the brain and spinal cord

asymmetry [æ'sɪmətrɪ] *noun* state where two sides of the body, of an organ are not closely similar to each other

asymptomatic [æsɪmptə'mætɪk] *adjective* which does not show any symptoms of disease

asynclitism [æ'sɪnklɪtɪzm] *noun* situation at childbirth, where the head of the baby enters the vagina at an angle

asynergia [æsɪ'nɜ:dʒə] *noun* awkward movements and bad coordination, caused by a disorder of the cerebellum (NOTE: also called **dyssynergia**)

asynergy [ə'sɪnədʒi] = ASYNERGIA

asystole [ə'sɪstəli] *noun* state where the heart has stopped beating

ataractic *or* **ataraxic** [ætə'ræktɪk or ætə'ræksɪk] *adjective* & *noun* (drug) which calms a patient

ataraxia *or* **ataraxis** [ætə'ræksiə or ætə'ræksɪs] *noun* being calm, not worrying

atavism ['ætəvɪzm] *noun* situation where a patient suffers from a condition which an ancestor was known to have suffered from, but not his immediate parents

ataxia [ə'tæksiə] *noun* lack of control of movements due to defects in the nervous system; **cerebellar ataxia** = disorder where the patient staggers and cannot speak clearly, due to a disease of the cerebellum; **locomotor ataxia** = TABES DORSALIS

ataxic [əˈtæksɪk] *adjective* referring to ataxia; *see also* GAIT

atelectasis [ætəˈlektəsɪs] *noun* collapse of a lung, where the lung fails to expand properly

atherogenic [æθərəʊˈdʒenɪk] *adjective* which may produce atheroma

atheroma [æθəˈrəʊmə] *noun* thickening of the walls of an artery by deposits of a fatty substance such as cholesterol

atherosclerosis [æθərəʊskləˈrəʊsɪs] *noun* condition where deposits of fats and minerals form on the walls of an artery (especially the aorta, the coronary arteries and the cerebral arteries) and prevent blood from flowing easily

atherosclerotic [æθərəʊskləˈrɒtɪk] *adjective* referring to atherosclerosis; **atherosclerotic plaque** = deposit on the walls of arteries

athetosis [æθəˈtəʊsɪs] *noun* repeated slow movements of the limbs, caused by a brain disorder such as cerebral palsy

athlete's foot [ˈæθliːts ˈfʊt] = TINEA PEDIS

atlas [ˈætləs] *noun* top vertebra in the spine, which supports the skull and pivots on the axis or second vertebra; *see illustration at* VERTEBRAL COLUMN

atmospheric pressure [ætməsˈferɪk ˈpreʃə] *noun* normal pressure of the air

COMMENT: disorders due to variations in atmospheric pressure include mountain sickness and caisson diseases

atomizer [ˈætəmaɪzə] *noun* instrument which sprays liquid in the form of very small drops like mist (NOTE: also called a **nebulizer**)

atony [ˈætəni] *noun* lack of tone or tension in the muscles

atopen [ˈætəpen] *noun* allergen which causes an atopy

atopic eczema *or* **atopic dermatitis** [əˈtɒpɪk ˈeksɪmə *or* əˈtɒpɪk dɜːməˈtaɪtɪs] *noun* type of eczema often caused by hereditary allergy

atopy [ˈætəpi] *noun* hereditary allergic reaction

ATP [ˈeɪ ˈtiː ˈpiː] = ADENOSINE TRIPHOSPHATE

atresia [əˈtriːziə] *noun* abnormal closing or absence of a tube in the body

atretic [əˈtretɪk] *adjective* referring to atresia; **atretic follicle** = scarred remains of an ovarian follicle

atrial [ˈeɪtriəl] *adjective* referring to the heart; **atrial fibrillation** = rapid uncoordinated fluttering of the atria of the heart, causing an irregular heartbeat

atrioventricular [eɪtriəʊvenˈtrɪkjʊlə] *adjective* referring to the atria and ventricles; **atrioventricular bundle** *or* **AV bundle** = bundle of modified cardiac muscle which conducts impulses from the atrioventricular node to the septum and then divides to connect with the ventricles (NOTE: also called **bundle of His**); **atrioventricular groove** = groove round the outside of the heart, showing the division between the atria and ventricles; **atrioventricular node** *or* **AV node** = mass of conducting tissue in the right atrium, which continues as the bundle of His and passes impulses from the atria to the ventricles

atrium [ˈeɪtriəm] *noun* (i) one of the two upper chambers in the heart; (ii) cavity in the ear behind the eardrum; *see illustration at* HEART (NOTE: the plural is **atria**)

COMMENT: the two atria in the heart both receive blood from veins; the right atrium receives venous blood from the superior and inferior vena cavae and the left atrium receives oxygenated blood from the pulmonary veins

atrophy [ˈætrəfi] **1** *noun* wasting of an organ or part of the body **2** *verb (of an organ or part of the body)* to waste away, become smaller

atropine [ˈætrəpiːn] *noun* alkaloid substance derived from belladonna, a poisonous plant, used, among other things, to enlarge the pupil of the eye, and to reduce salivary and bronchial secretions during anaesthesia, as a muscarinic antagonist

ATS [ˈeɪ ˈtiː ˈes] = ANTITETANUS SERUM

attach [əˈtætʃ] *verb* to fix, fasten; *the stomach is attached to the other organs by the greater and lesser omenta*

attachment [əˈtætʃmənt] *noun* (i) something which is attached; (ii) arrangement where a home nurse is attached to a particular general practice

attack [əˈtæk] *noun* sudden illness; *he had an attack of fever*; *she had two attacks of laryngitis during the winter*; **heart attack** = condition where the heart suffers from defective blood supply because one of the arteries becomes blocked by a blood clot (coronary thrombosis), causing myocardial ischaemia and myocardial infarction

attempt [əˈtemt] **1** *noun* try; *they made an attempt to treat the disease with antibiotics* **2** *verb* to try; *the surgeons attempted to sew the finger back on*

attend [əˈtend] *verb* **(a)** to be present at; *will you attend the meeting tomorrow?*; *seventeen patients are attending the antenatal clinic* **(b)** to look after (a patient); *he was attended by two doctors*; **attending physician** = doctor who is looking after a certain patient; *he was referred to the hypertension unit by his attending physician*

attend to [əˈtend ˈtʊ] *verb* to deal with; *the doctor is attending to his patients*

attention [əˈtenʃn] *noun* care in looking after a patient; *he has had the best medical attention*; *she needs urgent medical attention*; **attention deficit hyperactivity disorder** = disorder in children characterized by an inability to concentrate with disruptive behaviour

attract [əˈtrækt] *verb* to make something come nearer; *the solid attracts the gas to its surface*; *the patient is sexually attracted to both males and females*

attraction [əˈtrækʃn] *noun* act of attracting; **sexual attraction** = feeling of wanting to have sexual intercourse with someone

attributable risk (AR) [əˈtrɪbjutəbl ˈrɪsk] *noun* a measure of the excess risk of disease due to a particular exposure; *the excess risk of bacteriuria in oral contraceptive users attributable to the use of oral contraceptives is 1,566 per 100,000*

attrition [əˈtrɪʃn] *noun* wearing away, as may be caused by friction; *examination showed attrition of two extensor tendons*

Au *chemical symbol for* gold

audi(o)- [ˈɔːdi or ˈɔːdiəʊ] *prefix* referring to hearing, sound

audible [ˈɔːdəbl] *adjective* which can be heard; **audible limits** = upper and lower limits of sound frequencies which can be heard by humans

audiogram [ˈɔːdiəʊɡræm] *noun* graph drawn by an audiometer

audiometer [ɔːdiˈɒmɪtə] *noun* apparatus for testing hearing, for testing the range of sounds that the human ear can detect

audiometry [ɔːdiˈɒmətri] *noun* science of testing hearing

audit [ˈɔːdɪt] *noun* (i) analysis of the accounts of a hospital or doctor's practice to see if they are correct; (ii) analysis of statistics relating to a doctor's practice (such as the numbers of patients, the incidence of disease, the numbers of patients referred to specialists, etc.) for research purposes; **audit cycle** = cycle of selection of (medical) topic for review, observation and comparison with agreed standards and the implementation of change within a medical audit, eg. assessment of outpatient appointment system, prevention of bedsores, etc.; **medical audit** = systematic critical analysis of the quality of medical care including the procedures used for diagnosis and treatment, the use of resources and the resulting outcome and quality of life for the patient

auditory [ˈɔːdɪtri] *adjective* referring to hearing; **external auditory canal** *or* **external auditory meatus** = tube in the skull leading from the outer ear to the eardrum; **internal auditory meatus** = channel which takes the auditory nerve through the temporal bone; **auditory nerve** = the vestibulocochlear nerve, the eighth cranial nerve which governs hearing and balance; *see illustration at* EAR

Auerbach's plexus [ˈaʊəbɑːks ˈpleksəs] *noun* group of nerve fibres in the intestine wall

aura [ˈɔːrə] *noun* warning sensation of varying kinds which is experienced before an attack of epilepsy

aural [ˈɔːrəl] *adjective* (i) referring to the ear; (ii) like an aura; **aural polyp** = polyp in the middle ear; **aural surgery** = surgery on the ear

auricle [ˈɔːrɪkl] *noun* tip of each atrium in the heart

auriculae [ɔːˈrɪkjʊliː] *see* CONCHA

auricular [ɔːˈrɪkjʊlə] *adjective* (i) referring to the ear; (ii) referring to an auricle; **auricular veins** = veins which lead into the posterior facial vein

auriscope [ˈɔːrəskəʊp] *noun* instrument for examining the ear and eardrum (NOTE: also called an **otoscope**)

auscultation [ɔ:skəl'teɪʃn] *noun* listening to the sounds of the body using a stethoscope

auscultatory [ɔ:'skʌltətrɪ] *adjective* referring to auscultation

authority [ɔ:'θɒrəti] *noun* **(a)** power to act; **to abuse one's authority** = to use powers in an illegal, harmful way **(b)** official body which controls an area, region; *see also* DISTRICT, HEALTH, REGIONAL

autism ['ɔ:tɪzm] *noun* condition of children and adolescents where the patient has difficulty in social interaction, language and communication problems and shows obsessional repetitive behaviour; more common in boys than in girls

autistic [ɔ:'tɪstɪk] *adjective* (i) referring to autism; (ii) suffering from autism

auto- ['ɔ:təʊ] *prefix* meaning self

autoantibody [ɔ:təʊ'æntɪbɒdi] *noun* antibody formed to attack the body's own cells

autoclavable ['ɔ:təʊkleɪvəbl] *adjective* which can be sterilized in an autoclave; *waste should be put into autoclavable plastic bags*

autoclave ['ɔ:təʊkleɪv] **1** *noun* equipment for sterilizing surgical instruments using heat under high pressure **2** *verb* to sterilize using heat under high pressure; *autoclaving is the best method of sterilization*

autograft ['ɔ:təgrɑ:ft] *noun* graft, transplant made using parts of the patient's own body

autoimmune [ɔ:təʊ'mju:n] *adjective* referring to an immune reaction in a person to antigens in his own tissue; **autoimmune disease** = disease where the patient's own cells are attacked by autoantibodies; *rheumatoid arthritis is thought to be an autoimmune disease*

autoimmunity [ɔ:təʊɪ'mju:nəti] *noun* state where an organism produces autoantibodies to attack its own cells

autoinfection [ɔ:təʊɪn'fekʃn] *noun* infection by a germ already in the body; infection of one part of the body by another

autointoxication [ɔ:təʊɪntɒksɪ'keɪʃn] *noun* poisoning of the body by toxins produced in the body itself

autologous [ɔ:'tɒləgəs] *adjective* (graft, material) coming from the same source; **autologous transfusion** = blood transfusion where the blood is removed from the patient for later transfusion after an operation; *see also* TRANSFUSION

autolysis [ɔ:'tɒlɪsɪs] *noun* action of cells destroying themselves with their own enzymes

automatic [ɔ:tə'mætɪk] *adjective* which works by itself, without anyone giving instructions

automatically [ɔ:tə'mætɪkli] *adverb* by itself, without anyone giving instructions; *the heart beats automatically*

automatism [ɔ:'tɒmətɪzm] *noun* state where a person acts without consciously knowing that he is acting

COMMENT: automatic acts can take place after concussion or epileptic fits. In law, automatism can be a defence to a criminal charge when the accused states that he acted without knowing what he was doing

autonomic [ɔ:tə'nɒmɪk] *adjective* which governs itself independently; **autonomic nervous system** = nervous system formed of ganglia linked to the spinal column, which regulates the automatic functioning of the main organs of the body, such as the heart and lungs, and which works when a person is asleep or even unconscious; *see also* PARASYMPATHETIC SYSTEM, SYMPATHETIC SYSTEM

autonomy [ɔ:'tɒnəmi] *noun* being free to act as one wishes

autopsy ['ɔ:tɒpsi] *noun* post mortem, the examination of a dead body by a pathologist to find out the cause of death; *the autopsy showed that he had been poisoned*

autosomal [ɔ:təʊ'səʊməl] *adjective* referring to autosome

autosome ['ɔ:təʊsəʊm] *noun* one of a pair of similar chromosomes

autotransfusion [ɔ:təʊtræns'fju:ʒn] *noun* infusion into a patient of his own blood

auxiliary [ɔ:g'zɪliəri] **1** *adjective* which helps; *the hospital has an auxiliary power supply in case the electricity supply breaks down* **2** *noun* assistant; **nursing auxiliary** = helper who does general work in a hospital, clinic

AV bundle ['eɪ'vi: 'bʌndl] = ATRIOVENTRICULAR BUNDLE

AV node ['eɪ'vi: 'nəʊd] = ATRIOVENTRICULAR NODE

available [ə'veɪləbl] *adjective* which can be got; *the drug is available only on prescription*; *all available ambulances were rushed to the scene of the accident*

avascular [əˈvæskjʊlə] *adjective* with no blood vessels, with a deficient blood supply; **avascular necrosis** = condition where tissue cells die because their supply of blood has been cut

average [ˈævrɪdʒ] **1** *noun* **(a)** usual amount, size, rate, etc.; *her weight is above (the) average* **(b)** value calculated by adding together several quantities and then dividing the total by the number of quantities **2** *adjective* **(a)** usual, ordinary; *their son is of above average weight* **(b)** calculated by adding together several quantities and then dividing the total by the number of quantities; *their average age is 25*

aversion to [əˈvɜːʃn ˈtʊ] *noun* great dislike of; **aversion therapy** = treatment where the patient is cured of a type of behaviour by making him develop a great dislike for it

avitaminosis [ævɪtəmɪnˈəʊsɪs] *noun* disorder caused by lack of vitamins

avoid [əˈvɔɪd] *verb* to try not to do something such as not to eat a particular food; *you must try to avoid overexerting yourself*; *a patient on this diet should avoid alcohol*

avulse [əˈvʌls] *verb* to tear away

avulsion [əˈvʌlʃn] *noun* pulling away tissue by force; **nail avulsion** = pulling away an ingrowing toenail; **phrenic avulsion** = surgical removal of part of the phrenic nerve in order to paralyse the diaphragm; **avulsion fracture** = fracture where a tendon pulls away part of the bone to which it is attached

awake [əˈweɪk] **1** *verb* **(a)** to wake somebody up; *he was awoken by pains in his chest* **(b)** to wake up; *after the accident he awoke to find himself in hospital* (NOTE: **awaking - awoke - has awoken**) **2** *adjective* not asleep; *he was still awake at 2 o'clock in the morning*; *the patients were kept awake by shouts in the next ward*; **the baby is wide awake** = very awake (NOTE: **awake** cannot be used in front of a noun)

awaken [əˈweɪkn] *verb* to wake somebody up; to stimulate someone's senses

aware [əˈweə] *adjective* knowing, conscious enough to know what is happening; *she is not aware of what is happening around her*; *the surgeon became aware of a problem with the heart-lung machine*

awareness [əˈweənəs] *noun* being aware (especially of a problem)

doctors should use the increased public awareness of whooping cough during epidemics to encourage parents to vaccinate children

Health Visitor

awkward [ˈɔːkwəd] *adjective* difficult to reach or to find or to deal with; *the tumour is in a very awkward position for surgery*

awkwardly [ˈɔːkwədli] *adverb* in a way which is difficult to reach, to find, to deal with; *the tumour is awkwardly placed and not easy to reach*

axial [ˈæksɪəl] *adjective* referring to an axis; **axial skeleton** = trunk, the main part of the skeleton, formed of the spine, skull, ribs and breastbone; *compare* APPENDICULAR SKELETON; **computerized axial tomography (CAT)** = system of scanning a patient's body, where a narrow X-ray beam, guided by a computer, can photograph a thin section of the body or of an organ from several angles, using the computer to build up an image of the section

axilla [ækˈsɪlə] *noun* armpit, the hollow under the shoulder, between the upper arm and the body, where the upper arm joins the shoulder (NOTE: the plural is **axillae**)

axillary [ækˈsɪləri] *adjective* referring to the armpit; **axillary artery** = artery leading from the subclavian artery in the armpit; **axillary nodes** = part of the lymphatic system in the arm; **axillary temperature** = temperature in the armpit

COMMENT: the armpit contains several important blood vessels, lymph nodes and sweat glands

axis [ˈæksɪs] *noun* **(a)** imaginary line through the centre of the body **(b)** central vessel which divides into other vessels **(c)** second vertebra on which the atlas sits; *see illustration at* VERTEBRAL COLUMN (NOTE: the plural is **axes**)

axodendrite [æksəʊˈdendraɪt] *noun* appendage like a fibril on the axon of a nerve

axolemma [æksəˈlemə] *noun* membrane covering an axon

axon [ˈæksɒn] *noun* nerve fibre which sends impulses from one neurone to another, linking with the dendrites of the other neurone; **axon covering** = myelin sheath which covers a nerve; **postsynaptic axon** *or* **presynaptic axon** = nerves on either side of a synapse; *see illustration at* NEURONE

-azepam ['æzɪpæm] *suffix* used in names of benzodiazepines; *diazepam*

azidothymidine (AZT)
[eizaidəʊ'θaimidin] *noun* zidovudine, a drug used in the treatment of AIDS

COMMENT: there is no cure for AIDS but this drug may help to slow its progress

azo dyes ['eizəʊ 'daiz] *plural noun* artificial colouring additives derived from coal tar, added to food to give it colour

COMMENT: many of the azo dyes (such as tartrazine) provoke allergic reactions; some are believed to be carcinogenic

azoospermia [eizəʊə'spɜːmiə] *noun* absence of sperm

azotaemia [æzəʊ'tiːmiə] *noun* presence of urea or other nitrogen compounds in the blood

azoturia [æzəʊ'tjʊəriə] *noun* presence of urea or other nitrogen compounds in the urine, caused by kidney disease

AZT = AZIDOTHYMIDINE

azygos ['æzɪgəs] *adjective* single, not one of a pair; **azygos vein** = vein which brings blood back into the vena cava from the abdomen

Bb

B *chemical symbol for* boron

Vitamin B ['vɪtəmɪn 'biː] *noun* **Vitamin B complex** = group of vitamins which are soluble in water, including folic acid, pyridoxine, riboflavine and many others; **Vitamin B₁**= thiamine, vitamin found in yeast, liver, cereals and pork; **Vitamin B₂**= riboflavine, vitamin found in eggs, liver, green vegetables, milk and yeast; **Vitamin B₆**= pyridoxine, vitamin found in meat, cereals and molasses; **Vitamin B₁₂**= cyanocobalamin, vitamin found in liver and kidney, but not present in vegetables

COMMENT: lack of vitamins from the B complex can have different results: lack of thiamine causes beriberi; lack of riboflavine affects a child's growth, and can cause anaemia and inflammation of the tongue and mouth; lack of pyridoxine causes convulsions and vomiting in babies; lack of vitamin B₁₂ causes anaemia

Ba *chemical symbol for* barium

Babinski reflex *or* **Babinski test** [bə'bɪnskɪ 'riːfleks *or* bə'bɪnskɪ 'test] *noun* abnormal response of the toes to running a finger lightly across the sole of the foot; *see* PLANTAR REFLEX

COMMENT: the normal response is for all the toes to turn down, but in the case of the Babinski reflex, the big toe turns up while the others turn down and spread out, a sign of hemiplegia and pyramidal tract disease

baby ['beɪbɪ] *noun* very young child; *babies start to walk when they are about 12 months old*; **baby blues** = depression which affects a young mother soon after the birth of a baby; **baby care** = looking after babies; **baby clinic** = special clinic which deals with babies (NOTE: if you do not know the sex of a baby you can use **it: the baby was sucking its thumb**)

bacillaemia [bæsɪ'liːmɪə] *noun* infection of the blood by bacilli

bacillary [bə'sɪləri] *adjective* referring to bacillus; **bacillary dysentery** = dysentery caused by the bacillus *Shigella* in contaminated food

bacille Calmette-Guérin (BCG) [bæ'sɪl 'kælmet ge'ræn] *noun* vaccine which immunizes against tuberculosis

bacilluria [bæsɪ'ljʊərɪə] *noun* presence of bacilli in the urine

bacillus [bə'sɪləs] *noun* bacterium shaped like a rod (NOTE: the plural is **bacilli**)

back [bæk] *noun* **(a)** dorsum, the part of the body from the neck downwards to the waist, which is made up of the spine and the bones attached to it; *he complained of a pain in the back*; *he hurt his back lifting the piece of wood*; *she strained her back working in the garden*; **back muscles** = strong muscles in the back which help hold the body upright; **back pain** = pain in the back; **back strain** = condition where the muscles or ligaments in the back have been strained **(b)** other side to the front; *she has a swelling on the back of her hand*; *the calf muscles are at the back of the lower leg*

backache ['bækeɪk] *noun* pain in the back

COMMENT: backache can result from bad posture, a soft bed or muscle strain, but it can also be caused by rheumatism (lumbago), fevers such as typhoid fever, and osteoarthritis. Pains in the back can also be referred pains from gallstones or kidney disease

backbone ['bækbəʊn] *noun* rachis or spine, a series of bones (the vertebrae) linked together to form a flexible column running from the pelvis to the skull; *see also* SPINE, SPINAL COLUMN, VERTEBRAL COLUMN (NOTE: for other terms referring to the back, see words beginning with **dors-**)

baclofen ['bækləʊfen] *noun see* DRUGS TABLE IN SUPPLEMENT

bacteraemia [bæktə'riːmiə] *noun* blood poisoning, having bacteria in the blood

bacteria [bæk'tɪəriə] *plural noun* microscopic organisms, some of which are permanently present in the gut and can break down food tissue; many of them can cause disease (NOTE: the singular is **bacterium**)

> COMMENT: bacteria can be shaped like rods (bacilli), like balls (cocci) or have a spiral form (such as spirochaetes). Bacteria, especially bacilli and spirochaetes, can move and reproduce very rapidly

bacterial [bæk'tɪəriəl] *adjective* referring to bacteria or caused by bacteria; *children with sickle-cell anaemia are susceptible to bacterial infection*; **(subacute) bacterial endocarditis** = infection of the endocardium (the membrane covering the inner surfaces of the heart) by bacteria; **bacterial strain** = distinct variety of bacteria

bactericidal [bæktɪərɪ'saɪdl] *adjective* (substance) which destroys bacteria

bactericide [bæk'tɪərɪsaɪd] *noun* substance which destroys bacteria

bacteriological [bæktɪəriə'lɒdʒɪkl] *adjective* referring to bacteriology; **bacteriological warfare** = war where one side tries to kill or affect the people of the enemy side by infecting them with bacteria

bacteriologist [bæktɪəri'ɒlədʒɪst] *noun* doctor who specializes in the study of bacteria

bacteriology [bæktɪəri'ɒlədʒɪ] *noun* scientific study of bacteria

bacteriolysin [bæktɪəri'ɒlɪsiːn] *noun* protein, usually an immunoglobulin, which destroys bacterial cells

bacteriolysis [bæktɪəri'ɒlɪsɪs] *noun* destruction of bacterial cells

bacteriolytic [bæktɪəriə'lɪtɪk] *adjective* (substance) which can destroy bacteria, etc.

bacteriophage [bæk'tɪərɪəfeɪdʒ] *noun* virus which affects bacteria

bacteriostasis [bæktɪəriəʊ'steɪsɪs] *noun* action of stopping bacteria from multiplying

bacteriostatic [bæktɪəriəʊ'stætɪk] *adjective* (substance) which does not kill bacteria but stops them from multiplying

bacterium [bæk'tɪəriəm] *noun see* BACTERIA

bacteriuria [bæktɪəri'jʊəriə] *noun* presence of bacteria in the urine

bad [bæd] *adjective* **(a)** not good, not well; *he has a bad leg and can't walk fast*; **eating too much fat is bad for you** = it will make you ill; **bad breath** = halitosis, condition where a person has breath which smells unpleasant; **bad tooth** = tooth which has caries **(b)** unpleasant or quite serious; *she has got a bad cold*; *he had a bad attack of bronchitis* (NOTE: **bad - worse - worst**)

bag [bæg] *noun* something made of paper, cloth, plastic or tissue which can contain things; **colostomy bag** *or* **ileostomy bag** = bag attached to the opening made by a colostomy or an ileostomy, to collect faeces as they are passed out of the body; **sleeping bag** = comfortable warm bag for sleeping in; **bag of waters** = part of the amnion which covers an unborn baby in the uterus and contains the amniotic fluid

Baghdad boil *or* **Baghdad sore** ['bægdæd 'bɔɪl *or* 'bægdæd 'sɔː] *noun* Leishmaniasis, oriental sore, a skin disease of tropical countries caused by the parasite *Leishmania*

Baker's cyst ['beɪkəz 'sɪst] *noun* swelling filled with synovial fluid, at the back of the knee, caused by weakness of the joint membrane

baker's itch *or* **baker's dermatitis** ['beɪkəz 'ɪtʃ *or* 'beɪkəz dɜːmə'taɪtɪs] *noun* irritation of the skin caused by handling yeast

BAL ['biː 'eɪ 'el] = BRITISH ANTI-LEWISITE

balance ['bæləns] **1** *noun* **(a)** device for weighing, made with springs or weights; *he weighed the powder in a spring balance* **(b)** staying upright, not falling; **sense of balance** = feeling that keeps someone upright, governed by the fluid in the inner ear balance mechanism; **he stood on top of the fence and kept his balance** = he did not fall off **(c)** **balance of mind** = good mental state; **disturbed balance of mind** = state of mind when someone is for a time incapable of reasoned action (because of illness or depression) **(d)** proportions of substances as, for example, in the diet; *to maintain a healthy balance of vitamins in the diet*; **water balance** = state where the water lost by the body (in urine or perspiration, etc.) is made up by water absorbed from food and drink **2** *verb* to stand on something narrow without falling; *he was balancing on top of* *the fence*; *how long can you balance on one foot?*

balanced diet ['bælənst 'daɪət] *noun* diet which provides all the nutrients needed in the correct proportions

balanitis [bælə'naɪtɪs] *noun* inflammation of the glans of the penis

balanoposthitis [bælənəʊpɒs'θaɪtɪs] *noun* inflammation of the foreskin and the end of the penis

balantidiasis [bæləntɪ'daɪəsɪs] *noun* infestation of the large intestine by a parasite *Balantidium coli*, which causes ulceration of the wall of the intestine, giving diarrhoea and finally dysentery

balanus ['bælənəs] *noun* glans, the round end of the penis

bald [bɔːld] *adjective* with no hair, (person) who has no hair; **he is going bald** *or* **he is becoming bald** = he is beginning to lose his hair; *he went bald when he was still young*; *after the operation she became quite bald*

balding ['bɔːldɪŋ] *adjective* (man) who is losing his hair

baldness ['bɔːldnəs] *noun* alopecia, the state of not having any hair

Balkan frame *or* **Balkan beam** ['bɔːlkən 'freɪm *or* 'bɔːlkən 'biːm] *noun* frame fitted above a bed to which a leg in plaster can be attached

ball [bɔːl] *noun* (i) round object; (ii) soft part of the hand below the thumb; soft part of the foot below the big toe

ball and socket joint ['bɔːl ənd 'sɒkɪt 'dʒɔɪnt] *noun* joint where the round end of a long bone is attached to a cup-shaped hollow in another bone in such a way that the long bone can move in almost any direction

balloon [bə'luːn] *noun* bag of light material inflated with air or a gas (used to unblock arteries); *see also* ANGIOPLASTY

ballottement [bə'lɒtmənt] *noun* method of examining the body by tapping or moving a part, especially during pregnancy

balneotherapy [bælniəʊ'θerəpi] *noun* treatment of diseases by bathing in hot water or water containing certain chemicals

balsam ['bɔːlsəm] *noun* mixture of resin and oil, used to rub on sore joints or to put in hot water and use as an inhalant; *see also* FRIAR'S BALSAM

ban [bæn] *verb* to forbid or to say that something should not be done; *alcohol has been banned by his doctor* *or* *he has been banned alcohol by his doctor*; *smoking is banned in most restaurants*

band [bænd] *noun* **(a)** thin piece of material for tying things together; *the papers were held together with a rubber band* **(b)** part of the pattern in muscle tissue

bandage ['bændɪdʒ] **1** *noun* piece of cloth which is wrapped around a wound or an injured limb; *his head was covered with bandages*; *put a bandage round your knee*; **elastic bandage** = stretch bandage used to support a weak joint or for treatment of a varicose vein; **pressure bandage** = bandage which presses on a part of the body; **rolled bandage** *or* **roller bandage** = bandage in the form of a long strip of cloth which is rolled up from one or both ends; **spiral bandage** = bandage which is wrapped round a limb, each turn overlapping the one before; **T bandage** = bandage shaped like the letter T, used for bandaging the area between the legs; **triangular bandage** = bandage made of a triangle of cloth, used to make a sling for the arm; **tubular bandage** = bandage made of a tube of elastic cloth; *see also* ESMARCH'S 2 *verb* to wrap a piece of cloth around a wound; *she bandaged his leg*; *his arm is bandaged up*

Bandl's ring ['bændlz 'rɪŋ] = RETRACTION RING

bank [bæŋk] *noun* place where blood or organs from donors can be stored until needed; *see also* BLOOD BANK, EYE BANK, SPERM BANK

Bankart's operation ['bæŋkɑːts ɒpə'reɪʃn] *noun* operation to repair a recurrent dislocation of the shoulder

Banti's syndrome *or* **Banti's disease** ['bæntɪz 'sɪndrəʊm *or* 'bæntɪz dɪ'ziːz] *noun* splenic anaemia, type of anaemia where the patient has portal hypertension, an enlarged spleen and haemorrhages, caused by cirrhosis of the liver

Barbados leg [bɑː'beɪdɒs 'leg] *noun* form of elephantiasis, a large swelling due to a Filaria worm

barber's itch *or* **barber's rash** ['bɑːbəz 'ɪtʃ *or* 'bɑːbəz 'ræʃ] = SYCOSIS

barbital ['bɑːbɪtəl] *US* = BARBITONE

barbitone ['bɑːbɪtəʊn] *noun* type of barbiturate

barbiturate [bɑːˈbɪtʃʊrət] *noun* sedative drug; **barbiturate abuse** = repeated addictive use of barbiturates which in the end affects the brain; **barbiturate dependence** = being dependent on regularly taking barbiturate tablets; **barbiturate poisoning** = poisoning caused by an overdose of barbiturates

barbiturism [bɑːˈbɪtʃʊrɪzm] *noun* addiction to barbiturates

barbotage [bɑːbəˈtɑːʒ] *noun* method of spinal analgesia where cerebrospinal fluid is withdrawn and reinjected

bare [beə] *adjective* **(a)** not covered by clothes; *the children had bare feet*; *her dress left her arms bare* **(b) bare area of the liver** = large triangular part of the liver not covered with peritoneum

barium [ˈbeərɪəm] *noun* chemical element, forming poisonous compounds, used as a contrast when taking X-ray photographs of soft tissue; **barium enema** = liquid solution containing barium sulphate which is put into the rectum so that an X-ray can be taken of the lower intestine; **barium meal** *or* **barium solution** = liquid solution containing barium sulphate which a patient drinks to increase the contrast of an X-ray of the alimentary tract; **barium sulphate (BaSO₄)** = salt of barium not soluble in water and which shows as opaque in X-ray photographs (NOTE: chemical symbol is **Ba**)

Barlow's disease [ˈbɑːləʊz dɪˈziːz] *noun* scurvy in children, caused by lack of vitamin C

baroreceptor [bærəʊrɪˈseptə] *noun* one of a group of nerves near the carotid artery and aortic arch, which sense changes in blood pressure

barotrauma [bærəʊˈtrɔːmə] *noun* injury caused by a sharp increase in pressure

Barr body [ˈbɑː ˈbɒdi] *see* CHROMATIN

barrier [ˈbærɪə] *noun* thing which prevents contact; **barrier cream** = cream put on the skin to prevent the skin coming into contact with irritating substances; **barrier nursing** = nursing of a patient suffering from an infectious disease, while keeping him away from other patients and making sure that faeces and soiled bedclothes do not carry the infection to other patients; **placental barrier** = barrier which prevents the blood from the fetus and that of the mother from mixing, but allows water, oxygen, hormones, etc., to pass

from mother to fetus; *see also* SUNBARRIER

those affected by salmonella poisoning are being nursed in five isolation wards and about forty suspected sufferers are being barrier nursed in other wards

Nursing Times

bartholinitis [bɑːθɒlɪˈnaɪtɪs] *noun* inflammation of the Bartholin's glands

Bartholin's glands [ˈbɑːθəlɪnz ˈɡlændz] *plural noun* vestibular glands, two glands at the side of the vagina and between it and the vulva, which secrete a lubricating substance

basal [ˈbeɪsl] *adjective* extremely important; which affects a base; **basal cell** = cell from the stratum germinativum; *see also* STRATUM; **basal cell carcinoma** = RODENT ULCER; **basal ganglia** = masses of grey matter at the base of each cerebral hemisphere which receive impulses from the thalamus and influence the motor impulses from the frontal cortex; **basal metabolic rate (BMR)** = amount of energy used by a body in exchanging oxygen and carbon dioxide when at rest, i.e. energy needed to keep the body functioning and the temperature normal (formerly used as a way of testing the thyroid gland); **basal metabolism** = minimum amount of energy needed to keep the body functioning and the temperature normal when at rest; **basal narcosis** = making a patient completely unconscious by administering a narcotic before a general anaesthetic; **basal nuclei** = masses of grey matter at the bottom of each cerebral hemisphere

basale [bəˈseɪli] *see* STRATUM

basalis [bəˈseɪlɪs] *see* DECIDUA

base [beɪs] *noun* **1 (a)** bottom part; *the base of the spine*; **base of the brain** = bottom surface of the cerebrum **(b)** main ingredient of an ointment, as opposed to the active ingredient **(c)** substance which reacts with an acid to form a salt **2** *verb* to make, using a substance as a main ingredient; **cream based on zinc oxide** = cream which uses zinc oxide as a base

Basedow's disease [ˈbeɪzɪdəʊz dɪˈziːz] = THYROTOXICOSIS

basement membrane [ˈbeɪsmənt ˈmembreɪn] *noun* membrane at the base of an epithelium

basic ['beɪsɪk] *adjective* **(a)** very simple, from which everything else comes; *you should know basic maths if you want to work in a shop*; **basic structure of the skin** = the two layers of skin (the inner dermis and the outer epidermis) **(b)** (chemical substance) which reacts with an acid to form a salt; **basic salt** = chemical compound formed when an acid reacts with a base

basilar ['bæzɪlə] *adjective* referring to a base; **basilar artery** = artery which lies at the base of the brain; **basilar membrane** = membrane in the cochlea which transmits nerve impulses from sound vibrations to the auditory nerve

basilic [bə'sɪlɪk] *adjective* important or prominent; **basilic vein** = large vein running along the inside of the arm

basin ['beɪsən] *noun* large bowl

basis ['beɪsɪs] *noun* **(a)** main part of which something is formed; *water forms the basis of the solution*; *the basis of the treatment is quiet and rest* **(b)** main reason for deciding; *the basis for the diagnosis is the result of the test for the patient's blood sugar*

basophil *or* **basophilic granulocyte** ['beɪsəfɪl *or* beɪsə'fɪlɪk 'grænjʊləsaɪt] *noun* type of leucocyte or white blood cell which contains granules; **basophil leucocyte** = blood cell which carries histamines

basophilia [beɪsə'fɪlɪə] *noun* increase in the number of basophils in the blood

Batchelor plaster ['bætʃələ 'plɑːstə] *noun* plaster cast which keeps both legs apart

bath [bɑːθ] **1** *noun* **(a)** large container for water, in which you can wash your whole body; *there's a shower and a bath in the bathroom*; **hip bath** = small low bath in which a person can sit but not lie down **(b)** washing the whole body; *the patient was given a hot bath*; *he believes that a cold bath every morning is good for you*; **blanket bath** = washing a patient who is confined to bed; **medicinal bath** = treatment where the patient lies in a bath of hot water containing certain chemicals, in hot mud or in other substances; **sponge bath** = washing a patient in bed, using a sponge or damp cloth; *the nurse gave her a sponge bath* **(c)** **eye bath** = small dish into which a solution can be placed for bathing the eye **2** *verb* to wash with a lot of liquid; *he's bathing the baby*

bathe [beɪð] *verb* to wash (a wound); *he bathed his knee with boiled water*

bathroom ['bɑːθruːm] *noun* small room with a bath or shower and usually a toilet

bathtub ['bɑːθtʌb] *US* = BATH (a)

battered baby syndrome *or* **battered child syndrome** ['bætəd 'beɪbi *or* 'bætəd 'tʃaɪld 'sɪndrəʊm] *noun* condition where a baby or small child is frequently beaten by one or both of its parents, sustaining injuries such as multiple fractures

battledore placenta ['bætəldɔː plə'sentə] *noun* placenta where the umbilical cord is attached at the edge and not the centre

Bazin's disease ['beɪzɪnz dɪ'ziːz] = ERYTHEMA INDURATUM

BC ['biː 'siː] = BONE CONDUCTION; *see* CONDUCTION

B cell ['biː 'sel] = BETA CELL

BCG ['biː 'siː 'dʒiː] = BACILLE CALMETTE-GUERIN; *the baby had a BCG vaccination*; *we need some more BCG vaccine*

BCh ['biː 'siː'eɪtʃ] = BACHELOR OF SURGERY

BDA ['biː 'diː 'eɪ] = BRITISH DENTAL ASSOCIATION

Be *chemical symbol for* beryllium

beam [biːm] *noun* line of light or rays; *the X-ray beam is directed at the patient's jaw*

bearing down ['beərɪŋ 'daʊn] *noun* (*of a woman giving birth*) stage in childbirth when the woman starts to push out the baby from the uterus

beat [biːt] **1** *noun* regular sound which forms a rhythm; *the patient's heart had an irregular beat* **2** *verb* **(a)** to hit; **beat joint** (**beat elbow** *or* **beat knee**) = inflammation of a joint (such as the elbow or knee) caused by frequent sharp blows or other pressure **(b)** to make a regular sound; *his heart was beating fast* (NOTE: **beating - beat - has beaten**)

becquerel ['bekrəl] *noun* SI unit of measurement of radiation: 1 becquerel is the amount of radioactivity in a substance where one nucleus decays per second (NOTE: now used in place of the **curie**. See also **rad**. Becquerel is written **Bq** with figures: **200Bq**)

bed [bed] *noun* piece of furniture for sleeping on; *lie down on the bed if you're tired*; *she always goes to bed at 9 o'clock*; *he was sitting up in bed drinking a cup of coffee*; *she's in bed with a cold*; *ward with twenty beds*; *a 250-bed or 250-bedded hospital*; **hospital bed** = (i) special type of bed used in hospitals; (ii) place in a hospital which can be occupied by a patient; *a hospital bed is needed if the patient has to have traction; there will be no reduction in the number of hospital beds*; **bed occupancy rate** = number of beds occupied in a hospital shown as a percentage of all the beds in the hospital; *see also* AIRBED, RIPPLE BED, WATER BED

bedbug ['bedbʌg] *noun* small insect which lives in dirty bedclothes and sucks blood

bedclothes ['bedkləʊðz] *plural noun* sheets and blankets which cover a bed

bedpan ['bedpæn] *noun* dish into which a patient can urinate or defecate without getting out of bed

bedridden ['bedrɪdən] *adjective* (patient) who cannot get out of bed; *he is bedridden and has to be looked after by a nurse; she stayed at home to look after her bedridden mother*

bedroom ['bedruːm] *noun* room where you sleep

bedside manner ['bedsaɪd 'mænə] *noun* way in which a doctor behaves towards a patient, especially a patient who is in bed; **doctor with a good bedside manner** = doctor who comforts and reassures patients, especially those patients who are in bed

bedsore ['bedsɔː] *noun* inflamed patch of skin on a bony part of the body, which develops into an ulcer, caused by pressure of the part on the mattress after lying for some time in one position (NOTE: also called **pressure sore** *or* **decubitus ulcer**)

COMMENT: special types of mattresses can be used to try to prevent the formation of bedsores. See AIR BED, RIPPLE BED, WATER BED

bedtable ['bedteɪbl] *noun* specially designed table which can be used by a person sitting up in bed

bedtime ['bedtaɪm] *noun* time when someone (usually) goes to bed; *9 o'clock is the patients' bedtime; go to bed - it's past your bedtime*

bedwetting ['bedwetɪŋ] *noun* nocturnal enuresis, passing urine when asleep in bed at night (especially used of children)

Beer's knife ['bɪəz 'naɪf] *noun* knife with a triangular blade, used in eye operations

bee sting ['biː stɪŋ] *noun* sting by a bee

COMMENT: because a bee injects acid into the body, relief can be obtained by dabbing an alkaline solution onto a sting

behave [bɪ'heɪv] *verb* to act; *after she was ill she started to behave in a very strange way; the children behaved (themselves)* or *behaved very well when the doctor visited the ward*

behaviour *US* **behavior** [bɪ'heɪvjə] *noun* way of acting; *his behaviour was very strange; the behaviour of the patients in the mental ward is causing concern*; **behaviour therapy** = psychiatric treatment where the patient learns to improve his condition

behavioural *US* **behavioral** [bɪ'heɪvjərl] *adjective* referring to behaviour; **behavioural scientist** = person who specializes in the study of behaviour

behaviourism *US* **behaviorism** [bɪ'heɪvjərɪzm] *noun* psychological theory that only the patient's behaviour should be studied to discover his psychological problems

behaviourist *US* **behaviorist** [bɪ'heɪvjərɪst] *noun* psychologist who follows behaviourism

Behçet's syndrome ['beɪsets 'sɪndrəʊm] *noun* viral condition with no known cause, in which the patient has mouth ulcers and inflamed eyes accompanied by polyarthritis

bejel ['bedʒəl] *noun* endemic syphilis, non-venereal form of syphilis which is endemic among children in some areas of the Middle East and elsewhere and is caused by a spirochaete strain of bacteria

belch [beltʃ] **1** *noun* eructation, allowing air in the stomach to come up through the mouth **2** *verb* to make air in the stomach come up through the mouth (NOTE: with babies the word **burp** is used)

belladonna [belə'dɒnə] *noun* deadly nightshade, a poisonous plant which produces atropine

belle indifférence ['bel æn'dɪferɑːns] *noun* excessively calm state of a patient, when normally he should show emotion

Bellocq's cannula or **Bellocq's sound** [be'lɒks 'kænjʊlə or 'saʊnd] *noun* instrument used to control a nosebleed

Bell's mania ['belz 'meɪniə] *noun* form of acute mania with delirium

Bell's palsy ['belz 'pɔːlzi] *noun* facial paralysis, paralysis of one side of the face, preventing the patient from closing one eye, caused by a defect in the facial nerve

belly ['beli] *noun* **(a)** abdomen, the space in the front of the body below the diaphragm and above the pelvis, containing the stomach **(b)** fatter central part of a muscle

bellyache ['belieik] *noun* pain in the abdomen or stomach

belly button ['beli 'bʌtn] *noun (used mainly by children)* navel

belt [belt] *noun* long piece of leather or plastic, etc., which goes around the waist to keep trousers, etc., up, or to attach a coat; **seat belt** = belt in a car or in an aircraft which holds someone safely in his seat; **surgical belt** = fitted covering, worn to support part of the back, chest or abdomen

Bence Jones protein ['bens 'dʒəunz 'prəuti:n] *noun* protein found in the urine of patients suffering from myelomatosis, lymphoma, leukaemia and some other cancers

bend [bend] **1** *noun* curved shape; *the pipe under the washbasin has two bends in it* **2** *verb* **(a)** to make something curved; to be curved; *he bent the pipe into the shape of an S* **(b)** to lean towards the ground; *he bent down to tie up his shoe*; *she was bending over the table* (NOTE: **bending - bent - has bent**)

bends [bendz] *noun* **the bends** = CAISSON DISEASE

Benedict's solution ['benɪdɪkts sə'lu:ʃn] *noun* solution used to carry out Benedict's test

Benedict's test ['benɪdɪkts 'test] *noun* test to see if sugar is present in the urine

benign [bɪ'naɪn] *adjective* generally harmless; **benign tumour** *or* **benign growth** = tumour which will not grow again or spread to other parts of the body if it is removed surgically, but which can be fatal if not treated (NOTE: the opposite is **malignant**)

Bennett's fracture ['benɪts 'fræktʃə] *noun* fracture of the first metacarpal, the bone between the thumb and the wrist

benzodiazepine [benzəudaɪ'æzəpin] *noun* drug which acts on receptors in the central nervous system to relieve symptoms of anxiety and insomnia (NOTE: benzodiazepines have names ending in **-azepam: diazepam**)

COMMENT: indiscriminate prescription, prolonged use and abrupt withdrawal should be avoided

benzoin ['benzəuɪn] *noun* resin used to make friar's balsam

benzyl penicillin ['benzɪl penə'sɪlɪn] *noun see* DRUGS TABLE IN SUPPLEMENT

bereavement [bɪ'ri:vmənt] *noun* loss of someone you know, especially a close relative, through death

beriberi [beri'beri] *noun* disease of the nervous system caused by lack of vitamin B_1 **dry beriberi** = beriberi where the patient suffers loss of feeling and paralysis; **wet beriberi** = beriberi where the patient's body swells with oedema

COMMENT: beriberi is prevalent in tropical countries where the diet is mainly formed of white rice which is deficient in thiamine

berylliosis [bərɪli'əusɪs] *noun* poisoning caused by breathing in particles of beryllium oxide

beryllium [bə'rɪliəm] *noun* chemical element (NOTE: chemical symbol is **Be**)

Besnier's prurigo [beni'eɪz pru'raɪgəu] *see* PRURIGO

beta ['bi:tə] *noun* second letter of the Greek alphabet; **beta amyloid** = wax-like protein formed from amyloid precursor protein in nerve cells which aggregates in Alzheimer's disease to form plaques; **beta blocker** = drug which blocks the beta-adrenergic receptors and so reduces the activity of the heart (NOTE: beta blockers have names ending in **-olol: atenolol, propranolol hydrochloride**); **beta cell** = cell which produces insulin (NOTE: also called **B cell**)

betamethasone [bi:tə'meθəsəun] *noun* very strong corticosteroid drug

better ['betə] *adjective & adverb* healthy again, not as ill as before; *I had a cold last week but now I'm better*; *I hope you're better soon*; *she had flu but now she's feeling better*; **vegetables are better for you than sweets** = vegetables make you healthier

Bi *chemical symbol for* bismuth

bi- ['baɪ] *prefix meaning* two or twice

bias ['baɪəs] *noun* the systematic error in the design or conduct of a study which could explain the results (for example, if patients and controls are selected in a different way)

bicarbonate of soda (NaHCO₃)
[baɪˈkɑːbənət əv ˈsəʊdə] *noun* sodium salt used to treat acidity in the stomach

bicellular [baɪˈseljʊlə] *adjective* which has two cells

biceps [ˈbaɪseps] *noun* any muscle formed of two parts joined to form one tendon, especially the muscles in the front of the upper arm (biceps brachii) and the back of the thigh (biceps femoris); *compare* TRICEPS (NOTE: the plural is **biceps**)

bicipital [baɪˈsɪpɪtl] *adjective* (i) referring to a biceps muscle; (ii) with two parts

biconcave [baɪˈkɒŋkeɪv] *adjective* (lens) which is concave on both sides

biconvex [baɪˈkɒnveks] *adjective* (lens) which is convex on both sides

bicornuate [baɪˈkɔːnjuɪt] *adjective* which is divided into two parts (sometimes applied to a malformation of the uterus)

bicuspid [baɪˈkʌspɪd] **1** *adjective* with two points; **bicuspid valve** = mitral valve, the valve in the heart which allows blood to flow from the left atrium to the left ventricle but not in the opposite direction; *see illustration at* HEART **2** *noun* premolar tooth

b.i.d. *or* **bis in die** [ˈbiː ˈaɪ ˈdiː *or* ˈbɪs ɪn ˈdiːeɪ] *Latin phrase meaning* twice daily

bifid [ˈbaɪfɪd] *adjective* in two parts

bifida [ˈbɪfɪdə] *see* SPINA BIFIDA

bifocal lenses *or* **bifocals** *or* **bifocal glasses** [baɪˈfəʊkl ˈlenzɪz *or* baɪˈfəʊkəlz] *plural noun* type of spectacles where two lenses are combined in the same piece of glass, the top lens being for seeing at a distance and the lower lens for reading; *see also* TRIFOCAL

bifurcation [baɪfəˈkeɪʃn] *noun* place where something divides into two parts

bigeminy [baɪˈdʒemɪni] *noun* pulsus bigeminus, a double pulse with an extra ectopic beat

big toe [ˈbɪg ˈtəʊ] *noun* largest of the five toes, on the inside of the foot

bilateral [baɪˈlætrəl] *adjective* which affects both sides; **bilateral pneumonia** = pneumonia affecting both lungs; **bilateral vasectomy** = surgical operation to cut both vasa deferentia and so make the patient sterile

bile [baɪl] *noun* thick bitter brownish yellow fluid produced by the liver, stored in the gall bladder and used to digest fatty substances and to neutralize acids; **bile acids** = acids (such as cholic acid) found in bile; **bile canal** = very small vessel leading from a hepatic cell to the bile duct; **bile duct** = tube which links the cystic duct and the hepatic duct to the duodenum; **common bile duct** = duct leading to the duodenum, formed of the hepatic and cystic ducts together; **bile pigment** = colouring matter in bile; **bile salts** = sodium salts of bile acids (NOTE: for other terms referring to bile, see words beginning with **chol-**)

> COMMENT: in jaundice, excess bile pigments flow into the blood and cause the skin to turn yellow

Bilharzia [bɪlˈhɑːtsiə] *noun* Schistosoma, genus of fluke which enters the patient's bloodstream and causes bilharziasis

bilharziasis [bɪlhɑːˈtsaɪəsɪs] *noun* schistosomiasis, tropical disease caused by flukes in the intestine or bladder (NOTE: although strictly speaking, **Bilharzia** is the name of the fluke, it is also generally used for the name of the disease: **bilharzia patients; six cases of bilharzia**)

> COMMENT: the larvae of the fluke enter the skin through the feet and lodge in the walls of the intestine or bladder. They are passed out of the body in stools or urine and return to water, where they lodge and develop in the water snail, the secondary host, before going back into humans. Patients suffer from fever and anaemia

biliary [ˈbɪliəri] *adjective* referring to bile; **primary biliary cirrhosis** = cirrhosis of the liver caused by autoimmune disease; **secondary biliary cirrhosis** = cirrhosis of the liver caused by an obstruction of the bile ducts; **biliary colic** = pain in the abdomen caused by gallstones in the bile duct or by inflammation of the gall bladder; **biliary fistula** = opening which discharges bile onto the surface of the skin from the gall bladder, bile duct or liver

bilious [ˈbɪliəs] *adjective* (condition) caused by bile or where bile is brought up into the mouth; (any condition) where the patient suffers nausea; **he had a bilious attack** = he had indigestion together with nausea

biliousness [ˈbɪliəsnəs] *noun* feeling of indigestion and nausea

bilirubin [bɪliˈruːbɪn] *noun* red pigment in bile; **serum bilirubin** = bilirubin in serum, converted from haemoglobin as red blood cells are destroyed

bilirubinaemia [bɪliruːbɪ'niːmiə] *noun* excess of bilirubin in the blood

biliuria [bɪli'juəriə] *noun* presence of bile in the urine; *see* CHOLURIA

biliverdin [bɪli'vɜːdɪn] *noun* green pigment in bile, produced by oxidation of bilirubin (NOTE: for other terms referring to bile, see words beginning with **chol-**)

billion ['bɪljən] *noun* number equal to one thousand million or one million million (NOTE: in the USA it has always meant one thousand million, but in GB it formerly meant one million million, and it is still sometimes used with this meaning. With figures it is usually written **bn: 5bn**)

Billroth's operations ['bɪlrɒθs ɒpə'reɪʃnz] *plural noun* surgical operations where the lower part of the stomach is removed and the part which is left is linked to the duodenum (Billroth I) or jejunum (Billroth II)

bilobate [baɪ'ləʊbeɪt] *adjective* with two lobes

bimanual [baɪ'mænjʊəl] *adjective* done with two hands, needing both hands to be done

binary ['baɪnəri] *adjective* (i) made of two parts; (ii) (compound) made of two elements; **binary fission** = splitting into two parts (in some types of cell division)

binaural [baɪn'ɔːrl] *adjective* referring to both ears; using both ears

bind [baɪnd] *verb* to tie; to fasten; *she bound his sprained wrist with a wet cloth* (NOTE: **binding - bound - has bound**)

binder ['baɪndə] *noun* bandage which is wrapped round a limb to support it

Binet's test ['bɪneɪz 'test] *noun* intelligence test for children

binocular [bɪ'nɒkjʊlə] *adjective* referring to the two eyes; **binocular vision** = ability to see with both eyes at the same time, which gives a stereoscopic effect and allows a person to judge distances; *compare* MONOCULAR

binovular [bɪ'nɒvjʊlə] *adjective* (twins) which come from two different ova

binucleate [baɪ'njuːklieɪt] *adjective* with two nuclei

bio- ['baɪəʊ] *prefix* referring to living organisms

bioassay [baɪəʊə'seɪ] *noun* test of the strength of a drug, hormone, vitamin or serum, by examining the effect it has on living animals or tissue

bioavailability [baɪəʊəveɪlə'bɪləti] *noun* extent to which a nutrient or medicine can be taken up by the body

biochemical [baɪəʊ'kemɪkl] *adjective* referring to biochemistry

biochemist [baɪəʊ'kemɪst] *noun* scientist who specializes in biochemistry

biochemistry [baɪəʊ'kemɪstri] *noun* chemistry of living tissues

biocide ['baɪəʊsaɪd] *noun* substance which kills living organisms

biodegradable [bauəʊdɪ'greɪdəbl] *adjective* which can be easily decomposed by organisms such as bacteria or by the effect of sunlight, the sea, etc.

bioengineering [baɪəʊendʒɪ'nɪərɪŋ] *noun* science of manipulating and combining different genetic material to produce living organisms with particular characteristics

biofeedback [baɪəʊ'fiːdbæk] *noun* control of the autonomic nervous system by the patient's conscious thought (as he sees the results of tests or scans)

biogenesis [baɪəʊ'dʒenəsɪs] *noun* theory that living organisms can only develop from other living organisms

biological [baɪə'lɒdʒɪkl] *adjective* referring to biology; **biological clock** = circadian rhythm, the rhythm of daily activities and bodily processes (eating, defecating, sleeping, etc.) frequently controlled by hormones, which repeats every twenty-four hours; **biological warfare** = war where one side tries to kill or to affect the people of the enemy side by infecting them with living organisms or poison derived from living organisms

biologist [baɪ'ɒlədʒɪst] *noun* scientist who specializes in biology

biology [baɪ'ɒlədʒi] *noun* study of living organisms

biomaterial [baɪəʊmə'tɪəriəl] *noun* synthetic material which can be used as an implant in living tissue

biometry [baɪ'ɒmətri] *noun* science which studies biological variations and their effects; *(of the fetus)* measurement of key parameters of growth of the fetus by ultrasound; **biometry of the eye** = measurement of the eye by ultrasound

bionics [baɪˈɒnɪks] *noun* applying knowledge of biological systems to mechanical and electronic devices

biopsy [ˈbaɪɒpsi] *noun* taking a small piece of living tissue for examination and diagnosis; *the biopsy of the tissue from the growth showed that it was benign*

biorhythms [ˈbaɪəʊrɪðmz] *plural noun* recurring cycles of biological processes thought to affect a person's behaviour, sensitivity and intelligence

biostatistics [baɪəʊstəˈtɪstɪks] *plural noun* statistics used in medicine and the study of disease

biotechnology [baɪəʊtekˈnɒlədʒi] *noun* use of technology to manipulate and combine different genetic materials to produce living organisms with particular characteristics; *a biotechnology company is developing a range of new pesticides based on naturally occurring toxins*; *artificial insemination of cattle was one of the first examples of biotechnology*

biotin [ˈbaɪətɪn] *noun* type of vitamin B, found in egg yolks, liver and yeast

bipara [baɪˈpeərə or baɪˈpærə] *noun* woman who has been pregnant twice and each time has given birth normally

biparietal [baɪpəˈraɪətl] *adjective* referring to the two parietal bones

biparous [ˈbɪpərəs] *adjective* which produces twins

bipennate [baɪˈpeneɪt] *adjective* (muscle) with fibres which rise from either side of the tendon

bipolar [baɪˈpəʊlə] *adjective* with two poles; **bipolar disorder** = mental disorder where the patient moves from mania to depression; **bipolar neurone** = nerve cell with two processes, a dendrite and an axon (found in the retina); *see illustration at* NEURONE

birth [bɜːθ] *noun* being born; **date of birth** = date when a person was born; **to give birth** = to have a baby; *she gave birth to twins*; **breech birth** = birth where the baby's buttocks appear first; **live birth** = birth of a baby which is alive; *the number of live births has remained steady compared to last year*; **premature birth** = birth of a baby earlier than 37 weeks from conception; **birth canal** = uterus, vagina and vulva; **birth certificate** = official document giving details of a person's date and place of birth and parents; **birth control** = restricting the number of children born by using contraception; **birth control pill** = THE PILL; **birth defect** = congenital defect, a malformation which exists in a person's body from birth; **birth injury** = injury (such as brain damage) which a baby suffers during a difficult birth; **birth rate** = number of births per year, shown per thousand of the population; *a birth rate of 15 per thousand*; *there has been a severe decline in the birth rate*; **birth weight** = weight of a baby at birth

birthing chair [ˈbɜːθɪŋ ˈtʃeə] *noun* special chair in which a mother sits to give birth

birthmark [ˈbɜːθmɑːk] *noun* naevus, a mark on the skin which a baby has at birth and which cannot be removed

bisexual [baɪˈsekʃʊl] *adjective* (i) (person) who is sexually attracted to both males and females; (ii) (person) who has both male and female physical characteristics

bisexuality [baɪsekʃʊˈælɪti] *noun* (i) being sexually attracted to both males and females; (ii) having both male and female physical characteristics; *compare* AMBISEXUAL, HETEROSEXUAL, HOMOSEXUAL

bis in die [ˈbɪs ɪn ˈdiːeɪ] *see* B.I.D.

bismuth [ˈbɪzməθ] *noun* chemical element; **bismuth salts** = salts used to treat acid stomach and formerly used in the treatment of syphilis (NOTE: chemical symbol is **Bi**)

bistoury [ˈbɪstəri] *noun* sharp, thin surgical knife

bite [baɪt] **1** *verb* to cut into something with the teeth; *the dog bit the postman*; *he bit a piece out of the apple*; *she was bitten by an insect*; **to bite on something** = to hold onto something with the teeth; *the dentist told him to bite on the bite wing* (NOTE: **biting - bit - has bitten**) **2** *noun* action of biting or of being bitten; place where someone has been bitten; *animal bite*; *dog bite*; *insect bite*; *her arm was covered with bites*

bite wing [ˈbaɪt ˈwɪŋ] *noun* holder for dental X-ray film, which the patient holds between the teeth, so allowing an X-ray of both upper and lower teeth to be taken

Bitot's spots [ˈbitəʊz ˈspɒts] *plural noun* small white spots on the conjunctiva, caused by vitamin A deficiency

bitter [ˈbɪtə] *adjective* one of the four tastes, not sweet, sour or salt; *quinine is bitter but oranges are sweet; see illustration at* TONGUE

bivalve ['baɪvælv] *noun & adjective* (organ) which has two valves

black [blæk] *adjective & noun* having the very darkest colour which is the opposite of white; *the surgeon was wearing a black coat*; **black coffee** = coffee with no milk in it; **Black Death** = violent form of bubonic plague, a pandemic during the Middle Ages; **black eye** = bruising and swelling of the tissues round an eye, caused by a blow; *he got a black eye in the fight* (NOTE: **black - blacker - blackest**)

blackhead ['blækhed] *noun* comedo, a small point of dark, hard matter in a sebaceous follicle, often found associated with acne on the skin of adolescents; *see* ACNE

blackout ['blækaut] *noun* fainting fit, sudden loss of consciousness; *he must have had a blackout while driving*

black out ['blæk 'aut] *verb* to have a fainting fit, sudden loss of consciousness; *I suddenly blacked out and I can't remember anything more*

blackwater fever ['blækwɔːtə 'fiːvə] *noun* tropical disease, a form of malaria, where haemoglobin from red blood cells is released into plasma and makes the urine dark

bladder ['blædə] *noun* any sac in the body, especially the sac where the urine collects before being passed out of the body; *he is suffering from bladder trouble*; *she is taking antibiotics for a bladder infection*; **neurogenic bladder** = any disturbance of the bladder function caused by lesions in the nerve supply to the bladder; **urinary bladder** = sac where the urine collects from the kidneys through the ureters, before being passed out of the body through the urethra; *see illustrations at* KIDNEY, UROGENITAL SYSTEM; *see also* GALL BLADDER (NOTE: for other terms referring to the bladder, see words beginning with **cyst-**, **vesico-**)

bladder worm ['blædə 'wɜːm] *noun* cysticercus, the larva of a tapeworm found in pork, which is enclosed in a cyst, typical of *Taenia*

blade [bleɪd] *noun* thin flat piece of metal; *this bistoury has a very sharp blade*

Blalock's operation or **Blalock-Taussig operation** ['bleɪlɒks ɒpə'reɪʃn or 'bleɪlɒk'tɔːsɪg ɒpə'reɪʃn] *noun* surgical operation to connect the pulmonary artery to the subclavian artery, in order to increase blood flow to the lungs in a patient suffering from tetralogy of Fallot

bland [blænd] *adjective* (food) which is not spicy, not irritating or not acid; **bland diet** = diet in which the patient eats mainly milk-based foods, boiled vegetables and white meat, as a treatment for peptic ulcers

blank [blæŋk] *adjective* (paper) with nothing written on it; *the doctor took out a blank prescription form*

blanket ['blæŋkɪt] *noun* thick woollen cover which is put over a person to keep him warm when asleep or lying still; *he woke up when his blankets fell off*; **blanket bath** = washing a patient who is confined to bed

blast [blɑːst] *noun* **(a)** immature form of a cell before definite characteristics develop **(b)** wave of air pressure from an explosion, which can cause concussion; **blast injury** = severe injury to the chest following a blast

-blast [blæst] *suffix* referring to a very early stage in the development of a cell

blasto- ['blæstəu] *prefix* referring to a germ cell

blastocoele *US* **blastocele** ['blæstəusiːl] *noun* cavity filled with fluid in a morula

blastocyst ['blæstəusɪst] *noun* early stage in the development of an embryo

Blastomyces [blæstəu'maɪsiːz] *noun* type of parasitic fungus which affects the skin

blastomycosis [blæstəumaɪ'kəusɪs] *noun* infection caused by Blastomyces

blastula ['blæstjulə] *noun* first stage of the development of an embryo in animals

bleb [bleb] *noun* small blister; *compare* BULLA

bled [bled] *see* BLEED

bleed [bliːd] *verb* to lose blood; *his knee was bleeding*; *his nose began to bleed*; *when she cut her finger it bled*; *he was bleeding from a cut on the head* (NOTE: **bleeding - bled - has bled**)

bleeder ['bliːdə] *noun* person who suffers from haemophilia

bleeding ['bliːdɪŋ] *noun* abnormal loss of blood from the body through the skin or through an orifice or internally; **internal bleeding** = loss of blood inside the body (as from a wound in the intestine); **control of bleeding** = ways of stopping bleeding by applying pressure to blood vessels; **bleeding point** or **bleeding site** = place in the body where bleeding is taking place; **bleeding time** = test of clotting of a patient's blood, by timing the length of time it takes for the blood to congeal

COMMENT: blood lost through bleeding from an artery is bright red and can rush out because it is under pressure. Blood from a vein is darker red and flows more slowly

blenno- ['blenəʊ] *prefix* referring to mucus

blennorrhagia [blenəʊ'reɪdʒə] *noun* (i) discharge of mucus; (ii) gonorrhoea

blennorrhoea [blenəʊ'rɪə] *noun* (i) discharge of watery mucus; (ii) gonorrhoea

blephar(o)- ['blefə or 'blefərəʊ] *prefix* referring to the eyelid

blepharitis [blefə'raɪtɪs] *noun* inflammation of the eyelid

blepharon ['blefərɒn] *noun* eyelid

blepharoptosis [blefərɒp'təʊsɪs] *noun* condition where the upper eyelid is half closed because of paralysis of the muscle or nerve

blepharospasm ['blefərəʊspæzm] *noun* sudden contraction of the eyelid, as when a tiny piece of dust gets in the eye

blind [blaɪnd] **1** *adjective* **(a)** not able to see; *a blind man with a white stick*; *after her illness she became blind*; **colour blind** = not able to tell the difference between certain colours, especially red and green; **blind loop syndrome** = *see* LOOP; **blind spot** = point in the retina where the optic nerve joins it, which does not register light **(b)** **blind (study)** = an investigation to test an intervention (often a drug) in which the patient does not know if he has active medicine or a placebo; **double blind (study)** = an investigation to test an intervention in which neither the patient nor the doctor knows if the patient is receiving active medicine or placebo **2** *plural noun* **the blind** = people who are blind; **blind register** = official list of blind people **3** *verb* to make someone blind; *he was blinded in the accident*

blindness ['blaɪndnəs] *noun* not being able to see; **colour blindness** = being unable to tell the difference between certain colours; **day blindness** = hemeralopia, being able to see better in bad light than in ordinary daylight (usually a congenital condition); **night blindness** = nyctalopia, being unable to see in bad light; **snow blindness** = temporary painful blindness caused by bright sunlight shining on snow; **sun blindness** = PHOTORETINITIS

blink [blɪŋk] *verb* to close and open the eyelids rapidly several times or once; *he blinked in the bright light*

blister ['blɪstə] **1** *noun* (i) swelling on the skin containing serous liquid; (ii) substance which acts as a counterirritant **2** *verb* to have blisters; *after the fire his hands and face were badly blistered*

COMMENT: blisters contain serum or watery liquid from the blood. They can be caused by rubbing, burning or by a disease such as chickenpox. Blood blisters contain blood which has passed from broken blood vessels under the skin. Water blisters contain lymph

block [blɒk] **1** *noun* **(a)** stopping of a function; **caudal block** = local analgesia of the cauda equina nerves in the lower spine; **epidural block** = analgesia produced by injecting an analgesic solution into the space between the vertebral canal and the dura mater; **heart block** = slowing of the action of the heart because the impulses from the SA node to the ventricles are delayed or interrupted; **mental block** = temporary inability to remember something, caused by the effect of nervous stress on the mental processes; **nerve block** = stopping the function of a nerve by injecting an anaesthetic; **speech block** = temporary inability to speak, caused by the effect of nervous stress on the mental processes; **spinal block** analgesia produced by injecting the spinal cord with an anaesthetic **(b)** large piece; *a block of wood fell on his foot* **(c)** one of the different buildings forming a section of a hospital; *the patient is in Block 2, Ward 7*; *she is having treatment in the physiotherapy block* **2** *verb* to obstruct; *the artery was blocked by a clot*; *he swallowed a piece of plastic which blocked his oesophagus*

blockage ['blɒkɪdʒ] *noun* something which obstructs; being obstructed; *there is a blockage in the rectum*; *the blockage of the artery was caused by a blood clot*

blocker ['blɒkə] *noun* substance which blocks; **alpha/beta blocker** = drug which blocks the alpha/beta-adrenergic receptors, to relax smooth muscle (alpha blocker, such as alfuzosin hydrochloride) or to reduce blood pressure or the activity of the heart (beta blocker, such as atenolol)

blocking [ˈblɒkɪŋ] *noun* psychiatric disorder, where the patient suddenly stops one train of thought and switches to another

blood [blʌd] *noun* red liquid in the body; *the police followed the spots of blood to find the wounded man*; *blood was pouring from the cut in his hand*; *he suffered serious loss of blood or blood loss in the accident*; **blood bank** = section of a hospital where blood given by donors is stored for use in transfusions; **blood casts** = pieces of blood cells which are secreted by the kidneys in kidney disease; **blood cell** *or* **blood corpuscle** = red blood cell or white blood cell which is one of the parts of blood; **blood chemistry** *or* **chemistry of the blood** = (i) substances which make up blood, which can be analysed in blood tests, the results of which are useful in diagnosing disease; (ii) record of changes which take place in blood during disease and treatment; **blood clot** = thrombus, a soft mass of coagulated blood in a vein or an artery; **blood clotting** *or* **blood coagulation** = process where blood changes from being liquid to being semi- solid and so stops flowing; **blood count** = test to count the number and types of different blood cells in a certain tiny sample of blood, to give an indication of the condition of the patient's blood as a whole; **blood culture** = putting a sample of blood into a culture medium to see if foreign organisms in it grow; **blood donor** = person who gives blood which is then used in transfusions to other patients; **blood formation** = haemopoiesis, the continual production of blood cells and blood platelets by the bone marrow; **blood-letting** = phlebotomy or venesection, an operation where a vein or an artery is cut so that blood can be removed; **blood loss** = loss of blood from the body by bleeding; *US* **blood picture** = full blood count; **blood plasma** = yellow watery liquid which makes up the main part of blood; **blood platelet** = small blood cell which releases thromboplastin and which multiplies rapidly after an injury, encouraging the coagulation of blood; **blood poisoning** = septicaemia, a condition where bacteria are present in the blood and cause illness; **blood sample** = sample of blood, taken for testing; **blood serum** = yellowish watery liquid which separates from (whole) blood when the blood clots; **blood sugar level** = amount of glucose in the blood; **blood test** = laboratory test of a blood sample to analyse its chemical composition; **blood transfusion** = transferring blood from another person into a patient's vein; **blood type** = BLOOD GROUP; **blood typing** = analysis of blood for transfusion, factors and blood group; **blood urea** = urea present in the blood (a high level occurs following heart failure or kidney disease); **blood vessel** = any tube (artery, vein, capillary) which carries blood round the body (NOTE: for other terms referring to blood, see words beginning with **haem-, haemato-**. For other terms referring to blood vessels, see words beginning with **angio-**)

COMMENT: blood is formed of red and white corpuscles, platelets and plasma. It circulates round the body, going from the heart and lungs along arteries and returns to the heart through the veins. As it moves round the body it takes oxygen to the tissues and removes waste material which is cleaned out through the kidneys or exhaled through the lungs. It also carries hormones produced by glands to the various organs which need them. Each adult person has about six litres or ten pints of blood in his body.

blood-brain barrier [ˈblʌdbreɪn ˈbæriə] *noun* process by which certain substances are held back by the endothelium of cerebral capillaries (where in other parts of the body the same substances will diffuse from capillaries) so preventing these substances from getting into contact with the fluids round the brain

blood group [ˈblʌd ˈgruːp] *noun* one of the different types of blood by which groups of people are identified

COMMENT: blood is classified in various ways. The most common classifications are by the agglutinogens in red blood corpuscles (factors A and B) and by the Rhesus factor. Blood can therefore have either factor (Group A and Group B) or both factors (Group AB) or neither (Group O) and each of these groups can be Rhesus negative or positive

blood pressure [ˈblʌd ˈpreʃə] *noun* pressures (measured in millimetres of mercury) at which the blood is pumped round the body by the heart; **high blood pressure** *or* **raised blood pressure** = level of blood pressure which is higher than normal; *she suffers from high blood pressure*

COMMENT: blood pressure is measured using a sphygmomanometer, where a rubber tube is wrapped round the patient's arm and inflated. Two readings of blood pressure are taken: the systolic pressure, when the heart is contracting and so pumping out, and the diastolic pressure (which is always a lower figure) when the heart relaxes. Normal adult values are considered to be 160/95, unless the patient is diabetic or has heart disease, when lower target values are set

raised blood pressure may account for as many as 70% of all strokes. The risk of stroke rises with both systolic and diastolic blood pressure in the normotensive and hypertensive ranges. Blood pressure control reduces the incidence of first stroke and aspirin appears to reduce the risk of stroke after TIAs

British Journal of Hospital Medicine

bloodshot ['blʌdʃɒt] *adjective* (eye) with small specks of blood in it

bloodstained ['blʌdsteɪnd] *adjective* having blood in or on it; *he coughed up bloodstained sputum*; *the nurses took away the bloodstained sheets*

bloodstream ['blʌdstriːm] *noun* blood flowing round the body; *the antibiotics are injected into the bloodstream*; *hormones are secreted by the glands into the bloodstream*

blot [blɒt] *see* RORSCHACH TEST

blue [bluː] *adjective & noun* (of a) colour such as that of a clear unclouded sky in the daytime; *the sister was dressed in a blue uniform*; **blue baby** = baby suffering from congenital cyanosis, born either with a congenital heart defect or with atelectasis (a collapsed lung), which prevents an adequate supply of oxygen reaching the tissues, giving the baby's skin a bluish colour (NOTE: **blue - bluer - bluest**)

Blue Cross *or* **Blue Shield** ['bluː 'krɒs or 'bluː 'ʃiːld] *noun US* systems of private medical insurance

blueness *or* **blue disease** ['bluːnəs or 'bluː dɪ'ziːz] *noun* cyanosis, the blue colour of the skin, a symptom of lack of oxygen in the blood

blunt [blʌnt] *adjective* not sharp or which does not cut well; *he hurt his hand with a blunt knife*; *the surgeon's instruments must not be blunt* (NOTE: **blunt - blunter - bluntest**)

blurred [blɜːd] *adjective* not clear; **blurred vision** = condition where the patient does not see objects clearly

blurring of vision ['blɜːrɪŋ əv 'vɪʒn] *noun* condition where a patient does not see objects

clearly, caused by loss of blood or sometimes by inadequate diet

blush [blʌʃ] **1** *noun* rush of red colour to the skin of the face (caused by emotion) **2** *verb* to go red in the face because of emotion

BM ['biː 'em] = BACHELOR OF MEDICINE

BMA ['biː 'em 'eɪ] = BRITISH MEDICAL ASSOCIATION

BMI ['biː 'em 'aɪ] = BODY MASS INDEX

BMR ['biː 'em 'ɑː] = BASAL METABOLIC RATE; **BMR test** = test of thyroid function

BNF ['biː 'en 'ef] = BRITISH NATIONAL FORMULARY book listing key information on the prescribing, dispensing and administration of prescription drugs used in the UK

BO ['biː 'əʊ] = BODY ODOUR

board of directors ['bɔːd əv daɪ'rektəz] *noun* group of people (usually, consultants, heads of nursing staff and administrators) chosen to run a hospital trust

bodily ['bɒdɪli] *adjective* referring to the body; *the main bodily functions are controlled by the sympathetic nervous system*; *he suffered from several minor bodily disorders*

body ['bɒdi] *noun* **(a)** the trunk, the main part of a person, not including the head or arms and legs **(b)** all of a person (as opposed to the mind); *the dead man's body was found several days later*; **body fat** = adipose tissue, tissue where the cells contain fat, which replaces the normal fibrous tissue when too much food is eaten; **body fluids** = liquid in the body, including mainly water and blood; **body image** *or* **body schema** = mental image which a person has of his own body; **body odour** = unpleasant smell caused by perspiration; **body scan** = examination of the whole of a patient's body using ultrasound or other scanning techniques; **body temperature** = internal temperature of the human body (normally about 37°C) **(c)** mass, or piece of material (of any size); **cell body** = part of a nerve cell which surrounds the nucleus and from which the axon and dendrites begin; **ciliary body** = part of the eye which connects the iris to the choroid; **inclusion bodies** = very small particles found in cells infected by virus; **Nissl bodies** *or* **Nissl granules** = coarse granules surrounding the nucleus in the cytoplasm of nerve cells; **pineal body** *or* **pineal gland** = small cone-shaped gland situated below the corpus callosum in the brain, which produces melatonin and is believed to be associated with the circadian rhythm; *see illustration at* BRAIN **(d)** main part of something; **body of sternum** = main central part of the breastbone; **body of vertebra** = main part of a vertebra which supports the weight of the body; **body of the stomach** = main part of the stomach between the fundus and the pylorus; *see illustration at* STOMACH **(e) foreign body** = piece of material which is not part of the surrounding tissue and should not be there (such as sand in a cut, dust in the eye or pin which has been swallowed); *the X-ray showed the presence of a foreign body*; **swallowed foreign bodies** = anything (a pin, coin or button) which should not have been swallowed

body mass index (BMI) ['bɒdi 'mæs 'ɪndeks] *noun* figure obtained by dividing the weight in kilos (of a person) by the square of his or her height in metres; 19 - 25 is considered normal

> COMMENT: if a person is 1m 70 (ie 5' 7") and weighs 82kg (ie 180 pounds), his or her BMI is 28 (ie above normal)

Boeck's disease *or* **Boeck's sarcoid** ['beks dɪ'ziːz or 'beks 'saːkɔɪd] = SARCOIDOSIS

Bohn's nodules *or* **Bohn's epithelial pearls** ['bɔːnz 'nɒdjuːlz or 'bɔːnz epɪ'θiːliəl 'pɜːlz] *plural noun* tiny cysts found in the mouths of healthy infants

boil [bɔɪl] **1** *noun* furuncle, a tender raised mass of infected tissue and skin, usually caused by infection of a hair follicle by the bacterium *Staphylococcus aureus* **2** *verb* to heat water (or another liquid) until it changes into gas; *(of water, etc.)* to change into a gas because of heating; *can you boil some water so we can sterilize the instruments?*

bolus ['bəʊləs] *noun* food which has been chewed and is ready to be swallowed; mass of food passing along the intestine

bonding ['bɒndɪŋ] *noun* making a psychological link between the baby and its mother; *in autistic children bonding is difficult*

bone [bəʊn] *noun* **(a)** one of the calcified pieces of connective tissue which make the skeleton; *he fell over and broke a bone in his ankle*; *there are several small bones in the human ear*; **cranial bones** = bones in the skull; *see illustration at* SKULL; **metacarpal bone** = one of the five bones in

the hand; *see illustration at* HAND **(b)** hard substance which forms a bone; **cancellous bone** *or* **spongy bone** = light spongy bone tissue which forms the inner core of a bone and also the ends of long bones; **compact bone** *or* **dense bone** = type of bone tissue which forms the hard outer layer of a bone; *see illustration at* BONE STRUCTURE; **bone conduction;** *see* CONDUCTION; **bone graft** = piece of bone taken from one part of the body to repair a defect in another bone; **bone structure** = (i) system of jointed bones forming the body; (ii) arrangement of the various components of a bone (NOTE: for other terms referring to bone, see words beginning with **ost-, osteo-**)

> COMMENT: bones are formed of a hard outer layer (compact bone) which is made up of a series of layers of tissue (Haversian systems) and a softer inner part (cancellous bone *or* spongy bone) which contains bone marrow

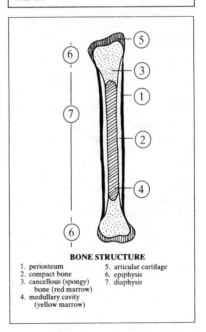

BONE STRUCTURE

1. periosteum
2. compact bone
3. cancellous (spongy) bone (red marrow)
4. medullary cavity (yellow marrow)
5. articular cartilage
6. epiphysis
7. diaphysis

bone marrow ['bəʊn 'mærəʊ] *noun* soft tissue in cancellous bone; **bone marrow transplant** = transplant of marrow from a donor to a recipient; *see illustration at* BONE STRUCTURE (NOTE: for other terms referring to bone marrow, see words beginning with **myel-, myelo-**)

COMMENT: two types of bone marrow are to be found: red bone marrow or myeloid tissue, which forms red blood cells and is found in cancellous bone in the vertebrae, the sternum and other flat bones; as a person gets older, fatty yellow bone marrow develops in the central cavity of long bones

Bonney's blue [ˈbɒnɪz ˈbluː] *noun* blue dye used as a disinfectant

bony [ˈbəʊnɪ] *adjective* (i) referring to bones; (ii) (part of the body) where the structure of the bones underneath can be seen; *she has long bony hands*; **bony labyrinth** = hard part of the temporal bone surrounding the membranous labyrinth in the inner ear

booster (injection) [ˈbuːstə ɪnˈdʒekʃn] *noun* repeat injection of vaccine given some time after the first injection so as to keep the immunizing effect

boot [buːt] *noun* strong shoe which goes above the ankle; **surgical boot** = specially made boot for a person who has a deformed foot; boot made to correct a deformity

boracic acid *or* **boric acid (H_3BO_3)** [bəˈræsɪk ˈæsɪd *or* ˈbɔːrɪk ˈæsɪd] *noun* soluble white powder used as a general disinfectant

borax [ˈbɔːræks] *noun* white powder used as a household cleaner and disinfectant

borborygmus [bɔːbəˈrɪgməs] *noun* rumbling noise in the abdomen, caused by gas in the intestine (NOTE: the plural is **borborygmi**)

border [ˈbɔːdə] *noun* edge; **vermill(l)ion border** = external red parts of the lips

Bordetella [bɔːdəˈtelə] *noun* bacteria of the family Brucellaceae (*Bordetella pertussis* causes whooping cough)

boric acid [ˈbɔːrɪk ˈæsɪd] *see* BORACIC ACID

born [bɔːn] *verb* **to be born** = to begin to live outside the mother's uterus; *he was born in Germany*; *she was born in 1963*; *the twins were both born blind* (NOTE: **born** is usually only used with **was** or **were** or **be**)

Bornholm disease *or* **epidemic pleurodynia** [ˈbɔːnhəʊm dɪˈziːz *or* epɪˈdemɪk pluərəʊˈdaɪnɪə] *see* PLEURODYNIA

boron [ˈbɔːrɒn] *noun* chemical element which is present in borax, and essential for healthy plant growth (NOTE: chemical symbol is **B**; atomic number is 5)

bother [ˈbɒðə] **1** *noun* something which is annoying or worrying; *the accident has caused a lot of bother* **2** *verb* (i) to take trouble to do something; (ii) to worry about something; *she didn't bother to send a telegram*; *don't bother about cleaning the room*; *smoke bothers him because he has asthma*

bottle [ˈbɒtl] *noun* glass container for liquids; *he drinks a bottle of milk a day*; *open another bottle of orange juice*; **baby's (feeding) bottle** = special bottle with a rubber teat, used for giving milk (or other liquids) to babies; **bottle feeding** = giving a baby milk from a bottle, as opposed to breast feeding; *compare* BREAST FEEDING

bottle-fed [ˈbɒtlfed] *adjective* (baby) which is fed from a bottle; *she was bottle-fed after the first two months*; *compare* BREASTFED

bottom [ˈbɒtəm] *noun* **(a)** lowest part; *there was some jam left in the bottom of the jar* **(b)** part of the body on which you sit; *see also* BUTTOCKS

botulism [ˈbɒtjʊlɪzm] *noun* type of food poisoning caused by a toxin of *Clostridium botulinum* in badly canned or preserved food

COMMENT: symptoms include paralysis of the muscles, vomiting and hallucinations. Botulism is often fatal. Small doses of toxin are used in the treatment of muscle spasm

bougie [ˈbuːʒiː] *noun* thin tube which can be inserted into passages in the body (such as the oesophagus or rectum) either to allow liquid to be introduced or simply to dilate the passage

bout [baʊt] *noun* sudden attack of a disease, especially one which recurs; *he is recovering from a bout of flu*; **bout of fever** = period when a patient is feverish; *she has recurrent bouts of malarial fever*

bovine spongiform encephalopathy (BSE) [ˈbəʊvaɪn ˈspʌndʒɪfɔːm enkefəˈlɒpəθi *or* ɪnsefəˈlɒpəθi] *noun* a fatal brain disease of cattle, also called 'mad cow disease'; *see comment at* ENCEPHALOPATHY

bowel *or* **bowels** [ˈbaʊəl *or* ˈbaʊəlz] *noun* the intestine, especially the large intestine; **to open the bowels** = to defecate, to have a bowel movement; **bowel movement** = defecation, the evacuation of solid waste matter from the bowel though the anus; *the patient had a bowel movement this* *morning*; **irritable bowel syndrome =** MUCOUS COLITIS

bowl [bəʊl] *noun* **(a)** wide container with higher sides than a plate, used for semi-liquids; *a bowl of soup or of cream*; **soup bowl** = bowl specially made for soup **(b)** the part of a sink, washbasin or toilet which contains water

bow-legged [ˈbəʊlegɪd] *adjective* with bow legs

bow legs [ˈbəʊ ˈlegz] *noun* genu varum, state where the ankles touch and the knees are apart when a person is standing straight; *compare* KNOCK KNEE

Bowman's capsule [ˈbəʊmənz ˈkæpsjuːl] *noun* Malpighian glomerulus, expanded end of a renal tubule, surrounding a glomerular tuft in the kidney, which filters plasma in order to reabsorb useful foodstuffs and eliminate waste

boy [bɔɪ] *noun* male child; *they have three children - two boys and a girl*; *the boys were playing in the field*

BP [ˈbiː ˈpiː] = BLOOD PRESSURE, BRITISH PHARMACOPOEIA

Bq [ˈbiː ˈkjuː] = BECQUEREL

Br *chemical symbol for* bromine

brace [breɪs] *noun* any type of splint or appliance worn for support, such as a metal support used on children's legs to make the bones straight or on teeth which are forming badly; *she wore a brace on her front teeth*

bracelet [ˈbreɪslət] *noun* chain or band which is worn around the wrist; **identity bracelet** = label attached to the wrist of a newborn baby or patient in hospital so that he or she can be identified

brachi(o)- [ˈbreɪki or ˈbreɪkiəʊ] *prefix* referring to the arm

brachial [ˈbreɪkiəl] *adjective* referring to the arm, especially the upper arm; **brachial artery** = artery running down the arm from the axillary artery to the elbow, where it divides into the radial and ulnar arteries; **brachial plexus** = group of nerves at the armpit and base of the neck which lead to the nerves in the arms and hands; injury to the brachial plexus at birth leads to Erb's palsy; **brachial pressure point** = point on the arm where pressure will stop bleeding from the brachial artery; **brachial veins** = veins accompanying the brachial artery, draining into the axillary vein

brachialis muscle [breɪkiˈeɪlɪs or breɪkiˈɑːlɪs ˈmʌsl] *noun* flexor of the elbow

brachiocephalic artery [ˈbreɪkiəʊsəˈfælɪk ˈɑːtəri] *noun* largest branch of the arch of the aorta, which continues as the right common carotid and right subclavian arteries

brachiocephalic veins [ˈbreɪkiəʊsəˈfælɪk ˈveɪnz] *plural noun* innominate veins, two veins which continue the subclavian and jugular veins to the superior vena cava

brachium [ˈbreɪkiəm] *noun* arm, especially the upper arm between the elbow and the shoulder (NOTE: the plural is **brachia**)

brachy- [ˈbræki] *prefix meaning* short

brachycephaly [bræki'sefəli] *noun* condition where the skull is shorter than normal

Bradford's frame [ˈbrædfədz ˈfreɪm] *noun* frame of metal and cloth, used to support a patient

brady- [ˈbrædi] *prefix meaning* slow

bradycardia [brædi'kɑːdiə] *noun* slow rate of heart contraction, shown by a slow pulse rate (less than 70 per minute)

bradykinesia [brædikaɪˈniːziə] *noun* walking slowly, making slow movements (because of disease)

bradypnoea *US* **bradypnea** [brædɪpˈniːə] *noun* abnormally slow breathing

Braille [breɪl] *noun* system of writing using raised dots on the paper to indicate letters, which allows a blind person to read by passing his fingers over the page; *she was reading a Braille book*; *the book has been published in Braille*

brain [breɪn] *noun* encephalon, cranial part of the central nervous system, situated inside the skull; **brain death** = condition where the nerves in the brain stem have died, and the patient can be certified as dead, although the heart may not have stopped beating; **brain haemorrhage** = bleeding inside the brain from a cerebral artery; *see also* FOREBRAIN, HINDBRAIN, MIDBRAIN (NOTE: for other terms referring to the brain, see words beginning with **cerebr-, encephal-**)

COMMENT: the main part of the brain is the cerebrum, formed of two sections or hemispheres, which relate to thought and to sensations from either side of the body; at the back of the head and beneath the cerebrum is the cerebellum which coordinates muscle reaction and balance. Also in the brain are the hypothalamus which governs body temperature, hunger, thirst and sexual urges, and the tiny pituitary gland which is the most important endocrine gland in the body

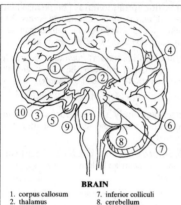

BRAIN

1. corpus callosum
2. thalamus
3. hypothalamus
4. pineal body
5. pituitary gland
6. superior colliculi
7. inferior colliculi
8. cerebellum
9. cerebral peduncle
10. fornix
11. pons

brain damage ['breɪn 'dæmɪdʒ] *noun* damage caused to the brain in an accident; *he suffered brain damage in the car crash*

brain-damaged ['breɪn'dæmɪdʒd] *adjective* (person) who has suffered brain damage; *she was brain-damaged from birth*

brain fever ['breɪn 'fiːvə] *noun* non-medical term for an infection which affects the brain (such as encephalitis or meningitis)

brain stem ['breɪn 'stem] *noun* lower part of the brain, shaped like a stem, which connects the brain to the spinal cord

brain tumour ['breɪn 'tjuːmə] *noun* tumour which grows in the brain

COMMENT: tumours may grow in any part of the brain. The symptoms of brain tumour are usually headaches and dizziness, and as the tumour grows it may affect the senses or mental faculties. Operations to remove brain tumours can be very successful

bran [bræn] *noun* outside covering of the wheat seed, removed to make white flour, but an important source of roughage, hence used in breakfast cereals

branch [brɑːnʃ] **1** *noun* (i) part of a tree growing out of the main trunk; (ii) any part which grows out of a main part **2** *verb* to split out into smaller parts; *the radial artery branches from the brachial artery at the elbow*

branchial cyst ['bræŋkiəl 'sɪst] *noun* cyst on the side of the neck of an embryo

branchial pouch ['bræŋkiəl 'pautʃ] *noun* pouch on the side of the neck of an embryo

Braun's frame *or* **Braun's splint** ['braunz 'freɪm *or* 'braunz 'splɪnt] *noun* metal splint and frame to which pulleys are attached, used for holding up a fractured leg while a patient is lying in bed

Braxton-Hicks contractions ['brækstən'hɪks kən'trækʃnz] *plural noun* contractions of the uterus which occur throughout the pregnancy and become more frequent and stronger towards the end

bread [bred] *noun* food made by baking flour and yeast

break [breɪk] **1** *noun* point at which a bone has broken; **clean break** = break in a bone which is not complicated and where the two parts will join again easily **2** *verb* to make something go to pieces; to go to pieces; *she fell off the wall and broke her leg*; *he can't play football with a broken leg* (NOTE: **breaking - broke - has broken**)

breakbone fever ['breɪkbəun 'fiːvə] = DENGUE

breakdown ['breɪkdaun] *noun* **(a) (nervous) breakdown** = non-medical term for a sudden illness where a patient becomes so depressed and worried that he is incapable of doing anything **(b) breakdown product** = substance which is produced when a compound is broken down into its parts

break down ['breɪk 'daun] *verb* **(a)** to reduce a compound to its parts **(b)** to collapse in a nervous state; *she broke down and cried as she described the symptoms to the doctor*

breakfast ['brekfəst] *noun* first meal of the day; *the patient had a boiled egg for breakfast*; *she didn't have any breakfast because she was due to have surgery later in the day*; *we have breakfast at 7.30 every day*

breast [brest] *noun* mamma, one of two glands in a woman which secrete milk; **breast augmentation** = surgical procedure to increase the size of the breast for cosmetic purposes; **breast cancer** = malignant tumour in the breast; **breast feeding** = feeding a baby from the mother's breast as opposed to from a bottle; *compare* BOTTLE FEEDING; **breast milk** = milk produced by a woman who has recently had a baby; **breast reduction** = reduction of the size of the breast for cosmetic purposes (NOTE: for other terms referring to the breast, see words beginning with **mamm-, mast-**)

breastbone ['brestbəʊn] *noun* sternum, bone which is in the centre of the front of the thorax and to which the ribs are connected

breastfed ['brestfed] *adjective* (baby) which is fed from the mother's breast; *she was breastfed for the first two months*

breath [breθ] *noun* air which goes in and out of the body when you breathe; *he ran so fast he was out of breath*; *stop for a moment to get your breath back*; *she took a deep breath and dived into the water*; **to hold your breath** = to stop breathing out, after having inhaled deeply; **short of breath** = unable to breathe quickly enough to supply the oxygen needed; **bad breath** = HALITOSIS; **breath sounds** = hollow sounds made by the lungs and heard through a stethoscope placed on a patient's chest, used in diagnosis

breathe [bri:ð] *verb* to inhale and exhale, to take air in and blow air out through the nose or mouth; *he could not breathe under water*; *the patient has begun to breathe normally*; **to breathe in** = to take air into your lungs; **to breathe out** = to let the air out of your lungs; *he breathed in the smoke from the fire and it made him cough*; *the doctor told him to take a deep breath and breathe out slowly*

COMMENT: children breathe about 20 to 30 times per minute, men 16-18 per minute, and women slightly faster. The breathing rate increases if the person is taking exercise or has a fever. Some babies hold their breath and go blue in the face, especially when crying or during a temper tantrum

breathing ['bri:ðɪŋ] *noun* respiration, taking air into the lungs and blowing it out again through the mouth or nose; *if breathing is difficult or has stopped, begin artificial ventilation immediately*; **breathing rate** = number of times a person breathes in and out; **laboured breathing** = difficult breathing (due to various causes, such as asthma, etc.) (NOTE: for other terms referring to breathing, see words beginning with **pneumo-**)

breathless ['breθləs] *adjective* (patient) who finds it difficult to breathe enough air; *after running upstairs she became breathless and had to sit down*

breathlessness ['breθləsnəs] *noun* difficulty in breathing enough air

26 patients were selected from the outpatient department on grounds of disabling breathlessness present for at least five years
Lancet

breech [bri:tʃ] *noun* buttocks; **breech birth** *or* **breech delivery** = birth where the baby's buttocks appear first; **breech presentation** = position of the baby in the uterus, where the buttocks will appear first

breed [bri:d] *verb* to reproduce and spread; *the bacteria breed in dirty water*; *insanitary conditons help to breed disease*

bregma ['bregmə] *noun* point at the top of the head where the soft gap between the bones of a baby's skull (the anterior fontanelle) hardens

bridge [brɪdʒ] *noun* **(a)** top part of the nose where it joins the forehead **(b)** *(for teeth)* artificial tooth (or teeth) which is joined to natural teeth which hold it in place **(c)** a part joining two or more other parts

Bright's disease ['braɪts dɪ'zi:z] *noun* glomerulonephritis, inflammation of the kidney, characterized by albuminuria and high blood pressure

brim [brɪm] *noun* edge; **pelvic brim** = line on the ilium which separates the false pelvis from the true pelvis

bring up ['brɪŋ 'ʌp] *verb* **(a)** to look after and educate a child; *he was brought up by his uncle in Scotland*; *I was brought up in the country*; *she has been badly brought up* **(b)** (i) to vomit, to force material from the stomach back into the mouth; (ii) to cough up material such as mucus from the lungs or throat; *he was bringing up mucus*

British ['brɪtɪʃ] *adjective* referring to Great Britain

British anti-lewisite (BAL) ['brɪtɪʃ 'æntɪ'lu:ɪsaɪt] *noun* antidote for blister gases, but also used to treat cases of poisoning, such as mercury poisoning

British Dental Association (BDA) ['brɪtɪʃ 'dentl əsəʊsɪ'eɪʃn] *noun* professional association of dentists

British Medical Association (BMA)
[ˈbrɪtɪʃ ˈmedɪkl əsəʊsɪˈeɪʃn] *noun* professional association of doctors

British National Formulary (BNF)
[ˈbrɪtɪʃ ˈnæʃnl ˈfɔːmjələri] *noun* book listing key information on the prescribing, dispensing and administration of prescription drugs used in the UK

British Pharmacopoeia (BP) [ˈbrɪtɪʃ fɑːməkəˈpiːə] *noun* book listing approved drugs and their dosages

COMMENT: drugs listed in the British Pharmacopoeia have the letters BP written after them on labels

brittle [ˈbrɪtl] *adjective* which breaks easily; *the bones of old people become brittle* (NOTE: the opposite is **ductile**)

brittle bone disease [ˈbrɪtl ˈbəʊn dɪˈziːz] *see* OSTEOGENESIS, OSTEOPOROSIS

broad [brɔːd] *adjective* wide in relation to length; **broad ligament** = peritoneal folds supporting the uterus on either side; **broad-spectrum antibiotic** = antibiotic used to control many types of bacteria (NOTE: **broad - broader - broadest;** opposite is **narrow**)

Broadbent's sign [ˈbrɔːdbents ˈsaɪn] *noun* movement of a patient's left side near the lower ribs at each beat of the heart, indicating adhesion between the diaphragm and pericardium in cases of pericarditis

Broca's aphasia [ˈbrəʊkəz əˈfeɪziə] *noun* being unable to speak or write, caused by damage to Broca's area

Broca's area [ˈbrəʊkəz ˈeəriə] *noun* area on the left side of the brain which governs the motor aspects of speaking

Brodie's abscess [ˈbrəʊdiz ˈæbses] *noun* abscess of a bone, caused by staphylococcal osteomyelitis

bromhidrosis [brɒmhɪˈdrəʊsɪs] *noun* condition where the perspiration has an unpleasant smell

bromides [ˈbrəʊmaɪdz] *plural noun* bromine salts, formerly used as depressants or sedatives

bromine [ˈbrəʊmiːn] *noun* chemical element (NOTE: chemical symbol is **Br**)

bromism *or* **bromide poisoning**
[ˈbrəʊmɪzm *or* ˈbrəʊmaɪd ˈpɔɪzənɪŋ] *noun* chronic ill health caused by excessive use of bromides

bronch- *or* **bronchi(o)-** [ˈbrɒŋk *or* ˈbrɒŋki] *prefix* referring to the windpipe

bronchi [ˈbrɒŋkaɪ] *plural noun* air passages leading from the trachea into the lungs, where they split into many bronchioles; **lobar bronchi** *or* **secondary bronchi** = air passages supplying a lobe of a lung; **main** *or* **primary bronchi** = two main air passages which branch from the trachea outside the lung; **segmental bronchi** *or* **tertiary bronchi** = air passages supplying a segment of a lung; *see illustration at* LUNGS (NOTE: the singular is **bronchus**)

bronchial [ˈbrɒŋkiəl] *adjective* referring to the bronchi; **bronchial asthma** = type of asthma mainly caused by an allergen or by exertion; **bronchial breath sounds** = distinctive breath sounds from the lungs which help diagnosis; **bronchial pneumonia** = BRONCHOPNEUMONIA; **bronchial tree** = system of tubes (bronchi and bronchioles) which take the air from the trachea into the lungs; **bronchial tubes** = bronchi, air tubes leading from the windpipe into the lungs

bronchiectasis [brɒŋkiˈektəsɪs] *noun* disorder of the bronchi which become wide, infected and filled with pus; the disorder can lead to pneumonia

bronchiolar [brɒŋkiˈəʊlə] *adjective* referring to the bronchioles

bronchiole [ˈbrɒŋkiəʊl] *noun* very small air tube in the lungs leading from a bronchus to the alveoli; *see illustration at* LUNGS

bronchiolitis [brɒŋkiəʊˈlaɪtɪs] *noun* inflammation of the bronchioles

bronchitic [brɒŋˈkɪtɪk] *adjective* (i) referring to bronchitis; (ii) (patient) suffering from bronchitis

bronchitis [brɒŋˈkaɪtɪs] *noun* inflammation of the mucous membrane of the bronchi; **acute bronchitis** = attack of bronchitis caused by a virus or by exposure to cold and wet

bronchoconstrictor [brɒŋkəʊkənˈstrɪktə] *noun* drug which narrows the bronchi

bronchodilator [brɒŋkəʊdaɪˈleɪtə] *noun* drug which makes the bronchi wider, used in the treatment of asthma and allergy, by stimulating -2 adrenoceptors or blocking muscarinic receptors, used in the treatment of asthma (NOTE: bronchodilators have names ending in **-terol**; however, the most common example is **salbutamol**)

19 children with mild to moderately severe perennial bronchial asthma were selected. These children gave a typical history of exercise-induced asthma and their symptoms were controlled with oral or aerosol bronchodilators

Lancet

bronchogram [ˈbrɒŋkəʊgræm] *noun* X-ray picture of the bronchial tubes after an opaque substance has been put into them

bronchography [brɒŋˈkɒgrəfi] *noun* X-ray examination of the lungs after an opaque substance has been put into the bronchi

bronchomediastinal trunk [brɒŋkəʊmiːdiəˈstaɪnəl ˈtrʌŋk] *noun* lymph nodes draining part of the chest

bronchomycosis [brɒŋkəʊmaɪˈkəʊsɪs] *noun* infection of the bronchi by a fungus

bronchophony [brɒŋˈkɒfəni] *noun* vibrations of the voice heard when the consolidation of the lungs produces a loud sound

bronchopleural [brɒŋkəʊˈplʊərl] *adjective* referring to a bronchus and pleura

bronchopneumonia [brɒŋkəʊnjuˈməʊniə] *noun* infectious inflammation of the bronchioles, which may lead to general infection of the lungs

bronchopulmonary [brɒŋkəʊˈpʌlmənri] *adjective* referring to the bronchi and the lungs

bronchoscope [ˈbrɒŋkəʊskəʊp] *noun* instrument which is passed down the trachea into the lungs, which a doctor can use to inspect the inside passages of the lungs

bronchoscopy [brɒŋˈkɒskəpi] *noun* examination of a patient's bronchi using a bronchoscope

bronchospasm [ˈbrɒŋkəʊspæzm] *noun* tightening of the bronchial muscles which causes the tubes to contract

bronchospirometer [brɒŋkəʊspaɪˈrɒmɪtə] *noun* instrument for measuring the volume of the lungs

bronchospirometry [brɒŋkəʊspaɪˈrɒmɪtri] *noun* measuring the volume of the lungs

bronchostenosis [brɒŋkəʊsteˈnəʊsɪs] *noun* abnormal constriction of the bronchial tubes

bronchotracheal [brɒŋkəʊtrəˈkiːəl] *adjective* referring to the bronchi and the trachea

bronchus [ˈbrɒŋkəs] *noun* air passage leading from the trachea into the lungs, where it splits into many bronchioles (NOTE: the plural is **bronchi**)

bronze diabetes [ˈbrɒnz daɪəˈbiːtiːz] = HAEMOCHROMATOSIS

broth [brɒθ] *noun* (i) light soup made from meat; (ii) medium in which bacteria can be cultivated

brother [ˈbrʌðə] *noun* male who has the same mother and father as another child; *he's my brother*; *that girl has three brothers*; *his brother's a doctor*

brow [braʊ] *noun* (i) forehead, the part of the face above the eyes; (ii) eyebrow, the line of hair above the eye

brown [braʊn] *adjective & noun* (of a) colour like the colour of earth or wood; *he has brown hair and blue eyes*; *you're very brown - you must have been sitting in the sun*; **brown bread** = bread made with flour which has not been refined; *brown bread is better for you than white*; **brown fat** = animal fat which can easily be converted to energy and is believed to offset the effects of ordinary white fat (NOTE: **brown - browner - brownest**)

Brown-Séquard syndrome [ˈbraʊnˈseɪkɑː ˈsɪndrəʊm] *noun* condition of a patient where the spinal cord has been partly severed or compressed, with the result that the lower half of the body is paralysed on one side and loses feeling in the other side

Brucella [bruˈselə] *noun* type of rod-shaped bacterium

brucellosis [bruːsɪˈləʊsɪs] *noun* disease which can be caught from cattle or goats or from drinking infected milk, spread by a species of the bacterium *Brucella* (NOTE: also called **undulant fever** or **Malta fever** or **mountain fever**)

COMMENT: symptoms include tiredness, arthritis, headache, sweating, irritability and swelling of the spleen

bruise [bruːz] **1** *noun* contusion, dark painful area on the skin, where blood has escaped under the skin following a blow; *see* *also* BLACK EYE **2** *verb* to make a bruise; *she bruised her knee on the corner of the table*; *the nurse put a compress on his bruised leg*; **she bruises easily** = even a soft blow will give her a bruise

bruising ['bruːzɪŋ] *noun* area of bruises; *the baby has bruising on the back and legs*

bruit [bruːt] *noun* abnormal noise heard through a stethoscope

Brunner's glands ['brʊnəz 'glændz] *plural noun* glands in the duodenum and jejunum

brush [brʌʃ] **1** *noun* stiff hairs or wire set in a hard base, used for cleaning; *you need a stiff brush to remove the dandruff from the scalp* **2** *verb* to clean with a brush; *have you brushed your hair?*; *remember to brush your teeth after a meal*

bruxism ['brʌksɪzm] *noun* grinding of the teeth, as a habit

bubble ['bʌbl] *noun* small amount of air or gas surrounded by a liquid; *air bubbles formed in the blood vessel, causing embolism*

bubo ['bjuːbəʊ] *noun* swelling of a lymph node in the groin or armpit

bubonic plague [bjuːˈbɒnɪk ˈpleɪg] *noun* usually fatal infectious disease caused by *Yersinia pestis* in the lymph system, transmitted to humans by fleas from rats

COMMENT: bubonic plague was the Black Death of the Middle Ages; its symptoms are fever, delirium, vomiting and swelling of the lymph nodes

buccal ['bʌkəl] *adjective* referring to the cheek; **buccal cavity** = the mouth; **buccal fat** = pad of fat separating the buccinator muscle from the masseter

buccinator (muscle) ['bʌksɪneɪtə] *noun* cheek muscle which helps the jaw to move when chewing

bud [bʌd] *noun* small appendage; **taste bud** = tiny sensory receptor in the vallate and fungiform papillae of the tongue and in part of the back of the mouth

Budd-Chiari syndrome ['bʌdkɪˈeəri 'sɪndrəʊm] *noun* disease of the liver, where thrombosis has occurred in the hepatic veins

Buerger's disease ['bɜːgəz dɪˈziːz] = THROMBOANGIITIS OBLITERANS

buffer ['bʌfə] **1** *noun* (i) substance that keeps a constant balance between acid and alkali; (ii) solution where the pH is not changed by adding acid or alkali; **buffer action** = balancing between acid and alkali **2** *verb* to prevent a solution from becoming acid; *buffered aspirin*

bug [bʌg] *noun* (*informal*) infectious disease; *he caught a bug on holiday*; *half the staff are sick with a stomach bug*

build [bɪld] *noun* general size of a person's body; *he has a heavy or strong build for his height*; *the girl has a slight build, but she can run very fast*

build-up ['bɪldʌp] *noun* gradual accumulation; *a build-up of fatty deposits on the walls of the arteries*

build up ['bɪld 'ʌp] *verb* to form gradually by accumulation (NOTE: **building - built - has built**)

built [bɪlt] *adjective* & *suffix* referring to the general size of a person's body; *she's slightly built*; *a heavily-built man*

bulb [bʌlb] *noun* round part at the end of an organ or bone; **olfactory bulb** = end of the olfactory tract, where the processes of the sensory cells in the nose are linked to the fibres of the olfactory nerve; **bulb of the penis** = round end of the penis (NOTE: also called **glans penis**)

bulbar ['bʌlbə] *adjective* referring to a bulb; referring to the medulla oblongata; **bulbar paralysis** *or* **bulbar palsy** = form of motor neurone disease which affects the muscles of the mouth, jaw and throat; **bulbar poliomyelitis** = type of polio affecting the brain stem, which makes it difficult for a patient to swallow or breathe

bulbospongiosus muscle [bʌlbəʊspʌndʒiˈəʊsəs 'mʌsəl] *noun* muscle in the perineum behind the penis

bulbourethral glands [bʌlbəʊjuˈriːθrl 'glændz] Cowper's glands; *see* GLAND

bulge [bʌldʒ] *verb* to swell out, to push out; *the wall of the abdomen becomes weak and part of the intestine bulges through*

bulging ['bʌldʒɪŋ] *adjective* swollen, protruding; *bulging eyes*

bulimia (nervosa) [bjuːˈlɪmiə nəˈvəʊsə] *noun* psychological condition where the patient eats too much and is incapable of controlling his eating

bulimic [bjuːˈlɪmɪk] *adjective* referring to bulimia; (person) suffering from bulimia

COMMENT: although the patient eats a large quantity of food, this is followed by vomiting which is induced by the patient himself, so that the patient does not in fact become overweight

bulla ['bʊlə] *noun* large blister (NOTE: the plural is **bullae**)

bump [bʌmp] **1** *noun* **(a)** slight knock against something; *the plane landed with a bump* **(b)** slightly swollen part on the skin, caused by a blow, sting, etc.; *she has a bump on the back of her head where the door hit her*; *the vaccination has left a little bump on her left arm* **2** *verb* to knock slightly; *she bumped her head on the door*

bumper fracture ['bʌmpə 'fræktʃə] *noun* fracture in the upper part of the tibia (so called, because it can be caused by a blow from the bumper of a car)

bundle ['bʌndl] *noun* (i) collection of things roughly fastened together; (ii) group of nerves running in the same direction; **bundle branch block** = defect in the heart's conduction tissue; **bundle of His** = atrioventricular bundle, a bundle of modified cardiac muscle which conducts impulses from the atrioventricular node to the septum and then divides to connect with the ventricles, causing synchronization of cardiac contraction

bunion ['bʌnjən] *noun* inflammation and swelling of the big toe, caused by tight shoes which force the toe sideways with a callus developing over the joint between the toe and the metatarsal

buphthalmos [bʌf'θælməs] *noun* type of congenital glaucoma occurring in infants

burial ['beriəl] *noun* putting a dead person's body into the ground; *he died on Monday and the burial took place on Friday*

Burkitt's tumour *or* **Burkitt's lymphoma** ['bɜːkɪts 'tjuːmə or lɪm'fəʊmə] *noun* malignant tumour, usually on the maxilla

COMMENT: Burkitt's tumour is found especially in children in Africa

burn [bɜːn] **1** *noun* injury to skin and tissue caused by light, heat, radiation, electricity or chemicals; **cold burn** = injury to the skin caused by exposure to extreme cold or by touching a very cold surface; **deep dermal burn** *or* **full thickness burn** = burn which is so severe that a graft will be necessary to repair the skin damage; **dry burn** = injury to

the skin caused by touching a very hot dry surface; **partial thickness burn** *or* **superficial thickness burn** = burn which leaves enough tissue for the skin to grow again; **wet burn** = scald, an injury to the skin caused by touching a very hot liquid or steam; **first-degree burn** = burn where the skin turns red because the epidermis has been affected; **second-degree burn** = burn where the skin becomes very red and blisters; **burns unit** = special department in a hospital which deals with burns **2** *verb* to destroy by fire; *she burnt her hand on the hot frying pan; most of his hair or his skin was burnt off* (NOTE: **burning - burnt/burned - has burnt/burned**)

COMMENT: burns were formerly classified by degrees and are still often referred to in this way. The modern classification is into two categories: deep and superficial

burning ['bɜːnɪŋ] *adjective* (sensation) similar to that of being hurt by fire; *he had a burning pain in his foot*

burnout ['bɜːnaʊt] *noun* feeling of depression, fatigue, lack of energy caused by stress and being overworked; *he suffered a burnout and had to go on leave*

burp [bɜːp] **1** *noun* allowing air in the stomach to come up through the mouth **2** *verb* to allow air in the stomach to come up through the mouth; **to burp a baby** = to pat a baby on the back until it burps (NOTE: used particularly of babies. For adults the word **belch** is used)

burr [bɜː] *noun* bit used with a drill to make holes in a bone (as in the cranium) or in a tooth

bursa ['bɜːsə] *noun* sac containing fluid, forming part of the normal structure of a joint such as the knee and elbow, where it protects against frequent pressure and rubbing; **adventitious bursa** = abnormal bursa which develops as a result of continued pressure or rubbing (NOTE: the plural is **bursae**)

bursitis [bɜː'saɪtɪs] *noun* inflammation of a bursa, especially in the shoulder; **prepatellar bursitis** = housemaid's knee, a condition where the bursa in the knee becomes inflamed, caused by kneeling on hard surfaces

burst [bɜːst] *verb* (*of a sac or blister*) to break open; *never use a needle to burst a blister*; *he was rushed to hospital with a burst appendix* (NOTE: **bursting - burst - has burst**)

bury ['beri] *verb* to put a dead person's body into the ground; *he died on Monday and was buried on Friday*

butter ['bʌtə] *noun* solid yellow edible fat made from cream; *he was spreading butter on a piece of bread; fry the onions in butter*

buttock ['bʌtək] *noun* one of the two fleshy parts below the back, on which a person sits, made up mainly of the gluteal muscles; *he had a boil on his right buttock* (NOTE: the buttocks are also called **nates)**

buttonhole surgery ['bʌtənhəʊl 'sɜːdʒri] *noun* surgical operation through a small hole in the body, using an endoscope

bypass ['baɪpɑːs] *noun* act of going round an obstruction; **cardiopulmonary bypass** = machine or method for artificially circulating the patient's blood during open-heart surgery, where the heart and lungs are cut off from the circulation and replaced by a pump; **heart bypass operation** *or* **coronary bypass surgery** = surgical operation to treat angina by grafting pieces of vein to go around the diseased part of a coronary artery

byssinosis [bɪsɪ'nəʊsɪs] *noun* lung disease (a form of pneumoconiosis) caused by inhaling cotton dust

Cc

C [siː] **1** *abbreviation for* Celsius and Centigrade **2** *chemical symbol for* carbon **3** *noun* **vitamin C** = ascorbic acid, vitamin which is soluble in water and is found in fresh fruit (especially oranges and lemons) and in raw vegetables, liver and milk

COMMENT: lack of vitamin C can cause anaemia and scurvy

c *symbol for* centi-

Ca *chemical symbol for* calcium

CABG [ˈsiː ˈeɪ ˈbiː ˈdʒiː] = CORONARY ARTERY BYPASS GRAFT

cabinet [ˈkæbɪnət] *noun* cupboard; *the drugs cabinet must be kept locked*; **medicine cabinet** = cupboard where drugs and medicine are kept

cachet [ˈkæʃeɪ] *noun* quantity of a drug wrapped in paper, to be swallowed

cachexia [kæˈkeksiə] *noun* state of ill health with wasting and general weakness

cadaver [kəˈdævə] *noun* dead body, especially one used for dissection

cadaveric *or* **cadaverous** [kəˈdævərɪk or kəˈdævərəs] *adjective* (person who is) thin or wasting away

cadmium [ˈkædmiəm] *noun* metallic element, which if present in soil can make plants poisonous (NOTE: chemical symbol is Cd)

caecostomy [siːˈkɒstəmi] *noun* surgical operation to make an opening between the caecum and the abdominal wall to allow faeces to be passed without going through the rectum and anus

caecum *US* **cecum** [ˈsiːkəm] *noun* wider part of the large intestine in the lower right-hand side of the abdomen at the point where the small intestine joins it and which has the appendix attached to it; *see illustration at* DIGESTIVE SYSTEM

Caesarean section *or* **caesarean** *US* **Cesarean section** *or* **cesarean** [sɪˈzeəriən ˈsekʃn] *noun* surgical operation to deliver a baby by cutting through the abdominal wall into the uterus (NOTE: the operation is correctly called **Caesarean section** but informally most people use **caesarean**: 'she had her baby by Caesarean section *or* she had a caesarean; the baby was delivered by caesarean')

COMMENT: Caesarean section is performed only when it appears that normal childbirth is impossible or might endanger mother or child, and only after the 28th week of gestation

caesium *US* **cesium** [ˈsiːziəm] *noun* radioactive element, used in treatment by radiation (NOTE: chemical symbol is Cs)

caffeine [ˈkæfiːn] *noun* alkaloid found in coffee, tea and chocolate, which acts as a stimulant

COMMENT: apart from acting as a stimulant, caffeine also helps in the production of urine. It can be addictive, and exists in both tea and coffee in about the same percentages as well as in chocolate and other drinks

caisson disease [ˈkeɪsən dɪˈziːz] *noun* condition where the patient suffers pains in the joints and stomach, and dizziness caused by nitrogen in the blood (NOTE: also called **decompression sickness** *or* **compressed air sickness**)

COMMENT: found when a person has moved rapidly from high atmospheric pressure to a lower pressure area, especially in divers who come back to the surface too quickly after a deep dive. The first symptoms, pains in the joints, are known as 'the bends'. The disease can be fatal

cal *abbreviation for* calorie

Cal *abbreviation for* Calorie or kilocalorie

calamine (lotion) [ˈkæləmaɪn ˈləʊʃn] *noun* lotion, based on zinc oxide, which helps relieve skin irritation (such as that caused by sunburn or chickenpox)

calc- *or* **calci-** [kælk *or* ˈkælsɪ] *prefix* referring to calcium

calcaemia [kælˈsiːmiə] *noun* condition where the blood contains an abnormally large amount of calcium

calcaneal [kælˈkeɪniəl] *adjective* referring to the calcaneus; **calcaneal tendon** = Achilles tendon, the tendon at the back of the ankle which connects the calf muscles to the heel and which acts to pull up the heel when the calf muscle is contracted

calcaneus *or* **calcaneum** [kælˈkeɪniəs *or* kælˈkeɪniəm] *noun* heel bone, situated underneath the talus; *see illustration at* FOOT

calcareous degeneration [kælˈkeəriəs dɪdʒenəˈreɪʃn] *noun* formation of calcium on bones or at joints in old age

calciferol [kælˈsɪfərɒl] *noun* vitamin D₂

calcification [kælsɪfɪˈkeɪʃn] *noun* hardening by forming deposits of calcium salts; *see also* PELLEGRINI-STIEDA'S DISEASE

COMMENT: calcification can be normal in the formation of bones, but can occur abnormally in joints, muscles and organs, where it is known as calcinosis

calcified [ˈkælsɪfaɪd] *adjective* made hard; *bone is calcified connective tissue*

calcinosis [kælsɪˈnəʊsɪs] *noun* abnormal condition where deposits of calcium salts form in joints, muscles and organs

calcitonin [kælsɪˈtəʊnɪn] *noun* thyrocalcitonin, hormone produced by the thyroid gland, which is believed to regulate the level of calcium in the blood

calcium [ˈkælsiəm] *noun* metallic chemical element which is a major component of bones and teeth and which is essential for various bodily processes such as blood clotting; **calcium deficiency** = lack of calcium in the bloodstream; **calcium phosphate (Ca₃(PO₄)₂)** = main constituent of bones; **calcium supplement** = addition of calcium to the diet, or as injections, to improve the level of calcium in the bloodstream (NOTE: chemical symbol is **Ca**)

COMMENT: calcium is an important element in a balanced diet. Milk, cheese, eggs and certain vegetables are its main sources. Calcium deficiency can be treated by injections of calcium salts

calcium blocker [ˈkælsiəm ˈblɒkə] *noun* drug which affects the smooth muscle of the cardiovascular system, used in the treatment of angina and hypertension (NOTE: calcium blockers have names ending in **-dipine**: **nifedipine**)

COMMENT: not to be used in heart failure as reduces cardiac function further

calculosis [kælkjʊˈləʊsɪs] *noun* condition where calculi exist in an organ

calculus [ˈkælkjʊləs] *noun* stone, a hard mass like a little piece of stone, which forms inside the body; **renal calculus** = stone in the kidney (NOTE: plural is **calculi** [ˈkælkjʊlaɪ])

COMMENT: calculi are formed of cholesterol and various inorganic substances, and are commonly found in the bladder, the gall bladder (gallstones) and various parts of the kidney

Caldwell-Luc operation [ˈkɔːldwelˈluːk ɒpəˈreɪʃn] *noun* surgical operation to drain the maxillary sinus by making an incision above the canine tooth

calf [kɑːf] *noun* muscular fleshy part at the back of the lower leg, formed by the gastrocnemius muscles (NOTE: plural is **calves**)

calibrate [ˈkælɪbreɪt] *verb* **(a)** to measure the inside diameter of a tube or passage **(b)** *(in surgery)* to measure the sizes of two parts of the body to be joined together **(c)** to adjust an instrument or piece of equipment against a known standard

calibrator [ˈkælɪbreɪtə] *noun* **(a)** instrument used to enlarge a tube or passage **(b)** instrument for measuring the diameter of a tube or passage

calibre *US* **caliber** [ˈkælɪbə] *noun* interior diameter of a tube, of a blood vessel, etc.

caliper [ˈkælɪpə] *noun* **(a)** instrument with two legs, used for measuring the width of the pelvic cavity **(b)** instrument with two sharp points which are put into a fractured bone and weights attached to cause traction **(c)** metal splints used to support an injured leg, made of a pair of rods attached to the thigh and to a special boot

call [kɔːl] **1** *noun* **(a)** speaking by telephone; *I want to make a (phone) call to Canada*;

there were three calls for you while you were out; **on call** = ready to be called for duty; *three nurses are on call during the night* (b) visit; *the district nurse makes a regular call every Thursday* **2** *verb* (a) to telephone; *if he comes, tell him I'll call him when I'm at the surgery*; *Mr Smith is out - shall I ask him to call you back?* (b) to visit; *the district nurse called at the house, but there was no one there*; *she called on the patient for the last time on Tuesday*

calliper ['kælɪpə] = CALIPER

callosity [kə'lɒsəti] *noun* hard patch on the skin (such as a corn) resulting from frequent pressure or rubbing (NOTE: also called **callus**)

callosum [kə'ləʊsəm] *see* CORPUS

callus ['kæləs] *noun* (a) = CALLOSITY (b) tissue which forms round a broken bone as it starts to mend, leading to consolidation; *callus formation is more rapid in children and young adults than in elderly patients*

calm [kɑːm] *adjective* quiet, not upset; *the patient was delirious but became calm after the injection*

calm down ['kɑːm 'daʊn] *verb* to become quiet; to make someone quiet; *he was soon calmed down or he soon calmed down when the nurse gave him an injection*

calomel (Hg₂Cl₂) ['kæləmel] *noun* mercurous chloride, poisonous substance used to treat pinworms in the intestine

calor ['kælə] *noun* heat

caloric [kə'lɒrɪk] *adjective* referring to calories; **caloric energy** = amount of energy shown as a number of calories; **caloric requirement** = amount of energy (shown in calories) which a person needs each day

calorie *or* **gram calorie** *or* **small calorie** ['kæləri] *noun* unit of measurement of heat or energy (the heat needed to raise the temperature of 1g of water by 1°C) (NOTE: the **joule** is now more usual; also written **cal** after figures: **2,500 cal**)

Calorie *or* **large calorie** ['kæləri] *noun* kilocalorie, 1,000 calories (the heat needed to raise the temperature of 1kg of water by 1°C) (NOTE: spelt with a capital; also written **Cal** and **kcal** after figures: **250 Cal, 360 kcal**)

COMMENT: one calorie is the amount of heat needed to raise the temperature of one gram of water by one degree Celsius. A Calorie or kilocalorie is the amount of heat needed to raise the temperature of one kilogram of water by one degree

Celsius. The Calorie is also used as a measurement of the energy content of food and to show the caloric requirement or amount of energy needed by an average person. The average adult in an office job requires about 3,000 Calories per day, supplied by carbohydrates and fats to give energy and proteins to replace tissue. More strenuous physical work needs more Calories. If a person eats more than the number of Calories needed by his energy output or for his growth, the extra Calories are stored in the body as fat

calorific value [kælə'rɪfɪk 'væljuː] *noun* heat value of a substance, the number of Calories which a certain amount of a substance (such as a certain food) contains; *the tin of beans has 250 calories or has a calorific value of 250 calories*

calvaria *or* **calvarium** [kæl'veəriə *or* kæl'veəriəm] *noun* top part of the skull

calyx ['keɪlɪks] *noun* part of the body shaped like a cup especially the tube leading to a renal pyramid (NOTE: plural is **calyces**); *see illustration at* KIDNEY

COMMENT: the renal pelvis is formed of three major calyces, which themselves are formed of several smaller minor calyces

camphor ['kæmfə] *noun* white crystals with a strong smell, made from a tropical tree, used to keep insects away or as a liniment; **camphor oil** *or* **camphorated oil** = mixture of 20% camphor and oil, used as a rub

canal [kə'næl] *noun* tube along which something flows; **alimentary canal** = tube in the body going from the mouth to the anus and including the throat, stomach, intestine, etc., through which food passes and is digested; **anal canal** = passage leading from the rectum to the anus; **auditory canals** = external and internal passages of the ear; **bile canal** = very small vessel leading from a hepatic cell to the bile duct; **central canal** = thin tube in the centre of the spinal cord containing cerebrospinal fluid; **cervical canal** *or* **cervicouterine canal** = tube running through the cervix from the point where the uterus joins the vagina to the entrance of the uterine cavity; **Eustachian canal** = passage through the porous bone forming the outside part of the Eustachian tube; **femoral canal** = inner tube of the sheath surrounding the femoral artery and vein; **Haversian canal** = fine canal which runs vertically through the Haversian systems in compact bone, containing blood vessels and lymph ducts;

inguinal canal = passage in the lower abdominal wall, carrying the spermatic cord in the male and the round ligament of the uterus in the female; **root canal** = canal in the root of a tooth through which the nerves and blood vessels pass; *see illustration at* TOOTH; **canal of Schlemm** *or* **Schlemm's canal** = circular canal in the sclera of the eye, which drains the aqueous humour; **semicircular canals** = three canals in the inner ear partly filled with fluid and which regulate the sense of balance; *see illustration at* EAR; **vertebral canal** = channel formed of the holes in the centre of each vertebra, through which the spinal cord passes; **Volkmann's canal** = canal running horizontally through compact bone, carrying blood to the Haversian systems

canaliculotomy [kænəlıkjʊˈlɒtəmi] *noun* surgical operation to open up a little canal

canaliculus [kænəˈlıkjʊləs] *noun* little canal, such as a canal leading to the Haversian systems in compact bone, or a canal leading to the lacrimal duct (NOTE: plural is **canaliculi**)

cancellous bone [ˈkænsɪləs ˈbəʊn] *noun* light spongy bone tissue which forms the inner core of a bone and also the ends of long bones; *see illustration at* BONE STRUCTURE

cancer [ˈkænsə] *noun* malignant growth, a tumour which develops in tissue and destroys it, which can spread by metastasis to other parts of the body and cannot be controlled by the body itself; *cancer cells developed in the lymph*; *he has been diagnosed as having lung cancer or as having cancer of the lung* (NOTE: used with **the** or **a** to indicate one particular tumour, and without **the** or **a** to indicate the disease: **doctors removed a cancer from her breast; she has breast cancer.** For other terms referring to cancer, see words beginning with **carcin-**)

COMMENT: cancers can be divided into cancers of the skin (carcinomas) or cancers of connective tissue, such as bone or muscle (sarcomas). Cancer can be caused by tobacco, radiation and many other factors. Many cancers are curable by surgery, by chemotherapy or by radiation, especially if they are detected early

cancerophobia [kænsərəʊˈfəʊbiə] *noun* fear of cancer

cancerous [ˈkænsərəs] *adjective* referring to cancer; *the X-ray revealed a cancerous growth in the breast*

cancrum oris [ˈkænkrəm ˈɔːrıs] *noun* noma, severe ulcers in the mouth, leading to gangrene

Candida [ˈkændıdə] *noun* Monilia, a type of fungus which causes mycosis; **Candida albicans** = one type of Candida which is normally present in the mouth and throat without causing any illness, but which can cause thrush

It is incorrect to say that oral candida is an infection. Candida is easily isolated from the mouths of up to 50% of healthy adults and is a normal commensal

Nursing Times

candidate [ˈkændıdət] *noun* **(a)** person who is applying for a job or for a promotion; *the board is interviewing the candidates for the post of administrator* **(b)** patient who could have an operation; *these types of patients may be candidates for embolization*; **candidate vaccine** = vaccine which is being tested for use in immunization

candidiasis *or* **candidosis** [kændıˈdaıəsıs or ˈkændıˈdəʊsıs] *noun* moniliasis, infection with Candida

COMMENT: when the infection occurs in the vagina or mouth it is known as 'thrush'. Thrush in the mouth usually affects small children

canicola fever [kəˈnıkələ ˈfiːvə] *noun* form of leptospirosis, giving high fever and jaundice

canine (tooth) [ˈkænaın ˈtuːθ] *noun* pointed tooth next to an incisor; *see illustration at* TEETH

COMMENT: there are four canines in all, two in the upper jaw and two in the lower; those in the upper jaw are referred to as the 'eyeteeth'

canities [kəˈnıʃiiːz] *noun* loss of pigments, which makes the hair turn white

canker [ˈkæŋkə] *noun* lesion of the skin

cannabis [ˈkænəbıs] *noun* **(a)** Indian hemp, a tropical plant from whose leaves or flowers an addictive drug is produced **(b)** marijuana, an addictive drug made from the dried leaves or flowers of the Indian hemp plant; **cannabis resin** = addictive drug, a purified extract made from the flowers of the Indian hemp plant

COMMENT: cannabis has analgesic properties, and the possibility that it should be legalized for therapeutic use in conditions of chronic pain is being debated

cannula ['kænjʊlə] *noun* tube with a trocar or blunt needle inside, inserted into the body to introduce fluids

canthal ['kænθəl] *adjective* referring to the corner of the eye

canthus ['kænθəs] *noun* corner of the eye

cap [kæp] *noun* **(a)** type of hat which fits tightly on the head; *the surgeons were wearing white caps* **(b)** top which covers something; *screw the cap back on the bottle*; **child-proof cap** = special top on a bottle containing a potentially dangerous substance, designed so that a young child cannot open it **(c)** covering which protects something; **Dutch cap** = vaginal diaphragm, a contraceptive device for women, which is placed over the cervix uteri before sexual intercourse **(d)** artificial hard covering for a damaged or broken tooth

capacity [kə'pæsəti] *noun (of a person)* ability to do something; *(of an organ)* ability to contain or absorb a substance

capillary [kə'pɪləri] *noun* (i) tiny blood vessel between the arterioles and the venules, which carries blood and nutrients into the tissues; (ii) any tiny tube carrying a liquid in the body; **capillary bleeding** = bleeding where blood oozes out from small blood vessels

capitate (bone) ['kæpɪteɪt 'bəʊn] *noun* largest of the eight small carpal bones in the wrist; *see illustration at* HAND

capitis [kə'paɪtɪs] *see* CORONA

capitulum [kə'pɪtjʊləm] *noun* round end of a bone, such as the distal end of the humerus, which articulates with another bone (NOTE: plural is **capitula**)

caplet ['kæplət] *noun* small oblong tablet covered with a casing which dissolves easily, and which (usually) cannot be broken in two

capsular ['kæpsjʊlə] *adjective* referring to a capsule

capsularis [kæpsjʊ'leərɪs] *see* DECIDUA

capsule ['kæpsjuːl] *noun* **(a)** membrane round an organ or joint; **fibrous capsule** *or* **renal capsule** = fibrous tissue surrounding a kidney; **joint capsule** = white fibrous tissue which surrounds and holds a joint together; **Tenon's capsule** = tissue which lines the

orbit of the eye **(b) internal capsule** = bundle of fibres linking the cerebral cortex and other parts of the brain **(c)** small hollow digestible case, filled with a drug to be swallowed by the patient; *she swallowed three capsules of painkiller*; *the doctor prescribed the drug in capsule form*; *see also* BOWMAN'S CAPSULE

capsulectomy [kæpsjʊ'lektəmi] *noun* surgical removal of the capsule round a joint

capsulitis [kæpsjʊ'laɪtɪs] *noun* inflammation of a capsule

caput ['kæpət] *noun* **(a)** the head **(b)** top of part of the body (NOTE: plural is **capita**)

carbohydrates [kɑːbəʊ'haɪdreɪts] *plural noun* organic compounds which derive from sugar and which are the main ingredients of many types of food

COMMENT: carbohydrates are compounds of carbon, hydrogen and oxygen. They are found in particular in sugar and starch, and provide the body with energy

carbolic acid [kɑː'bɒlɪk 'æsɪd] = PHENOL

carbon ['kɑːbən] *noun* one of the common non-metallic elements, an essential component of living matter and organic chemical compounds (NOTE: chemical symbol is **C**)

carbonated ['kɑːbəneɪtɪd] *adjective* (drink) with bubbles in it, because carbon dioxide has been added

carbon dioxide (CO₂) ['kɑːbən daɪ'ɒksaɪd] *noun* colourless gas produced by the body's metabolism as the tissues burn carbon, and breathed out by the lungs as waste

COMMENT: carbon dioxide can be solidified at low temperatures and is known as 'dry ice' or 'carbon dioxide snow', being used to remove growths on the skin

carbonic anhydrase [kɑː'bɒnɪk 'ænhaɪdreɪz] *noun* enzyme which acts as a buffer and regulates the body's water balance, including gastric acid secretion and aqueous humour production

carbon monoxide (CO) ['kɑːbən mə'nɒksaɪd] *noun* poisonous gas found in fumes from car engines, from burning gas and cigarette smoke; **carbon monoxide poisoning** = poisoning caused by breathing carbon monoxide

COMMENT: carbon monoxide exists in

tobacco smoke and in car exhaust fumes and is dangerous because it is easily absorbed into the blood and takes the place of the oxygen in the blood, combining with haemoglobin to form carboxyhaemoglobin, which has the effect of starving the tissues of oxygen. Carbon monoxide has no smell and people do not realize that they are being poisoned by it until they become unconscious, with a characteristic red colouring to the skin. Poisoning using car exhaust fumes is a method for suicide. The treatment for carbon monoxide poisoning is very rapid inhalation of fresh air together with carbon dioxide if this can be provided

carboxyhaemoglobin

[kɑː'bɒksɪhiːməʊ'gləʊbɪn] *noun* compound of carbon monoxide and haemoglobin formed when a person breathes in carbon monoxide from tobacco smoke or car exhaust fumes; **background carboxyhaemoglobin level** = level of carboxyhaemoglobin in the blood of a person living a normal existence without exposure to particularly high levels of carbon monoxide

carbuncle ['kɑːbʌŋkl] *noun* localized staphylococcal infection, which goes deep into the tissue

carcin- *or* **carcino-** ['kɑːsɪn *or* kɑː'sɪnəʊ] *prefix* referring to carcinoma or cancer

carcinogen [kɑː'sɪnədʒn] *noun* substance which produces carcinoma

COMMENT: carcinogens are found in pesticides such as DDT, in asbestos, tobacco, and aromatic compounds such as benzene, and radioactive substances

carcinogenesis [kɑːsɪnə'dʒenəsɪs] *noun* process of forming carcinoma in tissue

carcinogenic [kɑːsɪnə'dʒenɪk] *adjective* which produces carcinoma

carcinoid (tumour) ['kɑːsɪnɔɪd 'tjuːmə] *noun* type of intestinal tumour (especially in the appendix), which causes diarrhoea; **carcinoid syndrome** = group of symptoms which are associated with a carcinoid tumour

carcinoma [kɑːsɪ'nəʊmə] *noun* cancer of the epithelium or glands; **carcinoma in situ** = first stage in the development of a cancer, where the epithelial cells begin to change

carcinomatosis [kɑsɪnəʊmə'təʊsɪs] *noun* carcinoma which has spread to many sites in the body

carcinomatous [kɑːsɪ'nɒmətəs] *adjective* referring to carcinoma

card [kɑːd] *noun* stiff piece of paper which can carry information on it for reference; **filing card** = card with information written on it, used to classify information in correct order; **index card** = card used to make a card index; **punched card** = card with holes punched in it which a computer can read

cardi- *or* **cardio-** ['kɑːdi *or* 'kɑːdiəʊ] *prefix* referring to the heart

cardia ['kɑːdiə] *noun* **(a)** opening at the top of the stomach which joins it to the gullet; *see illustration at* STOMACH **(b)** the heart

cardiac ['kɑːdiæk] *adjective* (i) referring to the heart; (ii) referring to the cardia; **cardiac achalasia** = being unable to relax the cardia (the muscle at the entrance to the stomach), with the result that food cannot enter the stomach; *see also* CARDIOMYOTOMY; **cardiac arrest** = stopping of the heart, a condition where the heart muscle stops beating; **cardiac asthma** = difficulty in breathing caused by heart failure; **cardiac catheterization** = passing a catheter into the heart to take samples of tissue or to check blood pressure; **cardiac cirrhosis** = cirrhosis of the liver caused by heart disease; **cardiac compression** = compression of the heart by fluid in the pericardium; **cardiac conducting system** = nerve system in the heart which links an atrium to a ventricle, so that the two beat at the same rate; **cardiac cycle** = repeated beating of the heart, formed of the diastole and systole; **cardiac decompression** = removal of a haematoma or constriction of the heart; **cardiac glycoside** = drug (such as digoxin) used in the treatment of tachycardia and atrial fibrillation; **cardiac index** = cardiac output per square metre of body surface - it is normally between 3.1 and 3.8 $l/min/m^2$ (litres per minute per square metre); **cardiac failure** = heart failure, situation where the heart cannot function in a satisfactory way and is unable to circulate blood normally; **cardiac impression** = (i) concave area near the centre of the upper surface of the liver under the heart; (ii) depression on the mediastinal part of the lungs where they touch the pericardium; **external cardiac massage** = method of making a patient's heart start beating again by rhythmic pressing on the breastbone; **internal cardiac massage** = method of making a patient's heart start beating again by pressing on the heart itself; **cardiac monitor** = electrocardiograph, an apparatus for measuring and recording the electrical impulses of the muscles of the heart as it beats; **cardiac murmur** = abnormal sound made by the heart, heard through a stethoscope; **cardiac muscle** = special muscle which forms the heart; **cardiac neurosis** = da Costa's syndrome, condition where the patient suffers palpitations, breathlessness and dizziness, caused by effort or worry; **cardiac notch** = (i) point in the left lung, where the right inside wall is bent; (ii) notch at the point where the oesophagus joins the greater curvature of the stomach; **cardiac orifice** = opening where the oesophagus joins the stomach; **cardiac output** = volume of blood expelled by each ventricule in a given time - it is normally between 4.8 and 5.3 l/min (litres per minute); **cardiac pacemaker** = electronic device implanted on a patient's heart, or which a patient wears attached to his chest, which stimulates and regulates the heartbeat; *see also* PACEMAKER; **cardiac patient** = patient suffering from heart disorder; **cardiac reflex** = reflex which controls the heartbeat automatically; **cardiac surgery** = surgery to the heart; **cardiac tamponade** = pressure on the heart when the pericardial cavity fills with blood; **cardiac veins** = veins which lead from the myocardium to the right atrium

cardialgia [kɑːdiˈældʒiə] *noun* heartburn, pain in the chest from indigestion

card index [ˈkɑːd ˈɪndeks] *noun* series of cards with information written on them, kept in special order so that the information can be found easily; *the hospital records used to be kept on a card index, but have been transferred to the computer*; **card-index file** = information kept on filing cards

card-index [kɑːdˈɪndeks] *verb* to put information onto a card index

cardiogram [ˈkɑːdɪəgræm] *noun* graph showing the heartbeat, produced by a cardiograph

cardiograph [ˈkɑːdɪəgrɑːf] *noun* instrument which records the heartbeat

cardiographer [kɑːdiˈɒgrəfə] *noun* technician who operates a cardiograph

cardiography [kɑːdɪˈɒgrəfi] *noun* action of recording of the heartbeat

cardiologist [kɑːdɪˈɒlədʒɪst] *noun* heart specialist, a doctor who specializes in the study of the heart

cardiology [kɑːdɪˈɒlədʒi] *noun* study of the heart, its diseases and functions

cardiomegaly [kɑːdiəʊˈmegəli] *noun* enlarged heart

cardiomyopathy [kɑːdiəʊmaɪˈɒpəθi] *noun* disease of the heart muscle

cardiomyotomy [kɑːdiəʊmaɪˈɒtəmi] *noun* Heller's operation, an operation to treat cardiac achalasia by splitting the ring of muscles where the oesophagus joins the stomach

cardiopathy [kɑːdiˈɒpəθi] *noun* any kind of heart disease

cardiophone [ˈkɑːdiəfəʊn] *noun* microphone attached to a patient to record sounds (used to record the heart of an unborn baby)

cardiopulmonary bypass [kɑːdiəʊˈpʌlmənəri ˈbaɪpɑːs] *noun* machine or method for artificially circulating the patient's blood during open-heart surgery, where the heart and lungs are cut off from the circulation and replaced by a pump

cardiopulmonary resuscitation (CPR) [kɑːdiəʊˈpʌlmənəri rɪsʌsɪˈteɪʃn] *noun* method of resuscitation which stimulates both heart and lungs, consisting of a combination of external chest compression which serves to get the heart going again, and mouth-to-mouth ventilation to get the breathing going again

cardioscope [ˈkɑːdiəskəʊp] *noun* instrument formed of a tube with a light at the end, used to inspect the inside of the heart

cardiospasm [ˈkɑːdiəspæzm] *noun* = CARDIAC ACHALASIA

cardiothoracic [kɑːdiəʊθɒˈræsɪk] *adjective* referring to the heart and the chest region; *a cardiothoracic surgeon*

cardiotocography [kɑːdiəʊtɒˈkɒgrəfi] *noun* recording of the heartbeat of a fetus

cardiovascular [kɑːdiəʊˈvæskjʊlə] *adjective* referring to the heart and the blood circulation system; **cardiovascular disease** = any disease (such as hypertension) which affects the circulatory system; **cardiovascular system** = system of blood circulation

cardiovascular diseases remain the leading cause of death in the United States
Journal of American Medical Association

cardioversion [kɑːdiəʊˈvɜːʃn] *noun* defibrillation, correcting an irregular heartbeat by using an electric impulse

carditis [kɑːˈdaɪtɪs] *noun* inflammation of the connective tissue of the heart

care [keə] *noun* attention, general treatment (of a patient); *the patient is under the care of a cancer specialist*; *she is responsible for the care of patients in the outpatients' department*; **coronary care unit** = section of a hospital reserved to treat patients suffering from heart attacks; *a coronary care unit has been opened at a London hospital*; **intensive care** = continual supervision and treatment of a patient in a special section of a hospital; **intensive care unit (ICU)** = special section of a hospital which supervises seriously ill patients who need constant supervision; *she is in intensive care or in the intensive care unit*; *the patient was put in intensive care*; *he came out of intensive care and was moved to the general ward*; *see also* RESIDENTIAL

the experience of the ward sister is the most important factor in the standard of care
Nursing Times

care for [ˈkeə ˈfɔː] *verb* to look after; *nurses were caring for the injured people at the scene of the accident*; *severely handicapped children are cared for in special clinics*

care plan [ˈkeə ˈplæn] *noun* plan drawn up by the nursing staff for the treatment of an individual patient

all relevant sections of the nurses' care plan and nursing process had been left blank
Nursing Times

carer *or* **caregiver** [ˈkeərə *or* keəˈgɪvə] *noun* someone who looks after a sick or dependent person

most research has focused on those caring for older people or for adults with disability and chronic illness. Most studied are the carers of those who might otherwise have to stay in hospital for a long time
British Medical Journal

caries [ˈkeərɪz] *noun* decay in a tooth or bone; **dental caries** = decay in a tooth

carina [kəˈriːnə] *noun* structure shaped like the bottom of a boat, such as the cartilage at the point where the trachea branches into the bronchi

cariogenic [keərɪəʊˈdʒenɪk] *adjective* (substance) which causes caries

carminative [ˈkɑːmɪnətɪv] *adjective & noun* (substance) which relieves colic or indigestion

carotenaemia [kærətɪˈniːmɪə] *noun* xanthaemia, excessive amount of carotene in the blood as a result of eating mainly too many carrots or tomatoes, which gives the skin a yellow colour

carotene [ˈkærətiːn] *noun* orange or red pigment in carrots, egg yolk and some natural oils, which is converted by the liver into vitamin A

carotid [kəˈrɒtɪd] *noun* artery in the neck; **common carotid artery** *or* **carotid** = main artery running up each side of the lower part of the neck; **carotid body** = tissue in the carotid sinus which is concerned with cardiovascular reflexes; **carotid pulse** = pulse in the carotid artery at the side of the neck; **carotid sinus** = expanded part attached to the carotid artery, which monitors blood pressure in the skull

COMMENT: the common carotid artery is in the lower part of the neck and branches upwards into the external and internal carotids. The carotid body is situated at the point where the carotid divides

carp- *or* **carpo-** [kɑːp *or* ˈkɑːpəʊ] *prefix* referring to the wrist

carpal [ˈkɑːpl] *adjective & noun* referring to the wrist; **carpal bones** *or* **carpals** = the eight bones which make up the carpus or wrist; *see illustration at* HAND; **carpal tunnel syndrome** = condition (usually in women) where the fingers tingle and hurt at night, caused by compression of the median nerve; **carpal tunnel release** = operation to relieve the compression of the median nerve

carphology [kɑːˈfɒlədʒi] *noun* floccitation, pulling at the bedclothes (a sign of delirium in typhoid and other fevers)

carpometacarpal joints (CM joints) [ˈkɑːpəʊmetəˈkɑːpl ˈdʒɔɪnts] *plural noun* joints between the carpals and metacarpals

carpopedal spasm [kɑːpəʊˈpiːdl ˈspæzm] *noun* spasm in the hands and feet caused by lack of calcium

carpus [ˈkɑːpəs] *noun* wrist, the bones by which the lower arm is connected to the hand

COMMENT: the carpus is formed of eight small bones (the carpals): these are the capitate, hamate, lunate, pisiform, scaphoid, trapezium, trapezoid and triquetral

carrier ['kærɪə] *noun* **(a)** person who carries bacteria of a disease in his body and who can transmit the disease to others without showing any sign of it himself; *ten per cent of the population are believed to be unwitting carriers of the bacteria* **(b)** insect which carries disease and infects humans **(c)** healthy person who carries the chromosome defect of a hereditary disease (such as haemophilia or Duchenne muscular dystrophy)

carry out ['kærɪ 'aʊt] *verb* to perform (an operation)

carsick ['kɑːsɪk] *adjective* feeling sick because of the movement of a car

carsickness ['kɑːsɪknəs] *noun* sickness caused by the movement of a car

cart [kɑːt] *US* = TROLLEY

cartilage ['kɑːtəlɪdʒ] *noun* gristle, thick connective tissue which lines the joints and acts as a cushion and which forms part of the structure of an organ; **articular cartilage** = layer of cartilage at the end of a bone where it forms a joint with another bone; **costal cartilage** = cartilage which forms the end of each rib and either joins the rib to the breastbone or to the rib above; **cricoid cartilage** = ring-shaped cartilage in the lower part of the larynx; **elastic cartilage** = flexible cartilage such as that in the ear and epiglottis; **epiphyseal cartilage** = type of cartilage in the bones of children and adolescents which expands and hardens as the bones grow to full size; **hyaline cartilage** = type of cartilage found in the nose, larynx and joints; **thyroid cartilage** = large cartilage in the larynx, part of which forms the Adam's apple

COMMENT: cartilage in small children is the first stage in the formation of bones

cartilaginous [kɑːtə'lædʒɪnəs] *adjective* made of cartilage; **(primary) cartilaginous joint** = synchondrosis, a joint, as in children, where the bones are linked by cartilage, before the cartilage has changed to bone; **(secondary) cartilaginous joint** = symphysis, a point (such as the pubic symphysis) where two bones are joined by cartilage which makes the joint rigid (NOTE: for other terms referring to cartilage, see words beginning with **chondr-**); *see illustrations at* BONE STRUCTURE, JOINTS

caruncle [kə'rʌŋkl] *noun* small swelling; **lacrimal caruncle** = small red point at the inner corner of each eye

cascara (sagrada) [kæ'skɑːrə sə'grɑːdə] *noun* laxative made from the bark of a tropical tree

case [keɪs] *noun* (i) single occurrence of a disease; (ii) person who has a disease or who is undergoing treatment; *there were two hundred cases of cholera in the recent outbreak*; *the hospital is only admitting urgent cases*; *there is an appendicectomy case waiting for the operating theatre*; **case control study** = an investigation in which a group of patients with a disease (cases) are compared with a group without the disease in order to study possible causes; **case history** = details of what has happened to a patient undergoing treatment

casein ['keɪsiːn] *noun* protein found in milk

COMMENT: casein is precipitated when milk comes into contact with an acid and so makes milk form cheese

cast [kɑːst] *noun* **(a) plaster cast** = hard support made of bandage soaked in liquid plaster of Paris, which is allowed to harden after being wrapped round a broken limb and which prevents the limb moving while the bone heals **(b)** mass of material formed in a hollow organ or tube and excreted in fluid; **blood casts** = pieces of blood cells which are secreted by the kidneys in kidney disease

castor oil ['kɑːstər 'ɒɪl] *noun* vegetable oil which acts as a laxative

castrate [kæs'treɪt] *verb* to remove the sexual organs, usually referring to the testicles in males

castration [kæs'treɪʃn] *noun* surgical removal of the sexual organs, usually referring to the testicles in males

casualty ['kæʒʊlti] *noun* **(a)** person who has suffered an accident or who is suddenly ill; *the fire caused several casualties*; *the casualties were taken by ambulance to the nearest hospital*; **casualty department** *or* **hospital** *or* **ward** = department, hospital or ward which deals with accident victims **(b)** casualty department; *the accident victim was rushed to casualty*

CAT [kæt] = COMPUTERIZED AXIAL TOMOGRAPHY; **CAT scan** = scan where a narrow X-ray beam, guided by a computer, photographs a thin section of the body or an organ from different angles; the results are fed into the computer which analyses them and produces a picture of a slice of the body or organ

cata- ['kætə] *prefix* meaning downwards

catabolic [kætə'bɒlɪk] *adjective* referring to catabolism

catabolism [kə'tæbəlɪzm] *noun* breaking down of complex chemicals into simple chemicals

catalase ['kætəleɪs] *noun* enzyme present in the blood and liver which catalyses the breakdown of hydrogen peroxide into water and oxygen

catalepsy ['kætəlepsi] *noun* condition often associated with schizophrenia, where a patient becomes incapable of sensation, his body is rigid and he does not move for long periods

catalyse *US* **catalyze** ['kætəlaɪz] *verb* to act as a catalyst, to help make a chemical reaction take place

catalysis [kə'tæləsɪs] *noun* process where a chemical reaction is helped by a substance (the catalyst) which does not change during the process

catalyst ['kætəlɪst] *noun* substance which produces or helps a chemical reaction without itself changing; *an enzyme which acts as a catalyst in the digestive process*

catalytic [kætə'lɪtɪk] *adjective* referring to catalysis; **catalytic reaction** = chemical reaction which is caused by a catalyst which does not change during the reaction

catamenia [kætə'miːniə] *noun* menstruation

cataplexy ['kætəpleksi] *noun* condition where the patient's muscles become suddenly rigid and he falls without losing consciousness, possibly caused by a shock

cataract ['kætərækt] *noun* condition where the lens of the eye gradually becomes hard and opaque; **congenital cataract** = cataract which is present from birth; **diabetic cataract** = cataract which develops in people suffering from diabetes; **senile cataract** = cataract which occurs in an elderly person; **cataract extraction** = surgical removal of a cataract from the eye

COMMENT: cataracts form most often in people after the age of 50. They are sometimes caused by a blow or an electric shock. Cataracts can easily and safely be removed by surgery

cataractous [kætə'ræktəs] *adjective* **cataractous lens** = lens on which a cataract has formed

catarrh [kə'tɑː] *noun* inflammation of mucous membranes in the nose and throat, creating an excessive amount of mucus; *he suffers from catarrh in the winter*; *is there anything I can take to relieve my catarrh?*

catarrhal [kə'tɑːrəl] *adjective* referring to catarrh; *a catarrhal cough*

catatonia [kætə'təʊniə] *noun* condition where a psychiatric patient is either motionless or shows violent reactions to stimulation

catatonic [kætə'tɒnɪk] *adjective* (behaviour) where the patient is either motionless or extremely violent; **catatonic schizophrenia** = type of schizophrenia where the patient is alternately apathetic or very active and disturbed

catch [kætʃ] *verb* to get a disease; *he caught a cold after standing in the rain*; *she caught mumps* (NOTE: **catching - caught - has caught**)

catching ['kætʃɪŋ] *adjective* infectious; *is the disease catching?*

catchment area ['kætʃmənt 'eəriə] *noun* area around a hospital which is served by that hospital

catecholamines [kætə'kɒləmiːnz] *plural noun* the hormones adrenaline and noradrenaline which are released by the adrenal glands

category ['kætəgri] *noun* classification, the way in which things can be classified; *his condition is of a non-urgent category*

catgut ['kætgʌt] *noun* thread made from part of the intestines of sheep and other animals, now usually artificially hardened, used to sew up incisions made during surgery

COMMENT: catgut is slowly dissolved by fluids in the body after the wound has healed and therefore does not need to be removed. Ordinary catgut will dissolve in 5 to 10 days; hardened catgut takes up to three or four weeks

catharsis [kə'θɑːsɪs] *noun* purgation of the bowels

cathartic [kə'θɑːtɪk] *adjective* laxative or purgative

catheter ['kæθɪtə] *noun* tube passed into the body along one of the passages in the body; **cardiac catheter** = catheter passed through a vein into the heart, to take blood samples, to record pressure or to examine the interior of the heart before surgery; **ureteric catheter** = catheter passed through the ureter to the kidney, to inject an opaque solution into the kidney before taking an X-ray; **urinary** *or* **urethral catheter** = catheter passed up the urethra to allow urine to flow out of the bladder, used to empty the bladder before an abdominal operation

catheterization [kæθɪtəraɪ'zeɪʃn] *noun* putting a catheter into a patient's body; **cardiac catheterization** = passing a catheter into the heart to take samples of tissue or to check blood pressure

> high rates of disconnection of closed urine drainage systems, lack of hand washing and incorrect positioning of urine drainage bags have been highlighted in a new report on urethral catheterization
> *Nursing Times*

> the technique used to treat aortic stenosis is similar to that for any cardiac catheterization. A catheter introduced through the femoral vein is placed across the aortic valve and into the left ventricle
> *Journal of the American Medical Association*

catheterize ['kæθɪtəraɪz] *verb* to insert a catheter into a patient

cat scratch fever ['kæt 'skrætʃ 'fiːvə] *noun* viral fever with inflammation of the lymph glands, caught from being scratched by a cat's claws or by other sharp points

cauda equina ['kɔːdə ɪ'kwaɪnə] *noun* group of nerves which go from the spinal cord to the lumbar region and the coccyx

caudal ['kɔːdl] *adjective (in animals)* referring to the tail; *(in humans)* referring to the cauda equina; **caudal analgesia** = technique often used in childbirth, where an analgesic is injected into the extradural space at the base of the spine to remove feeling in the lower part of the trunk; **caudal block** = local analgesia of the cauda equina nerves

caudate ['kɔːdeɪt] *adjective* like a tail; *(of the liver)* **caudate lobe** = posterior lobe, lobe at the back of the liver, behind the right and left lobes

caul [kɔːl] *noun* **(a)** membrane which sometimes covers a baby's head at birth **(b)** = OMENTUM

cauliflower ear [kɒli'flauər 'ɪə] *noun* permanently swollen ear, caused by blows (in boxing)

causalgia [kɔː'zældʒə] *noun* burning pain in a limb, caused by a damaged nerve

caustic ['kɔːstɪk] *adjective & noun* (chemical substance) which destroys tissues which it touches

cauterization [kɔːtəraɪ'zeɪʃn] *noun* act of cauterizing; *the growth was removed by cauterization*

cauterize ['kɔːtəraɪz] *verb* to use burning, radiation or laser beams to remove tissue or to stop bleeding

cautery ['kɔːtəri] *noun* surgical instrument used to cauterize a wound; **cold cautery** = removal of a skin growth using carbon dioxide snow; *see also* ELECTROCAUTERY, GALVANOCAUTERY

cava ['keɪvə] *see* VENA CAVA

cavernous ['kævənəs] *adjective* hollow; **cavernous breathing** *or* **breath sounds** = hollow sounds made by the lungs and heard through a stethoscope placed on a patient's chest, used in diagnosis; **cavernous haemangioma** = tumour in connective tissue with wide spaces which contain blood; **cavernous sinus** = *see* SINUS

cavernosa [kævə'nəusə] *see* CORPUS

cavitation [kævɪ'teɪʃn] *noun* forming of a cavity

cavity ['kævəti] *noun* (i) hole or space inside the body; (ii) hole in a tooth; **abdominal cavity** = space in the body below the chest; **buccal cavity** = the mouth; **cerebral cavity** = ventricles in the brain; **chest cavity** = space in the body containing the heart, lungs and diaphragm; **cranial cavity** = space inside the bones of the cranium, in which the brain is situated; **glenoid cavity** = socket in the shoulder joint into which the head of the humerus fits; *see illustration at* SHOULDER; **medullary cavity** = hollow centre of a long bone, containing bone marrow; *see illustration at* BONE STRUCTURE; **nasal cavity** = cavity behind the nose between the cribriform plates above and the hard palate below, divided in two by the nasal septum and leading to the nasopharynx; *see illustration at* THROAT; **oral cavity** = the mouth; **pelvic cavity** = space below the abdominal cavity, above the pelvis; **peritoneal cavity** = space between the layers of the peritoneum, containing the major organs of the abdomen; **pleural cavity** = space between the inner and outer pleura of the chest; **pulp cavity** = centre of a tooth containing soft tissue; *see illustration at* TOOTH; **synovial cavity** = space inside a synovial joint; **thoracic cavity** = space in the body containing the heart, lungs and diaphragm

cavus ['keɪvəs] *see* PES

CBC ['si: 'bi: 'si:] = COMPLETE BLOOD COUNT

cc ['si: 'si:] = CUBIC CENTIMETRE

CCU ['si: 'si: 'ju:] = CORONARY CARE UNIT

Cd *chemical symbol for* cadmium

CDH ['si: 'di: 'eɪtʃ] = CONGENITAL DISLOCATION OF THE HIP

cecum ['si:kəm] *noun US* = CAECUM

-cele [si:l] *suffix* referring to a swelling

celi- ['si:li] *see* COELI-

celiac ['si:lɪæk] *US* = COELIAC

cell [sel] *noun* tiny unit of matter which is the base of all plant and animal tissue; **alpha cell** = one of the types of cells in glands (such as the pancreas) which have more than one type of cell; **beta cell** = cell which produces insulin; **blood cell** = corpuscle, any type of cell found in the blood; **daughter cell** = one of the cells which develop by mitosis from a single parent cell; **goblet cell** = tube-shaped cell in the epithelium which secretes mucus; **mast cell** = large cell in connective tissue, which carries histamine and reacts to allergens; **mother cell** *or* **parent cell** = original cell which splits into daughter cells by mitosis; **mucous cell** = cell which contains mucinogen which secretes mucin; **oxyntic cell** *or* **parietal cell** = cell in the gastric gland which secretes hydrochloric acid; **receptor cell** = cell which senses a change (such as cold or heat) in the surrounding environment or in the body and reacts to it by sending an impulse to the central nervous system; **cell body** = part of a nerve cell which surrounds the nucleus and from which the axon and dendrites begin; **cell division** = way in which a cell reproduces itself by mitosis; **cell membrane** = membrane enclosing the cytoplasm of a cell; *see also* COLUMNAR, TARGET

COMMENT: the cell is a unit which can reproduce itself. It is made up of a jelly-like substance (cytoplasm) which surrounds a nucleus and contains many other small organisms which are different according to the type of cell. Cells reproduce by division (mitosis) and their process of feeding and removing waste products is metabolism. The division and reproduction of cells is how the human body is formed.

cellular ['seljʊlə] *adjective* **(a)** referring to cells; formed of cells **(b)** made of many similar parts connected together; **cellular tissue** = form of connective tissue with large spaces (NOTE: for other terms referring to cells, see words beginning with **cyt-, cyto-**)

cellulite ['seljʊlaɪt] *noun* lumpy deposits of subcutaneous fat, especially in the thighs and buttocks

cellulitis [seljʊ'laɪtɪs] *noun* usually bacterial inflammation of connective tissue or of the subcutaneous tissue

cellulose ['seljʊləʊs] *noun* carbohydrate which makes up a large percentage of plant matter

COMMENT: cellulose is not digestible and is passed through the digestive system as roughage

Celsius ['selsiəs] *noun* scale of temperature where the freezing and boiling points of water are 0° and 100° (NOTE: used in many countries, except in the USA, where the Fahrenheit system is still preferred. Normally written as a **C** after the degree sign: **52ºC** (say: 'fifty-two degrees Celsius'). Also called **centigrade**)

COMMENT: to convert Celsius temperatures to Fahrenheit, multiply by 1.8 and add 32. So 20°C is equal to 68°F

cement [sə'ment] *noun* **(a)** adhesive used in dentistry to attach a crown to the base of a tooth **(b)** = CEMENTUM

cementum [sə'mentəm] *noun* layer of thick hard material which covers the roots of teeth; *see illustration at* TOOTH

centi- ['senti] *prefix* meaning one hundredth (10^{-2} (NOTE: symbol is **c**)

centigrade ['sentɪgreɪd] *noun* scale of temperature where the freezing and boiling points of water are 0° and 100°; *see note at* CELSIUS

centilitre *US* **centiliter** ['sentɪli:tə] *noun* unit of measurement of liquid (= one hundredth of a litre) ((NOTE: with figures usually written **cl**)

centimetre *US* **centimeter** ['sentɪmiːtə] *noun* unit of measurement of length (= one hundredth of a metre) (NOTE: with figures usually written **cm: 10cm: 'the appendix is about 6cm (six centimetres) in length'**)

central ['sentrl] *adjective* referring to the centre; **central canal** = thin tube in the centre of the spinal cord containing cerebrospinal fluid; **central line** = line inserted through the neck used to monitor central venous pressure in conditions such as shock where fluid balance is severely upset; **central nervous system (CNS)** = the brain and spinal cord which link together all the nerves; **central sulcus** = one of the grooves which divide a cerebral hemisphere into lobes; **central vein** = vein in the liver; **central venous pressure** = blood pressure in the right atrium, which can be measured by means of a catheter

centralis [sen'treɪlɪs] *see* FOVEA

centre *US* **center** ['sentə] *noun* **(a)** middle point, main part; *the aim of the examination is to locate the centre of infection* **(b)** large building; **medical centre** = place where several different doctors and specialists practise **(c)** point where a group of nerves come together; **vision centre** = point in the brain where the nerves relating to the eye come together

centrifugal [sentrɪ'fjuːgl] *adjective* which goes away from the centre

centrifugation *or* **centrifuging** [sentrɪfjuː'geɪʃn *or* 'sentrɪfjuːdʒɪŋ] *noun* separating the components of a liquid in a centrifuge

centrifuge ['sentrɪfjuːdʒ] *noun* device to separate the components of a liquid by rapid spinning

centriole ['sentrɪəʊl] *noun* small structure found in the cytoplasm of a cell, which forms asters during cell division

centripetal [sen'trɪpɪtl] *adjective* which goes towards the centre

centromere ['sentrəmɪə] *noun* kinetochore, constricted part of a cell, seen as the cell divides

centrosome ['sentrəsəʊm] *noun* structure of the cytoplasm in a cell, near the nucleus, and containing the centrioles

centrum ['sentrəm] *noun* centre, central part of an organ (NOTE: plural is **centra**)

cephal- *or* **cephalo-** ['sefəl *or* 'sefələʊ] *prefix* referring to the head

cephalalgia [sefə'lældʒə] *noun* headache, a pain in the head

cephalhaematoma [sefəlhiːmə'təʊmə] *noun* swelling found mainly on the head of babies delivered with forceps

cephalic [sə'fælɪk] *adjective* referring to the head; **cephalic index** = measurement of the shape of the skull; **cephalic presentation** = normal position of a baby in the uterus, where the baby's head will appear first; **cephalic version** = turning a wrongly positioned fetus round in the uterus, so that the head will appear first at birth

cephalocele ['sefələʊsiːl] *noun* swelling caused by part of the brain passing through a weak point in the bones of the skull

cephalogram ['sefələʊgræm] *noun* X-ray photograph of the bones of the skull

cephalometry [sefə'lɒmɪtri] *noun* measurement of the head

cephalopelvic [sefələʊ'pelvɪk] *adjective* referring to the head of the fetus and the pelvis of the mother; **cephalopelvic disproportion** = condition where the pelvic opening of the mother is not large enough for the head of the fetus

cephalosporin [sefələʊ'spɔːrɪn] *noun* drug (such as cefaclor) used in the treatment of bacterial infection

cerea ['sɪərɪə] *see* FLEXIBILITAS CEREA

cereal ['sɪərɪəl] *noun* **(a)** plant whose seeds are used for food, especially to make flour; *the European Union grows large quantities of cereals or of cereal crops* **(b)** food made of seeds of corn, etc. which is usually eaten at breakfast; *he ate a bowl of cereal*; *put milk and sugar on your cereal*

cerebellar [serə'belə] *adjective* referring to the cerebellum; **cerebellar ataxia** = disorder where the patient staggers and cannot speak clearly, due to a disease of the cerebellum; **cerebellar gait** = way of walking where the patient staggers along, caused by a disease of the cerebellum; **cerebellar peduncle** = band of nerve tissue connecting parts of the cerebellum; **cerebellar syndrome** = disease affecting the cerebellum, the symptoms of which are lack of muscle coordination, spasms in the eyeball and impaired speech

cerebellum [serə'beləm] *noun* section of the hindbrain, located at the back of the head beneath the back part of the cerebrum; *see illustration at* BRAIN; **tentorium cerebelli** =

part of the dura mater which separates the cerebellum from the cerebral hemispheres

COMMENT: the cerebellum is formed of two hemispheres with the vermis in the centre. Fibres go into or out of the cerebellum through the peduncles. The cerebellum is the part of the brain where voluntary movements are coordinated and is associated with the sense of balance

cerebr- or **cerebro-** ['serəbr or 'serəbrəu] *prefix* referring to the cerebrum

cerebral ['serəbrl] *adjective* referring to the cerebrum or to the brain in general; **cerebral aqueduct** or **aqueduct of Sylvius** = canal connecting the third and fourth ventricles in the brain; **cerebral arteries** = main arteries which take blood into the brain; **cerebral cavity** = ventricles in the brain; **cerebral cortex** = outer layer of grey matter which covers the cerebrum; **cerebral decompression** = removal of part of the skull to relieve pressure on the brain; **cerebral haemorrhage** = bleeding inside the brain from a cerebral artery; **cerebral hemisphere** = one of the two halves of the cerebrum; **cerebral peduncle** = mass of nerve fibres connecting the cerebral hemispheres to the midbrain; **cerebral thrombosis** = stroke, condition where a blood clot enters and blocks a brain artery

cerebral palsy ['serəbrl 'pɔːlzi] *noun* disorder of the brain, mainly due to brain damage occurring before birth, or due to lack of oxygen during birth

COMMENT: cerebral palsy is the disorder affecting spastics. The patient may have bad coordination of muscular movements, impaired speech, hearing and sight, and sometimes mental retardation. Premature babies are at higher risk

cerebration [serə'breɪʃn] *noun* working of the brain

cerebrospinal [serəbrəu'spaɪnl] *adjective* referring to the brain and the spinal cord; **cerebrospinal fever** or **cerebrospinal meningitis** = meningococcal meningitis or spotted fever, the commonest epidemic form of meningitis, caused by a bacterium *Neisseria meningitidis,* where the meninges become inflamed causing headaches and fever; **cerebrospinal fluid (CSF)** = fluid which surrounds the brain and the spinal cord; **cerebrospinal tracts** = main motor pathways in the anterior and lateral white columns of the spinal cord

COMMENT: CSF is found in the space between the arachnoid mater and pia mater of the brain, within the ventricles of the brain and in the central canal of the spinal cord. CSF consists mainly of water, with some sugar and sodium chloride. Its function is to cushion the brain and spinal cord and it is continually formed and absorbed to maintain the correct pressure

cerebrovascular [serəbrəu'væskjulə] *adjective* referring to the blood vessels in the brain; **cerebrovascular accident (CVA)** = stroke, a sudden blocking of or bleeding from a blood vessel in the brain resulting in temporary or permanent paralysis or death; **cerebrovascular disease** = disease of the blood vessels in the brain

cerebrum [sə'riːbrəm] *noun* main part of the brain; **falx cerebri** = fold of the dura mater between the two hemispheres of the cerebrum; *see illustration at* BRAIN

COMMENT: the cerebrum is the largest part of the brain, formed of two sections (the cerebral hemispheres) which run along the length of the head. The cerebrum controls the main mental processes, including the memory

certificate [sə'tɪfɪkət] *noun* official paper which states something; **birth certificate** = official document giving details of a person's date and place of birth and parents; **death certificate** = official document signed by a doctor, stating that a person has died and giving details of the person and the cause of death; **medical certificate** = official document signed by a doctor, giving a patient permission to be away from work or not to do certain types of work

certify ['sɜːtɪfaɪ] *verb* to make an official statement in writing; *he was certified dead on arrival at hospital* (NOTE: formerly used to refer to patients sent to a mental hospital)

cerumen [sə'ruːmen] *noun* wax which forms inside the ear

ceruminous glands [sə'ruːmɪnəs 'glændz] *noun* glands which secrete earwax; *see illustration at* EAR

cervic- or **cervico-** ['sɜːvɪk or sə'vaɪkəu] *prefix* (i) referring to a neck; (ii) referring to the cervix of the uterus

cervical [sə'vaɪkl or 'sɜːvɪkl] *adjective* (i) referring to any neck; (ii) referring to the cervix of the uterus; **cervical canal** = tube running through the cervix from the point where the uterus joins the vagina to the entrance of the uterine cavity; **cervical cancer** = cancer of the cervix of the uterus; **cervical cap** = DUTCH CAP; **cervical collar** = special strong orthopaedic collar to support the head of a patient with neck injuries or a condition such as cervical spondylosis; **cervical ganglion** = one of the bundles of nerves in the neck; **cervical (lymph) node** = lymph node in the neck; **cervical nerves** = spinal nerves in the neck; **cervical rib** = extra rib sometimes found attached to the vertebrae above the other ribs and which may cause thoracic inlet syndrome; **cervical smear** = test for cervical cancer, where cells taken from the mucus in the cervix of the uterus are examined; **cervical spondylosis** = degenerative change in the neck bones; *see also* SPONDYLOSIS; **deep cervical vein** = vein in the neck, which drains into the vertebral vein; **cervical vertebrae** = the seven bones which form the neck; *see illustration at* VERTEBRAL COLUMN

cervicectomy [sɜ:vɪˈsektəmi] *noun* surgical removal of the cervix uteri

cervicitis [sɜ:vɪˈsaɪtɪs] *noun* inflammation of the cervix uteri

cervicography [sɜ:vɪˈkɒgrəfi] *noun* photographing the cervix uteri: used as a method of screening for cervical cancer

cervicouterine canal [sɜ:vɪkəʊˈjuːtəraɪn kəˈnæl] = CERVICAL CANAL

cervix [ˈsɜ:vɪks] *noun* (i) any narrow neck of an organ; (ii) neck of the uterus, the narrow lower part of the uterus leading into the vagina (NOTE: cervix means 'neck' and can refer to any neck; it is most usually used to refer to the narrow part of the uterus and is then referred to as the **cervix uteri**)

cestode [ˈsestəʊd] *noun* type of tapeworm

CFT [ˈsiː ˈef ˈtiː] = COMPLEMENT FIXATION TEST

chafe [tʃeɪf] *verb* to rub, especially to rub against the skin; *the rough cloth of the collar chafed the patient's neck*

chafing [ˈtʃeɪfɪŋ] *noun* irritation of the skin due to rubbing; *she was experiencing chafing of the thighs*

Chagas' disease [ˈʃɑːgəs dɪˈziːz] *noun* type of sleeping sickness found in South America, transmitted by insect bites which pass trypanosomes into the bloodstream

COMMENT: the first symptom is an inflamed spot at the place of the insect bite, followed later by fever, swelling of the liver and spleen and swelling of tissues in the face. Children are mainly affected and if untreated the disease can cause fatal heart block in early adult life

chain [tʃeɪn] *noun* (i) number of metal rings attached together to make a line; (ii) number of components linked together or number of connected events; **chain reaction** = reaction where each stage is started by the one before it

chair [tʃeə] *noun* piece of furniture for sitting on; *a badly made chair can affect the posture*; **dentist's chair** = special chair which can be made to tip backwards, used by dentists when operating on patients' teeth; *see also* BIRTHING

chalasia [tʃəˈleɪziə] *noun* excessive relaxation of the oesophageal muscles, which causes regurgitation

chalazion [kəˈleɪziən] *noun* meibomian cyst, a swelling of a sebaceous gland in the eyelid

chalone [ˈkeɪlɒn or ˈkæləʊn] *noun* hormone which stops a secretion, as opposed to those hormones which stimulate secretion

chamber [ˈtʃeɪmbə] *noun* hollow space; atrium or ventricle in the heart where blood is collected; **anterior** *or* **posterior chambers of the eye** = parts of the aqueous chamber of the eye which are in front of or behind the iris; **collection chambers** = sections of the heart where blood collects before being pumped out; **pumping chambers** = sections of the heart where blood is pumped

chancre [ˈʃæŋkə] *noun* sore on the lip, penis or eyelid which is the first symptom of syphilis

chancroid [ˈʃæŋkrɔɪd] *noun* soft chancre, venereal sore with a soft base, situated in the groin or on the genitals and caused by the bacterium *Haemophilus ducreyi*

change [tʃeɪndʒ] **1** *noun* being different; *we will try a change of treatment*; *this patient needs a change of bedclothes*; **change of life** = MENOPAUSE **2** *verb* (a) to make something different; to become different; *treatment of tuberculosis has changed a lot in the past few years*; *he's changed so much since his illness that I hardly recognized him*; *the doctor decided to change the dosage* (b) to put on different clothes, bedclothes or bandages; *she changed into her uniform* *before going into the ward; the nurses change the bedclothes every day; make sure the dressing on the wound is changed every morning*

channel ['tʃænl] *noun* tube or passage through which fluid flows

chaplain ['tʃæplɪn] *noun* **hospital chaplain** = religious minister attached to a hospital, who visits and comforts patients and their families and gives them the sacraments when necessary

chapped [tʃæpt] *adjective* (skin) which is cracked due to cold; *put some cream on your chapped lips*

chapping ['tʃæpɪŋ] *noun* cracking of the skin due to cold; *cream will prevent your hands chapping*

character ['kærəktə] *noun* way in which a person thinks and behaves

characteristic [kærəktə'rɪstɪk] **1** *adjective* typical or special; *the inflammation is characteristic of shingles; symptoms characteristic of anaemia* **2** *noun* difference which makes something special; *cancer destroys the cell's characteristics*

characterize ['kærəktəraɪz] *verb* to make something typical or special; *the disease is characterized by the development of coarse features*

charcoal ['tʃɑːkəʊl] *noun* black substance, an impure form of carbon, formed when wood is burnt in the absence of oxygen

COMMENT: charcoal tablets can be used to relieve diarrhoea or flatulence

Charcot's joint ['ʃɑːkəʊz 'dʒɔɪnt] *noun* joint which becomes deformed because the patient cannot feel pain in it when the nerves have been damaged by syphilis, diabetes or leprosy

charge nurse ['tʃɑːdʒ 'nɜːs] *noun* nurse in charge of a group of patients

charleyhorse ['tʃɑːlihɔːs] *noun US (not a technical term)* painful cramp in a leg or thigh

chart [tʃɑːt] *noun* diagram, record of information shown as a series of lines or points on graph paper; *a chart showing the rise in cases of whooping cough during the first five months of 1993*; **temperature chart** = chart showing changes in a patient's temperature over a period of time

ChB = BACHELOR OF SURGERY

CHC ['siː 'eɪtʃ 'siː] = CHILD HEALTH CLINIC, COMMUNITY HEALTH COUNCIL

CHD ['siː 'eɪtʃ 'diː] = CORONARY HEART DISEASE

checkup ['tʃekʌp] *noun* test to see if someone is fit; general examination by a doctor or dentist; *he had a heart checkup last week; she has entered hospital for a checkup; he made an appointment with the dentist for a checkup*

cheek [tʃiːk] *noun* one of two fleshy parts of the face on each side of the nose; *a little girl with red cheeks*

cheekbone ['tʃiːkbəʊn] *noun* zygomatic bone or malar bone, the bone which forms the prominent part of the cheek and the lower part of the eye socket

cheil- *or* **cheilo-** ['kaɪl or 'kaɪləʊ] *prefix* referring to lips

cheilitis [kaɪ'laɪtɪs] *noun* inflammation of the lips

cheilosis [kaɪ'ləʊsɪs] *noun* swelling and cracks on the lips and corners of the mouth caused by lack of vitamin B

cheir- *or* **cheiro-** ['keɪr or 'keɪrəʊ] *prefix meaning* hand

chelating agent ['kiːleɪtɪŋ 'eɪdʒnt] *noun* chemical compound which can combine with certain metals, used as a treatment for metal poisoning

cheloid ['kiːlɔɪd] = KELOID

chem- *or* **chemo-** ['kem or 'keməʊ] *prefix* referring to chemistry or to chemicals

chemical ['kemɪkl] **1** *adjective* referring to chemistry **2** *noun* substance produced by a chemical process or formed of chemical elements

The MRI body scanner is able to provide a chemical analysis of tissues without investigative surgery

Health Services Journal

chemist ['kemɪst] *noun* **(a)** scientist who specializes in the study of chemistry **(b) dispensing chemist** = pharmacist who prepares and sells drugs according to doctors' prescriptions; **a chemist's** = shop where you can buy medicine, toothpaste, soap, etc.; *go to the chemist's to get some cough medicine; the tablets are sold at all chemists'; there's a chemist's on the corner*

chemistry ['kemɪstri] *noun* study of substances, elements and compounds and their reactions with each other; **blood chemistry** *or* **chemistry of the blood** = (i) substances which make up blood, which can be analysed in blood tests, the results of which are useful in diagnosing disease; (ii) record of changes which take place in blood during disease and treatment

chemo- ['ki:məʊ] *prefix* referring to chemistry

chemoreceptor [ki:məʊrɪ'septə] *noun* cell which responds to the presence of a chemical compound by activating a nerve (such as a taste bud reacting to food or cells in the carotid body reacting to lowered oxygen and raised carbon dioxide in the blood); *see also* EXTEROCEPTOR, INTEROCEPTOR, RECEPTOR

chemosis [ki:'məʊsɪs] *noun* swelling of the conjunctiva

chemotaxis [ki:məʊ'tæksɪs] *noun* movement of a cell which is attracted to or repelled by a chemical substance

chemotherapeutic agent [ki:məʊθerə'pju:tɪk 'eɪdʒnt] *noun* chemical substance used to treat a disease

chemotherapy [ki:məʊ'θerəpi] *noun* using chemical drugs (such as antibiotics, painkillers or antiseptic lotions) to fight a disease, especially using toxic chemicals to destroy rapidly developing cancer cells

chest [tʃest] *noun* thorax, the cavity in the top part of the front of the body above the abdomen, containing the diaphragm, heart and lungs and surrounded by the rib cage; *he placed the stethoscope on the patient's chest or he listened to the patient's chest; she is suffering from chest pains; after the fight he was rushed to hospital with chest wounds; a day unit set up for disabled chest patients; she has a cold in the chest* = she coughs badly; **chest cavity** = space in the body containing the heart, lungs and diaphragm; **chest examination** = examination of the patient's chest by percussion, stethoscope or X-rays; **chest muscle** = pectoral muscle, one of two muscles which lie across the chest and control movements of the shoulder and arm (NOTE: for other terms referring to the chest, see words beginning with **pecto-, steth-, thorac-**)

chew [tʃu:] *verb* to masticate, to crush food with the teeth; *he was chewing a piece of meat; food should be chewed slowly*

COMMENT: the action of chewing grinds the food into small pieces and mixes it with saliva to start the process of breaking down the food to extract nutrients from it

chewing gum ['tʃu:ɪŋ 'gʌm] *noun* sweet substance which you can chew for a long time but not swallow

Cheyne-Stokes respiration *or* **breathing** ['tʃeɪn'stəʊks respə'reɪʃn *or* 'bri:ðɪŋ] *noun* condition (usually of unconscious patients) where breathing is irregular, with short breaths gradually increasing to deep breaths, then reducing again, until breathing appears to stop; caused by a disorder of the brain centre which controls breathing

chiasm *or* **chiasma** ['kaɪæzm *or* kaɪ'æzmə] *noun* cross-shaped crossing of fibres; **optic chiasma** = structure where some of the optic nerves from each eye partially cross each other in the hypothalamus

chickenpox ['tʃɪkɪn 'pɒks] *noun* varicella, infectious disease of children, with fever and red spots which turn into itchy blisters

COMMENT: chickenpox is caused by a herpesvirus. In later life, shingles is usually a re-emergence of a dormant chickenpox virus and an adult with shingles can infect a child with chickenpox

chigger ['tʃɪgə] *noun* harvest mite, a tiny insect which bites and causes irritation; its larva also can enter the skin near a hair follicle and travel under the skin causing intense irritation

chilblain ['tʃɪlbleɪn] *noun* erythema pernio, condition where the skin of the fingers, toes, nose or ears becomes red, swollen and itchy because of exposure to cold; *he has chilblains on his toes*

child [tʃaɪld] *noun* young boy or girl; *here is a photograph of my father as a child; all the children were playing out in the field; when do the children come out of school?; they have six children* = they have six sons or daughters; **child abuse** = bad treatment of children, including sexual interference; **children's hospital** = hospital which specializes in treating children (NOTE: plural is **children** ['tʃɪldrən]. Note also that **child** is the legal term for a person under 14 years of age. For other terms referring to children, see words beginning with **paed-** *or* **ped-**)

childbearing ['tʃaɪldbeərɪŋ] *noun* giving birth

childbirth ['tʃaɪldbɜːθ] *noun* parturition, the act of giving birth; **natural childbirth** = childbirth where the mother is not given any pain-killing drugs or anaesthetic but is encouraged to give birth after having prepared herself through relaxation and breathing exercises and a new psychological outlook

child care ['tʃaɪld 'keə] *noun* care of young children and study of their special needs

child health clinic (CHC) *or* **child development clinic** ['tʃaɪld 'helθ 'klɪnɪk or 'tʃaɪld dɪ'veləpmənt 'klɪnɪk] *noun* special clinic for checking the health and development of small children under school age

childhood ['tʃaɪldhʊd] *noun* time when a person is a child; *he had a happy childhood in the country*; *she spent her childhood in Canada*; **childhood illnesses** *or* **disorders** = disorders which mainly affect children and not adults

child-proof ['tʃaɪldpruːf] *adjective* which a child cannot use; *the pills are sold in bottles with child-proof lids*

chill [tʃɪl] *noun* feeling cold and shivering, usually the sign of the beginning of a fever, of flu or a cold; *he caught a chill on the train*

chin [tʃɪn] *noun* bottom part of the face, beneath the mouth; *she hit him on the chin*; *he rested his chin on his hand while he was thinking*

Chinese restaurant syndrome ['tʃaɪniːz 'restərɒnt 'sɪndrəʊm] *noun* allergic condition which gives people violent headaches after eating food flavoured with monosodium glutamate

chiropodist [kɪ'rɒpədɪst] *noun* person who specializes in treatment of minor disorders of the feet; *see also* PODIATRIST, PODIATRY

chiropody [kɪ'rɒpədi] *noun* study and treatment of minor diseases and disorders of the feet

chiropractic [kaɪrə'præktɪk] *noun* treatment of disorders by manipulating the bones of the spine

chiropractor ['kaɪrəpræktə] *noun* person who treats disorders by manipulating the bones of the spine

chlamydia [klə'mɪdɪə] *noun* type of parasite, which is transmitted to humans by insects, causing psittacosis and trachoma

chloasma [kləʊ'æzmə] *noun* presence of brown spots on the skin from various causes

chlor- *or* **chloro-** ['klɔːr or 'klɔːrəʊ] *prefix* (i) referring to chlorine; (ii) referring to the colour green

chloride ['klɔːraɪd] *noun* a salt of hydrochloric acid; **sodium chloride (NaCl)** = common salt

chlorination [klɔːrɪ'neɪʃn] *noun* sterilizing by adding chlorine

> COMMENT: chlorination is used to kill bacteria in drinking water, in swimming pools and sewage farms, and has many industrial applications such as sterilization in food processing

chlorinator ['klɔːrɪneɪtə] *noun* apparatus for adding chlorine to water

chlorine ['klɔːriːn] *noun* powerful greenish gas, used to sterilize water (NOTE: chemical symbol is Cl)

chloroform (CHCl₃) ['klɒrəfɔːm] *noun* powerful drug formerly used as an anaesthetic

chloroma [klɔː'rəʊmə] *noun* bone tumour associated with acute leukaemia

chlorophyll ['klɒrəfɪl] *noun* green pigment in plants, also used in deodorants and toothpaste

chloroquine ['klɔːrəkwɪn] *noun* *see* DRUGS TABLE IN SUPPLEMENT

chlorosis [klɔː'rəʊsɪs] *noun* type of severe anaemia due to iron deficiency, affecting mainly young girls

chlorpromazine [klɔː'prəʊməziːn] *noun; see* DRUGS TABLE IN SUPPLEMENT

ChM = MASTER OF SURGERY

choana ['kəʊənə] *noun* any opening shaped like a funnel, especially that leading from the nasal cavity to the pharynx (NOTE: plural is **choanae**)

choke [tʃəʊk] *verb* to stop breathing because the windpipe becomes blocked by a foreign body or by inhalation of water; **to choke on something** = to take something into the windpipe instead of the gullet, so that the breathing is interrupted; *he choked on a piece of bread or a piece of bread made him choke*

choking ['tʃəʊkɪŋ] **1** *noun* asphyxia, a condition where someone is prevented from breathing **2** *adjective* (smoke) which makes you choke; *the room filled with choking black smoke*

chol- [kɒl] *prefix* referring to bile

cholaemia [kəˈliːmiə] *noun* presence of abnormal amount of bile in the blood

cholagogue [ˈkɒləgɒg] *noun* drug which encourages the production of bile

cholangiography [kɒlændʒiˈɒgrəfi] *noun* X-ray examination of the bile ducts and gall bladder

cholangiolitis [kɒlændʒiəʊˈlaɪtɪs] *noun* inflammation of the small bile ducts

cholangitis [kəʊlænˈdʒaɪtɪs] *noun* inflammation of the bile ducts

chole- [ˈkɒlɪ] *prefix* referring to bile

cholecystectomy [kɒlɪsɪˈstektəmi] *noun* surgical removal of the gall bladder

cholecystitis [kɒlɪsɪˈstaɪtɪs] *noun* inflammation of the gall bladder

cholecystoduodenostomy [kɒlɪsɪstədjuːədɪˈnɒstəmi] *noun* surgical operation to join the gall bladder to the duodenum to allow bile to pass into the intestine when the main bile duct is blocked

cholecystogram [kɒlɪˈsɪstəgræm] *noun* X-ray photograph of the gall bladder

cholecystography [kɒlɪsɪˈstɒgrəfi] *noun* X-ray examination of the gall bladder

cholecystotomy [kɒlɪsɪˈstɒtəmi] *noun* surgical operation to make a cut in the gall bladder, usually to remove gallstones

choledoch- [kəˈledɒk] *prefix* referring to the common bile duct

choledochotomy [kəledɒˈkɒtəmi] *noun* surgical operation to make a cut in the common bile duct to remove stones

cholelithiasis *or* **choledocholithiasis** [kɒlɪlɪˈθaɪəsɪs *or* kəledɒkəlɪˈθaɪəsɪs] *noun* condition where gallstones form in the gall bladder or bile ducts

cholelithotomy [kɒlɪlɪˈθɒtəmi] *noun* surgical removal of gallstones by cutting into the gall bladder

cholera [ˈkɒlərə] *noun* serious bacterial disease spread through food or water which has been infected by *Vibrio cholerae*; *he caught cholera while on holiday*; *a cholera epidemic broke out after the flood*; **cholera vaccine** = vaccine used to prevent cholera

COMMENT: the infected person suffers diarrhoea, cramp in the intestines and dehydration. The disease is often fatal and vaccination is only effective for a relatively short period

choleresis [kəˈliərəsɪs] *noun* production of bile by the liver

choleretic [kɒlɪˈretɪk] *adjective* (substance) which increases the production and flow of bile

cholestasis [kɒlɪˈsteɪsɪs] *noun* condition where all bile does not pass into the intestine but some remains in the liver and causes jaundice

cholesteatoma [kɒlɪstɪəˈtəʊmə] *noun* cyst containing some cholesterol found in the middle ear and also in the brain

cholesterol [kəˈlestərɒl] *noun* fatty substance found in fats and oils, also produced by the liver and forming an essential part of all cells

COMMENT: cholesterol is found in brain cells, the adrenal glands, liver and bile acids. High levels of cholesterol in the blood are found in diabetes. Cholesterol is formed by the body, and high blood cholesterol levels are associated with diets rich in animal fat (such as butter and fat meat). Excess cholesterol can be deposited in the walls of arteries, causing atherosclerosis

cholesterolaemia [kəlestərəˈleɪmiə] *noun* (high) level of cholesterol in the blood

cholesterosis [kɒlestəˈrəʊsɪs] *noun* inflammation of the gall bladder with deposits of cholesterol

cholic acid [ˈkəʊlɪk ˈæsɪd] *noun* one of the bile acids

choline [ˈkəʊliːn] *noun* compound involved in fat metabolism and the precursor for acetylcholine

cholinergic [kəʊlɪˈnɜːdʒɪk] *adjective* (neurone or receptor) responding to acetylcholine

cholinesterase [kəʊlɪˈnestəreɪz] *noun* enzyme which breaks down a choline ester

choluria [kəʊˈljʊəriə] *noun* bile in the urine

chondr- [ˈkɒndr] *prefix* referring to cartilage

chondritis [kɒnˈdraɪtɪs] *noun* inflammation of a cartilage

chondroblast [ˈkɒndrəʊblæst] *noun* cell from which cartilage develops in an embryo

chondrocalcinosis [kɒndrəʊkælsɪˈnəʊsɪs] *noun* condition where deposits of calcium phosphate are found in articular cartilage

chondrocyte ['kɒndrəusaɪt] *noun* mature cartilage cell

chondrodysplasia [kɒndrəudɪs'pleɪziə] *noun* hereditary disorder of cartilage which is linked to dwarfism

chondrodystrophy [kɒndrəu'dɪstrəfi] *noun* general term for disorders of the cartilage

chondroma [kɒn'drəumə] *noun* tumour formed of cartilaginous tissue

chondromalacia [kɒndrəumə'leɪʃə] *noun* degeneration of the cartilage of a joint

chondrosarcoma [kɒndrəusɑː'kəumə] *noun* malignant, rapidly growing tumour involving cartilage cells

chorda ['kɔːdə] *noun* cord or tendon; **chordae tendineae** = tiny fibrous ligaments in the heart which attach the edges of some of the valves to the walls of the ventricles (NOTE: plural is **chordae**)

chordee ['kɔːdiː] *noun* painful condition where the erect penis is curved; a complication of gonorrhoea

chorditis [kɔː'daɪtɪs] *noun* inflammation of the vocal cords

chordotomy [kɔː'dɒtəmi] *noun* surgical operation to cut any cord, such as a nerve pathway in the spinal cord, to relieve intractable pain

chorea [kɔː'rɪə] *noun* sudden severe twitching (usually of the face and shoulders), symptom of disease of the nervous system; **Huntington's chorea** = progressive hereditary disease which affects adults, where the outer layer of the brain degenerates and the patient makes involuntary jerky movements and develops progressive dementia; **Sydenham's chorea** = temporary chorea affecting children, frequently associated with endocarditis and rheumatism

chorion ['kɔːrɪən] *noun* membrane covering the fertilized ovum

chorionic [kɔːrɪ'ɒnɪk] *adjective* referring to the chorion; **(human) chorionic gonadotrophin (hCG)** = hormone produced by the placenta, which suppresses the mother's normal menstrual cycle during pregnancy; it is found in the urine during pregnancy; it can be given by injection to encourage ovulation and help a woman to become pregnant

chorionic villi [kɔːrɪ'ɒnɪk 'vɪlaɪ] *noun* tiny finger-like folds in the chorion

choroid ['kɔːrɔɪd] *noun* middle layer of tissue which forms the eyeball, between the sclera and the retina; **choroid plexus** = part of the pia mater, a network of small blood vessels in the ventricles of the brain which produce cerebrospinal fluid; *see illustration at* EYE

choroiditis [kɔːrɔɪ'daɪtɪs] *noun* inflammation of the choroid in the eyeball

Christmas disease ['krɪsməs dɪ'ziːz] *noun* haemophilia B, clotting disorder of the blood, similar to haemophilia A, but in which the blood coagulates badly due to deficiency of Factor IX

COMMENT: haemophilia A is caused by deficiency of Factor VIII

Christmas factor ['krɪsməs 'fæktə] *noun* Factor IX, one of the coagulating factors in the blood

chrom- *or* **chromo-** ['krəum or 'krəuməu] *prefix* referring to colour

chromatid ['krəumətɪd] *noun* one of two parallel filaments making up a chromosome

chromatin ['krəumətɪn] *noun* network which forms the nucleus of a cell and can be stained with basic dyes; **sex chromatin** = Barr body, chromatin found only in female cells, which can be used to identify the sex of a baby before birth

chromatography [krəumə'tɒgrəfi] *noun* method of separating chemicals through a porous medium and analysing compounds; **gas chromatography** = chromatography where chemicals are passed through a gas before being analysed

chromatophore [krəu'mætəfɔː] *noun* any pigment-bearing cell in the eyes, hair and skin

chromicized catgut ['krəuməsaɪzd 'kætgʌt] *noun* catgut which is hardened with chromium to make it slower to dissolve in the body

chromium ['krəumiəm] *noun* metallic trace element (NOTE: chemical symbol is **Cr**)

chromosomal [krəumə'səuml] *adjective* referring to chromosomes; **chromosomal aberration** = CHROMOSOME ABERRATION; **chromosomal deletion** = abnormality in which a part of the chromosome is lost or removed

chromosome ['krəuməsəum] *noun* rod-shaped structure in the nucleus of a cell, formed of DNA which carries the genes;

chromosome aberration = abnormality in the number, arrangement, etc. of chromosomes; *see also* MAPPING

COMMENT: each human cell has 46 chromosomes, 23 inherited from each parent. The female has one pair of X chromosomes, and the male one pair of XY chromosomes, which are responsible for the sexual difference. Sperm from a male have either an X or a Y chromosome; if a Y chromosome sperm fertilizes the female's ovum the child will be male

chronic ['krɒnɪk] *adjective* (disease or condition) which lasts for a long time; *he has a chronic chest complaint*; *she is a chronic asthma sufferer*; **chronic fatigue syndrome** = MYALGIC ENCEPHALOMYELITIS; **chronic obstructive pulmonary disease (COPD)** = a group of progressive respiratory disorders such as emphysema and chronic bronchitis where patients experience loss of lung function which has little or no response to steroid or bronchodilator drug treatments (NOTE: the opposite is **acute**)

chrysotherapy [kraɪsəʊ'θerəpi] *noun* treatment which involves gold injections

chyle [kaɪl] *noun* fluid in the lymph vessels in the intestine which contains fat, especially after a meal

chylomicron [kaɪləʊ'maɪkrən] *noun* particle of chyle present in the blood

chyluria [kaɪ'ljʊəriə] *noun* presence of chyle in the urine

chyme [kaɪm] *noun* semi-liquid mass of food and gastric juices which passes from the stomach to the intestine

chymotrypsin [kaɪmə'trɪpsɪn] *noun* enzyme which digests protein

Ci *abbreviation for* curie

cicatrix ['sɪkətrɪks] *noun* scar, a mark on the skin, left when a wound or surgical incision has healed

-ciclovir ['sɪkləvɪə] *suffix* used for antiviral drugs; *aciclovir*

-cide [saɪd] *suffix* referring to killing

cilia ['sɪliə] *see* CILIUM

ciliary ['sɪliəri] *adjective* (i) referring to cilia; (ii) referring to the eyelid or eyelashes; **ciliary body** = part of the eye which connects the iris to the choroid; **ciliary muscle** = muscle which makes the lens of the eye change its shape to focus on objects at different distances; *see illustration at* EYE;

ciliary processes = series of ridges behind the iris to which the lens of the eye is attached

ciliated epithelium ['sɪlieɪtɪd epɪ'θiːliəm] *noun* simple epithelium where the cells have tiny hairs or cilia

cilium ['sɪliəm] *noun* **(a)** eyelash **(b)** one of many tiny hair-like processes which line cells in passages in the body and by moving backwards and forwards drive particles or fluid along the passage (NOTE: plural is **cilia**)

-cillin ['sɪlɪn] *suffix* used in names of penicillin drugs; *amoxycillin*

-cin [sɪn] *suffix* used for aminoglycosides; *gentamicin*

cinematics [sɪnə'mætɪks] *noun* science of movement, especially of body movements

cineplasty ['sɪnɪplæsti] *noun* amputation where the muscles of the stump of the amputated limb are used to operate an artificial limb

cineradiography [sɪnɪreɪdi'ɒgrəfi] *noun* taking a series of X-ray photographs for diagnosis, or to show how something moves or develops in the body

cinesiology [sɪniːsi'ɒlədʒi] *noun* study of muscle movements, particularly in relation to treatment

cingulectomy [sɪŋgju'lektəmi] *noun* surgical operation to remove the cingulum

cingulum ['sɪŋgjʊləm] *noun* long curved bundle of nerve fibres in the cerebrum (NOTE: plural is **cingula**)

circadian rhythm [sɜː'keɪdiən 'rɪðm] *noun* rhythm of daily activities and bodily processes (eating, defecating, sleeping, etc.) frequently controlled by hormones, which repeats every twenty-four hours

circle of Willis ['sɜːkl əv 'wɪlɪs] *noun* circle of branching arteries at the base of the brain formed by the basilar, anterior and posterior cerebral, anterior and posterior communicating, and internal carotid arteries

circular ['sɜːkjʊlə] *adjective* in the form of a circle; **circular fold** = large transverse fold of mucous membrane in the small intestine

circulate ['sɜːkjʊleɪt] *verb* (*of fluid*) to move around; *blood circulates around the body*; *bile circulates from the liver to the intestine through the bile ducts*

circulation [sɜːkjʊ'leɪʃn] *noun* **circulation (of the blood)** = movement of blood around the body from the heart through the arteries to the capillaries and back to the heart through the veins; *she has poor circulation in her legs*; *rub your hands to get the circulation going*; **collateral circulation** = enlargement of certain secondary blood vessels, as a response when the main vessels become slowly blocked; **pulmonary circulation** *or* **lesser circulation** = circulation of blood from the heart through the pulmonary arteries to the lungs for oxygenation and back to the heart through the pulmonary veins; **systemic circulation** *or* **greater circulation** = circulation of blood around the whole body (except the lungs) starting with the aorta and returning through the venae cavae

COMMENT: blood circulates around the body, carrying oxygen from the lungs and nutrients from the liver through the arteries and capillaries to the tissues; the capillaries exchange the oxygen for waste matter such as carbon dioxide which is taken back to the lungs to be expelled. At the same time the blood obtains more oxygen in the lungs to be taken to the tissues. The circulation pattern is as follows: blood returns through the veins to the right atrium of the heart; from there it is pumped through the right ventricle into the pulmonary artery, and then into the lungs. From the lungs it returns through the pulmonary veins to the left atrium of the heart and is pumped from there through the left ventricle into the aorta and from the aorta into the other arteries

circulatory [sɜːkjuˈleɪtri] *adjective* referring to the circulation of the blood; **circulatory system** = system of arteries and veins, together with the heart, which makes the blood circulate around the body

circumcise [ˈsɜːkəmsaɪz] *verb* to remove the foreskin of the penis

circumcision [sɜːkəmˈsɪʒn] *noun* surgical removal of the foreskin of the penis

circumduction [sɜːkəmˈdʌkʃn] *noun* moving a part in a circular motion

circumflex [ˈsɜːkəmfleks] *adjective* bent or curved; **circumflex arteries** = branches of the femoral artery in the upper thigh; **circumflex nerve** = sensory and motor nerve in the upper arm

circumvallate papillae [sɜːkəmˈvæleɪt pəˈpɪliː] *noun* large papillae at the base of the tongue, which have taste buds

cirrhosis [səˈrəʊsɪs] *noun* **cirrhosis of the liver** = hepatocirrhosis, condition where some cells of the liver die and are replaced by hard fibrous tissue

COMMENT: cirrhosis can have many causes: the commonest cause is alcoholism (alcoholic cirrhosis or Laennec's cirrhosis); it can also be caused by heart disease (cardiac cirrhosis), by viral hepatitis (postnecrotic cirrhosis), by autoimmune disease (primary biliary cirrhosis), or by obstruction or infection of the bile ducts (biliary cirrhosis)

cirrhotic [səˈrɒtɪk] *adjective* referring to cirrhosis; *the patient had a cirrhotic liver*

cirsoid [ˈsɜːsɔɪd] *adjective* dilated (as of a varicose vein); **cirsoid aneurysm** = condition where arteries become swollen and twisted

cistern *or* **cisterna** [ˈsɪstən or sɪˈstɜːnə] *noun* space containing fluid; **cisterna magna** = large space containing cerebrospinal fluid, situated underneath the cerebellum and behind the medulla oblongata; **lumbar cistern** = subarachnoid space in the spinal cord, where the dura mater ends, filled with cerebrospinal fluid

citric acid [ˈsɪtrɪk ˈæsɪd] *noun* acid found in fruit such as oranges, lemons and grapefruit

citric acid cycle [ˈsɪtrɪk ˈæsɪd ˈsaɪkl] *noun* Krebs cycle, an important series of events concerning amino acid metabolism, taking place in the mitochondria in the cell

citrullinaemia [sɪtrʊlɪˈniːmiə] *noun* deficiency of an enzyme which helps break down proteins

citrulline [ˈsɪtrʊliːn or ˈsɪtrʊlaɪn] *noun* an amino acid

CJD [ˈsiː ˈdʒeɪ ˈdiː] = CREUTZFELDT-JAKOB DISEASE; **new variant CJD** *or* **vCJD** = form of CJD which was observed first in the 1980s, especially affecting younger patients

Cl *chemical symbol for* chlorine

cl = CENTILITRE

clamp [klæmp] **1** *noun* surgical instrument to hold something tightly (such as a blood vessel during an operation) **2** *verb* to hold something tightly

clap [klæp] *noun* *(slang)* = GONORRHOEA

classic [ˈklæsɪk] *adjective* typically well-known (symptom); *she showed classic heroin withdrawal symptoms: sweating, fever, sleeplessness and anxiety*

classification [klæsɪfɪˈkeɪʃn] *noun* putting references or components into order so as to be able to refer to them again and identify them easily; *the ABO classification of blood*

classify ['klæsɪfaɪ] *verb* **(a)** to put references or components into order so as to be able to refer to them again and identify them easily; *the medical records are classified under the surname of the patient*; *blood groups are classified according to the ABO system* **(b)** to make information secret; *doctors' reports on patients are classified and may not be shown to the patients themselves*

claudication [klɔːdɪˈkeɪʃn] *noun* limping or being lame; **intermittent claudication** = condition caused by impairment of the arteries

COMMENT: at first, the patient limps after having walked a short distance, then finds walking progressively more difficult and finally impossible. The condition improves after rest

claustrophobia [klɔːstrəˈfəubiə] *noun* being afraid of enclosed spaces or crowded rooms

claustrophobic [klɔːstrəˈfəubik] *adjective* (room) which causes claustrophobia; (person) suffering from claustrophobia (NOTE: the opposite is **agoraphobia**)

clavicle ['klævɪkl] *noun* collarbone, one of two long thin bones which join the shoulder blades to the breastbone; *see illustration at* SHOULDER

clavicular [kləˈvɪkjulə] *adjective* referring to the clavicle

clavus ['kleɪvəs] *noun* **(a)** corn (on the foot) **(b)** severe pain in the head, like a nail being driven in

claw foot ['klɔː 'fut] *noun* pes cavus, deformed foot with the toes curved towards the instep and with a very high arch

claw hand ['klɔː 'hænd] *noun* deformed hand with the fingers (especially the ring finger and little finger) bent towards the palm, caused by paralysis of the muscles

clean [kliːn] **1** *adjective* not dirty; *the beds have clean sheets every morning*; *these plates aren't clean*; *the report suggested the hospital kitchens were not as clean as they should have been* (NOTE: clean - cleaner - cleanest) **2** *verb* to make clean by taking away dirt; *the nurses have to make sure the wards are cleaned before the inspection*; *have you cleaned your teeth today?*; *she was cleaning the patients' bathroom*

cleanliness ['klenlɪnəs] *noun* state of being clean; *the report criticized the cleanliness of the hospital kitchen*

cleanse [klenz] *verb* to make very clean

cleanser ['klenzə] *noun* powder or liquid which cleanses

clear [klɪə] **1** *adjective* **(a)** easily understood; *the doctor made it clear that he wanted the patient to have a home help*; *the words on the medicine bottle are not very clear* **(b)** which is not cloudy and which you can easily see through; *a clear glass bottle*; *the urine sample was clear, not cloudy* **(c)** **clear of** = free from; *the area is now clear of infection* (NOTE: clear - clearer - clearest) **2** *verb* to take away a blockage; *the inhalant will clear your blocked nose*; *he is on antibiotics to try to clear the congestion in his lungs*

clearance ['klɪərəns] *noun;* **renal clearance** = measurement of the rate at which kidneys filter impurities from blood

clearly ['klɪəli] *adverb* plainly or obviously; *the swelling is clearly visible on the patient's neck*

clear up ['klɪər 'ʌp] *verb* to get better; *his infection should clear up within a few days*; *I hope your cold clears up before the holiday*

cleavage ['kliːvɪdʒ] *noun* repeated division of cells in an embryo

cleft lip ['kleft 'lɪp] *noun* = HARELIP

cleft foot ['kleft 'fut] *noun* = TALIPES

cleft palate ['kleft 'pælət] *noun* congenital defect, where there is a fissure in the hard palate allowing the mouth and nasal cavities to be linked

COMMENT: a cleft palate is usually associated with a harelip. Both are due to incomplete fusion of the maxillary processes. Both can be successfully corrected by surgery

clerking ['klɑːkɪŋ] *noun (informal)* writing down the details of a patient on admission to a hospital

client ['klaɪənt] *noun* person visited by a health visitor or social worker

climacteric [klaɪˈmæktərɪk] *noun* **(a)** = MENOPAUSE **(b)** period of diminished sexual activity in a man who reaches middle age

clinic ['klɪnɪk] *noun* **(a)** small hospital or department in a large hospital which deals only with walking patients or which specializes in the treatment of certain conditions; *he is being treated in a private clinic*; *she was referred to an antenatal clinic*; **antenatal clinic** *or* **maternity clinic** = clinic where expectant mothers are taught how to look after babies, do exercises and have medical checkups; **physiotherapy clinic** = clinic where patients can have physiotherapy **(b)** group of students under a doctor or surgeon who examine patients and discuss their treatment

clinical ['klınıkl] *adjective* **(a)** (i) referring to a clinic; (ii) referring to a physical examination of patients by doctors (as opposed to a surgical operation, a laboratory test or experiment); **clinical effectiveness** = the ability of an intervention (procedure or treatment) to achieve the desired outcome; **clinical governance** = the responsibility given to doctors to co-ordinate audit, research, education, use of guidelines and risk management to develop a strategy to raise the quality of medical care; **clinical medicine** = treatment of patients in a hospital ward or in the doctor's surgery (as opposed to the operating theatre or laboratory); **clinical nurse specialist** = nurse who specializes in a particular branch of clinical care; **clinical thermometer** = thermometer for taking a patient's body temperature; **clinical trial** = trial carried out in a medical laboratory on a patient or on tissue from a patient **(b)** referring to instruction given to students at the bedside of patients as opposed to class instruction with no patient present

we studied 69 patients who met the clinical and laboratory criteria of definite MS

Lancet

the allocation of students to clinical areas is for their educational needs and not for service requirements

Nursing Times

clinically ['klınıkli] *adverb* using information gathered from the treatment of patients in a hospital ward or in the doctor's surgery; *smallpox is now clinically extinct*

clinician [klı'nıʃn] *noun* doctor, usually not a surgeon, who has considerable experience in treating patients

clip [klıp] **1** *noun* piece of metal with a spring, used to attach things together; **Michel's clips** = clips used to suture a wound **2** *verb* to attach together; *the case notes are*

clipped together with the patient's record card

clitoris ['klıtərıs] *noun* small erectile female sex organ, a structure in females, situated at the anterior angle of the vulva, which can be excited by sexual activity; *see illustrations at* UROGENITAL SYSTEM (FEMALE)

cloaca [kləu'eıkə] *noun* end part of the hindgut in an embryo

clone [kləun] **1** *noun* group of cells derived from a single cell by asexual reproduction and so identical to the first cell **2** *verb* to reproduce an individual organism by asexual means

clonic ['klɒnık] *adjective* (i) referring to clonus; (ii) having spasmodic contractions

cloning ['kləunıŋ] *noun* reproduction of an individual organism by asexual means

clonorchiasis [kləunə'kaıəsıs] *noun* liver condition, common in the Far East, caused by the fluke *Clonorchis sinensis*

clonus ['kləunəs] *noun* rhythmic contraction and relaxation of a muscle (usually a sign of upper motor neurone lesions)

close [kləuz] *verb (of wound)* to be covered with new tissue

Clostridium [klɒ'strıdıəm] *noun* type of bacteria

COMMENT: species of Clostridium cause botulism, tetanus and gas gangrene

clot [klɒt] **1** *noun* soft mass of coagulated blood in a vein or an artery; *the doctor diagnosed a blood clot in the brain*; *blood clots occur in thrombosis* **2** *verb* to coagulate, to change from liquid to semi-solid; *his blood does not clot easily* (NOTE: **clotting - clotted**)

clothes [kləuðz] *noun* things worn to cover the body and keep a person warm; *all his clothes had to be destroyed*; *you ought to put some clean clothes on*; **bedclothes** = sheets and blankets which cover a bed

clotting ['klɒtıŋ] *noun* action of coagulating; **clotting factors** = coagulation factors, substances (called Factor I, Factor II, and so on) in plasma which act one after the other to make the blood coagulate when a blood vessel is damaged; **clotting time** = coagulation time, the time taken for blood to coagulate under normal conditions

COMMENT: deficiency in one or more of the clotting factors results in haemophilia

cloud [klaʊd] *noun* **(a)** (i) light white or grey mass of water vapour or ice particles in the sky which can produce rain; (ii) mass of particles suspended in the air; *I think it is going to rain - look at those grey clouds*; *clouds of smoke were pouring out of the house* **(b)** disturbed sediment in a liquid

cloudy ['klaʊdi] *adjective* (i) (sky) which is covered with clouds; (ii) (liquid) which is not transparent but which has an opaque substance in it; *the patient is passing cloudy urine*

clubbing ['klʌbɪŋ] *noun* thickening of the ends of the fingers and toes, a sign of many different diseases

club foot ['klʌb 'fʊt] *noun* talipes, a congenitally deformed foot

COMMENT: the most usual form (talipes equinovarus) is where the person walks on the toes, because the foot is permanently bent forward; in other forms, the foot either turns towards the inside (talipes varus), towards the outside (talipes valgus) or upwards (talipes calcaneus) at the ankle so that the patient cannot walk on the sole of the foot

cluster ['klʌstə] *noun* group of small items which cling together; **cluster headache** = headache which occurs behind one eye for a short period

Clutton's joint ['klʌtənz 'dʒɔɪnt] *noun* swollen knee joint occurring in congenital syphilis

cm = CENTIMETRE

CMV = CYTOMEGALOVIRUS

C/N = CHARGE NURSE

CNS ['si: 'en 'es] = CENTRAL NERVOUS SYSTEM

Co *chemical symbol for* cobalt

coagulant [kəʊ'ægjʊlənt] *noun* substance which can make blood clot

coagulase [kəʊ'ægjʊleɪz] *noun* enzyme produced by Staphylococci which makes blood plasma clot

coagulate [kəʊ'ægjʊleɪt] *verb* to clot, to change from liquid to semi-solid; *his blood does not coagulate easily*

COMMENT: blood coagulates with the conversion into fibrin of fibrinogen, a

protein in the blood, under the influence of the enzyme thromboplastin

coagulation [kəʊægjʊ'leɪʃn] *noun* action of clotting; **coagulation factors** = CLOTTING FACTORS; **coagulation time** = CLOTTING TIME

coagulum [kəʊ'ægjʊləm] *noun* blood clot, mass of clotted blood

coalescence [kəʊə'lesəns] *noun (of wound edges)* coming together when healing

coarctation [kəʊɑːk'teɪʃn] *noun* narrowing; **coarctation of the aorta** = congenital narrowing of the aorta which results in high blood pressure in the upper part of the body and low blood pressure in the lower part

coarse [kɔːs] *adjective* rough, not fine; *coarse hair grows on parts of the body at puberty*; *disease characterized by coarse features*

coat [kəʊt] **1** *noun* layer of material covering an organ or a cavity; **muscle coats** = two layers of muscle forming part of the lining of the intestine **2** *verb* to cover

coating ['kəʊtɪŋ] *noun* covering; *pill with a sugar coating*

cobalt ['kəʊbɒlt] *noun* metallic element; **cobalt 60** = radioactive isotope which is used in radiotherapy to treat cancer (NOTE: chemical symbol is **Co**)

cocaine [kə'keɪn] *noun* alkaloid from the coca plant, sometimes used as a local anaesthetic but not generally used because its use leads to addiction

coccidioidomycosis [kɒksɪdɪɔɪdəʊmaɪ'kəʊsɪs] *noun* lung disease, caused by inhaling spores of the fungus *Coccidioides immitis*

coccus ['kɒkəs] *noun* bacterium shaped like a ball (NOTE: plural is **cocci**)

COMMENT: cocci grow together in groups: either in groups (staphylococci) or in long chains (streptococci)

coccy- ['kɒksi] *prefix* referring to the coccyx

coccydynia *or* **coccygodynia** [kɒksi'dɪnɪə or kɒksɪgəʊ'dɪnɪə] *noun* sharp pain in the coccyx, usually caused by a blow

coccygeal vertebrae [kɒk'sɪdʒɪəl 'vɜːtɪbreɪ] *noun* fused bones in the coccyx

coccyx ['kɒksɪks] *noun* lowest bones in the backbone (NOTE: plural is **coccyges**); *see illustration at* VERTEBRAL COLUMN

COMMENT: the coccyx is a rudimentary tail made of four bones which have fused together into a bone in the shape of a triangle

cochlea ['kɒkliə] *noun* spiral tube, shaped like a snail shell, inside the inner ear, which is the essential organ of hearing; *see illustration at* EAR

COMMENT: sounds are transmitted as vibrations to the cochlea from the ossicles through the oval window. The lymph fluid in the cochlea passes the vibrations to the organ of Corti which in turn is connected to the auditory nerve

cochlear ['kɒkliə] *adjective* referring to the cochlea; **cochlear duct** = spiral channel in the cochlea; **cochlear implant** = type of hearing aid for profound hearing loss; **cochlear nerve** = division of the auditory nerve

code [kəʊd] **1** *noun* signs which have a hidden meaning; **genetic code** = characteristics which exist in the DNA of a cell and are passed on when the cell divides and so are inherited by a child from a parent **2** *verb* to give a meaning; *genes are sequences of DNA that code for specific proteins*; **coding gene** = gene which carries a particular genetic code

codeine ['kəʊdi:n] *noun; see* DRUGS TABLE IN SUPPLEMENT

cod liver oil ['kɒd 'lɪvə 'ɔɪl] *noun* oil from the liver of codfish, which is rich in calories and vitamins A and D

codon ['kəʊdɒn] *noun* group of three of the four basic elements in DNA (adenine, cytosine, guanine and thymine) which translates into a specific amino acid and so determines protein structure

-coele [si:l] *suffix* referring to a hollow

coeli- *or* **coelio** ['si:li or 'si:liəʊ] *prefix* referring to a hollow, usually the abdomen (NOTE: words beginning **coeli-** are spelled **celi-** in American English)

coeliac ['si:liæk] *adjective* referring to the abdomen; **coeliac artery** *or* **coeliac axis** *or* **coeliac trunk** = main artery in the abdomen leading from the abdominal aorta and dividing into the left gastric, hepatic and splenic arteries; **coeliac disease** = gluten enteropathy or malabsorption syndrome, an allergic disease (mainly affecting children) in which the lining of the intestine is sensitive to gluten, preventing the small intestine from digesting fat; **adult coeliac disease** = condition in adults where the villi in the intestine become smaller and so reduce the surface which can absorb nutrients; **coeliac plexus** = network of nerves in the abdomen, behind the stomach

COMMENT: symptoms of coeliac disease include a swollen abdomen, pale diarrhoea, abdominal pains and anaemia

coelioscopy [si:li'ɒskəpi] *noun* examining the peritoneal cavity by inflating the abdomen with sterile air and passing an endoscope through the abdominal wall

coelom ['si:ləm] *noun* body cavity in an embryo, which divides to form the thorax and abdomen

coffee ground vomit ['kɒfi 'graʊnd 'vɒmɪt] *noun* vomit containing dark pieces of blood, indicating that the patient is bleeding from the stomach or upper intestine

cognitive ['kɒgnɪtɪv] *adjective* referring to the mental processes of perception, memory, judgement and reasoning; *a cognitive disorder or impairment*

cohort study ['kəʊhɔ:t 'stʌdi] *noun* an investigation in which a group of people (a cohort) without the disease are classified according to their exposure to a certain risk and are studied over a period of time to see if they develop the disease, in order to study links between risk and disease;

coil [kɔɪl] *noun* spiral metal wire fitted into a woman's uterus as a contraceptive

coiled [kɔɪld] *adjective* spiral, twisted round and round; *a coiled tube at the end of a nephron*

coital ['kəʊɪtl] *adjective* referring to coitus

coition [kəʊ'ɪʃn] *noun* sexual intercourse

coitus ['kəʊɪtəs] *noun* sexual intercourse; **coitus interruptus** = form of contraception where the penis is removed from the vagina before ejaculation

COMMENT: this is not a safe method of contraception

cold [kəʊld] **1** *adjective* not warm, not hot; *he always has a cold shower in the morning*; *the weather is colder than last week and they say it will be even colder tomorrow*; *many old people suffer from hypothermia in cold weather*; *cold drinks give him colic pains*; **cold burn** = injury to the skin caused by exposure to extreme cold or by touching a very cold surface; **cold compress** = wad of cloth soaked in cold water, used to relieve a headache or bruise; **cold sore** = herpes simplex, a burning sore, usually on the lips **2** *noun;* **common cold** *or* **cold in the head** = coryza, an illness, with inflammation of the nasal passages, in which the patient sneezes and coughs and has a blocked and running nose; *he caught a cold by standing in the rain; she's got a cold so she can't go out; mother's in bed with a cold; don't come near me - I've got a cold and you may catch it*

COMMENT: a cold usually starts with a virus infection which causes inflammation of the mucous membrane in the nose and throat. Symptoms include running nose, cough and loss of taste and smell; there is no cure for a cold at present, though the coronavirus which causes a cold has been identified

colectomy [kə'lektəmi] *noun* surgical removal of the whole or part of the colon

coli ['kəʊlaɪ] *see* TAENIA

colic ['kɒlɪk] *noun* (a) enteralgia, pain in any part of the intestinal tract; **biliary colic** = pain in the abdomen caused by gallstones in the bile duct or by inflammation of the gall bladder; **mucous colic** = inflammation of the colon, with painful spasms in the muscles of the walls of the colon; **renal colic** = sudden pain caused by kidney stone or stones in the ureter (b) **right colic** *or* **middle colic** = arteries which lead from the superior mesenteric artery

COMMENT: although colic can refer to pain caused by indigestion, it can also be caused by stones in the gall bladder or kidney

colicky ['kɒlɪki] *adjective* referring to colic; *he had colicky pains in his abdomen*

coliform bacteria ['kəʊlifɔːm bæk'tɪərɪə] *plural noun* bacteria which are similar to *Bacterium coli*

colitis [kə'laɪtɪs] *noun* inflammation of the colon; **mucous colitis** = irritable bowel syndrome, inflammation of the mucous membrane in the intestine, where the patient suffers pain caused by spasms in the muscles of the walls of the colon; **ulcerative colitis** = severe pain in the colon, with diarrhoea and ulcers in the rectum, often with a psychosomatic cause

collagen ['kɒlədʒən] *noun* bundles of protein fibres, which form the connective tissue, bone and cartilage; **collagen disease** = any of several diseases of the connective tissue; **collagen fibre** = fibre which is the main component of fasciae, tendons and ligaments, and is essential in bone and cartilage

COMMENT: collagen diseases include rheumatic fever, rheumatoid arthritis, periarteritis nodosa, scleroderma and dermatomyositis. Collagen diseases can be treated with cortisone

collagenous [kə'lædʒɪnəs] *adjective* (i) containing collagen; (ii) referring to collagen disease

collapse [kə'læps] **1** *noun* condition where a patient is extremely exhausted or semi-conscious; *he was found in a state of collapse* **2** *verb* **(a)** to fall down in a semi-conscious state; *after running to catch his train he collapsed* **(b)** to become flat, to lose air; **collapsed lung** = *see* PNEUMOTHORAX

collar ['kɒlə] *noun* part of a coat, shirt, etc. which goes round the neck; *my shirt collar's too tight; she turned up her coat collar because of the wind*; **cervical collar** *or* **neck collar** *or* **orthopaedic collar** *or* **surgical collar** = special strong collar to support the head of a patient with neck injuries or a condition such as cervical spondylosis

collarbone ['kɒləbəʊn] *noun* clavicle, one of two long thin bones which join the shoulder blades to the breastbone; **collarbone fracture** = fracture of the collarbone (one of the most frequent fractures in the body)

collateral [kə'lætərəl] *adjective* secondary or less important; **collateral circulation** = enlargement of certain secondary blood vessels, as a response when the main vessels become slowly blocked

embolization of the coeliac axis is an effective treatment for severe bleeding in the stomach or duodenum, localized by endoscopic examination. A good collateral blood supply makes occlusion of a single branch of the coeliac axis safe

British Medical Journal

collect [kə'lekt] *verb* to bring various things together; to come together; *fluid collects in the tissues of patients suffering from heart or kidney failure*

collecting duct [kəˈlektɪŋ ˈdʌkt] *noun* part of the system by which urine is filtered in the kidney

collection [kəˈlekʃn] *noun* bringing together of various things; *the hospital has a collection of historical surgical instruments*

college [ˈkɒlɪdʒ] *noun* place of further education where people study after they have left secondary school; *I'm going to college to study pharmacy*

Colles' fracture [ˈkɒlɪsɪz ˈfræktʃə] *see* FRACTURE

colliculus [kəˈlɪkjʊləs] *noun* one of four small projections (the superior and inferior colliculi) in the midbrain; *see illustration at* BRAIN (NOTE: the plural is **colliculi**)

collodion [kəˈləʊdiən] *noun* liquid used to paint on a clean wound, where it dries to form a flexible covering

collyrium [kəˈlɪriəm] *noun* solution used to bathe the eyes

colo- [ˈkɒləʊ] *prefix meaning* colon

coloboma [kɒləʊˈbəʊmə] *noun* condition where part of the eye, especially part of the iris, is missing

colon [ˈkəʊlən] *noun* the main part of the large intestine (running from the caecum at the end of the small intestine to the rectum); **ascending colon** = first part of the colon which goes up the right side of the body from the caecum; **descending colon** = third section of the colon which goes down the left side of the body; **sigmoid colon** *or* **pelvic colon** = fourth section of the colon which continues as the rectum; **transverse colon** = second section of the colon which crosses the body below the stomach; **irritable** *or* **spastic colon** = MUCOUS COLITIS; *see illustration at* DIGESTIVE SYSTEM

> COMMENT: the colon is about 1.35 metres in length, and rises from the end of the small intestine up the right side of the body, then crosses beneath the stomach and drops down the left side of the body to end as the rectum. In the colon, water is extracted from the waste material which has passed through the small intestine, leaving only the faeces which are pushed forward by peristaltic movements and passed out of the body through the rectum

colonic [kəʊˈlɒnɪk] *adjective* referring to the colon; **colonic irrigation** = washing out of the large intestine

colonoscope [kəˈlɒnəskəʊp] *noun* surgical instrument for examining the interior of the colon

colonoscopy [kɒləˈnɒskəpi] *noun* examination of the inside of the colon, using a colonoscope passed through the rectum

colony [ˈkɒləni] *noun* group or culture of microorganisms

colostomy [kəˈlɒstəmi] *noun* surgical operation to make an opening (stoma) between the colon and the abdominal wall to allow faeces to be passed out without going through the rectum

> COMMENT: a colostomy is carried out when the colon or rectum is blocked, or where part of the colon or rectum has had to be removed

colostomy bag [kəˈlɒstəmi ˈbæg] *noun* bag attached to the opening made by a colostomy, to collect faeces as they are passed out of the body

colostrum [kəˈlɒstrəm] *noun* fluid rich in antibodies and low in fat, secreted by the breasts at the birth of a baby, but before the true milk starts to flow

colour *US* **color** [ˈkʌlə] **1** *noun* differing wavelengths of light (red, blue, yellow, etc.) which are reflected from objects and sensed by the eyes; *what is the colour of a healthy liver?*; *the diseased parts are shown by the colour red on the chart*; *he looks unwell, and his face has no colour* **2** *verb* to give colour to; *the arteries are coloured red on the diagram*; *bile colours the urine yellow*

colour-blind [ˈkʌləˈblaɪnd] *adjective* not able to tell the difference between certain colours; *several of the students are colour-blind*

colour blindness [ˈkʌlə ˈblaɪndnəs] *noun* being unable to tell the difference between certain colours

> COMMENT: colour blindness is a condition which almost never occurs in women. The commonest form is the inability to tell the difference between red and green. The Ishihara test is used to test for colour blindness

colouring (matter) [ˈkʌlərɪŋ ˈmætə] *noun* substance which colours an organ

colourless [ˈkʌlələs] *adjective* with no colour; *a colourless fluid was discharged from the sore*

colp- *or* **colpo-** ['kɒlp *or* 'kɒlpəʊ] *prefix* referring to the vagina

colpocele ['kɒlpəsiːl] = COLPOPTOSIS

colpocystitis [kɒlpəsɪs'taɪtɪs] *noun* inflammation of both the vagina and the urinary bladder

colpocystopexy [kɒlpə'sɪstəpeksi] *noun* surgical operation to lift and stitch the vagina and bladder to the abdominal wall

colpopexy ['kɒlpəpeksi] *noun* surgical operation to fix a prolapsed vagina to the abdominal wall

colpoplasty ['kɒlpəplæsti] *noun* surgical operation to repair a damaged vagina

colpoptosis [kɒlpə'təʊsɪs] *noun* prolapse of the walls of the vagina

colporrhaphy [kɒl'pɒrəfi] *noun* surgical operation to suture a prolapsed vagina

colposcope ['kɒlpəʊskəʊp] *noun* surgical instrument used to examine the inside of the vagina

colposcopy [kɒl'pɒskəpi] *noun* examination of the inside of the vagina

colpotomy [kɒl'pɒtəmi] *noun* any surgical operation to make a cut in the vagina

column ['kɒləm] *noun* usually circular mass standing upright like a tree; **spinal column** *or* **vertebral column** = backbone, the series of bones and discs which forms a flexible column running from the pelvis to the skull

columnar [kə'lʌmnə] *adjective* shaped like a column; **columnar cell** = type of epithelial cell

coma ['kəʊmə] *noun* state of unconsciousness from which a person cannot be awakened by external stimuli; *he went into a coma and never regained consciousness*; *she has been in a coma for four days*; **diabetic coma** = unconsciousness caused by untreated diabetes

COMMENT: a coma can have many causes: head injuries, diabetes, stroke, drug overdose. A coma is often fatal, but a patient may continue to live in a coma for a long time, even several months, before dying or regaining consciousness

comatose ['kəʊmətəʊs] *adjective* (i) unconscious, in a coma; (ii) like a coma

combat ['kɒmbæt] *verb* to fight against; *the medical team is combating an outbreak of* diphtheria; *what can we do to combat the spread of the disease?*

combination [kɒmbɪ'neɪʃn] *noun* act of joining together; *actomyosin is a combination of actin and myosin*

combine [kəm'baɪn] *verb* to join together

comedo ['kɒmɪdəʊ] *noun* blackhead, a small point of dark, hard matter in a sebaceous follicle, often found associated with acne on the skin of adolescents (NOTE: the plural is **comedones**)

comfort ['kʌmfət] *verb* to make relaxed, to help make a patient less miserable; *the paramedics comforted the injured until the ambulance arrived*

commensal [kə'mensl] *noun & adjective* (plant or animal) which lives on another plant or animal, but does not harm it in any way and both may benefit from the association; *Candida is a normal commensal in the mouths of 50% of healthy adults* (NOTE: if it causes harm it is a **parasite**)

comminuted fracture ['kɒmɪnjuːtɪd 'fræktʃə] *noun* fracture where the bone is broken in several places

commissure ['kɒmɪsjʊə] *noun* structure which joins two tissues of similar material, such as a group of nerves which crosses from one part of the central nervous system to another; **grey commissure** *or* **white commissure** = parts of grey and white matter in the spinal cord nearest the central canal; *see also* CORPUS CALLOSUM

commode [kə'məʊd] *noun* special chair with a removable basin used as a toilet by patients with limited mobility

common ['kɒmən] *adjective* (a) ordinary or not exceptional; which happens very frequently; *accidents are quite common on this part of the motorway*; *it's a common mistake to believe that cancer is always fatal*; **common cold** = coryza, a virus infection which causes inflammation of the mucous membrane in the nose and throat (b) (in) **common** = belonging to more than one thing or person; *haemophilia and Christmas disease have several symptoms in common*; **common bile duct** = duct leading to the duodenum, formed of the hepatic and cystic ducts; **common carotid artery** = large artery in the lower part of the neck; **common hepatic duct** = duct from the liver formed when the right and left hepatic ducts join; **common iliac arteries** = arteries which branch from the aorta and divide into the internal and external iliac arteries; **common iliac veins** = veins draining the legs, pelvis and abdomen, which unite to form the inferior vena cava; **final common pathway** = linked neurones which take all impulses from the central nervous system to a muscle

commonly ['kɒmənli] *adverb* which happens often; *a cold winter commonly brings a flu epidemic*

communicable disease [kə'mjuːnɪkəbl dɪ'ziːz] *noun* disease which can be passed from one person to another or from an animal to a person; *see also* CONTAGIOUS, INFECTIOUS

communicate [kə'mjuːnɪkeɪt] *verb* to pass a message to someone or something; *autistic children do not communicate, even with their parents*; **communicating arteries** = arteries which connect the blood supply from each side of the brain, forming part of the circle of Willis

community [kə'mjuːnəti] *noun* group of people who live and work in a district; *the health services serve the local community*; *community care is an important part of primary health care*; **community health council (CHC)** = statutory body of interested lay people charged with putting forward the patients' point of view on local health issues; *(public health medicine)* **community medicine** = study of medical practice which examines groups of people and the health of the community, including housing, pollution and other environmental factors; **community nurse** = nurse who treats patients in a local community; **community physician** = doctor who specializes in community medicine; **Community Psychiatric Nurse (CPN)** = psychiatric nurse who works in a district, visiting various patients in the area; **community services** = nursing services which are available to the community

compact bone ['kɒmpækt 'bəʊn] *noun* type of bone tissue which forms the hard outer layer of a bone; *see illustration at* BONE STRUCTURE

compatibility [kəmpætə'bɪləti] *noun* (i) ability of two drugs not to interfere with each other when administered together; (ii) ability of a body to accept organs, tissue or blood from another person and not to reject them

compatible [kəm'pætəbl] *adjective* able to work together without being rejected; *the surgeons are trying to find a compatible donor or a donor with a compatible blood group*

compensate ['kɒmpenseɪt] *verb (of an organ)* to make good the failure of another organ; *the heart has to beat more strongly to compensate for the narrowing of the arteries*

complain [kəm'pleɪn] *verb* to say that something is not good; *the patients have complained about the food*; *he is complaining of pains in his legs*

complaint [kəm'pleɪnt] *noun* **(a)** illness; *he is suffering from a nervous complaint* **(b)** saying that something is wrong; *the hospital administrator wouldn't listen to the complaints of the consultants*

complement ['kɒmplɪmənt] *noun* substance which forms part of blood plasma and is essential to the work of antibodies and antigens; **complement fixation test (CFT)** = test to measure the amount of complement in antibodies and antigens

complete blood count (CBC) [kəm'pliːt 'blʌd 'kaʊnt] *noun* test to find the exact numbers of each type of blood cell in a certain amount of blood

complex ['kɒmpleks] **1** *noun* **(a)** *(in psychiatry)* group of ideas which are based on the experience a person has had in the past, and which influence the way he behaves; **Electra complex** = condition where a woman feels sexually attracted to her father and sees her mother as an obstacle; **inferiority complex** = condition where the person feels he is inferior to others; **OEdipus complex** = condition where a man feels sexually attracted to his mother and sees his father as an obstacle; **superiority complex** = condition where the person feels he is superior to others and pays little attention to them **(b)** group of items, buildings or organs; *he works in the new laboratory complex*; **primary complex** = first lymph node to be infected by TB; **Vitamin B complex** = group of vitamins such as folic acid, riboflavine and thiamine **(c)** syndrome, a group of signs and symptoms due to a particular cause **2** *adjective* complicated; *a gastrointestinal fistula can cause many complex problems, including fluid depletion*

complexion [kəm'plekʃn] *noun* general colour of the skin on the face; *he has a red complexion*; *she has a fine pink complexion*; *people with fair complexions burn easily in the sun*

compliance [kɒm'plaɪəns] *noun* the agreement of a patient to co-operate with a treatment

complicated fracture ['kɒmplɪkeɪtɪd 'fræktʃə] *noun* fracture with an associated injury of tissue, as where the bone has punctured an artery

complication [kɒmplɪ'keɪʃn] *noun* **(a)** condition where two or more diseases exist in a patient, and are not always connected **(b)** situation where a patient develops a second disease which changes the course of treatment for the first; *he was admitted to hospital suffering from pneumonia with complications*; *she appeared to be improving, but complications set in and she died in a few hours*

sickle cell chest syndrome is a common complication of sickle cell disease, presenting with chest pain, fever and leucocytosis

British Medical Journal

venous air embolism is a potentially fatal complication of percutaneous venous catheterization

Southern Medical Journal

component [kəm'pəʊnənt] *noun* substance or element which forms part of a complete item

compose [kəm'pəʊz] *verb* to make up; *the lotion is composed of oil, calamine and camphor*

composition [kɒmpə'zɪʃn] *noun* way in which a compound is formed; **chemical composition** = the chemicals which make up a substance; *they analysed the blood samples to find out their chemical composition*

compos mentis ['kɒmpɒs 'mentɪs] *Latin phrase meaning* of sound mind, sane; *the patient was non compos mentis when he attacked the doctor*

compound ['kɒmpaʊnd] *noun* chemical substance made up of two or more components

compound fracture ['kɒmpaʊnd 'fræktʃə] *noun* fracture where the skin surface is damaged or where the broken bone penetrates the surface of the skin

compress 1 ['kɒmpres] *noun* wad of cloth soaked in hot or cold liquid and applied to the skin to relieve pain or to force pus out of an infected wound **2** [kəm'pres] *verb* to squeeze, to press; **compressed air sickness** = CAISSON DISEASE

compression [kəm'preʃn] *noun* **(a)** squeezing, pressing; *the first aider applied compression to the chest of the casualty*; **compression stockings** = strong elastic stockings worn to support a weak joint in the knee or to hold varicose veins tightly; **compression syndrome** = pain in muscles after strenuous exercise **(b)** serious condition where the brain is compressed by blood or cerebrospinal fluid accumulating in it or by a fractured skull

compulsive [kəm'pʌlsɪv] *adjective* (feeling) which cannot be stopped; *she has a compulsive desire to steal*; **compulsive eating** = psychological condition where the patient has a continual desire to eat; *see also* BULIMIA

computer [kəm'pju:tə] *noun* machine programmed to receive, store or process data

computerized axial tomography (CAT) *or* **computed tomography (CT)** [kəm'pju:təraɪzd 'æksɪəl tə'mɒgrəfi] *noun* system of scanning a patient's body, where a narrow X-ray beam, guided by a computer, can photograph a thin section of the body or of an organ from several angles, using the computer to build up an image of the section

-conazole ['kɒnəzəʊl] *suffix* used for antifungal drugs; *fluconazole*

concave ['kɒnkeɪv] *adjective* which curves towards the inside; *a concave lens*

conceive [kən'si:v] *verb* **(a)** *(of woman)* to become pregnant; *see* CONCEPTION **(b)** *(of child)* **to be conceived** = to start existence; *our son was conceived during our holiday in Italy*

concentrate ['kɒnsəntreɪt] **1** *noun* **(a)** strength of a solution **(b)** way of showing amounts of a substance in body tissues and fluids **(c)** strong solution which is to be diluted **2** *verb* **(a) to concentrate on** = to examine something in particular **(b)** to reduce a solution and increase its strength by evaporation

conception [kən'sepʃn] *noun* point at which a woman becomes pregnant and the development of a baby starts

COMMENT: conception is usually taken to be the moment when the sperm cell fertilizes the ovum, or a few days later, when the fertilized ovum attaches itself to the wall of the uterus

conceptus [kən'septəs] *noun* result of the fertilized ovum which will develop into an embryo and fetus

concha ['kɒŋkə] *noun* part of the body shaped like a shell; **concha auriculae** = part of the outer ear; **nasal conchae** = little projections of bone which form the sides of the nasal cavity (NOTE: the plural is **conchae**)

concretion [kən'kri:ʃn] *noun* mass of hard material which forms in the body (such as a gallstone or deposits on bone in arthritis)

concussed [kən'kʌst] *adjective* (person) who has been hit on the head and has lost and then regained consciousness; *he was walking around in a concussed state*

concussion [kən'kʌʃn] *noun* **(a)** applying force to any part of the body **(b)** disturbance of the brain, loss of consciousness for a short period, caused by a blow to the head

concussive [kən'kʌsɪv] *adjective* which causes concussion

condensed [kən'denst] *adjective* made compact or more dense

condition [kən'dɪʃn] *noun* **(a)** state (of health or of cleanliness); *the arteries are in very · good condition; he is ill, and his condition is getting worse; conditions in the hospital are very bad* **(b)** illness, injury or disorder; *he is being treated for a heart condition*

conditioned reflex [kən'dɪʃnd 'ri:fleks] *noun* automatic reaction by a person to a stimulus, a normal reaction to a normal stimulus which comes from past experience

condom ['kɒndəm] *noun* rubber sheath worn on the penis during intercourse as a contraceptive and also as a protection against sexually transmitted disease; **female condom** = rubber sheath inserted into the vagina before intercourse, covering the walls of the vagina and the cervix

conducting system [kən'dʌktɪŋ 'sɪstəm] *noun* nerve system in the heart which links an atrium to a ventricle, so that the two beat at the same rate

conduction [kən'dʌkʃn] *noun* passing of heat, sound or nervous impulses from one part of the body to another; **conduction fibres** = fibres (as in the bundle of His) which transmit impulses; **air conduction** = conduction of sounds from the outside to the inner ear through the auditory meatus; **bone conduction** = osteophony, conduction of

sound waves to the inner ear through the bones of the skull; *see also* RINNE'S TEST

conductive [kən'dʌktɪv] *adjective* referring to conduction; **conductive deafness** *or* **conductive hearing loss** = deafness caused by a disorder in the conduction of sound into the inner ear, rather than a disorder of the hearing nerves

conduit ['kɒndjuɪt] *noun* channel or passage along which a fluid flows; **ileal conduit** = using a loop of the ileum to which one or both ureters are anastomosed, in order to drain urine from the body

condyle ['kɒndaɪl] *noun* rounded end of a bone which articulates with another; **occipital condyle** = round part of the occipital bone which joins it to the atlas

condyloid process ['kɒndɪlɔɪd 'prəuses] *noun* projecting part at each end of the lower jaw which forms the head of the jaw, joining the jaw to the skull

condyloma [kɒndɪ'ləumə] *noun* growth usually found on the vulva

cone [kəun] **1** *noun* one of two types of cell in the retina of the eye which is sensitive to light; *see also* ROD **2** *verb* (life-threatening process) to undergo rapid deterioration of neurological status due to herniation of the midbrain through the foramen magnum in the skull, caused by raised intracranial pressure

COMMENT: cones are sensitive to bright light and colours and do not function in bad light

confidentiality [kɒnfɪdenʃi'æləti] *noun* obligation not to reveal professional information

confined [kən'faɪnd] *adjective* kept in a place; *she was confined to bed with pneumonia; since his accident he has been confined to a wheelchair*

confinement [kən'faɪnmənt] *noun* period when a woman stays in (hospital) from the beginning of labour and until some time after the birth of her baby (this period is very short nowadays)

confirm [kən'fɜ:m] *verb* to agree officially that something is true; *X-rays confirmed the presence of a tumour; the number of confirmed cases of the disease has doubled*

confounding factor [kən'faundɪŋ 'fæktə] *noun* factor which has an association with both a disease and an exposure and thus interferes with the true association between disease and exposure, such as an association found between coffee drinking and myocardial infarction could be explained by the effect of smoking, which is associated with both coffee drinking and with myocardial infarction

confuse [kən'fju:z] *verb* to make someone think wrongly; to make things difficult for someone to understand; *the patient was confused by the physiotherapist's instructions*

confused [kən'fju:zd] *adjective (of patient)* not clearly aware of where one is or what one is doing; *old people can easily become confused if they are moved from their homes; many severely confused patients do not respond to spoken communication*

confusion [kən'fju:ʒn] *noun* being confused; *he has attacks of mental confusion; the absence of any effective treatment for confusion*

congeal [kən'dʒi:l] *verb (of fat or blood)* to become solid

congenita [kən'dʒenɪtə] *see* AMYOTONIA

congenital [kən'dʒenɪtl] *adjective* which exists at or before birth; **congenital defect** *or* **anomaly** = birth defect, a malformation which exists in a person's body from birth; **congenital dislocation of the hip (CDH)** = condition where a baby is born with weak ligaments in the hip, so that the femur does not stay in position in the pelvis; **congenital heart disease** = heart trouble caused by defects present in the heart at birth

COMMENT: a congenital condition is not always inherited from a parent through the genes, as it may be due to abnormalities which develop in the fetus because of factors such as a disease which the mother has (as in the case of German measles) or a drug which she has taken

congenitally [kən'dʒenɪtli] *adverb* at or before birth; *the baby is congenitally incapable of absorbing gluten*

congested [kən'dʒestɪd] *adjective* with blood or fluid inside; **congested face** = red face, caused by blood rushing to the face

congestion [kən'dʒestʃn] *noun* accumulation of blood in an organ; **nasal congestion** = blocking of the nose by inflammation as a response to a cold or other infection

congestive [kən'dʒestɪv] *adjective* (heart failure) caused by congestion

conization [kɒnaɪ'zeɪʃn] *noun* surgical removal of a cone-shaped piece of tissue

conjoined twins [kən'dʒɔɪnd 'twɪnz] *see* SIAMESE TWINS

conjugate *or* **true conjugate** *or* **conjugate diameter** ['kɒndʒʊgət daɪ'æmɪtə] *noun* measurements of space in the pelvis, used to calculate if normal childbirth is possible

conjunctiva [kɒndʒʌŋk'taɪvə] *noun* membrane which covers the front of the eyeball and the inside of the eyelids

conjunctival [kɒndʒʌŋk'taɪvl] *adjective* referring to the conjunctiva

conjunctivitis [kəndʒʌŋktɪ'vaɪtɪs] *noun* inflammation of the conjunctiva; *see also* PINK EYE

connect [kə'nekt] *verb* to join; *the lungs are connected to the mouth by the trachea; the pulmonary artery connects the heart to the lungs; the biceps is connected to both the radius and the scapula*

connection [kə'nekʃn] *noun* something which joins

connective tissue [kə'nektɪv 'tɪʃu:] *noun* tissue which forms the main part of bones and cartilage, ligaments and tendons, in which a large proportion of fibrous material surrounds the tissue cells

Conn's syndrome ['kɒnz 'sɪndrəʊm] *noun* condition caused by excessive production of aldosterone

consanguinity [kɒnsæŋ'gwɪnəti] *noun* blood relationship between people

conscious ['kɒnʃəs] *adjective* awake and knowing what is happening; *he became conscious in the recovery room two hours after the operation; it was two days after the accident before she became conscious*

consciously ['kɒnʃəsli] *adverb* in a conscious way

consciousness ['kɒnʃəsnəs] *noun* being mentally awake and knowing what is happening; **to lose consciousness** = to become unconscious, to become unable to respond to stimulation by the senses; **to regain consciousness** = to become conscious after being unconscious

consent [kən'sent] *noun* agreement; *the parents gave their consent for their son's heart to be used in the transplant operation;*

the nurses checked the patient's identity bracelet and that his consent had been given; **consent form** = form which a patient signs to show he agrees to have the operation; **informed consent** = agreement given by a patient or the guardians of a patient after they have been given all the necessary information, that an operation can be carried out

conserve [kən'sɜːv] *verb* to keep, not to waste; *the body needs to conserve heat in cold weather*

consolidation [kənsɒlɪ'deɪʃn] *noun* (i) stage in mending a broken bone, where the callus formed at the break changes into bone; (ii) condition where part of the lung becomes solid (as in pneumonia)

constant ['kɒnstənt] *adjective* **(a)** continuous, not stopping; *patients with Alzheimer's disease need constant supervision* **(b)** level, not varying; *his blood pressure remained constant during the operation*

constipated ['kɒnstɪpeɪtɪd] *adjective* unable to pass faeces often enough

constipation [kɒnstɪ'peɪʃn] *noun* difficulty in passing faeces

COMMENT: constipated bowel movements are hard, and may cause pain in the anus. Constipation may be caused by worry or by a diet which does not contain enough roughage or by lack of exercise, as well as more serious diseases of the intestine

constituent [kən'stɪtjuənt] *noun* substance which forms part of something; *the chemical constituents of nerve cells*

constitution [kɒnstɪ'tjuːʃn] *noun* general health and strength of a person; *she has a strong constitution or a healthy constitution*; *he has a weak constitution and is often ill*

constitutional [kɒnstɪ'tjuːʃənl] *adjective* referring to a person's constitution

constitutionally [kɒnstɪ'tjuːʃənli] *adverb* in a person's constitution; *he is constitutionally incapable of feeling tired*

constrict [kən'strɪkt] *verb* to squeeze, to make a passage narrower

constriction [kən'strɪkʃn] *noun* stenosis, becoming narrow

constrictive [kən'strɪktɪv] *adjective* which constricts; **constrictive pericarditis** = condition where the pericardium becomes

thickened and prevents the heart from functioning normally

constrictor [kən'strɪktə] *noun* muscle which squeezes an organ or which makes an organ contract

consult [kən'sʌlt] *verb* to ask someone for his opinion; *he consulted an eye specialist*

consultancy [kən'sʌltənsi] *noun* post of consultant; *she was appointed to a consultancy with a London hospital*

consultant [kən'sʌltnt] *noun* (i) doctor who is a senior specialist in a particular branch of medicine and who is consulted by a GP; (ii) senior specialized doctor in a hospital; *she was referred to the consultant orthopaedist*

consultation [kɒnsəl'teɪʃn] *noun* (i) discussion between two doctors about a case; (ii) meeting with a doctor who examines the patient, discusses his condition with him, and prescribes treatment

consulting room [kən'sʌltɪŋ 'ruːm] *noun* room where a doctor sees his patients

consumption [kən'sʌmpʃn] *noun* **(a)** taking food or liquid into the body; *the patient's increased consumption of alcohol* **(b)** former name for pulmonary tuberculosis

consumptive [kən'sʌmptɪv] *adjective* referring to consumption; (patient) suffering from consumption

contact ['kɒntækt] **1** *noun* **(a)** touching someone or something; **to have (physical) contact with someone** *or* **something** = to actually touch someone or something; **to be in contact with someone** = to be near someone, to touch someone; *the hospital is anxious to trace anyone who may have come into contact with the patient*; **direct contact** = actually touching an infected person or object; **indirect contact** = catching a disease by inhaling germs or by being in contact with a vector; **contact dermatitis** = inflammation of the skin, caused by touch (as in the case of some types of plant, soap, etc.) **(b)** person who has been in contact with a person suffering from an infectious disease; *now that Lassa fever has been diagnosed, the authorities are anxious to trace all contacts which the* patient may have met **2** *verb* to meet, to get in touch with (someone)

contact lens ['kɒntækt 'lenz] *noun* tiny plastic or glass lens which fits over the eyeball (worn instead of spectacles)

contagion [kən'teɪdʒn] *noun* spreading of a disease by touching an infected person or objects which an infected person has touched; *the contagion spread through the whole school*

contagious [kən'teɪdʒəs] *adjective* (disease) which can be transmitted by touching an infected person or objects which an infected person has touched; **contagious stage** = period when a disease (such as chickenpox) is contagious and can be transmitted to someone else

contaminant [kən'tæmɪnənt] *noun* substance which contaminates

contaminate [kən'tæmɪneɪt] *verb* **(a)** to spread infection **(b)** to make something impure by touching it or by adding something to it; *supplies of drinking water were contaminated by refuse from the factories; the whole group of tourists fell ill after eating contaminated food*

contamination [kəntæmɪ'neɪʃn] *noun* action of contaminating; *the contamination resulted from polluted water*

content ['kɒntent] *noun* proportion of a substance in something; *these foods have a high starch content; dried fruit has a higher sugar content than fresh fruit*

continual [kən'tɪnjul] *adjective* which goes on all the time without stopping; which happens again and again; *he suffered continual recurrence of the disease*

continually [kən'tɪnjuli] *adverb* all the time; *the intestine is continually infected*

continuation [kəntɪnju'eɪʃn] *noun* part which continues; *the radial artery is a continuation of the brachial artery*

continue [kən'tɪnjuː] *verb* to go on doing something; to do something which was being done before; *the fever continued for three days; they continued eating as if nothing had happened; the doctor recommended that the treatment should be continued for a further period*

continuous [kən'tɪnjuəs] *adjective* which continues without breaks or stops; **continuous positive airways pressure (CPAP)** = method used in intensive care which forces air into the lungs of patients with lung collapse

contraception [kɒntrə'sepʃn] *noun* prevention of pregnancy by using devices (such as a condom or an IUD) or drugs (such as the contraceptive pill) or by other means; *see also* BIRTH CONTROL

contraceptive [kɒntrə'septɪv] **1** *adjective* which prevents conception; *a contraceptive device* or *contraceptive drug* **2** *noun* drug or condom which prevents pregnancy; **oral contraceptive** = contraceptive pill which is taken through the mouth

contract [kən'trækt] *verb* **(a)** *(of muscle)* to become smaller and tighter; *as the muscle contracts the limb moves*; *the diaphragm acts to contract the chest* **(b)** to contract a disease = to catch a disease; *he contracted Lassa fever*

contractility [kɒntræk'tɪləti] *adjective* the capacity to contract

contractile tissue [kən'træktaɪl 'tɪʃuː] *noun* tissue in muscle which makes the muscle contract

contraction [kən'trækʃn] *noun* (i) tightening movement which makes a muscle shorter, which makes the pupil of the eye smaller or which makes the skin wrinkle; (ii) movement of the muscles of the uterus, marking the beginning of labour

contracture [kən'træktʃə] *noun* permanent tightening of a muscle caused by fibrosis; **Dupuytren's contracture** = condition where the palmar fascia becomes thicker, causing the fingers to bend forwards; **Volkmann's contracture** = tightening and fibrosis of the muscles of the forearm because blood supply has been restricted, leading to deformity of the fingers

contraindication [kɒntrəɪndɪ'keɪʃn] *noun* something which suggests that a patient should not be treated with a certain drug or not continue to be treated in the same way as at present, because circumstances make that treatment unsuitable

contralateral [kɒntrə'lætərl] *adjective* affecting the side of the body opposite the one referred to

contrast medium ['kɒntrɑːst 'miːdiəm] *noun* radio-opaque dye or sometimes gas, put into an organ or part of the body so that it will show clearly in an X-ray photograph

```
comparing the MRI scan and the
CT  scan:  in  the  first  no
contrast medium is required; in
the    second    iodine-based
contrast  media  are  often
required
```
Nursing 87

contrecoup ['kɒntrəkuː] *noun* injury to one point of an organ (for example, the brain) caused by a blow received on an opposite point of the organ

control [kən'trəʊl] **1** *noun* power, keeping in order; *the manager has no control over the consultants working in the hospital*; **the specialists brought the epidemic under control** = they stopped it from spreading; **the epidemic rapidly got out of control** = it spread quickly; *(in experiments)* **control group** = group of people who are not being treated, but whose test data are used as a comparison **2** *verb* to keep in order; *the medical authorities are trying to control the epidemic*; *certain drugs help to control the convulsions*; *he controls his asthma with a bronchodilator*

controlled [kə'trəʊld] *adjective* **controlled drugs** *or* **dangerous drugs** = drugs which are on the official list of drugs which are harmful and are not available to the general public; **controlled respiration** = control of a patient's breathing by an anaesthetist during an operation, when normal breathing has stopped

contused wound [kən'tjuːzd 'wuːnd] *noun* wound caused by a blow where the skin is bruised as well as torn and bleeding

contusion [kən'tjuːʒn] *noun* bruise, a dark painful area on the skin, where blood has escaped into the tissues but not through the skin, following a blow

conus ['kəʊnəs] *noun* structure shaped like a cone

convalesce [kɒnvə'les] *verb* to get back to good health gradually after an illness or operation

convalescence [kɒnvə'lesəns] *noun* period of time when a patient is convalescing

convalescent [kɒnvə'lesənt] *adjective & noun* referring to convalescence; **convalescent patients** *or* **convalescents** = people who are convalescing; **convalescent home** = type of hospital where patients can recover from illness or surgery

converge [kən'vɜːdʒ] *verb (of rays)* to come together at a point

convergent strabismus [kən'vɜːdʒnt strə'bɪzməs] *noun* squint, condition where a person's eyes look towards the nose

conversion [kən'vɜːʃn] *noun* change; *the conversion of nutrients into tissue*

convert [kən'vɜːt] *verb* to change something into something else; *keratinization is the process of converting cells into horny tissue*

convex ['kɒnveks] *adjective* which curves towards the outside; *a convex lens*

convoluted ['kɒnvəluːtɪd] *adjective* folded and twisted; **convoluted tubules** = coiled parts of a nephron

convolution [kɒnvə'luːʃn] *noun* twisted shape; *the convolutions of the surface of the cerebrum*

convulsion [kən'vʌlʃn] *noun* fit, the rapid involuntary contracting and relaxing of the muscles in several parts of the body (NOTE: often used in the plural: **the child had convulsions**)

> COMMENT: convulsions in children may be caused by brain disease, such as meningitis, but can often be found at the beginning of a disease (such as pneumonia) which is marked by a sudden rise in body temperature. In adults, convulsions are usually associated with epilepsy

convulsive [kən'vʌlsɪv] *adjective* referring to convulsions; *he had a convulsive seizure*; *see also* **ELECTROCONVULSIVE THERAPY**

cool [kuːl] **1** *adjective* not very warm, quite cold; *the patient should be kept cool*; *keep this bottle in a cool place* (NOTE: **cool - cooler - coolest**) **2** *verb* to become cool

Cooley's anaemia ['kuːliz ə'niːmiə] = **THALASSAEMIA**

Coombs' test ['kuːmz 'test] *noun* test for antibodies in red blood cells, used as a test for erythroblastosis fetalis and other haemolytic syndromes

coordinate [kəʊ'ɔːdɪneɪt] *verb* to make things work together; *he was unable to coordinate the movements of his arms and legs*

> there are four recti muscles and two oblique muscles in each eye, which coordinate the movement of the eyes and enable them to work as a pair
> *Nursing Times*

coordination [kəʊɔːdɪ'neɪʃn] *noun* ability to work together; *the patient showed lack of coordination between eyes and hands*

> Alzheimer's disease is a progressive disorder which sees a gradual decline in intellectual functioning and

deterioration of physical coordination

Nursing Times

COPD = CHRONIC OBSTRUCTIVE PULMONARY DISEASE

cope with ['kəʊp wɪð] *verb* to deal with, to manage; *a hospital administrator has to cope with a lot of forms*; *he walks with crutches and has difficulty in coping with the stairs*

copper ['kɒpə] *noun* metallic trace element (NOTE: the chemical symbol is **Cu**)

coprolith ['kɒprəlɪθ] *noun* hard faeces in the bowel

coproporphyrin [kɒprə'pɔːfərɪn] *noun* porphyrin excreted by the liver

copulate ['kɒpjʊleɪt] *verb* to have sexual intercourse

copulation [kɒpjʊ'leɪʃn] *noun* coitus, sexual intercourse

cor [kɔː] *noun* the heart; **cor pulmonale** = pulmonary heart disease where the right ventricle is enlarged

coraco-acromial [kɒrəkəʊə'krəʊmiəl] *adjective* referring to the coracoid process and the acromion

coracobrachialis [kɒrəkəʊbræki'eɪlɪs] *noun* muscle on the medial side of the upper arm, below the armpit

coracoid process ['kɒrəkɔɪd 'prəʊses] *noun* projecting part on the shoulder blade

cord [kɔːd] *noun* long flexible structure in the body like a thread; **spermatic cord** = cord formed of the vas deferens, the blood vessels, nerves and lymphatics of the testis, running from the testis to the abdomen; **spinal cord** = part of the central nervous system, running from the medulla oblongata to the filum terminale, in the vertebral canal of the spine; **umbilical cord** = cord containing two arteries and one vein which links the fetus inside the uterus to the placenta; *(vocal folds)* **true vocal cords** = cords in the larynx which can be brought together to make sounds as air passes between them; *see also* FOLD

cordectomy [kɔː'dektəmi] *noun* surgical removal of a vocal cord

cordotomy [kɔː'dɒtəmi] = CHORDOTOMY

core [kɔː] *noun* central part

corectopia [kɔːrek'təʊpiə] *noun* ectopia of the pupil

corium ['kɔːriəm] *noun* dermis, layer of living tissue beneath the epidermis

corn [kɔːn] *noun* heloma, a hard painful lump of skin usually on the foot or hand, where something (such as tight shoe) has rubbed or pressed on the skin

cornea ['kɔːniə] *noun* transparent part of the front of the eyeball (NOTE: plural is **corneae**)

corneal ['kɔːniəl] *adjective* referring to a cornea; *corneal tissue from donors is used in grafting to replace a damaged cornea*; **corneal abrasion** = scratch on the cornea, caused by something sharp getting into the eye; **corneal bank** = place where eyes of dead donors can be kept ready for use in corneal grafts

corneal graft *or* **transplant** ['kɔːniəl 'grɑːft or traːnzplaːnt] *noun* keratoplasty, corneal tissue from a donor or from a dead person, grafted in place of diseased tissue (NOTE: for terms referring to the cornea, see words beginning with **kerat-**)

corneum ['kɔːniəm] *see* STRATUM

cornification [kɔːnɪfɪ'keɪʃn] *noun* keratinization, process of converting cells into horny tissue

cornu ['kɔːnjuː] *noun* structure in the body which is shaped like a horn; **cornua of the thyroid** = four processes of the thyroid cartilage (NOTE: the plural is **cornua**)

corona [kə'rəʊnə] *noun* structure in the body which is shaped like a crown; **corona capitis** = the crown of the head, the top part of the skull

coronal ['kɒrənl] *adjective* (i) referring to a corona; (ii) referring to the crown of a tooth; **coronal plane** = plane at right angles to the median plane, dividing the body into dorsal and ventral halves; **coronal suture** = horizontal joint across the top of the skull between the parietal and frontal bones; *see illustration at* SKULL

coronary ['kɒrənri] **1** *noun (non-medical term)* coronary thrombosis, a blood clot in the coronary arteries which leads to a heart attack; *he had a coronary and was rushed to hospital* **2** *adjective* referring to any structure shaped like a crown, but especially to the arteries which supply blood to the heart muscles; **coronary arteries** = arteries which supply blood to the heart muscles; **coronary artery bypass graft (CABG)** *or* **surgery** =

surgical operation to treat angina by grafting pieces of vein to go around the diseased part of a coronary artery; **coronary care unit (CCU)** = section of a hospital caring for patients with heart disorders or who have had heart surgery; **coronary circulation** = blood circulation through the arteries and veins of the heart muscles; **coronary heart disease (CHD)** = any disease affecting the coronary arteries, which can lead to strain on the heart or a heart attack; **coronary ligament** = folds of peritoneum connecting the back of the liver to the diaphragm; **coronary obstruction** *or* **coronary occlusion** = thickening of the walls of the coronary arteries, a blood clot in the coronary arteries, which prevents blood reaching the heart muscles and leads to heart failure; **coronary sinus** = vein which takes most of the venous blood from the heart muscles to the right atrium; **coronary thrombosis** = blood clot which blocks the coronary arteries, leading to a heart attack

coronary heart disease (CHD) patients spend an average of 11.9 days in hospital. Among primary health care services, 1.5% of all GP consultations are due to CHD

Health Services Journal

apart from death, coronary heart disease causes considerable morbidity in the form of heart attack, angina and a number of related diseases

Health Education Journal

coronavirus [kəˈrəʊnəvaɪrəs] *noun* virus which causes the common cold

coroner [ˈkɒrənə] *noun* public official (either a doctor or a lawyer) who investigates sudden or violent deaths; **coroner's court** = court where a coroner is the chairman; **coroner's inquest** = inquest carried out by a coroner into a death

COMMENT: coroners investigate deaths which are caused by poison, violence, neglect or privation, from unnatural causes, during the post-operative recovery period and when the doctor feels unable to give a reliable cause of death. They investigate deaths which are violent or not expected, deaths which may be murder or manslaughter, deaths of prisoners and deaths involving the police

coronoid process [ˈkɒrənɔɪd ˈprəʊses] *noun* (i) projecting piece of bone on the ulna; (ii) projecting piece on each side of the lower jaw

corpse [kɔːps] *noun* body of a dead person

corpus [ˈkɔːpəs] *noun* any mass of tissue; **corpus albicans** = scar tissue which replaces the corpus luteum in the ovary; **corpus callosum** = tissue which connects the two cerebral hemispheres; *see illustration at* BRAIN; **corpus cavernosum** = part of the erectile tissue in the penis and clitoris; *see illustration at* UROGENITAL SYSTEM (MALE); **corpus haemorrhagicum** = blood clot formed in the ovary where a Graafian follicle has ruptured; **corpus luteum** = body which forms in the ovary after a Graafian follicle has ruptured (the corpora lutea secrete the hormone progesterone to prepare the uterus for implantation of the fertilized ovum); **corpus spongiosum** = part of the penis round the urethra, forming the glans; **corpus striatum** = part of a cerebral hemisphere (NOTE: the plural is **corpora**)

corpuscle [ˈkɔːpʌsl] *noun* any small round mass; **red corpuscle** = erythrocyte, red blood cell which contains haemoglobin and carries oxygen to the tissues and takes carbon dioxide from them; **white corpuscle** = leucocyte, white blood cell, a colourless cell which contains a nucleus but has no haemoglobin; **Krause corpuscles** = encapsulated nerve endings in mucous membrane of mouth, nose, eyes and genitals; **Meissner's corpuscle** = sensory nerve ending in the skin which is sensitive to touch; **Pacinian corpuscle** = sensory nerve ending in the skin which is sensitive to touch and vibrations; *see illustration at* SKIN & SENSORY RECEPTORS; **renal corpuscle** *or* **Malpighian corpuscle** = part of a nephron in the cortex of a kidney (NOTE: also called **Malpighian body**); **Ruffini corpuscles** = branching nerve endings in the skin, which are thought to be sensitive to heat (NOTE: also called **Ruffini nerve endings**); *see illustration at* SKIN & SENSORY RECEPTORS

correct [kəˈrekt] *verb* to put faults right, to make something work properly; *she wears a brace to correct the growth of her teeth*; *doctors are trying to correct his speech defect*

correction [kəˈrekʃn] *noun* showing the mistake in something; making something correct

corrective [kəˈrektɪv] *noun* drug which changes the harmful effect of another drug

Corrigan's pulse [ˈkɒrɪɡənz ˈpʌls] *noun* type of pulse, where there is a visible rise in pressure followed by a sudden collapse, of the arterial pulse in the neck, caused by aortic regurgitation

corrosive [kəˈrəʊsɪv] *adjective & noun* (substance, such as acid or alkali) which destroys tissue

corrugator muscles [ˈkɒrəɡeɪtə ˈmʌslz] *noun* muscles which produce vertical wrinkles on the forehead when frowning

corset [ˈkɔːsɪt] *noun* piece of stiff clothing, worn on the chest or over the trunk to support the body as after a back injury

cortex [ˈkɔːteks] *noun* outer layer of an organ, as opposed to the soft inner medulla; **adrenal cortex** = firm outside layer of the adrenal or suprarenal glands, which secretes various hormones, including cortisone; **cerebellar cortex** = outer covering of grey matter which covers the cerebellum; **cerebral cortex** = outer layer of grey matter which covers the cerebrum; **olfactory cortex** *or* **visual cortex** = parts of the cerebral cortex which receive information about smell or sight; **renal cortex** = outer covering of a kidney, immediately beneath the capsule, containing glomeruli; *see illustration at* KIDNEY; **sensory cortex** = area of the cerebral cortex which receives information from nerves in all parts of the body (NOTE: the plural is **cortices**)

Corti [ˈkɔːti] *see* ORGAN

cortical [ˈkɔːtɪkl] *adjective* referring to a cortex; **(suprarenal) cortical hormones** = hormones (such as cortisone) secreted by the cortex of the adrenal glands; **subcortical** = beneath the cortex

corticospinal [kɔːtɪkəʊˈspaɪnl] *adjective* referring to both the cerebral cortex and the spinal cord

corticosteroid [kɔːtɪkəʊˈstɪərɔɪd] *noun* **(a)** any steroid hormone produced by the cortex of the adrenal glands **(b)** drug (such as beclomethasone dipropionate) which reduces inflammation, used in asthma, gastro-intestinal disease and in adreno-cortical insufficiency

corticosterone [kɔːtɪkəʊˈstɪərəʊn] *noun* hormone secreted by the cortex of the adrenal glands

corticotrophin *US* **corticotropin** [kɔːtɪkəʊˈtrəʊfɪn or ˈtrɒpɪn] *noun* adrenocorticotrophic hormone (ACTH), hormone produced by the anterior pituitary gland, which causes the cortex of the adrenal glands to release corticosteroids

cortisol [ˈkɔːtɪsɒl] *noun* hydrocortisone, steroid hormone produced by the cortex of the adrenal glands

COMMENT: cortisol is used by the body to maintain blood pressure, connective tissue and break down carbohydrates. It also reduces the body's immune response to infection.

cortisone [ˈkɔːtɪzəʊn] *noun* hormone secreted in small quantities by the adrenal cortex; *the doctor gave her a cortisone injection in the ankle*; **cortisone treatment** = treatment of conditions by injections of cortisone

COMMENT: Synthetic cortisone is used in the treatment of arthritis, asthma and skin disorders, but can have powerful side-effects on some patients and is less often used

Corynebacterium [kəʊraɪniːbækˈtɪəriəm] *noun* genus of bacteria which includes the bacterium which causes diphtheria

coryza [kəˈraɪzə] *noun* nasal catarrh, common cold or cold in the head, an illness, with inflammation of the nasal passages, in which the patient sneezes and coughs and has a blocked and running nose

cosmetic surgery [kɒzˈmetɪk ˈsɜːdʒəri] *noun* surgical operation carried out to improve the appearance of the patient

COMMENT: whereas plastic surgery may be prescribed by a doctor to correct skin or bone defects or the effect of burns or after a disfiguring operation, cosmetic surgery is carried out on the instructions of the patient to remove wrinkles, enlarge breasts, etc.

cost- *or* **costo-** [kɒst or kɒstəʊ] *prefix* referring to the ribs

costal [ˈkɒstl] *adjective* referring to the ribs; **costal cartilage** = cartilage which forms the end of each rib and either joins the rib to the breastbone or to the rib above; **costal pleura** = part of the pleura lining the walls of the chest

costive [ˈkɒstɪv] **1** *adjective* constipated, suffering from difficulty in passing bowel movements **2** *noun* drug which causes constipation

costocervical trunk [ˌkɒstəʊˈsɜːvɪkl ˈtrʌŋk] *noun* large artery in the chest

costodiaphragmatic [ˌkɒstəʊdaɪəfrægˈmætɪk] *adjective* referring to the ribs and the diaphragm

costovertebral joints [ˌkɒstəʊˈvɜːtɪbrl ˈdʒɔɪnts] *noun* joints between the ribs and the vertebral column

cot death US **crib death** [ˈkɒt ˈdeθ or ˈkrɪb ˈdeθ] *noun* sudden infant death syndrome, the sudden death of a baby in bed, without any identifiable cause

COMMENT: occurs in very young children, up to the age of about 12 months; the causes are still being investigated, but may be related to the position of the baby, in particular whether it is lying on its back or front

co-trimoxazole [ˌkəʊtraɪˈmɒksəzəʊl] *noun* drug used to combat bacteria in the urinary tract

cottage hospital [ˈkɒtɪdʒ ˈhɒspɪtl] *noun* small local hospital sometimes set in pleasant gardens in the country

cotton [ˈkɒtn] *noun* fibres from a tropical plant; cloth made from cotton thread; *she wore a cotton shirt*; **cotton bud** = little stick with some cotton wool usually at both ends, used for cleaning cavities

cotton wool [ˈkɒtn ˈwʊl] *noun* purified fibres from the cotton plant used as a dressing on wounds, etc.; *she dabbed the cut with cotton wool soaked in antiseptic*; *the nurse put a pad of cotton wool over the sore* (NOTE: also called **absorbent cotton**)

cotyledon [ˌkɒtɪˈliːdn] *noun* one of the divisions of a placenta

cotyloid cavity [ˈkɒtɪlɔɪd ˈkævəti] *noun* acetabulum, part of the pelvic bone shaped like a cup, into which the head of the femur fits to form the hip joint

couch [kaʊtʃ] *noun* long bed on which a patient lies when being examined by a doctor in a surgery

couching [ˈkaʊtʃɪŋ] *noun* in treatment of cataract, surgical operation to displace the opaque lens of an eye

cough [kɒf] **1** *noun* reflex action, caused by irritation in the throat, when the glottis is opened and air is sent out of the lungs suddenly; *he gave a little cough to attract the nurse's attention*; *she has a bad cough and cannot make the speech*; **cough medicine** *or*

cough linctus = liquid taken to soothe the irritation which causes a cough; **barking cough** = loud noisy dry cough; **dry cough** = cough where no phlegm is produced; **hacking cough** = continuous short dry cough; **productive cough** = cough where phlegm is produced **2** *verb* to send air out of the lungs suddenly because the throat is irritated; *the smoke made him cough*; *he has a cold and keeps on coughing and sneezing*; **coughing fit** = sudden attack of coughing

cough suppressant [ˈkɒf səˈpresənt] *noun* opioid or sedative antihistamine drug (such as pholcodine) which suppresses the cough reflex

cough up [ˈkɒf ˈʌp] *verb* to cough hard to produce a substance from the trachea; *he coughed up phlegm*; *she became worried when the girl started coughing up blood*

council [ˈkaʊnsl] *noun* group of people elected to manage something; **town council** = elected committee which manages a town; **General Medical Council (GMC)** = body which registers all practising doctors (without such registration, a doctor cannot practise)

counselling [ˈkaʊnslɪŋ] *noun* method of treating especially psychiatric disorders, where a specialist advises and talks with a patient about his condition and how to deal with it

counsellor [ˈkaʊnslə] *noun* person who advises and talks with someone about his problems

count [kaʊnt] **1** *verb* **(a)** to say numbers in order; *the little girl can count up to ten*; *hold your breath and count to twenty to try to stop a hiccup* **(b)** to add up to see how many things there are; *count the number of tablets left in the bottle* **(c)** to include; *there were thirty people in the ward if you count the visitors* **2** *noun* act of adding things to see how many there are; **blood count** = test to count the number and types of different blood cells in a certain tiny sample of blood, to give an indication of the condition of the patient's blood as a whole; **platelet count** = test to see the quantity of platelets in a patient's blood

the normal platelet count during pregnancy is described as 150,000 to 400,000 per cu mm
Southern Medical Journal

counteract [ˌkaʊntəˈrækt] *verb* to act against something, to reduce the effect of something; *the lotion should counteract the irritant effect of the spray on the skin*

counteraction [kaʊntər'ækʃn] *noun (in pharmacy)* action of one drug which acts against another drug

counterextension [kaʊntərɪk'stenʃn] *noun* orthopaedic treatment, where the upper part of a limb is kept fixed and traction is applied to the lower part of it

counterirritant [kaʊntər'ɪrɪtnt] *noun* substance which alleviates the pain in an internal organ, by irritating an area of skin whose sensory nerves are close to those of the organ in the spinal cord

counterirritation [kaʊntərɪrɪ'teɪʃn] *noun* skin irritation, applied artificially to alleviate the pain in another part of the body

counterstain ['kaʊntəsteɪn] **1** *noun* stain used to identify tissue samples, such as red dye used to identify Gram-negative bacteria **2** *verb* to stain specimens with a counterstain, as bacteria with a red stain after having first stained them with violet dye; *see also* GRAM

course [kɔːs] *noun* **(a)** passing of time; *his condition has deteriorated in the course of the last few weeks* **(b)** series of lessons; *I'm taking a course in physiotherapy; she's taking a hospital administration course* **(c)** series of drugs to be taken, series of sessions of treatment; *we'll put you on a course of antibiotics*; **course of treatment** = series of applications of a treatment (such as a series of injections or physiotherapy); **to put someone on a course of drugs** *or* **of antibiotics** *or* **of injections** = to decide that a patient should take a drug, an antibiotic or should have a number of injections regularly over a certain period of time

court [kɔːt] *noun* place where a trial is heard or where a legal judgement is reached; **court order** = order made by a court telling someone to do, or not to do, something; *he was sent to a mental institution by court order*

cover ['kʌvə] **1** *noun* **(a)** thing put over something to keep it clean, etc.; *keep a cover on the petri dish*; **cover test** = test for a squint, where an eye is covered and its movements are checked when the cover is taken off **(b)** doing work for someone who is absent; *out-of-hours cover is provided by the other GPs in the practice* **2** *verb* **(a)** to put something over something to keep it clean, etc.; *you should cover the table with a plastic sheet before you start to mix the mouthwash; the fetus is covered with a membrane* **(b)** to be available to work in place of someone who is absent; *the other GPs will cover for him while he is on holiday*

covering ['kʌvərɪŋ] *noun* layer which covers or protects something; **brain covering** = the meninges

Cowper's glands ['kuːpəz 'glændz] *noun* bulbourethral glands, two glands at the base of the penis which secrete into the urethra

cowpox ['kaʊpɒks] *noun* vaccinia, infectious viral disease of cattle

COMMENT: the virus can be transmitted to man, and is used as a constituent of the vaccine for smallpox

coxa ['kɒksə] *noun* the hip joint

coxalgia [kɒk'sældʒə] *noun* pain in the hip joint

Coxsackie virus [kɒk'sæki 'vaɪrəs] *noun* one of a group of enteroviruses which enter the cells of the intestines but can cause diseases such as aseptic meningitis and Bornholm disease

CPAP ['siː 'piː 'eɪ 'piː] = CONTINUOUS POSITIVE AIRWAYS PRESSURE

CPR ['siː 'piː 'ɑː] = CARDIOPULMONARY RESUSCITATION

Cr *chemical symbol for* chromium

crab (louse) ['kræb 'laʊs] *noun* pubic louse, a louse *Phthirius pubis* which infests the pubic region and other parts of the body with coarse hair

crack [kræk] **1** *noun* thin break; *there's a crack in one of the bones in the skull* **2** *verb* to make a thin break in something; to split; *she cracked a bone in her leg*; **cracked lips** = lips where the skin has split because of cold or dryness

cradle ['kreɪdl] *noun* **(a)** metal frame put over a patient in bed to keep the weight of the bedclothes off the body **(b)** carrying an injured child by holding him with one arm under the thigh and the other above the waist; **cradle cap** = yellow deposit on the scalp of babies, caused by seborrhoea

cramp [kræmp] *noun* painful involuntary spasm in the muscles, where the muscle may stay contracted for some time; *he went swimming and got cramp in the cold water*; **menstrual cramps** = cramp in the muscles around the uterus during menstruation; **stomach cramp** = sharp spasm of the stomach muscles; **swimmer's cramp** = spasms in arteries and muscles caused by cold water, or swimming soon after a meal; **writer's cramp** = spasms and pain in the muscles of the wrist and hand, caused by holding a pen for long periods

crani- or **cranio-** ['kreɪni or 'kreɪniəʊ] *prefix* referring to the skull

cranial ['kreɪniəl] *adjective* referring to the skull; **cranial bone** = one of the bones in the skull; **cranial cavity** = space inside the bones of the cranium, in which the brain is situated; **cranial nerve** = one of the nerves, twelve on each side, which are connected directly to the brain, governing mainly the structures of the head and neck; *see* NERVE

craniometry [kreɪni'ɒmetri] *noun* measuring skulls to find differences in size and shape

craniopharyngioma
[kreɪniəʊfərɪndʒi'əʊmə] *noun* tumour in the brain originating in hypophyseal duct

craniostenosis or **craniosynostosis** [kreɪniəʊste'nəʊsɪs or kreɪniəʊsɪnəʊ'stəʊsɪs] *noun* early closing of the bones in a baby's skull, so making the skull contract

craniotabes [kreɪniəʊ'teɪbiːz] *noun* thinness of the bones in the occipital region of a child's skull, caused by rickets, marasmus or syphilis

craniotomy [kreɪni'ɒtəmi] *noun* any surgical operation on the skull, especially cutting away part of the skull

cranium ['kreɪniəm] *noun* skull, the group of eight bones which surround the brain

COMMENT: the cranium consists of the occipital bone, two parietal bones, two temporal bones and the frontal, ethmoid and sphenoid bones. See also SUTURE. The cranial nerves are: **I**: olfactory. **II**: optic. **III**: oculomotor. **IV**: trochlear. **V**: trigeminal (ophthalmic, maxillary, mandibular). **VI**: abducent. **VII**: facial. **VIII**: auditory (vestibular, cochlear). **IX**: glossopharyngeal. **X**: vagus. **XI**: accessory. **XII**: hypoglossal.

cranky ['kræŋki] *adjective US (informal)* bad-tempered or difficult (child)

crash [kræʃ] **1** *noun* accident where cars, planes, etc. are damaged; *he was killed in a car crash*; *none of the passengers was hurt in the crash*; **crash helmet** = hard hat worn by motorcyclists, etc. **2** *verb (of vehicles)* to hit something and be damaged; *the car*

crashed into the wall; *the plane crashed* = the plane hit the ground and was damaged **3** *adjective* rapid; *she took a crash course in physiotherapy* = a course to learn physiotherapy very quickly

cream [kriːm] *noun* medicinal oily substance, used to rub on the skin; **cold cream** = mixture of almond oil and borax

create [kri'eɪt] *verb* to make

creatine ['kriːətiːn] *noun* compound of nitrogen found in the muscles and produced by protein metabolism, and excreted as creatinine; **creatine phosphate** = store of energy-giving phosphate in muscles

creatinine [kri'ætəniːn] *noun* substance which is the form in which creatine is excreted; **creatinine clearance** = removal of creatinine from the blood by the kidneys

creatinuria [kriəæti'njʊəriə] *noun* excess creatine in the urine

creatorrhoea [kriətə'riːə] *noun* presence of undigested muscle fibre in the faeces, occurring in some pancreatic diseases

Credé's method [kreɪ'deɪz 'meθəd] *noun* **(a)** method of extracting a placenta, by massaging the uterus through the abdomen **(b)** putting silver nitrate solution into the eyes of a baby born to a mother suffering from gonorrhoea, in order to prevent gonococcal conjunctivitis

creeping eruption ['kriːpɪŋ ɪ'rʌpʃn] *noun* itching skin complaint, caused by larvae of various parasites which creep under the skin

crepitation [krepɪ'teɪʃn] *noun* rale, abnormal soft crackling sound heard in the lungs through a stethoscope

crepitus ['krepɪtəs] *noun* (i) harsh crackling sound heard through a stethoscope in a patient with inflammation of the lungs; (ii) scratching sound made by a broken bone or rough joint

crest [krest] *noun* long raised part on a bone; **crest of ilium** or **iliac crest** = curved top edge of the ilium

cretin ['kretɪn] *noun* patient suffering from congenital hypothyroidism

cretinism ['kretɪnɪzm] *noun* condition of being a cretin

COMMENT: the condition is due to a defective thyroid gland and affected children, if not treated, develop more slowly than normal, are mentally retarded and have coarse facial features

Creutzfeldt-Jakob disease (CJD)
['krɔɪtsfelt'dʒækɒb dɪ'ziːz] *noun* disease of the nervous system, caused by a slow-acting virus, which eventually affects the brain; it may be linked to BSE in cows; **new variant CJD** *or* **vCJD** = form of CJD which was observed first in the 1980s, especially affecting younger patients

crib death ['krɪb 'deθ] *noun US* = COT DEATH

cribriform plate ['krɪbrɪfɔːm 'pleɪt] *noun* top part of the ethmoid bone which forms the roof of the nasal cavity, and part of the roof of the eye sockets

cricoid cartilage ['kraɪkɔɪd 'kɑːtəlɪdʒ] *noun* ring-shaped cartilage in the lower part of the larynx; *see illustration at* LUNGS

cripple ['krɪpl] **1** *verb* to make someone physically handicapped; *she was crippled by arthritis*; *he was crippled in a car crash* **2** *noun* person who is physically disabled; **cardiac cripple** = person who has a cardiac disease which makes him unable to work normally

crippling ['krɪplɪŋ] *adjective* (disease) which makes someone physically handicapped; *arthritis is a crippling disease*

crisis ['kraɪsɪs] *noun* **(a)** turning point in a disease, after which the patient may start to become better or very much worse **(b)** important point or time; **mid-life crisis** = MENOPAUSE (NOTE: plural is **crises**)

> COMMENT: many diseases progress to a crisis and then the patient rapidly gets better; the opposite situation where the patient gets better very slowly is called lysis

crista ['krɪstə] *noun* crest; **crista galli** = projection from the ethmoid bone

critical ['krɪtɪkl] *adjective* **(a)** referring to crisis **(b)** extremely serious; *he was taken to hospital in a critical condition*; *the hospital spokesman said that three of the accident victims were still on the critical list* **(c)** which criticizes; *the report was critical of the state of aftercare provision*

critically ['krɪtɪkəli] *adverb* in a way which criticizes; **critically ill** = very seriously ill, where it is not known if the patient will get better

criticize ['krɪtɪsaɪz] *verb* to say what is wrong with something; *the report criticized the state of the hospital kitchens*

CRNA = CERTIFIED REGISTERED NURSE ANAESTHETIST

Crohn's disease ['krəʊnz dɪ'ziːz] *see* ILEITIS

cross [krɒs] *noun* **(a)** shape made with an upright line with another going across it, used as a sign of the Christian church; *(in anatomy)* any cross-shaped structure; **the Red Cross** = international organization which provides emergency medical help **(b)** mixture of two different breeds

cross eye ['krɒs 'aɪ] *noun* condition where a person's eyes both look towards the nose (NOTE: also called **convergent strabismus**)

cross-eyed ['krɒs'aɪd] *adjective* strabismal, with eyes looking towards the nose

cross-infection ['krɒsɪn'fekʃn] *noun* infection passed from one patient to another in hospital, either directly or from nurses, visitors or equipment

crossmatch [krɒs'mætʃ] *verb (in transplant surgery)* to match a donor to a recipient as closely as possible to avoid tissue rejection; *see* BLOOD GROUP

crossmatching [krɒs'mætʃɪŋ] *noun* matching a donor to a recipient as closely as possible to avoid tissue rejection

cross-resistance [krɒsrɪ'zɪstəns] *noun* ability of two organisms not to be affected by each other

cross-section ['krɒs'sekʃn] *noun* **(a)** sample cut across a specimen for examination under a microscope; *he examined a cross-section of the lung tissue* **(b)** small part of something, taken to be representative of the whole; *the team consulted a cross-section of hospital ancillary staff*

crotch [krɒtʃ] *noun* point where the legs meet the body, where the genitals are

croup [kruːp] *noun* children's disease, acute infection of the upper respiratory passages which blocks the larynx

> COMMENT: the patient's larynx swells, and he breathes with difficulty and has a barking cough. Attacks usually occur at night. They can be fatal if the larynx becomes completely blocked

crown [kraʊn] **1** *noun* (i) top part of a tooth (above the level of the gums); (ii) artificial top attached to a tooth; (iii) top part of the head; *see illustration at* TOOTH **2** *verb* to put an artificial crown (on a tooth)

crowning ['kraʊnɪŋ] *noun* (i) putting an artificial crown on a tooth; (ii) stage in childbirth, where the top of the baby's head becomes visible

cruciate ligament ['kruːʃiət 'lɪgəmənt] *noun* any ligament shaped like a cross, especially the ligaments behind the knee, which prevent the knee from bending forwards

crural ['krʊərəl] *adjective* referring to the thigh, leg or shin

crus [krʌs] *noun* long projecting part; **crus cerebri** = one of the nerve tracts between the cerebrum and the medulla oblongata; **crus of penis** = part of corpus cavernosum attached to the pubic arch; **crura cerebri** = CEREBRAL PEDUNCLES; **crura of the diaphragm** = long muscle fibres joining the diaphragm to the lumbar vertebrae (NOTE: plural is **crura**)

crush [krʌʃ] *verb* to squash or to injure with a heavy weight; *he was crushed by falling stones*

crush syndrome ['krʌʃ 'sɪndrəʊm] *noun* condition where the limb of a patient has been crushed, as in an accident

COMMENT: the condition causes kidney failure and shock

crutch [krʌtʃ] *noun* **(a)** strong support for a patient with an injured leg, formed of a stick with either a holding bar and elbow clasp or with a T-bar which fits under the armpit; **elbow crutch** = crutch with clamps to hold the arms; **human crutch** = method of helping an injured person to walk, where the patient puts his arm round the shoulders of a first aider **(b)** = CROTCH

cry [kraɪ] **1** *noun* sudden vocal sound **2** *verb* to produce tears because of pain, shock, fear, etc.; *she cried when she heard her mother had been killed; the pain made him cry; the baby started crying when it was time for its feed*

cry- *or* **cryo-** [kraɪ *or* 'kraɪəʊ] *prefix* referring to cold

cryaesthesia [kraɪiːs'θiːziə] *noun* being sensitive to cold

cryoprecipitate [kraɪəʊprɪ'sɪpɪtət] *noun* precipitate (such as that from blood plasma) which separates out on freezing and thawing

COMMENT: cryoprecipitate from plasma contains Factor VIII and is used to treat haemophiliacs

cryoprobe ['kraɪəʊprəʊb] *noun* instrument used in cryosurgery, where the tip is kept very cold to destroy tissue

cryosurgery [kraɪəʊ'sɜːdʒəri] *noun* surgery which uses extremely cold instrument to destroy tissue

cryotherapy [kraɪəʊ'θerəpi] *noun* treatment using extreme cold (as in removing a wart with dry ice)

crypt [krɪpt] *noun* small cavity in the body; **crypts of Lieberkuhn** = tubular glands found in the mucous membrane of the small and large intestine, especially those between the bases of the villi in the small intestine (NOTE: also called **Lieberkuhn's glands**)

crypto- ['krɪptəʊ] *prefix* hidden

cryptococcal meningitis [krɪptə'kɒkl menɪn'dʒaɪtɪs] *noun* form of meningitis caused by infection with a Cryptococcus fungus, occurring in persons who are immunodeficient

Cryptococcus [krɪptə'kɒkəs] *noun* one of several single-celled yeasts, which exist in the soil and can cause disease (NOTE: plural is **Cryptococci**)

cryptomenorrhoea [krɪptəmenə'riːə] *noun* retention of menstrual flow probably caused by an obstruction

cryptorchidism *or* **cryptorchism** [krɪp'tɔːkɪdɪzm *or* krɪp'tɔːkɪzm] *noun* undescended testicle(s), condition in a young male where the testicles do not move down into the scrotum

crystal ['krɪstl] *noun* chemical formation of hard regular-shaped solids

crystalline ['krɪstəlaɪn] *adjective* clear like pure crystal

crystal violet ['krɪstl 'vaɪələt] *noun* gentian violet, blue antiseptic dye used to paint on skin infections

Cs *chemical symbol for* caesium

CSF ['siː 'es 'ef] = CEREBROSPINAL FLUID

CT ['siː 'tiː] = COMPUTERIZED (AXIAL) TOMOGRAPHY, COMPUTED TOMOGRAPHY; **CT scan** = scan where a narrow X-ray beam, guided by a computer, photographs a thin section of the body or an organ from different angles; the results are fed into the computer which analyses them and produces a picture of a slice of the body or organ; **CT scanner** = device which directs a narrow X-ray beam at a thin section of the body from various angles, using a computer to build up a complete picture of the cross-section (NOTE: also abbreviated to **CAT**)

Cu *chemical symbol for* copper

cubital ['kjuːbɪtl] *adjective* referring to the ulna; **cubital fossa** = depression in the front of the elbow joint

cuboidal [kjuː'bɔɪdl] *adjective;* **cuboidal cell** = cube-shaped epithelial cell

cuboid bone ['kjuːbɔɪd 'bəʊn] *noun* one of the tarsal bones in the foot; *see illustration at* FOOT

cuff [kʌf] *noun* (i) inflatable ring put round a patient's arm and inflated when blood pressure is being measured; (ii) inflatable ring put round an endotracheal tube to close the passage

cuirass respirator [kwɪ'ræs 'respəreɪtə] *noun* type of artificial respirator, which surrounds only the patient's chest

culdoscope ['kʌldəʊskəʊp] *noun* instrument used to inspect the interior of the female pelvis, introduced through the vagina

culdoscopy [kʌl'dɒskəpi] *noun* examination of the interior of a woman's pelvis, using a culdoscope

cultivate ['kʌltɪveɪt] *verb* to make something grow; *agar is used as a culture medium to cultivate bacteria in a laboratory*

culture ['kʌltʃə] **1** *noun* bacteria or tissues grown in a laboratory; **culture medium** = agar, liquid or gel used to grow bacteria or tissue; **stock culture** = basic culture of bacteria from which other cultures can be taken **2** *verb* to grow bacteria in a culture medium; *see also* SUBCULTURE

cumulative ['kjuːmjʊlətɪv] *adjective* which grows by adding; **cumulative action** = effect of a drug which is given more often than it can be excreted, and so accumulates in the tissues

cuneiform bones *or* **cuneiforms** ['kjuːnɪfɔːm 'bəʊn *or* 'kjuːnɪfɔːmz] *noun* three of the tarsal bones in the foot; *see illustration at* FOOT

cupola ['kjuːpələ] *noun* (i) cap; (ii) piece of cartilage in a semicircular canal which is moved by the fluid in the canal and connects with the vestibular nerve

curable ['kjuːərəbl] *adjective* which can be cured; *a curable form of cancer*; *see also* INCURABLE

curare [kjuə'rɑːri] *noun* drug derived from South American plants, antagonist to acetylcholine and used surgically as an anaesthetic to paralyse muscles during operations

COMMENT: curare is the poison used to make poison arrows

curative ['kjuːərətɪv] *adjective* which can cure

curdle ['kɜːdl] *verb (of milk)* to coagulate

cure [kjuə] **1** *noun* particular way of making a patient well or of stopping an illness; *scientists are trying to develop a cure for the common cold*; *this is the only cure for tuberculosis* **2** *verb* to make a patient healthy; *he was completely cured*; *can the doctors cure his bad circulation?*; *some forms of cancer can't be cured*

curettage *or* **curettement** [kjuə'retɪdʒ *or* kjuə'retmənt] *noun* scraping the inside of a hollow organ to remove a growth or tissue for examination (often used in connection with the uterus); *see also* D AND C, DILATATION AND CURETTAGE

curette *US* **curet** [kjuə'ret] **1** *noun* surgical instrument like a long thin spoon, used for scraping the inside of an organ **2** *verb* to scrape with a curette

curie ['kjuːəri] *noun* unit of measurement of radioactivity (NOTE: with figures usually written as **Ci: 25 Ci**)

curvature ['kɜːvətʃə] *noun* way in which something bends from a straight line; **curvature of the spine** = abnormal bending of the spine forwards or sideways; **greater** *or* **lesser curvature of the stomach** = longer outside convex line of the stomach *or* shorter inside concave line of the stomach

curve [kɜːv] **1** *noun* line which bends round **2** *verb* to make a round shape; to bend something round

curved [kɜːvd] *adjective* with a shape which is not straight or flat; *a curved line*; *a curved scalpel*

cushingoid ['kʊʃɪŋɔɪd] *adjective* showing symptoms of Cushing's syndrome

Cushing's disease *or* **Cushing's syndrome** ['kʊʃɪŋz dɪ'ziːz *or* 'kʊʃɪŋz 'sɪndrəʊm] *noun* condition where the adrenal cortex produces too many corticosteroids

COMMENT: the syndrome is caused either by a tumour in the adrenal gland, by excessive stimulation of the adrenals by the basophil cells of the pituitary gland, or by a corticosteroid-secreting tumour. The syndrome causes swelling of the face and trunk, the muscles weaken, the blood pressure rises and the body retains salt and water

cusp [kʌsp] *noun* **(a)** pointed tip of a tooth **(b)** flap of membrane forming a valve in the heart

cuspid ['kʌspɪd] *noun* a canine tooth, one of the four pointed teeth next to the incisors (two in the top jaw and two in the lower jaw)

cut [kʌt] **1** *noun* place where the skin has been penetrated by a sharp instrument; *she had a bad cut on her left leg*; *the nurse will put a bandage on your cut* **2** *verb* **(a)** to make an opening using a knife, scissors, etc.; *the surgeon cut the diseased tissue away with a scalpel*; *she got tetanus after cutting her finger on the broken glass* **(b)** to reduce the number of something; *accidents have been cut by 10%* (NOTE: **cutting - cut - has cut**)

cutaneous [kju'teɪnɪəs] *adjective* referring to the skin; **cutaneous leishmaniasis** = form of skin disease caused by the tropical parasite *Leishmania*

cuticle ['kju:tɪkl] *noun* (i) epidermis, the outer layer of skin; (ii) strip of epidermis attached at the base of a nail

cutis ['kju:tɪs] *noun* skin; **cutis anserina** = goose flesh or goose pimples, reaction of the skin to being cold or frightened, where the skin is raised into many little bumps by the action of the arrector pili muscles

CVA ['si: 'vi: 'eɪ] = CEREBROVASCULAR ACCIDENT

cyanide ['saɪənaɪd] *noun* prussic acid, salt of hydrocyanic acid, a poison which kills very rapidly when drunk or inhaled

cyan- *or* **cyano-** ['saɪən or 'saɪənəʊ] *prefix* blue

cyanocobalamin [saɪənəʊkəʊ'bæləmɪn] = VITAMIN B$_{12}$

cyanosed ['saɪənəʊst] *adjective* with blue skin; *the patient was cyanosed round the lips*

cyanosis [saɪə'nəʊsɪs] *noun* blue colour of the peripheral skin and mucous membranes, symptom of lack of oxygen in the blood (as in a blue baby)

cyanotic [saɪə'nɒtɪk] *adjective* suffering from cyanosis; **cyanotic congenital heart disease** = cyanosis

cyclandelate [sɪ'klændəleɪt] *noun* drug used to treat cerebrovascular disease

cycle ['saɪkl] *noun* **(a)** series of events which recur regularly; **menstrual cycle** = period (usually 28 days) during which the endometrium develops, a woman ovulates, and menstruation takes place; **ovarian cycle** = regular changes in the ovary during reproductive life **(b)** bicycle, a vehicle with two wheels; **exercise cycle** = type of cycle which is fixed to the floor, so that someone can pedal on it for exercise

cyclical ['sɪklɪkl] *adjective* referring to cycles; **cyclical vomiting** = repeated attacks of vomiting

-cycline ['saɪklɪn] *suffix* used in names of several antibiotics; *tetracycline*

cyclitis [sɪ'klaɪtɪs] *noun* inflammation of the ciliary body in the eye

cyclizine ['saɪklɪziːn] *noun see* DRUGS TABLE IN SUPPLEMENT

cyclo- ['saɪkləʊ] *prefix* meaning cyclical, referring to cycles

cyclodialysis [saɪkləʊdaɪ'æləsɪs] *noun* surgical operation to connect the anterior chamber of the eye and the choroid, as treatment of glaucoma

cycloplegia [saɪkləʊ'pliːdʒə] *noun* paralysis of the ciliary muscle which makes it impossible for the eye to focus properly

cyclothymia [saɪkləʊ'θaɪmɪə] *noun* mild form of manic depression, where the patient suffers from alternating depression and excitement

cyclotomy [saɪ'klɒtəmi] *noun* surgical operation to make a cut in the ciliary body

cyesis [saɪ'iːsɪs] *noun* pregnancy, condition where a woman is carrying an unborn child in her uterus

cylinder ['sɪlɪndə] *see* OXYGEN

cyst [sɪst] *noun* abnormal growth in the body shaped like a pouch, containing liquid or semi-liquid substances; **branchial cyst** = cyst on the side of the neck of an embryo; **dental cyst** = cyst near the root of a tooth; **dermoid cyst** = cyst found under the skin, usually in the midline, containing hair, sweat glands and sebaceous glands; **ovarian cyst** = cyst which develops in the ovaries; **parasitic cyst** = cyst produced by a parasite, usually in the liver; **pilonidal cyst** = cyst at the bottom of the spine near the buttocks; **sebaceous cyst** = cyst which forms in a sebaceous gland (NOTE: also called a **wen**)

cyst- [sɪst] *prefix* referring to the bladder

cystadenoma [sɪstədɪˈnəʊmə] *noun* adenoma in which fluid-filled cysts form

cystalgia [sɪˈstældʒə] *noun* pain in the urinary bladder

cystectomy [sɪˈstektəmi] *noun* surgical operation to remove all or part of the urinary bladder

cystic [ˈsɪstɪk] *adjective* **(a)** referring to cysts **(b)** referring to a bladder; **cystic artery** = artery leading from the hepatic artery to the gall bladder; **cystic duct** = duct which takes bile from the gall bladder to the common bile duct; **cystic vein** = vein which drains the gall bladder

cystica [ˈsɪstɪkə] *see* SPINA BIFIDA

cysticercosis [sɪstɪsɜːˈkəʊsɪs] *noun* disease caused by infestation of tapeworm larvae from pork

cysticercus [sɪstɪˈsɜːkəs] *noun* bladder worm, the larva of a tapeworm found in pork, which is enclosed in a cyst, typical of *Taenia*

cystic fibrosis [ˈsɪstɪk faɪˈbrəʊsɪs] *noun* fibrocystic disease of the pancreas or mucoviscidosis, hereditary disease in which there is malfunction of the exocrine glands, such as the pancreas, in particular those which secrete mucus, causing respiratory difficulties, male infertility and malabsorption of food from the GI tract

COMMENT: the thick mucous secretions cause blockage of ducts and many serious secondary effects in the intestines and lungs. Symptoms include loss of weight, abnormal faeces and bronchitis. If diagnosed early, cystic fibrosis can be controlled with vitamins, physiotherapy and pancreatic enzymes

cystine [ˈsɪstiːn] *noun* amino acid found in protein: it can cause stones to form in the urinary system of patients suffering from a rare inherited metabolic disorder

cystinosis [sɪstɪˈnəʊsɪs] *noun* defective absorption of amino acids, which results in excessive amounts of cystine accumulating in the kidneys

cystinuria [sɪstɪˈnjʊəriə] *noun* cystine in the urine

cystitis [sɪˈstaɪtɪs] *noun* inflammation of the urinary bladder, which makes a patient pass water often and giving a burning sensation

cystocele [ˈsɪstəsiːl] *noun* hernia of the urinary bladder into the vagina

cystogram [ˈsɪstəgræm] *noun* X-ray photograph of the urinary bladder

cystography [sɪˈstɒgrəfi] *noun* examination of the urinary bladder by X-rays after radio-opaque dye has been introduced

cystolithiasis [sɪstəlɪˈθaɪəsɪs] *noun* condition where stones are formed in the urinary bladder

cystometer [sɪˈstɒmɪtə] *noun* apparatus which measures the pressure in the bladder

cystometry [sɪˈstɒmetrɪ] *noun* measurement of the pressure in the bladder

cystopexy [sɪˈstɒpeksi] *noun* vesicofixation, surgical operation to fix the bladder in a different position

cystoscope [ˈsɪstəskəʊp] *noun* instrument made of a long tube with a light at the end, used to inspect the inside of the bladder

cystoscopy [sɪˈstɒskəpi] *noun* examination of the bladder using a cystoscope

cystostomy [sɪˈstɒstəmi] *noun* vesicostomy, surgical operation to make an opening between the bladder and the abdominal wall to allow urine to pass without going through the urethra

cystotomy [sɪˈstɒtəmi] *noun* vesicotomy, surgical operation to make a cut in a bladder

cyt- *or* **cyto-** [sɪt *or* ˈsaɪtəʊ] *prefix* referring to cells

cytochemistry [saɪtəʊˈkemɪstrɪ] *noun* study of the chemical activity of living cells

cytodiagnosis [saɪtəʊdaɪəgˈnəʊsɪs] *noun* diagnosis after examination of cells

cytogenetics [saɪtəʊdʒəˈnetɪks] *noun* branch of genetics, which studies the structure and function of cells, especially the chromosomes

cytokinesis [saɪtəʊkɪˈniːsɪs] *noun* changes in the cytoplasm of a cell during division

cytological smear [saɪtəˈlɒdʒɪkl ˈsmɪə] *noun* sample of tissue taken for examination under a microscope

cytology [saɪˈtɒlədʒɪ] *noun* study of the structure and function of cells

cytolysis [saɪˈtɒləsɪs] *noun* breaking down of cells

cytomegalovirus (CMV) [saɪtəʊmegələʊˈvaɪrəs] *noun* virus (one of the herpesviruses) which can cause serious congenital disorders in a fetus if it infects the pregnant mother

cytometer [saɪˈtɒmɪtə] *noun* instrument attached to a microscope, used for measuring and counting the number of cells in a specimen

cytopenia [saɪtəʊˈpiːniə] *noun* deficiency of cellular elements in blood or tissue

cytoplasm [ˈsaɪtəʊplæzm] *noun* substance inside the cell membrane, which surrounds the nucleus of a cell

cytoplasmic [saɪtəʊˈplæzmɪk] *adjective* referring to the cytoplasm of a cell

cytosine [ˈsaɪtəʊsiːn] *noun* one of the four basic elements of DNA

cytosome [ˈsaɪtəʊsəʊm] *noun* body of a cell, not including the nucleus

cytotoxic drug [saɪtəʊˈtɒksɪk ˈdrʌg] *noun* drug which reduces the reproduction of cells, and is used to treat cancer

cytotoxin [saɪtəʊˈtɒksɪn] *noun* substance which has a toxic effect on cells of certain organs

Dd

Vitamin D ['vɪtəmɪn 'diː] *noun* vitamin which is soluble in fat, and is found in butter, eggs and fish; it is also produced by the skin when exposed to sunlight

COMMENT: Vitamin D helps in the formation of bones, and lack of it causes rickets in children

d *symbol for* deci-

da *symbol for* deca-

dab [dæb] *verb* to touch lightly; *he dabbed the cut with a piece of absorbent cotton*

da Costa's syndrome [dɑːˈkɒstəz ˈsɪndrəʊm] *noun* disordered action of the heart, a condition where the patient suffers palpitations, breathlessness and dizziness, caused by effort or worry

dacryo- [ˈdækriəʊ] *prefix* referring to tears

dacryoadenitis [dækriəʊædeˈnaɪtɪs] *noun* inflammation of the lacrimal gland

dacryocystitis [dækriəʊsɪˈstaɪtɪs] *noun* inflammation of the lacrimal sac when the tear duct, which drains into the nose, becomes blocked

dacryocystography [dækriəʊsɪˈstɒgrəfi] *noun* contrast radiography to determine the site of an obstruction in the tear ducts

dacryocystorhinostomy (DCR) [dækriəʊsɪstɔːraɪˈnɒstəmi] *noun* surgical operation to bypass a blockage from the tear duct which takes tears into the nose

dacryolith [ˈdækriəʊlɪθ] *noun* stone in the lacrimal sac

dacryoma [dækriˈəʊmə] *noun* benign swelling in one of the tear ducts

dactyl- *or* **dactylo-** [ˈdæktɪl *or* ˈdæktɪləʊ] *prefix meaning* fingers or toes

dactyl [ˈdæktɪl] *noun* finger or toe

dactylitis [dæktɪˈlaɪtɪs] *noun* inflammation of the fingers or toes, caused by bone infection or rheumatic disease

dactylology [dæktɪˈlɒlədʒi] *noun* deaf and dumb language, signs made with the fingers, used in place of words when talking to a deaf and dumb person, or when a deaf and dumb person wants to communicate

dactylomegaly [dæktɪləʊˈmegəli] *noun* condition where a person has longer fingers than normal

DAH [ˈdiː ˈeɪ ˈeɪtʃ] = DISORDERED ACTION OF THE HEART

daily [ˈdeɪli] **1** *adjective* which happens every day; *you should do daily exercises to keep fit* **2** *adverb* every day; *take the medicine twice daily*; **three times daily** = three times every day

Daltonism [ˈdɔːltənɪzm] *noun* protanopia, the commonest form of colour blindness, where the patient cannot see red; *compare* DEUTERANOPIA, TRITANOPIA

damage [ˈdæmɪdʒ] **1** *noun* harm done to things; *the disease caused damage to the brain cells*; **bone damage** *or* **tissue damage** = damage caused to a bone or to tissue **2** *verb* to harm something; *his hearing* or *his sense of balance was damaged in the accident*; *a surgical operation to remove damaged tissue*

damp [dæmp] *adjective* slightly wet; *you should put a damp compress on the bruise*

D and C [ˈdiː ən ˈsiː] = DILATATION AND CURETTAGE

dandruff [ˈdændrəf] *noun* pityriasis capitis or scurf, pieces of dead skin which form on the scalp and fall out when the hair is combed

D and V [ˈdiː ən ˈviː] = DIARRHOEA AND VOMITING

danger [ˈdeɪndʒə] *noun* possibility of harm or death; *unless the glaucoma is treated quickly, there's a danger that the patient will lose his eyesight* or *a danger of the patient losing his eyesight;* **the doctors say she's out of danger** = she is not likely to die

dangerous ['deɪndʒrəs] *adjective* which can cause harm or death; *don't touch the electric wires - they're dangerous*; *cigarettes are dangerous to health*; **dangerous drugs** = drugs (such as morphine or heroin) which are harmful and are not available to the general public, and also poisons which can only be sold to certain persons

dark [dɑːk] **1** *adjective* **(a)** with very little light; *switch the lights on - it's getting too dark to read*; *in the winter it gets dark early*; **dark adaptation** = change in the retina and pupil of the eye to adapt to dim light after being in normal light **(b)** with black or brown hair; *he's dark, but his sister is fair* (NOTE: **dark - darker - darkest) 2** *noun* lack of light; *she is afraid of the dark*; *cats can see in the dark*

darkening ['dɑːknɪŋ] *noun* becoming darker in colour; *darkening of the tissue takes place after bruising*

darkroom ['dɑːkruːm] *noun* room with no light, in which photographic film can be developed; *the X-rays are in the darkroom, so they should be ready soon*; *he hopes to get a job as a darkroom technician*

data ['deɪtə] *noun* any information (in words or figures) about a certain subject, especially information which is available on computer; **data bank** *or* **bank of data** = store of information in a computer; *the hospital keeps a data bank of information about possible kidney donors*; **Data Protection Act** = British Parliament (1984), by which any owner of a database that contains personal details must register with a central Government agency; it ensures that all information is stored securely and allows individuals to have access to their entries

date [deɪt] *noun* number of a day or year, name of a month (when something happened); *what's the date today?*; *what is the date of your next appointment*; *do you remember the date of your last checkup?*; **up-to-date** = very modern, using very recent information or equipment; *the new hospital is provided with the most up-to-date equipment*; **out-of-date** = not modern; *the surgeons have to work with out-of-date equipment*

daughter ['dɔːtə] *noun* girl child of a parent; *they have two sons and one daughter*; **daughter cell** = one of the cells which develop by mitosis from a single parent cell

day [deɪ] *noun* **(a)** (i) period of 24 hours; (ii) period from morning until night, when it is light; *he works all day in the office, and then visits patients in the hospital in the evening*; *take two tablets three times a day*; *she's attending a day unit for disabled patients*; **day hospital** = hospital where patients are treated during the day and go home in the evenings; **day nursery** = place where small children can be looked after during the daytime, while their parents are at work; **day patient** *or* **day case** = patient who is in hospital for treatment for a day (i.e. one who does not stay overnight); **day recovery ward** = ward where day patients who have had minor operations can recover before going home; **day surgery** = surgical operation which does not require the patient to stay overnight in hospital

> paediatric day-surgery patients spend on average between 2 and 8 hours in hospital
>
> *British Journal of Nursing*

day blindness ['deɪ 'blaɪndnəs] = HEMERALOPIA

daylight ['deɪlaɪt] *noun* light during the day

daytime ['deɪtaɪm] *noun* period of light between morning and night; *he works at night and sleeps during the daytime*

dazed [deɪzd] *adjective* confused in the mind; *she was found walking about in a dazed condition*; *he was dazed after the accident*

dB ['diː 'biː] = DECIBEL

DCR ['diː 'siː 'ɑ] = DACRYOCYSTORHINOSTOMY

DDS ['diː 'diː 'es] *US* = DOCTOR OF DENTAL SURGERY

DDT ['diː 'diː 'tiː] = DICHLORODIPHENYLTRICHLOROETHANE

de- *prefix* meaning removal or loss

dead [ded] *adjective* **(a)** not alive; *my grandparents are both dead*; *when the injured man arrived at hospital he was found to be dead*; *the woman was rescued from the crash, but was certified dead on arrival at the hospital* **(b)** not sensitive; *the nerve endings are dead*; *his fingers went dead* **(c) dead space** = breath in the last part of the inspiration which does not get further than the bronchial tubes

deaden ['dedn] *verb* to make (pain or noise) less strong; *the doctor gave him an injection to deaden the pain*

deadly ['dedli] *adjective* likely to kill; *cyanide is a deadly poison*; **deadly nightshade** = BELLADONNA

dead (man's) fingers ['ded 'mænz 'fɪŋgəz] = RAYNAUD'S DISEASE

deaf [def] **1** *adjective* not able to hear; *you have to speak slowly and clearly when you talk to Mr Jones because he's quite deaf*; **totally deaf** *or* **completely deaf** *or* **stone deaf** = unable to hear any sound at all; **partially deaf** = able to hear some sounds but not all; **deaf and dumb** = not able to hear or to speak; **deaf and dumb language** = signs made with the fingers, used instead of words when talking to a trained deaf and dumb person, or when a deaf and dumb person wants to communicate (NOTE: also called **sign language** *or* **dactylology**) **2** *noun* **the deaf** = people who are deaf; *hearing aids can be of great use to the partially deaf*

deafen ['defn] *verb* to make (someone) deaf for a time; *he was deafened by the explosion*

deafness ['defnəs] *noun* loss of hearing; being unable to hear; **conductive deafness** = deafness caused by defective conduction of sound into the inner ear; **partial deafness** = (i) being able to hear some tones, but not all; (ii) general dulling of the whole range of hearing; **perceptive deafness** *or* **sensorineural deafness** = deafness caused by a disorder in the auditory nerves, the cochlea or the brain centres which receive impulses from the nerves; **progressive deafness** = condition, common in people as they get older, where a person gradually becomes more and more deaf; **total deafness** = being unable to hear any sound at all; *see also* HEARING LOSS

COMMENT: deafness has many degrees and many causes: old age, viruses, exposure to continuous loud noise or intermittent loud explosions, and diseases such as German measles

deaminate [diːˈæmɪneɪt] *verb* to remove an amino group from an amino acid, forming ammonia

deamination [diːæmɪˈneɪʃn] *noun* removal of an amino group from an amino acid, forming ammonia

COMMENT: after deamination, the ammonia which is formed is converted to urea by the liver, while the remaining carbon and hydrogen from the amino acid provide the body with heat and energy

death [deθ] *noun* dying; end of life; *his sudden death shocked his friends*; *he met his death in a car crash*; **death certificate** = official document signed by a doctor, stating that a person has died and giving details of the person and the cause of death; **death rate** = number of deaths per year per thousand of population; *the death rate from cancer of the liver has remained stable*; **brain death** = condition where the nerves in the brain stem have died, and the patient can be certified as dead, although the heart may not have stopped beating; **cot death,** *US* **crib death** = sudden death of a baby in bed, with no identifiable cause (NOTE: for terms referring to death see words beginning with **necro-**)

debilitate [dɪˈbɪlɪteɪt] *verb* to make weak; *he was debilitated by a long illness*; **debilitating disease** = disease which makes the patient weak

debility [dɪˈbɪləti] *noun* general weakness

debridement [dɪˈbriːdmənt] *noun* removal of dirt or dead tissue from a wound to help healing

deca- ['dekə] *prefix meaning* ten (NOTE: symbol is **da**)

decaffeinated [diːˈkæfɪneɪtɪd] *adjective* (coffee) with the caffeine removed

decalcification [diːkælsɪfɪˈkeɪʃn] *noun* loss of calcium salts from teeth and bones

decapsulation [diːkæpsjuˈleɪʃn] *noun* surgical operation to remove a capsule from an organ, especially from a kidney

decay [dɪˈkeɪ] **1** *noun* **(a)** process by which tissues become rotten, caused by the action of microbes and oxygen **(b)** *(of teeth)* dental caries, rotting of a tooth **2** *verb (of tissue)* to rot; *the surgeon removed decayed matter from the wound*

deci- ['desɪ] *prefix meaning* one tenth (10^{-1} (NOTE: symbol is **d**)

decibel ['desɪbel] *noun* unit of measurement of the loudness of sound, used to compare different levels of sound (NOTE: usually written **dB** with figures: **20dB:** say 'twenty decibels')

COMMENT: normal conversation is at about 50dB. Very loud noise with a value of over 120dB (such as aircraft engines) can cause pain

decidua [dɪˈsɪdjuə] *noun* membrane which lines the uterus after fertilization

COMMENT: the decidua is divided into several parts: the decidua basalis, where the embryo is attached, the decidua capsularis, which covers the embryo and the decidua vera which is the rest of the decidua not touching the embryo; it is expelled after the birth of the baby

deciduous [dɪˈsɪdjuəs] *adjective* **deciduous teeth** = milk teeth, a child's first twenty teeth, which are gradually replaced by the permanent teeth

decilitre *US* **deciliter** [ˈdesɪliːtə] *noun* unit of measurement of liquid (= one tenth of a litre) (NOTE: with figures usually written **dl**)

decimetre *US* **decimeter** [ˈdesɪmiːtə] *noun* unit of measurement of length (= one tenth of a metre) (NOTE: with figures usually written **dm**)

decompensation [diːkɒmpənˈseɪʃn] *noun* condition where an organ such as the heart cannot cope with extra stress placed on it (and so is unable to circulate the blood properly)

decompose [diːkəmˈpəuz] *verb* to rot, to become putrefied

decomposition [diːkɒmpəˈzɪʃn] *noun* process where dead matter is rotted by the action of bacteria or fungi

decompression [diːkəmˈpreʃn] *noun* **(a)** reduction of pressure; **cardiac decompression** = removal of a haematoma or constriction of the heart; **cerebral decompression** = removal of part of the skull to relieve pressure on the brain **(b)** controlled reduction of atmospheric pressure which occurs as a diver returns to the surface; **decompression sickness** = CAISSON DISEASE

decongestant [diːkənˈdʒestənt] *adjective & noun* (drug) which reduces congestion and swelling, sometimes used to unblock the nasal passages

decortication [diːkɔːtɪˈkeɪʃn] *noun* surgical removal of the cortex of an organ; **decortication of a lung** = pleurectomy, a surgical operation to remove part of the pleura which has been thickened or made stiff by chronic empyema

decrease 1 [ˈdiːkriːs] *noun* lowering in numbers, becoming less; *a decrease in the numbers of new cases being notified* **2** [diːˈkriːs] *verb* to become less, to make something less; *his blood pressure has decreased to a more normal level*; *the pressure in the vessel is gradually decreased*

decubitus [dɪˈkjuːbɪtəs] *noun* position of a patient who is lying down; **decubitus ulcer** = BEDSORE

decussation [diːkʌˈseɪʃn] *noun* chiasma, crossing of nerve fibres in the central nervous system

deep [diːp] *adjective* **(a)** which goes a long way down; *be careful - the water is very deep here*; *the wound is several millimetres deep*; **take a deep breath** = to inhale a large amount of air **(b)** inside the body, further from the skin; *the internal intercostal muscle is deep to the external*; **deep vein** = vein which is inside the body near a bone, as opposed to a superficial vein near the skin; **deep-vein thrombosis (DVT)** = phlebothrombosis, thrombus in the deep veins of a leg or the pelvis, also called 'economy class syndrome' because it affects many air travellers who have not enough leg room in economy class during long-haul flights because airlines have reduced the space between seats (or pitch); (passengers are recommended to walk up and down the aisle at least once every hour during a long flight); **deep facial vein** = small vein which drains from the pterygoid process behind the cheek into the facial vein (NOTE: the opposite is **superficial**. Note also that a part is **deep to** another part)

deeply [ˈdiːpli] *adverb* (breathing) which takes in a large amount of air; *he was breathing deeply*

defaecate *US* **defecate** [ˈdefəkeɪt] *verb* to pass faeces from the bowels

defaecation *US* **defecation** [defəˈkeɪʃn] *noun* passing out faeces from the bowels

defecate, defecation *US* *see* DEFAECATE, DEFAECATION

defect [ˈdiːfekt] *noun* (i) wrong formation, something which is badly formed; (ii) lack of something which is necessary; **birth defect** *or* **congenital defect** = malformation which exists in a person's body from birth

defective [dɪˈfektɪv] **1** *adjective* which works badly, which is wrongly formed; *the surgeons operated to repair a defective heart valve* **2** *noun* person suffering from severe mental subnormality

defence *US* **defense** [dɪˈfens] *noun* (i) resistance against an attack of a disease; (ii) behaviour of a person which is aimed at protecting him from harm; **muscular defence** = rigidity of muscles associated with inflammation such as peritonitis; **defence**

mechanism = subconscious reflex by which a person prevents himself from showing emotion

defense *US* = DEFENCE

deferens ['defərənz] *see* VAS DEFERENS

deferent ['defərənt] *adjective* (i) which goes away from the centre; (ii) referring to the vas deferens

defervescence [defɜː'vesns] *noun* period during which a fever is subsiding

defibrillation [diːfɪbrɪ'leɪʃn] *noun* cardioversion, correcting an irregular heartbeat by using an electric impulse

defibrillator [diː'fɪbrɪleɪtə] *noun* apparatus used to apply an electric impluse to the heart to make it beat regularly

defibrination [diːfaɪbrɪ'neɪʃn] *noun* removal of fibrin from a blood sample to prevent clotting

deficiency [dɪ'fɪʃənsi] *noun* lack, not having enough of something; **deficiency disease** = disease caused by lack of an essential element in the diet (such as vitamins, essential amino and fatty acids, etc.); **iron-deficiency anaemia** = anaemia caused by lack of iron in red blood cells; **vitamin deficiency** = lack of vitamins; **immunodeficiency** = lack of immunity to a disease

deficient [dɪ'fɪʃnt] *adjective* **deficient in something** = not containing the necessary amount of something; *his diet is deficient in calcium or he has a calcium-deficient diet*

deficit ['defɪsɪt] *noun* deficiency

defloration [diːflɔː'reɪʃn] *noun* breaking the hymen of a virgin usually at the first sexual intercourse

deflorescence [diːflɔː'resns] *noun* disappearance of a rash

deformans [diː'fɔːməns] *see* OSTEITIS

deformation [diːfɔː'meɪʃn] *noun* becoming deformed; *the later stages of the disease are marked by bone deformation*

deformed [dɪ'fɔːmd] *adjective* not shaped or formed in a normal way

deformity [dɪ'fɔːməti] *noun* abnormal shape of part of the body

degenerate [dɪ'dʒenəreɪt] *verb* to change so as not to be able to function; *his brain degenerated so much that he was incapable of looking after himself*

degeneration [dɪdʒenə'reɪʃn] *noun* change in the structure of a cell or organ so that it no longer works properly; **adipose degeneration** *or* **fatty degeneration** = accumulation of fat in the cells of an organ (such as the heart or liver), making the organ less able to perform; **calcareous degeneration** = deposits of calcium which form at joints in old age; **fibroid degeneration** = change of normal tissue to fibrous tissue (as in cirrhosis of the liver)

degenerative [dɪ'dʒenərətɪv] *adjective* **degenerative disease** *or* **degenerative disorder** = disease or disorder where there is progressive loss of function of a part of the body or a part of the body wears and fails to repair

> The weight-bearing joints, such as the spine, hip and knees, are the most frequent sites of degenerative disease
> *British Journal of Nursing*

deglutition [diːglu'tɪʃn] *noun* swallowing, the action of passing food or liquid (sometimes also air) from the mouth into the oesophagus

degree [dɪ'griː] *noun* **(a)** *(in science)* unit of measurement; *a circle has 360°; the temperature is only 20° Celsius* (NOTE: the word **degree** is written ° after figures: **40°C**: say: 'forty degrees Celsius') **(b)** title given by a university or college to a person who has successfully completed a course of studies; *he has a medical degree from London University*; *she was awarded a first-class degree in pharmacy* **(c)** level of how important or serious something is; **to a minor degree** = in a small way; **degree of burn** = the amount of damage done to the skin and tissue by light, heat, radiation, electricity or chemicals; **first-degree burn** = burn where the skin turns red because the epidermis has been affected; **second-degree burn** = burn where the skin becomes very red and blisters; *see also* BURN

COMMENT: burns were formerly classified by degrees and are still often referred to in this way. The modern classification is into two categories: deep and superficial

dehisced [dɪ'hɪst] *adjective* (wound) which has split open again

dehiscence [dɪ'hɪsns] *noun* opening wide; **wound dehiscence** = splitting open of a surgical incision

dehydrate [di:'haɪdreɪt] *verb* to lose water; *after two days without food or drink, he became dehydrated*

dehydration [di:haɪ'dreɪʃn] *noun* loss of water

COMMENT: water is more essential than food for a human being's survival. If someone drinks during the day less liquid than is passed out of the body in urine and sweat, he begins to dehydrate

an estimated 60-70% of diarrhoeal deaths are caused by dehydration
Indian Journal of Medical Sciences

déjà vu ['deɪʒɑ: 'vu:] *noun* illusion that a new situation is a previous one being repeated, usually caused by a disease of the brain

deletion [dɪ'li:ʃn] *noun* **chromosomal deletion** = chromosomal aberration in which a part of the chromosome is lost or removed

Delhi boil ['deli 'bɔɪl] *noun* cutaneous Leishmaniasis, a tropical skin disease caused by the parasite Leishmania

delicate ['delɪkət] *adjective* (i) easily broken or harmed; (ii) easily falling ill; *the bones of a baby's skull are very delicate*; *the eye is covered by a delicate membrane*; *the surgeons carried out a delicate operation to join the severed nerves*; *his delicate state of health means that he is not able to work long hours*

delirious [dɪ'lɪriəs] *adjective* suffering from delirium

COMMENT: a person can become delirious because of shock, fear, drugs or fever

delirium [dɪ'lɪriəm] *noun* mental state where the patient is confused, excited, restless and has hallucinations; **delirium tremens (DTs)** *or* **delirium alcoholicum** = state of mental disturbance, especially including hallucinations about insects, trembling and excitement, usually found in chronic alcoholics who attempt to give up alcohol consumption

deliver [dɪ'lɪvə] *verb* to bring something to someone; **to deliver a baby** = to help a mother in childbirth; *the twins were delivered by the midwife*

delivery [dɪ'lɪvri] *noun* birth of a child; *the delivery went very smoothly*; **breech delivery** = birth where the baby's buttocks appear first; **face delivery** = birth where the baby's face appears first; **forceps delivery** *or* **instrumental delivery** = childbirth where the doctor uses forceps to help the baby out of the mother's uterus; **spontaneous delivery** = delivery which takes place naturally, without any medical or surgical help; **vertex delivery** = normal birth, where the baby's head appears first; **delivery bed** = special bed on which a mother lies to give birth

delta ['deltə] *noun* fourth letter of the Greek alphabet; **delta hepatitis** *or* **hepatitis delta** = severe form of hepatitis caused by the delta virus in conjunction with HBV; **delta virus** = virus which causes hepatitis delta

deltoid (muscle) ['deltɔɪd 'mʌsl] *noun* big triangular muscle covering the shoulder joint and attached to the humerus, which lifts the arm sideways; **deltoid tuberosity** = raised part of the humerus to which the deltoid muscle is attached

delusion [dɪ'lu:ʒn] *noun* false belief which a person holds which cannot be changed by reason; *he suffered from the delusion that he was wanted by the police*

dementia [dɪ'menʃə] *noun* loss of mental ability and memory, causing disorientation and personality changes, due to organic disease of the brain; **AIDS dementia** = form of mental degeneration resulting from infection with HIV; **dementia of the Alzheimer's type** = form of mental degeneration probably due to Alzheimer's disease; **Lewy body dementia** = disease which affects the mental processes similar to Alzheimer's disease, but with the presence of Lewy bodies in the brain and patients are more prone to hallucinations and delusions; **multi-infarct dementia** = form of mental degeneration due to small strokes; **vascular dementia** = form of mental degeneration due to disease of the blood vessels in the brain; **dementia paralytica** = mental degeneration at the tertiary stage of syphilis; **dementia praecox** = (formerly) schizophrenia

AIDS dementia is a major complication of HIV infection, occurring in 70-90% of patients
British Journal of Nursing

dementing [dɪ'mentɪŋ] *adjective* (patient) suffering from dementia

demographic [demə'græfɪk] *adjective* referring to demography; **demographic forecasts** = forecasts of the numbers of people of different ages and sexes in an area at some time in the future

demography [di'mɒgrəfi] *noun* study of populations and environments or changes affecting populations

demonstrate ['demənstreɪt] *verb* to show how something is done or is used; *the surgeon demonstrated how to make the incision or demonstrated the incision*

demonstrator ['demənstreɪtə] *noun* person who demonstrates, especially in a laboratory or surgical department

demulcent [dɪ'mʌlsnt] *noun* soothing substance which relieves irritation in the stomach

demyelination *or* **demyelinating** [di:maɪəlɪ'neɪʃn *or* di:'maɪəlɪneɪtɪŋ] *noun* destruction of the myelin sheath round nerve fibres

COMMENT: can be caused by injury to the head, or is the main result of multiple sclerosis

denatured alcohol [di:'neɪtʃəd 'ælkəhɒl] *see* ALCOHOL

dendrite ['dendraɪt] *noun* branched process of a nerve cell, which receives impulses from nerve endings of axons of other neurones at synapses; *see illustration at* NEURONE

dendritic [den'drɪtɪk] *adjective* referring to a dendrite; **dendritic ulcer** = branching ulcer on the cornea, caused by herpesvirus; *see also* AXODENDRITE

denervation [di:nɜ:'veɪʃn] *noun* stopping or cutting of the nerve supply to a part of the body

dengue ['deŋgi] *noun* breakbone fever, tropical disease caused by an arbovirus, transmitted by mosquitoes, where the patient suffers a high fever, pains in the joints, headache and rash

Denis Browne splint ['denɪs 'braun 'splɪnt] *noun* metal splint used to correct a club foot

dens [dens] *noun* tooth; something shaped like a tooth

dense [dens] *adjective* compact, tightly pressed together; **dense bone** = type of bone tissue which forms the hard outer layer of a bone

density ['densəti] *noun* **(a)** amount of mass of a substance per unit of volume **(b)** number of things in a certain area

dent- [dent] *prefix meaning* tooth or teeth

dental ['dentl] *adjective* referring to teeth or to a dentist; **dental auxiliary** = person who helps a dentist; **dental care** = looking after teeth; **dental caries** *or* **dental decay** = rotting of a tooth; **dental cyst** = cyst near the root of a tooth; **dental floss** = soft thread used to clean between the teeth; **dental hygienist** = qualified assistant who cleans teeth and gums; **dental plaque** = hard smooth bacterial deposit on teeth, which is the probable cause of caries; **dental practice** = office and patients of a dentist; **dental pulp** = soft tissue inside a tooth; **dental surgeon** = dentist, qualified doctor who practises surgery on teeth; **dental surgery** = (i) office and operating room of a dentist; (ii) surgery carried out on teeth; **dental technician** = person who makes dentures

dentifrice ['dentɪfrɪs] *noun* paste or powder used with a toothbrush to clean teeth

dentine *US* **dentin** ['denti:n] *noun* hard substance which surrounds the pulp of teeth, beneath the enamel; *see illustration at* TOOTH

dentist ['dentɪst] *noun* trained doctor who looks after teeth and gums; *I must go to the dentist - I've got toothache*; *she had to wait for an hour at the dentist's*; *I hate going to see the dentist*

dentistry ['dentɪstri] *noun* profession of a dentist; branch of medicine dealing with teeth and gums

dentition [den'tɪʃn] *noun* number, arrangement and special characteristics of all the teeth in a person's jaws; **adult** *or* **permanent dentition** = the thirty-two teeth which an adult has; **milk** *or* **deciduous dentition** = the twenty teeth which a child has, and which are gradually replaced by the permanent teeth

COMMENT: children have incisors, canines and molars. These are replaced over a period of years by the permanent teeth, which are eight incisors, four canines, eight premolars and twelve molars (the last four molars being called the wisdom teeth)

denture ['dentʃə] *noun* set of false teeth, fixed to a plate which fits inside the mouth; **partial denture** = part of a set of false teeth, replacing only a few teeth

deodorant [dɪ'əudərənt] *adjective & noun* (substance) which hides or prevents unpleasant smells

deoxygenate [diːˈɒksɪdʒəneɪt] *verb* to remove oxygen; **deoxygenated blood** = venous blood, blood from which most of the oxygen has been removed by the tissues and is darker than arterial oxygenated blood

deoxyribonuclease [diːɒksɪraɪbəʊˈnjuːkliːeɪz] *noun* enzyme which breaks down DNA

deoxyribonucleic acid (DNA) [diːɒksɪraɪbəʊnjuːˈkliːɪk ˈæsɪd] *noun* one of the nucleic acids, the basic genetic material present in the nucleus of each cell; *see also* RNA

department [dɪˈpaːtmənt] *noun* **(a)** part of a large organization (such as a hospital); *if you want treatment for that cut, you must go to the outpatients department*; *she is in charge of the physiotherapy department* **(b) Department of Health (DOH)** = section of the British government which is in charge of the National Health Service; **Department of Social Security (DSS)** = section of British government which is in charge of national insurance, sickness and unemployment benefits, pensions, etc.

depend [dɪˈpend] *verb* **to depend on something** *or* **someone** = to be sure that something will happen or that someone will do something; to rely on something; *we depend on the nursing staff in the running of the hospital*; *he depends on drugs to relieve the pain*; *the blood transfusion service depends on a large number of donors*

dependant [dɪˈpendnt] *noun* person who is looked after or supported by someone else; *he has to support a family of six children and several dependants*

dependence [dɪˈpendns] *noun* being dependent on or addicted to (a drug); **drug dependence** = being addicted to a drug and unable to exist without taking it regularly; **physical drug dependence** = state where a person is addicted to a drug (such as heroin) and suffers physical effects if he stops or reduces the drug; **psychological drug dependence** = state where a person is addicted to a drug (such as cannabis or alcohol) but suffers only mental effects if he stops taking it

dependent [dɪˈpendnt] *adjective* **(a)** relying on (a person); **dependent relative** = person who is looked after by another member of the family **(b)** addicted to (a drug); *he is physically dependent on*

amphetamines **(c)** (part of the body) which is hanging down

depersonalization [diːpɜːsənlaɪˈzeɪʃn] *noun* psychiatric state where the patient does not believe he is real

depilation [depɪˈleɪʃn] *noun* removal of hair

depilatory [dɪˈpɪlətri] *adjective & noun* (substance) which removes hair

deplete [dɪˈpliːt] *verb* **(i)** to exhaust the strength or the numbers of something; **(ii)** to remove a component from a substance; *venous blood is depleted of oxygen by the tissues and returns to the lungs for oxygenation*; *our nursing staff has been depleted by illness, and the outpatients' unit has had to be closed*

depletion [dɪˈpliːʃn] *noun* being depleted, lacking something; **salt depletion** = loss of salt from the body, by sweating or vomiting, which causes cramp

depolarization [diːpəʊləraɪˈzeɪʃn] *noun* electrochemical reaction which takes place when an impulse travels along a nerve

deposit [dɪˈpɒzɪt] **1** *noun* substance which is attached to part of the body; *some foods leave a hard deposit on teeth*; *a deposit of fat forms on the walls of the arteries* **2** *verb* to attach a substance to part of the body; *fat is deposited on the walls of the arteries*

depress [dɪˈpres] *verb* to make someone miserable; *the grey winter weather always depresses her*

depressant [dɪˈpresnt] *noun* drug (such as a tranquillizer) which reduces the activity of part of the body; **thyroid depressant** = drug which reduces the activity of the thyroid gland

depressed [dɪˈprest] *adjective* **(a)** feeling miserable and worried; *he was depressed after his exam results*; *she was depressed for some weeks after the death of her husband* **(b)** (metabolic rate, freezing point, etc.) which is operating below the normal level

depressed fracture [dɪˈprest ˈfræktʃə] *noun* fracture of a flat bone, such as those in the skull, where part of the bone has been pushed down lower than the surrounding parts

depression [dɪˈpreʃn] *noun* **(a)** mental state where the patient feels miserable and hopeless; **pathological depression** = abnormally severe state of depression, possibly leading to suicide **(b)** hollow on the surface of a part of the body

depressive [dɪˈpresɪv] *adjective & noun* (substance) which causes mental depression; (state of) depression; *he is in a depressive state*; **manic-depressive** = person suffering from a psychological condition where he moves from mania to depression

depressor [dɪˈpresə] *noun* (i) muscle which pulls part of the body downwards; (ii) nerve which inhibits the activity of an organ such as the heart and lowers the blood pressure; **tongue depressor** = instrument, usually a thin piece of wood, used by a doctor to hold the patient's tongue down while his throat is being examined

deprivation [deprɪˈveɪʃn] *noun* (i) needing something; (ii) loss of something which is needed; **maternal deprivation** = psychological condition caused when a child does not have a proper relationship with a mother

deradenitis [dɪrædəˈnaɪtɪs] *noun* inflammation of the lymph nodes in the neck

deranged [dɪˈreɪnʒd] *adjective* **mentally deranged** = suffering from a mental illness

derangement [dɪˈreɪnʒmənt] *noun* disorder; **internal derangement of the knee (IDK)** = condition where the knee cannot function properly because of a torn meniscus

Derbyshire neck [ˈdɑːbɪʃə ˈnek] *noun* endemic goitre, a form of goitre which was once widespread in Derbyshire

Dercum's disease [ˈdɜːkəmz dɪˈziːz] = ADIPOSIS DOLOROSA

derealization [diːrɪələˈzeɪʃn] *noun* psychological state where the patient feels the world around him is not real

derivative [dɪˈrɪvətɪv] *noun* substance which is derived from another substance; *what are the derivatives of petroleum?*; *see also* PURIFIED

derive [dɪˈraɪv] *verb* to start from, to come into existence from; *compounds which derive from or are derived from sugar*; *the sublingual region has a rich supply of blood derived from the carotid artery*

derm- *or* **derma-** *or* **dermato-** *or* **dermo-** [ˈdɜːm *or* ˈdɜːmə *or* ˈdɜːˈmætəʊ *or* ˈdɜːməʊ] *prefix meaning* skin

dermal [ˈdɜːml] *adjective* referring to the skin

dermatitis [dɜːməˈtaɪtɪs] *noun* inflammation of the skin; **contact dermatitis** = dermatitis caused by touching something (such as certain types of plant or

soap); **eczematous dermatitis** = itchy inflammation or irritation of the skin due to an allergic reaction to a substance which a person has touched or absorbed; **exfoliative dermatitis** = typical form of dermatitis where the skin becomes red and comes off in flakes; **occupational dermatitis** = dermatitis caused by materials touched at work; **dermatitis artefacta** = injuries to the skin caused by the patient himself; **dermatitis herpetiformis** = type of dermatitis where large itchy blisters form on the skin

various types of dermal reaction to nail varnish have been noted. Also contact dermatitis caused by cosmetics such as toothpaste, soap, shaving creams

Indian Journal of Medical Sciences

dermatoglyphics [dɜːmətəʊˈglɪfɪks] *noun* study of the patterns of lines and ridges on the palms of the hands and the soles of the feet

dermatographia [dɜːmətəʊˈgræfiə] *noun; see* DERMOGRAPHIA

dermatological [dɜːmətəˈlɒdʒɪkl] *adjective* referring to dermatology

dermatologist [dɜːməˈtɒlədʒɪst] *noun* doctor who specializes in the study and treatment of the skin

dermatology [dɜːməˈtɒlədʒi] *noun* study and treatment of the skin and diseases of the skin

dermatome [ˈdɜːmətəʊm] *noun* **(a)** special knife used for cutting thin sections of skin for grafting **(b)** area of skin supplied by one spinal nerve

dermatomycosis [dɜːmətəʊmaɪˈkəʊsɪs] *noun* skin infections caused by a fungus

dermatomyositis [dɜːmətəʊmaɪəʊˈsaɪtɪs] *noun* collagen disease with a wasting inflammation of the skin and muscles

dermatophyte [ˈdɜːmətəʊfaɪt] *noun* fungus which affects the skin

dermatophytosis [dɜːmətəʊfaɪˈtəʊsɪs] *noun* fungus infection of the skin

dermatoplasty [ˈdɜːmətəʊplæsti] *noun* skin graft, replacing damaged skin by skin taken from another part of the body or from a donor

dermatosis [dɜːməˈtəʊsɪs] *noun* any skin disease

dermis [ˈdɜːmɪs] *noun* corium, thick layer of living skin beneath the epidermis; *see* *illustrations at* SKIN & SENSORY RECEPTORS

dermographia [dɜːməˈgræfiə] swelling on the skin produced by pressing with a blunt instrument, usually an allergic reaction (NOTE: also called **dermatographia**)

dermoid [ˈdɜːmɔɪd] *adjective* referring to the skin, like skin; **dermoid cyst** = cyst found under the skin, usually in the midline, containing hair, sweat glands and sebaceous glands

Descemet's membrane [deʃəˈmets ˈmembreɪn] *noun* one of the deep layers of the cornea

descend [dɪˈsend] *verb* to go down; **descending aorta** = second part of the aorta as it goes downwards after the aortic arch; **descending colon** = third section of the colon which goes down the left side of the body; *see illustration at* DIGESTIVE SYSTEM; **descending tract** = tract of nerves which take impulses away from the head

describe [dɪˈskraɪb] *verb* to say or write what something or someone is like; *can you describe the symptoms?*; *she described how her right leg suddenly became inflamed*

description [dɪˈskrɪpʃn] *noun* saying or writing what something or someone is like; *the patient's description of the symptoms*

desensitization [diːsensətaɪˈzeɪʃn] *noun* (i) removal of sensitivity; (ii) treatment of an allergy by giving the patient injections of small quantities of the substance to which he is allergic over a period of time until he becomes immune to it

desensitize [diːˈsensətaɪz] *verb* (i) to deaden a nerve, to remove sensitivity; (ii) to treat a patient suffering from an allergy by giving graduated injections of the substance to which he is allergic over a period of time until he becomes immune to it; *the patient was prescribed a course of desensitizing injections*

desire [dɪˈzaɪə] *noun* wanting greatly to do something; *he has a compulsive desire to steal*

desquamate [ˈdeskwəmeɪt] *verb (of skin)* to peel off

desquamation [deskwəˈmeɪʃn] *noun* (i) continual process of losing the outer layer of dead skin; (ii) peeling off of the epithelial part of a structure

destroy [dɪˈstrɔɪ] *verb* to ruin or kill completely; *the nerve cells were destroyed by the infection*

destruction [dɪˈstrʌkʃn] *noun* ruining or killing of something completely; *the destruction of the tissue or the cells by infection*; *the destruction of bacteria by phagocytes*

detach [dɪˈtætʃ] *verb* to separate one thing from another; *an operation to detach the cusps of the mitral valve*; **detached retina** = condition where the retina is partially detached from the choroid (NOTE: also called **retinal detachment**)

COMMENT: a detached retina can be caused by a blow to the eye, or simply is a condition occurring in old age; if left untreated the eye will become blind. A detached retina can sometimes be attached to the choroid again using lasers

detachment [dɪˈtætʃmənt] *noun* **retinal detachment** = *see* DETACHED RETINA

detect [dɪˈtekt] *verb* to sense or to notice (usually something which is very small or difficult to see); *an instrument to detect microscopic changes in cell structure*; *the nurses detected a slight improvement in the patient's condition*

detection [dɪˈtekʃn] *noun* action of detecting something; *the detection of sounds by nerves in the ears*; *the detection of a cyst using an endoscope*

detergent [dɪˈtɜːdʒnt] *noun* cleaning substance which removes grease and bacteria

COMMENT: most detergents are not allergenic but some biological detergents which contain enzymes to remove protein stains can cause dermatitis

deteriorate [dɪˈtɪəriəreɪt] *verb* to become worse; *the patient's condition deteriorated rapidly*

deterioration [dɪtɪəriəˈreɪʃn] *noun* becoming worse; *the nurses were worried by the deterioration in the patient's mental state*

determine [dɪˈtɜːmɪn] *verb* to find out something correctly; *health inspectors are trying to determine the cause of the outbreak of Salmonella poisoning*

detoxication *or* **detoxification** [diːtɒksɪˈkeɪʃn *or* diːtɒksɪfɪˈkeɪʃn] *noun* removal of toxic substances to make a poisonous substance harmless

detrition [dɪ'trɪʃn] *noun* wearing away by rubbing or use

detritus [dɪ'traɪtəs] *noun* rubbish produced when something disintegrates

detrusor muscle [dɪ'truːzə 'mʌsl] *noun* muscular coat of the urinary bladder

detumescence [diːtjuˈmesns] *noun* (of penis or clitoris after an erection or orgasm) becoming limp; (of a swelling) going down

deuteranopia [djuːtərə'nəupiə] *noun* form of colour blindness, a defect in vision, where the patient cannot see green; *compare* DALTONISM, TRITANOPIA

develop [dɪ'veləp] *verb* **(a)** to grow or to make grow; to mature; *the embryo developed quite normally, in spite of the mother's illness*; *a swelling developed under the armpit*; *the sore throat developed into an attack of meningitis* **(b)** to start to get; *she developed a cold*; *he developed complications and was rushed to hospital*

```
rheumatoid  arthritis  is  a
chronic  inflammatory  disease
which  can  affect  many  systems
in  the  body,  but  mainly  the
joints.  70%  of  sufferers
develop  the  condition  in  the
metacarpophalangeal  joints
                        Nursing Times
```

development [dɪ'veləpmənt] *noun* thing which develops or is being developed; action of becoming mature; *the development of the embryo takes place in the uterus*

developmental [dɪveləp'mentl] *adjective* referring to the development of an embryo

deviance ['diːvɪəns] *noun* abnormal sexual behaviour

deviation [diːvɪ'eɪʃn] *noun* variation from normal; abnormal position of a joint or of the eye (such as strabismus)

device [dɪ'vaɪs] *noun* instrument or piece of equipment; *a device for weighing very small quantities of powder*; *he used a device for examining the interior of the ear*

Devic's disease [də'vɪks dɪ'ziːz] = NEUROMYELITIS OPTICA

dextro- ['dekstrəu] *prefix* referring to the right side of the body, to the right hand

dextrocardia [dekstrəu'kɑːdiə] *noun* congenital condition where the apex of the heart is towards the right of the body instead of the left; *compare* LAEVOCARDIA

dextrose ['dekstrəus] *noun* glucose, simple sugar found in fruit, also broken down in the body from white sugar or carbohydrate and absorbed into the body or excreted by the kidneys

DHA ['diː 'eɪtʃ 'eɪ] = DISTRICT HEALTH AUTHORITY

dhobie itch ['dəubi 'ɪtʃ] *noun* contact dermatitis (believed to be caused by an allergy to the marking ink used by laundries)

DI = DONOR INSEMINATION

diabetes [daɪə'biːtiːz] *noun* one of a group of diseases, but most commonly used to refer to diabetes mellitus; **diabetes insipidus** = rare disease caused by a disorder of the pituitary gland, making the patient pass large quantities of urine and want to drink more than normal; **diabetes mellitus** = disease where the body cannot control sugar absorption because the pancreas does not secrete enough insulin; **bronze diabetes** = haemochromatosis, hereditary disease where the body absorbs and stores too much iron, giving a dark colour to the skin; **gestational diabetes** = diabetes which develops in a pregnant woman; **insulin-dependent diabetes** = diabetes caused by inadequate production or utilization of insulin (Type 1)

COMMENT: diabetes mellitus has two forms: Type 1 may have a viral trigger caused by an infection which affects the cells in the pancreas which produce insulin; Type 2 is common in older people and is caused by a lower sensitivity to insulin and is associated with obesity. Symptoms of diabetes mellitus are tiredness, abnormal thirst, frequent passing of water and sweet-smelling urine. Blood and urine tests will reveal high levels of sugar. Treatment for Type 2 diabetes involves keeping to a strict diet and reducing weight, and the use of oral hypoglycaemic drugs such as glibenclamide, and can involve oral medication. Type 1 diabetes must be treated with regular injections of insulin

diabetic [daɪə'betɪk] **1** *adjective* **(a)** referring to diabetes mellitus; **diabetic coma** = state of unconsciousness caused by untreated diabetes; **diabetic diet** = diet which is low in carbohydrates and sugar; **diabetic retinopathy** = defect in vision caused by diabetes **(b)** (food) which contains few carbohydrates and sugar; *he bought some diabetic chocolate*; *she lives on diabetic soups* **2** *noun* person suffering from diabetes

diabetologist [daɪəbe'tɒlədʒɪst] *noun* physician specializing in the treatment of diabetes mellitus

diaclasia [daɪə'kleɪzɪə] *noun* fracture made by a surgeon to repair a earlier fracture which has set badly, or to correct a deformity

diadochokinesis [daɪædəkɒkaɪ'niːsɪs] *noun* normal ability to make muscles move limbs in opposite directions

diagnose ['daɪəgnəʊz] *verb* to identify a patient's condition or illness, by examining the patient and noting symptoms; *the doctor diagnosed appendicitis*

diagnosis [daɪəg'nəʊsɪs] *noun* (i) act of diagnosing a patient's condition or illness; (ii) the conclusion reached about a condition; *the doctor's diagnosis was cancer, but the patient asked for a second opinion*; *they found it difficult to make a diagnosis*; **differential diagnosis** = identification of one particular disease from other similar diseases by comparing the range of symptoms of each; **antenatal** *or* **prenatal diagnosis** = medical examination of a pregnant woman to see if the fetus is developing normally (NOTE: plural is **diagnoses**)

diagnostic [daɪəg'nɒstɪk] *adjective* referring to diagnosis; **diagnostic imaging** = scanning for the purpose of diagnosis, as of a pregnant woman to see if the fetus is healthy; **diagnostic process** = method of making a diagnosis; **diagnostic test** = test which helps a doctor diagnose an illness; *compare* PROGNOSIS

diagonal [daɪ'ægənl] *adjective* going across at an angle

diagonally [daɪ'ægənli] *adverb* crossing at an angle

diagram ['daɪəgræm] *noun* chart or drawing which records information as lines or points; *the book gives a diagram of the circulation of blood*; *the diagram shows the occurrence of cancer in the southern part of the town*

dialyse ['daɪəlaɪz] *verb* to treat (a patient) using a kidney machine

dialyser ['daɪəlaɪzə] *noun* apparatus which uses a membrane to separate solids from liquids, especially a kidney machine

dialysis [daɪ'æləsɪs] *noun* using a membrane as a filter to separate soluble waste substances from the blood; **kidney dialysis** = haemodialysis, removing waste matter from a patient's blood by passing it through a kidney machine or dialyser;

peritoneal dialysis = removing waste matter from the blood by introducing fluid into the peritoneum which then acts as the filter membrane

diameter [daɪ'æmɪtə] *noun* distance across a circle (such as a tube or blood vessel); *they measured the diameter of the pelvic girdle*

diapedesis [daɪəpɪ'diːsɪs] *noun* movement of white blood cells through the walls of the capillaries into tissues in inflammation

diaper ['daɪəpə] *noun* US cloth used to wrap round a baby's bottom and groin, to keep clothing clean and dry; **diaper rash** = sore red skin on a baby's buttocks and groin, caused by long contact with ammonia in a wet diaper (NOTE: British English is **nappy**)

diaphoresis [daɪəfə'riːsɪs] *noun* excessive perspiration

diaphoretic [daɪəfə'retɪk] *adjective* (drug) which causes sweating

diaphragm ['daɪəfræm] *noun* **(a)** thin layer of tissue stretched across an opening, especially the flexible sheet of muscle and fibre which separates the chest from the abdomen, and moves to pull air into the lungs in respiration; **pelvic diaphragm** = sheet of muscle between the pelvic cavity and the peritoneum; **urogenital diaphragm** = fibrous layer beneath the prostate gland through which the urethra passes **(b)** **vaginal diaphragm** = circular contraceptive device for women, which is inserted into the vagina and placed over the neck of the uterus before sexual intercourse

COMMENT: the diaphragm is a muscle which in breathing expands and contracts with the walls of the chest. The normal rate of respiration is about 16 times a minute

diaphragmatic [daɪəfræg'mætɪk] *adjective* referring to a diaphragm; like a diaphragm; **diaphragmatic hernia** = condition where a membrane and organ in the abdomen pass through an opening in the diaphragm into the chest; **diaphragmatic pleura** = part of the pleura which covers the diaphragm; **diaphragmatic pleurisy** = inflammation of the pleura which covers the diaphragm

diaphyseal [daɪə'fɪzɪəl] *adjective* referring to a diaphysis

diaphysis [daɪ'æfəsɪs] *noun* shaft, the long central part of a long bone; *compare* EPIPHYSIS, METAPHYSIS; *see illustration at* BONE STRUCTURE

diaphysitis [daɪəfə'zaɪtɪs] *noun* inflammation of the diaphysis, often associated with rheumatic disease

diarrhoea *US* **diarrhea** [daɪə'rɪə] *noun* condition where a patient frequently passes liquid faeces; *he had an attack of diarrhoea after going to the restaurant*; *she complained of mild diarrhoea*; **traveller's diarrhoea** = diarrhoea that affects people who travel to foreign countries and which is due to a different type of E. coli than the one they are used to; *see also* ELECTROLYTE MIXTURE

COMMENT: diarrhoea can have many causes: types of food or allergy to food; contaminated or poisoned food; infectious diseases, such as dysentery; sometimes worry or other emotions

diarrhoeal [daɪə'rɪəl] *adjective* referring to or caused by diarrhoea

diarthrosis [daɪɑː'θrəʊsɪs] *noun* synovial joint, a joint which moves freely

diastase ['daɪəsteɪz] *noun* enzyme which breaks down starch and converts it into sugar

diastasis [daɪə'steɪsɪs] *noun* (i) condition where a bone separates into parts; (ii) dislocation of bones at an immovable joint

diastole [daɪ'æstəli] *noun* phase in the beating of the heart between two contractions, where the heart dilates and fills with blood; *the period of diastole (normally 95 mmHg) lasts about 0.4 seconds in a normal heart rate*

diastolic pressure [daɪə'stɒlɪk 'preʃə] *noun* blood pressure taken at the diastole; *compare* SYSTOLE, SYSTOLIC

COMMENT: diastolic pressure is always lower than systolic

diathermy [daɪə'θɜːmi] *noun* using high frequency electric current to produce heat in body tissue; **medical diathermy** = using heat produced by electricity for treatment of muscle and joint disorders (such as rheumatism); **surgical diathermy** = using a knife or electrode which is heated by a strong electric current until it coagulates tissue; **diathermy knife** *or* **diathermy needle** = instrument used in surgical diathermy

COMMENT: the difference between medical and surgical uses of diathermy is in the size of the electrodes used. Two large electrodes will give a warming effect over a large area (medical diathermy); if

one of the electrodes is small, the heat will be concentrated enough to coagulate tissue (surgical diathermy)

diathesis [daɪ'æθəsɪs] *noun* general inherited constitution of a person, with his susceptibility to certain diseases or allergies

dichlorodiphenyltrichloroethane (DDT) [dɪklɒrəʊdaɪ'fiːnɪltraɪklɒrəʊ'eθeɪn] *noun* higly toxic insecticide, formerly commonly used, but now banned in many countries

dichromatic [daɪkrəʊ'mætɪk] *adjective* seeing only two of the three primary colours; *compare* TRICHROMATIC

Dick test ['dɪk 'test] *noun* test to show if a patient is immune to scarlet fever

dicrotic pulse *or* **dicrotic wave** [daɪ'krɒtɪk 'pʌls *or* daɪ'krɒtɪk 'weɪv] *noun* pulse which beats twice

dicrotism ['daɪkrətɪzm] *noun* condition where the pulse dilates twice with each heartbeat

didelphys [daɪ'delfɪs] *noun* **uterus didelphys** = double uterus, a condition where the uterus is divided in two by a membrane

die [daɪ] **1** *noun* cast of the patient's mouth taken by a dentist before making a denture **2** *verb* to stop living; *his father died last year*; *she died in a car crash* (NOTE: **dying - died - has died**)

diencephalon [daɪen'sefəlɒn *or* daɪen'kefəlɒn] *noun* central part of the forebrain, formed of the thalamus, hypothalamus, pineal gland and third ventricle

diet ['daɪət] **1** *noun* (i) amount and type of food eaten; (ii) measured amount of food eaten, usually to try to lose weight; *he lives on a diet of bread and beer*; *the doctor asked her to follow a strict diet*; *he has been on a diet for some weeks, but still hasn't lost enough weight*; **diet sheet** = list of suggestions for quantities and types of food given to a patient to follow; **balanced diet** = diet which contains the right quantities of basic nutrients; **bland diet** = diet in which the patient eats mainly milk-based foods, boiled vegetables and white meat, as a treatment for peptic ulcers; **diabetic diet** = diet which is low in carbohydrates and sugar; **low-calorie diet** = diet which provides less than the normal number of calories; **low salt diet** = diet which includes very little salt; **salt-free diet** = diet which does not contain any salt at all; *see also* SLIMMING **2** *verb* to reduce the quantity of food eaten, to change the type of food eaten in order to become thinner or healthier; *she dieted for two weeks before going on holiday*; *he is dieting to try to lose weight*

dietary ['daɪətrɪ] **1** *noun* system of nutrition and energy; *the nutritionist supervised the dietaries for the patients* **2** *adjective* referring to a diet; **dietary fibre** = roughage, fibrous matter in food, which cannot be digested

COMMENT: dietary fibre is found in cereals, nuts, fruit and some green vegetables. It is believed to be necessary to help digestion and avoid developing constipation, obesity and appendicitis

dietetic [daɪə'tetɪk] *adjective* referring to diet; **dietetic principles** = rules concerning the body's needs in food, vitamins or trace elements

dietetics [daɪə'tetɪks] *noun* study of food, nutrition and health, especially when applied to the food intake

dieting ['daɪətɪŋ] *noun* attempting to reduce weight by reducing the amount of food eaten

dietitian [daɪə'tɪʃn] *noun* person who specializes in the study of diet, especially an officer in a hospital who supervises dietaries as part of the medical treatment of patients

Dietl's crisis ['diːtəlz 'kraɪsɪs] *noun* painful blockage of the ureter, causing back pressure on the kidney which fills with urine, and swells

difference ['dɪfrns] *noun* way in which two things are not the same; *can you tell the difference between butter and margarine?*

different ['dɪfrnt] *adjective* not the same; *living in the country is very different from living in the town*; *he looks quite different since he had the operation*

differential [dɪfə'renʃl] *adjective* referring to a difference; **differential diagnosis** = identification of one particular disease from other similar diseases by comparing the range of symptoms of each; **differential blood count** *or* **differential white cell count** = showing the amounts of different types of (white) blood cell in a blood sample

differentiate [dɪfə'renʃɪeɪt] *verb* to tell the difference between; to be different from; **the tumour is clearly differentiated** = the tumour can be easily identified from the surrounding tissue

differentiation [dɪfərenʃɪ'eɪʃn] *noun* development of specialized cells during the early embryo stage

difficult ['dɪfɪkʌlt] *adjective* hard to do, not easy; *the practical examination was very difficult - half the students failed*; *the heart-lung transplant is a particularly difficult operation*; *the doctor had to use forceps because the childbirth was difficult*

difficulty ['dɪfɪkʌltɪ] *noun* problem, thing which is not easy; *she has difficulty in breathing* *or* *in getting enough vitamins*

diffuse 1 [dɪ'fjuːz] *verb* to spread through tissue; *some substances easily diffuse through the walls of capillaries* **2** [dɪ'fjuːs] *adjective* (disease) which is widespread in the body, or which affects many organs or cells

diffusion [dɪ'fjuːʒn] *noun* (i) mixing a liquid with another liquid, or a gas with another gas; (ii) passing of a liquid or gas through a membrane

digest [daɪ'dʒest] *verb* to break down food in the alimentary tract and convert it into elements which are absorbed into the body

digestible [daɪ'dʒestəbl] *adjective* which can be digested; *glucose is an easily digestible form of sugar*

digestion [daɪ'dʒestʃn] *noun* process by which food is broken down in the alimentary tract into elements which can be absorbed by the body

digestive [daɪ'dʒestɪv] *adjective* referring to digestion; **digestive enzymes** = enzymes which encourage digestion; **digestive system** = all the organs in the body (such as the liver and pancreas) which are associated with the digestion of food; **digestive tract** = the alimentary tract, the passage from the mouth to the rectum, down which food passes and is digested; *US* **digestive tube** = ALIMENTARY CANAL

COMMENT: the digestive tract is formed of the mouth, throat, oesophagus stomach and small and large intestines. Food is broken down by digestive juices in the mouth, stomach and small intestine, water is removed in the large intestine, and the remaining matter is passed out of the body as faeces

digit ['dɪdʒɪt] *noun* (a) a finger or a toe (b) a number

digital ['dɪdʒɪtl] *adjective* (a) referring to fingers or toes; **digital veins** = veins draining the fingers or toes (b) **digital computer** =

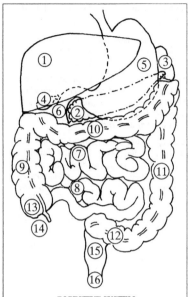

DIGESTIVE SYSTEM

1. liver	9. ascending colon
2. pancreas	10. transverse colon
3. spleen	11. descending colon
4. gall bladder	12. sigmoid colon
5. stomach	13. caecum
6. duodenum	14. appendix
7. jejunum	15. rectum
8. ileum	16. anus

computer which calculates on the basis of numbers

digitalin *or* **digitalis** [dɪdʒɪˈteɪlɪn or dɪdʒɪˈteɪlɪs] *noun* poisonous drug extracted from the foxglove plant, used in small doses to treat heart conditions, the active form is digoxin; *see also* DRUGS TABLE IN SUPPLEMENT

digitalize [ˈdɪdʒɪtəlaɪz] *verb* to treat with digoxin (for the treatment of heart failure)

digoxin [daɪˈgɒksɪn] *noun* the active form of digitalis

dilatation *or* **dilation** [daɪleɪˈteɪʃn or daɪˈleɪʃn] *noun* (i) expansion of a hollow space or a passage in the body; (ii) expansion of the pupil of the eye as a reaction to bad light or to drugs; *dilatation of the cervix during labour*; **dilatation and curettage (D & C)** = surgical operation to scrape the interior of the uterus to obtain a tissue sample or to remove products of miscarriage

dilate [daɪˈleɪt or dɪˈleɪt] *verb* to swell; *the veins in the left leg have become dilated*; *the drug is used to dilate the pupil of the eye*

dilator [daɪˈleɪtə or dɪˈleɪtə] *noun* (i) instrument used to widen the entrance to a cavity; (ii) drug used to make part of the body expand; **dilator pupillae muscle** = muscle in the iris which pulls the iris back and so dilates the pupil

diluent [ˈdɪljuənt] *noun* substance (such as water) which is used to dilute a liquid

dilute [daɪˈluːt or dɪˈluːt] **1** *adjective* with water added; *bathe the wound in a solution of dilute antiseptic* **2** *verb* to add water to a liquid to make it weaker; *the disinfectant must be diluted in four parts of water before it can be used on the skin*

dilution [daɪˈluːʃn or dɪˈluːʃn] *noun* (i) action of diluting; (ii) liquid which has been diluted

dimetria [daɪˈmiːtriə] *noun* condition where a woman has a double uterus; *see also* DIDELPHYS

dioptre US **diopter** [daɪˈɒptə] *noun* unit of measurement of refraction of a lens

> COMMENT: a one dioptre lens has a focal length of one metre; the greater the dioptre, the shorter the focal length

dioxide [daɪˈɒksaɪd] *see* CARBON

DIP = DISTAL INTERPHALANGEAL JOINT

diphtheria [dɪfˈθɪəriə] *noun* serious infectious disease of children, caused by the bacillus *Corynebacterium diphtheriae,* with fever and the formation of a fibrous growth like a membrane in the throat which restricts breathing

> COMMENT: infants in the UK are immunized against diphtheria. Symptoms begin usually with a sore throat, followed by a slight fever, rapid pulse and swelling of glands in the neck. The 'membrane' which forms can close the air passages, and the disease is often fatal, either because the patient is asphyxiated or because the heart becomes fatally weakened. The disease is also highly infectious, and all contacts of the patient must be tested. The Schick test is used to test if a person is immune or susceptible to diphtheria

diphtheroid [ˈdɪfθərɔɪd] *adjective* (bacterium) like the diphtheria bacterium

-dipine [ˈdɪpɪn] *suffix* used in names of calcium blockers; *nifedipine*

dipl- *or* **diplo-** [dɪpl *or* ˈdɪpləʊ] *prefix* meaning double

diplacusis [dɪpləˈkjuːsɪs] *noun* (i) condition where a patient hears double sounds; (ii) condition where a patient hears the same sound in a different way in each ear

diplegia [daɪˈpliːdʒə] *noun* paralysis of a similar part on both sides of the body (such as both arms)

diplegic [daɪˈpledʒɪk] *adjective* referring to diplegia; *compare* HEMIPLEGIA

diplococcus   [dɪpləʊˈkɒkəs]   *noun* bacterium which occurs in pairs (NOTE: plural is **diplococci**)

diploe [ˈdɪpləʊiː] *noun* layer of spongy bone tissue filled with red bone marrow, between the inner and outer layers of the skull

diploid [ˈdɪplɔɪd] *adjective* (cell) where each chromosome (except the sex chromosome) occurs twice; *compare*   HAPLOID, POLYPLOID

diploma [dɪˈpləʊmə] *noun* certificate showing that a person has successfully finished a course of specialized training; *he has a diploma from a College of Nursing*; *she is taking her diploma exams next week*

diplopia [dɪˈpləʊpiə] *noun* double vision, a condition where a patient sees single objects as double; *compare* POLYOPIA

dipsomania   [dɪpsəʊˈmeɪniə]   *noun* uncontrollable desire to drink alcohol

direct [dəˈrekt *or* dɪˈrekt *or* daɪˈrekt] **1** *adjective & adverb* straight, with nothing intervening; *his dermatitis is due to direct contact with irritants* **2** *verb* to tell someone what to do or how to go somewhere; *the police directed the ambulances to the scene of the accident*; *can you direct me to the outpatients' unit?*; *she spent two years directing the work of the research team*

direction [daɪˈrekʃn] *noun (on bottle of medicine, etc.)* **directions (for use)** = instructions showing how to use something and how much of it to use

directly [dəˈrektlɪ *or* dɪˈrektlɪ *or* daɪˈrektlɪ] *adverb* straight, with nothing in between; *the endocrine or ductless glands secrete hormones directly into the bloodstream*; *the dressing should not be placed directly on the burn*

director [dəˈrektə *or* dɪˈrektə *or* daɪˈrektə] *noun* **(a)** person in charge of a department; *he is the director of the burns unit* **(b)**

instrument used to limit the incision made with a surgical knife

dirt [dɜːt] *noun* material which is not clean, like mud, dust, earth, etc.; *he allowed dirt to get into the wound which became infected*

dirty [ˈdɜːti] *adjective* not clean; *dirty sheets are taken off the beds every morning*; *everyone concerned with patient care has to make sure that the wards are not dirty* (NOTE: **dirty - dirtier - dirtiest**)

disability [dɪsəˈbɪləti] *noun* condition where part of the body does not function normally; *deafness is a disability which affects old people*; *people with severe disabilities can claim grants from the government*; *see also* LEARNING DISABILITY

> disability – any restriction or lack (resulting from an impairment) of ability to perform an activity in the manner or within the range considered normal for a human being
>
> *WHO*

disable [dɪsˈeɪbl] *verb* to make someone unable to do some normal activity; *he was disabled by the lung disease*; *a hospital for disabled soldiers*; **disabling disease** = disease which makes it impossible for a person to do some normal activity; **the disabled** = people suffering from a physical or mental handicap which prevents them from doing some normal activity

disablement   [dɪsˈeɪbəlmənt]   *noun* condition where a person has a physical or mental handicap

disarticulation   [dɪsɑːtɪkjuˈleɪʃn]   *noun* amputation of a limb at a joint, which does not involve dividing a bone

disc [dɪsk] *noun* flat round structure like a plate; **intervertebral disc** = round plate of cartilage which separates two vertebrae in the spinal column; **displaced intervertebral disc** *or* **prolapsed intervertebral disc** *or* **slipped disc** = condition where an intervertebral disc becomes displaced or where the soft centre of a disc passes through the hard cartilage outside and presses on a nerve; *see illustrations at* JOINTS, VERTEBRAL COLUMN; **Merkel's discs** = receptor cells in the lower part of the epidermis; *see illustration at* SKIN AND SENSORY RECEPTORS

discharge 1 ['dɪstʃɑːdʒ] *noun* **(a)** (i) secretion of liquid from an opening; (ii) release of nervous energy; **vaginal discharge** = flow of liquid from the vagina **(b)** sending a patient away from a hospital because the treatment has ended; **discharge rate** = number of patients with a certain type of disorder who are sent away from hospitals in a certain area (shown as a number per 10,000 of population) **2** [dɪs'tʃɑːdʒ] *verb* **(a)** to secrete liquid out of an opening; *the wound discharged a thin stream of pus* **(b)** to send a patient away from hospital because the treatment has ended; *he was discharged from hospital last week*; **she discharged herself** = she decided to leave hospital and stop taking the treatment provided

discoloration [dɪskʌlə'reɪʃn] *noun* change in colour

discolour *US* **discolor** [dɪs'kʌlə] *verb* to change the colour of something; *his teeth were discoloured from smoking cigarettes*

COMMENT: teeth can be discoloured in fluorosis; if the skin on the lips is discoloured it may indicate that the patient has swallowed a poison

discomfort [dɪs'kʌmfət] *noun* feeling of not being comfortable or not being completely well; *she experienced some discomfort after the operation*

discontinue [dɪskən'tɪnjuː] *verb* to stop doing something; *the doctors decided to discontinue the treatment*; *the use of the drug has been discontinued because of the possibility of side-effects*

discontinued [dɪskən'tɪnjuːd] *adjective* no longer made; *the drug is discontinued*

discover [dɪs'kʌvə] *verb* to find something which was hidden or not known before; *scientists are trying to discover a cure for this disease*

discoverer [dɪ'skʌvrə] *noun* person who discovers something; *who was the discoverer of penicillin?*

discovery [dɪ'skʌvri] *noun* finding something which was not known before; *the discovery of penicillin completely changed hospital treatment*; *new medical discoveries are reported each week*

discrete [dɪ'skriːt] *adjective* separate, not joined together; **discrete rash** = rash which is formed of many separate spots, which do not join together into one large red patch

disease [dɪ'ziːz] *noun* illness (of people, animals, plants, etc.) where the body functions abnormally; *he caught a disease in the tropics*; *she is suffering from a very serious disease of the kidneys or from a serious kidney disease*; *he is a specialist in occupational diseases or in diseases which affect workers*

diseased [dɪ'ziːzd] *adjective* (person or part of the body) affected by an illness, not whole or normal; *the doctor cut away the diseased tissue* (NOTE: although a particular disease may have few visible characteristic symptoms, the term 'disease' is applied to all physical and mental reactions which make a person ill. Diseases with distinct characteristics have names. For terms referring to disease, see words beginning with **path-** or **patho-**)

disfigure [dɪs'fɪgə] *verb* to change someone's appearance so as to make it less pleasant; *her legs were disfigured by scars*

disinfect [dɪsɪn'fekt] *verb* to make a place free from microbes; *she disinfected the skin with surgical spirit*; *all the patient's clothes have to be disinfected*

disinfectant [dɪsɪn'fektənt] *noun* substance used to kill microbes

disinfection [dɪsɪn'fekʃn] *noun* removal of infection caused by microbes (NOTE: the words **disinfect** and **disinfectant** are used for substances which destroy microbes on instruments, objects or the skin; substances used to kill microbes inside infected people are **antibiotics, drugs, etc.**)

disintegrate [dɪs'ɪntɪgreɪt] *verb* to come to pieces; *in holocrine glands the cells disintegrate as they secrete*

disintegration [dɪsɪntɪ'greɪʃn] *noun* act of disintegrating

disk [dɪsk] *see* DISC

dislike [dɪs'laɪk] **1** *noun* not liking something; *he has a strong dislike of cats* **2** *verb* not to like something; *she dislikes going to the dentist*

dislocate ['dɪsləkeɪt] *verb* to displace a bone from its normal position at a joint; *he fell and dislocated his elbow*; *the shoulder joint dislocates easily or is easily dislocated*

dislocation [dɪslə'keɪʃn] *noun* luxation, condition where a bone is displaced from its normal position at a joint; **pathological dislocation** = dislocation of a diseased joint

dislodge [dɪsˈlɒdʒ] *verb* to move something which is stuck; *by coughing he managed to dislodge the bone stuck in his throat*

disorder [dɪsˈɔːdə] *noun* (i) illness or sickness; (ii) state where part of the body is not functioning correctly; *the doctor specializes in disorders of the kidneys or in kidney disorders*; *the family has a history of mental disorder*; **cognitive disorder** = impairment of any of the mental processes of perception, memory, judgement and reasoning; **motor disorder** = impairment of the nerves or neurons that cause muscles to contract to produce movement

disordered [dɪsˈɔːdəd] *adjective* (i) not functioning correctly; (ii) (organ) affected by a disease; **disordered action of the heart (DAH)** = da Costa's syndrome, condition where the patient suffers palpitations, breathlessness and dizziness, caused by effort or worry

disorientated [dɪsˈɔːrɪənteɪtɪd] *adjective* (patient) who is confused and does not know where he is

disorientation [dɪsɔːrɪənˈteɪʃn] *noun* condition where the patient is not completely conscious of space, time or place

dispensary [dɪˈspensri] *noun* place (part of a chemist's shop or department of a hospital) where drugs are prepared or mixed and given out according to a doctor's prescription

dispensing chemist [dɪˈspensɪŋ ˈkemɪst] *noun* pharmacist who prepares and provides drugs according to a doctor's prescription

> COMMENT: in the UK, prescriptions can only be dispensed by qualified and registered pharmacists who must keep accurate records

displace [dɪsˈpleɪs] *verb* to put out of the usual place; **displaced intervertebral disc** = disc which has moved slightly, so that the soft interior passes through the tougher exterior and causes pressure on a nerve

displacement [dɪsˈpleɪsmənt] *noun* movement out of the normal position; *fracture of the radius together with displacement of the wrist*

disposable [dɪsˈpəʊzəbl] *adjective* (item) which can be thrown away after use; *disposable syringes*; *disposable petri dishes*

disproportion [dɪsprəˈpɔːʃn] *noun* lack of proper relationships between two things; **cephalopelvic disproportion** = condition

where the pelvic opening of the mother is not large enough for the head of the fetus

dissecans [ˈdɪsəkæns] *see* OSTEOCHONDRITIS

dissect [dɪˈsekt or daɪˈsekt] *verb* to cut and separate tissues in a body to examine them; **dissecting aneurysm** = aneurysm which occurs when the inside wall of the aorta is torn, and blood enters the membrane

dissection [dɪˈsekʃn or daɪˈsekʃn] *noun* cutting and separating parts of a body or an organ as part of a surgical operation, as part of an autopsy or as part of a course of study

```
renal dissection usually takes
from 40 - 60 minutes, while
liver and pancreas dissections
take from one to three hours.
Cardiac dissection takes about
20 minutes and lung dissection
takes 60 to 90 minutes
```
Nursing Times

disseminated [dɪˈsemɪneɪtɪd] *adjective* occurring in every part of an organ or in the whole body; **disseminated sclerosis** = MULTIPLE SCLEROSIS; **disseminated lupus erythematosus (DLE)** = inflammatory disease where the skin rash is associated with widespread changes in the central nervous system, the cardiovascular system and many organs

dissemination [dɪsemɪˈneɪʃn] *noun* being widespread throughout the body

dissociate [dɪˈsəʊsɪeɪt] *verb* (i) to separate parts or functions; (ii) to separate part of the conscious mind from the rest; **dissociated anaesthesia** = loss of sensitivity to heat, pain or cold

> COMMENT: patients will dissociate their delusion from the real world around them as a way of escaping from the facts of the real world

dissociation [dɪsəʊʃɪˈeɪʃn] *noun* **(a)** separating of parts or functions **(b)** *(in psychiatry)* condition where part of the consciousness becomes separated from the rest and becomes independent

dissociative disorder [dɪˈsəʊsɪətɪv dɪsˈɔːdə] *noun* type of hysteria where the subject shows psychological rather than physical troubles (split personality, amnesia, etc.)

dissolve [dɪˈzɒlv] *verb* to absorb or disperse something in liquid; *the gut used in sutures slowly dissolves in the body fluids*

distal ['dɪstl] *adjective* further away from the centre of a body; **distal interphalangeal joint (DIP)** = joint nearest the end of the finger or toe; **distal phalanges** = bones nearest the ends of the fingers and toes; **distal convoluted tubule** = part of the kidney filtering system before the collecting ducts (NOTE: the opposite is **proximal.** Note also that you say that a part is distal **to** another part)

distally ['dɪstli] *adverb* placed further away from the centre or point of attachment

distend [dɪs'tend] *verb* to swell by pressure

distended [dɪs'tendɪd] *adjective* made larger by gas such as air, by liquid such as urine, or by a solid; **distended bladder** = bladder which is full of urine

distension [dɪs'tenʃn] *noun* condition where something is swollen; *distension of the veins in the abdomen is a sign of blocking of the portal vein*; **abdominal distension** = swelling of the abdomen (because of gas or fluid)

distil [dɪ'stɪl] *verb* to separate the component parts of a liquid by boiling and collecting the condensed vapour; **distilled water** = purified water, water which has been made pure by distillation

distillation [dɪstɪ'leɪʃn] *noun* action of distilling a liquid

distinct [dɪ'stɪŋkt] *adjective* separate, not to be confused; *the colon is divided into four distinct sections*

distinctive [dɪ'stɪŋktɪv] *adjective* easily noticed, characteristic; *mumps is easily diagnosed by distinctive swellings on the side of the face*

distort [dɪ'stɔːt] *verb* to twist something into an abnormal shape; *his lower limbs were distorted by the disease*

distortion [dɪ'stɔːʃn] *noun* twisting of part of the body out of its normal shape

distress [dɪ'stres] *noun* suffering caused by pain or worry; *attempted suicide is often a sign of the person's mental distress*; **fetal distress** = condition (heart problems, respiratory problems, etc.) of a fetus which may not survive if the condition is not monitored and corrected; **infant respiratory distress syndrome** = condition of newborn babies where the lungs do not function properly

district ['dɪstrɪkt] *noun* area or part of the country or town; **district general hospital** = hospital which serves the needs of the population of a district; **District Health Authority (DHA)** = administrative unit in the National Health Service which is responsible for all health services provided in a district; **district nurse** = nurse who visits patients in their homes in a certain area

disturb [dɪ'stɜːb] *verb* to worry someone, to stop someone working by talking, etc.; *don't disturb him when he's working*; *his sleep was disturbed by the other patients in the ward*

disturbance [dɪ'stɜːbns] *noun* being disturbed; *the blow to the head caused disturbance to the brain*

diuresis [daɪjuˈriːsɪs] *noun* increase in the production of urine

diuretic [daɪjuˈretɪk] *adjective & noun* (substance, such as frusemide) which makes the kidneys produce more urine, used in the treatment of oedema and hypertension

diurnal [daɪˈɜːnl] *adjective* happening in the daytime, happening every day

divalent ['daɪveɪlənt] *adjective* having a valency of two

divergent strabismus [daɪˈvɜːdʒnt strəˈbɪzməs] *noun* condition where a person's eyes both look away from the nose

diverticular disease [daɪvəˈtɪkjulə dɪˈziːz] *noun* disease of the large intestine, where the colon thickens and diverticula form in the walls, causing the patient pain in the lower abdomen

diverticulitis [daɪvətɪkjuˈlaɪtɪs] *noun* inflammation of diverticula formed in the wall of the colon

diverticulosis [daɪvətɪkjuˈləusɪs] *noun* condition where diverticula form in the intestine but are not inflamed (in the small intestine, this can lead to blind loop syndrome)

diverticulum [daɪvəˈtɪkjuləm] *noun* little sac or pouch which develops in the wall of the intestine or other organ; **Meckel's diverticulum** = congenital formation of a diverticulum in the ileum (NOTE: the plural is **diverticula**)

divide [dɪ'vaɪd] *verb* to separate into parts; *the common carotid divides into two smaller arteries*

division [dɪ'vɪʒn] *noun* cutting into parts, splitting into parts; **cell division** = way in which a cell reproduces itself by mitosis

divulsor [dɪˈvʌlsə] *noun* surgical instrument used to expand a passage

dizygotic twins [daɪzaɪˈgɒtɪk ˈtwɪnz] = FRATERNAL TWINS

dizziness [ˈdɪzinəs] *noun* feeling that everything is going round because the sense of balance has been affected

dizzy [ˈdɪzi] *adjective* having the sense of balance affected, feeling that everything is going round; *after standing in the sun, she became dizzy and had to lie down*; *he suffers from dizzy spells*

dl = DECILITRE

DLE [ˈdiː ˈel ˈiː] = DISSEMINATED LUPUS ERYTHEMATOSUS

dm = DECIMETRE

DMD [ˈdiː ˈem ˈdiː] *US* = DOCTOR OF DENTAL MEDICINE

DNA [ˈdiː ˈen ˈeɪ] = DEOXYRIBONUCLEIC ACID

DOA [ˈdiː ˈəʊ ˈeɪ] = DEAD ON ARRIVAL

doctor [ˈdɒktə] *noun* **(a)** person who has trained in medicine and is qualified to examine people when they are ill to find out what is wrong with them and to prescribe a course of treatment; *his son is training to be a doctor*; *if you have a pain in your chest, you ought to see a doctor*; *he has gone to the doctor's*; *do you want to make an appointment with the doctor?*; **family doctor** = general practitioner, a doctor who looks after the health of people in his area; **hospital doctor** = doctor who works only in a hospital and does not receive patients in his own surgery **(b)** title given to a qualified person who is registered with the General Medical Council; *I have an appointment with Dr Jones* (NOTE: **doctor** is shortened to **Dr** when written before a name. In the UK surgeons are traditionally not called 'Doctor', but are addressed as 'Mr', 'Mrs', etc. The title 'doctor' is also applied to persons who have a high degree from a university in a non-medical subject. So 'Dr Jones' may have a degree in music, or in any other subject without a connection with medicine)

Döderlein's bacillus [ˈdɜːdəlaɪnz bəˈsɪlʌs] *noun* bacterium usually found in the vagina

DOH [ˈdiː ˈəʊ ˈeɪtʃ] = DEPARTMENT OF HEALTH

dolichocephalic [dɒlɪkəʊseˈfælɪk] *adjective* (person) with a long skull

dolichocephaly [dɒlɪkəʊˈsefəli] *noun* condition of a person who has a skull which is longer than normal

COMMENT: in dolichocephaly, the measurement across the skull is less than 75% of the length of the head from front to back

dolor [ˈdɒlə] *noun* pain

dolorimetry [dɒləˈrɪmətri] *noun* measuring of pain

dolorosa [dɒləˈrəʊsə] *see* ADIPOSIS

domicile [ˈdɒmɪsaɪl] *noun* (*in official use*) home, place where someone lives

domiciliary [dɒmɪˈsɪliəri] *adjective* at home or in the home; **the doctor made a domiciliary visit** = he visited the patient at home; **domiciliary midwife** = nurse with special qualification in midwifery, who can assist in childbirth at home; **domiciliary services** = nursing services which are available to patients in their homes

dominance [ˈdɒmɪnəns] *noun* being more powerful; **cerebral dominance** = normal condition where the centres for various functions are located in one cerebral hemisphere; **ocular dominance** = condition where a person uses one eye more than the other

dominant [ˈdɒmɪnənt] *adjective & noun* (genetic trait) which is more powerful than other recessive genes

COMMENT: since each physical trait is governed by two genes, if one is recessive and the other dominant, the resulting trait will be that of the dominant gene

donor [ˈdəʊnə] *noun* person who gives his own tissue or organs for use in transplants; **blood donor** = person who gives blood which is then used in transfusions to other patients; **kidney donor** = person who gives one of his kidneys as a transplant; **sperm donor** = male who gives sperm (for a fee) to allow a childless woman to bear a child; **universal donor** = subject with group O blood, whose blood may, in theory, be given to anyone; **donor card** = card carried by a person stating that he approves of his organs being used for transplanting after he has died; *see also* INSEMINATION

dopamine [ˈdəʊpəmiːn] *noun* substance found in the medulla of the adrenal glands, which also acts as a neurotransmitter, lack of which is associated with Parkinson's disease;

see also DRUGS TABLE IN SUPPLEMENT

dopaminergic [dəʊpəmɪˈnɜːdʒɪk] *adjective* (neurones, receptors) stimulated by dopamine

doppler transducer [ˈdɒplə trænzˈdjuːsə] *noun* device to measure blood flow, commonly used to monitor foetal heart rate

dormant [ˈdɔːmənt] *adjective* inactive for a time; *the virus lies dormant in the body for several years*

dorsal [ˈdɔːsl] *adjective* (i) referring to the back; (ii) referring to the back of the body; **dorsal vertebrae** = twelve vertebrae in the back, between the cervical vertebrae and the lumbar vertebrae (NOTE: the opposite is **ventral**)

dorsi- *or* **dorso-** [ˈdɔːsi *or* ˈdɔːsəʊ] *prefix* referring to the back

dorsiflexion [dɔːsɪˈflekʃn] *noun* flexion towards the back of part of the body (such as raising the foot at the ankle, as opposed to plantar flexion)

dorsoventral [dɔːsəʊˈventrl] *adjective* (i) referring to the back of the body and the front; (ii) extending from the back of the body to the front

dorsum [ˈdɔːsəm] *noun* back of any part of the body

dosage [ˈdəʊsɪdʒ] *noun* **(a)** correct amounts of a drug calculated by a doctor to be necessary for a patient; *the doctor decided to increase the dosage of antibiotics*; *the dosage for children is half that for adults* **(b)** quantity of a drug, etc., prescribed; *he prescribed an incorrect dosage*

dose [dəʊs] **1** *noun* measured quantity of a drug or radiation which is to be administered to a patient at a time; *it is dangerous to exceed the prescribed dose*; **effective dose** = dose which will produce the effect required; **safe dose** = amount of a drug which can be given without being harmful to the patient **2** *verb* **to dose with** = to give a patient a drug; *she dosed her son with aspirin and cough medicine before he went to his examination*; *the patient has been dosing herself with laxatives*

dosimeter [dəʊˈsɪmɪtə] *noun* instrument which measures the amount of X-rays or other radiation received

dosimetry [dəʊˈsɪmətri] *noun* measuring the amount of X-rays or radiation received, using a dosimeter

double [ˈdʌbl] *adjective* with two similar parts; **double figures** = numbers from 10 to 99; **double pneumonia** = pneumonia in both lungs; **double uterus** = DIDELPHYS; **bent double** = bent over completely so that the face is towards the ground; *he was bent double with arthritis*

double-blind [ˈdʌblˈblaɪnd] *noun* **double blind** *or* **double-blind study** = way of testing a new drug, where neither the people taking the test, nor the people administering it know which patients have had the real drug and which have had the placebo

double-jointed [ˈdʌblˈdʒɔɪntɪd] *adjective* able to bend joints to an abnormal degree

double vision [ˈdʌbl ˈvɪʒn] = DIPLOPIA

douche [duːʃ] *noun* liquid forced into the body to wash out a cavity; device used for washing out a cavity; **vaginal douche** = device or liquid for washing out the vagina

Douglas [ˈdʌgləs] *noun* **Douglas bag** = bag used for measuring the volume of air breathed out of the lungs; **Douglas' pouch** = the rectouterine peritoneal recess

douloureux [duːluːˈruː] *see* TIC

Down's syndrome [ˈdaʊnz ˈsɪndrəʊm] *noun* trisomy 21, a congenital defect, due to existence of an extra third chromosome at number 21; in which the patient has slanting eyes, a wide face, speech difficulties and is usually mentally retarded to some extent (NOTE: formerly called 'mongolism' because of the shape of the eyes)

doze [dəʊz] *verb* to sleep a little, to sleep lightly; *she dozed off for a while after lunch*

dozy [ˈdəʊzi] *adjective* sleepy; *these antihistamines can make you feel dozy*

DPT [ˈdiː ˈpiː ˈtiː] = DIPHTHERIA, WHOOPING COUGH (Pertussis), TETANUS; **DPT vaccine** *or* **DPT immunization** = combined vaccine or immunization against the three diseases given to infants in the UK

drachm [dræm] *noun* measure used in pharmacy (dry weight equals 3.8g, liquid measure equals 3.7ml)

dracontiasis *or* **dracunculiasis** [drækɒnˈtaɪəsɪs *or* drəkʌŋkjuˈlaɪəsɪs] *noun* tropical disease caused by the guinea worm *Dracunculus medinensis* which enters the body from infected drinking water and forms blisters on the skin, frequently leading to secondary arthritis, fibrosis and cellulitis

Dracunculus [drə'kʌŋkjuləs] *noun* the guinea worm, a parasitic worm which enters the body and rises to the skin to form a blister

dragee ['dræʒeɪ] *noun* sugar-coated drug tablet or pill

drain [dreɪn] **1** *noun* **(a)** pipe for carrying waste water from a house; *the report of the health inspectors was critical of the drains* **(b)** tube to remove liquid from the body **2** *verb* to remove liquid from something; *an operation to drain the sinus*; *they drained the pus from the abscess*

drainage ['dreɪnɪdʒ] *noun* **(a)** removal of liquid from the site of an operation, pus from an abscess by means of a tube or wick left in the body for a time **(b)** removal of waste water

drape [dreɪp] *noun* thin material used to place over a patient about to undergo surgery, leaving the operation site uncovered

draw-sheet ['drɔːʃiːt] *noun* sheet under a patient in bed, folded so that it can be pulled out as it becomes soiled

dream [driːm] **1** *noun* images which a person sees when asleep; *I had a bad dream about spiders* **2** *verb* to think you see something happening while you are asleep; *he dreamt he was attacked by spiders* (NOTE: **dreaming - dreamed** *or* **dreamt**)

drepanocyte ['drepənəusaɪt] = SICKLE CELL

drepanocytosis [drepənəusaɪ'təusɪs] = SICKLE-CELL ANAEMIA

dress [dres] *verb* **(a)** to put on clothes; *he (got) dressed and then had breakfast*; *the surgeon was dressed in a green gown*; *you can get dressed again now* **(b)** to clean a wound and put a covering over it; *nurses dressed the wounds of the accident victims*

dressing ['dresɪŋ] *noun* covering or bandage applied to a wound to protect it; *the patient's dressings need to be changed every two hours*; **gauze dressing** = dressing of thin light material; **sterile dressing** = dressing which is sold in a sterile pack, ready for use; **adhesive dressing** = *see* ADHESIVE

dribble ['drɪbl] *verb* to let liquid flow slowly out of an opening, especially saliva out of the mouth; *the baby dribbled over her dress*

dribbling ['drɪblɪŋ] *noun* (i) letting saliva flow out of the mouth; (ii) incontinence, being unable to keep back the flow of urine

drill [drɪl] **1** *noun* tool which rotates very rapidly to make a hole; surgical instrument used in dentistry to remove caries **2** *verb* to make a hole with a drill; *a small hole is drilled in the skull*; *the dentist drilled one of her molars*

drink [drɪŋk] **1** *noun* **(a)** liquid which is swallowed; *have a drink of water*; *always have a hot drink before you go to bed*; **soft drinks** = drinks (like orange juice) with no alcohol in them **(b)** alcoholic drink **2** *verb* **(a)** to swallow liquid; *he drinks two cups of coffee for breakfast*; *you need to drink at least five pints of liquid a day* **(b)** to drink alcoholic drinks; *do you drink a lot?* (NOTE: **drinking - drank - has drunk**)

Drinker respirator ['drɪŋkə 'respɪreɪtə] *noun* iron lung, a machine which encloses the whole of a patient's body except the head, and in which air pressure is increased and decreased, so forcing the patient to breathe in and out

drip [drɪp] *noun* method of introducing liquid slowly and continuously into the body, where a bottle of liquid is held above the patient and the fluid flows slowly down a tube into a needle in a vein or into the stomach; *the patient was put on a drip*; **intravenous drip** = drip which goes into a vein; **saline drip** = drip containing salt solution; **drip feed** = drip containing nutrients

drop [drɒp] **1** *noun* **(a)** small quantity of liquid; *a drop of water fell on the floor*; *the optician prescribed her some drops for the eyes* **(b)** reduction or fall in quantity of something; **drop in pressure** = sudden reduction in pressure **2** *verb* to fall, to let something fall; *pressure in the artery dropped suddenly*

drop attack ['drɒp ə'tæk] *noun* condition where a person suddenly falls down, though he is not unconscious, caused by sudden weakness of the spine

drop foot ['drɒp 'fʊt] *noun* condition, caused by muscular disorder, where the ankle is not strong, and the foot hangs limp

droplet ['drɒplət] *noun* very small drop of liquid

drop off ['drɒp 'ɒf] *verb* to fall asleep; *she dropped off in front of the TV*

dropper ['drɒpə] *noun* small glass or plastic tube with a rubber bulb at one end, used to suck up and expel liquid in drops

dropsy ['drɒpsi] *noun* old term for the swelling of part of the body because of accumulation of fluid in the tissues

COMMENT: dropsy is usually caused by kidney failure or heart failure, leading to bad circulation. The legs (especially the ankles) and the arms become very swollen

drop wrist ['drɒp 'rɪst] *noun* condition, caused by muscular disorder, where the wrist is not strong, and the hand hangs limp

drown [draʊn] *verb* to die by inhaling liquid; *he fell into the sea and (was) drowned; six people drowned when the boat sank*

drowning ['draʊnɪŋ] *noun* act of dying by inhaling liquid; *the autopsy showed that death was due to drowning*; **dry drowning** = death where the patient's air passage has been constricted because he is under water, though he does not inhale any water

drowsiness ['draʊzɪnəs] *noun* sleepiness; *the medicine is likely to cause drowsiness*

drowsy ['draʊzi] *adjective* sleepy; *the injection will make you feel drowsy; (especially of cough medicine containing antihistamine)* **non drowsy** = which will not cause drowsiness

drug [drʌg] *noun* **(a)** chemical substance (either natural or synthetic) which is used in medicine and affects the way in which organs or tissues function; *the doctors are trying to cure him with a new drug; she was prescribed a course of pain-killing drugs; the drug is being monitored for possible side-effects*; **drug dependence** = being addicted to a drug and unable to exist without taking it regularly (can also apply to habit-forming substances not used in medicine) **(b)** habit-forming substance; *he has been taking drugs for several months; the government is trying to stamp out drug pushing; when he was arrested he was high on drugs*; **drug abuse** = taking habit-forming drugs; **drug abuser** = person who is addicted to a drug; **a high rate of drug-related deaths** = of deaths associated with the taking of drugs; **controlled drugs, US controlled substances** = drugs which are not freely available, which are restricted by law, and which are classified (Class A, B, C), and of which possession may be an offence; **dangerous drugs** = drugs which may be harmful to people who take them, and so can be prohibited from import and general sale; *see also* ABUSE, ADDICT, ADDICTION

COMMENT: there are three classes of controlled drugs: **Class 'A' drugs:** (cocaine, heroin, crack, LSD, etc.); **Class 'B' drugs:** (amphetamines, cannabis, codeine, etc.); and **Class 'C' drugs:** (drugs which are related to the amphetamines, such as benzphetamine). The drugs are covered by five schedules under the Misuse of Drugs Regulations: **Schedule 1:** drugs which are not used medicinally, such as cannabis and LSD, for which possession and supply are prohibited; **Schedule 2:** drugs which can be used medicinally, such as heroin, morphine, cocaine, and amphetamines: these are fully controlled as regards prescriptions by doctors, safe custody in pharmacies, registering of sales, etc. **Schedule 3:** barbiturates, which are controlled as regards prescriptions, but need not be kept in safe custody; **Schedule 4:** benzodiazepines, which are controlled as regards registers of purchasers; **Schedule 5:** other substances for which invoices showing purchase must be kept

drugstore ['drʌgstɔː] *noun US* shop where medicines and drugs can be bought (as well as many other goods)

drum [drʌm] *see* EARDRUM

drunk [drʌŋk] *adjective* intoxicated with too much alcohol

drunken ['drʌŋkn] *adjective* intoxicated; *the doctors had to get help to control the drunken patient* (NOTE: drunken is only used in front of a noun, and drunk is usually used after the verb to be: **a drunken patient; that patient is drunk**)

dry [draɪ] **1** *adjective* not wet, with the smallest amount of moisture; *the surface of the wound should be kept dry; she uses a cream to soften her dry skin*; **dry burn** = burn caused by touching a very hot dry surface; **dry eye** = XEROSIS; **dry gangrene** = condition where the blood supply has been cut off and the tissue becomes black; **dry ice** = CARBON DIOXIDE; *(dentistry)* **dry socket** = inflammation or infection of the socket of a tooth which has just been removed (NOTE: **dry - drier - driest**) **2** *verb* to remove moisture from something; to wipe something until it is dry

dryness ['draɪnəs] *noun* state of being dry; *she complained of dryness in her mouth; dryness in the eyes, accompanied by rheumatoid arthritis*

dry out ['draɪ 'aʊt] *verb* (i) to dry completely; (ii) *(informal)* to treat someone for alcoholism

DSS = DEPARTMENT OF SOCIAL SECURITY

DTs ['diː 'tiːz] = DELIRIUM TREMENS

Duchenne muscular dystrophy [duːˈʃen ˈmʌskjulə ˈdɪstrəfi] *noun* hereditary disease of the muscles where some muscles (starting with the legs) swell and become weak

COMMENT: usually found in young boys. It is carried in the mother's genes

Ducrey's bacillus [duːˈkreɪz bəˈsɪləs] *noun* type of bacterium found in the lungs, causing chancroid

duct [dʌkt] *noun* tube which carries liquids, especially one which carries secretions; **duct gland** = exocrine gland; **bile duct** = tube which links the cystic duct and the hepatic duct to the duodenum; **common bile duct** = duct leading to the duodenum, formed of the hepatic and cystic ducts together; **cystic duct** = duct which takes bile from the gall bladder to the common bile duct; **hepatic duct** = duct which links the liver to the bile duct leading to the duodenum; **common hepatic duct** = duct from the liver formed when the right and left hepatic ducts join; **cochlear duct** = spiral channel in the cochlea; **collecting duct** = part of the kidney filtering system; **efferent duct** = duct which carries liquid away from an organ; **ejaculatory ducts** = two ducts formed by the seminal vesicles and vas deferens, which go through the prostate and end in the urethra; *see illustration at* UROGENITAL SYSTEM (MALE); **lacrimal duct** *or* **nasolacrimal duct** *or* **tear duct** = canal which takes tears from the lacrimal sac into the nose; **right lymphatic duct** = one of the main terminal channels for carrying lymph, draining the right side of the head and neck and entering the junction of the right subclavian and internal jugular veins. It is the smaller of the two main discharge points of the lymphatic system into the venous system, the larger being the thoracic duct; **pancreatic ducts** = ducts leading through the pancreas to the duodenum; **semicircular ducts** = ducts in the semicircular canals in the ear; *see illustration at* EAR; **tear duct** = lacrimal duct, the canal which takes tears from the lacrimal sac to the nose; **thoracic duct** = one of the main terminal ducts carrying lymph, on the left side of the neck

ductile [ˈdʌktaɪl] *adjective* soft, which can bend (NOTE: the opposite is **brittle**)

ductless gland [ˈdʌktləs ˈglænd] *noun* endocrine gland, gland without a duct which produces hormones which are introduced directly into the bloodstream (such as the pituitary gland, thyroid gland, the adrenals, and the gonads); *see illustration at* GLAND

ductule [ˈdʌktjuːl] *noun* very small duct

ductus [ˈdʌktəs] *noun* duct; **ductus arteriosus** = in a fetus, the blood vessel connecting the left pulmonary artery to the aorta so that blood does not pass through the lungs; **ductus deferens** = one of two tubes along which sperm passes from the epididymis to the prostate gland (NOTE: also called **vas deferens**); *see illustration at* UROGENITAL SYSTEM (MALE); **ductus venosus** = in a fetus, the blood vessel connecting the portal sinus to the inferior vena cava

dull [dʌl] **1** *adjective* (pain) which is not sharp, but continuously painful; *she complained of a dull throbbing pain in her head*; *he felt a dull pain in the chest* **2** *verb* to make less sharp; *his senses were dulled by the drug*

dumb [dʌm] *adjective* not able to speak

dumbness [ˈdʌmnəs] *noun* being unable to speak

dummy [ˈdʌmi] *noun* rubber teat given to a baby to suck, to prevent it crying (NOTE: American English is **pacifier**)

dumping syndrome [ˈdʌmpɪŋ ˈsɪndrəum] *noun* rapid passing of the contents of the stomach and duodenum into the jejunum, causing fainting, diarrhoea and sweating in patients who have had a gastrectomy

duoden- [ˈdjuːəudiːn] *prefix* referring to the duodenum

duodenal [djuːəuˈdiːnl] *adjective* referring to the duodenum; **duodenal papillae** = small projecting parts in the duodenum where the bile duct and pancreatic duct open; **duodenal ulcer** = ulcer in the duodenum

duodenoscope [djuːəuˈdiːnəuskəup] *noun* instrument used to examine the inside of the duodenum

duodenostomy [djuːəudɪˈnɒstəmi] *noun* permanent opening made between the duodenum and the abdominal wall

duodenum [djuːəuˈdiːnəm] *noun* first part of the small intestine, going from the stomach to the jejunum; *see illustrations at* DIGESTIVE SYSTEM, STOMACH

COMMENT: the duodenum is the shortest part of the small intestine, about 250 mm long. It takes bile from the gall bladder and pancreatic juice from the pancreas and continues the digestive processes started in the mouth and stomach

Dupuytren's contracture [du'pwiːtrənz kən'træktʃə] *noun* condition where the palmar fascia becomes thicker, causing the fingers (usually the middle and ring fingers) to bend forwards

dural [djuərl] *adjective* referring to the dura mater

dura mater ['djuərə 'meɪtə] *noun* thicker outer meninx covering the brain and spinal cord

Dutch cap ['dʌtʃ 'kæp] *noun* vaginal diaphragm, a contraceptive device for women, which is placed over the cervix uteri before sexual intercourse

duty ['djuːti] *noun* requirement for a particular job, something which has to be done (especially in a particular job), work which a person has to do; *what are the duties of a night sister?*; **to be on duty** = to be doing official work at a special time; **night duty** = work done at night; *Nurse Smith is on night duty this week*; **duty nurse** = nurse who is on duty; **a doctor owes a duty of care to his patient** = the doctor has to treat a patient in a proper way, as this is part of the work of being a doctor

d.v.t. *or* **DVT** ['diː 'viː 'tiː] = DEEP VEIN THROMBOSIS

dwarf [dwɔːf] *noun* person who is much smaller than normal

dwarfism ['dwɔːfɪzm] *noun* condition where the growth of a person has stopped leaving him much smaller than normal

COMMENT: may be caused by achondroplasia, where the long bones in the arms and legs do not develop fully but the trunk and head are of normal size. Dwarfism can have other causes, such as rickets or deficiency in the pituitary gland

dynamometer [daɪnə'mɒmɪtə] *noun* instrument for measuring the force of muscular contraction

-dynia ['dɪniə] *suffix* meaning pain

dys- [dɪs] *prefix* meaning difficult or defective

dysaesthesia [dɪsiːs'θiːziə] *noun* (i) impairment of a sense, in particular the sense of touch; (ii) unpleasant feeling of pain experienced when the skin is touched lightly

dysarthria [dɪs'ɑːθriə] *noun* difficulty in speaking words clearly, caused by damage to the central nervous system

dysbarism ['dɪsbɑːrɪzm] *noun* any disorder caused by differences between the atmospheric pressure outside the body and the pressure inside

dysbasia [dɪs'beɪziə] *noun* difficulty in walking, especially when caused by a lesion to a nerve

dyschezia [dɪs'kiːziə] *noun* difficulty in passing faeces

dyschondroplasia [dɪskɒndrəʊ'pleɪziə] *noun* abnormal shortness of the long bones

dyscoria [dɪs'kɔːriə] *noun* (i) abnormally shaped pupil of the eye; (ii) abnormal reaction of the pupil

dyscrasia [dɪs'kreɪziə] *noun* old term for any abnormal body condition

dysdiadochokinesia [dɪsdaɪædəʊkɒkaɪ'niːsiə] *noun* inability to carry out rapid movements, caused by a disorder or lesion of the cerebellum

dysenteric [dɪsən'terɪk] *adjective* referring to dysentery

dysentery ['dɪsəntri] *noun* infection and inflammation of the colon, causing bleeding and diarrhoea

COMMENT: dysentery occurs mainly in tropical countries. The symptoms include diarrhoea, discharge of blood and pain in the intestines. There are two main types of dysentery: bacillary dysentery, caused by the bacterium *Shigella* in contaminated food; and amoebic dysentery or amoebiasis, caused by a parasitic amoeba *Entamoeba histolytica* spread through contaminated drinking water

dysfunction [dɪs'fʌŋkʃn] *noun* abnormal functioning of an organ

dysfunctional uterine bleeding [dɪs'fʌŋkʃənl 'juːtəraɪn 'bliːdɪŋ] *noun* bleeding in the uterus, not caused by a menstrual period

dysgenesis [dɪs'dʒenəsɪs] *noun* abnormal development

dysgerminoma [dɪsdʒɜːmɪ'nəʊmə] *noun* malignant tumour of the ovary or testicle

dysgraphia [dɪs'græfiə] *noun* (i) difficulty in writing caused by a brain lesion; (ii) writer's cramp

dyskinesia [dɪskaɪ'niːziə] *noun* inability to control voluntary movements

dyslalia [dɪsˈleɪlɪə] *noun* disorder of speech, caused by abnormal formation of the tongue

dyslexia [dɪsˈleksɪə] *noun* disorder of development, where a person is unable to read or write properly and confuses letters

COMMENT: caused either by an inherited disability or by a brain lesion; dyslexia does not suggest any lack of normal intelligence

dyslexic [dɪsˈleksɪk] **1** *adjective* referring to dyslexia **2** *noun* person suffering from dyslexia

dyslipidaemia [dɪslɪpɪˈdiːmɪə] *noun* imbalance of lipids

dyslogia [dɪsˈləʊdʒə] *noun* difficulty in putting ideas in words

dysmenorrhoea [dɪsmenəˈriːə] *noun* pain experienced at menstruation; **primary** *or* **essential dysmenorrhoea** = dysmenorrhoea which occurs at the first menstrual period; **secondary dysmenorrhoea** = dysmenorrhoea which starts at some time after the first menstruation

dysostosis [dɪsɒsˈtəʊsɪs] *noun* defective formation of bones

dyspareunia [dɪspæˈruːnɪə] *noun* difficult or painful sexual intercourse in a woman

dyspepsia [dɪsˈpepsɪə] *noun* condition where a person feels pains or discomfort in the stomach, caused by indigestion

dyspeptic [dɪsˈpeptɪk] *adjective* referring to dyspepsia

dysphagia [dɪsˈfeɪdʒɪə] *noun* difficulty in swallowing

dysphasia [dɪsˈfeɪzɪə] *noun* difficulty in speaking and putting words into the correct order

dysphemia [dɪsˈfiːmɪə] = STAMMERING

dysphonia [dɪsˈfəʊnɪə] *noun* difficulty in speaking caused by impairment of the voice or vocal cords, or by laryngitis

dysplasia [dɪsˈpleɪzɪə] *noun* abnormal development of tissue

dyspnoea [dɪspˈniːə] *noun* difficulty or pain in breathing; **paroxysmal dyspnoea** = attack of breathlessness at night, caused by heart failure

dyspnoeic [dɪspˈniːɪk] *adjective* where breathing is difficult or painful

dyspraxia [dɪsˈpræksɪə] *noun* difficulty in carrying out coordinated movements

dysrhythmia [dɪsˈrɪðmɪə] *noun* abnormal rhythm (either in speaking or in electrical impulses in the brain)

dyssynergia [dɪsɪˈnɜːdʒɪə] = ASYNERGIA

dystocia [dɪsˈtəʊsɪə] *noun* difficult childbirth; **fetal dystocia** = difficult childbirth caused by an abnormality or malpresentation of the fetus; **maternal dystocia** = difficult childbirth caused by an abnormality in the mother

dystonia [dɪsˈtəʊnɪə] *noun* disordered muscle tone, causing involuntary contractions which make the limbs deformed

dystrophia *or* **dystrophy** [dɪsˈtrəʊfɪə or ˈdɪstrəfi] *noun* wasting of an organ, muscle or tissue due to lack of nutrients in that part of the body; **dystrophia adiposogenitalis** = FRÖHLICH'S SYNDROME; **dystrophia myotonica** = hereditary disease with muscle stiffness followed by atrophy of the face and neck muscles; **muscular dystrophy** = condition where the tissue of the muscles wastes away

dysuria [dɪsˈjʊərɪə] *noun* difficulty in passing urine

Ee

Vitamin E [ˈvɪtəmɪn ˈiː] *noun* vitamin found in vegetables, vegetable oils, eggs and wholemeal bread

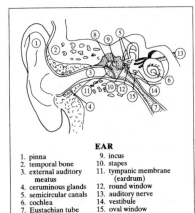

EAR

1. pinna
2. temporal bone
3. external auditory meatus
4. ceruminous glands
5. semicircular canals
6. cochlea
7. Eustachian tube
8. malleus
9. incus
10. stapes
11. tympanic membrane (eardrum)
12. round window
13. auditory nerve
14. vestibule
15. oval window

ear [ɪə] *noun* organ which is used for hearing; *if your ears are blocked, ask a doctor to syringe them*; *he has gone to see an ear specialist about his deafness*; **inner ear** = part of the ear inside the head containing the vestibule, the cochlea and the semicircular canals; **middle ear** = part of the ear between the eardrum and the inner ear, containing the ossicles; **outer ear** *or* **external ear** = the pinna, the ear on the outside of the head together with the passage leading to the eardrum; **ear canal** = one of several passages in or connected to the ear, especially the external auditory meatus, the passage from the outer ear to the eardrum; **ear ossicle** = auditory ossicle, one of three small bones (the malleus, the incus and the stapes) in the middle ear (NOTE: for terms referring to the ear, see words beginning with **auric-**, **ot-** or **oto-**)

COMMENT: the outer ear is shaped in such a way that it collects sound and channels it to the eardrum. Behind the eardrum, the three ossicles in the middle ear vibrate with sound and transmit the vibrations to the cochlea in the inner ear. From the cochlea, the vibrations are passed by the auditory nerve to the brain

earache [ˈɪəreɪk] *noun* otalgia, pain in the ear

eardrum [ˈɪədrʌm] *noun* myringa or tympanum, the membrane at the end of the external auditory meatus leading from the outer ear, which vibrates with sound and passes the vibrations on to the ossicles in the middle ear (NOTE: for terms referring to the eardrum, see words beginning with **auric-** or **tympan-**)

early [ˈɜːli] **1** *adjective* **(a)** which happens at the beginning of a period of time; **early diagnosis** = diagnosis made at the onset of an illness; **early treatment** = treatment given almost as soon as the illness has started **(b)** *(of condition or illness)* in its first stage; **during early pregnancy** = within the first couple of months of pregnancy; **early synovitis** = point at which synovitis first starts **2** *adverb* at the beginning of a period of time; *if the condition is diagnosed early*

Ear, Nose & Throat (ENT) [ˈɪə ˈnəʊz ən ˈθrəʊt] *noun* otorhinolaryngology, the study of the ear, nose and throat; **ENT department** = department of otorhinolaryngology; **ENT doctor** = otorhinolaryngologist

earwax [ˈɪəwæks] *noun* cerumen, wax which forms inside the ear

ease [iːz] *verb* to make (pain or worry) less; *she had an injection to ease the pain in her leg*; *the surgeon tried to ease the patient's fears about the results of the scan*

eat [iːt] *verb* to chew and swallow food; *I haven't eaten anything since breakfast*; *the patient must not eat anything for twelve* *hours before the operation*; **eating disorders** = illnesses (such as anorexia or bulimia) which are associated with eating; **eating habits** = types of food and quantities of food regularly eaten by a person; *the dietitian advised her to change her eating habits* (NOTE: eating - ate - has eaten)

eburnation [iːbəˈneɪʃn] *noun* conversion of cartilage into a hard mass with a shiny surface like bone

EB virus [ˈiː ˈbiː ˈvaɪrəs] = EPSTEIN-BARR VIRUS

ecbolic [ekˈbɒlik] *adjective & noun* (substance) which produces contraction of the uterus and so induces childbirth or abortion

ecchondroma [ekənˈdrəʊmə] *noun* benign tumour on the surface of cartilage or bone

ecchymosis [ekiˈməʊsis] *noun* bruise or contusion, dark area on the skin, made by blood which has escaped into the tissues after a blow

eccrine [ˈekrin] *adjective* (gland, especially a sweat gland) which does not disintegrate and remains intact during secretion (NOTE: also called **merocrine**)

eccyesis [eksaɪˈiːsis] = ECTOPIC PREGNANCY

ecdysis [ˈekdɪsis] *noun* desquamation, continuous process of losing the outer layer of dead skin

ECG [ˈiː ˈsiː ˈdʒiː] = ELECTROCARDIOGRAM

echinococciasis *or* **echinococcosis** [ɪkaɪnəʊkɒˈkaɪəsis or ɪkaɪnəʊkəˈkəʊsis] *noun* disorder caused by a tapeworm *Echinococcus* which forms hydatid cysts in the lungs, liver, kidney or brain

Echinococcus granulosus [ɪkaɪnəʊˈkɒkəs grænjuˈləʊsəs] *noun* type of tapeworm, usually found in animals, but sometimes transmitted to humans, causing hydatid cysts

echo- [ˈekəʊ] *prefix* referring to sound

echocardiogram [ekəʊˈkaːdɪəgræm] *noun* recording of heart movements using ultrasound

echocardiography [ekəʊkaːdiˈɒgrəfi] *noun* ultrasonography of the heart

echoencephalography [ekəʊensefəˈlɒgrəfi] *noun* ultrasonography of the brain

echography [eˈkɒgrəfi] *noun* ultrasonography, passing ultrasound waves through the body and recording echoes to show details of internal organs

echokinesis [ekəʊkaɪˈniːsis] *noun* meaningless imitating of another person's actions

echolalia [ekəʊˈleɪliə] *noun* repeating words spoken by another person

echopraxia [ekəʊˈpræksiə] *noun* imitating another person's actions

echovirus [ekəʊˈvaɪrəs] *noun* one of a group of viruses which can be isolated from the intestine and which can cause serious illnesses such as aseptic meningitis, gastroenteritis and respiratory infection in small children; *compare* REOVIRUS

eclabium [ɪˈkleɪbiəm] *noun* turning the lips outwards, eversion of the lips

eclampsia [ɪˈklæmpsiə] *noun* serious condition of pregnant women at the end of pregnancy, where the patient has convulsions and high blood pressure and may go into a coma, caused by toxaemia of pregnancy; *see also* PRE-ECLAMPSIA

ecmnesia [ekˈniːziə] *noun* not being able to remember recent events, while remembering clearly events which happened some time ago

E. coli [ˈiː ˈkəʊlaɪ] *see* ESCHERICHIA

ecological [iːkəˈlɒdʒɪkl] *adjective* referring to ecology

ecologist [ɪˈkɒlədʒɪst] *noun* scientist who studies ecology

ecology [ɪˈkɒlədʒi] *noun* study of the environment and the relationship of living organisms to it; **human ecology** = study of man's place in the natural world

economy class syndrome [ɪˈkɒnəmi ˈklaːs ˈsɪndrəʊm] *noun* non-medical term for DEEP-VEIN THROMBOSIS

ECR = EXTRA-CONTRACTUAL REFERRAL

écraseur [eɪkraːˈzɜː] *noun* surgical instrument (usually with a wire loop) used to cut a part or a growth off at its base

ecstasy [ˈekstəsi] *noun* **(a)** feeling of extreme happiness **(b)** *(informal)* methylenedioxymethamphetamine, an illegal, powerful stimulant and hallucinatory drug

ECT ['iː 'siː 'tiː] = ELECTROCONVULSIVE THERAPY (electroshock treatment)

ect- or **ecto-** ['ekt or 'ektəʊ] *prefix* meaning outside

ectasia [ek'teɪziə] *noun* dilatation of a passage

ecthyma [ek'θaɪmə] *noun* skin disorder, a serious form of impetigo which penetrates deep under the skin and leaves scars

ectoderm or **embryonic ectoderm** ['ektəʊdɜːm or embri'ɒnɪk 'ektəʊdɜːm] *noun* outer layer of an early embryo

ectodermal [ektəʊ'dɜːml] *adjective* referring to the ectoderm

ectomorph ['ektəʊmɔːf] *noun* type of person who tends to be quite thin; *compare* ENDOMORPH, MESOMORPH

ectomorphic [ektə'mɔːfik] *adjective* referring to an ectomorph

-ectomy ['ektəmi] *suffix* referring to the removal of a part by surgical operation; **appendicectomy** = operation to remove the appendix

ectoparasite [ektəʊ'pærəsaɪt] *noun* parasite which lives on the skin; *compare* ENDOPARASITE

ectopia [ek'təʊpiə] *noun* condition where an organ or part of the body is not in its normal position

ectopic [ek'tɒpɪk] *adjective* abnormal, not in the normal position; **ectopic heart beat** = abnormal extra beat of the heart which originates from a point other than the sinoatrial node; **ectopic pregnancy** or **extrauterine pregnancy** or **eccyesis** = pregnancy where the fetus develops outside the uterus, often in one of the Fallopian tubes (tubal pregnancy) (NOTE: the opposite is entopic)

ectoplasm ['ektəplæzm] *noun (in cells)* outer layer of cytoplasm which is the densest part of the cytoplasm

ectro- ['ektrəʊ] *prefix* meaning absence or lack of something (usually congenital)

ectrodactyly [ektrəʊ'dæktɪli] *noun* congenital absence of all or part of a finger

ectrogeny [ek'trɒdʒəni] *noun* congenital absence of a part at birth

ectromelia [ektrəʊ'miːliə] *noun* congenital absence of one or more limbs

ectropion [ek'trəʊpiən] *noun* eversion, turning of the edge of an eyelid outwards

eczema ['eksɪmə] *noun* non-contagious inflammation of the skin, with itchy rash and blisters; **atopic eczema** = type of eczema often caused by hereditary allergy; **endogenous eczema** = eczema which is caused internally; **seborrhoeic eczema** = type of eczema where scales form on the skin, usually on the scalp, and then move down the body; **varicose eczema** or **hypostatic eczema** = eczema which develops on the legs, caused by bad circulation

eczematous [ek'semətəs] *adjective* referring to eczema; **eczematous dermatitis** = itchy inflammation or irritation of the skin due to an allergic reaction to a substance which a person has touched or absorbed

EDD ['iː 'diː 'diː] = EXPECTED DATE OF DELIVERY

edema [ɪ'diːmə] *US* = OEDEMA

edentulous [ɪ'dentjuləs] *adjective* having lost all teeth

edge [edʒ] *noun* side of something flat; *the edge of a wound*

edible ['edəbəl] *adjective* which can be eaten; **edible fungi** = fungi which can be eaten and are not poisonous

EEG ['iː 'iː 'dʒiː] = ELECTROENCEPHALOGRAM

effect [ɪ'fekt] **1** *noun* result of a drug, a treatment or an action; *the effect of the disease is to make the patient blind*; *the antiseptic cream has had no effect on the rash*; *radiotherapy has a positive effect on cancer cells* **2** *verb* to make something happen; *the doctors effected a cure*

effective [ɪ'fektɪv] *adjective* which has an effect; *his way of making the children keep quiet is very effective*; *embolization is an effective treatment for severe haemoptysis*

effector [ɪ'fektə] *noun* special nerve ending in muscles or glands which is activated to produce contraction or secretion

efferens ['efərns] *see* VAS EFFERENS

efferent ['efərnt] *adjective* carrying away from part of the body or from the centre; **efferent duct** = duct which carries a secretion away from a gland; **efferent vessel** = vessel which drains lymph from a gland (NOTE: the opposite is afferent)

efficient [ɪ'fɪʃnt] *adjective* which works well, which functions correctly; *the new* *product is an efficient antiseptic; the ward sister is extremely efficient*

efficiently [ɪˈfɪʃntli] *adverb* in an efficient way; *she manages all her patients very efficiently*

effleurage [eflu:ˈrɑ:ʒ] *noun* form of massage where the skin is stroked in one direction to increase blood flow

effort [ˈefət] *noun* using power, either mental or physical; *he made an effort and lifted his hands above his head; it took a lot of effort to walk even this short distance; if he made an effort he would be able to get out of bed;* **effort syndrome** = da Costa's syndrome, disordered action of the heart, condition where the patient suffers palpitations caused by worry

effusion [ɪˈfju:ʒn] *noun* (i) discharge of blood, fluid or pus into or out of an internal cavity; (ii) fluid, blood or pus which is discharged; **pericardial effusion** = excess of fluid which forms in the pericardial sac; **pleural effusion** = excess of fluid formed in the pleural sac

egg [eg] *noun* **(a)** reproductive cell produced in the female body by the ovary, and which, if fertilized by the male sperm, becomes an embryo; **egg cell** = immature ovum or female cell **(b)** hen's egg = egg with a hard shell, laid by a hen, which is used for food; *he is allergic to eggs*

ego [ˈi:gəʊ or ˈegəʊ] *noun (in psychology)* part of the mind which is consciously in contact with the outside world and is influenced by experiences of the world; *compare* ID, SUBCONSCIOUS, SUPEREGO

Egyptian ophthalmia [ɪˈdʒɪpʃn ɒfˈθælmiə] *see* TRACHOMA

EHO [ˈi: ˈeɪtʃ ˈəʊ] = ENVIRONMENTAL HEALTH OFFICER

EIA [ˈi: ˈaɪ ˈeɪ] = EXERCISE-INDUCED ASTHMA

eidetic imagery [aɪˈdetɪk ˈɪmɪdʒri] *noun* recalling extremely clear pictures in the mind

Eisenmenger syndrome [ˈaɪsenmeŋgə ˈsɪndrəʊm] *noun* heart disease caused by a septal defect between the ventricles, with pulmonary hypertension

ejaculate [ɪˈdʒækjuleɪt] *verb* to send out semen from the penis

ejaculation [ɪdʒækjuˈleɪʃn] *noun* sending out of semen from the penis; **premature**

ejaculation = situation where the man ejaculates too early during sexual intercourse

ejaculatio praecox [ɪˈdʒækjuˈleɪʃiəʊ ˈpri:kɒks] *noun* situation where the man ejaculates too early during sexual intercourse

ejaculatory [ɪˈdʒækjulətri] *adjective* referring to ejaculation; **ejaculatory ducts** = two ducts, leading from the seminal vesicles and vas deferens, which go through the prostate and end in the urethra; *see illustration at* UROGENITAL SYSTEM (MALE)

eject [ɪˈdʒekt] *verb* to send out something with force; *blood is ejected from the ventricle during systole*

ejection [ɪˈdʒekʃn] *noun* sending out something with force

EKG [ˈi: ˈkeɪ ˈdʒi:] US = ELECTROCARDIOGRAM (NOTE: British English is **ECG**)

elastic [ɪˈlæstɪk] *adjective* which can be stretched and compressed and return to its former shape; **elastic bandage** = stretch bandage used to support a weak joint or for treatment of a varicose vein; **elastic cartilage** *or* **yellow elastic fibrocartilage** = flexible cartilage such as that in the ear and epiglottis; **elastic fibres** = yellow fibres, basic components of elastic cartilage, also found in the skin and the walls of arteries or the lungs; **elastic tissue** = connective tissue, as in the walls of arteries or of the alveoli in the lungs, which contains elastic fibres

elasticity [i:læsˈtɪsəti] *noun* being able to expand and be compressed and to return to the former shape

elastin [ɪˈlæstɪn] *noun* protein which occurs in elastic fibres

elation [ɪˈleɪʃn] *noun* being stimulated and excited

elbow [ˈelbəʊ] *noun* hinged joint where the arm bone (humerus) joins the forearm bones (radius and ulna); **tennis elbow** *or* **golf elbow,** US **pitcher's elbow** = inflammation of the tendons of the extensor muscles in the hand which are attached to the bone near the elbow (NOTE: for other terms referring to the elbow, see **cubital**)

elderly [ˈeldəli] **1** *adjective* old, aged over 65; *she looks after her two elderly parents; a home for elderly single women* **2** *noun* **the elderly** = old people, people aged over 65

elective [ɪˈlektɪv] *adjective* (i) (chemical substance) which tends to combine with one particular substance rather than another; (ii) (part of a course in a college or university) which a student can choose to take rather than another; **elective surgery** *or* **elective treatment** = surgery or treatment which a patient can choose to have but is not urgently necessary to save his life

Electra complex [ɪˈlektrə ˈkɒmpleks] *noun (in psychology)* condition where a girl feels sexually attracted to her father and sees her mother as an obstacle

electric [ɪˈlektrɪk] *adjective* worked by electricity; used for carrying electricity; **electric shock** = sudden passage of electricity into the body, causing a nervous spasm or, in severe cases, death; **electric shock treatment** = treatment of a disorder by giving the patient light electric shocks; *see also* ELECTROSHOCK

electricity [ɪlekˈtrɪsəti] *noun* electron energy which can be converted to light, heat or power; *the motor is run by electricity*; *electricity is used to administer shocks to a patient*

electro- [ɪˈlektrəʊ] *prefix* referring to electricity

electrocardiogram (ECG) [ɪlektrəʊˈkɑːdiəgræm] *noun* chart which records the electrical impulses in the heart muscle (NOTE: American English is **EKG**)

electrocardiograph [ɪlektrəʊˈkɑːdiəgrɑːf] *noun* apparatus for measuring and recording the electrical impulses of the muscles of the heart as it beats

electrocardiography [ɪlektrəʊkɑːdɪˈɒgrəfi] *noun* process of recording the electrical impulses of the heart

electrocardiophonography [ɪlektrəʊkɑːdiəfəˈnɒgrəfi] *noun* process of electrically recording the sounds of the heartbeats

electrocautery [ɪlektrəʊˈkɔːtri] = GALVANOCAUTERY

electrochemical [ɪlektrəʊˈkemɪkl] *adjective* referring to electricity and chemicals and their interaction

electrocoagulation [ɪlektrəʊkəʊæɡjuˈleɪʃn] *noun* control of haemorrhage in surgery by coagulation of divided blood vessels by passing a high-frequency electric current through them

electroconvulsive therapy (ECT) *or* **electroplexy** [ɪlektrəʊkənvʌlsɪv ˈθerəpi *or* ɪˈlektrəʊpleksi] *noun* treatment of severe

depression and some mental disorders by giving the patient small electric shocks in the brain to make him have convulsions

electrode [ɪˈlektrəʊd] *noun* conductor of an electrical apparatus which touches the body and carries an electric shock

electrodesiccation [ɪlektrəʊdesɪˈkeɪʃn] *noun* fulguration, the destruction of tissue (such as the removal of a wart) by burning with an electric needle

electroencephalogram (EEG) [ɪlektrəʊɪnˈsefələgræm] *noun* chart on which are recorded the electrical impulses in the brain

electroencephalograph [ɪlektrəʊɪnˈsefələgrɑːf] *noun* apparatus which records the electrical impulses in the brain

electroencephalography [ɪlektrəʊɪnsefəˈlɒgrəfi] *noun* process of recording the electrical impulses in the brain

electrolysis [ɪlekˈtrɒləsɪs] *noun* destruction of tissue (such as removing unwanted hair) by applying an electric current

electrolyte [ɪˈlektrəlaɪt] *noun* **(a)** chemical solution of a substance which can conduct electricity **(b)** *(to prevent dehydration by diarrhoea)* **electrolyte mixture** = a pint (0.56 of a litre) of boiled water with a teaspoonful of sugar and a generous pinch of table salt

electrolytic [ɪlektrəˈlɪtɪk] *adjective* referring to electrolytes or to electrolysis

electromyogram (EMG) [ɪlektrəˈmaɪəʊgræm] *noun* chart showing the electric currents in muscles in action

electromyography [ɪlektrəʊmaɪˈɒgrəfi] *noun* study of electric currents in active muscles

electron [ɪˈlektrɒn] *noun* negative particle in an atom; **electron microscope (EM)** = microscope which uses a beam of electrons instead of light

electronic [ɪlekˈtrɒnɪk] *adjective* referring to electrons, working with electrons; **electronic stethoscope** = stethoscope fitted with an amplifier

electronystagmography [elektrəʊnɪstægˈmɒgrəfi] *noun* measuring of nystagmus

electro-oculogram [ɪlektrəʊˈɒkjuːləgræm] *noun* a record of the electric currents round the eye, induced by eye movements

electro-oculography [ɪlektrəʊɒkjuˈlɒgrəfi] *noun* recording the electric currents round the eye, induced by eye movements

electrophoresis [ɪlektrəʊfə'riːsɪs] *noun* analysis of a substance by the movement of charged particles towards an electrode in a solution

electroplexy [ɪ'lektrəpleksɪ] *noun; see* ELECTROCONVULSIVE THERAPY

electroretinogram (ERG) [ɪkektrəʊre'tɪnəgræm] *noun* printed result of electroretinography

electroretinography [ɪlektrəʊretɪ'nɒɡrəfɪ] *noun* process of recording electrical changes in the retina when stimulated by light

electroshock therapy *or* **electroshock treatment** [ɪ'lektrəʊʃɒk 'θerəpɪ or ɪ'lektrəʊʃɒk 'triːtmənt] *noun* electroplexy or electroconvulsive therapy, the treatment of some mental disorders by giving the patient electric shocks in the brain to make him have convulsions

electrotherapy [ɪlektrəʊ'θerəpɪ] *noun* treatment of a disorder, such as some forms of paralysis, using low-frequency electric current to try to revive the muscles

element ['elɪmənt] *noun* basic simple chemical substance which cannot be broken down to a simpler substance; **trace element** = substance which is essential to the human body, but only in very small quantities

elephantiasis [elɪfən'taɪəsɪs] *noun* oedematous condition where parts of the body swell and the skin becomes hardened, frequently caused by filariasis (infestation with various species of the parasitic worm *Filaria*)

elevate ['elɪveɪt] *verb* to raise or to lift up

elevation [elɪ'veɪʃn] *noun* raised part; **elevation sling** = sling tied round the neck, used to hold the arm in a high position to prevent bleeding

elevator ['elɪveɪtə] *noun* **(a)** muscle which raises part of the body **(b)** (i) surgical instrument used to lift part of a broken bone; (ii) instrument used by a dentist to remove a tooth or part of a tooth; **periosteum elevator** = surgical instrument used to remove the periosteum from a bone

elicit [ɪ'lɪsɪt] *verb* to make happen, to provoke; *muscle tenderness was elicited in the lower limbs*

eliminate [ɪ'lɪmɪneɪt] *verb* to get rid of waste matter from the body; *the excess salts are eliminated through the kidneys*

elimination [ɪlɪmɪ'neɪʃn] *noun* removal of waste matter from the body; **elimination diet** = structured diet where different foods are eliminated one at a time in order to see the effect on symptoms, used in conditions such as allergies and attention deficit hyperactivity disorder

elixir [ɪ'lɪksə] *noun* sweet liquid which hides the unpleasant taste of a drug

elliptocytosis [ɪlɪptəʊsaɪ'təʊsɪs] *noun* condition where abnormal oval-shaped red cells appear in the blood

EM ['iː 'em] = ELECTRON MICROSCOPE

EmA = IgA ANTIENDOMYSIAL ANTIBODY

emaciated [ɪ'meɪʃieɪtɪd] *adjective* very thin, extremely underweight; *anorexic patients become emaciated and may need hospitalization*

emaciation [ɪmeɪsɪ'eɪʃn] *noun* being extremely thin; wasting away of body tissue

emaculation [ɪmækju'leɪʃn] *noun* removing spots from the skin

emasculation [ɪmæskju'leɪʃn] *noun* (i) removal of the penis; (ii) loss of male characteristics

embalm [ɪm'bɑːm] *verb* to preserve a dead body by using special antiseptic chemicals to prevent decay

embolectomy [embə'lektəmi] *noun* surgical operation to remove a blood clot

embolism ['embəlɪzm] *noun* blocking of an artery by a mass of material (usually a blood clot), preventing the flow of blood; **air embolism** = interference with the flow of blood in vessels by bubbles of air; **pulmonary embolism** = blockage of the pulmonary artery

embolization [embəlaɪ'zeɪʃn] *noun* using emboli inserted down a catheter into a blood vessel to treat internal bleeding

once a bleeding site has been located, a catheter is manipulated as near as possible to it, so that embolization can be carried out. Many different materials are used as the embolus

British Medical Journal

embolus ['embələs] *noun* mass of material (such as a blood clot, air bubble or fat globule) which blocks a blood vessel (NOTE: plural is **emboli**)

embrocation [embrə'keɪʃn] *noun* liniment, oily liquid rubbed on the skin, which eases the pain or stiffness of a sprain or bruise by acting as a vasodilator or counterirritant

embryo ['embriəʊ] *noun* unborn baby during the first eight weeks after conception (NOTE: after eight weeks, the unborn baby is called a **fetus**)

embryological [embriə'lɒdʒɪkl] *adjective* referring to embryology

embryology [embri'ɒlədʒi] *noun* study of the early stages of the development of the embryo

embryonic [embri'ɒnɪk] *adjective* (i) referring to an embryo; (ii) in an early stage of development; **embryonic membranes** = skins around an embryo providing protection and food supply (the amnion and chorion)

emergency [ɪ'mɜːdʒənsi] *noun* situation where immediate action has to be taken; *US* **emergency medical technician (EMT)** = trained paramedic who gives care to victims at the scene of an accident or in an ambulance; **emergency ward** = hospital ward which deals with urgent cases (such as accident victims)

emesis ['eməsɪs] *noun* vomiting

emetic [ɪ'metɪk] *adjective & noun* (substance) which causes vomiting; *the doctor administered an emetic*

EMG ['iː 'em 'dʒiː] = ELECTROMYOGRAM

eminence ['emɪnəns] *noun* something which protrudes from a surface, such as a lump on a bone or swelling on the skin; *see also* HYPOTHENAR, THENAR

emissary veins ['emɪsəri 'veɪnz] *noun* veins through the skull which connect the venous sinuses with the scalp veins

emission [ɪ'mɪʃn] *noun* discharge or release of fluid; **nocturnal emission** = production of semen from the penis while a man is asleep

emmenagogue [ɪ'menəgɒg] *noun* drug which will help increase menstrual flow

emmetropia [emɪ'trəʊpiə] *noun* normal vision, the correct focusing of light rays by the eye onto the retina; *compare* AMETROPIA

emollient [ɪ'mɒliənt] *adjective & noun* (substance) which smooths the skin

emotion [ɪ'məʊʃn] *noun* strong feeling

emotional [ɪ'məʊʃənl] *adjective* showing strong feeling; **emotional disorder** = disorder due to worry, stress, etc.

empathy ['empəθi] *noun* being able to understand the problems and feelings of another person

emphysema [emfɪ'siːmə] *noun* condition where the alveoli of the lungs become enlarged, rupture or break down, with the result that the surface available for gas exchange is reduced, so reducing the oxygen level in the blood and making it difficult for the patient to breathe (NOTE: also called **pulmonary emphysema**)

COMMENT: emphysema can be caused by smoking or by living in a polluted environment, by old age, asthma or whooping cough

empirical [ɪm'pɪrəkl] *adjective* **empirical treatment** = treatment which is based on symptoms and clinical experience rather than on a thorough knowledge of the cause of the disorder

employ [ɪm'plɔɪ] *verb* **(a)** to use; *the dentist usually has to employ force to extract a tooth* **(b)** to pay a person for regular work; *the local health authority employs a staff of two thousand*; *she is employed by the dentist as a hygienist*; *a practice nurse is employed by the practice, not by the health authority*

empty ['empti] **1** *adjective* with nothing inside; *the medicine bottle is empty*; *take this empty bottle and provide a urine sample*; *the children's ward is never empty* **2** *verb* to take everything out of something; *she emptied the water out of the bottle*

empyema [empaɪ'iːmə] *noun* pyothorax, collection of pus in a cavity, especially in the pleural cavity

EMT ['iː 'em 'tiː] *US* = EMERGENCY MEDICAL TECHNICIAN

emulsion [ɪ'mʌlʃn] *noun* mixture of liquids which do not normally mix (such as oil and water)

EN ['iː 'en] = ENROLLED NURSE

enamel [ɪ'næml] *noun* hard white shiny outer covering of the crown of a tooth; *see illustration at* TOOTH

enanthema [enən'θiːmə] *noun* rash on a mucous membrane, as in the mouth or vagina, produced by the action of toxic substances on small blood vessels

enarthrosis [enɑː'θrəʊsɪs] *noun* ball and socket joint, such as the hip joint

ENB ['iː 'en 'biː] = ENGLISH NATIONAL BOARD

encapsulated [ɪn'kæpsjuleɪtɪd] *adjective* enclosed in a capsule or in a sheath of tissue

encephal- *or* **encephalo-** [enkɪ'fæl or ensɪ'fæl or en'kefələʊ or en'sefələʊ] *prefix* referring to the brain

encephalin *US* **enkephalin** [en'sefəlɪn or en'kefəlɪn] *noun* peptide produced in the brain; *see also* ENDORPHIN

encephalitis [enkefə'laɪtɪs or ensefə'laɪtɪs] *noun* inflammation of the brain; **encephalitis lethargica** *or* **lethargic encephalitis** = common type of encephalitis occurring in epidemics in the 1920s

COMMENT: encephalitis is caused by any of several viruses (viral encephalitis) and is also associated with infectious viral diseases such as measles or mumps; the variant St Louis encephalitis is transmitted by mosquitoes

encephalocele [en'kefələʊsiːl or en'sefələʊsiːl] *noun* condition where the brain protrudes through a congenital or traumatic gap in the skull bones

encephalogram *or* **encephalograph** [en'kefələɡræm or en'kefələɡrɑːf or en'sefələ-] *noun* X-ray photograph of the ventricles and spaces of the brain taken after air has been injected into the cerebrospinal fluid by lumbar puncture

encephalography [enkefə'lɒɡrəfi or ensefə'lɒɡrəfi] *noun* pneumoencephalography, an X-ray examination of the ventricles and spaces of the brain taken after air has been injected into the cerebrospinal fluid by lumbar puncture

COMMENT: the air takes the place of the cerebrospinal fluid and makes it easier to photograph the ventricles clearly. This technique has been superseded by CAT and MRI

encephaloid [en'kefələɪd or en'sefələɪd] **1** *adjective* which looks like brain tissue **2** *noun* large carcinoma of the breast

encephaloma [enkefə'ləʊmə] *noun* tumour of the brain

encephalomalacia [enkefələʊmə'leɪʃiə or ensefələʊ-] *noun* softening of the brain

encephalomyelitis [enkefələʊmaɪə'laɪtɪs or ensefələʊ-] *noun* group of diseases which cause inflammation of the brain and the spinal cord; **acute disseminated encephalomyelitis** = late reaction to a vaccination or disease; **myalgic encephalomyelitis (ME)** = postviral fatigue syndrome, a long-term condition affecting the nervous system, where the patient feels tired and depressed and has pain and weakness in the muscles

encephalomyelopathy [enkefələʊmaɪə'lɒpəθi or ensefələʊ-] *noun* any condition where the brain and spinal cord are diseased

encephalon [en'kefəlɒn or en'sefəlɒn] *noun* the brain, the contents of the head

encephalopathy [enkefə'lɒpəθi or ensefə'lɒpəθi] *noun* any disease of the brain; **bovine spongiform encephalopathy (BSE)** = a fatal brain disease of cattle, also called 'mad cow disease'; *see also* CREUTZFELDT, WERNICKE'S ENCEPHALOPATHY

COMMENT: caused by the use of ruminant-based additives in cattle feed, by which 'scrapie' (a disease of sheep) infects cattle. BSE-infected meat is believed to be the cause of a new strain of Creutzfeldt-Jakob disease in humans

enchondroma [enkən'drəʊmə] *noun* tumour formed of cartilage growing inside a bone

enchondromatosis [enkəndrɒmə'təʊsɪs] *noun* condition where a tumour formed of cartilage grows inside a bone

enclose [ɪn'kləʊz] *verb* to surround, to keep something inside; *the membrane enclosing the cytoplasm*

encopresis [enkəʊ'priːsɪs] *noun* faecal incontinence, being unable to control the faeces

encounter group [ɪn'kaʊntə 'gruːp] *noun* form of treatment of psychological disorders, where people meet and talk about their problems in a group

encourage [ɪn'kʌrɪdʒ] *verb* to persuade someone that he should do something; *the surgeon encouraged her to get out of bed and start trying to walk*; *children should not be encouraged to take medicines by themselves*

encysted [en'sɪstɪd] *adjective* enclosed in a capsule like a cyst

end- *or* **endo-** [end or 'endəʊ] *prefix* meaning inside

end [end] **1** *noun* last part of something; **end artery** = last section of an artery which does not divide into smaller arteries and does not anastomose with other arteries; **end organ** = nerve ending with encapsulated nerve filaments; **end piece** = last part of the tail of a spermatazoon; **end plate** = end of a motor nerve, where it joins muscle fibre **2** *verb* to finish; to come to an end; *he ended his talk by showing a series of slides of diseased parts*

endanger [ɪn'deɪndʒə] *verb* to put at risk; *the operation may endanger the life of the patient*

endarterectomy [endɑːtə'rektəmi] *noun* surgical removal of the lining of a blocked artery (NOTE: also called a **rebore**)

endarteritis [endɑːtə'raɪtɪs] *noun* inflammation of the inner lining of an artery; **endarteritis obliterans** = condition where inflammation in an artery is so severe that it blocks the artery

endemic [en'demɪk] *adjective* (any disease) which is very common in certain places; *this disease is endemic to Mediterranean countries*; **endemic syphilis** = BEJEL; *see also* EPIDEMIC, PANDEMIC

endemiology [endiːmi'ɒlədʒi] *noun* study of endemic diseases

end-expiratory [endɪk'spaɪrətri] *see* POSITIVE

ending ['endɪŋ] *noun* last part of something; **nerve ending** = last part of a nerve, especially of a peripheral nerve; *see illustration at* SKIN & SENSORY RECEPTORS

endo- ['endəʊ] *prefix* meaning inside

endobronchial [endəʊ'brɒŋkiəl] *adjective* inside the bronchi

endocardial [endəʊ'kɑːdiəl] *adjective* referring to the endocardium; **endocardial pacemaker** = pacemaker attached to the lining of the heart muscle

endocarditis [endəʊkɑː'daɪtɪs] *noun* inflammation of the endocardium, the membrane lining of the heart; **(subacute) infective endocarditis** *or* **(subacute) bacterial endocarditis** = infection of the endocardium (the membrane covering the inner surfaces of the heart) by bacteria

endocardium [endəʊ'kɑːdiəm] *noun* membrane which lines the heart; *see illustration at* HEART

endocervicitis [endəʊsɜːvɪ'saɪtɪs] *noun* inflammation of the membrane in the neck of the uterus

endocervix [endəʊ'sɜːvɪks] *noun* membrane which lines the neck of the uterus

endochondral [endəʊ'kɒndrl] *adjective* inside a cartilage

endocrine gland ['endəʊkraɪn 'glænd] *noun* ductless gland, gland without a duct which produces hormones which are introduced directly into the bloodstream (such as the pituitary gland, thyroid gland, the adrenals, and the gonads); **endocrine system** = system of related ductless glands

```
the endocrine system releases
hormones in response to a change
in concentration of trigger
substances in the blood or other
body fluids
                        Nursing 87
```

endocrinologist [endəʊkrɪ'nɒlədʒɪst] *noun* doctor who specializes in the study of endocrinology

endocrinology [endəʊkrɪ'nɒlədʒi] *noun* study of the endocrine system, its function and effects

endoderm *or* **entoderm** ['endəʊdɜːm *or* 'entəʊdɜːm] *noun* inner of three layers surrounding an embryo

COMMENT: the endoderm gives rise to most of the epithelium of the respiratory system, the alimentary tract, some of the ductless glands the bladder and part of the urethra

endodermal *or* **entodermal** [endəʊ'dɜːml *or* entəʊ'dɜːml] *adjective* referring to the endoderm

endodontia [endəʊ'dɒntiə] *noun* treatment of chronic toothache by removing the roots of a tooth

endogenous [en'dɒdʒənəs] *adjective* developing or being caused by something inside an organism; **endogenous depression** = depression caused by something inside the body; **endogenous eczema** = eczema which is caused by no obvious external factor; *compare* EXOGENOUS

endolymph ['endəʊlɪmf] *noun* fluid inside the membranous labyrinth in the inner ear

endolymphatic duct [endəʊlɪm'fætɪk 'dʌkt] *noun* duct which carries the endolymph inside the membranous labyrinth

endolysin [en'dɒlɪsɪn] *noun* substance present in cells, which kills bacteria

endometrial [endəʊ'miːtrɪəl] *adjective* referring to the endometrium; **endometrial laser ablation** = gynaecological surgical procedure using a laser to treat fibroids or other causes of thickening of the lining of the uterus

endometriosis [endəʊmiːtri'əʊsɪs] *noun* condition affecting women, where tissue similar to the tissue of the uterus is found in other parts of the body

endometritis [endəʊmɪ'traɪtɪs] *noun* inflammation of the lining of the uterus

endometrium [endəʊ'miːtrɪəm] *noun* mucous membrane lining the uterus part of which is shed at each menstruation

endomorph ['endəʊmɔːf] *noun* type of person who tends to be quite fat with large intestines and small muscles; *see also* ECTOMORPH, MESOMORPH

endomorphic [endəʊ'mɔːfɪk] *adjective* referring to an endomorph

endomyocarditis [endəʊmaɪəʊkɑː'daɪtɪs] *noun* inflammation of the muscle and inner membrane of the heart

endomysium [endəʊ'mɪsɪəm] *noun* connective tissue around and between muscle fibres

endoneurium [endəʊ'njʊərɪəm] *noun* fibrous tissue between the nerve fibres in a nerve trunk

endoparasite [endəʊ'pærəsaɪt] *noun* parasite which lives inside its host (as in the intestines); *compare* ECTOPARASITE

endophthalmitis [endɒfθæl'maɪtɪs] *noun* inflammation of the interior of the eyeball

endoplasm ['endəʊplæzm] *noun* inner layer of the cytoplasm, which is less dense than the rest

endoplasmic reticulum (ER) [endəʊ'plæzmɪk rɪ'tɪkjʊləm] *noun* network of vessels forming a membrane in a cytoplasm

endorphin [en'dɔːfɪn] *noun* peptide produced by the brain which acts as a natural pain killer; *see also* ENCEPHALIN

endoscope ['endəskəʊp] *noun* instrument used to examine the inside of the body, made of a thin tube which is passed into the body down a passage (the tube has a fibre optic light, and may have small surgical instruments attached)

endoscopic retrograde cholangiopancreatography (ERCP) [endəʊ'skɒpɪk 'retrəgreɪd kəlendʒiəʊpænkriə'tɒgrəfi] *noun* method used to examine the pancreatic duct and bile duct for possible obstructions

endoscopy [en'dɒskəpi] *noun* examination of the inside of the body using an endoscope

endoskeleton [endəʊ'skelɪtn] *noun* inner structure of bones and cartilage in an animal; *compare* EXOSKELETON

endospore ['endəʊspɔː] *noun* spore formed inside a special spore case

endosteum [en'dɒstɪəm] *noun* membrane lining the bone marrow cavity inside a long bone

endothelial [endəʊ'θiːlɪəl] *adjective* referring to the endothelium

endothelioma [endəʊθiːli'əʊmə] *noun* malignant tumour originating inside the endothelium

endothelium [endəʊ'θiːlɪəm] *noun* membrane of special cells which lines the heart, the lymph vessels, the blood vessels and various body cavities; *compare* EPITHELIUM

endotoxin [endəʊ'tɒksɪn] *noun* toxic substance released after the death of certain bacterial cells

endotracheal [endəʊ'treɪkɪəl] *adjective* inside the trachea; **endotracheal tube** = tube passed down the trachea (through either the nose or mouth) in anaesthesia or to help the patient breathe

enema ['enəmə] *noun* liquid substance put into the rectum to introduce a drug into the body, to wash out the colon before an operation or for diagnosis; **enema bag** = bag containing the liquid, attached to a tube into the rectum; **barium enema** = enema made of barium sulphate, injected into the rectum so as to show up the bowel in X-rays (NOTE: the plural is **enemas** or **enemata**)

energetic [enə'dʒetɪk] *adjective* full of energy, using energy; *the patient should not do anything energetic*

energy ['enədʒi] *noun* force or strength to carry out activities; *you need to eat certain types of food to give you energy*; **energy value** = calorific value, the heat value of food, the number of Calories which a certain amount of a certain food contains; *the tin of beans has an energy value of 250 calories*

COMMENT: energy is measured in calories, one calorie being the amount of heat needed to raise the temperature of one gram of water by one degree Celsius. The kilocalorie or Calorie is also used as a measurement of the energy content of food, and to show the amount of energy needed by an average person

enervate ['enəveɪt] *verb* to deprive someone of nervous energy

enervation [enə'veɪʃn] *noun* (i) general nervous weakness; (ii) surgical operation to resect a nerve

EN(G) = ENROLLED NURSE (GENERAL)

engagement [ɪn'geɪdʒmənt] *noun (in obstetrics)* moment where the presenting part of the fetus (usually the head) enters the pelvis at the beginning of labour

engineering [endʒɪ'nɪərɪŋ] *noun* **genetic engineering** = techniques used to change the genetic composition of a cell so as to change certain characteristics which can be inherited; *see also* BIOENGINEERING

English National Board (ENB) ['ɪŋlɪʃ 'næʃnl 'bɔːd] *noun* official body responsible for training nurses, for setting nursing examinations and for approving nursing schools

engorged [ɪn'gɔːdʒd] *adjective* filled with liquid (usually blood)

engorgement [ɪn'gɔːdʒmənt] *noun* congestion, the excessive filling of a vessel with blood

enkephalin [en'kefəlɪn] *see* ENCEPHALIN

enlarge [ɪn'lɑːdʒ] *verb* to make larger or wider; *operation to enlarge a defective vessel*

enlargement [ɪn'lɑːdʒmənt] *noun* (i) widening; (ii) point where something becomes wider; **lumbar enlargement** = point where the spinal cord widens in the lower part of the spine

EN(M) = ENROLLED NURSE (MENTAL)

EN(MH) = ENROLLED NURSE (MENTAL HANDICAP)

enophthalmos [enɒf'θælməs] *noun* condition where the eyes are very deep in their sockets

enostosis [enə'stəʊsɪs] *noun* benign growth inside a bone (usually in the skull or in a long bone)

enrolled [ɪn'rəʊld] *adjective* registered on an official list; **(State) Enrolled Nurse (SEN)** = nurse who has passed examinations successfully in one of the special courses of study

COMMENT: Enrolled Nurses follow a two year course to qualify in general nursing, mental nursing or nursing mentally handicapped patients. On qualifying, they are classified according to their area of specialization: **EN(G)** = Enrolled Nurse (General); **EN(M)** = Enrolled Nurse (Mental); **EN(MH)** = Enrolled Nurse (Mental Handicap))

ensiform ['ensifɔːm] *adjective* shaped like a sword; **ensiform cartilage** = bottom part of the breastbone, which in young people is formed of cartilage, but becomes bone by middle age (NOTE: also called the **xiphoid process**)

ensure [en'ʃɔː] *verb* to make sure of something; *please ensure that the patient takes his medicine*

ENT ['iː 'en 'tiː] = EAR, NOSE & THROAT; *she was sent to see an ENT specialist*

Entamoeba [entə'miːbə] *noun* genus of amoeba which lives in the intestine; **Entamoeba coli** = harmless intestinal parasite; **Entamoeba gingivalis** = amoeba living in the gums and tonsils, and causing gingivitis; **Entamoeba histolytica** = intestinal amoeba which causes amoebic dysentery

enter- *or* **entero-** ['entə *or* 'entrəʊ] *prefix* referring to the intestine

enteral ['entərl] *adjective* (i) referring to the intestine; (ii) (drug or food) which is taken through the intestine; **enteral nutrition** *or* **feeding** = feeding of a patient by a nasogastric tube or directly into the intestine; *compare* PARENTERAL

Standard nasogastric tubes are usually sufficient for enteral feeding in critically ill patients

British Journal of Nursing

enteralgia [entər'ældʒə] = COLIC

enterally ['entərli] *adverb* (to feed a patient) by nasogastric tube or directly into the intestine

All patients requiring nutrition are fed enterally, whether nasogastrically or directly into the small intestine

British Journal of Nursing

enterectomy [entər'ektəmi] *noun* surgical removal of part of the intestine

enteric [en'terɪk] *adjective* referring to the intestine; **enteric fever** = (i) any one of three fevers (typhoid, paratyphoid A and paratyphoid B); (ii) *US* any febrile disease of the intestines

enteric-coated [en'terɪk'kəʊtɪd] *adjective* (pill) with a coating which prevents it from being digested in the stomach, so that it goes through whole into the intestine and can release the drug there

enteritis [entə'raɪtɪs] *noun* inflammation of the mucous membrane of the intestine; **infective enteritis** = enteritis caused by bacteria; **post-irradiation enteritis** = enteritis caused by X-rays; **regional enteritis** = Crohn's disease; *see also* GASTROENTERITIS

Enterobacteria [entərəʊbæk'tɪəriə] *noun* important family of bacteria, including Salmonella, Shigella, Escherichia and Klebsiella

enterobiasis [entərəʊ'baɪəsɪs] *noun* oxyuriasis, infection with *Enterobius vermicularis*, a common children's disease, caused by threadworms in the large intestine which give itching round the anus

Enterobius [entə'rəʊbiəs] *noun* threadworm, a small thin nematode which infests the large intestine and causes itching round the anus

enterocele ['entərəʊsiːl] *noun* = HYDROCELE

enterocentesis [entərəʊsen'tiːsɪs] *noun* surgical puncturing of the intestines where a hollow needle is pushed through the abdominal wall into the intestine to remove gas or fluid

enterococcus [entərəʊ'kɒkəs] *noun* streptococcus in the intestine

enterocoele [enterəʊ'siːl] *noun* the abdominal cavity

enterocolitis [entərəʊkə'laɪtɪs] *noun* inflammation of the colon and small intestine

enterogastrone [entərəʊ'gæstrəʊn] *noun* hormone released in the duodenum, which controls secretions of the stomach

enterogenous [entərəʊ'dʒiːnəs] *adjective* originating in the intestine

enterolith ['entərəʊlɪθ] *noun* calculus, stone in the intestine

enteron ['entərɒn] *noun* the whole intestinal tract

enteropathy [entə'rɒpəθi] *noun* any disorder of the intestine; **gluten-induced enteropathy (coeliac disease)** = (i) allergic disease (mainly affecting children) in which the lining of the intestine is sensitive to gluten, preventing the small intestine from digesting fat; (ii) condition in adults where the villi in the intestine become smaller and so reduce the surface which can absorb nutrients

enteropeptidase [entərəʊ'peptɪdeɪz] *noun* enzyme produced by glands in the small intestine

enteroptosis [entərɒp'təʊsɪs] *noun* condition where the intestine is lower than normal in the abdominal cavity

enterorrhaphy [entə'rɔːrəfi] *noun* surgical operation to stitch up a perforated intestine

enterospasm ['entərəʊspæzm] *noun* irregular painful contractions of the intestine

enterostomy [entə'rɒstəmi] *noun* surgical operation to make an opening between the small intestine and the abdominal wall

enterotomy [entə'rɒtəmi] *noun* surgical incision of the intestine

enterotoxin [entərəʊ'tɒksɪn] *noun* bacterial exotoxin which particularly affects the intestine

enterovirus [entərəʊ'vaɪrəs] *noun* virus which prefers to live in the intestine

COMMENT: the enteroviruses are an important group of viruses, and include poliomyelitis virus, Coxsackie viruses and the echoviruses

enterozoon [enterəʊ'zəʊɒn] *noun* parasite which infests the intestine (NOTE: the plural is **enterozoa**)

entoderm ['entəʊdɜːm] *noun* inner of three layers surrounding an embryo

entodermal [entəʊ'dɜːml] *adjective* referring to the entoderm; *see comment at* ENDODERM

entopic [ɪn'tɒpɪk] *adjective* in the normal place (NOTE: the opposite is **ectopic**)

entropion [ɪn'trəʊpɪən] *noun* turning of the edge of the eyelid towards the inside

enucleate [ɪ'njuːklɪeɪt] *verb* to remove an eyeball

enucleation [ɪnjuːklɪ'eɪʃn] *noun* (i) surgical removal of all of a tumour; (ii) surgical removal of the whole eyeball

E number ['iː nʌmbə] classification of additives to food according to the European Union

COMMENT: additives are classified as follows: colouring substances: E100 - E180; preservatives: E200 - E297; antioxidants: E300 - E321; emulsifiers and stabilizers: E322 - E495; acids and bases: E500 - E529; anti-caking additives: E530 - E578; flavour enhancers and sweeteners: E620 - E637

enuresis [enjʊə'riːsɪs] *noun* involuntary passing of urine; **nocturnal enuresis** = bedwetting, passing urine when asleep in bed at night (especially used of children)

enuretic [enju'retɪk] *adjective* referring to enuresis, causing enuresis

envenomation [ɪnvenə'meɪʃn] *noun* using snake venom as part of a therapeutic treatment

environment [ɪn'vaɪrənmənt] *noun* conditions and influences under which an organism lives

COMMENT: man's environment can be the country or town, house or room where he lives; a parasite's environment can be the intestine or the scalp and different parasites have different environments

environmental [ɪnvaɪrən'mentl] *adjective* referring to the environment; **Environmental Health Officer (EHO)** = official of a local authority who examines the environment and tests for air pollution, bad sanitation, noise pollution, etc.

enzymatic [enzaɪ'mætɪk] *adjective* referring to enzymes

enzyme ['enzaɪm] *noun* protein substance produced by living cells which catalyses a biochemical reaction in the body (NOTE: the names of enzymes mostly end with the suffix **-ase**)

COMMENT: many different enzymes exist in the body, working in the digestive system, in the metabolic processes and helping the synthesis of certain compounds

eosin ['iːəʊsɪn] *noun* red dye used in staining tissue samples

eosinopenia [iːəʊsɪnə'piːnɪə] *noun* reduction in the number of eosinophils in the blood

eosinophil [iːəʊ'sɪnəfɪl] *noun* type of cell which can be stained with eosin

eosinophilia [iːəʊsɪnə'fɪlɪə] *noun* having an excess of eosinophils in the blood

eparterial [iːpɑː'tɪərɪəl] *adjective* situated over or on an artery

ependyma [ɪ'pendɪmə] *noun* thin membrane which lines the ventricles of the brain and the central canal of the spinal cord

ependymal [ɪ'pendɪml] *adjective* referring to the ependyma; **ependymal cell** = one of the cells which form the ependyma

ependymoma [ɪpendɪ'məʊmə] *noun* tumour in the brain originating in the ependyma

epi- ['epɪ] *prefix* meaning on or over

epiblepharon [epɪ'blefərɒn] *noun* abnormal fold of skin over the eyelid, which may press the eyelashes against the eyeball

epicanthus *or* **epicanthic fold** [epɪ'kænθəs *or* epɪ'kænθɪk 'fəʊld] *noun* large fold of skin in the inner corner of the eye, common in babies, and Mongoloid races

epicardial [epɪ'kɑːdɪəl] *adjective* referring to the epicardium; **epicardial pacemaker** = pacemaker attached to the surface of the ventricle

epicardium [epɪ'kɑːdɪəm] *noun* inner layer of the pericardium which lines the walls of the heart, outside the myocardium

epicondyle [epɪ'kɒndaɪl] *noun* projecting part of the round end of a bone above the condyle; **lateral epicondyle (of the humerus)** = lateral projection on the condyle of the humerus; **medial epicondyle (of the humerus)** = medial projection on the condyle of the humerus

epicondylitis [epɪkɒndɪ'laɪtɪs] *noun* = TENNIS ELBOW

epicranium [epɪ'kreɪnɪəm] *noun* the five layers of the scalp, the skin and hair on the head covering the skull

epicranius [epɪ'kreɪnɪəs] *noun* a scalp muscle

epicritic [epɪˈkrɪtɪk] *adjective* referring to the nerves which govern the fine senses of touch and temperature; *see also* PROTOPATHIC

epidemic [epɪˈdemɪk] *adjective & noun* (infectious disease) which spreads quickly through a large part of the population; *the disease rapidly reached epidemic proportions*; *the health authorities are taking steps to prevent an epidemic of cholera or a cholera epidemic*; epidemic pleurodynia (Bornholm disease) = *see* PLEURODYNIA; *see also* ENDEMIC, PANDEMIC

epidemiological [epɪdiːmɪəˈlɒdʒɪkl] *adjective* concerning epidemiology

epidemiologist [epɪdiːmɪˈɒlədʒɪst] *noun* person who specializes in the study of diseases in groups of people

epidemiology [epɪdiːmɪˈɒlədʒi] *noun* study of diseases in the community, in particular how they spread and how they can be controlled

epidermal [epɪˈdɜːml] *adjective* referring to the epidermis

epidermis [epɪˈdɜːmɪs] *noun* outer layer of skin, including the dead skin on the surface; *see illustration at* SKIN & SENSORY RECEPTORS

epidermolysis [epɪdəˈmɒlɪsɪs] *noun* loose condition of the epidermis

Epidermophyton [epɪdəˈmɒfɪtən] *noun* fungus which grows on the skin and causes athlete's foot among other disorders

epidermophytosis [epɪdɜːməʊfaɪˈtəʊsɪs] *noun* fungus infection of the skin, such as athlete's foot

epididymal [epɪˈdɪdəml] *adjective* referring to the epididymis

epididymis [epɪˈdɪdəmɪs] *noun* long twisting thin tube at the back of the testis, which forms part of the efferent duct of the testis, and in which spermatozoa are stored before ejaculation; *see illustration at* UROGENITAL SYSTEM (MALE)

epididymitis [epɪdɪdɪˈmaɪtɪs] *noun* inflammation of the epididymis

epididymo-orchitis [epɪˈdɪdəməʊɔːˈkaɪtɪs] *noun* inflammation of the epididymis and the testes

epidural [epɪˈdjʊərl] *adjective* on the outside of the dura mater; epidural anaesthesia = local anaesthesia (used in childbirth) in which anaesthetic is injected into the space between the vertebral canal and the dura mater; epidural block = analgesia produced by injecting an analgesic solution into the space between the vertebral canal and the dura mater; epidural space = space in the spinal cord between the vertebral canal and the dura mater (NOTE: also called **extradural**)

epigastric [epɪˈgæstrɪk] *adjective* referring to the upper abdomen; *the patient complained of pains in the epigastric area*

epigastrium [epɪˈgæstriəm] *noun* pit of the stomach, the part of the upper abdomen between the ribcage and the navel

epigastrocele [epɪˈgæstrəʊsiːl] *noun* hernia in the upper abdomen

epiglottis [epɪˈglɒtɪs] *noun* cartilage at the root of the tongue which moves to block the windpipe when food is swallowed, so that the food does not go down the trachea; *see illustration at* THROAT

epiglottitis [epɪglɒˈtaɪtɪs] *noun* inflammation and swelling of the epiglottis

epilation [epɪˈleɪʃn] *noun* removing hair by destroying the hair follicles

epilepsy [ˈepɪlepsi] *noun* disorder of the nervous system in which there are convulsions and loss of consciousness due to disordered discharge of cerebral neurones; focal epilepsy = epilepsy arising from a localized area of the brain; Jacksonian epilepsy = form of epilepsy where the jerking movements start in one part of the body before spreading to others; idiopathic epilepsy = epilepsy not caused by lesions of the brain; psychomotor epilepsy or temporal lobe epilepsy = epilepsy caused by abnormal discharges from the temporal lobe; *see also* TEMPORAL

COMMENT: the commonest form of epilepsy is major epilepsy or 'grand mal', where the patient loses consciousness and falls to the ground with convulsions. A less severe form is minor epilepsy or 'petit mal', where attacks last only a few seconds, and the patient appears simply to be hesitating or thinking deeply

epileptic [epɪˈleptɪk] *adjective & noun* referring to epilepsy, (person) suffering from epilepsy; epileptic fit = attack of convulsions (and sometimes unconsciousness) due to epilepsy

epileptiform [epɪˈleptɪfɔːm] *adjective* similar to epilepsy

epileptogenic [epɪleptəʊ'dʒenɪk] *adjective* which causes epilepsy

epiloia [epɪ'lɔɪə] *noun* hereditary disease of the brain, where the child is mentally retarded, suffers from epilepsy and has tumours on the kidney and heart

epimenorrhagia [epɪmenə'reɪdʒə] *noun* very heavy bleeding during menstruation occurring at very short intervals

epimenorrhoea [epɪmenə'riːə] *noun* menstruation at shorter intervals than twenty-eight days

epimysium [epɪ'maɪsɪəm] *noun* connective tissue binding striated muscle fibres

epinephrine [epɪ'nefrɪn] *noun* US adrenaline, hormone secreted by the medulla of the adrenal glands which has an effect similar to stimulation of the sympathetic nervous system

epineurium [epɪ'njʊərɪəm] *noun* sheath of connective tissue round a nerve

epiphenomenon [epɪfə'nɒmɪnən] *noun* strange symptom which may not be caused by a disease

epiphora [e'pɪfərə] *noun* condition where the eye fills with tears either because the lacrimal duct is blocked or because excessive tears are being secreted

epiphyseal [epɪ'fɪzɪəl] *adjective* referring to an epiphysis; **epiphyseal cartilage** = type of cartilage in the bones of children and adolescents, which expands and hardens as the bone grows to full size; **epiphyseal line** = plate of epiphyseal cartilage separating the epiphysis and the diaphysis of a long bone

epiphysis [e'pɪfəsɪs] *noun* end part of a long bone, the centre of bone growth which is separated from the main part of the bone by cartilage until bone growth stops; **epiphysis cerebri** = pineal gland; *see illustration at* BONE STRUCTURE

epiphysitis [epɪfɪ'saɪtɪs] *noun* inflammation of an epiphysis; *compare* DIAPHYSIS, METAPHYSIS

epiplo- [e'pɪpləʊ] *prefix* referring to the omentum

epiplocele [e'pɪpləʊsiːl] *noun* hernia containing part of the omentum

epiploic [epɪ'pləʊɪk] *adjective* referring to the omentum

epiploon [e'pɪpləʊɒn] = OMENTUM

episcleritis [epɪsklə'raɪtɪs] *noun* inflammation of the outer surface of the sclera in the eyeball

episio- [ə'pɪzɪəʊ] *adjective* referring to the vulva

episiorrhaphy [əpɪzɪ'ɔːrəfi] *noun* stitching of torn labia majora

episiotomy [əpɪzɪ'ɒtəmi] *noun* surgical incision of the perineum near the vagina to prevent tearing during childbirth

episode ['epɪsəʊd] *noun* separate occurrence of an illness

episodic [epɪ'sɒdɪk] *adjective* (asthma) which occurs in separate attacks

epispadias [epɪ'speɪdɪəs] *noun* congenital defect where the urethra opens on the top of the penis and not at the end; *compare* HYPOSPADIAS

epispastic [epɪ'spæstɪk] = VESICANT

epistaxis [epɪ'stæksɪs] *noun* nosebleed

epithalamus [epɪ'θæləməs] *noun* part of the forebrain containing the pineal body

epithelial [epɪ'θiːlɪəl] *adjective* referring to the epithelium; **epithelial layer** = the epithelium; **epithelial tissue** = epithelial cells arranged as a continuous sheet consisting of one or several layers

epithelialization [epɪθiːlɪəlaɪ'zeɪʃn] *noun* growth of skin over a wound

epithelioma [epɪθiːli'əʊmə] *noun* tumour arising from epithelial cells

epithelium [epɪ'θiːlɪəm] *noun* layer(s) of cells covering an organ, including the skin and the lining of all hollow cavities except blood vessels, lymphatics and serous cavities; *see also* ENDOTHELIUM, MESOTHELIUM

COMMENT: epithelium is classified according to the shape of the cells and the number of layers of cells which form it. The types of epithelium according to the number of layers are: **simple epithelium** (epithelium formed of a single layer of cells) and **stratified epithelium** (epithelium formed of several layers of cells). The main types of epithelial cells are: **columnar epithelium** (simple epithelium with long narrow cells, forming the lining of the intestines); **ciliated epithelium** (simple epithelium where the cells have little hairs, forming the lining of air passages); **cuboidal epithelium** (with cube-shaped cells, forming the lining of glands and intestines); **squamous epithelium** *or*

pavement epithelium (with flat cells like scales, which forms the lining of pericardium, peritoneum and pleura)

epituberculosis [epɪtjuːbɜːkjuˈləʊsɪs] *noun* swelling of the lymph node in the thorax, due to tuberculosis

eponym [ˈepənɪm] *noun* procedure, disease or part of the body which is named after a person

COMMENT: an eponym can refer to a disease or condition (Dupuytren's contracture, Guillain-Barré syndrome), a part of the body (circle of Willis), an organism (Leishmania), a surgical procedure (Trendelenburg's operation) or an appliance (Kirschner wire); *see* list of names in SUPPLEMENT

eponymous [ɪˈpɒnɪməs] *adjective* named after a person

Epsom salts [ˈepsəm ˈsɔːlts] *noun* magnesium sulphate (MgSO$_4$7H$_2$O), white powder which when diluted in water is used as a laxative

Epstein-Barr virus (EB virus) [ˈepstaɪnˈbɑː ˈvaɪrəs] *noun* virus which probably causes glandular fever (mononucleosis)

epulis [ɪˈpjuːlɪs] *noun* small fibrous swelling on a gum

equal [ˈiːkwəl] **1** *adjective* exactly the same in quantity, size, etc. as something else; *the twins are of equal size and weight* **2** *verb* to be exactly the same as something

equilibrium [iːkwɪˈlɪbriəm] *noun* state of balance

equina [ɪˈkwaɪnə] *see* CAUDA EQUINA

equinovarus [ɪkwaɪnəʊˈveərəs] *see* TALIPES

equip [ɪˈkwɪp] *verb* to provide the necessary apparatus; *the operating theatre is equipped with the latest scanning devices*

equipment [ɪˈkwɪpmənt] *noun* apparatus or tools which are required to do something; *the centre urgently needs surgical equipment*; *the surgeons complained about the out-of-date equipment in the hospital* (NOTE: no plural: for one item say: **a piece of equipment**)

ER [ˈiː ˈɑː] = ENDOPLASMIC RETICULUM

eradicate [ɪˈrædɪkeɪt] *verb* to wipe out, to remove completely; *international action to eradicate tuberculosis*

eradication [ɪrædɪˈkeɪʃn] *noun* removing completely

Erb's palsy *or* **Erb's paralysis** [ˈɜːbz ˈpɔːlzi *or* ˈɜːbz pəˈræləsɪs] *see* PALSY

ERCP [ˈiː ˈɑː ˈsiː ˈpiː] = ENDOSCOPIC RETROGRADE CHOLANGIOPANCREATOGRAPHY

erect [ɪˈrekt] *adjective* stiff and straight

erectile [ɪˈrektaɪl] *adjective* which can become erect; **erectile tissue** = vascular tissue which can become erect and stiff when engorged with blood (as the corpus cavernosum in the penis)

erection [ɪˈrekʃn] *noun* state where a part, such as the penis, becomes swollen because of engorgement with blood

erector pili [ɪˈrektə ˈpaɪlaɪ] *noun* small muscle attached to a hair follicle, which makes the hair stand upright and also forms goose pimples (NOTE: often called **arrector pili**)

erector spinae [ɪˈrektə ˈspaɪniː] *noun* large muscle starting at the base of the spine, and dividing as it runs up the spine

erepsin [ɪˈrepsɪn] *noun* mixture of enzymes produced by the glands in the intestine, used in the production of amino acids

erethism [ˈerəθɪzm] *noun* abnormal irritability

erg [ɜːg] *noun* unit of measurement of work or energy

ergograph [ˈɜːgəʊgrɑːf] *noun* apparatus which records the work of one or several muscles

ergometrine [ɜːgəʊˈmetrɪn] *noun; see* DRUGS TABLE IN SUPPLEMENT

ergonomics [ɜːgəˈnɒmɪks] *noun* study of man at work

ergot [ˈɜːgət] *noun* fungus which grows on rye

ergotism [ˈɜːgətɪzm] *noun* poisoning by eating rye which has been contaminated with ergot

COMMENT: the symptoms are muscle cramps and dry gangrene in the fingers and toes

erode [ɪˈrəʊd] *verb* to wear away, to break down

erogenous [ɪˈrɒdʒənəs] *noun* which produces sexual excitement; **erogenous zone** = part of the body which, if stimulated, produces sexual excitement (such as penis, clitoris, nipples, etc.)

erosion [ɪˈrəʊʒn] *noun* wearing away of tissue, breaking down of tissue; **cervical erosion** = condition where the epithelium of the mucous membrane lining the cervix uteri extends outside the cervix

ERPC = EVACUATION OF RETAINED PRODUCTS OF CONCEPTION

eructation [iːrʌkˈteɪʃn] *noun* belching, allowing air in the stomach to come up through the mouth

erupt [ɪˈrʌpt] *verb* to break through the skin; *the permanent incisors erupt before the premolars*

eruption [ɪˈrʌpʃn] *noun* (i) something which breaks through the skin (such as a rash or pimple); (ii) appearance of a new tooth in a gum

ery- *or* **erythr(o)-** [ˈerɪ *or* eˈrɪθrəʊ] *prefix* meaning red

erysipelas [erɪˈsɪpələs] *noun* contagious skin disease, where the skin on the face becomes hot and red and painful, caused by *Streptococcus pyogenes*

erysipeloid [erɪˈsɪpəlɔɪd] *noun* bacterial skin infection caused by touching infected fish or meat

erythema [erɪˈθiːmə] *noun* redness on the skin, caused by hyperaemia of the blood vessels near the surface; **erythema ab igne** = pattern of red lines on the skin caused by exposure to heat; **erythema induratum** = tubercular disease where ulcerating nodules appear on the legs of young women (NOTE: also called **Bazin's disease**); **erythema multiforme** = sudden appearance of inflammatory red patches and sometimes blisters on the skin; **erythema nodosum** = inflammatory disease where red swellings appear on the front of the legs; **erythema pernio** = CHILBLAIN; **erythema serpens** = bacterial skin infection caused by touching infected fish or meat

erythematosus [erɪθiːməˈtəʊsɪs] *see* DISSEMINATED, LUPUS

erythraemia [erɪˈθriːmiə] *noun* polycythaemia vera, a blood disorder where the number of red blood cells increases sharply, together with an increase in the number of white cells, making the blood thicker and slower to flow

erythrasma [erɪˈθræzmə] *noun* chronic bacterial skin condition in a fold in the skin or where two skin surfaces touch (such as between the toes), caused by a Corynebacterium

erythroblast [ɪˈrɪθrəblæst] *noun* cell which forms an erythrocyte or red blood cell

erythroblastosis [ɪrɪθrəʊblæˈstəʊsɪs] *noun* presence of erythroblasts in the blood, usually found in haemolytic anaemia; **erythroblastosis fetalis** = blood disease affecting newborn babies, caused by a reaction between the rhesus factor of the mother and the fetus

COMMENT: usually this occurs where the mother is rhesus negative and has developed rhesus positive antibodies, which are passed into the blood of a rhesus positive fetus

erythrocyanosis [ɪrɪθrəsaɪəˈnəʊsɪs] *noun* red and purple patches on the skin of the thighs, often accompanied by chilblains and made worse by cold

erythrocyte [ɪˈrɪθrəsaɪt] *noun* mature non-nucleated red blood cell, a blood cell which contains haemoglobin and carries oxygen; **erythrocyte sedimentation rate (ESR)** = diagnostic test to see how fast erythrocytes settle in a sample of blood plasma

anemia may be due to insufficient erythrocyte production, in which case the corrected reticulocyte count will be low, or it may be due to hemorrhage or hemolysis, in which cases there should be reticulocyte response

Southern Medical Journal

erythrocytosis [ɪrɪθrəsaɪˈtəʊsɪs] *noun* increase in the number of red blood cells in the blood

erythroderma [ɪrɪθrəˈdɜːmə] *noun* condition where the skin becomes red and flakes off

erythroedema [ɪrɪθrəɪˈdiːmə] *noun* pink disease, a disease of infants where the child's hands and feet swell and become pink, with a fever and loss of appetite, probably formerly caused by allergic reaction to mercury in lotions

erythrogenesis or **erythropoiesis**
[ɪrɪθrə'dʒenəsɪs or ɪrɪθrəpɔɪ'iːsɪs] *noun*
formation of red blood cells in red bone
marrow

erythromelalgia [ɪrɪθrəmel'ældʒə] *noun*
painful swelling of blood vessels in the
extremities

erythromycin [ɪrɪθrə'maɪsɪn] *noun; see*
DRUGS TABLE IN SUPPLEMENT

erythropenia [ɪrɪθrə'piːniə] *noun* condition
where a patient has a low number of
erythrocytes in his blood

erythropoiesis [ɪrɪθrəpɔɪ'iːsɪs] =
ERYTHROGENESIS

erythropoietin [ɪrɪθrə'pɔɪətɪn] *noun*
hormone which regulates the production of
red blood cells

COMMENT: erythropoietin can now be
produced by genetic techniques and is
being used to increase the production of
red blood cells in anaemia

erythropsia [erɪ'θrɒpsiə] *noun* condition
where the patient sees things as if coloured
red

Esbach's albuminometer ['esbɑːks
ælbjuːmɪ'nɒmɪtə] *noun* glass for measuring
albumin in urine, using Esbach's method

eschar ['eskɑː] *noun* dry scab, such as one
on a burn

escharotic [eskə'rɒtɪk] *noun* substance
which produces an eschar

Escherichia [eʃə'rɪkiə] *noun* one of the
Enterobacteria commonly found in faeces;
Escherichia coli or **E. coli** = Gram-negative
bacillus associated with acute gastroenteritis
in infants

escort [ɪ'skɔːt] *verb* to go with someone,
especially to go with a patient to make sure
he arrives at the right place; **escort nurse** =
nurse who goes with patients to the operating
theatre and back again to the ward

Esmarch's bandage ['esmɑːks 'bændɪdʒ]
noun rubber band wrapped round a limb as a
tourniquet before a surgical operation and left
in place during the operation so as to keep the
site free of blood

eso- ['iːsəʊ] *US* = OESO-

esophagus [iː'sɒfəgəs] *US* =
OESOPHAGUS

esotropia [esə'trəʊpiə] *noun* convergent
strabismus, a type of squint, where the eyes
both look towards the nose

espundia [ɪ'spuːndiə] *see*
LEISHMANIASIS

ESR ['iː 'es 'ɑː] = ERYTHROCYTE
SEDIMENTATION RATE

essence ['esəns] *noun* concentrated oil
from a plant, used in cosmetics, and
sometimes as analgesics or antiseptics

essential [ɪ'senʃl] *adjective* **(a)** idiopathic,
(disease) with no obvious cause; **essential
hypertension** = high blood pressure without
any obvious cause; **essential uterine
haemorrhage** = heavy uterine bleeding for
which there is no obvious cause **(b)**
extremely important or necessary; **essential
amino acid** = amino acid which is necessary
for growth but which cannot be synthesized
and has to be obtained from the food supply;
essential elements = chemical elements
(such as carbon, oxygen, hydrogen, nitrogen
and many others) which are necessary to the
body's growth or function; **essential fatty
acid (EFA)** = unsaturated fatty acid which is
necessary for growth and health; **essential
oils** = volatile oils, concentrated oils from a
scented plant used in cosmetics or as
antiseptics

COMMENT: the essential amino acids are:
isoleucine, leucine, lysine, methionine,
phenylalanine, threonine, tryptophan and
valine. The essential fatty acids are linoleic
acid, linolenic acid and arachidonic acid

estrogen ['iːstrədʒn] *US* = OESTROGEN

ethanol ['eθənɒl] *noun* ethyl alcohol, a
colourless liquid, present in drinking alcohols
(whisky, gin, vodka, etc.) and also used in
medicines and as a disinfectant

ether ['iːθə] *noun* anaesthetic substance,
now rarely used

ethical ['eθɪkl] *adjective* (i) concerning
ethics; (ii) (drug) available on prescription
only; **ethical committee** = group of
specialists who monitor experiments
involving human beings or who regulate the
way in which members of the medical
profession conduct themselves

ethically ['eθɪkli] *adverb* concerning ethics

ethics ['eθɪks] *noun* **medical ethics** = code
of working which shows how a professional
group (such as doctors and nurses) should
work, and in particular what type of
relationship they should have with their
patients

ethmoid or **ethmoidal** [eθ'mɔɪd or
eθ'mɔɪdl] *adjective* referring to the ethmoid

bone, near to the ethmoid bone; **ethmoidal sinuses** = air cells inside the ethmoid bone

ethmoid bone ['eθmɔɪd 'bəʊn] *noun* bone which forms the top of the nasal cavity and part of the orbits

ethmoiditis [eθmɔɪ'daɪtɪs] *noun* inflammation of the ethmoid bone or of the ethmoidal sinuses

ethyl alcohol ['eθɪl 'ælkəhɒl] *see* ALCOHOL

ethylene *or* **ethene** ['eθəliːn *or* 'iːθiːn] *noun* gas used as an anaesthetic

etiology, etiological [iːti'ɒlədʒi *or* iːtiə'lɒdʒɪkl] *US* = AETIOLOGY, AETIOLOGICAL

eu- ['juː] *prefix* meaning good

eubacteria [juːˈbækˈtɪərɪə] *noun* true bacteria with rigid cell walls

eucalyptol [juːkəˈlɪptəl] *noun* substance obtained from eucalyptus oil

eucalyptus [juːkəˈlɪptəs] *noun* genus of tree growing mainly in Australia, from which a strongly smelling oil is distilled

COMMENT: eucalyptus oil is used in pharmaceutical products especially to relieve congestion in the respiratory passages

eugenics [juːˈdʒenɪks] *noun* study of how to improve the human race by genetic selection

eunuch ['juːnək] *noun* castrated male

eupepsia [juːˈpepsɪə] *noun* good digestion

euphoria [juːˈfɔːrɪə] *noun* feeling of extreme happiness

euplastic [juːˈplæstɪk] *adjective* (tissue) which heals well

Eustachian tube [juːˈsteɪʃn 'tjuːb] *noun* syrinx or pharyngotympanic tube, the tube which connects the pharynx to the middle ear; *see illustration at* EAR

COMMENT: the Eustachian tubes balance the air pressure on either side of the eardrum. When a person swallows or yawns, air is allowed into the Eustachian tubes and equalizes the pressure with the normal atmospheric pressure outside the body. The tubes can be blocked by an infection (as in a cold) or by pressure differences (as inside an aircraft) and if they are blocked, the hearing is impaired

euthanasia [juːθəˈneɪzɪə] *noun* mercy killing, the killing of a sick person to put an end to his suffering

euthyroidism *or* **euthyroid state** [juːˈθaɪrɔɪdɪzm *or* juːˈθaɪrɔɪd 'steɪt] *noun* having a normal thyroid gland

eutocia [juːˈtəʊsɪə] *noun* normal childbirth

evacuant [ɪˈvækjuənt] *noun* medicine which makes a person have a bowel movement

evacuate [ɪˈvækjueɪt] *verb* to discharge faeces from the bowel, to have a bowel movement

evacuation [ɪvækjuˈeɪʃn] *noun* removing the contents of something, especially discharging faeces from the bowel; **evacuation of retained products of conception (ERPC)** = D & C operation performed after an abortion or miscarriage to ensure the uterus is left empty

evacuator [ɪˈvækjueɪtə] *noun* instrument used to empty a cavity such as the bladder or bowel

evaluate [ɪˈvæljueɪt] *verb* to examine and calculate the quantity or level of something; to examine a patient and calculate the treatment required; *the laboratory is still evaluating the results of the tests*

all patients were evaluated and followed up at the hypertension unit

British Medical Journal

evaluation [ɪvæljuˈeɪʃn] *noun* examining and calculating; *in further evaluation of these patients no side-effects of the treatment were noted*

evaluation of fetal age and weight has proved to be of value in the clinical management of pregnancy, particularly in high-risk gestations

Southern Medical Journal

evaporate [ɪˈvæpəreɪt] *verb* to convert liquid into vapour

evaporation [ɪvæpəˈreɪʃn] *noun* converting liquid into vapour

eversion [ɪˈvɜːʃn] *noun* turning towards the outside, turning inside out; **eversion of the cervix** = condition after laceration during childbirth, where the edges of the cervix sometimes turn outwards

evertor [ɪˈvɜːtə] *noun* muscle which makes a limb turn outwards

evidence-based ['evidəns'beist] *adjective* (medicine) practice based on the results of well designed trials of specific interventions for specific conditions

evisceration [ɪvɪsə'reɪʃn] *noun* (i) surgical removal of the abdominal viscera; (ii) removal of the contents of an organ; **evisceration of the eye** = surgical removal of the contents of an eyeball

evolution [i:və'lu:ʃn] *noun* changes in organisms which take place over a long period involving many generations

Ewing's tumour or **Ewing's sarcoma** ['ju:ɪŋz 'tju:mə or 'ju:ɪŋz sɑ:'kəʊmə] *noun* malignant tumour in the marrow of a long bone

ex- or **exo-** ['eks or 'eksəʊ] *prefix* meaning out of

exacerbate [ɪgz'æsəbeit] *verb* to make a condition more severe; *the cold damp weather will only exacerbate his chest condition*

exacerbation [ɪgzæsə'beɪʃn] *noun* making a condition worse; period when a condition becomes worse

```
patients     were     re-examined
regularly    or    when    they felt
they    might    be    having    an
exacerbation.    Exacerbation
rates    were    calculated    from the
number    of    exacerbations during
the study
                                    Lancet
```

exact [ɪg'zækt] *adjective* correct or precise

exaltation [egzɔ:l'teɪʃn] *noun* sense of being extremely cheerful and excited

examination [ɪgzæmɪ'neɪʃn] *noun* **(a)** (i) looking at someone or something carefully; (ii) looking at a patient to find out what is wrong with him or her; *from the examination of the X-ray photographs, it seems that the tumour has not spread; the surgeon carried out a medical examination before operating*; **manual examination** = examination using the hands and fingers **(b)** written or oral test to see if a student is progressing satisfactorily; *there will be a written and an oral examination in German* (NOTE: in this sense often abbreviated to **exam**)

examine [ɪg'zæmɪn] *verb* (i) to look at or to investigate someone or something carefully; (ii) to look at and test a patient to find what is wrong with him or her; *the doctor examined*

the patient's heart; the tissue samples were examined in the laboratory

exanthem [ɪg'zænθəm] *noun* skin rash found with infectious diseases like measles or chickenpox; **exanthem subitum** = ROSEOLA INFANTUM

exanthematous [eksæn'θemətəs] *adjective* referring to an exanthem, like an exanthem

excavator ['ekskəveɪtə] *noun* surgical instrument shaped like a spoon

excavatum ['ekskəveɪtəm] *see* PECTUS

exceed [ɪk'si:d] *verb* to do more than, to be more than; *his pulse rate exceeded 100*; **do not exceed the stated dose** = do not take more than the stated dose

exceptional [ɪk'sepʃənl] *adjective* strange, not common; *in exceptional cases, treatment can be carried out in the patient's home*

excess [ɪk'ses] *noun* too much of a substance; *the gland was producing an excess of hormones; the body could not cope with an excess of blood sugar*; **in excess of** = more than; *short men who weigh in excess of 100 kilos are very overweight*

excessive [ɪk'sesɪv] *adjective* more than normal; *the patient was passing excessive quantities of urine; the doctor noted an excessive amount of bile in the patient's blood*

excessively [ɪk'sesɪvli] *adverb* too much; *he has an excessively high blood pressure; if the patient sweats excessively, it may be necessary to cool his body with cold compresses*

exchange [ɪks'tʃeɪnʒ] **1** *noun* giving one thing and taking another; **gas exchange** = process where oxygen in air is exchanged in the lungs for waste carbon dioxide from the blood; **exchange transfusion** = method of treating leukaemia or erythroblastosis in newborn babies, where almost all the abnormal blood is removed from the body and replaced by normal blood **2** *verb* to take something away and give something in its place; *in the lungs, carbon dioxide in the blood is exchanged for oxygen from the air*

excipient [ɪk'sɪpiənt] *noun* substance added to a drug so that it can be made into a pill

excise [ɪk'saɪz] *verb* to cut out

excision [ɪk'sɪʒn] *noun* operation by a surgeon to cut and remove part of the body (such as a growth); *compare* INCISION

excitation [eksɪ'teɪʃn] *noun* state of being mentally or nervously aroused

excitatory [ɪk'saɪtətri] *adjective* which tends to excite

excite [ɪk'saɪt] *verb* to stimulate, to give an impulse to a nerve or muscle

excited [ɪk'saɪtɪd] *adjective* (i) very lively and happy; (ii) aroused

excitement [ɪk'saɪtmənt] *noun* **(a)** being excited **(b)** second stage of anaesthesia

excoriation [ɪkskɔːri'eɪʃn] *noun* raw skin surface or mucous membrane after rubbing or burning

excrement ['ekskrəmənt] *noun* faeces

excrescence [ɪk'skresns] *noun* growth on the skin

excreta [ɪk'skriːtə] *plural noun* waste material from the body (such as faeces)

excrete [ɪk'skriːt] *verb* to pass waste matter out of the body, especially to discharge faeces; *the urinary system separates waste liquids from the blood and excretes them as urine*

excretion [ɪk'skriːʃn] *noun* passing waste matter (faeces, urine or sweat) out of the body

excruciating [ɪk'skruːʃieɪtɪŋ] *adjective* (pain) which is extremely painful; *he had excruciating pains in his head*

exenteration [eksentə'reɪʃn] = EVISCERATION

exercise ['eksəsaɪz] **1** *noun* physical or mental activity; active use of the muscles as a way of keeping fit, to correct a deformity or to strengthen a part; *regular exercise is good for your heart*; *you should to do five minutes' exercise every morning*; *he doesn't do or take enough exercise - that's why he's too fat*; **exercise cycle** = cycle which is fixed to the floor so that you can pedal on it to get exercise; **exercise-induced asthma (EIA)** = asthma which is caused by exercise such as running or cycling **2** *verb* to take exercise; *he exercises twice a day to keep fit*

exert [ɪg'zɜːt] *verb* to use (force or pressure)

exertion [ɪg'zɜːʃn] *noun* physical activity

exfoliation [eksfəuli'eɪʃn] *noun* losing layers of tissue (such as sunburnt skin)

exfoliative [eks'fəulieɪtɪv] *adjective* referring to exfoliation; **exfoliative**

dermatitis = condition where the skin becomes red and flakes off

exhalation [ekshə'leɪʃn] *noun* (i) expiration, breathing out; (ii) air which is breathed out (NOTE: the opposite is **inhalation**)

exhale [eks'heɪl] *verb* to breathe out (NOTE: the opposite is **inhale**)

exhaust [ɪg'zɔːst] *verb* to tire someone out; to drain energy; *he was exhausted by his long walk*; *the patient was exhausted after the second operation*

exhaustion [ɪg'zɔːstʃn] *noun* extreme tiredness or fatigue; **heat exhaustion** = collapse caused by physical exertion in hot conditions

exhibit [ek'sɪbɪt] *verb* to show signs of; *the patient exhibited significant mental and psychological impairment*

exhibitionism [eksɪ'bɪʃənɪzm] *noun* sexual aberration in which there is a desire to show the genitals to a person of the opposite sex

exo- ['eksəu] *prefix* meaning outside

exocrine gland ['eksəkraɪn 'glænd] *noun* gland (such as the liver, the sweat glands, the pancreas and the salivary glands) with ducts which channel secretions to particular parts of the body; **exocrine secretions of the pancreas** = enzymes carried from the pancreas to the second part of the duodenum

exogenous [ek'sɒdʒənəs] *adjective* developing or caused by something outside the organism; *compare* ENDOGENOUS

exomphalos [ek'sɒmfələs] = UMBILICAL HERNIA

exophthalmic goitre [eksɒf'θælmɪk 'gɔɪtə] *see* THYROTOXICOSIS (NOTE: also called **Graves' disease**)

exophthalmos [eksɒf'θælməs] *noun* protruding eyeballs

exoskeleton [eksə'skelɪtn] *noun* outer skeleton of some animals such as insects; *compare* ENDOSKELETON

exostosis [eksə'stəusɪs] *noun* benign growth on the surface of a bone

exotic [ɪg'zɒtɪk] *adjective* (disease) which is not native, which comes from a foreign country

exotoxin [eksəu'tɒksɪn] *noun* poison produced by bacteria, which affects parts of the body away from the place of infection (such as the toxins which cause botulism or tetanus)

COMMENT: diphtheria is caused by a bacillus; the exotoxin released causes the generalized symptoms of the disease (such as fever and rapid pulse) while the bacillus itself is responsible for the local symptoms in the patient's upper throat

exotropia [eksəu'trəupiə] *noun* divergent strabismus, a form of squint where both eyes look away from the nose

expand [ɪk'spænd] *verb* to spread out; *the chest expands as the person breathes in*

expansion [ɪk'spænʃn] *noun* growing larger or becoming swollen

expect [ɪk'spekt] *verb* to think or to hope that something is going to happen; *she's expecting a baby in June* = she is pregnant and the baby is due to be born in June; **expected date of delivery** = day on which a doctor calculates that the birth will take place; **expected death** = death of a patient who was undergoing care for a terminal disease

expectant [ɪk'spektnt] *noun* **expectant woman** *or* **expectant mother** = pregnant woman

expectorant [ɪk'spektərnt] *noun* drug which helps the patient to expectorate, to cough up phlegm

expectorate [ɪk'spektəreɪt] *verb* to cough up phlegm or sputum from the respiratory passages

expectoration [ɪkspektə'reɪʃn] *noun* coughing up fluid or phlegm from the respiratory tract

expel [ɪk'spel] *verb* to send out of the body; *air is expelled from the lungs when a person breathes out*

experience [ɪk'spɪəriəns] **1** *noun* **(a)** having worked in many types of situation, and so knowing how to cope with different problems; *he has had six years' experience in tropical medicine*; *his research is based on his experience as a nurse in a teaching hospital* **(b)** something which has happened to someone; *he told the complaints board about his experiences as an outpatient* **2** *verb* to live through a situation; *she experienced acute mental disturbance*; *he is experiencing pains in his right upper leg*

experienced [ɪk'spɪəriənst] *adjective* (person) who has lived through many situations and has learnt how to deal with problems; *she is the most experienced member of our nursing staff*; *we require an experienced nurse to take charge of a geriatric ward*

experiment [ɪk'sperɪmənt] *noun* scientific test conducted under set conditions; *the scientists did some experiments to try the new drug on a small sample of people*

expert ['eksp3:t] **1** *noun* person who is trained or who has experience in a certain field; *he was referred to an expert in tropical diseases*; *she is an expert in the field of optics*; *they asked for a second expert opinion* **2** *adjective* done well, showing experience; *the clinic offers expert treatment of sexually transmitted diseases*

expiration [ekspə'reɪʃn] *noun* **(a)** breathing out, pushing air out of the lungs; *expiration takes place when the chest muscles relax and the lungs become smaller* (NOTE: the opposite is **inspiration**) **(b)** dying

expire [ɪk'spaɪə] *verb* **(a)** to breathe out **(b)** to die

explain [ɪk'spleɪn] *verb* to give reasons for something; to make something clear; *the doctors cannot explain why he suddenly got better*; *she tried to explain her symptoms to the doctor*

explanation [eksplə'neɪʃn] *noun* reason for something; *the staff of the hospital could not offer any explanation for the strange behaviour of the consultant*

explant [eks'plɑ:nt] **1** *noun* tissue taken from a body and grown in a culture in a laboratory **2** *verb* **(a)** to take tissue from a body and grow it in a culture in a laboratory **(b)** to remove an implant

explantation [eksplɑ:n'teɪʃn] *noun* **(a)** taking tissue from a body and growing it in a culture in a laboratory **(b)** removal of an implant

exploration [eksplə'reɪʃn] *noun* procedure or surgical operation where the aim is to discover the cause of the symptoms or the nature and extent of the illness

exploratory [ɪk'splɔ:rətri] *adjective* referring to an exploration; **exploratory surgery** = surgical operations in which the aim is to discover the cause of the patient's symptoms or the nature and extent of the illness

expose [ɪk'spəuz] *verb* **(a)** to show something which was hidden; *the operation exposed a generalized cancer*; *the report exposed a lack of medical care on the part of some of the hospital staff* **(b)** to place something or someone under the influence of something; *he was exposed to the disease for two days*; *she was exposed to a lethal dose of radiation*

exposure [ɪk'spəʊʒə] *noun* **(a)** being exposed; *his exposure to radiation* **(b)** being damp, cold and with no protection from the weather; *the survivors of the crash were all suffering from exposure after spending a night in the snow*

express [ɪk'spres] *verb* to squeeze out; *to express pus*

expression [ɪk'spreʃn] *noun* **(a)** look on a person's face which shows his emotions, what he thinks and feels; *his expression showed that he was annoyed* **(b)** pushing something out of the body; *the expression of the fetus and placenta during childbirth*

exquisitely tender [ɪk'skwɪzɪtli 'tendə] *adjective* producing a sharp localized pain or tenderness when touched

exsanguinate [ɪk'sæŋgwɪneɪt] *verb* to drain blood from the body

exsanguination [ɪksæŋgwɪ'neɪʃn] *noun* removal of blood from the body

exsufflation [eksə'fleɪʃn] *noun* forcing breath out of the body

extend [ɪk'stend] *verb* to stretch out; *the patient is unable to extend his arms fully*

extension [ɪk'stenʃn] *noun* **(a)** (i) stretching or straightening out of a joint; (ii) stretching of a joint by traction **(b)** something built on afterwards; *the hospital has had an extension built to house its new X-ray equipment*

extensor (muscle) [ɪk'stensə] *noun* muscle which makes a joint become straight; *compare* FLEXOR

exterior [ɪk'stɪəriə] *noun* the outside; *the interior of the disc has passed through the tough exterior and is pressing on a nerve*

exteriorization [ɪkstɪəriərɑɪ'zeɪʃn] *noun* surgical operation to bring an internal organ to the outside surface of the body

externa [ɪk'stɜːnə] *see* OTITIS

external [ɪk'stɜːnl] *adjective* which is outside, especially outside the surface of the body; *the lotion is for external use only* = it should only be used on the outside of the body; **external auditory meatus** = tube in the skull leading from the outer ear to the eardrum; **external cardiac massage** *or* **external chest** *or* **cardiac compression** =

method of making a patient's heart start beating again by rhythmic pressing on the breastbone; **external jugular** = main jugular vein in the neck, leading from the temporal vein; **external oblique** = outer muscle covering the abdomen; *compare* INTERNAL

externally [ɪk'stɜːnli] *adverb* on the outside of the body; *the ointment should only be used externally*; *compare* INTERNALLY

exteroceptor [ekstərəʊ'septə] *noun* sensory nerve such as those in the eye or ear, which is affected by stimuli from outside the body; *see also* CHEMORECEPTOR, INTEROCEPTOR, RECEPTOR

extirpate ['ekstɜːpeɪt] *verb* to remove by surgery

extirpation [ekstɜː'peɪʃn] *noun* total removal of a structure, an organ or growth by surgery

extra- ['ekstrə] *prefix* meaning outside

extracapsular [ekstrə'kæpsjʊlə] *adjective* outside a capsule; **extracapsular fracture** = fracture of the upper part of the femur, but which does not involve the capsule round the hip joint

extracellular [ekstrə'seljʊlə] *adjective* outside cells; **extracellular fluid** = fluid which surrounds cells

extra-contractual referral (ECR) [ekstrəkən'træptjʊəl rɪ'fɜːrəl] *noun* referral of a patient (usually by a GP) to a hospital outside normal referral patterns and which therefore incurs additional cost and may be subject to review by a PCG

extract 1 ['ekstrækt] *noun* preparation made by removing water or alcohol from a substance, leaving only the essence; **liver extract** = concentrated essence of liver **2** [ɪk'strækt] *verb* (i) to take out; (ii) to remove the essence from a liquid; (iii) to pull out a tooth; *adrenaline extracted from the animal's adrenal glands is used in the treatment of asthma*

all the staff are RGNs, partly because they do venesection, partly because they work in plasmapheresis units which extract plasma and return red blood cells to the donor
Nursing Times

extraction [ɪk'strækʃn] *noun* (i) removal of part of the body, especially a tooth; (ii) in obstetrics, delivery, usually a breech presentation, which needs medical assistance;

cataract extraction = surgical removal of a cataract from the eye; **vacuum extraction** = pulling on the head of the baby with a suction instrument to aid birth

extradural [ekstrə'djuərl] *adjective* epidural, lying on the outside of the dura mater; **extradural haematoma** = blood clot which forms in the head outside the dura mater, caused by a blow; **extradural haemorrhage** = serious condition where bleeding occurs between the dura mater and the skull

extraembryonic [ekstrəembri'ɒnɪk] *adjective* (part of a fertilized ovum, such as the amnion, allantois and chorion) which is not part of the embryo

extrapleural [ekstrə'pluərl] *adjective* outside the pleural cavity

extrapyramidal [ekstrəpɪ'ræmɪdl] *adjective* outside the pyramidal tracts; **extrapyramidal system** *or* **tracts** = motor system which carries motor nerves outside the pyramidal system

extrasystole [ekstrə'sɪstli] *noun* ectopic beat, an abnormal extra heartbeat which originates from a point other than the sinoatrial node

extrauterine pregnancy [ekstrə'juːtəraɪn 'pregnənsi] *noun* ectopic pregnancy, pregnancy where the embryo develops outside the uterus, often in one of the Fallopian tubes

extravasation [ekstrævə'seɪʃn] *noun* escaping of bodily fluid (such as blood or secretions) into tissue

extravert, extraversion ['ekstrəvɜːt or ekstrə'vɜːʃn] *noun* = EXTROVERT, EXTROVERSION

extreme [ɪks'triːm] *adjective* very severe; *extreme forms of the disease can cause blindness*

extremities [ɪk'stremətiz] *noun* parts of the body at the ends of limbs, such as the fingers, toes, nose and ears

extrinsic [eks'trɪnsɪk] *adjective* external, which originates outside a structure; **extrinsic allergic alveolitis** = condition where the lungs are allergic to fungus and other allergens; **extrinsic factor** = former term for vitamin B_{12} which is necessary for the production of red blood cells; **extrinsic ligament** = ligament between the bones in a joint which is separate from the joint capsule; **extrinsic muscle** = muscle which is some

way away from the part of the body (such as the eye) which it operates

extroversion [ekstrə'vɜːʃn] *noun* **(a)** *(in psychology)* condition where a person is mainly interested in people and things other than himself **(b)** congenital turning of an organ inside out

extrovert ['ekstrəvɜːt] *noun* person who is interested in people and things apart from himself

extroverted ['ekstrəvɜːtɪd] *adjective* **(a)** *(person)* interested in people and things apart from himself **(b)** *(organ)* turned inside out; *compare* INTROVERSION, INTROVERT

exudate ['eksjudeɪt] *noun* fluid which is deposited on the surface of tissue as the result of a condition or disease

exudation [eksju'deɪʃn] *noun* escape of exudate into tissue as a defence mechanism

eye [aɪ] *noun* part of the body with which a person sees; *she has blue eyes*; *shut your eyes while the doctor gives you an injection*; *he has got a speck of dust in his eye*; *she has been having trouble with her eyes* or *she has been having eye trouble*; *he is an outpatient at the local eye hospital*; **black eye** = darkening and swelling of the tissues round an eye, caused by a blow; *he got two black eyes in the fight*; **glass eye** = artificial eye made of glass; **pink eye** *or* **red eye** = epidemic conjunctivitis, common in schools, and caused by the Koch-Weeks bacillus; **eye bath** = small dish into which a solution can be placed for bathing the eye; **eye drops** =

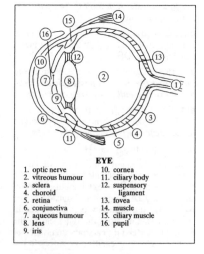

EYE

1. optic nerve	10. cornea
2. vitreous humour	11. ciliary body
3. sclera	12. suspensory
4. choroid	ligament
5. retina	13. fovea
6. conjunctiva	14. muscle
7. aqueous humour	15. ciliary muscle
8. lens	16. pupil
9. iris	

medicine in liquid form which is put into the eye in small amounts; **eye ointment** = smooth oily medicinal preparation which is put into or around the eye; *the doctor prescribed some eye drops or eye ointment*; **eye specialist** = ophthalmologist, a doctor who specializes in the study of the eye and its diseases; **eye test** = examination of the inside of an eye to see if it is working correctly, and if the patient needs glasses (NOTE: For other terms referring to the eye, see words beginning with **oculo-**, **ophth-** and **opt-**)

eyeball ['aɪbɔːl] *noun* the receptor part of the eye, a round ball of tissue through which light passes and which is controlled by various muscles

COMMENT: light rays enter the eye through the cornea, pass through the pupil and are refracted through the aqueous humour onto the lens, which then focuses the rays through the vitreous humour onto the retina at the back of the eyeball. Impulses from the retina pass along the optic nerve to the brain

eye bank ['aɪ 'bæŋk] *noun* place where parts of eyes given by donors can be kept for use in grafts

eyebath ['aɪbɑːθ] *noun* small dish into which a solution can be put for bathing the eye

eyebrow ['aɪbraʊ] *noun* arch of skin with a line of hair above the eye; **he raised his eyebrows** = he looked surprised

eyeglasses ['aɪglɑːsɪz] *noun US* glasses, spectacles

eyelash ['aɪlæʃ] *noun* small hair which grows out from the edge of the eyelid

eyelid ['aɪlɪd] *noun* piece of skin which covers the eye (NOTE: also called the **blepharon** or **palpebra**. For terms referring to the eyelids, see words beginning with **blepharo-**)

eyesight ['aɪsaɪt] *noun* being able to see; *he has got very good eyesight*; *failing eyesight is common in old people*

eyestrain ['aɪstreɪn] *noun* asthenopia, tiredness in the muscles of the eye, with a headache, caused by reading in bad light, watching television, working on a computer screen, etc.

eyetooth ['aɪtuːθ] *noun* canine tooth in the upper jaw, one of a pair of pointed teeth next to the incisors (NOTE: plural is **eyeteeth**)

Ff

F 1 *abbreviation for* Fahrenheit **2** *chemical symbol for* fluorine

face [feɪs] **1** *noun* front part of the head, where the eyes, nose and mouth are placed; *don't forget to wash the patient's face*; **face delivery** = birth where the baby's face appears first; *(in cosmetic surgery)* **face lift** *or* **face-lifting operation** = surgical operation to remove wrinkles on the face and neck; *she's gone into hospital for a face lift*; **face mask** = (i) rubber mask that fits over the patient's nose and mouth and is used to administer an anaesthetic; (ii) piece of gauze which fits over the mouth and nose to prevent droplet infection; **face presentation** = position of a baby in the uterus where the face will appear first at birth **2** *verb* to have your face towards or to look towards; *please face the screen*; *the hospital faces east*

COMMENT: the fourteen bones which make up the face are: two maxillae forming the upper jaw; two nasal bones forming the top part of the nose; two lacrimal bones on the inside of the orbit near the nose; two zygomatic or malar bones forming the sides of the cheeks; two palatine bones forming the back part of the top of the mouth; two nasal conchae or turbinate bones which form the sides of the nasal cavity; the mandible or lower jaw; and the vomer in the centre of the nasal septum

facet [ˈfæsɪt] *noun* flat surface on a bone; **facet syndrome** = condition where a joint in the vertebrae becomes dislocated

facial [ˈfeɪʃəl] *adjective* referring to the face; *the psychiatrist examined the patient's facial expression*; **facial bones** = the fourteen bones which form the face; **facial artery** = artery which branches off the external carotid into the face and mouth; **facial nerve** = seventh cranial nerve, which governs the muscles of the face, the taste buds on the front of the tongue, and the salivary and lacrimal glands; **facial paralysis** = BELL'S PALSY; **facial vein** = vein which

drains down the side of the face into the internal jugular vein; **deep facial vein** = small vein which drains from behind the cheek into the facial vein

-facient [ˈfeɪʃənt] *prefix* which makes; **abortifacient** = drug or instrument which produces an abortion

facies [ˈfeɪʃiːz] *noun* facial appearance of a patient, used as a guide to diagnosis

facilitate [fəˈsɪləteɪt] *verb* to help, to make something easy

facilitation [fəsɪləˈteɪʃn] *noun* act where several slight stimuli help a neurone to be activated

facilities [fəˈsɪlətiz] *plural noun* equipment, counselling or rooms which can be used to do something; *provision of aftercare facilities*

fact [fækt] *noun* something which is real and true; *it is a fact that the disease is rarely fatal*; *tell me all the facts of your son's illness so that I can decide what to do*; **the facts of life** = description of how sexual intercourse is performed and how conception takes place, given to children

factor [ˈfæktə] *noun* **(a)** something which has an influence, which makes something else take place; **extrinsic factor** = form of vitamin B_{12} **growth factor** = chemical substance produced in one part of the body which encourages the growth of a type of cell (such as red blood cells); **intrinsic factor** = protein produced in the gastric glands which controls the absorption of extrinsic factor, and the lack of which causes pernicious anaemia **(b)** substance (called Factor I, Factor II, etc.) in the plasma which makes the blood coagulate when a blood vessel is injured; **Factor VIII** = substance in plasma which is lacking in haemophiliacs; **Christmas factor** *or* **Factor IX** = substance in plasma, the lack of which causes Christmas disease; **Hageman factor** *or* **Factor XII** = protein substance in plasma, one of the blood clotting factors; **von Willebrand's factor** = protein substance in plasma involved in platelet aggregation

faculty ['fækəltɪ] *noun* ability to do something; **mental faculties** = power of the mind to think or decide; *a reduction in blood supply to the brain can have a lasting effect on the mental faculties*

faecal *US* **fecal** ['fiːkl] *adjective* referring to faeces; **faecal matter** = solid waste matter from the bowels

faeces *US* **feces** ['fiːsiːz] *plural noun* stools or bowel movements, solid waste matter passed from the bowels through the anus (NOTE: for other terms referring to faeces, see words beginning with **sterco-**)

Fahrenheit ['færənhaɪt] *noun* scale of temperatures where the freezing and boiling points of water are 32° and 212°; *compare* CELSIUS, CENTIGRADE (NOTE: used in the USA, but less common in the UK. Normally written with an **F** after the degree sign: **32°F** (say: **thirty-two degrees Fahrenheit**))

fail [feɪl] *verb* not to be successful in doing something, not to succeed or not to do something which you are trying to do; *the doctor failed to see the symptoms*; *she has failed her pharmacy exams*; *he failed his medical and was rejected by the police force*

failing ['feɪlɪŋ] *adjective* weakening, becoming closer to death

failure ['feɪljə] *noun* not a success; *the operation to correct the bone defect was a failure*; **heart failure** = situation where the heart cannot function in a satisfactory way and is unable to circulate blood normally; **kidney failure** = situation where a kidney does not function properly; **failure to thrive** = wasting disease of small children who have difficulty in absorbing nutrients or who are suffering from malnutrition

faint [feɪnt] **1** *verb* to lose consciousness, to stop being conscious for a short time; *she fainted when she saw the blood*; *it was so hot standing in the sun that he fainted* **2** *noun* loss of consciousness for a short period, caused by a temporary reduction in the flow of blood to the brain; *he collapsed in a faint* **3** *adjective* not very clear, difficult to see or hear; *he could detect a faint improvement in the patient's condition*; *there's a faint smell of apples in the urine* (NOTE: **faint - fainter - faintest**)

fainting ['feɪntɪŋ] *noun* syncope, becoming unconscious for a short time; **fainting fit** *or*

fainting spell = becoming unconscious for a short time; *she often had fainting fits when she was dieting*

COMMENT: a fainting spell happens when the supply of blood to the brain is reduced for a short time, and this can be due to many causes, including lack of food, heat exhaustion, standing upright for a long time, and fear

fair [feə] *adjective* light-coloured (hair or skin); *she's got fair hair*; *he's dark, but his sister is fair*

Fairbanks' splint ['feəbæŋks 'splɪnt] *noun* special splint used for correcting Erb's palsy

fair-haired ['feə'heəd] *adjective* (person) with light-coloured hair

fairly ['feəlɪ] *adverb* quite; *I'm fairly certain I have met him before*; *he has been working as a doctor only for a fairly short time*

falciform ['fælsɪfɔːm] *adjective* in the shape of a sickle; **falciform ligament** = tissue which separates the two lobes of the liver and attaches it to the diaphragm

fall [fɔːl] **1** *noun* losing balance and going onto the ground; *she had a fall and hurt her back*; *he broke a bone in his hip after a fall* **2** *verb* **(a)** to drop down onto the ground; *he fell down the stairs*; *she fell off the wall*; *don't put the baby's bottle on the cushion - it will fall over* **(b)** **to fall pregnant** = to become pregnant (NOTE: **falling - fell - has fallen**)

fall asleep ['fɔːl ə'sliːp] *verb* to go to sleep; *he fell asleep in front of the TV*

fall ill ['fɔːl 'ɪl] *verb* to get ill or to start to have an illness; *he fell ill while on holiday and had to be flown home*

fall off ['fɔːl 'ɒf] *verb* to become less; *the number of admissions has fallen off this month*

Fallopian tube [fæ'ləupɪən 'tjuːb] *noun* one of two tubes which connect the ovaries to the uterus; *see illustration at* UROGENITAL SYSTEM (FEMALE) (NOTE: also called **oviduct** *or* **salpinx** *or* **uterine tube**. For other terms referring to Fallopian tubes, see words beginning with **salping-**)

COMMENT: once a month, ova (unfertilized eggs) leave the ovaries and move down the Fallopian tubes to the uterus; at the point where the Fallopian tubes join the uterus an ovum may be fertilized by a sperm cell. Sometimes fertilization and development of the embryo take place in the Fallopian tube itself

Fallot's tetralogy ['fæləts te'trælədʒi] *see* TETRALOGY, WATERSTON'S OPERATION

false [fɔːls] *adjective* not true or not real; **false pains** = pains which appear to be labour pains but are not; **false ribs** = ribs which are not attached to the breastbone; **false teeth** = dentures, artificial teeth, which fit in the mouth and take the place of teeth which have been extracted

falx (cerebri) ['fælks 'serəbri] *noun* fold of the dura mater between the two hemispheres of the cerebrum

familial [fə'miliəl] *adjective* referring to a family; **familial adenomatous polyposis (FAP)** = hereditary disorder where polyps develop in the small intestine; **familial disorder** = hereditary disorder which affects several members of the same family

family ['fæmli] *noun* group of people who are related to each other, especially mother, father and children; *John is the youngest in our family*; *they have a very big family - two sons and three daughters*; **family doctor** = general practitioner, especially one who looks after all the members of a family; **family planning** = using contraception to control the number of children in a family; **family planning clinic** = clinic which gives advice on contraception; **family therapy** = type of psychotherapy where members of the family of a person with a disorder meet a therapist to discuss the condition and help come to terms with it

Fanconi syndrome [fæn'kəuni 'sindrəum] *noun* kidney disorder where amino acids are present in the urine

fantasize ['fæntəsaiz] *verb* to imagine that things have happened

fantasy ['fæntəsi] *noun* series of imaginary events which a patient believes really took place

FAP = FAMILIAL ADENOMATOUS POLYPOSIS

farcy ['fɑːsi] *noun* form of glanders which affects the lymph nodes

farinaceous [færi'neiʃəs] *adjective* referring to flour, containing starch; **farinaceous foods** = foods (such as bread) which are made of flour and have a high starch content

farm [fɑːm] *noun* land used for growing crops and keeping animals; *he's going to work on the farm during the holidays*; *you can buy eggs and vegetables at the farm*

farmer ['fɑːmə] *noun* man who looks after or owns a farm; **farmer's lung** = type of asthma caused by an allergy to rotting hay

farsighted [fɑː'saitid] *adjective* US longsighted, able to see things which are far away but not those which are near

farsightedness [fɑː'saitidnəs] *noun* US longsightedness or hypermetropia or hypertropia, condition where the patient sees clearly objects which are a long way away but cannot see objects which are close (NOTE: the opposite is **shortsightedness** or **myopia**)

fascia ['feiʃə] *noun* fibrous tissue covering a muscle or an organ; **fascia lata** = wide sheet of tissue covering the thigh muscles (NOTE: the plural is **fasciae**)

fasciculation [fəsikju'leiʃn] *noun* small muscle movements which appear as trembling skin

fasciculus [fə'sikjuləs] *noun* bundle of nerve fibres (NOTE: plural is **fasciculi**)

Fasciolopsis [fæsiəu'lɒpsis] *noun* type of liver fluke, often found in the Far East, which is transmitted to humans through contaminated waterplants

fast [fɑːst] **1** *adjective* quick, not slow; *this is a very fast-acting drug* **2** *noun* going without food (either to lose weight or for religious reasons); *he went on a fast to lose some weight* **3** *verb* to go without food; *the patient should fast from midnight of the night before an operation*

fastigium [fæ'stidʒiəm] *noun* highest temperature during a bout of fever

fat [fæt] **1** *adjective* big and round in the body; *you ought to eat less - you're getting too fat*; *that fat man has a very thin wife*; *he's the fattest boy in the class* (NOTE: **fat - fatter - fattest**) **2** *noun* **(a)** white oily substance in the body, which stores energy and protects the body against cold; **body fat** = adipose tissue, tissue where the cells contain fat, which replaces the normal fibrous tissue when too much food is eaten; **brown fat** = animal fat which can easily be converted to energy, and is believed to offset the effects of ordinary white fat; **saturated fat** = fat which has the largest amount of hydrogen possible; **unsaturated fat** = fat which does not have a large amount of hydrogen, and so can be broken down more easily **(b)** type of food which supplies protein and Vitamins A and D, especially that part of meat which is white, solid substances (like lard or butter) produced from animals and used for cooking or liquid substances like oil; *if you don't like the fat on the meat, cut it off; fry the eggs in some fat* (NOTE: **fat** has no plural when it means the substance; the plural **fats** is used to mean different types of fat. For other terms referring to fats, see also **lipid** and words beginning with **steato-**)

COMMENT: fat is a necessary part of diet because of the vitamins and energy-giving calories which it contains. Fat in the diet comes from either animal fats or vegetable fats. Animal fats such as butter, fat meat or cream, are saturated fatty acids. It is believed that the intake of unsaturated and polyunsaturated fats (mainly vegetable fats and oils, and fish oil) in the diet, rather than animal fats, helps keep down the level of cholesterol in the blood and so lessens the risk of atherosclerosis. A low-fat diet does not always help to reduce weight

fatal ['feɪtl] *adjective* which causes or results in death; *he had a fatal accident*; *cases of bee stings are rarely fatal*

fatality [fə'tæləti] *noun* case of death; *there were three fatalities during the flooding*

fatally ['feɪtli] *adverb* in a way which causes death; *his heart was fatally weakened by the lung disease*

father ['fɑːðə] *noun* man who has a son or daughter; *ask your father if you can borrow his car*; *she is coming to tea with her father and mother*

fatigue [fə'tiːg] **1** *noun* very great tiredness; **muscle fatigue** *or* **muscular fatigue** = tiredness in the muscles after strenuous exercise; **chronic fatigue syndrome** = MYALGIC ENCEPHALOMYELITIS **2** *verb* to tire someone out; *he was fatigued by the hard work*

fat-soluble ['fæt'sɒljʊbl] *adjective* which can dissolve in fat; *Vitamin D is fat-soluble*

fatty ['fæti] *adjective* containing fat; **fatty acid** = acid (such as stearic acid) which is an important substance in the body; **essential fatty acid** = unsaturated fatty acid which is essential for growth but cannot be synthesized by the body and has to be obtained from the food supply; **fatty degeneration** = accumulation of fat in the cells of an organ (such as the liver or heart), making the organ less able to perform

fauces ['fɔːsiːz] *noun* opening between the tonsils at the back of the throat, leading to the pharynx

favism ['feɪvɪzm] *noun* type of inherited anaemia caused by an allergy to beans

favus ['feɪvəs] *noun* highly contagious type of ringworm caused by a fungus which attacks the scalp

FDA ['ef 'diː 'eɪ] *US* = FOOD AND DRUG ADMINISTRATION

Fe *chemical symbol for* iron

fear [fɪə] *noun* state where a person is afraid of something happening; *he has a morbid fear of flying or of spiders*

features ['fiːtʃəz] *noun* appearance of a person's face; *he has heavy features*

febricula [fe'brɪkjʊlə] *noun* low fever

febrifuge ['febrɪfjuːdʒ] *adjective & noun* (drug such as aspirin) which prevents or lowers a fever

febrile ['fiːbraɪl] *adjective* referring to a fever, caused by a fever; **febrile disease** = disease which is accompanied by fever

feces, fecal ['fiːsiːz *or* 'fiːkl] *US* = FAECES, FAECAL

feeble ['fiːbl] *adjective* very weak; *she is old and feeble*; *some of the patients in the geriatric ward are very feeble*

feebleminded ['fiːbl'maɪndɪd] *adjective* being less than normally intelligent

feeblemindedness ['fiːbl'maɪndɪdnəs] *noun* state of less than normal intelligence

feed [fiːd] *verb* to give food (to someone or an animal); *he has to be fed with a spoon*; *the baby has reached the stage when she can feed herself* (NOTE: **feeding - fed - has fed**)

feedback ['fiːdbæk] *noun* linking of the result of an action back to the action itself; **negative feedback** = situation where the result represses the process which caused it; **positive feedback** = situation where the result stimulates the process again

feeding ['fiːdɪŋ] *noun* action of giving someone something to eat; **feeding cup** = special cup with a spout, used for feeding patients who cannot feed themselves; *see also* BREAST FEEDING, BOTTLE FEEDING, INTRAVENOUS FEEDING

feel [fiːl] *verb* **(a)** to touch (usually with your finger); *feel how soft the cushion is*; *when the lights went out we had to feel our way to the door* **(b)** to give a sensation when touched; *the knife felt cold*; *the floor feels hard* **(c)** to have a sensation; *I felt the table move*; *did you feel the lift go down suddenly?*; *he felt ill after eating the fish*;

when she saw the report she felt better (**d**) to believe or to think; to have an opinion; *he feels it would be wrong to leave the children alone in the house*; *the police felt that the accident was the fault of the driver of the car*; *the doctor feels the patient is well enough to be moved out of intensive care* (NOTE: **feeling - felt - felt**)

feeling ['fiːlɪŋ] *noun* sensation, something which you feel; *I had a feeling that someone was watching me*; *she had an itchy feeling inside her stomach*

Fehling's solution ['feɪlɪŋz səˈluːʃn] *noun* solution used to detect sugar in urine

felon ['felən] = WHITLOW

Felty's syndrome ['feltiːz 'sɪndrəʊm] *noun* condition where the spleen is enlarged, and the number of white blood cells increases, associated with rheumatoid arthritis

female ['fiːmeɪl] *adjective & noun* (animal or plant) of the same sex as a woman or girl; animal which produces ova and bears young; *a female cat*; *a condition found more often in females aged 40 - 60*

feminization [femənaɪˈzeɪʃn] *noun* development of female characteristics in a male

femoral ['femərl] *adjective* referring to the femur or to the thigh; **femoral artery =** continuation of the external iliac artery, which runs down the front of the thigh and then crosses to the back; **femoral canal =** inner tube of the sheath surrounding the femoral artery and vein; **femoral head =** head of the femur, the rounded projecting end part of the thigh bone which joins the acetabulum at the hip; **femoral neck =** neck of the femur, the narrow part between the head and the diaphysis of the femur; **femoral hernia =** hernia of the bowel at the top of the thigh; **femoral nerve =** nerve which governs the muscle at the front of the thigh; **femoral triangle** *or* **Scarpa's triangle =** slight hollow at the side of the thigh; **femoral vein =** vein running up the upper leg, a continuation of the popliteal vein

femoris ['femərɪs] *noun see* BICEPS, RECTUS

femur ['fiːmə] *noun* thighbone, the bone in the top part of the leg which joins the acetabulum at the hip and the tibia at the knee; *see illustration at* PELVIS (NOTE: plural is **femora**)

-fen [fen] *suffix* used in names of non-steroidal anti-inflammatory drugs; *ibuprofen*

fenestra [fəˈnestrə] *noun* small opening in the ear; **fenestra ovalis** *or* **fenestra vestibuli** = oval opening between the middle ear and the inner ear, closed by a membrane and covered by the stapes (NOTE: also called the **oval window**) ; **fenestra rotunda** *or* **fenestra cochleae** = round opening between the middle ear and the cochlea, and closed by a membrane (NOTE: also called the **round window**)

fenestration [fenəˈstreɪʃn] *noun* surgical operation to relieve deafness by making a small opening in the inner ear

fennel ['fenl] *noun* herb which tastes of aniseed and is used to treat flatulence

fermentation [fɜːmenˈteɪʃn] *noun* zymosis, process where carbohydrates are broken down by enzymes from yeast and produce alcohol

fertile ['fɜːtaɪl *US* 'fɜːtl] *adjective* able to bear fruit or to produce children

fertility [fəˈtɪləti] *noun* being fertile; **fertility rate** = number of births per year, per thousand females aged between 15 and 44

fertilization [fɜːtəlaɪˈzeɪʃn] *noun* joining of an ovum and a sperm to form a zygote and so start the development of an embryo

fertilize ['fɜːtəlaɪz] *verb*; *(of a sperm)* to join with an ovum (NOTE: the opposites are **sterile, sterility, sterilize**)

fester ['festə] *verb*; *(of an infected wound)* to become inflamed and produce pus; *his legs were covered with festering sores*

festination [festɪˈneɪʃn] *noun* way of walking where the patient takes short steps, seen in patients suffering from Parkinson's disease

fetal *or* **foetal** ['fiːtl] *adjective* referring to a fetus; *a sample of fetal blood was examined*; *fetal movements can be felt quite early in the pregnancy*; **fetal alcohol syndrome** = damage caused to the fetus by alcohol in the blood of the mother, including growth of the embryo, its facial development, etc.; women are recommended not to drink alcohol during pregnancy; **fetal heart** = the heart of the fetus; **fetal position** = position where a person lies curled up on his side, like a fetus in the uterus

fetalis ['fiːtɑːlɪs] *see* ERYTHROBLASTOSIS

fetishism or **fetichism** ['fetɪʃɪzm] noun psychological disorder where the patient gets sexual satisfaction from touching objects

fetishist or **fetichist** ['fetɪʃɪst] noun person suffering from fetishism

fetoprotein [fiːtəʊ'prəʊtiːn] see ALPHA

fetor or **foetor** ['fiːtə] noun bad smell

fetoscope ['fiːtəskəʊp] noun US stethoscope used in fetoscopy

fetoscopy [fɪ'tɒskəpi] noun examination of a fetus inside the uterus, taking blood samples to diagnose blood disorders

fetus or **foetus** ['fiːtəs] noun unborn baby in the uterus (NOTE: **fetus** is used to refer to unborn babies from two months after conception until birth. Before then, the baby is an **embryo**)

fever ['fiːvə] noun pyrexia (i) rise in the body temperature; (ii) sickness when the temperature of the body is higher than normal; *she is running a slight fever*; *you must stay in bed until the fever has gone down*; **intermittent fever** = fever which rises and falls regularly, as in malaria; **relapsing fever** = disease caused by a bacterium, where attacks of fever recur from time to time; **remittent fever** = fever which goes down for a period each day, as in typhoid fever; **fever sore** or **fever blister** = cold sore or burning sore, usually on the lips

COMMENT: normal oral body temperature is about 98.6ºF or 37ºC and rectal temperature is about 99ºF or 37.2ºC. A fever often makes the patient feel cold, and is accompanied by pains in the joints. Most fevers are caused by infections; infections which result in fever include cat scratch fever, dengue, malaria, meningitis, psittacosis, Q fever, rheumatic fever, Rocky mountain spotted fever, scarlet fever, septicaemia, typhoid fever, typhus, and yellow fever

feverfew ['fiːvəfjuː] noun herb, formerly used to reduce fevers, but now used to relieve migraine

feverish ['fiːvrɪʃ] adjective with a fever; *he felt feverish and took an aspirin*; *she is in bed with a feverish chill*

fibr- ['faɪbr] prefix referring to fibres, fibrous

-fibrate ['faɪbreɪt] suffix used in names of lipid-lowering drugs; *bezafibrate*

fibre US **fiber** ['faɪbə] noun **(a)** structure in the body shaped like a thread; **collagen fibre** = fibre which is the main component of fasciae, tendons and ligaments and is essential in bones and cartilage; **elastic fibres** or **yellow fibres** = fibres which can expand easily and are found in elastic cartilage, the skin and the walls of arteries and the lungs; **nerve fibre** = thread-like structure (axon or dendron) leading from a nerve cell and carrying nerve impulses **(b) optical fibres** = artificial fibres which carry light or images **(c) dietary fibre** = fibrous matter in food, which cannot be digested; **high fibre diet** = diet which contains a high percentage of cereals, nuts, fruit and vegetables

COMMENT: dietary fibre is found in cereals, nuts, fruit and some green vegetables. There are two types of fibre in food: insoluble fibre (in bread and cereals) which is not digested and soluble fibre (in vegetables and pulses). Foods with the highest proportion of fibre are bread, beans and dried apricots. Fibre is thought to be necessary to help digestion and avoid developing constipation, obesity and appendicitis

fibre optics or **fibreoptics** ['faɪbər 'ɒptɪks] noun examining internal organs using thin fibres which conduct light and images

fibrescope ['faɪbəskəʊp] noun device made of bundles of optical fibres which is passed into the body, used for examining internal organs

fibril ['faɪbrɪl] noun very small fibre

fibrillating ['faɪbrɪleɪtɪŋ or 'fɪbrɪleɪtɪŋ] adjective with a fluttering of a muscle; *they applied a defibrillator to correct a fibrillating heart beat*

fibrillation [faɪbrɪ'leɪʃn or fɪbrɪ'leɪʃn] noun fluttering of a muscle; **atrial fibrillation** = rapid uncoordinated fluttering of the atria of the heart, causing an irregular heartbeat; **ventricular fibrillation** = serious heart condition where the ventricular muscles flutter and the heart no longer beats to pump blood

Cardiovascular effects may include atrial arrhythmias but at 30°C there is the possibility of spontaneous ventricular fibrillation

British Journal of Nursing

fibrin ['faɪbrɪn] noun protein produced by fibrinogen, which helps make blood coagulate; **fibrin foam** = white material made artificially from fibrinogen, used to prevent bleeding

COMMENT: removal of fibrin from a blood sample is called defibrination

fibrinogen [faɪˈbrɪnədʒn] *noun* substance in blood plasma which produces fibrin when activated by thrombin

fibrinolysin [faɪbrɪˈnɒləsɪn] *noun* plasmin, an enzyme which digests fibrin

fibrinolysis [faɪbrɪˈnɒləsɪs] *noun* removal of blood clots from the system by the action of plasmin on fibrin

fibro- [ˈfaɪbrəu] *prefix* referring to fibres

fibroadenoma [faɪbrəuædɪˈnəumə] *noun* benign tumour formed of fibrous and glandular tissue

fibroblast [ˈfaɪbrəublæst] *noun* long flat cell found in connective tissue, which develops into collagen

fibrocartilage [faɪbrəuˈkɑːtəlɪdʒ] *noun* cartilage and fibrous tissue combined

COMMENT: fibrocartilage is found in the discs of the spine. It is elastic like cartilage and pliable like fibre

fibrochondritis [faɪbrəukɒnˈdraɪtɪs] *noun* inflammation of the fibrocartilage

fibrocyst [ˈfaɪbrəusɪst] *noun* benign tumour of fibrous tissue

fibrocystic [faɪbrəuˈsɪstɪk] *adjective* referring to a fibrocyst; **fibrocystic disease (of the pancreas)** = cystic fibrosis, hereditary disease in which there is malfunction of the exocrine glands such as the pancreas, and in particular those which secrete mucus

fibrocyte [ˈfaɪbrəusaɪt] *noun* cell which derives from a fibroblast and is found in connective tissue

fibroelastosis [faɪbrəuiːlæˈstəusɪs] *noun* deformed growth of the elastic fibres, especially in the ventricles of the heart

fibroid [ˈfaɪbrɔɪd] *adjective & noun* like fibre; **fibroid degeneration** = changing of normal tissue into fibrous tissue (as in cirrhosis of the liver); **a fibroid** *or* **fibroid tumour** *or* **fibromyoma** *or* **uterine fibroma** = benign tumour in the muscle fibres of the uterus

fibroma [faɪˈbrəumə] *noun* small benign tumour formed in connective tissue

fibromuscular [faɪbrəuˈmʌskjulə] *adjective* referring to fibrous tissue and muscular tissue

fibromyoma [faɪbrəumaɪˈəumə] *noun* benign tumour in the muscle fibres of the uterus

fibroplasia [faɪbrəuˈpleɪzɪə] *see* RETROLENTAL

fibrosa [faɪˈbrəusə] *see* OSTEITIS

fibrosarcoma [faɪbrəusɑːˈkəumə] *noun* malignant tumour of the connective tissue, common in the legs

fibrosis [faɪˈbrəusɪs] *noun* replacing damaged tissue by scar tissue; **cystic fibrosis** = FIBROCYSTIC DISEASE

fibrositis [faɪbrəˈsaɪtɪs] *noun* painful inflammation of the fibrous tissue which surrounds muscles and joints, especially the muscles of the back

fibrous [ˈfaɪbrəs] *adjective* made of fibres, like fibre; **fibrous capsule** = fibrous tissue surrounding a kidney; **fibrous joint** = joint where fibrous tissue holds two bones together so that they cannot move (as in the bones of the skull); **fibrous pericardium** = outer part of the pericardium which surrounds the heart, and is attached to the main blood vessels; **fibrous tissue** = tissue made of collagen fibres; *muscles are attached to bones by bands of strong fibrous tissue called tendons*

COMMENT: fibrous tissue is the strong white tissue which makes tendons and ligaments; also forms scar tissue

fibula [ˈfɪbjulə] *noun* long thin bone running between the ankle and the knee, the other thicker bone in the lower leg is the tibia (NOTE: plural is **fibulae**)

fibular [ˈfɪbjulə] *adjective* referring to the fibula

field [fiːld] *noun* (a) area of interest; *he specializes in the field of community medicine; don't see that specialist with your breathing problems - his field is obstetrics* (b) **field of vision** = area which can be seen without moving the eye

fil- [fɪl] *prefix* like a thread

filament [ˈfɪləmənt] *noun* long thin structure like a thread

filamentous [fɪləˈmentəs] *adjective* like a thread

Filaria [fɪˈleərɪə] *noun* thin parasitic worm which is found especially in the lymph system, and is passed to humans by mosquitoes (NOTE: plural is **Filariae**)

COMMENT: infestation with Filariae in the lymph system causes elephantiasis

filariasis [filəˈraɪəsɪs] *noun* tropical disease caused by parasitic threadworms in the lymph system, transmitted by mosquito bites

filiform [ˈfilifɔːm] *adjective* shaped like a thread; **filiform papillae** = papillae on the tongue which are shaped like threads, and have no taste buds; *see illustration at* TONGUE

filipuncture [ˈfilipʌntʃə] *noun* putting a wire into an aneurysm to cause blood clotting

fill [fil] *verb* (a) to make something full; *she was filling the bottle with water* (b) **to fill a tooth** = to put metal, amalgam,etc., into a hole in a tooth after it has been drilled

filling [ˈfiliŋ] *noun* (i) surgical operation carried out by a dentist to fill a hole in a tooth with amalgam; (ii) amalgam, metallic mixture put into a hole in a tooth by a dentist; *I had to have two fillings when I went to the dentist's*

film [film] *noun* (a) roll of material which is put into a camera for taking photographs; *I must buy a film before I go on holiday*; *do you want a colour film or a black and white one?* (b) very thin layer of a substance, especially on the surface of a liquid; *a film of oil on the surface of water*

filter [ˈfiltə] **1** *noun* piece of paper or cloth through which a liquid is passed to remove solid substances in it **2** *verb* to pass a liquid through a membrane, piece of paper or cloth to remove solid substances; *impurities are filtered from the blood by the kidneys*

filtrate [ˈfiltreɪt] *noun* substance which has passed through a filter

filtration [filˈtreɪʃn] *noun* passing a liquid through a filter

filum [ˈfaɪləm] *noun* structure which is shaped like a thread; **filum terminale** = thin end section of the pia mater in the spinal cord

fimbria [ˈfimbriə] *noun* fringe, especially the fringe of hair-like processes at the end of a Fallopian tube near the ovaries (NOTE: plural is **fimbriae**)

final [ˈfaɪnl] *adjective* last; *this is your final injection*; **final common pathway** = lower motor neurones, linked neurones which take all motor impulses from the spinal cord to a muscle

fine [faɪn] *adjective* (a) healthy; *he was ill last week, but he's feeling fine now* (b) (hair, thread, etc.) which is very thin; *there is a growth of fine hair on the back of her neck*; *fine sutures are used for delicate operations*

finger [ˈfiŋgə] *noun* one of the five parts at the end of the hand, but usually not including the thumb; *he touched the switch with his finger*; **finger-nose test** = test of coordination, where the patients is asked to close his eyes, stretch out his arm and then touch his nose with his index finger (NOTE: the names of the fingers are **little finger, third finger** or **ring finger, middle finger, forefinger** or **index finger** (and the **thumb**))

COMMENT: each finger is formed of three finger bones (the phalanges), but the thumb has only two

fingernail [ˈfiŋgəneɪl] *noun* hard thin growth covering the end of a finger; *she painted her fingernails red*

fingerprint [ˈfiŋgəprɪnt] *noun* mark left by a finger when you touch something; *the police found fingerprints near the broken window*; *see also* GENETIC

fingerprinting [ˈfiŋgəprɪntɪŋ] *noun; see* GENETIC

fingerstall [ˈfiŋgəstɔːl] *noun* cover for an infected finger, attached to the hand with strings

fireman's lift [ˈfaɪəmənz ˈlift] *noun* way of carrying an injured person by putting him over one's shoulder

firm [fɜːm] *noun (informal)* group of doctors and consultants in a hospital (especially one to which a trainee doctor is attached during clinical studies)

first [fɜːst] *adjective* coming before everything else; **first-degree relative** = relative with whom an individual shares 50% of their genes (father, mother, sibling, child); **first-ever stroke** = stroke which a patient has for the first time in his life; **first intention** = healing of a clean wound where the tissue forms again rapidly and no prominent scar is left

cerebral infarction (embolic or thrombolic) accounts for about 80% of first-ever strokes
British Journal of Hospital Medicine

first aid [ˈfɜːst ˈeɪd] *noun* help given by an ordinary person to someone who is suddenly ill or hurt, given until full-scale medical treatment can be given; *she ran to the man* who had been knocked down and gave him first aid until the ambulance arrived; **first-aid kit** = box with bandages and dressings kept ready to be used in an emergency; **first-aid post** *or* **station** = special place where injured people can be taken for immediate attention

first-aider ['fɜːstˈeɪdə] *noun* person who gives first aid to someone who is suddenly ill or injured

fish [fɪʃ] *noun* cold-blooded animal which swims in water, eaten for food; *they live on a diet of fish and rice* (NOTE: no plural when referring to the food: **you should eat some fish every week**)

> COMMENT: fish are high in protein, phosphorus, iodine and vitamins A and D. White fish has very little fat. Certain constituents of fish oil are thought to help prevent the accumulation of cholesterol on artery walls

fissile ['fɪsaɪl] *adjective* which can split or can be split

fission ['fɪʃn] *noun* splitting (as of the cells of bacteria)

fissure ['fɪʃə] *noun* crack or groove in the skin, tissue or an organ; **anal fissure** *or* **rectal fissure** *or* **fissure in ano** = crack in the mucous membrane wall of the anal canal; **horizontal and oblique fissures** = grooves between the lobes of the lungs; *see illustration at* LUNGS; **lateral fissure** = groove along the side of each cerebral hemisphere; **longitudinal fissure** = groove separating the two cerebral hemispheres

fist [fɪst] *noun* hand which is tightly closed; *the baby held the spoon in its fist; he hit the nurse with his fist*

fistula ['fɪstjʊlə] *noun* passage or opening which has been made abnormally between two organs, often near the rectum or anus; **anal fistula** *or* **fistula in ano** = fistula which develops between the rectum and the outside of the body after an abscess near the anus; **biliary fistula** = opening which discharges bile on to the surface of the skin from the gall bladder, bile duct or liver; **vesicovaginal fistula** = abnormal opening between the bladder and the vagina

fit [fɪt] **1** *adjective* strong and physically healthy; *the manager is not a fit man; you'll have to get fit before the football match; she exercises every day to keep fit; the doctors decided the patient was not fit for surgery; he isn't fit enough to work* = he is still too ill to work (NOTE: **fit - fitter - fittest**) **2** *noun*

sudden attack of a disorder, especially convulsions and epilepsy; *she had a fit of coughing; he had an epileptic fit; the baby had a series of fits* **3** *verb* **(a)** to be the right size or shape; *he's grown so tall that his trousers don't fit him any more; these shoes don't fit me - they're too tight* **(b)** to attach an appliance correctly; *the surgeons fitted the artificial hand to the patient's arm* or *fitted the patient with an artificial hand* (NOTE: you fit someone **with** an appliance) **(c)** to have convulsions; *the patient has fitted twice*

fitness ['fɪtnəs] *noun* being healthy; *he had to pass a fitness test to join the police force; being in the football team demands a high level of physical fitness*

fix [fɪks] *verb* **(a)** (i) to fasten or to attach; (ii) to treat a specimen on a slide for study through a microscope; *the slide is fixed with an alcohol solution*; **fixed oils** = liquid fats, especially those used as food **(b)** to arrange; *the meeting has been fixed for next week*

fixated [fɪkˈseɪtɪd] *adjective* (person) with a fixation on a parent

fixation [fɪkˈseɪʃn] *noun* **(a)** psychological disorder where a person does not develop beyond a certain stage; **mother-fixation** = condition where a person's development has been stopped at a stage where he remains like a child, dependent on his mother **(b)** way of preserving a specimen on a slide for study through a microscope **(c)** **surgical fixation** = method of immobilizing something, such as a bone, either externally by the use of a splint or internally by a metal plate and screws

fixative ['fɪksətɪv] *noun* chemical used in the preparation of samples on slides

flab [flæb] *noun; (informal)* soft fat flesh; *he's doing exercises to try to fight the flab*

flabby ['flæbi] *adjective* with soft flesh; *she has got flabby from sitting at her desk all day*

flaccid ['flæksɪd or 'flæsɪd] *adjective* soft or flabby

flagellate ['flædʒəlɪt] *noun* type of parasitic protozoan which uses whip-like hairs to swim (such as Leishmania)

flagellum [fləˈdʒeləm] *noun* tiny growth on a microorganism, shaped like a whip (NOTE: the plural is **flagella**)

flail chest ['fleɪl 'tʃest] *noun* condition where the chest is not stable, because several ribs have been broken

flake [fleɪk] **1** *noun* thin piece of tissue; *dandruff is formed of flakes of dead skin on the scalp*; **flake fracture** = fracture where thin pieces of bone come off **2** *verb* **to flake off** = to fall off as flakes

flap [flæp] *noun* flat piece, especially a piece of skin or tissue still attached to the body at one side and used in grafts

flare [fleə] *noun* red colouring of the skin at an infected spot or in urticaria

flat [flæt] *adjective & adverb* level, not curved; *spread the paper out flat on the table*; **flat foot** *or* **flat feet** = pes planus, condition where the soles of the feet lie flat on the ground instead of being arched as normal

flatulence [ˈflætjʊləns] *noun* gas or air which collects in the stomach or intestines causing discomfort

flatulent [ˈflætjʊlənt] *adjective* caused by flatulence

COMMENT: flatulence is generally caused by indigestion, but can be made worse if the patient swallows air (aerophagy)

flatus [ˈfleɪtəs] *noun* air and gas which collects in the intestines and is painful

flatworm [ˈflætwɜːm] *noun* any of several types of parasitic worm with a flat body (such as a tapeworm)

flea [fliː] *noun* tiny insect which sucks blood and is a parasite on animals and humans

COMMENT: fleas can transmit disease, most especially bubonic plague which is transmitted by infected rat fleas

flesh [fleʃ] *noun* tissue containing blood, forming the part of the body which is not skin, bone or organs; **flesh wound** = wound which only affects the fleshy part of the body; *she had a flesh wound in her leg*

fleshy [ˈfleʃi] *adjective* **(a)** made of flesh **(b)** fat

flex [fleks] *verb* to bend; **to flex a joint** = to use a muscle to make a joint bend

flexibilitas cerea [fleksɪˈbɪlɪtəs ˈsɪəriə] *noun* condition where if a patient's arms or legs are moved, they remain in that set position for some time

flexible [ˈfleksəbl] *adjective* which bends easily

flexion [ˈflekʃn] *noun* bending of a joint; **plantar flexion** = bending of the toes downwards

Flexner's bacillus [ˈfleksnəz bəˈsɪləs] *noun* bacterium which causes bacillary dysentery

flexor [ˈfleksə] *noun* muscle which makes a joint bend; *compare* EXTENSOR

flexure [ˈflekʃə] *noun* bend in an organ; fold in the skin; **hepatic flexure** = bend in the colon, where the ascending and transverse colons join; **splenic flexure** = bend in the colon where the transverse colon joins the descending colon

float [fləʊt] *verb* to lie on top of a liquid, not to sink; *the unborn baby floats in amniotic fluid*; **floating kidney** = NEPHROPTOSIS; **floating ribs** = the two lowest ribs on each side, which are not attached to the breastbone

floaters [ˈfləʊtəz] *noun* cellular or blood debris present in the vitreous of the eye, common in old age but if a sudden event can be a symptom of retinal haemorrhage (NOTE: formally called **muscae volitantes**)

floccitation [flɒksɪˈteɪʃn] = CARPHOLOGY

flooding [ˈflʌdɪŋ] *noun* menorrhagia, very heavy bleeding during menstruation

floppy baby syndrome [ˈflɒpi ˈbeɪbi ˈsɪndrəʊm] = AMYOTONIA CONGENITA

flora [ˈflɔːrə] *noun* bacteria which exist in a certain part of the body; *intestinal flora*

floss [flɒs] **1** *noun* **dental floss** = soft thread which can be pulled between the teeth to help keep them clean **2** *verb* to clean the teeth with floss

flow [fləʊ] **1** *noun* **(a)** movement of liquid or gas; *they used a tourniquet to try to stop the flow of blood* **(b)** amount of liquid or gas which is moving; *the meter measures the flow of water through the pipe* **2** *verb (of liquid)* to move past; *the water flowed down the pipe*; *blood was flowing from the wound*

flowmeter [ˈfləʊmiːtə] *noun* meter attached to a pipe (as in anaesthetic equipment) to measure the speed at which a liquid or gas moves in the pipe

flu [fluː] *noun* influenza, common viral illness like a bad cold, but with a fever; *he's in bed with flu*; *she caught flu and had to stay at home*; *there is a lot of flu about this winter*; **Asian flu** = type of flu which originated in Asia; **gastric flu** = general term for any mild stomach disorder; **twenty-four hour flu** = type of flu which lasts for a short period (NOTE: sometimes written ʼflu to show it is a short form of **influenza**)

fluctuation [flʌktʃuˈeɪʃn] *noun* feeling of movement of liquid inside part of the body or inside a cyst when pressed by the fingers

fluid [ˈfluːɪd] *noun* liquid substance; **amniotic fluid** = fluid in the amnion in which an unborn baby floats; **cerebrospinal fluid (CSF)** = fluid which surrounds the brain and the spinal cord; **pleural fluid** = fluid which forms between the layers of pleura in pleurisy

fluke [fluːk] *noun* parasitic flatworm which settles inside the liver (liver flukes), in the blood stream (Schistosoma), and other parts of the body

fluorescence [flɔːˈresəns] *noun* sending out of light from a substance which is receiving radiation

fluorescent [flɔːˈresənt] *adjective* (substance) which sends out light

fluoridate [fluːərɪˈdeɪt] *verb* to add fluoride to a substance, usually to drinking water, in order to help prevent tooth decay

fluoridation [fluːərɪˈdeɪʃn] *noun* adding fluoride to a substance, usually to drinking water, in order to help prevent tooth decay

fluoride [ˈfluəraɪd] *noun* chemical compound of fluorine and sodium, potassium or tin; *fluoride toothpaste*

COMMENT: fluoride will reduce decay in teeth and is often added to drinking water or to toothpaste. Some people object to fluoridation and it is thought that too high a concentration (such as that achieved by highly fluoridated water and the use of a highly fluoridated toothpaste) may damage the teeth of children

fluorine [ˈfluəriːn] *noun* chemical element found in bones and teeth (NOTE: chemical symbol is F)

fluoroscope [ˈfluərəskəup] *noun* apparatus which projects an X-ray image of a part of the body on to a screen, so that the part of the body can be examined as it moves

fluoroscopy [flɔːˈrɒskəpi] *noun* examination of the body using X-rays projected onto a screen

fluorosis [flɔːˈrəusɪs] *noun* condition caused by excessive fluoride in drinking water

COMMENT: at a low level, fluorosis causes discoloration of the teeth, and as the level of fluoride rises, ligaments can become calcified

flush [flʌʃ] **1** *noun* red colour in the skin; **hot flush** = condition in menopausal women, where the patient becomes hot, and sweats, often accompanied by redness of the skin **2** *verb* **(a)** to wash a wound with liquid **(b)** *(of person)* to turn red

flushed [flʌʃt] *adjective* with red skin (due to heat, emotion or overeating); *his face was flushed and he was breathing heavily*

flutter *or* **fluttering** [ˈflʌtə *or* ˈflʌtərɪŋ] *noun* rapid movement, especially of the atria of the heart, which is not controlled by impulses from the SA node

flux [flʌks] *noun* excessive production of liquid from the body

fly [flaɪ] *noun* small insect with two wings, often living in houses; *flies can walk on the ceiling*; *flies can carry infection onto food*

focal [ˈfəukl] *adjective* referring to a focus; **focal distance** *or* **focal length** = distance between the lens of the eye and the point behind the lens where light is focused; **focal epilepsy** = form of epilepsy arising from a localized area of the brain; **focal myopathy** = destruction of muscle tissue caused by the substance injected in an intramuscular injection

focus [ˈfəukəs] **1** *noun* **(a)** point where light rays converge through a lens **(b)** centre of an infection (NOTE: plural is **foci** [ˈfəusaɪ]) **2** *verb* to change the lens of an eye so that you see clearly at different distances; *he has difficulty in focusing on the object* **3** *adjective* **focus group** = discussion group of lay people brought together under professional guidance to discuss issues such as care

foetor [ˈfiːtə] = FETOR

foetus, foetal [ˈfiːtəs *or* ˈfiːtl] = FETUS, FETAL

folacin [ˈfəuləsɪn] = FOLIC ACID

fold [fəuld] **1** *noun* part of the body which is bent so that it lies on top of another part; **circular fold** = large transverse fold of mucous membrane in the small intestine; **vestibular folds** = folds in the larynx above the vocal folds, which are not used for speech (sometimes called 'false vocal cords'); **vocal folds** = VOCAL CORDS *see* CORD **2** *verb* to bend something so that part of it is on top of the rest; *he folded the letter and put it in an envelope*; **to fold your arms** = to rest one arm on the other across your chest

folic acid ['fəʊlɪk or 'fɒlɪk 'æsɪd] *noun* vitamin in the Vitamin B complex found in milk, liver, yeast and green vegetables like spinach, which is essential for creating new blood cells

COMMENT: lack of folic acid can cause anaemia and neural tube defects in the developing foetus; it can also be caused by alcoholism

folie à deux ['fɒlɪ æ 'dɜː] *noun* rare condition where a psychological disorder is communicated between two people who live together

follicle ['fɒlɪkl] *noun* tiny hole or sac in the body; **atretic follicle** = scarred remains of an ovarian follicle; **Graafian follicle** *or* **ovarian follicle** = cell which contains the ovum; **hair follicle** = tiny hole in the skin with a gland from which a hair grows

COMMENT: an ovarian follicle goes through several stages in its development. The first stage is called a primordial follicle, which then develops into a primary follicle and becomes a mature follicle by the sixth day of the period. This follicle secretes oestrogen until the ovum has developed to the point when it can break out, leaving the corpus luteum behind

follicle-stimulating hormone (FSH) ['fɒlɪkl'stɪmjʊleɪtɪŋ 'hɔːməʊn] *noun* hormone produced by the pituitary gland which stimulates ova in the ovaries and sperm in the testes

follicular *or* **folliculate** [fə'lɪkjʊlə or fə'lɪkjʊlət] *adjective* referring to follicles; **follicular tumour** = tumour in a follicle

folliculin [fə'lɪkjʊlɪn] *noun* oestrone, a type of oestrogen; *she is undergoing folliculin treatment*

folliculitis [fəlɪkju'laɪtɪs] *noun* inflammation of the hair follicles, especially where hair has been shaved

follow (up) ['fɒləʊ 'ʌp] *verb* to check on a patient who has been examined before in order to assess the progress of the disease or the results of treatment

follow-up ['fɒləʊʌp] *noun* check on a patient who has been examined before

length of follow-ups varied from three to 108 months. Thirteen patients were followed for less than one

year, but the remainder were seen regularly for periods from one to nine years
New Zealand Medical Journal

fomentation [fəʊmen'teɪʃn] = POULTICE

fomites ['fəʊmɪtiːz] *plural noun* objects (such as bedclothes) touched by a patient with a communicable disease which can therefore pass on the disease to others

fontanelle *US* **fontanel** [fɒntə'nel] *noun* soft cartilage between the bony sections of a baby's skull; **anterior fontanelle** = cartilage at the top of the head where the frontal bone joins the two parietals; **posterior fontanelle** = cartilage at the back of the head where the parietal bones join the occipital; *see also* BREGMA

COMMENT: the fontanelles gradually harden over a period of months and by the age of 18 months the bones of the baby's skull are usually solid

food [fuːd] *noun* things which are eaten; *this restaurant is famous for its food*; *do you like Chinese food?*; *this food tastes funny*; **health food** = food with no additives, food consisting of natural cereals, dried fruit and nuts; **food allergies** = allergies which are caused by food (the commonest are oranges, eggs, tomatoes, strawberries); **food canal** = alimentary canal, the passage from the mouth to the rectum through which food passes and is digested; **food poisoning** = illness caused by eating food which is contaminated with bacteria; *the hospital had to deal with six cases of food poisoning*; *all the people at the party went down with food poisoning* (NOTE: **food** is usually used in the singular, but can sometimes be used in the plural)

Food and Drug Administration (FDA) ['fuːd ən drʌg ədmɪnɪs'treɪʃn] *noun* US government agency responsible for the safety of food as well as medicines

foot [fʊt] *noun* end part of the leg on which a person stands; *he has got big feet*; *you stepped on my foot*; **athlete's foot** = infectious skin disorder between the toes, caused by a fungus; **drop foot** *or* **foot drop** = being unable to keep the foot at right angles to the leg; **flat foot** *or* **feet** = *see* FLAT; **Madura foot** = *see* MADUROMYCOSIS; **trench foot** *or* **immersion foot** = condition, caused by exposure to cold and damp, where the skin of the foot becomes red and blistered and in severe cases turns black when gangrene sets in. (The condition was common among soldiers serving in the trenches during the First World War) (NOTE: the plural is **feet**)

COMMENT: the foot is formed of 26 bones: 14 phalanges in the toes, five metatarsals in the main part of the foot and seven tarsals in the heel

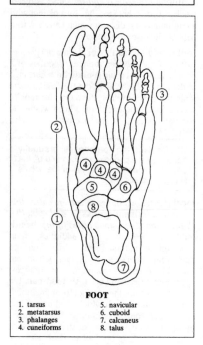

FOOT

1. tarsus   5. navicular
2. metatarsus   6. cuboid
3. phalanges   7. calcaneus
4. cuneiforms   8. talus

footpump ['fʊtpʌmp] *noun* device to reduce the risk of post-operative deep vein thrombosis by mechanical use of leg muscles

foramen [fə'reɪmən] *noun* natural opening inside the body, such as the opening in a bone through which veins or nerves pass; **foramen magnum** = the hole at the bottom of the skull where the brain is joined to the spinal cord; **intervertebral foramen** = space between two vertebrae; **vertebral foramen** = hole in the centre of a vertebra which links with others to form the vertebral canal through which the spinal cord passes; **foramen ovale** = opening between the two parts of the heart in a fetus (NOTE: plural is **foramina**)

COMMENT: the foramen ovale normally closes at birth, but if it stays open the blood from the veins can mix with the blood going to the arteries, causing cyanosis (blue baby disease)

forbid [fə'bɪd] *verb* to tell someone not to do something; *smoking is forbidden in the cinema*; *the health committee has forbidden any contact with the press*; *she has been forbidden all starchy food*; *the doctor forbade him to go back to work* (NOTE: **forbidding - forbade - has forbidden**)

force [fɔːs] **1** *noun* strength; *the tree was blown down by the force of the wind* **2** *verb* to make someone do something; *they forced him to lie down on the floor*; *she was forced to do whatever they wanted*

forceps ['fɔːseps] *noun* surgical instrument like a pair of scissors, made in different sizes and with differently shaped ends, used for holding and pulling; **obstetrical forceps** = type of large forceps used to hold a baby's head during childbirth; **forceps delivery** = birth of a baby done with the help of forceps

fore- [fɔː] *prefix* in front

forearm ['fɔːrɑːm] *noun* lower part of the arm from the elbow to the wrist; **forearm bones** = the ulna and the radius

forebrain ['fɔːbreɪn] *noun* cerebrum, the front part of the brain in an embryo

forefinger ['fɔːfɪŋgə] *noun* first finger on the hand, next to the thumb

foregut ['fɔːgʌt] *noun* front part of the gut in an embryo

forehead ['fɔːhed or 'fɒrɪd] *noun* part of the face above the eyes

foreign ['fɒrən] *adjective* not belonging to your own country; *he speaks several foreign languages*; **foreign body** = piece of material which is not part of the surrounding tissue and should not be there (such as sand in a cut, dust in the eye, a pin which has been swallowed); *the X-ray showed the presence of a foreign body*; **swallowed foreign bodies** = anything (a pin, coin or button) which should not have been swallowed

foreigner ['fɒrənə] *noun* person who comes from another country

forensic medicine [fə'rensɪk 'medsɪn] *noun* medical science concerned with finding solutions to crimes against people (such as autopsies on murdered people or taking blood samples from clothes)

foreskin ['fɔːskɪn] *noun* prepuce, skin covering the top of the penis, which can be removed by circumcision

forewaters ['fɔːwɔːtəz] *noun* fluid which comes out of the vagina at the beginning of childbirth when the amnion bursts

forget [fə'get] *verb* not to remember to do something, not to remember a piece of information; *old people start to forget names*; *she forgot to take the tablets*; *he forgot his appointment with the specialist* (NOTE: forgetting - forgot - has forgotten)

forgetful [fə'getful] *adjective* (person) who often forgets things; *she became very forgetful, and had to be looked after by her sister*

forgetfulness [fə'getflnəs] *noun* condition where someone often forgets things; *increasing forgetfulness is a sign of old age*

form [fɔːm] **1** *noun* **(a)** shape; *she has a ring in the form of the letter A* **(b)** paper with blank spaces which you have to write in; *you have to fill in a form when you are admitted to hospital* **(c)** state or condition; *our team was in good form and won easily*; **he's in good form today** = he is very amusing, is doing things well; **off form** = not very well, slightly ill **2** *verb* to make or to be the main part of; *calcium is one the elements which forms bones or bones are mainly formed of calcium*; *an ulcer formed in his duodenum*; *in diphtheria a membrane forms across the larynx*

formaldehyde [fɔː'mældɪhaɪd] *noun* strong antiseptic derived from formic acid

formalin ['fɔːməlɪn] *noun* solution of formaldehyde in water used to preserve specimens

formation [fɔː'meɪʃn] *noun* action of forming something; *drinking milk helps the formation of bones*

formication [fɔːmɪ'keɪʃn] *noun* itching feeling where the skin feels as if it were covered with insects

formula ['fɔːmjʊlə] *noun* **(a)** way of indicating a chemical compound using letters and numbers (such as H_2SO_4 **(b)** instructions on how to prepare a drug **(c)** *US* powdered milk for babies (NOTE: plural is **formulae** ['fɔːmjʊliː])

formulary ['fɔːmjʊləri] *noun* book containing formulae for making drugs

fornix ['fɔːnɪks] *noun* arch; **fornix cerebri** = section of white matter in the brain between the hippocampus and the hypothalamus; *see illustration at* BRAIN; **fornix of the vagina** = space between the cervix of the uterus and the vagina (NOTE: plural is **fornices**)

fortification figures [fɔːtɪfɪ'keɪʃn 'fɪgəz] *noun* patterns of coloured light, seen as part of the aura before a migraine attack occurs

fossa ['fɒsə] *noun* shallow hollow in a bone or the skin; **cubital fossa** = depression in the front of the elbow joint; **glenoid fossa** = socket in the shoulder joint into which the humerus fits; **iliac fossa** = depression on the inner side of the hip bone; **pituitary fossa** = hollow in the upper surface of the sphenoid bone in which the pituitary gland sits; **temporal fossa** = depression in the side of the head, in the temporal bone above the zygomatic arch (NOTE: plural is **fossae**)

Fothergill's operation ['fɒðəgɪlz ɒpə'reɪʃn] *noun* surgical operation to correct prolapse of the uterus

fourchette [fʊə'ʃet] *noun* fold of skin at the back of the vulva

fovea (centralis) ['fəʊvɪə sen'trɑːlɪs] *noun* depression in the retina which is the point where the eye sees most clearly; *see illustration at* EYE

FP10 ['ef'piː 'ten] *noun* NHS prescription from a GP

fracture ['fræktʃə] **1** *verb* **(a)** to break a bone; *he fractured his wrist* **(b)** *(of bone)* to break; *the tibia fractured in two places* **2** *noun* break in a bone; *facial fracture or nasal fracture or skull fracture*; *rib fracture or fracture of a rib*; *breastbone fracture or fracture of the breastbone*; **simple** *or* **closed fracture** = fracture where the skin surface around the damaged bone has not been broken and the broken ends of the bone are close together; **Bennett's fracture** = *see* BENNETT'S; **Colles' fracture** = fracture of the lower end of the radius with displacement of the wrist backwards, usually when someone has stretched out his hand to try to break a fall; **comminuted fracture** = fracture where the bone is broken in several places; **complicated fracture** = fracture with an associated injury of tissue, as where the bone has punctured an artery; **compound fracture** *or* **open fracture** = fracture where the skin surface is damaged or where the broken bone penetrates the surface of the skin; **crush fracture** = fracture by compression of the bone; **extracapsular fracture** = fracture of the upper part of the femur, but which does not involve the capsule round the hip joint; **fatigue fracture** = *see* STRESS FRACTURE; **greenstick fracture** = fracture occurring in children, where a long bone bends but does not break completely;

impacted fracture = fracture where the broken parts of the bones are pushed into each other; **march fracture** = a type of fatigue fracture, the fracture of one of the metatarsal bones in the foot, caused by too much exercise; **multiple fracture** = condition where a bone is broken in several places; **oblique fracture** = fracture where the bone is broken diagonally; **pathological fracture** = fracture of a diseased bone; **Pott's fracture** = fracture of the end of the fibula together with the end of the malleolus; **stellate fracture** = fracture of the kneecap shaped like a star; **stress fracture** or **fatigue fracture** = fracture of a bone caused by excessive force, as in certain types of sport; **transverse fracture** = fracture where the bone is broken straight across; *see also* AVULSION, DEPRESSED, FLAKE

fractured ['fræktʃəd] *adjective* broken (bone); *he had a fractured skull; she went to hospital to have her fractured leg reset*

fragile ['frædʒaɪl] *adjective* easily broken; *old people's bones are more fragile than those of adolescents*; **fragile-X syndrome** = hereditary condition where part of an X chromosome is defective, causing mental defects

fragilitas [frə'dʒɪlɪtəs] *noun* being fragile or brittle; **fragilitas ossium** = hereditary condition where the bones are brittle and break easily (NOTE: also called **osteogenesis imperfecta**)

frail [freɪl] *adjective* weak, easily broken; *grandfather is getting frail, and we have to look after him all the time; the baby's bones are still very frail*

framboesia [fræm'biːziə] = YAWS

frame [freɪm] *noun* (a) main part of a building, ship or bicycle, etc., which holds it together; *the bicycle has a very light frame; I've broken the frame of my glasses* (b) solid support; **walking frame** or **Zimmer frame** = metal frame used by patients who have difficulty in walking

framework ['freɪmwɜːk] *noun* main bones which make up the structure of part of the body

fraternal twins [frə'tɜːnl 'twɪnz] *noun* dizygotic twins, twins who are not identical (and not always of the same sex) because they come from two different ova fertilized at the same time; *compare* IDENTICAL, MONOZYGOTIC

freckled ['frekəld] *adjective* with brown spots on the skin

freckles ['frekəlz] *plural noun* brown spots on the skin, often found in people with fair hair

freeze [friːz] *verb* (a) to be so cold that water turns to ice; *it is freezing outside; they say it will freeze tomorrow*; **I'm freezing** = I'm very cold (b) to make something very cold, to become very cold; *the surgeon froze the tissue with dry ice* (NOTE: **freezing - froze - has frozen**)

freeze dry ['friːz 'draɪ] *verb* to freeze rapidly then dry in a vacuum

freeze drying ['friːz 'draɪɪŋ] *noun* method of preserving food or tissue specimens by freezing rapidly and drying in a vacuum

Freiberg's disease ['fraɪbɜːgz dɪ'ziːz] *noun* osteochondritis of the head of the second metatarsus

Frei test ['fraɪ 'test] *noun* test for the venereal disease lymphogranuloma inguinale

fremitus ['fremɪtəs] *noun* trembling or vibrating (of part of a patient's body, felt by the doctor's hand or heard through a stethoscope); **friction fremitus** = scratching felt when the hand is placed on the chest of a patient suffering from pericarditis; **vocal fremitus** = vibration of the chest when a person speaks or coughs

French letter ['frentʃ 'letə] *noun; (informal)* = CONDOM

Frenkel's exercises ['frenkəlz 'eksəsaɪzɪz] *plural noun* exercises for patients suffering from locomotor ataxia, to teach coordination of the muscles and limbs

frenulum or **frenum** ['frenjʊləm or 'friːnəm] *noun* fold of mucous membrane (under the tongue or by the clitoris)

frequency ['friːkwənsi] *noun* (a) the number of times something takes place in a given time; *the frequency of micturition* (b) rate of vibration in oscillations

fresh [freʃ] *adjective* (a) not used, not dirty; *I'll get some fresh towels; she put some fresh sheets on the bed*; **fresh air** = open air; *they came out of the mine into the fresh air* (b) recently made; *fresh bread*; **fresh frozen plasma** = plasma made from freshly donated blood, and kept frozen (c) not tinned or frozen; *fresh fish; fresh fruit salad; fresh vegetables are expensive in winter*

fretful ['fretfʊl] *adjective* (baby) which cries, cannot sleep or seems unhappy

friar's balsam ['fraɪəz 'bɒlsəm] *noun* mixture of various plant oils, including benzoin and balsam, which can be inhaled as a vapour to relieve bronchitis or congestion

friction ['frɪkʃn] *noun* rubbing together of two surfaces; **friction fremitus** = scratching felt when the hand is placed on the chest of a patient suffering from pericarditis; **friction murmur** = scratching sound around the heart, heard with a stethoscope in patients suffering from pericarditis

Friedländer's bacillus ['friːdlendəz bəˈsɪləs] *noun* bacterium *Klebsiella pneumoniae* which can cause pneumonia

Friedman's test ['friːdmənz 'test] *noun* test for pregnancy

Friedreich's ataxia ['friːdraɪks əˈtæksiə] *noun* inherited nervous disease which affects the spinal cord (ataxia is associated with club foot, and makes the patient walk unsteadily and speak with difficulty)

frighten ['fraɪtn] *verb* to make someone afraid; *the noise frightened me*; *she watched a frightening film about insects which eat people*

frightened ['fraɪtnd] *adjective* afraid; *I'm frightened of spiders*; *don't leave the patient alone - she's frightened of the dark*

frigid ['frɪdʒɪd] *adjective* (woman) who cannot experience orgasm or sexual pleasure

frigidity [frɪˈdʒɪdəti] *noun* being unable to experience orgasm, sexual pleasure or who does not feel sexual desire

fringe medicine ['frɪnʒ 'medsɪn] *noun* types of medicine which are not part of normal treatment taught in medical schools (such as homeopathy, acupuncture, etc.)

frog [frɒg] *noun* small animal with no tail, which lives in water or on land and can jump; **frog plaster** = plaster cast made to keep the legs in a correct position after an operation to correct a dislocated hip

Fröhlich's syndrome ['frɜːlɪks 'sɪndrəum] *noun* dystrophia adiposogenitalis, condition where the patient becomes obese and the genital system does not develop, caused by an adenoma of the pituitary gland

front [frʌnt] *noun* part of something which faces forwards; *the front of the hospital faces south*; *he has a rash on the front of his leg*; *the Adam's apple is visible in the front of the neck*

frontal ['frʌntl] *adjective* referring to the forehead or to the front of the head; **frontal bone** = bone which the front of the upper part of the skull that forms the forehead; *see illustration at* SKULL; **frontal lobe** = front lobe of each cerebral hemisphere; **frontal lobotomy** = surgical operation on the brain to treat mental illness by removing part of the frontal lobe; **frontal sinus** = one of two sinuses in the front of the face above the eyes and near the nose (NOTE: the opposite is **occipital**)

frost [frɒst] *noun* freezing weather when the temperature is below the freezing point of water. (It may lead to a deposit of crystals of ice on surfaces); *there was a frost last night*

frostbite ['frɒstbaɪt] *noun* injury caused by very severe cold which freezes tissue

frostbitten ['frɒstbɪtn] *adjective* suffering from frostbite

COMMENT: in very cold conditions, the outside tissue of the fingers, toes, ears and nose can freeze, becoming white and numb. Thawing of frostbitten tissue can be very painful and must be done very slowly. Severe cases of frostbite may require amputation because the tissue has died and gangrene has set in

frozen shoulder ['frəuzn 'ʃəuldə] *noun* stiffness and pain in the shoulder, caused by inflammation of the membranes of the shoulder joint after injury or after the shoulder has been immobile for a time, when deposits may be forming in the tendons

fructose ['frʌktəuz] *noun* fruit sugar found in honey and some fruit, which together with glucose forms sucrose

fructosuria [frʌktəʊˈsjuəriə] *noun* presence of fructose in the urine

fruit [fruːt] *noun* usually sweet part of a plant which contains the seeds, and is eaten as food; *a diet of fresh fruit and vegetables* (NOTE: no plural when referring to the food: **you should eat a lot of fruit**)

COMMENT: fruit contains fructose and is a good source of vitamin C and some dietary fibre. Dried fruit have a higher sugar content but less vitamin C than fresh fruit

FSH ['ef 'es 'eɪtʃ] = FOLLICLE-STIMULATING HORMONE

fugax ['fjuːgæks] *see* AMAUROSIS

-fuge [fjuːdʒ] *suffix* which drives away; **vermifuge** = substance which removes worms

fugue [fjuːg] *noun* condition where the patient loses his memory and leaves home

fulguration [fʌlgəˈreɪʃn] *noun* electrodesiccation, removal of a growth (such as a wart) by burning with an electric needle

full [ful] *adjective* complete, with no empty space; *the hospital cannot take in any more patients - all the wards are full*; *my appointments book is full for the next two weeks*

full-scale [ˈfulˈskeɪl] *adjective* complete, going into all details; *the doctors put him through a full-scale medical examination*; *the local health authority has ordered a full-scale inquiry into the case*

full term [ˈful ˈtɜːm] *noun* complete pregnancy of forty weeks; *she has had several pregnancies but none has reached full term*

fully [ˈfuli] *adverb* completely; *the fetus was not fully developed*; *is the muscle fully relaxed?*

fulminant *or* **fulminating** [ˈfulmɪnənt or ˈfulmɪneɪtɪŋ] *adjective* (dangerous disease) which develops very rapidly

the major manifestations of pneumococcal infection in sickle-cell disease are septicaemia, meningitis and pneumonia. The illness is frequently fulminant

The Lancet

fumes [fjuːmz] *plural noun* gas or smoke; **toxic fumes** = poisonous gases or smoke given off by a substance or a machine

fumigate [ˈfjuːmɪgeɪt] *verb* to kill microbes or insects by using gas

fumigation [fjuːmɪˈgeɪʃn] *noun* killing microbes or insects by gas

function [ˈfʌŋkʃn] **1** *noun* particular work done by an organ; *what is the function of the pancreas?*; *the function of an ovary is to form ova* **2** *verb* to work in a particular way; *the heart and lungs were functioning normally*; *his kidneys suddenly stopped functioning*

insulin's primary metabolic function is to transport glucose into muscle and fat cells, so that it can be used for energy

Nursing '87

the AIDS virus attacks a person's immune system and damages the ability to fight other disease. Without a functioning immune system to ward off other germs, the patient becomes vulnerable to becoming infected

Journal of American Medical Association

functional [ˈfʌŋʃənl] *adjective* (disorder or illness) which does not have a physical cause and may have a psychological cause, as opposed to an organic disorder; **functional enuresis** = bedwetting which has a psychological cause

fund [fʌnd] **1** *noun* sum of money set aside for a special purpose **2** *verb* to pay for; **how will the new health centre be funded?** = who will provide the money to pay for it?

fundus [ˈfʌndəs] *noun* (i) bottom of a hollow organ (such as the uterus); (ii) top section of the stomach (above the body of the stomach); *see illustration at* STOMACH; **optic fundus** = back part of the inside of the eye, opposite the lens

fungal [ˈfʌŋgl] *adjective* referring to fungi; *he had a case of fungal skin infection*

fungicide [ˈfʌŋgɪsaɪd] *adjective & noun* (substance) used to kill fungi

fungiform papillae [ˈfʌŋgɪfɔːm pəˈpɪli] *noun* rounded papillae on the tip and sides of the tongue, which have taste buds; *see illustration at* TONGUE

fungoid [ˈfʌŋgɔɪd] *adjective* like a fungus

fungus [ˈfʌŋgəs] *noun* simple plant organism with thread-like cells (such as yeast, mushrooms, mould), and without green chlorophyll; **fungus disease** = disease caused by a fungus; **fungus poisoning** = poisoning by eating a poisonous fungus (NOTE: plural is **fungi**. For other terms referring to fungi, see words beginning with **myc-**)

COMMENT: some fungi can become parasites of man, and cause diseases such as thrush. Other fungi, such as yeast, react with sugar to form alcohol. Some antibiotics (such as penicillin) are derived from fungi

funiculitis [fjunɪkjuˈlaɪtɪs] *noun* inflammation of the spermatic cord

funiculus [fjuˈnɪkjuləs] *noun* one of the three parts (lateral, anterior and posterior funiculus) of the white matter in the spinal cord

funis [ˈfjuːnɪs] *noun* umbilical cord

funnel chest [ˈfʌnl ˈtʃest] *noun* pectus excavatum, congenital deformity, where the chest is depressed in the centre because the lower part of the breastbone is curved backwards

funny [ˈfʌni] *adjective (informal)* unwell; *she felt funny after she had eaten the fish*; **he had a funny turn** = he had a dizzy spell; **funny bone** = part of the elbow where the ulnar nerve passes by the internal condyle of the humerus, which gives a painful tingling sensation when hit by accident

fur [fɜː] *verb (of the tongue)* to feel as if covered with soft hair

COMMENT: the tongue is furred when a patient is feeling unwell, and the papillae on the tongue become covered with a whitish coating

furfuraceous [fɜːfjəˈreɪʃəs] *adjective* scaly (skin)

Furley stretcher [ˈfɜːli ˈstretʃə] *see* STRETCHER

furor [ˈfjʊərɔː] *noun* attack of wild violence (especially when mentally deranged)

furuncle [ˈfjʊərʌŋkl] *noun* boil, a tender raised mass of infected tissue and skin, usually caused by infection of a hair follicle by the bacterium *Staphylococcus aureus*

furunculosis [fjʊərʌŋkjəˈləʊsɪs] *noun* condition where several boils appear at the same time

fuse [fjuːz] *verb* to join together to form a single structure; *the bones of the joint fused*

fusiform [ˈfjuːzɪfɔːm] *adjective* (muscles, etc.) shaped like a spindle, with a wider middle section which becomes narrower at each end

fusion [ˈfjuːʒn] *noun* joining, especially a surgical operation to join the bones at a joint permanently so that they cannot move and so relieve pain in the joint; **spinal fusion** = surgical operation to join two vertebrae together to make the spine more rigid

Gg

g [dʒiː] = GRAM

GABA ['gæbə] = GAMMA AMINOBUTYRIC ACID

gag [gæg] **1** *noun* instrument placed between a patient's teeth to stop him closing his mouth **2** *verb* to choke, to try to vomit but be unable to do so; *he gagged on his food*; *every time the doctor tries to examine her throat, she gags*; *he started gagging on the endotracheal tube*

gain [geɪn] **1** *noun* act of adding or increasing; *the baby showed a gain in weight of 25g or showed a weight gain of 25g* **2** *verb* to add or to increase; *to gain in weight or to gain weight*

gait [geɪt] *noun* way of walking; **ataxic gait** = way of walking where the patient walks unsteadily due to a disorder of the nervous system; **cerebellar gait** = way of walking where the patient staggers along, caused by a disease of the cerebellum; **spastic gait** = way of walking where the legs are stiff and the feet not lifted off the ground; *see also* FESTINATION

galact- [gə'lækt] *prefix* referring to milk

galactagogue [gə'læktəgɒg] *noun* substance which stimulates the production of milk

galactocele [gə'læktəsiːl] *noun* breast tumour which contains milk

galactorrhoea [gəlæktə'rɪə] *noun* excessive production of milk

galactosaemia [gəlæktə'siːmiə] *noun* congenital defect where the liver is incapable of converting galactose into glucose, with the result that a baby's development may be affected

COMMENT: the treatment is to remove galactose from the diet

galactose [gə'læktəʊz] *noun* sugar which forms part of milk, and is converted into glucose by the liver

galea ['geɪliə] *noun* **(a)** any part of the body shaped like a helmet, especially the loose band of tissue in the scalp **(b)** type of bandage wrapped round the head

gall [gɔːl] *noun* bile, thick bitter yellowish-brown fluid secreted by the liver and stored in the gall bladder or passed into the stomach, used to digest fatty substances and to neutralize acids

gall bladder ['gɔːl 'blædə] *noun* sac situated underneath the liver, in which bile produced by the liver is stored; *see illustration at* DIGESTIVE SYSTEM

COMMENT: bile is stored in the gall bladder until required by the stomach. If fatty food is present in the stomach, bile moves from the gall bladder along the bile duct to the stomach. Since the liver also secretes bile directly into the duodenum, the gall bladder is not an essential organ and can be removed by surgery

Gallie's operation ['gæliz ɒpə'reɪʃn] *noun* surgical operation where tissues from the patient's thigh are used to hold a hernia in place

gallipot ['gælipɒt] *noun* little pot for ointment

gallon ['gælən] *noun* measurement of liquids which equals eight pints or 4.5 litres; *the bucket can hold four gallons*; *the body contains about two gallons of blood*

gallop rhythm ['gæləp 'rɪðm] *noun* rhythm of heart sounds, three to each cycle, when a patient is experiencing tachycardia

gallstone ['gɔːlstəʊn] *noun* calculus, small stone formed from insoluble deposits from bile in the gall bladder

COMMENT: gallstones can be harmless, but some cause pain and inflammation and a serious condition can develop if a gallstone blocks the bile duct. Sudden pain going from the right side of the stomach towards the back indicates that a gallstone is passing through the bile duct

galvanism ['gælvənɪzm] *noun* treatment using low voltage electricity

galvanocautery [gælvnə'kɔːtəri] *noun* electrocautery, removal of diseased tissue using an electrically heated needle or loop of wire

gamete ['gæmiːt] *noun* sex cell, either a spermatozoon or an ovum

gametocide [gə'miːtəʊsaɪd] *noun* drug which kills gametocytes

gametocyte [gə'miːtəʊsaɪt] *noun* cell which is developing into a gamete

gametogenesis [gəmiːtəʊ'dʒenəsɪs] *noun* process by which a gamete is formed

gamgee tissue ['gæmdʒiː 'tɪʃuː] *noun* surgical dressing, formed of a layer of cotton wool between two pieces of gauze

gamma ['gæmə] *noun* third letter of the Greek alphabet

gamma aminobutyric acid (GABA)
['gæmə əmiːnəʊbjuː'tɪrɪk 'æsɪd] *noun* amino acid neurotransmitter

gamma camera ['gæmə 'kæmrə] *noun* camera for taking photographs of parts of the body into which radioactive isotopes have been introduced

gamma globulin [gæmə'glɒbjulɪn] *noun* protein found in plasma, forming antibodies as protection against infection

COMMENT: gamma globulin injections are sometimes useful as a rapid source of protection against a wide range of diseases

gamma rays ['gæmə 'reɪz] *noun* rays which are shorter than X-rays and are given off by radioactive substances

ganglion ['gæŋgliən] *noun* (a) mass of nerve cell bodies and synapses usually covered in connective tissue, found along the peripheral nerves with the exception of the basal ganglia; **basal ganglia** = masses of grey matter at the base of each cerebral hemisphere which receive impulses from the thalamus and influence the motor impulses from the frontal cortex; **ciliary ganglion** = parasympathetic ganglion in the orbit of the eye, supplying the intrinsic eye muscles;

coeliac ganglion = ganglion on each side of the origins of the diaphragm, connected with the coeliac plexus; **mesenteric ganglion** = plexus of sympathetic nerve fibres and ganglion cells around the superior mesenteric artery; **otic ganglion** = ganglion associated with the mandibular nerve where it leaves the skull; **pterygopalatine ganglion** *or* **sphenopalatine ganglion** = ganglion in the pterygopalatine fossa associated with the maxillary nerve (postganglionic fibres going to the nose, palate, pharynx and lacrimal glands); **spinal ganglion** = cone-shaped mass of cells on the posterior root, the main axons of which form the posterior root of the spinal nerve; **stellate ganglion** = group of nerve cells in the neck, shaped like a star; **submandibular ganglion** = ganglion associated with the lingual nerve, relaying impulses to the submandibular and sublingual salivary glands; **superior ganglion** = small collection of cells in the jugular foramen; **trigeminal ganglion** *or* **Gasserian ganglion** = sensory ganglion containing the cells of origin of the sensory fibres in the fifth cranial nerve; **vertebral ganglion** = ganglion in front of the origin of the vertebral artery **(b)** cyst of a tendon sheath or joint capsule (usually at the wrist) which results in a painless swelling containing fluid (NOTE: plural is **ganglia** ['gæŋgliə])

ganglionectomy [gæŋgliə'nektəmi] *noun* surgical removal of a ganglion

ganglionic [gæŋgli'ɒnɪk] *adjective* referring to a ganglion; *see also* POSTGANGLIONIC

gangrene ['gæŋgriːn] *noun* condition where tissues die and decay, as a result of bacterial action, because the blood supply has been lost through injury or disease of the artery; *after he had frostbite, gangrene set in and his toes had to be amputated*; **dry gangrene** = condition where the blood supply is cut off and the limb becomes black; **gas gangrene** = complication of severe wounds in which the bacterium *Clostridium welchii* breeds in the wound and then spreads to healthy tissue which is rapidly decomposed with the formation of gas; **hospital gangrene** = gangrene caused by insanitary hospital conditions; **moist gangrene** = condition where dead tissue decays and swells with fluid because of infection and the tissues have an unpleasant smell

gangrenous ['gæŋgrənəs] *adjective* referring to gangrene

Ganser state [ˈgænsə ˈsteɪt] = PSEUDODEMENTIA

gap [gæp] *noun* space; *there is a gap between his two front teeth*; *the muscle has passed through a gap in the mucosa*

gargle [ˈgɑːgl] **1** *noun* mildly antiseptic solution used to clean the mouth; *if diluted with water, the product makes a useful gargle* **2** *verb* to put some antiseptic liquid solution into the back of the mouth and throat and then breathe out air through it; *the doctor recommended gargling twice a day with a saline solution*

gargoylism [ˈgɑːgɔɪlɪzm] *noun* Hurler's syndrome, congenital defect of a patient's metabolism which causes polysaccharides and fat cells to accumulate in the body, resulting in mental defects, swollen liver and coarse features

gas [gæs] *noun* **(a)** (i) state of matter in which particles occupy the whole space in which they occur; (ii) substance often produced from coal or found underground, and used to cook or heat; *a gas cooker*; *we heat our house by gas*; **gas exchange** = process by which oxygen in air is exchanged in the lungs for waste carbon dioxide carried by the blood; **gas gangrene** = complication of severe wounds in which the bacterium *Clostridium welchii* breeds in the wound and then spreads to healthy tissue which is rapidly decomposed with the formation of gas; **gas poisoning** = poisoning by breathing in carbon monoxide or other toxic gas **(b)** gas which accumulates in the stomach or alimentary canal and causes pain; **gas pains** = flatus, excessive formation of gas in the stomach or intestine which is painful (NOTE: the plural **gases** is only used to mean different types of gas)

gash [gæʃ] **1** *noun* long cut, as made with a knife; *she had to have three stitches in the gash in her thigh* **2** *verb* to make a long cut; *she gashed her hand on the broken glass*

gasp [gɑːsp] **1** *noun* trying to breathe, breath taken with difficulty; *his breath came in short gasps* **2** *verb* to try to breathe taking quick breaths; *she was gasping for breath*

Gasserian ganglion [gæˈsɪərɪən ˈgæŋglɪən] *noun* trigeminal ganglion, sensory ganglion containing the cells of origin of the sensory fibres in the fifth cranial nerve

gastr(o)- [ˈgæstr or ˈgæstrəu] *prefix* referring to the stomach

gastralgia [gæˈstrældʒə] *noun* pain in the stomach

gastrectomy [gæˈstrektəmi] *noun* surgical removal of the stomach; **partial gastrectomy** = surgical removal of only the lower part of the stomach; **subtotal gastrectomy** = surgical removal of all but the top part of the stomach in contact with the diaphragm

gastric [ˈgæstrɪk] *adjective* referring to the stomach; **gastric acid** = hydrochloric acid secreted into the stomach by acid-forming cells; **gastric artery** = artery leading from the coeliac trunk to the stomach; **gastric flu** = general term for any mild stomach disorder; **gastric juices** = mixture of hydrochloric acid, pepsin, intrinsic factor and mucus secreted by the cells of the lining membrane of the stomach to help the digestion of food; *the walls of the stomach secrete gastric juices*; **gastric pit** = deep hollow in the mucous membrane forming the walls of the stomach; **gastric ulcer** = ulcer in the stomach; **gastric vein** = vein which follows the gastric artery

gastrin [ˈgæstrɪn] *noun* hormone which is released into the bloodstream from cells in the lower end of the stomach, stimulated by the presence of protein, and which in turn stimulates the flow of acid from the upper part of the stomach

gastritis [gæˈstraɪtɪs] *noun* inflammation of the stomach

gastrocele [ˈgæstrəusiːl] *noun* stomach hernia, a condition where part of the stomach wall becomes weak and bulges out

gastrocnemius [gæstrɒkˈniːmɪəs] *noun* large calf muscle

gastrocolic reflex [gæstrəuˈkɒlɪk ˈriːfleks] *noun* sudden peristalsis of the colon produced when food is taken into an empty stomach

gastroduodenal [gæstrəudjuːˈdiːnl] *adjective* referring to the stomach and duodenum; **gastroduodenal artery** = artery leading from the gastric artery towards the pancreas

gastroduodenostomy [gæstrəudjuːəudɪˈnɒstəmi] *noun* surgical operation to join the duodenum to the stomach so as to bypass a blockage in the pylorus

gastroenteritis [gæstrəuentəˈraɪtɪs] *noun* inflammation of the membrane lining the intestines and the stomach, caused by a viral infection and resulting in diarrhoea and vomiting

gastroenterologist
[gæstrəʊentə'rɒlədʒɪst] *noun* doctor who specializes in disorders of the stomach and intestine

gastroenterology [gæstrəʊentə'rɒlədʒi] *noun* study of the stomach, intestine and other parts of the digestive system and their disorders

gastroenterostomy
[gæstrəʊentə'rɒstəmi] *noun* surgical operation to join the small intestine directly to the stomach so as to bypass a peptic ulcer

gastroepiploic [gæstrəʊepɪ'plɔɪk] *adjective* referring to the stomach and greater omentum; **gastroepiploic artery** = artery linking the gastroduodenal artery to the splenic artery

gastroileac reflex [gæstrəʊ'ɪliæk 'riːfleks] *noun* automatic relaxing of the ileocaecal valve when food is present in the stomach

gastrointestinal (GI) [gæstrəʊɪn'testɪnl] *adjective* referring to the stomach and intestine; *he experienced some gastrointestinal (GI) bleeding*

gastrojejunostomy
[gæstrəʊdʒɪdʒu'nɒstəmi] *noun* surgical operation to join the jejunum to the stomach

gastrolith ['gæstrəʊlɪθ] *noun* stone in the stomach

gastro-oesophageal reflux
['gæstrəʊəsɒfə'dʒiəl 'riːflʌks] *noun* return of bitter-tasting, partly digested food from the stomach to the oesophagus when the patient has indigestion

gastropexy ['gæstrəʊpeksi] *noun* attaching the stomach to the wall of the abdomen

gastroplasty ['gæstrəʊplæsti] *noun* surgery to correct a deformed stomach

gastroptosis [gæstrəʊ'təʊsɪs] *noun* condition where the stomach hangs down

gastrorrhoea [gæstrə'rɪə] *noun* excessive flow of gastric juices

gastroscope ['gæstrəskəʊp] *noun* instrument formed of a tube or bundle of glass fibres with a lens attached, by which a doctor can examine the inside of the stomach (it is passed down into the stomach through the mouth)

gastroscopy [gæ'strɒskəpi] *noun* examination of the stomach using a gastroscope

gastrostomy [gæ'strɒstəmi] *noun* surgical operation to create an opening into the stomach from the wall of the abdomen, so that food can be introduced without passing through the mouth and throat

gastrotomy [gæ'strɒtəmi] *noun* surgical operation to open up the stomach

gastrula [gæ'struːlə] *noun* second stage of the development of an embryo

gather ['gæðə] *verb* **(a)** to bring together or to collect; *she was gathering material for the study of children suffering from rickets*; *pus had gathered round the wound*; *the lecturer gathered up his papers*; *a group of students gathered round the professor of surgery as he demonstrated the incision* **(b)** to understand; *did you gather who will be speaking at the ceremony?*

Gaucher's disease ['gəʊʃeɪz dɪ'ziːz] *noun* enzyme disease where fatty substances accumulate in the lymph glands, spleen and liver

COMMENT: symptoms are anaemia, a swollen spleen and darkening of the skin; the disease can be fatal in children

gauze [gɔːz] *noun* thin light material used to make dressings; *she put a gauze dressing on the wound*; *the dressing used was a light paraffin gauze*

gavage [gɑː'vɑːʒ] *noun* forced feeding of a patient who cannot eat or who refuses to eat

GC ['dʒiː 'siː] = GONORRHOEA

GDC ['dʒiː 'diː 'siː] = GENERAL DENTAL COUNCIL

Gehrig's disease ['geɪrɪgz dɪ'ziːz] = AMYOTROPHIC LATERAL SCLEROSIS

Geiger counter ['gaɪgə 'kaʊntə] *noun* instrument for detection and measurement of radiation

gel [dʒel] *noun* substance that has coagulated to form a jelly-like solid

gelatin ['dʒelətɪn] *noun* protein which is soluble in water, made from collagen

COMMENT: gelatin is used in foodstuffs (such as desserts or meat jellies) and is also used to make capsules in which to put medicine

gelatinous [dʒə'lætɪnəs] *adjective* like jelly

gemellus [dʒɪˈmeləs] *noun* twin or double; **gemellus superior muscle** *or* **gemellus inferior muscle** = two muscles arising from the ischium

gender [ˈdʒendə] *noun* sex of a person, being male or female; *she's just had a baby but I don't know what gender it is*; **gender reorientation** = the alteration of a person's sex through surgical and drug treatment

gene [dʒiːn] *noun* unit of DNA on a chromosome which governs the synthesis of one protein, usually an enzyme, and may combine with other genes to determine a particular characteristic; **allele gene** = one of two or more alternative forms of a gene, which can imitate each other's form: they are situated in the same area of a pair of chromosomes and produce different characteristics; **gene amplification** = a method for the repeated duplication of a specific length of DNA to produce an amount suitable for gene analysis, usually using the technique polymerase chain reaction (PCR) and used to test for genetic defects such as from a single cell from an embryo; **gene replacement therapy** = the treatment of disease caused by a genetic defect by manipulating the gene outside the body and replacing the repaired gene into the individual; **gene tracking** = the method used to trace the inheritance of a particular gene through a family, such as cystic fibrosis or Huntington's Chorea, in order to diagnose and predict genetic disorders; *see* GENETIC

COMMENT: genes are either dominant, where the characteristic is always passed on to the child, or recessive, where the characteristic only appears if both parents have contributed the same gene. Gene replacement therapy has been used successfully in animals, and is in the early stages of research in humans, but may be useful in the future treatment of cystic fibrosis, thalassaemia and other genetic disorders

general [ˈdʒenrəl] *adjective* not particular; which concerns everything or everybody; **general amnesia** = sudden and complete loss of memory, state where a person does not even remember who he is; **general anaesthesia** = loss of feeling and loss of sensation, after having been given an anaesthetic; **general anaesthetic** = substance given to make a patient lose consciousness so that a major surgical operation can be carried out; **general paralysis of the insane (GPI)** = old term for widespread damage of the nervous system, marking the final stages of untreated syphilis; **general practice** = doctor's practice where patients from a district are treated for all types of illness; *she qualified as a doctor and went into general practice*

General Dental Council (GDC) [ˈdʒenrəl ˈdentl ˈkaʊnsəl] official body which registers and supervises dentists in the UK

generalized [ˈdʒenrəlaɪzd] *adjective* occurring throughout the body; *the cancer became generalized* (NOTE: the opposite is localized)

generally [ˈdʒenrəli] *adverb* normally

General Medical Council (GMC) [ˈdʒenrəl ˈmedɪkl ˈkaʊnsəl] official body which registers and supervises doctors in the UK

General Optical Council (GOC) [ˈdʒenrəl ˈɒptɪkl ˈkaʊnsəl] official body which registers and supervises opticians in the UK

general practitioner (GP) [ˈdʒenrəl prækˈtɪʃənə] *noun* doctor who provides first-line medical care for a list of people who live in one community and treats all types of illness, refers patients to hospital and encourages health promotion (NOTE: plural is GPs)

COMMENT: a GP has a medical degree (MBChB) and then undergoes an additional three-year training in hospital and in general practice; he or she may hold additional specialist qualifications in areas such as obstetrics and family planning and care of the elderly

generation [dʒenəˈreɪʃn] *noun* all people born at about the same period

generic [dʒəˈnerɪk] *adjective* (i) referring to a genus; (ii) (name) given to a drug generally, as opposed to a proprietary name used by the manufacturer

genetic [dʒəˈnetɪk] *adjective* referring to the genes; **genetic code** = information which determines the characteristics for synthesis; **genetic disorder** = disorder or disease caused by a defective gene and often inherited; **genetic engineering** = techniques used to change the genetic composition of a cell so as to change certain characteristics which can be inherited; **genetic fingerprint** = the pattern of sequences of genetic material unique to an individual; **genetic fingerprinting** = method of revealing an individual's genetic fingerprint, used in paternity queries and criminal investigation; **genetic screening** = testing large numbers of people to see if anyone has a certain genetic disorder

geneticist [dʒə'netɪsɪst] *noun* person who specializes in the study of the way in which characteristics and diseases are inherited through the genes

genetics [dʒə'netɪks] *noun* study of genes, and of the way characteristics and diseases are inherited through the genes

-genic ['dʒenɪk] *suffix* produced by, which produces; **photogenic** = produced by light, which produces light

genicular [dʒe'nɪkjʊlə] *adjective* referring to the knee

genital ['dʒenɪtl] *adjective* referring to reproductive organs; **genital herpes** = venereal infection, caused by a herpesvirus, which forms blisters in the genital region and can have a serious effect on a fetus; **genital organs** *or* **genitals** = external organs for reproduction (penis and testicles in male, vulva in female)

genitalia [dʒenɪ'teɪliə] *noun* genital organs

genitourinary [dʒenɪtəʊ'jʊərɪnəri] *adjective* referring to both reproductive and urinary systems; **genitourinary system** = organs of reproduction and urination, including the kidneys

genome ['dʒiːnəʊm] *noun* (i) complete basic set of genes in each chromosome of a person; (ii) set of genes which are inherited from one parent

genomic imprinting ['dʒə'nɒmɪk ɪm'prɪntɪŋ] *noun* fixing of the complete set of genes from a parent in a person's chromosomes

genotype ['dʒenətaɪp] *noun* genetic composition of an organism; *compare* PHENOTYPE

gentian violet ['dʒenʃn 'vaɪələt] *noun* antiseptic blue dye used to paint on skin infections; dye used to stain specimens

gentle ['dʒentl] *adjective* soft; kind; *the doctor has gentle hands*; *you must be gentle when you are holding a little baby*; *use a gentle antiseptic on the rash* (NOTE: **gentle - gentler - gentlest**)

genu ['dʒə'nuː] *noun* the knee

genual ['dʒenjʊəl] *adjective* referring to the knee

genupectoral position [dʒenjuː'pektərl pə'zɪʃn] *noun* position of a patient when kneeling with the chest on the floor

genus ['dʒiːnəs] *noun* main group of related living organisms; *a genus is divided into different species* (NOTE: plural is **genera** ['dʒenərə])

genu valgum [dʒə'nuː 'vælgəm] *noun* knock knee, a state where the knees touch and the ankles are apart when a person is standing straight

genu varum ['dʒiːnjuː 'veərəm] *noun* bow legs, a state where the ankles touch and the knees are apart when a person is standing straight

geriatric [dʒeri'ætrɪk] *adjective* referring to old people; **geriatric unit** *or* **ward** *or* **hospital** = unit, ward or hospital which specializes in the treatment of old people

geriatrician [dʒeriə'trɪʃn] *noun* doctor who specializes in the treatment or study of diseases of old people

geriatrics [dʒeri'ætrɪks] *noun* study of the diseases and disorders of old people; *compare* PAEDIATRICS

germ [dʒɜːm] *noun* **(a)** microbe (such as a virus or bacterium) which causes a disease; *germs are not visible to the naked eye*; **germ free** = sterile, without any microbes present (NOTE: in this sense 'germ' is not a medical term) **(b)** part of an organism which develops into a new organism; **germ cell** = gonocyte, a cell which is capable of developing into a spermatozoon or ovum; **germ layers** = two or three layers of cell in animal embryos which form the organs of the body

German measles ['dʒɜːmən 'miːzlz] *noun* rubella, common infectious viral disease of children with mild fever, swollen lymph nodes and rash; *compare* MEASLES, RUBEOLA

COMMENT: German measles can cause stillbirth or malformation of an unborn baby if the mother catches the disease while pregnant. It is advisable that girls should catch the disease in childhood, or should be immunized against it

germicide ['dʒɜːmɪsaɪd] *adjective & noun* (substance) which can kill germs

germinal ['dʒɜːmɪnl] *adjective* (i) referring to a germ; (ii) referring to an embryo; **germinal epithelium** = outer layer of the ovary

gerontologist [dʒrən'tɒlədʒɪst] *noun* specialist in gerontology

gerontology [dʒerɒn'tɒlədʒi] *noun* study of the process of ageing and the diseases of old people

Gerstmann's syndrome ['gɜːstmænz 'sɪndrəʊm] *noun* condition where a patient no longer recognises his body image, cannot tell the difference between left and right, cannot recognise his different fingers and is unable to write

gestate [dʒe'steɪt] *verb* to carry a baby in the uterus from conception to birth

gestation [dʒe'steɪʃn] *noun* pregnancy, period (usually 266 days) from conception to birth, during which the baby develops in the mother's uterus

evaluation of fetal age and weight has proved to be of value in the clinical management of pregnancy, particularly in high-risk gestations

Southern Medical Journal

gestational diabetes [dʒe'steɪʃənl daɪə'biːtiːz] *noun* form of diabetes mellitus which develops in a pregnant woman

get [get] *verb* **(a)** to become; *the muscles get flabby from lack of exercise; she got fat from eating too much; waiting lists for operations are getting longer* **(b)** (i) to make something happen; (ii) to pay someone to do something; (iii) to persuade someone to do something; *he got the hospital to admit the patient as an emergency case; did you get the sister to fill in the form?; he got the doctor to repeat the prescription;* **to have got to** = must; *you have got to be at the surgery before 9.30; he is leaving early because he has got to drive a long way; has she got to take the tablets every day?* **(c)** to catch (a disease); *I think I'm getting a cold; she can't go to work because she's got flu*

get along ['get ə'lɒŋ] *verb* to manage, to work; *we seem to get along quite well without any electricity*

get around ['get ə'raʊnd] *verb* to move about; *since she had the accident she gets around on two sticks*

get better ['get 'betə] *verb* to become well again after being ill; *he was seriously ill, but seems to be getting better; her cold has got better; his flu has not got any better, so he will have to stay in bed*

get dressed ['get 'drest] *verb* to put your clothes on; *he got dressed quickly because he didn't want to be late for work; she was getting dressed when the phone rang; the patient has to be helped to get dressed*

get on ['get 'ɒn] *verb* **(a)** to go into (a bus, etc.); *we got on the bus at the post office; she got on her bike and rode away* **(b)** to become old; *he's getting on and is quite deaf*

get on with ['get 'ɒn wɪð] **(a)** to be friendly with someone; *he gets on very well with everyone; I didn't get on with the boss* **(b)** to continue to do some work; *I must get on with the blood tests*

get over ['get 'əʊvə] *verb* to become better after an illness or a shock; *he got over his cold; she never got over her mother's death*

get up ['get 'ʌp] *verb* to stand up; to get out of bed; *he got up from his chair and walked out of the room; at what time did you get up this morning?*

get well ['get 'wel] *verb* to become healthy again after being ill; *we hope your mother will get well soon;* **get well card** = card sent to a person who is ill, with good wishes for a rapid recovery

GH ['dʒiː 'eɪtʃ] = GROWTH HORMONE

Ghon's focus ['gɒnz 'fəʊkəs] *noun* spot on the lung produced by the tuberculosis bacillus

GI ['dʒiː'aɪ] = GASTROINTESTINAL; *they diagnosed a GI disease; operation on a GI fistula*

giant ['dʒaɪənt] *noun* very tall person; **giant cell** = very large cell such as an osteoclast or megakaryocyte; **giant hives** = large flat white blisters caused by an allergic reaction; *see also* ARTERITIS, GIGANTISM

Giardia [dʒiː'ɑːdiə] *noun* microscopic protozoan parasite in the intestine which causes giardiasis

giardiasis [dʒiː'ɑː'daɪəsɪs] *noun* lambliasis, disorder of the intestine caused by the parasite *Giardia lamblia,* usually with no symptoms, but in heavy infections the absorption of fat may be affected, causing diarrhoea

gibbosity *or* **gibbus** [gɪ'bɒsəti *or* 'gɪbəs] *noun* sharp angle in the curvature of the spine caused by the weakening of a vertebra by tuberculosis of the backbone

giddiness ['gɪdinəs] *noun* condition in which someone feels that everything is turning around, and so cannot stand up; *he* *began to suffer attacks of giddiness*; *see note at* LABYRINTH

giddy ['gɪdi] *adjective* feeling that everything is turning round; *she has had a giddy spell*

gigantism [dʒaɪ'gæntɪzm] *noun* condition in which the patient grows very tall, caused by excessive production of growth hormone by the pituitary gland

Gilliam's operation ['gɪliəmz ɒpə'reɪʃn] *noun* surgical operation to correct retroversion of the uterus

gingiva [dʒɪn'dʒaɪvə] *noun* gum, the soft tissue covering the part of the jaw which surrounds the teeth; *see illustration at* TOOTH

gingivalis [dʒɪndʒɪ'vælɪs] *see* ENTAMOEBA

gingivectomy [dʒɪndʒɪ'vektəmi] *noun* surgical removal of excess gum tissue

gingivitis [dʒɪndʒɪ'vaɪtɪs] *noun* inflammation of the gums as a result of bacterial infection; **ulcerative** *or* **ulceromembranous gingivitis** = ulceration of the gums which can also affect the membrane of the mouth

ginglymus ['dʒɪŋglɪməs] *noun* hinge joint, a joint (like the knee or elbow) which allows movement in two directions only

gippy tummy ['dʒɪpi 'tʌmi] *noun* (*informal*) diarrhoea which affects people travelling in foreign countries as a result of eating unwashed fruit or drinking water which has not been boiled

girdle ['gɜːdl] *noun* set of bones making a ring or arch; **hip girdle** *or* **pelvic girdle** = the sacrum and the two hip bones to which the thigh bones are attached; **pectoral girdle** *or* **shoulder girdle** = the shoulder bones (scapulae and clavicles) to which the upper arm bones are attached

Girdlestone's operation ['gɜːdəlstəunz ɒpə'reɪʃn] *noun* surgical operation to relieve osteoarthritis of the hip

girl [gɜːl] *noun* female child; *she's only got a little girl*; *they have three children - two boys and a girl*

give [gɪv] *verb* (**a**) to pass something to someone; *he was given a pain-killing injection*; *the surgeons have given him a new pacemaker* (**b**) to allow someone time; **the doctors have only given her two weeks**

to live = the doctors say she will die in two weeks' time (NOTE: **giving - gave - has given**)

give up ['gɪv 'ʌp] *verb* not to do something any more; *he was advised to give up smoking*; *she has given up eating chocolate*

glabella [glə'belə] *noun* flat area of bone in the forehead between the eyebrows

gladiolus [glædi'əuləs] *noun* middle section of the sternum

gland [glænd] *noun* (**a**) organ in the body containing cells which secrete substances which act elsewhere (such as a hormone, sweat or saliva); **endocrine gland** = gland without a duct which produces hormones which are introduced directly into the bloodstream (such as pituitary gland, thyroid gland, the pancreas, the adrenals, the gonads, the thymus); **exocrine gland** = gland with a duct down which its secretions pass to a particular part of the body (such as the liver, the sweat glands, the salivary glands); **adrenal glands** *or* **suprarenal glands** = two endocrine glands at the top of the kidneys which secrete cortisone, adrenaline and other hormones; *see illustration at* KIDNEY; **bulbourethral glands** *or* **Cowper's glands** = two glands at the base of the penis which secrete into the urethra; **ceruminous glands** = glands which secrete earwax; *see illustration at* EAR; **lacrimal gland** *or* **tear gland** = gland which secretes tears; **Lieberkühn's glands** = small glands between the bases of the villi in the small intestine; **mammary gland** = gland in female mammals which produces milk; **meibomian gland** = sebaceous gland on the edge of the eyelid which secretes the liquid which lubricates the eyelid; **parathyroid glands** = four glands in the neck near the thyroid gland, which secrete a hormone which regulates the level of calcium in blood plasma; **parotid gland** = one of the glands which produce saliva, situated in the neck behind the joint of the jaw; *see illustration at* THROAT; **pineal gland** = small cone-shaped gland near the midbrain, which produces melatonin and is believed to be associated with Circadian rhythms (NOTE: also called **pineal body**); *see illustration at* BRAIN; **pituitary gland** = hypophysis cerebri, the main endocrine gland, about the size of a pea, situated in the sphenoid bone below the hypothalamus, which secretes hormones which stimulate other glands; *see illustration at* BRAIN; **salivary gland** = gland which secretes saliva; **sebaceous gland** = gland which secretes oil at the base of each hair follicle; **sublingual**

gland = salivary gland under the tongue; *see illustration at* THROAT; **submandibular gland** = salivary gland in the lower jaw; *see illustration at* THROAT; **sweat gland** = gland which produces sweat, situated beneath the dermis and connected to the skin surface by a sweat duct; **thymus gland** = endocrine gland in the front of the top of the thorax, behind the breastbone; **thyroid gland** = endocrine gland in the neck, which secretes a hormone which regulates the body's metabolism; **greater vestibular glands** *or* **Bartholin's glands** = two glands at the side of the entrance to the vagina, which secrete a lubricating substance **(b) lymph** *or* **lymphatic glands** = glands situated in various points of the lymphatic system (especially under the armpits and in the groin) through which lymph passes

glanders ['glændəz] *noun* bacterial disease of horses, which can be caught by humans, with symptoms of high fever and inflammation of the lymph nodes; *see also* FARCY

glandular ['glændjʊlə] *adjective* referring to glands

glandular fever ['glændjʊlə 'fiːvə] *noun* infectious mononucleosis, an infectious disease where the body has an excessive number of white blood cells

COMMENT: the symptoms include sore throat, fever and swelling of the lymph glands in the neck. Glandular fever is probably caused by the Epstein-Barr virus. The test for glandular fever is the Paul-Bunnell reaction

glans *or* **glans penis** ['glænz 'piːnɪs] *noun* bulb at the end of the penis; *see illustration at* UROGENITAL SYSTEM (MALE)

glass [glɑːs] *noun* **(a)** material which you can see through, used to make windows; *the doors are made of glass*; *the specimen was kept in a glass jar* (NOTE: no plural **some glass, a piece of glass**) **(b)** thing to drink out of, usually made of glass; *she poured the mixture into a glass* **(c)** the contents of a glass; *he drinks a glass of milk every evening*; *you may drink a small glass of wine with your evening meal* (NOTE: plural is **glasses** for (b) and (c))

glasses [glɑːsɪz] *plural noun* two pieces of glass or plastic, made into lenses, which are worn in front of the eyes to help the patient see better; *she was wearing dark glasses*; *he has glasses with gold frames*; *she needs glasses to read*

glaucoma [glɔːˈkəumə] *noun* condition of the eyes, caused by abnormally high pressure of fluid inside the eyeball, resulting in disturbances of vision and blindness; **angle-closure glaucoma** *or* **acute glaucoma** = abnormally high pressure of fluid inside the eyeball caused by pressure of the iris against the lens, trapping the aqueous humour; **open-angle glaucoma** *or* **chronic glaucoma** = abnormally high pressure of fluid inside the eyeball caused by a blockage in the channel through which the aqueous humour drains

gleet [gliːt] *noun* thin discharge from the vagina, penis, a wound or an ulcer

glenohumeral [gliːnəʊˈhuːmərl] *adjective* referring to both the glenoid cavity and the humerus; **glenohumeral joint** = shoulder joint

glenoid cavity *or* **glenoid fossa** ['gliːnɔɪd 'kævəti *or* 'gliːnɔɪd 'fɒsə] *noun* socket in the shoulder joint into which the head of the humerus fits; *see illustration at* SHOULDER

glia *or* **glial tissue** ['gliːə *or* 'gliːəl 'tɪʃuː] *noun* neuroglia, connective tissue of the central nervous system, surrounding cell bodies, axons and dendrites

glial cells ['gliːəl 'selz] *noun* cells in the glia

glio- ['glaɪəʊ] *prefix* referring to brain tissue

glioblastoma [glaɪəʊblæˈstəumə] *noun* spongioblastoma, rapidly developing malignant brain tumour in the glial cells

glioma [glaɪˈəumə] *noun* any tumour of the glial tissue in the brain or spinal cord

gliomyoma [glaɪəumaɪˈəumə] *noun* tumour of both the nerve and muscle tissue

Glisson's capsule ['glɪsənz 'kæpsjuːl] *noun* tissue sheath in the liver containing the blood vessels

globin ['gləubɪn] *noun* protein which combines with other substances to form compounds such as haemoglobin and myoglobin

globule ['glɒbjuːl] *noun* round drop (of fat)

globulin ['glɒbjʊlɪn] *noun* class of protein, present in blood, including antibodies; **gamma globulin** = immunoglobulin, a protein found in plasma, and which forms antibodies as protection against infection

globulinuria [glɒbjʊlɪˈnjʊəriə] *noun* presence of globulins in the urine

globus ['gləubəs] *noun* any ball-shaped part of the body; **globus hystericus** = lump in the throat, feeling of not being able to swallow caused by worry or embarrassment

glomangioma [gləmændʒi'əumə] *noun* tumour of the skin at the ends of the fingers and toes

glomerular [gləu'merjulə] *adjective* referring to a glomerulus; **glomerular capsule** = Bowman's capsule, the expanded end of a renal tubule, surrounding a glomerular tuft; **glomerular tuft** = group of blood vessels in the kidney which filter the blood

glomerulitis [gləumerju'laɪtɪs] *noun* inflammation causing lesions of glomeruli in the kidney

glomerulonephritis
[gləumerjulauni'fraɪtɪs] *noun* form of nephritis where the glomeruli in the kidneys are inflamed

glomerulus [gləu'merjuləs] *noun* group of blood vessels which filter waste matter from the blood in a kidney; *see also* MALPIGHIAN (NOTE: plural is **glomeruli**)

gloss- ['glɒs] *prefix* referring to the tongue

glossa ['glɒsə] *noun* the tongue

glossectomy [glɒ'sektəmi] *noun* surgical removal of the tongue

Glossina [glɒ'saɪnə] *noun* genus of African flies (such as the tsetse fly), which cause trypanosomiasis

glossitis [glɒ'saɪtɪs] *noun* inflammation of the surface of the tongue

glossodynia [glɒsəu'dɪniə] *noun* pain in the tongue

glossopharyngeal nerve
[glɒsəufærɪn'dʒiːəl 'nɜːv] *noun* ninth cranial nerve which controls the pharynx, the salivary glands and part of the tongue

glossoplegia [glɒsəu'pliːdʒə] *noun* paralysis of the tongue

glossotomy [glɒ'sɒtəmi] *noun* surgical incision into the tongue

glottis ['glɒtɪs] *noun* opening in the larynx between the vocal cords, which forms the entrance to the main airway from the pharynx

glove [glʌv] *noun* piece of clothing which you wear on your hand; *the doctor was wearing rubber gloves or surgical gloves*

gluc- [gluːk] *prefix* referring to glucose

glucagon ['gluːkəgɒn] *noun* hormone secreted by the islets of Langerhans in the pancreas, which increases the level of blood sugar by stimulating the breakdown of glycogen

glucocorticoid [gluːkəu'kɔːtɪkɔɪd] *noun* any corticosteroid which breaks down carbohydrates and fats for use by the body, produced by the adrenal cortex

glucose ['gluːkəuz] *noun* dextrose, simple sugar found in some fruit, but also broken down from white sugar or carbohydrate and absorbed into the body or secreted by the kidneys; **blood-glucose level** = amount of glucose present in the blood; *the normal blood-glucose level stays at about 60 to 100 mg of glucose per 100 ml of blood*; **glucose tolerance test** = test for diabetes mellitus, where the patient eats glucose and his urine and blood are tested at regular intervals

COMMENT: combustion of glucose with oxygen to form carbon dioxide and water is the body's main source of energy

glucuronic acid [gluːkju'rɒnɪk 'æsɪd] *noun* acid formed by glucose and which acts on bilirubin

glue [gluː] **1** *noun* material which sticks things together; **glue-sniffing** = type of solvent abuse where a person is addicted to inhaling the toxic fumes given off by certain types of glue **2** *verb* to stick things together with glue

glue ear ['gluː 'ɪə] *noun* secretory otitis media, condition where fluid forms behind the eardrum and causes deafness

glutamic acid [gluː'tæmɪk 'æsɪd] *noun* amino acid in protein

glutaminase [gluː'tæmɪneɪz] *noun* enzyme in the kidneys, which helps to break down glutamine

glutamine ['gluːtəmiːn] *noun* amino acid in protein

gluteal ['gluːtɪəl] *adjective* referring to the buttocks; **superior** *or* **inferior gluteal artery** = arteries supplying the buttocks; **superior** *or* **inferior gluteal vein** = veins draining the buttocks; **gluteal muscles** = muscles in the buttocks; *see also* GLUTEUS

gluten ['gluːtən] *noun* protein found in certain cereals, which makes a sticky paste when water is added; **gluten enteropathy** = (i) allergic disease (mainly affecting children) in which the lining of the intestine is sensitive to gluten, preventing the small intestine from digesting fat; (ii) condition in adults where the villi in the intestine become smaller, and so reduce the surface which can absorb nutrients (NOTE: also called **coeliac disease**); **gluten-free diet** = diet including only food containing no gluten

gluteus ['glu:tiəs] *noun* one of three muscles in the buttocks, responsible for movements of the hip (the largest is the gluteus maximus, while gluteus medius and minimus are smaller)

glyc- [glɪs] *prefix* referring to sugar

glycaemia [glaɪ'si:miə] *noun* normal level of glucose found in the blood; *see also* HYPOGLYCAEMIA, HYPERGLYCAEMIA

glycerin(e) *or* **glycerol** ['glɪsrɪn or 'glɪsərɒl] *noun* colourless viscous sweet-tasting liquid present in all fats

COMMENT: synthetic glycerine is used in various medicinal preparations and also as a lubricant in toothpaste, cough medicines, etc. A mixture of glycerine and honey is useful to soothe a sore throat

glycine ['glaɪsi:n] *noun* amino acid in protein

glycocholic acid [glaɪkəu'kɒlɪk 'æsɪd] *noun* one of the bile acids

glycogen ['glaɪkədʒən] *noun* type of starch, converted from glucose by the action of insulin, and stored in the liver as a source of energy

glycogenesis [glaɪkəu'dʒenəsɪs] *noun* process by which glucose is converted into glycogen in the liver

glycogenolysis [glaɪkəudʒə'nɒləsɪs] *noun* process by which glycogen is broken down to form glucose

glycosuria [glaɪkəu'sjuəriə] *noun* high level of sugar in the urine, a symptom of diabetes mellitus

GMC ['dʒi: 'em 'si:] = GENERAL MEDICAL COUNCIL

gnathoplasty ['næθəuplæsti] *noun* plastic surgery to correct a defect in the jaw

goal [gəul] *noun* that which is expected to be achieved by a certain treatment

goblet cell ['gɒblət 'sel] *noun* tube-shaped cell in the epithelium which secretes mucus

GOC ['dʒi: 'əu 'si:] = GENERAL OPTICAL COUNCIL

go down ['gəu 'daun] *verb* to become smaller; *when the blood sugar level goes down*; *the swelling has started to go down*

goitre *US* **goiter** ['gɔɪtə] *noun* excessive enlargement of the thyroid gland, seen as a swelling round the neck, caused by a lack of iodine; **exophthalmic goitre** = form of goitre caused by hyperthyroidism, where the heart beats faster, the thyroid gland swells, the eyes protrude and the limbs tremble (NOTE: also called **Graves' disease**)

goitrogen ['gɔɪtrədʒən] *noun* substance which causes goitre

gold [gəuld] *noun* soft yellow-coloured precious metal, used as a compound in various drugs, and sometimes as a filling for teeth; **gold injections** = injections of a solution containing gold, used to relieve rheumatoid arthritis; **gold standard** = the best measure of a disease against which screening tests, diagnostic methods, etc., are compared (NOTE: the chemical symbol is **Au**)

golden ['gəuldən] *adjective* coloured like gold; **golden eye ointment** = yellow ointment, made of an oxide of mercury, used to treat inflammation of the eyelids

Golgi apparatus ['gɒldʒi æpə'reɪtəs] *noun* folded membranous structure inside the cell cytoplasm which stores and transports enzymes and hormones

Golgi cell ['gɒldʒi 'sel] *noun* type of nerve cell in the central nervous system, either with long axons (Golgi type 1) or without axons (Golgi type 2)

gomphosis [gɒm'fəusɪs] *noun* joint which cannot move, like a tooth in a jaw

gonad ['gəunæd] *noun* sex gland which produces gametes (the testicles produce spermatozoa in males, and the ovaries produce ova in females) and also sex hormones

gonadotrophic hormones [gəunədəu'trɒfɪk 'hɔ:məunz] *plural noun* hormones (the follicle-stimulating hormone (FSH) and the luteinizing hormone (LH)) produced by the anterior pituitary gland which have an effect on the ovaries in females and on the testes in males

gonadotrophin *US* **gonadotropin** [gəunədəu'trəufɪn or -trɒpɪn] *noun* any of a group of hormones produced by the pituitary gland which stimulates the sex glands at puberty; *see also* CHORIONIC

gonagra [gɒˈnægrə] *noun* form of gout which occurs in the knees

goni- [ˈgəʊni] *prefix* meaning angle

goniopuncture [gəʊniəʊˈpʌntʃə] *noun* surgical operation for draining fluid from the eyes of a patient who has glaucoma

gonioscope [ˈgəʊniəskəʊp] *noun* lens for measuring the angle of the front part of the eye

goniotomy [gəʊniˈɒtəmi] *noun* surgical operation to treat glaucoma by cutting Schlemm's canal

gonococcal [gɒnəˈkɒkl] *adjective* referring to gonococcus

gonococcus [gɒnəˈkɒkəs] *noun* type of bacterium, *Neisseria gonorrhoea*, which produces gonorrhoea (NOTE: plural is **gonococci**)

gonocyte [ˈgɒnəsaɪt] *noun* germ cell, a cell which is able to develop into a spermatozoon or an ovum

gonorrhoea [gɒnəˈrɪə] *noun* sexually transmitted disease, which produces painful irritation of the mucous membrane and a watery discharge from the vagina or penis

gonorrhoeal [gɒnəˈrɪəl] *adjective* referring to gonorrhoea

Goodpasture's syndrome [gʊdˈpɑːstʃəz ˈsɪndrəʊm] *noun* rare lung disease where the patient coughs up blood, is anaemic, and which may result in kidney failure

goose flesh *or* **goose pimples** US **goose bumps** [ˈguːs fleʃ or ˈguːs ˈpɪmplz or ˈguːs ˈbʌmps] *noun* reaction of the skin to being cold or frightened, where the skin is raised into many little bumps by the action of the erector pili muscles (NOTE: formally called **cutis anserina**)

Gordh needle [ˈgɔːd ˈniːdl] *noun* needle with a bag attached, so that several injections can be made one after the other

gorget [ˈgɔːdʒɪt] *noun* surgical instrument used to remove stones from the bladder

gouge [gaʊdʒ] *noun* surgical instrument like a chisel used to cut bone

goundou [ˈguːnduː] *noun* condition caused by yaws, in which growths form on either side of the nose

gout [gaʊt] *noun* podagra, disease in which abnormal quantities of uric acid are produced and precipitated as crystals in the cartilage round joints

COMMENT: formerly associated with drinking strong wines such as port, but now believed to arise in three ways: excess uric acid in the diet, excess uric acid synthesized by the body and defective excretion of uric acid. It is likely that both overproduction and defective excretion are due to inherited biochemical abnormalities. Excess intake of alcohol can provoke an attack by interfering with the excretion of uric acid

gown [gaʊn] *noun* long robe worn over other clothes to protect them; *the surgeons were wearing green gowns*; *the patient lay on his bed in a theatre gown, ready to go to the operating theatre*

GP [ˈdʒiː ˈpiː] *noun* general practitioner (NOTE: plural is **GPs**)

GPI [ˈdʒiː ˈpiː ˈaɪ] = **GENERAL PARALYSIS OF THE INSANE**

gr = GRAIN

Graafian follicle [ˈgræfiən ˈfɒlɪkl] *see* FOLLICLE

gracilis [ˈgreɪsɪlɪs] *noun* thin muscle running down the inside of the leg from the top of the leg down to the top of the tibia

graduate 1 [ˈgrædʒuət] *noun* person who has completed a university course and has a degree; *she is a graduate from the School of Tropical Medicine* **2** [ˈgrædʒueɪt] *verb* to finish a course of study at a university and have a degree; *he graduated in Pharmacy last year*

graduated [ˈgrædʒueɪtɪd] *adjective* with marks showing various degrees or levels; *a graduated measuring jar*

Graefe's knife [ˈgreɪfəz ˈnaɪf] *noun* sharp knife used in operations on cataracts

graft [grɑːft] **1** *noun* (i) act of transplanting an organ (heart, lung or kidney) or tissue (bone or skin) to replace an organ or tissue which is not functioning or which is diseased; (ii) organ or tissue which is transplanted; *she had to have a skin graft*; *the corneal graft was successful*; *the patient was given drugs to prevent the graft being rejected*; **graft versus host disease** = condition which develops when cells from the grafted tissue react against the patient's own tissue, causing skin disorders; *see also* AUTOGRAFT, HOMOGRAFT **2** *verb* to take a healthy organ or tissue and transplant it into a patient in place of diseased or defective organ or tissue; *the surgeons grafted a new section of bone at the side of the skull*

grain [greɪn] *noun* measure of weight equal to .0648 grams (NOTE: when used with numbers, **grain** is usually written **gr**)

gram [græm] measure of weight; *a thousand grams make one kilogram*; *I need 5 g of morphine* (NOTE: when used with numbers, **gram** is usually written **g: 50 g** say 'fifty grams')

-gram [græm] *suffix* meaning a record in the form of a picture; **cardiogram** = X-ray picture of the heart

Gram's stain ['græmz 'steɪn] *noun* method of staining bacteria so that they can be identified; **Gram-positive bacterium** = bacterium which retains the first dye and appears blue-black when viewed under the microscope; **Gram-negative bacterium** = bacterium which takes up the red counterstain, after the alcohol has washed out the first violet dye

COMMENT: the tissue sample is first stained with a violet dye, treated with alcohol, and then counterstained with a red dye

grandchild ['græntʃaɪld] *noun* child of a son or daughter (NOTE: plural is **grandchildren**)

granddaughter ['grændɔːtə] *noun* daughter of a son or daughter

grandes ['grændɪs] *see* MULTIPARA

grandfather ['grænfɑːðə] *noun* father of a mother or father

grand mal ['grɑː 'mal] *noun* major epilepsy, a type of epilepsy, in which the patient becomes unconscious and falls down, while the muscles become stiff and twitch violently

grandmother ['grænmʌðə] *noun* mother of a mother or father

grandparents ['grænpeərənts] *plural noun* parents of a mother or father

grandson ['grænsʌn] *noun* son of a son or daughter

granular ['grænjʊlə] *adjective* like grains; **granular cast** = cast composed of cells filled with protein and fatty granules; **granular leucocytes** *or* **granulocytes** = leucocytes with granules (basophils, eosinophils, neutrophils); **nongranular leucocytes** = leucocytes without granules (lymphocytes, monocytes)

granulation [grænjuˈleɪʃn] *noun* formation of rough red tissue on the surface of a wound or site of infection, the first stage in the healing process; **granulation tissue** *or*

granulations = soft tissue, consisting mainly of tiny blood vessels and fibres, which forms over a wound

granule ['grænjuːl] *noun* small particle or grain; **Nissl granules** = coarse granules surrounding the nucleus in the cytoplasm of nerve cells (NOTE: also called **Nissl bodies**)

granulocyte ['grænjuːləsaɪt] *noun* type of leucocyte or white blood cell which contains granules (such as basophils, eosinophils and neutrophils)

granulocytopenia [grænjuːləsaɪtəʊˈpiːnɪə] *noun* usually fatal disease caused by the lowering of the number of granulocytes in the blood due to a defect in the bone marrow

granuloma [grænjuˈləʊmə] *noun* mass of granulation tissue which forms at the site of bacterial infections; **granuloma inguinale** = tropical venereal disease affecting the anus and genitals in which the skin becomes covered with ulcers (NOTE: plural is **granulomata** or **granulomas**)

granulomatosis [grænjuːləʊməˈtəʊsɪs] *noun* chronic inflammation leading to the formation of nodules; **Wegener's granulomatosis** = disease of the connective tissue in which the nasal passages and lungs are inflamed and ulcerated

granulomatous [grænjuˈləʊmətəs] *adjective* **chronic granulomatous disease** = type of inflammation where macrophages are converted into epithelial-like cells as a result of infection, as in tuberculosis or sarcoidosis

granulopoiesis [grænjuːləʊpɔɪˈiːsɪs] *noun* normal production of granulocytes in the bone marrow

graph [grɑːf] *noun* diagram which shows the relationship between quantities as a line; **temperature graph** = graph showing how a patient's temperature rises and falls over a period of time

-graph [grɑːf] *suffix* meaning a machine which records as pictures

-grapher [grəfə] *suffix* meaning a technician who operates a machine which records; **radiographer** = technician who operates an X-ray machine

-graphy [grəfi] *suffix* meaning the technique of study through pictures; **radiography** = X-ray examination of part of the body

grattage [græˈtɑːʒ] *noun* scraping the surface of an ulcer which is healing slowly, in order to make it heal more quickly

grave [greɪv] *noun* place where a dead person is buried; *his grave is covered with flowers*

gravel ['grævl] *noun* small stones which pass from the kidney to the urinary system, causing pain in the ureter

Graves' disease ['greɪvz dɪ'ziːz] = THYROTOXICOSIS (NOTE: also called **exophthalmic goitre**)

gravid ['grævɪd] *adjective* pregnant; **hyperemesis gravidarum** = vomiting in pregnancy; **gravides multiparae** = women who have given birth to at least four live babies

Grawitz tumour ['grɑːvɪts 'tjuːmə] *noun* malignant tumour in kidney cells

gray [greɪ] **1** *adjective* US = GREY **2** *noun* SI unit of measurement of absorbed radiation equal to 100 rads; *see also* RAD (NOTE: **gray** is written **Gy** with figures)

graze [greɪz] **1** *noun* scrape on the skin surface, making some blood flow **2** *verb* to scrape the skin surface

great [greɪt] *adjective* large; **great cerebral vein** = median vein draining the choroid plexuses of the lateral and third ventricles; **great toe** = big toe, largest of the five toes, near the inside of the foot (NOTE: **great - greater - greatest**)

greater ['greɪtə] *adjective* larger; **greater curvature** = convex line of the stomach; *see also* OMENTUM, TROCHANTER

greatly ['greɪtli] *adverb* very much

greedy ['griːdi] *adjective* always wanting to eat a lot of food (NOTE: **greedy - greedier - greediest**)

green [griːn] *adjective & noun* of a colour like the colour of leaves; *when he saw the blood he turned green*

green monkey disease ['griːn 'mʌŋki dɪ'ziːz] = MARBURG DISEASE

greenstick fracture ['griːnstɪk 'fræktʃə] *noun* type of fracture occurring in children, where a long bone bends, but is not completely broken

grey US **gray** [greɪ] *adjective & noun* of a colour between black and white; *his hair is quite grey*; *a grey-haired man*; **grey commissure** = part of the grey matter nearest to the central canal of the spinal cord, where axons cross over each other; **grey matter** = nervous tissue of a dark grey

colour, formed of cell bodies and occurring in the central nervous system

COMMENT: in the brain, grey matter encloses the white matter, but in the spinal cord, white matter encloses grey matter

grief [griːf] *noun* feeling of great sadness felt when someone dies; **grief counsellor** = person who helps someone to cope with the feelings they have when someone, such as a close relative, dies

Griffith's types ['grɪfiθs 'taɪps] *noun* various types of haemolytic streptococci, classified according to the antigens present in them

gripe [graɪp] *noun* pains in the abdomen; **gripe water** = solution of glucose and alcohol, used to relieve gripe in babies

grippe [grɪp or griːp] *noun* influenza

gristle ['grɪsl] *noun* cartilage

grocer ['grəʊsə] *noun* person who sells sugar, butter, tins of food, etc.

grocer's itch ['grəʊsəz 'ɪtʃ] *noun* form of dermatitis on the hands caused by handling flour and sugar

groin [grɔɪn] *noun* junction at each side of the body where the lower abdomen joins the top of the thighs; *he had a dull pain in his groin* (NOTE: for other terms referring to the groin, see **inguinal**)

grommet ['grɒmɪt] *noun* tube which can be passed from the external auditory meatus into the middle ear, usually to allow fluid to drain off, as in a patient suffering from glue ear (secretory otitis media)

groove [gruːv] *noun* long shallow depression in a surface; **atrioventricular groove** = groove round the outside of the heart, showing the division between the atria and the ventricles

gross anatomy ['grəʊs ə'nætəmi] *noun* study of the structure of the body which can be seen without the use of a microscope

ground [graʊnd] *noun* **(a)** soil or earth **(b)** surface of the earth

ground substance ['graʊnd 'sʌbstəns] *noun* matrix, amorphous mass of cells forming the basis of connective tissue

group [gruːp] **1** *noun* **(a)** several people, animals or things which are all close together; *a group of patients were waiting in the surgery*; **group practice** = practice where several doctors or dentists share the same office building and support services; **group therapy** = type of psychotherapy where a group of people with the same disorder meet together with a therapist to discuss their condition and try to help each other **(b)** way of putting similar things together; **age group** = all people of a certain age; **blood group** = *see* BLOOD **2** *verb* to bring together in a group; *the drugs are grouped under the heading 'antibiotics'*; **blood grouping** = classifying patients according to their blood groups

grow [grəʊ] *verb* **(a)** to become taller or bigger; *your son has grown since I last saw him*; *he grew three centimetres in one year* **(b)** to become; *it's growing colder at night now*; *she grew weak with hunger* (NOTE: growing - grew - grown)

growing pains ['grəʊɪŋ peɪnz] *noun* pains associated with adolescence, which can be a form of rheumatic fever

grown-up ['grəʊnʌp] *noun* adult; *there are three grown-ups and ten children*

growth [grəʊθ] *noun* **(a)** increase in size; *the disease stunts children's growth*; *the growth in the population since 1960*; **growth factor** = chemical substance produced in the body which encourages a type of cell (such as a blood cell) to grow; **growth hormone (GH)** = somatotrophin, a hormone secreted by the pituitary gland during deep sleep, which stimulates growth of the long bones and protein synthesis (NOTE: no plural for this meaning) **(b)** lump of tissue which is not natural, a cyst or a tumour; *the doctor found she had a cancerous growth on the left breast*; *he had an operation to remove a small growth from his chin*

grumbling appendix ['grʌmblɪŋ ə'pendɪks] *noun* *(informal)* chronic appendicitis, condition where the vermiform appendix is always slightly inflamed

GU ['dʒiː 'juː] = GASTRIC ULCER, GENITOURINARY

guanine ['gwɑːniːn] *noun* one of the nitrogen-containing bases in DNA

gubernaculum [guːbə'nækjʊləm] *noun* fibrous tissue connecting the testes in a fetus (the gonads) to the groin

guide [gaɪd] **1** *noun* person or book which shows you how to do something or what to do; *read this guide to services offered by the local authority*; *the council has produced a*

guide for expectant mothers **2** *verb* to show someone where to go or how to do something

guide dog ['gaɪd 'dɒg] *noun* dog which shows a blind person where to go

guidelines ['gaɪdlaɪnz] *noun* a set of recommendations to advise doctors on how to manage clinical conditions

Guillain-Barré syndrome ['giːjænbə'reɪ 'sɪndrəʊm] *noun* nervous disorder, in which after a non-specific infection, demyelination of the spinal roots and peripheral nerves takes place, leading to generalized weakness and sometimes respiratory paralysis

guillotine ['gɪlətiːn] *noun* surgical instrument for cutting out tonsils

guinea worm ['gɪni 'wɜːm] = DRACUNCULUS

gullet ['gʌlɪt] *noun* oesophagus, the tube down which food and drink passes from the mouth to the stomach; *she had a piece of bread stuck in her gullet*

gum [gʌm] *noun* gingiva, part of the mouth, the soft epithelial tissue covering the part of the jaw which surrounds the teeth; *his gums are red and inflamed*; *a build-up of tartar can lead to gum disease*

gumboil ['gʌmbɔɪl] *noun* abscess on the gum near a tooth (NOTE: for other terms referring to the gums, see words beginning with **gingiv-, ul(o)-**)

gumma ['gʌmə] *noun* abscess of dead tissue and overgrown scar tissue, which develops in the later stages of syphilis

gustation [gʌ'steɪʃn] *noun* act of tasting

gustatory ['gʌstətri] *noun* referring to the sense of taste

gut [gʌt] *noun* **(a)** *(informal* guts*)* digestive tract, alimentary canal or the intestines, the tubular organ for the digestion and absorption of food; *he complained of having a pain in his gut* or *he said he had gut pain* **(b)** type of thread, made from the intestines of sheep, used to sew up internal incisions; it dissolves slowly so does not need to be removed; *see also* CATGUT

Guthrie test ['gʌθri 'test] *noun* test used on babies to detect the presence of phenylketonuria

gutta ['gʌtə] *noun* drop of liquid (as used in treatment of the eyes) (NOTE: plural is **guttae**)

gutter splint ['gʌtə splɪnt] *noun* shaped container in which a broken limb can rest without being completely surrounded

Gy *abbreviation for* gray

gyn- [gaɪn] *prefix* referring to (i) woman; (ii) the female reproductive system

gynaecological [gaɪnɪkə'lɒdʒɪkl] *adjective* referring to the treatment of diseases of women

gynaecologist [gaɪnɪ'kɒlədʒɪst] *noun* doctor who specializes in the treatment of diseases of women

gynaecology [gaɪnɪ'kɒlədʒi] *noun* study of female sex organs and the treatment of diseases of women in general

gynaecomastia [gaɪnɪkə'mæstiə] *noun* abnormal development of breasts in a male (NOTE: words beginning with **gynae-** are spelled **gyne-** in American English)

gyrus ['dʒaɪərəs] *noun* raised part of the cerebral cortex between the sulci; **postcentral gyrus** = sensory area of the cerebral cortex, which receives impulses from receptor cells and senses pain, heat, touch, etc.; **precentral gyrus** = motor area of the cerebral cortex (NOTE: plural is **gyri**)

Hh

H *chemical symbol for* hydrogen

HA ['eɪtʃ 'eɪ] = HEALTH AUTHORITY

habit ['hæbɪt] *noun* **(a)** action which is an automatic response to a stimulus **(b)** regular way of doing something; *he got into the habit of swimming every day before breakfast*; *she's got out of the habit of taking any exercise*; **from force of habit** = because you do it regularly; *I wake up at 6 o'clock from force of habit*

habit-forming ['hæbɪt'fɔːmɪŋ] *adjective* which makes someone addicted, which makes someone get into the habit of taking something; **habit-forming drugs** = drugs which are addictive

habitual [hə'bɪtʃul] *adjective* which is done frequently or as a matter of habit; **habitual abortion** = condition where a woman has abortions (miscarriages) with successive pregnancies

habituation [həbɪtʃu'eɪʃn] *noun* being psychologically but not physically addicted to or dependent on (a drug, alcohol, etc.); *his habituation to nicotine*

habitus ['hæbɪtəs] *noun* general physical appearance of the person (including build and posture)

hacking cough ['hækɪŋ 'kɒf] *noun* continuous short dry cough

haem [hiːm] *noun* molecule containing iron which binds proteins to form haemoproteins such as haemoglobin and myoglobin

haem- [hiːm] *prefix* referring to blood (NOTE: words beginning with the prefix **haem-** are written **hem-** in American English)

haemangioma [hiːmændʒɪ'əumə] *noun* benign tumour which forms in blood vessels and appears on the skin as a birthmark; **cavernous haemangioma** = tumour in connective tissue with wide spaces which contain blood (NOTE: plural is **haemangiomata**)

haemarthrosis [hiːmɑː'θrəusɪs] *noun* pain and swelling caused by blood getting into a joint

haematemesis [hiːmɑː'teməsɪs] *noun* vomiting of blood (usually because of internal bleeding)

haematic [hiː'mætɪk] *adjective* referring to blood

haematin ['hiːmətɪn] *noun* substance which forms from haemoglobin when bleeding takes place

haematinic [hiːmə'tɪnɪk] *noun* drug, such as an iron compound, which increases haemoglobin in blood, used to treat anaemia

haematocoele ['hiːmətəusiːl] *noun* swelling caused by blood getting into an internal cavity

haematocolpos [hiːmətəu'kɒlpəs] *noun* condition where the vagina is filled with blood at menstruation because the hymen has no opening

haematocrit ['hiːmətəukrɪt] *noun* (i) volume of red blood cells in a patient's blood, shown as a percentage of the total blood volume; (ii) instrument for measuring haematocrit

haematocyst ['hiːmətəusɪst] *noun* cyst which contains blood

haematogenous [hiːmə'tɒdʒənəs] *adjective* (i) which produces blood; (ii) which is produced by blood

haematological [hiːmətəu'lɒdʒɪkl] *adjective* referring to haematology

haematologist [hiːmə'tɒlədʒɪst] *noun* doctor who specializes in haematology

haematology [hiːmə'tɒlədʒi] *noun* scientific study of blood, its formation and its diseases

haematoma [hiːmə'təumə] *noun* mass of blood under the skin caused by a blow or by the effects of an operation; **extradural**

haematoma = haematoma in the head, between the dura mater and the skull; **intracerebral haematoma** = haematoma inside the cerebrum; **perianal haematoma** = haematoma in the anal region; **subdural haematoma** = blood plasma, clot between the dura mater and the arachnoid, which displaces the brain, caused by a blow on the head (NOTE: plural is **haematomata**)

haematometra [hiːmə'tɒmɪtrə] *noun* (i) excessive bleeding in the uterus; (ii) swollen uterus, caused by haematocolpos

haematomyelia [hiːmətəʊmaɪ'iːliə] *noun* condition where blood gets into the spinal cord

haematopoiesis [hiːmətəʊpɔɪ'iːsɪs] = HAEMOPOIESIS

haematoporphyrin [hiːmətəʊ'pɔːfərɪn] *noun* porphyrin produced from haemoglobin

haematosalpinx [hiːmətəʊ'sælpɪŋks] = HAEMOSALPINX

haematospermia [hiːmætəʊ'spɜːmiə] *noun* presence of blood in the sperm

haematozoon [hiːmətəʊ'zəʊɒn] *noun* parasite living in the blood (NOTE: plural is **haematozoa**)

haematuria [hiːmə'tjʊəriə] *noun* abnormal presence of blood in the urine, as a result of injury or disease of the kidney or bladder

haemochromatosis [hiːməʊkrəʊmə'təʊsɪs] *noun* bronze diabetes, hereditary disease in which the body absorbs and stores too much iron, causing cirrhosis of the liver, and giving the skin a dark colour

haemoconcentration [hiːməʊkɒnsən'treɪʃn] *noun* increase in the percentage of red blood cells because the volume of plasma is reduced; *opposite is* HAEMODILUTION

haemocytoblast [hiːməʊ'saɪtəʊblæst] *noun* embryonic blood cell in the bone marrow from which red and white blood cells and platelets develop

haemocytometer [hiːməʊsaɪ'tɒmɪtə] *noun* glass jar in which a sample of blood is diluted and the blood cells counted

haemodialysis [hiːməʊdaɪ'æləsɪs] *noun* removing waste matter from blood using a dialyser (kidney machine)

haemodialyse [hiːməʊ'daɪəlaɪz] *verb* to remove waste matter from the blood using a dialyser (kidney machine)

haemodialysed [hiːməʊ'daɪəlaɪzd] *adjective* **haemodialysed patient** = patient who has undergone haemodialysis

haemodilution [hiːməʊdaɪ'luːʃn] *noun* decrease in the percentage of red blood cells because the volume of plasma has increased; *opposite is* HAEMOCONCENTRATION

haemoglobin (Hb) [hiːməʊ'gləʊbɪn] *noun* red respiratory pigment (formed of haem and globin) in red blood cells which gives blood its red colour; *see also* OXYHAEMOGLOBIN

COMMENT: haemoglobin absorbs oxygen in the lungs and carries it in the blood to the tissues

haemoglobinaemia [hiːməʊgləʊbɪ'niːmiə] *noun* haemoglobin in the plasma

haemoglobinopathy [hiːməʊgləʊbɪ'nɒpəθi] *noun* inherited disease where production of haemoglobin is abnormal

haemoglobinuria [hiːməʊgləʊbɪ'njʊəriə] *noun* condition where haemoglobin is found in the urine

haemogram ['hiːməʊgræm] *noun* printed result of a blood test

haemolysin [hiːmɒ'laɪsɪn] *noun* protein which destroys red blood cells

haemolysis [hiː'mɒləsɪs] *noun* destruction of red blood cells

haemolytic [hiːməʊ'lɪtɪk] *adjective* (substance, such as snake venom) which destroys red blood cells; **haemolytic anaemia** = condition where the destruction of red blood cells is about six times the normal rate, and the supply of new cells from the bone marrow cannot meet the demand; **haemolytic disease of the newborn** = condition where the red blood cells of the fetus are destroyed because antibodies in the mother's blood react against the blood of the fetus in the uterus; **haemolytic jaundice** = jaundice caused by haemolysis of red blood cells; **haemolytic uraemic syndrome** = condition in which haemolytic anaemia damages the kidneys

haemopericardium [hiːməʊperɪ'kɑːdiəm] *noun* blood in the pericardium

haemoperitoneum [hiːməʊperitə'niːəm] *noun* blood in the peritoneal cavity

haemophilia [hiːməʊ'filiə] *noun* **haemophilia A** = familial disease, in which inability to synthesize Factor VIII (a clotting factor), means that patient's blood clots very slowly, prolonged bleeding occurs from the slightest wound and internal bleeding can occur without any cause; **haemophilia B** = clotting disorder of the blood, similar to haemophilia A, but in which the blood coagulates badly due to deficiency of Factor IX (NOTE: also called **Christmas disease**)

COMMENT: because haemophilia A is a sex-linked recessive characteristic, it is found only in males, but females are carriers. It can be treated by injections of Factor VIII

haemophiliac [hiːməʊˈfɪlɪək] *noun* person who suffers from haemophilia

haemophilic [hiːməʊˈfɪlɪk] *adjective* referring to haemophilia

Haemophilus [hiːˈmɒfɪləs] *noun* genus of bacteria, which need certain factors in the blood to grow; **Haemophilus influenzae** = bacterium which lives in healthy throats, but if the patient's resistance is lowered by a bout of flu, then it can cause pneumonia; **Haemophilus influenzae type b (Hib)** = bacterium which causes meningitis

haemophthalmia [hiːmɒfˈθælmɪə] *noun* blood in the eye

haemopneumothorax [hiːməʊnjuːməʊˈθɔːræks] = PNEUMOHAEMOTHORAX

haemopoiesis [hiːməʊpɔɪˈiːsɪs] *noun* continual production of blood cells and blood platelets by the bone marrow

haemopoietic [hiːməʊpɔɪˈetɪk] *adjective* referring to the formation of blood

haemoptysis [hiːˈmɒptəsɪs] *noun* condition where the patient coughs blood from the lungs, caused by a serious illness such as anaemia, pneumonia, tuberculosis or cancer; **endemic haemoptysis** = PARAGONIMIASIS

haemorrhage [ˈhemərɪdʒ] **1** *noun* bleeding where a large quantity of blood is lost, especially bleeding from a burst blood vessel; *she had a haemorrhage and was rushed to hospital; he died of a brain haemorrhage*; **arterial haemorrhage** = haemorrhage of bright red blood from an artery; **brain haemorrhage** *or* **cerebral haemorrhage** = bleeding inside the brain from a cerebral artery; **extradural haemorrhage** = serious condition where bleeding occurs between the dura mater and the skull; **internal haemorrhage** =

haemorrhage which takes place inside the body; **primary haemorrhage** = haemorrhage which occurs immediately after an injury is suffered; **secondary haemorrhage** = haemorrhage which occurs some time after the injury, due to infection of the wound; **venous haemorrhage** = haemorrhage of dark blood from a vein **2** *verb* to bleed heavily; *the injured man was haemorrhaging from the mouth*

haemorrhagic [heməˈrædʒɪk] *adjective* referring to heavy bleeding; **haemorrhagic disease of the newborn** = disease of babies, which makes them haemorrhage easily, caused by temporary lack of prothrombin; **haemorrhagic disorders** = disorders (such as haemophilia) where haemorrhages occur; **haemorrhagic stroke** = stroke caused by a burst blood vessel

haemorrhoidal [heməˈrɔɪdəl] *adjective* referring to haemorrhoids

haemorrhoidectomy [hemərɔɪˈdektəmi] *noun* surgical removal of haemorrhoids

haemorrhoids [ˈhemərɔɪdz] *plural noun* piles, swollen veins in the anorectal passage; **external haemorrhoids** = haemorrhoids in the skin just outside the anus; **internal haemorrhoids** = swollen veins inside the anus; **first-degree haemorrhoids** = haemorrhoids which remain in the rectum; **second-degree haemorrhoids** = haemorrhoids which protrude into the anus but return into the rectum automatically; **third-degree haemorrhoids** = haemorrhoids which protrude into the anus permanently

haemosalpinx [hiːməʊˈsælpɪŋks] *noun* blood accumulating in the Fallopian tubes

haemosiderosis [hiːməʊsɪdəˈrəʊsɪs] *noun* disorder in which iron forms large deposits in the tissue, causing haemorrhaging and destruction of red blood cells

haemostasis [hiːməʊˈsteɪsɪs] *noun* stopping bleeding, slowing the movement of blood

haemostat [ˈhiːməʊstæt] *noun* device, such as a clamp, which stops bleeding

haemostatic [hiːməʊˈstætɪk] *adjective & noun* (drug) which stops bleeding

haemothorax [hiːməʊˈθɔːræks] *noun* blood in the pleural cavity

hair [heə] *noun* **(a)** long thread growing on the body of an animal, from a small pit in the skin called a follicle (hair is mainly made up of a dense form of keratin); *he's beginning to* *get a few grey hairs*; *hairs are growing on his chest*; **hair follicle** = tube of epidermal cells containing the root of a hair; **hair papilla** = part of the skin containing capillaries which feed blood to the hair ; *see illustration at* SKIN & SENSORY RECEPTORS (NOTE: plural in this meaning is **hairs**) **(b)** mass of hairs growing on the head; *she's got long black hair*; *you ought to wash your hair*; *his hair is too long*; *he is going to have his hair cut*; **superfluous** *or* **unwanted hair** = hair which is growing in places where it is not thought to be beautiful (NOTE: no plural in this sense. For other terms referring to hair, see words beginning with **pilo-, tricho-**) **(c)** *(on the organ of Corti of the ear)* **hair cell** = receptor cell which converts fluid pressure changes into nerve impulses carried in the auditory nerve

COMMENT: hair is dead tissue and grows out of hair follicles. The follicles are tubes leading into the skin and lined with sebaceous glands which secrete the oil which covers the hair. Hair grows on almost all parts of the body, but is thicker and stronger on the head (the scalp, the eyebrows, inside the nose and ears). After puberty, hair becomes thicker on other parts of the body (the chin, chest and limbs in men, the pubic region and the armpits in both men and women). Hair on the head stops growing in many men in middle age, giving various degrees of baldness. Certain treatments, especially chemotherapy, can cause the hair to fall out. In later middle age, hair loses its natural pigmentation and becomes grey or white

hairline fracture ['heəlaɪn 'fræktʃə] *noun* fracture with a very thin crack

hairy ['heəri] *adjective* covered with hair; *he's got hairy arms*; **hairy cell leukaemia** = form of leukaemia with abnormal white blood cells with thread-like process on them

half-life ['hɑːf'laɪf] *noun* **(a)** time taken for half the atoms in a radioactive isotope to decay; *(of drug)* measurement of the period which shows that the concentration of a drug has reached half of what it was when it was administered

COMMENT: radioactive substances decay in a constant way and each has a different half-life: strontium-90 has a half-life of 28 years, radium-226 one of 1,620 years and plutonium-239 has a half-life of 24,360 years

halitosis [hæli'təʊsɪs] *noun* condition where a person has breath which smells unpleasant

COMMENT: halitosis can have several causes: caries in the teeth, infection of the gums, and indigestion are the most usual. The breath can also have an unpleasant smell during menstruation, or in association with certain diseases such as diabetes mellitus and uraemia

hallucinate [hə'luːsɪneɪt] *verb* to have hallucinations; *the patient was hallucinating*

hallucination [həluːsɪ'neɪʃn] *noun* seeing an imaginary scene or hearing an imaginary sound as clearly as if it were really there; *he had hallucinations and went into a coma*

hallucinatory [hə'luːsɪnətri] *adjective* (drug, such as cannabis or LSD) which causes hallucinations

hallucinogen [hælu'sɪnədʒn] *noun* drug which causes hallucinations (such as cannabis or LSD)

hallucinogenic [həluːsɪnə'dʒenɪk] *adjective* (substance) which produces hallucinations; *a hallucinogenic fungus*

hallux ['hæləks] *noun* big toe; **hallux valgus** = deformity of the foot, where the big toe turns towards the other toes and a bunion is formed on the protruding joint (NOTE: plural is **halluces)**

hamamelis [hæmə'miːlɪs] *see* WITCH HAZEL

hamartoma [hæmɑː'təʊmə] *noun* benign tumour containing tissue from any organ

hamate (bone) ['heɪmeɪt 'bəʊn] *noun* unciform bone, one of the eight small carpal bones in the wrist, shaped like a hook; *see illustration at* HAND

hammer ['hæmə] *noun* **(a)** heavy metal tool for knocking nails into wood, etc.; *he hit his thumb with the hammer*; **hammer toe** = toe where the middle joint is permanently bent downwards **(b)** malleus, one of the three ossicles in the middle ear

hamstring ['hæmstrɪŋ] *noun* group of tendons behind the knee, which link the thigh muscles to the bones in the lower leg; **hamstring muscles** = group of muscles at the back of the thigh, which flex the knee and extend the gluteus maximus

hand [hænd] **1** *noun* terminal part of the arm, beyond the wrist, which is used for holding things; *he injured his hand with a saw*; *the commonest hand injuries occur at work*; **hand, foot and mouth disease** = viral infection causing redness **2** *verb* to pass; *can you hand me that book?*; *he handed me the key to the cupboard*

COMMENT: the hand is formed of twenty-seven bones: fourteen phalanges (in the fingers), five metacarpals in the main part of the hand, and eight carpals in the wrist

HAND

1. carpus	8. trapezium
2. metacarpus	9. trapezoid
3. phalanges	10. capitate
4. scaphoid	11. hamate
5. lunate	12. ulna
6. triquetrum	13. radius
7. pisiform	14. wrist

handicap [ˈhændɪkæp] **1** *noun* physical or mental disability, condition which prevents someone from doing some normal activity; *in spite of her handicaps, she tries to live as normal a life as possible*; *after having both legs amputated, he fought to overcome the handicap* **2** *verb* to prevent someone from doing a normal activity; *he is handicapped by only having one arm*

handicap - disadvantage for a given individual, resulting from an impairment or a disability, that limits or prevents the fulfilment of a role that is normal for that individual

WHO

handicapped [ˈhændɪkæpt] *adjective* (person) who suffers from a handicap; **the physically handicapped** = people with physical disabilities; **the mentally handicapped** = people with impaired behavioural reactions

Hand-Schüller Christian disease

[ˈhɑntˈʃuːlə ˈkrɪʃən dɪˈziːz] *noun* disturbance of cholesterol metabolism in young children which causes defects in membranous bone, mainly in the skull, exophthalmos, diabetes insipidus, and a yellow-brown colour of the skin

hang [hæŋ] *verb* to attach (something) above the ground (to a nail or hook, etc.); to be attached above the ground (to a nail or hook, etc); *hang your coat on the hook; she hung the photograph over her bed; his hand was almost severed, it was hanging by a band of flesh* (NOTE: **hanging - hung - has hung**)

hangnail [ˈhæŋneɪl] *noun* piece of torn skin at the side of a nail

hangover [ˈhæŋəʊvə] *noun* condition after having drunk too much alcohol, with dehydration caused by inhibition of the antidiuretic hormone in the kidneys

COMMENT: the symptoms of a hangover are pain in the head, inability to stand noise and trembling of the hands

Hansen's bacillus [ˈhænsənz bəˈsɪləs] *noun Mycobacterium leprae,* the bacterium which causes leprosy

Hansen's disease [ˈhænsənz dɪˈziːz] = LEPROSY

haploid [ˈhæplɔɪd] *adjective* (cell, such as a gamete) with a single set of unpaired chromosomes; *compare* DIPLOID, POLYPLOID

happen [ˈhæpən] *verb* **(a)** to take place; *the accident happened at the corner of the street; how did it happen?*; **what's happened to his brother?** = what is his brother doing now? **(b)** to be or to do something (by chance); *she happened to be standing near the cooker when the fire started; luckily a doctor happened to be passing in the street when the baby fell out of the window; do you happen to have an antidote for snake bites?*

hapten ['hæptən] *noun* substance which causes an allergy, probably by changing a protein so that it becomes antigenic

harbour *US* **harbor** ['hɑːbə] *verb* to hold and protect; **to harbour a disease** = to hold germs or bacteria and allow them to breed and spread disease; *soiled clothing can harbour dysentery*; *stagnant water harbours malaria mosquitoes*

hard [hɑːd] **1** *adjective* **(a)** not soft; *this bed is not too hard - a hard bed is good for someone suffering from back problems*; *if you have a slipped disc, you will be made to lie on a hard surface for several weeks*; **hard mass** = lump which feels hard, not soft, when touched; **hard palate** = front part of the roof of the mouth between the upper teeth; **hard water** = tap water which contains a high percentage of calcium **(b)** difficult; *if the exam is too hard, nobody will pass*; **he's hard of hearing** = he's rather deaf **(c) a hard winter** = a very cold winter; *in a hard winter, old people can suffer from hypothermia* (NOTE: **hard - harder - hardest**) **2** *adverb* with a lot of effort; *hit the nail hard with the hammer*; *if we all work hard, we'll soon overcome the disease*

harden ['hɑːdən] *verb* to make hard, to become hard

hardened arteries *or* **hardening of the arteries** ['hɑːdənd 'ɑːtəriz *or* 'hɑːdnɪŋ əv ðɪ 'ɑːtəriz] = ARTERIOSCLEROSIS

harelip [heə'lɪp] *noun* defect in the upper lip occurring at birth, where the lip is split

COMMENT: a harelip is often associated with a cleft palate. Both can be successfully corrected by surgery

harm [hɑːm] **1** *noun* damage (especially to a person); *walking to work every day won't do you any harm*; **there's no harm in taking the tablets only for one week** = there will be no side effects if you take the tablets for a week **2** *verb* to damage or to hurt; *walking to work every day won't harm you*

harmful ['hɑːmfʊl] *adjective* which causes damage; *bright light can be harmful to your eyes*; *sudden violent exercise can be harmful*

harmless ['hɑːmləs] *adjective* which causes no damage; *these herbal remedies are quite harmless*

Harrison's sulcus *or* **Harrison's groove** ['hærisənz 'sʌlkəs *or* 'gruːv] *noun* hollow on either side of the chest which

develops in children who have rickets and breathe in with difficulty

Harris's operation ['hærisiz ɒpə'reiʃən] *noun* surgical removal of the prostate gland

Hartmann's solution ['hɑːtmənz sə'luːʃn] *noun* chemical solution used in drips to replace body fluids lost in dehydration, particularly as a result of infantile gastroenteritis

Hartnup disease ['hɑːtnəp dɪ'ziːz] *noun* condition caused by a hereditary defect in amino acid metabolism, producing thick skin and retarded mental development

harvest ['hɑːvəst] *verb* to take a piece of skin for a graft

harvest mite *or* **harvest tick** ['hɑːvəst 'mait *or* 'tik] = CHIGGER

Hashimoto's disease [hæʃɪ'məutəz dɪ'ziːz] *noun* type of goitre in middle-aged women, where the patient is sensitive to secretions from her own thyroid gland, and, in extreme cases, the face swells and the skin turns yellow

hashish ['hæʃiːʃ] *noun* cannabis or marijuana, an addictive drug made from the leaves or flowers of the Indian hemp plant

haustrum ['hɔːstrəm] *noun* sac on the outside of the colon (NOTE: plural is **haustra**)

HAV ['eitʃ 'ei 'viː] = HEPATITIS A VIRUS

Haversian canal [hə'vɜːʃn kə'næl] *noun* fine canal which runs vertically through the Haversian systems in compact bone, containing blood vessels and lymph ducts

Haversian system [hə'vɜːʃn 'sistəm] *noun* osteon, unit of compact bone built around a Haversian canal, made of a series of bony layers which form a cylinder

hay fever ['hei 'fiːvə] *noun* allergic rhinitis, a form of pollinosis, inflammation in the nasal passage and eyes caused by an allergic reaction to plant pollen; *when he has hay fever, he has to stay indoors*; *the hay fever season starts in May*

Hb = HAEMOGLOBIN

H band ['eitʃ 'bænd] *noun* part of pattern in muscle tissue, a light band in the dark A band, seen through a microscope

HBV ['eitʃ 'biː 'viː] = HEPATITIS B VIRUS

hCG ['eitʃ 'siː 'dʒiː] = HUMAN CHORIONIC GONADOTROPHIN

HDL ['eitʃ 'diː 'el] = HIGH DENSITY LIPOPROTEIN

He *chemical symbol for* helium

head [hed] **1** *noun* **(a)** top part of the body, which contains the eyes, nose, mouth, brain, etc; *can you stand on your head?*; *he hit his head on the low branch*; **he shook his head** = he moved his head from side to side to mean 'no'; **head lice** = small insects of the *Pediculus* genus, which live on the scalp and suck the blood of the host (NOTE: for other terms referring to the head, see words beginning with **cephal-**) **(b)** first place; *he stood at the head of the queue*; *who's name is at the head of the list?* **(c)** (i) rounded top part of a bone which fits into a socket; (ii) round main part of a spermatozoon; *head of humerus*; *head of radius*; *the head of a sperm*; **head of femur** = rounded projecting end part of the thigh bone which joins the acetabulum at the hip **(d)** most important person; *he's the head of the anatomy department*; *she was head of the research unit for some years* **2** *verb* **(a)** to be the first, to lead; *his name heads the list* **(b)** to go towards; *they are heading north*; *he headed for the administrator's office*

headache ['hedeɪk] *noun* pain in the head, caused by changes in pressure in the blood vessels feeding the brain which act on the nerves; *I must lie down - I've got a headache*; *she can't come with us because she has got a headache*; **cluster headache** = headache which occurs behind one eye for a short period; **migraine headache** = very severe throbbing headache which can be accompanied by nausea, vomiting, visual disturbance and vertigo; **tension headache** *or* **muscular contraction headache** = headache over all the head, caused by worry or stress, and thought to result from chronic contraction of the muscles of the scalp and neck

COMMENT: headaches can be caused by a blow to the head, by lack of sleep or food, by eye strain, sinus infections and many other causes. Mild headaches can be treated with an analgesic and rest. Severe headaches which recur may be caused by serious disorders in the head or nervous system

heal [hi:l] *verb (of wound)* to mend, to become better; *after six weeks, his wound had still not healed*; *a minor cut will heal faster if it is left without a bandage*

healing ['hi:lɪŋ] *noun* process of getting better; *a substance which will accelerate the healing process*

health [helθ] *noun* being well, not being ill; state of being free from physical or mental disease; *he's in good health*; *she had suffered from bad health for some years*; *the council said that fumes from the factory were a danger to public health*; *all cigarette packets carry a government health warning*; **Medical Officer of Health (MOH)** = formerly, a local government official in charge of the health services in an area; **Health and Safety at Work Act** = Act of Parliament which rules how the health of workers should be protected by the companies they work for; **District Health Authority (DHA** *or* **HA)** = administrative unit in the National Health Service which is responsible for health services in a district; **Regional Health Authority (RHA)** = administrative unit in the National Health Service which is responsible for planning the health service in a region; **health care** = general treatment of patients, especially using preventive measures to stop a disease from occurring; **health centre** = public building in which a group of doctors practise, which contains a children's clinic, etc.; **health education** = teaching people (school children and adults) to do things to improve their health, such as taking more exercise, stopping smoking, etc.; **health insurance** = insurance which pays the cost of treatment for illness, especially when travelling abroad; *US* **Health Maintenance Organization (HMO)** = private doctors' practice offering health care to patients who pay a regular subscription; **Environmental Health Officer (EHO)** *or* **Public Health Inspector** = official of a local authority who examines the environment and tests for air pollution, bad sanitation, noise pollution, etc.; **health service** = organization in a district or country which is in charge of doctors, hospitals, etc.; **National Health Service (NHS)** = British organization which provides medical services free of charge or at a low cost, to the whole population; **Health Service Commissioner** *or* **Health Service Ombudsman** = official who investigates complaints from the public about the National Health Service; **health tax** = tax which will be used to help fund the health service; *they have proposed a health tax on tobacco*; **health visitor** = registered nurse with qualifications in obstetrics, midwifery and preventive medicine, who visits babies and sick patients at home and advises on treatment

---

large numbers of women are dying of cervical cancer in health authorities where the longest backlog of smear tests exists

Nursing Times

---

the HA told the Health Ombudsman that nursing staff and students now received full training in the use of the nursing process

Nursing Times

---

in the UK, the main screen is carried out by health visitors at 6-10 months

Lancet

---

healthy [ˈhelθi] *adjective* (i) well, not ill; (ii) likely to make you well; *being a farmer is a healthy job*; *people are healthier than they were fifty years ago*; *this town is the healthiest place in England*; *if you eat a healthy diet and take plenty of exercise there is no reason why you should fall ill* (NOTE: **healthy - healthier - healthiest**)

hear [hɪə] *verb* **(a)** to sense sounds with the ears; *can you hear footsteps?*; *I can't hear what you're saying because of the noise of the aircraft*; *I heard her shut the front door*; *he must be getting deaf, because often he doesn't hear the telephone* **(b)** to get information; *have you heard that the Prime Minister has died?*; *where did you hear about the new drug for treating AIDS?* (NOTE: **hearing - heard - has heard**)

hearing [ˈhɪərɪŋ] *noun* ability to hear; function performed by the ear of sensing sounds and sending sound impulses to the brain; *his hearing is failing*; *she suffers from bad hearing*; **hearing aid** = tiny electronic device fitted into or near the ear, to improve the hearing of a deaf person by making sounds louder; **hearing loss** = deafness; **conductive hearing loss** = deafness caused by defective conduction of sound into the inner ear; **sensorineural hearing loss** = perceptive deafness, deafness caused by a disorder in the auditory nerves or the brain centres which receive impulses from the nerves; *see also* HARD (NOTE: for other terms referring to hearing, see words beginning with **audi-**)

heart [hɑːt] *noun* main organ in the body, which maintains the circulation of the blood around the body by its pumping action; *the doctor listened to his heart*; *she has heart trouble*; **chambers of the heart** = the two sections (an atrium and a ventricle) of each side of the heart; **heart block** = slowing of the action of the heart because the impulses from the SA node to the ventricles are delayed or interrupted; **heart disease** = any disease of the heart in general; *he has a long history of heart disease*; **heart failure** = failure of the heart to maintain the output of blood to meet the demands of the body; **heart massage** = treatment to make a heart which has stopped beating start working again; **heart murmur** = abnormal sound made by turbulent flow, usually the result of an abnormality in the structure of the heart; **heart rate** = number of times the heart beats per minute; **heart sounds** = two different sounds made by the heart as it beats; *see* LUBB-DUPP; **heart stoppage** = situation where the heart has stopped beating; **heart surgeon** = surgeon who specializes in operations on the heart; **heart surgery** = surgical operation to remedy a condition of the heart; **heart transplant** = surgical operation to transplant a heart into a patient

---

COMMENT: the heart is situated slightly to the left of the central part of the chest, between the lungs. It is divided into two parts by a vertical septum; each half is itself divided into an upper chamber (the atrium) and a lower chamber (the ventricle). The veins bring blood from the body into the right atrium; from there it passes into the right ventricle and is pumped into the pulmonary artery which takes it to the lungs. Oxygenated blood returns from the lungs to the left atrium, passes to the left ventricle and from there is pumped into the aorta for circulation round the arteries. The heart expands and contracts by the force of the heart muscle (the myocardium) under impulses from the sinoatrial node, and a normal heart beats about 70 times a minute; the contracting beat as it pumps blood out (the systole) is followed by a weaker diastole, where the muscles relax to allow blood to flow back into the heart. In a heart attack, part of the myocardium is deprived of blood because of a clot in a coronary artery; this has an effect on the rhythm of the heartbeat and can be fatal. In heart block, impulses from the sinoatrial node fail to reach the ventricles properly; there are either longer impulses (first degree block) or missing impulses (second degree block) or no impulses at all (complete heart block), in which case the ventricles continue to beat slowly and independently of the SA node

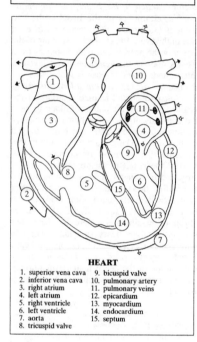

HEART

1. superior vena cava
2. inferior vena cava
3. right atrium
4. left atrium
5. right ventricle
6. left ventricle
7. aorta
8. tricuspid valve
9. bicuspid valve
10. pulmonary artery
11. pulmonary veins
12. epicardium
13. myocardium
14. endocardium
15. septum

heart attack ['hɑːt ə'tæk] *noun* condition where the heart suffers from defective blood supply because one of the arteries becomes blocked by a blood clot (coronary thrombosis), causing myocardial ischaemia and myocardial infarction

heartbeat ['hɑːtbiːt] *noun* regular noise made by the heart as it pumps blood

heartburn ['hɑːtbɜːn] *noun* pyrosis or indigestion, causing a burning feeling in the stomach and oesophagus, and a flow of acid saliva into the mouth

heart-lung ['hɑːtlʌŋ] *noun* referring to both the heart and the lungs; **heart-lung machine** = cardiopulmonary bypass, a machine used to pump blood round the body of a patient and maintain the supply of oxygen to the blood during heart surgery; **heart-lung transplant** = operation to transplant a new heart and lungs into a patient (NOTE: for other terms referring to the heart, see also words beginning with **card-** or **cardi-**)

heat [hiːt] **1** *noun* being hot; *the heat of the sun made the road melt*; **heat cramp** = cramp produced by loss of salt from the body in very hot conditions; **heat exhaustion** = collapse due to overexertion in hot conditions; **heat rash** = MILIARIA; **heat spots** = little red spots which develop on the face in very hot weather; **heat treatment** *or* **heat therapy** = using heat (from hot lamps or hot water) to treat certain conditions, such as arthritis and bad circulation **2** *verb* to make hot; *the solution should be heated to 25°C*

COMMENT: heat exhaustion involves loss of salt and body fluids; heat stroke is also caused by high outside temperatures, but in this case the body is incapable of producing sweat and the body temperature rises, leading to headaches, stomach cramps and sometimes loss of consciousness

heatstroke ['hiːtstrəuk] *noun* condition where the patient becomes too hot and his body temperature rises abnormally

heavily ['hevɪli] *adverb* strongly; *she was breathing heavily*; *he was heavily sedated*

heavy ['hevi] *adjective* **(a)** which weighs a lot; *this box is so heavy I can hardly lift it*; *people with back trouble should not lift heavy weights*; *he got a slipped disc from trying to lift a heavy box* **(b)** strong; in large quantities; *don't go to bed after you've had a heavy meal*; *she has a heavy cold and has to stay in bed*; *the patient was under heavy sedation*; **heavy drinker** = person who drinks a large amount of alcohol; **heavy smoker** = person who smokes large numbers of cigarettes (NOTE: **heavy - heavier - heaviest**)

hebephrenia *or* **hebephrenic schizophrenia** [hiːbɪ'friːniə or hiːbɪ'frenɪk skɪtsəu'friːniə] *noun* condition where the patient (usually an adolescent) has hallucinations, delusions, and deterioration of personality, talks rapidly and generally acts in a strange manner

Heberden's node ['hiːbədənz 'nəud] *noun* small bony lump which develops on the terminal phalanges of fingers in osteoarthritis

hebetude ['hebɪtjuːd] *noun* stupidity, dullness of the senses during acute fever, being uninterested in one's surroundings and not responding to stimuli

hectic ['hektɪk] *adjective* which recurs regularly; **hectic fever** = attack of fever which occurs each day in patients suffering from tuberculosis

heel [hiːl] *noun* **(a)** back part of the foot; **heel bone** = calcaneus, the bone forming the heel, beneath the talus **(b)** block under the back part of a shoe; *she wore shoes with very high heels*

Hegar's sign ['heɪgəz 'saɪn] *noun* way of detecting pregnancy, by inserting the fingers into the uterus and pressing with the other hand on the pelvic cavity to feel if the neck of the uterus has become soft

height [haɪt] *noun* **(a)** measurement of how tall or how high someone or something is; *he is of above average height*; *the patient's height is 1.23m* **(b)** high place; *he has a fear of heights*

helcoplasty ['helkəʊplæsti] *noun* skin graft to cover an ulcer to aid healing

Helicobacter pylori ['helikəʊbæktə paɪ'lɔːriː] *noun* bacterium found in gastric secretions strongly associated with duodenal ulcers and possibly with gastric carcinoma

heliotherapy [hiːləʊ'θerəpi] *noun* treatment of patients by sunlight or sunbathing

helium ['hiːliəm] *noun* very light gas used in combination with oxygen, especially to relieve asthma or sickness caused by decompression (NOTE: chemical symbol is **He**)

helix ['hiːlɪks] *noun* curved outer edge of the ear

Heller's operation ['heləz ɒpə'reɪʃn] = CARDIOMYOTOMY

Heller's test ['heləz 'test] *noun* test for protein in the urine

helminth ['helmɪnθ] *noun* general term for a parasitic worm (such as a tapeworm or fluke)

helminthiasis [helmɪn'θaɪəsɪs] *noun* infestation with parasitic worms

heloma [hɪ'ləʊmə] *noun* corn, hard lump of skin, usually on the foot or hand where something has pressed or rubbed against the skin

help [help] **1** *noun* **(a)** something which makes it easier for you to do something; *he cut his nails with the help of a pair of scissors*; *do you need any help with the patients?*; **home help** = person who helps an invalid or handicapped person in their house by doing housework **(b)** making someone safe; *they went to his help* = they went to rescue him; *she was calling for help*; *they phoned the police for help* **2** *verb* **(a)** to make it easier for someone to do something;

she has a home help to help her with the housework; *she got another nurse to help put the patients to bed*; *he helped the old lady across the street* **(b)** (used with **cannot**) not to be able to stop doing something; *she can't help dribbling*; *he can't help it if he's deaf* **3** *interjection* **help!** = call showing that someone is in difficulties; *help! help! call a doctor quickly! help, the patient is vomiting blood!*

helper ['helpə] *noun* person who helps

helpful ['helpfʊl] *adjective* which helps

helping hand ['helpɪŋ 'hænd] *noun* handle or grip fitted to a wall, bath side, etc., to help a patient to stand up, etc.

helpless ['helpləs] *adjective* not able to do anything

hem- [hiːm] *US see* HAEM-

hemeralopia [hemərə'ləʊpiə] *noun* day blindness, being able to see better in bad light than in ordinary daylight (usually a congenital condition)

hemi- ['hemi] *prefix* meaning half

hemianopia [hemiə'nəʊpiə] *noun* state of partial blindness, where the patient has only half the normal field of vision in each eye

hemiatrophy [hemi'ætrəfi] *noun* condition where half of the body or half of an organ or part is atrophied

hemiballismus [hemibə'lɪzməs] *noun* sudden movement of the limbs on one side of the body, caused by a disease of the basal ganglia

hemicolectomy [hemikə'lektəmi] *noun* surgical removal of part of the colon

hemicrania [hemi'kreɪniə] *noun* headache, migraine in one side of the head

hemimelia [hemi'miːliə] *noun* congenital condition where the patient has excessively short or defective arms and legs

hemiparesis [hemipə'riːsɪs] *noun* slight paralysis of the muscles of one side of the body

hemiplegia [hemi'pliːdʒə] *noun* severe paralysis affecting one side of the body due to damage of the central nervous system; *compare* DIPLEGIA

hemiplegic [hemi'pliːdʒɪk] *adjective* referring to paralysis of one side of the body

hemisphere ['hemɪsfɪə] *noun* half of a sphere; **cerebral hemisphere** = one of the two halves of the cerebrum

hemo- ['hi:məʊ] *see* HAEMO-

hemp [hemp] *see* INDIAN HEMP

Henle's loop ['henli:z 'lu:p] *see* LOOP

Henoch's purpura ['henəks 'pɜːpjʊrə] *noun* blood disorder of children, where the skin becomes dark blue and they suffer abdominal pains

heparin ['hepərɪn] *noun* anticoagulant substance found in the liver and lungs, and also produced artificially for use in the treatment of thrombosis

hepat- *or* **hepato-** [hɪ'pæt *or* 'hepətəʊ] *prefix* referring to the liver

hepatalgia [hepə'tældʒə] *noun* pain in the liver

hepatectomy [hepə'tektəmi] *noun* surgical removal of part of the liver

hepatic [hɪ'pætɪk] *adjective* referring to the liver; **hepatic artery** = artery which takes the blood to the liver; **hepatic cells** = epithelial cells of the liver acini; **hepatic duct** = duct which links the liver to the bile duct leading to the duodenum; **common hepatic duct** = duct from the liver formed when the right and left hepatic ducts join; **hepatic flexure** = bend in the colon, where the ascending and transverse colons join; **hepatic portal system** = group of veins linking to form the portal vein, which brings blood from the pancreas, spleen, gall bladder and the abdominal part of the alimentary canal to the liver; **hepatic vein** = vein which takes blood from the liver to the inferior vena cava

hepaticostomy [hɪpætɪ'kɒstəmi] *noun* surgical operation to make an opening in the hepatic duct taking bile from the liver

hepatis ['hepətɪs] *see* PORTA

hepatitis [hepə'taɪtɪs] *noun* inflammation of the liver through disease or drugs; **infectious virus hepatitis** *or* **infective hepatitis** *or* **hepatitis A** = hepatitis transmitted by a carrier through food or seawater; **hepatitis A virus (HAV)** = virus which causes hepatitis A; **serum hepatitis** *or* **hepatitis B** *or* **B viral hepatitis** = serious form of hepatitis transmitted by infected blood, unsterilized surgical instruments, shared needles or sexual intercourse; **hepatitis B virus (HBV)** = virus which causes hepatitis B

COMMENT: infectious hepatitis and serum hepatitis are caused by different viruses (called A and B), and having had one does not give immunity against an attack of the other. Hepatitis B is more serious than the

A form, and can vary in severity from a mild gastrointestinal upset to severe liver failure and death. Hepatitis C and D have also been identified

hepatoblastoma [hepətəʊblæ'stəʊmə] *noun* malignant tumour in the liver, made up of epithelial-type cells often with areas of immature cartilage and embryonic bone

hepatocele ['hepətəʊsi:l] *noun* hernia of the liver through the diaphragm or the abdominal wall

hepatocellular [hepətəʊ'seljʊlə] *adjective* referring to liver cells; **hepatocellular jaundice** = jaundice caused by injury to or disease of the liver cells

hepatocirrhosis [hepətəʊsə'rəʊsɪs] = CIRRHOSIS OF THE LIVER

hepatocolic ligament [hepətəʊ'kɒlɪk 'lɪgəmənt] *noun* ligament which links the gall bladder and the right flexure of the colon

hepatocyte ['hepətəʊsaɪt] *noun* liver cell which synthesizes and stores substances, and produces bile

hepatolenticular degeneration [hepətəʊlen'tɪkjʊlə dɪdʒenə'reɪʃn] = WILSON'S DISEASE

hepatoma [hepə'təʊmə] *noun* malignant tumour of the liver formed of mature cells, especially found in patients with cirrhosis

hepatomegaly [hepətəʊ'megəli] *noun* condition where the liver becomes very large

hepatotoxic [hepətəʊ'tɒksɪk] *adjective* which destroys the liver cells

herald patch ['herəld 'pætʃ] *noun* small spot of a rash (such as pityriasis rosea) which appears some time before the main rash

herb [hɜːb] *noun* plant which can be used as a medicine, to give a certain taste to food or to give a certain scent

herbal ['hɜːbl] *adjective* referring to herbs; **herbal remedies** = remedies made from plants, such as infusions made from dried leaves or flowers in hot water

herbalism ['hɜːbəlɪzm] *noun* science of treatment of illnesses or disorders by medicines extracted from plants

herbalist ['hɜːbəlɪst] *noun* person who treats illnesses or disorders by medicine extracted from plants

hereditary [hə'redətri] *adjective* which is transmitted from parents to children

heredity [hə'redəti] *noun* occurrence of physical or mental characteristics in children which are inherited from their parents

> COMMENT: the characteristics which are most commonly inherited are the pigmentation of skin and hair, eyes (including pigmentation, shortsightedness and other eye defects), blood grouping, and disorders which are caused by defects in blood composition, such as haemophilia

Hering-Breuer reflex ['herɪŋ'brɔɪə 'riːfleks] *noun* reflex which regulates breathing

hermaphrodite [hɜː'mæfrədaɪt] *noun* person with both male and female characteristics

hermaphroditism [hɜː'mæfrədaɪtɪzm] *noun* condition where a person has both male and female characteristics

hernia ['hɜːniə] *noun* condition where an organ bulges through a hole or weakness in the wall which surrounds it; **diaphragmatic hernia** = condition where the abdominal contents pass through an opening in the diaphragm into the chest (NOTE: also called in US English **upside-down stomach**); **femoral hernia** = hernia of the bowel at the top of the thigh; **hiatus hernia** = hernia where the stomach bulges through the opening in the diaphragm muscle through which the oesophagus passes; **incisional hernia** = hernia which breaks through the abdominal wall at a place where a surgical incision was made during an operation; **inguinal hernia** = hernia where the intestine bulges through the muscles in the groin; **irreducible hernia** = hernia where the organ cannot be returned to its normal position; **reducible hernia** = hernia where the organ can be pushed back into place without an operation; **reduction of a hernia** = putting a hernia back into the correct position; **strangulated hernia** = condition where part of the intestine is squeezed in a hernia and the supply of blood to it is cut off; **umbilical hernia** = exomphalos, hernia which bulges at the navel, usually in young children

hernial ['hɜːniəl] *adjective* referring to a hernia; **hernial sac** = sac formed where a membrane has pushed through a cavity in the body

herniated ['hɜːnieɪtɪd] *adjective* (organ) which has developed a hernia; **herniated disc** = slipped disc

herniation [hɜːni'eɪʃn] *noun* development of a hernia

hernioplasty ['hɜːniəʊplæsti] *noun* surgical operation to reduce a hernia

herniorrhaphy [hɜːni'ɔːrəfi] *noun* radical surgical operation to repair a hernia

herniotomy [hɜːni'ɒtəmi] *noun* surgical operation to relieve a hernia which results in its reduction

heroin ['herəʊɪn] *noun* narcotic drug, a white powder derived from morphine

herpangina [hɜːpæn'dʒaɪnə] *noun* infectious disease of children, where the tonsils and back of the throat become inflamed and ulcerated, caused by a Coxsackie virus

herpes ['hɜːpiːz] *noun* inflammation of the skin or mucous membrane, caused by a virus, where small blisters are formed; **herpes simplex (Type I)** = cold sore, a burning sore, usually on the lips; **herpes simplex (Type II)** *or* **genital herpes** = sexually transmitted disease which forms blisters in the genital region; **herpes zoster** = inflammation of a sensory nerve, characterized by pain along the nerve causing a line of blisters to form on the skin, usually found mainly on the abdomen or back, or on the face (NOTE: also called **shingles** *or* **zona**)

herpesvirus [hɜːpiːz'vaɪrəs] *noun* one of a group of viruses which cause herpes and chickenpox (herpesvirus Type I), and genital herpes (herpesvirus Type II)

> COMMENT: because the same virus causes herpes and chickenpox, anyone who has had chickenpox as a child carries the dormant herpesvirus in his bloodstream and can develop shingles in later life. It is not known what triggers the development of shingles, though it is known that an adult suffering from shingles can infect a child with chickenpox

herpetic [hɜː'petɪk] *adjective* referring to herpes; **post herpetic neuralgia** = pains felt after an attack of shingles

herpetiformis [həpetɪ'fɔːmɪs] *see* DERMATITIS

hetero- ['hetərəʊ] *prefix* meaning different

heterochromia [hetərəʊ'krəʊmiə] *noun* condition where the irises of the eyes are different colours

heterogametic [hetərəʊgə'metɪk] *adjective* (person) who produces gametes with different sex chromosomes (as a human male); *see note at* SEX

heterogeneous [hetərə'dʒiːniəs] *adjective* having different characteristics or qualities (NOTE: do not confuse with **heterogenous**)

heterogenous [hetə'rɒdʒinəs] *adjective* coming from a different source (NOTE: do not confuse with **heterogeneous**)

heterograft ['hetərəugrɑːft] *noun* tissue taken from one species and grafted onto an individual of another species; *see also* XENOGRAFT

heterologous [hetə'rɒləgʌs] *adjective* different, not homologous

heterophoria [hetərəu'fɔːriə] *noun* condition where if an eye is covered it tends to squint

heteroplasty ['hetərəuplæsti] *noun* = HETEROGRAFT

heteropsia [hetə'rɒpsiə] *noun* condition where the two eyes see differently

heterosexual [hetərə'sekʃuəl] **1** *adjective* referring to the normal relation of the two sexes **2** *noun* person who is sexually attracted to persons of the opposite sex

heterosexuality [hetərəsekʃu'æləti] *noun* condition where a person has sexual attraction towards persons of the opposite sex; *compare* BISEXUAL, HOMOSEXUAL

heterosis [hetə'rəusıs] *noun* hybrid vigour, the increase in size, rate of growth, fertility or resistance to disease found in offspring of a cross between two species

heterotopia [hetərəu'təupiə] *noun* state where an organ is placed in a different position from normal or is malformed or deformed; development of tissue which is not natural to the part in which it is produced

heterotropia [hetərəu'trəupiə] *noun* strabismus, a condition where the two eyes focus on different points

HFEA = HUMAN FERTILIZATION AND EMBRYOLOGY AUTHORITY

Hg *chemical symbol for* mercury

hGH = HUMAN GROWTH HORMONE

hiatus [haı'eıtəs] *noun* opening or space; **hiatus hernia** *US* **hiatal hernia** = hernia where the stomach bulges through the opening in the diaphragm muscle through which the oesophagus passes; **oesophageal hiatus and aortic hiatus** = openings in the diaphragm through which the oesophagus and aorta pass

Hib [hıb] *noun* haemophilus influenzae type b, bacterium which causes meningitis; **Hib vaccine** = vaccine used to inoculate against the Hib bacterium in order to prevent meningitis

hiccup *or* **hiccough** ['hıkʌp] **1** *noun* singultus, a spasm in the diaphragm which causes a sudden inhalation of breath followed by sudden closure of the glottis which makes a characteristic sound; *she had an attack of hiccups or a hiccuping attack*; *he got the hiccups from laughing too much, and found he couldn't stop them* **2** *verb* to make a hiccup; *she patted him on the back when he suddenly started to hiccup*; *do you know how to stop someone hiccuping?*; *he hiccuped so loudly that everyone in the restaurant looked at him*

COMMENT: many cures have been suggested for hiccups, but the main treatment is to try to get the patient to think about something else. A drink of water, holding the breath and counting, breathing into a paper bag, are all recommended

hidr- [haıdr] *prefix* meaning sweat

hidradenitis [haıdrədə'naıtıs] *noun* inflammation of the sweat glands

hidrosis [haı'drəusıs] *noun* (especially excessive) sweating

hidrotic [haı'drɒtık] **1** *adjective* referring to sweating **2** *noun* substance which makes someone sweat

Higginson's syringe ['hıgınsənz sı'rınʒ] *noun* syringe with a rubber bulb in the centre that allows flow in one direction only (used mainly to give enemas)

high [haı] *adjective* **(a)** tall, reaching far from the ground level; *the hospital building is 60 m high*; *the operating theatre has a high ceiling* **(b)** *(referring to numbers)* big; *the patient has a very high temperature*; *there was a high level of glucose in the patient's blood*; **high blood pressure** = hypertension, condition where the pressure of blood in the arteries is too high, causing the heart to strain; **high-energy foods** = foods containing a large number of calories, such as fats or carbohydrates, which give a lot of energy when they are broken down; **high temperature short time (HTST) method** = usual method of pasteurizing milk, where the milk is heated to 72°C for 15 seconds and then rapidly cooled (NOTE: **high - higher - highest**)

highly strung ['haɪli 'strʌŋ] *adjective* very nervous and tense; *she is highly strung, so don't make comments about her appearance, or she will burst into tears*

Highmore ['haɪmɔː] *noun* **antrum of Highmore** = MAXILLARY SINUS

high-risk ['haɪ'rɪsk] *adjective* (person) who is very likely to catch or develop a disease, develop a cancer or suffer an accident; *high-risk categories of worker*; **high-risk patient** = patient who has a high risk of catching an infection or developing a disease

hilar ['haɪlə] *adjective* referring to a hilum

hilum ['haɪləm] *noun* hollow where blood vessels or nerve fibres enter an organ such as a kidney or lung (NOTE: the plural is **hila**)

hindbrain ['haɪndbreɪn] *noun* part of brain of an embryo, from which the medulla oblongata, the pons and the cerebellum eventually develop

hindgut ['haɪndgʌt] *noun* part of an embryo which develops into the colon and rectum

hinge joint ['hɪndʒ 'dʒɔɪnt] *noun* synovial joint (like the knee) which allows two bones to move in one direction only; *compare* BALL AND SOCKET JOINT

hip [hɪp] *noun* ball and socket joint where the thigh bone or femur joins the acetabulum of the hip bone; **hip bath** = small low bath in which a person can sit but not lie down; **hip bone** = the innominate bone, a bone made of the ilium, the ischium and the pubis which are fused together, forming part of the pelvic girdle; **hip fracture** = fracture of the ball at the top of the femur; **hip girdle** = pelvic girdle, the sacrum and the two hip bones; **hip joint** = joint where the rounded end of the femur joins a socket in the acetabulum; *see illustration at* PELVIS; **hip replacement** = surgical operation to replace the whole ball and socket joint with an artificial one

Hippel-Lindau ['hɪpəl'lɪndaʊ] *see* VON HIPPEL-LINDAU

hippocampal formation [hɪpə'kæmpl fɔː'meɪʃn] *noun* curved pieces of cortex inside each part of the cerebrum

hippocampus [hɪpə'kæmpəs] *noun* long rounded elevation projecting into the lateral ventricle in the brain

Hippocratic oath [hɪpə'krætɪk 'əʊθ] *noun* oath sworn by medical students when they become doctors, in which they swear not to do anything to harm their patients and not to tell anyone the details of each patient's case

hippus ['hɪpəs] *noun* alternating rapid contraction and dilatation of the pupil of the eye

Hirschsprung's disease ['hɪrʃsprʌŋz dɪ'ziːz] *noun* congenital condition where parts of the lower colon lack nerve cells, making peristalsis impossible, so that food accumulates in the upper colon which becomes swollen

hirsutism ['hɜːsjuːtɪzm] *noun* having excessive hair, especially condition where a woman grows hair on the body in the same way as a man

hirudin [hɪ'ruːdɪn] *noun* anticoagulant substance produced by leeches, which is injected into the bloodstream while the leech is feeding

His [hɪs] *noun* **bundle of His** = atrioventricular bundle, a bundle of modified cardiac muscle which conducts impulses from the atrioventricular node to the septum and then divides to connect with the ventricles, causing synchronization of cardiac contraction

histamine ['hɪstəmiːn] *noun* substance released from mast cells throughout the body which stimulates tissues in various ways; *excess of histamine causes inflammation of the tissues*; *the presence of substances to which a patient is allergic releases large amounts of histamine into the* blood; **histamine receptor** = cell which is stimulated by histamine, H1 found in mast cells involved in allergic reactions, H2 in the stomach involved in gastric acid secretion; **histamine test** = test to determine the acidity of gastric juice; *US* **histamine headache** = HISTAMINIC HEADACHE

COMMENT: histamines dilate the blood vessels (giving nettlerash) or constrict the muscles of the bronchi (giving asthmatic attacks)

histaminic [hɪstə'mɪnɪk] *adjective* referring to histamines; **histaminic headache** = headache affecting the region over the external carotid artery, caused by release of histamines (and associated with rise in temperature and watery eyes) (NOTE: also called **Horton's disease**)

histidine ['hɪstədiːn] *noun* amino acid which may be a precursor of histamine

histiocyte [ˈhɪstiəʊsaɪt] *noun* macrophage of the connective tissue, involved in tissue defence

histiocytoma [hɪstiəʊsaɪˈtəʊmə] *noun* tumour containing histiocytes

histiocytosis [hɪstiəʊsaɪˈtəʊsɪs] *noun* condition where histiocytes are present in the blood; **histiocytosis X** = any form of histiocytosis (such as Hand-Schüller-Christian disease) where the cause is not known

histo- [ˈhɪstəʊ] *prefix* referring to tissue

histochemistry [hɪstəʊˈkemɪstri] *noun* study of the chemical constituents of cells and tissues and also their function and distribution, using a light or electron microscope to evaluate the stains

histocompatibility [hɪstəʊkəmpætəˈbɪləti] *noun* compatibility between antigens of donors and recipients of transplanted tissues

histocompatible [hɪstəʊkəmˈpætɪbl] *adjective* (two organisms) which have tissues which are antigenically compatible

histogenesis [hɪstəʊˈdʒenəsɪs] *noun* formation and development of tissue from the embryological germ layer

histoid [ˈhɪstɔɪd] *adjective* made of or developed from a particular tissue; like normal tissue

histological [hɪstəˈlɒdʒɪkl] *adjective* referring to histology

histology [hɪˈstɒlədʒi] *noun* study of anatomy of tissue cells and minute cellular structure, done using a microscope after the cells have been stained

histolysis [hɪˈstɒləsɪs] *noun* disintegration of tissue

histolytica [hɪstəˈlɪtɪkə] *see* ENTAMOEBA

histoplasmosis [hɪstəʊplæzˈməʊsɪs] *noun* lung disease caused by infection with a fungus *Histoplasma*

history [ˈhɪstri] *noun* study of what happened in the past; *he has a history of serious illness or a history of Parkinsonism*; **case history** = details of what has happened to a patient undergoing treatment; **medical history** = details of a patient's medical records over a period of time; **to take a patient's history** = to ask a patient to tell his case history in his own words on being admitted to hospital

these children gave a typical history of exercise-induced asthma

Lancet

the need for evaluation of patients with a history of severe heart disease

Southern Medical Journal

histotoxic [hɪstəʊˈtɒksɪk] *adjective* (substance) which is poisonous to tissue

HIV [ˈeɪtʃ ˈaɪ ˈviː] = HUMAN IMMUNODEFICIENCY VIRUS; **HIV-negative** = (patient) who has been tested and shown not to have HIV; **HIV-positive** = (patient) who has been tested and shown to have HIV; *tests showed that he was HIV-positive*; *the hospital is carrying out screening tests for HIV infection*; *HIV-infected patients need careful counselling*

COMMENT: HIV is the virus which causes AIDS. Two strains of HIV virus have been identified: HIV-1 and HIV-2; a third, HIV-3, is claimed to exist but it is, as yet, unconfirmed

HIV-associated dementia is characterized by psychomotor slowing and inattentiveness

British Journal of Nursing

hives [haɪvz] *noun* urticaria or nettlerash, an affliction of the skin where white, pink or red patches are formed which itch or sting; **giant hives** = ANGIONEUROTIC OEDEMA

HLA [ˈeɪtʃ ˈel ˈeɪ] = HUMAN LEUCOCYTE ANTIGEN

HLA system [ˈeɪtʃ ˈel ˈeɪ ˈsɪstəm] *noun* system of HLA antigens on the surface of cells which need to be histocompatible to allow transplants to take place

COMMENT: HLA-A is the most important of the antigens responsible for rejection of transplants

HMO [ˈeɪtʃ ˈem ˈəʊ] *US* = HEALTH MAINTENANCE ORGANIZATION

hoarse [hɔːs] *adjective* (voice) which is harsh and rough; *he became hoarse after shouting too much*; *she spoke in a hoarse whisper*

hoarseness [ˈhɔːsnəs] *noun* harsh and rough sound of the voice, often caused by laryngitis

hobnail liver [ˈhɒbneɪl ˈlɪvə] *noun* atrophic cirrhosis, advanced portal cirrhosis in which the liver has become considerably smaller, where clumps of new cells are formed on the surface of the liver where fibrous tissue has replaced damaged liver cells

Hodgkin's disease [ˈhɒdʒkɪnz dɪˈziːz] *noun* malignant disease in which the lymph glands are enlarged and there is an increase in the lymphoid tissues in the liver, spleen and other organs; *see also* PEL-EBSTEIN FEVER

> COMMENT: the lymph glands swell to a very large size, and the disease can then attack the liver, spleen and bone marrow. It is frequently fatal if not treated early

hoist [hɔɪst] *noun* device with pulleys and wires for raising a bed or a patient

hole [həʊl] *noun* opening or space in something; **hole in the heart** = congenital defect where a hole exists in the wall between the two halves of the heart and allows blood to flow abnormally through the heart and lungs

Holger-Nielsen method [ˈhɒlgəˈnɪlsən ˈmeθəd] *noun* method of giving artificial ventilation by hand, where the patient lies face down and the first-aider alternately presses on his back and pulls his arms outwards

holistic [hɒˈlɪstɪk] *adjective* (method of treatment) involving all the patient's mental and family circumstances rather than just dealing with the condition from which he is suffering

hollow [ˈhɒləʊ] **1** *adjective* (space) which is empty, with nothing inside; *the surgeon inserted a hollow tube into the lung*; *the hollow cavity filled with pus* **2** *noun* recess or place which is lower than the rest of the surface

holocrine [ˈhɒləkraɪn] *adjective* (gland) which is secretory only and where the secretion is made up of disintegrated cells of the gland itself

Homans' sign [ˈhəʊmənz ˈsaɪn] *noun* pain in the calf when the foot is bent back, a sign of deep vein thrombosis

home [həʊm] **1** *noun* **(a)** place where you live; house which you live in; *are you going to be at home tomorrow?*; *the doctor told her to stay at home instead of going to work*; **home help** = person who does housework for an invalid or handicapped

person; **home nurse** = district nurse, a nurse who visits patients in their homes **(b)** house where people are looked after; *an old people's home*; **children's home** = house where children with no parents are looked after; **convalescent home** = type of hospital where patients can recover from illness or surgery; **nursing home** = house where convalescents or old people can live under medical supervision by a qualified nurse **2** *adverb* towards the place where you usually live; *I'm going home*; *I'll take it home with me*; **I usually get home at 7 o'clock** = I reach the house where I live; **she can take the bus home** = she can go to where she lives by bus (NOTE: used without a preposition: **he went home, she's coming home**)

homeo- *or* **homoeo-** [ˈhəʊmɪəʊ] *prefix* meaning like or similar

homeopathic *or* **homoeopathic** [həʊmɪəˈpæθɪk] *adjective* **(a)** referring to homeopathy; *a homeopathic clinic*; *she is having a course of homeopathic treatment* **(b)** (drug) given in very small quantities

homeopathist *or* **homoeopathist** [həʊmɪˈɒpəθɪst] *noun* person who practises homeopathy

homeopathy *or* **homoeopathy** [həʊmɪˈɒpəθi] *noun* treatment of a condition by giving the patient very small quantities of a substance which, when given to a healthy person, would cause symptoms like those of the condition being treated; *compare* ALLOPATHY

homeostasis [həʊmɪəʊˈsteɪsɪs] *noun* process by which the functions and chemistry of a cell or internal organ are kept stable, even when external conditions vary greatly

homo- [ˈhəʊməʊ] *prefix* meaning the same

homogenize [həˈmɒdʒənaɪz] *verb* to make something all the same, to give something a uniform nature; **homogenized milk** = milk where the cream has been mixed up into the milk to give the same consistency throughout

homograft [ˈhɒməgrɑːft] *noun* allograft, graft of an organ or tissue from a donor to a recipient of the same species (as from one person to another); *compare* AUTOGRAFT; *see also* ALLOGRAFT

homoiothermic [həʊmɔɪəˈθɜːmɪk] *adjective* (animal) with warm blood, warm-blooded (animal); *compare* POIKILOTHERMIC

COMMENT: warm-blooded animals are able to maintain a constant body temperature whatever the outside temperature

homologous [hɒ'mɒləgəs] *adjective* (chromosomes) which form a pair

homonymous [hə'mɒnɪməs] *adjective* affecting the two eyes in the same way; **homonymous hemianopia** = condition where the same half of the field of vision is lost in each eye

homophobia [həʊmə'fəʊbiə] *noun* fear of and hostility towards homosexuals

homoplasty ['həʊməʊplæsti] *noun* surgery to replace lost tissues by grafting similar tissues from another person

homosexual [həʊmə'sekʃuəl] **1** *adjective* referring to homosexuality **2** *noun* person who is sexually attracted to people of the same sex, especially a man who experiences sexual attraction for other males

homosexuality [həʊməsekʃu'æləti] *noun* condition where a person experiences sexual attraction for persons of the same sex, has sexual relations with persons of the same sex; *compare* BISEXUAL, HETEROSEXUAL, LESBIAN (NOTE: although **homosexual** can apply to both males and females, it is commonly used for males only, and **lesbian** is used for females)

hook [hʊk] **1** *noun* surgical instrument with a bent end used for holding structures apart in operations **2** *verb* to attach something with a hook

hookworm ['hʊkwɜːm] = ANCYLOSTOMA; **hookworm disease** = ANCYLOSTOMIASIS

hordeolum [hɔː'dɪələm] *noun* stye, an infection of the gland at the base of an eyelash

horizontal [hɒrɪ'zɒntl] *adjective* which is lying flat or at a right angle to the vertical; **horizontal plane** = TRANSVERSE PLANE

hormonal [hɔː'məʊnl] *adjective* referring to hormones

hormone ['hɔːməʊn] *noun* substance which is produced by one part of the body, especially the endocrine glands and is carried to another part of the body by the bloodstream where it has particular effects or functions; **growth hormone** = hormone which stimulates the growth of long bones;

sex hormones = oestrogens and androgens which promote the growth of secondary sexual characteristics; **female sex hormone** = OESTROGEN; **male sex hormone** = ANDROGEN; **hormone replacement therapy (HRT)** *or* **hormone therapy** = (i) treatment for a patient whose endocrine glands have been removed; (ii) generally, treatment to relieve the symptoms of the menopause by supplying oestrogen and reducing the risk of osteoporosis

horn [hɔːn] *noun* **(a)** *(in animals)* hard tissue which protrudes from the head **(b)** *(in humans)* (i) tissue which grows out of an organ; (ii) one of the H-shaped limbs of grey matter seen in a cross-section of the spinal cord; (iii) extension of the pulp chamber of a tooth towards the cusp

Horner's syndrome ['hɔːnəz 'sɪndrəum] *noun* condition caused by paralysis of the sympathetic nerve in one side of the neck, making the patient's eyelids hang down and the pupils contract

horny ['hɔːni] *adjective* like horn, hard (skin) (NOTE: for terms referring to horny tissue, see words beginning with **kerat-**)

horseshoe kidney ['hɔːsʃuː 'kɪdni] *noun* congenital defect of the kidney, where sometimes the upper but usually the lower parts of both kidneys are joined together

Horton's disease *or* **Horton's headache** ['hɔːtənz dɪ'ziːz *or* 'hɔːtənz 'hedeɪk] *noun (temporal arteritis)* headache repeatedly affecting the region over the temporal artery (a branch of the carotid artery)

hose [həʊz] *noun* **(a)** long rubber or plastic tube **(b)** stocking; **surgical** *or* **elastic hose** = special stocking worn to support and relieve varicose veins

hospice ['hɒspɪs] *noun* hospital which cares for terminally ill patients

hospital ['hɒspɪtl] *noun* place where sick or injured people are looked after; *she's so ill she has been sent to hospital*; *he's been in hospital for several days*; *the children's hospital is at the end of our street*; **cottage hospital** = small local hospital set in pleasant gardens in the country; **day hospital** = hospital where the patients are treated during the day and go home in the evenings; **general hospital** = hospital which cares for all types of patient; **geriatric hospital** = hospital which specializes in the treatment of old people; **isolation hospital** = hospital where patients suffering from dangerous infectious diseases can be isolated; **mental hospital** = hospital for the treatment of mentally ill patients; **private hospital** = hospital which takes only paying patients; **teaching hospital** = hospital attached to a medical school where student doctors work and study as part of their training; **Hospital Activity Analysis** = regular detailed report on patients in hospitals, including information about treatment, length of stay, death rate, etc.; **hospital bed** = (i) special type of bed used in hospitals; (ii) place in a hospital which can be occupied by a patient; *a hospital bed is needed if the patient has to have traction*; *there will be no reduction in the number of hospital beds*; **hospital care** = hospitalization, treatment in hospital; **hospital trust** = self-governing hospital, a hospital which earns its revenue from services provided to the District Health Authorities and family doctors

hospitalization [hɒspɪtlaɪˈzeɪʃn] *noun* sending someone to hospital; *the doctor recommended immediate hospitalization*

hospitalize [ˈhɒspɪtlaɪz] *verb* to send someone to hospital; *he is so ill that he has had to be hospitalized*

host [həʊst] *noun* person or animal on which a parasite lives

hot [hɒt] *adjective* very warm; of a high temperature; *the water in my bath is too hot*; *if you're hot, take your coat off*; *affected skin will feel hot*; **hot flush** = condition in menopausal women, where the patient becomes hot and sweats, often accompanied by redness of the skin (NOTE: **hot - hotter - hottest)**

hour [ˈaʊə] *noun* period of time lasting sixty minutes; *there are 24 hours in a day*; *the hours of work are from 9 to 5*; *when is your lunch hour?* = when do you stop work for lunch?; **I'll be ready in a quarter of an hour** *or* **in half an hour** = in 15 minutes or 30 minutes

hourglass contraction [ˈaʊəglɑːs kənˈtrækʃn] *noun* condition where an organ (such as the stomach) is constricted in the centre

hourly [ˈaʊəli] *adjective* happening every hour; *repeat the treatment hourly*

house [haʊs] *noun* building which someone lives in; *he has a flat in the town and a house in the country*; *all the houses in our street look the same*; *his house has*

six bedrooms; **house mite** = small insect living in houses, which can cause an allergic reaction; **house officer** = doctor who works in a hospital (as house surgeon or house physician) during the final year of training before registration by the GMC

housemaid's knee [ˈhaʊsmeɪdz ˈniː] *noun* prepatellar bursitis, a condition where the fluid sac in the knee becomes inflamed, caused by kneeling on hard surfaces

houseman [ˈhaʊsmən] *noun* house surgeon or house physician (NOTE: the American English is **intern**)

HRT [ˈeɪtʃ ˈɑː ˈtiː] = HORMONE REPLACEMENT THERAPY

HTST method [ˈeɪtʃ ˈtiː ˈes ˈtiː ˈmeθəd] = HIGH TEMPERATURE SHORT TIME METHOD

Huhner's test [ˈhuːnəz ˈtest] *noun* test carried out several hours after sexual intercourse to determine the number and motility of spermatozoa

human [ˈhjuːmən] **1** *adjective* referring to any man, woman or child; **a human being** = a person; **human chorionic gonadotrophin (hCG)** = hormone produced by the placenta, which suppresses the mother's normal menstrual cycle during pregnancy; it is found in the urine during pregnancy; it can be given by injection to encourage ovulation and help a woman to become pregnant; **human immunodeficiency virus (HIV)** = virus which causes AIDS; *see* AIDS, HIV; **human leucocyte antigen (HLA)** = any of the system of antigens on the surface of cells which need to be histocompatible to allow transplants to take place; *see* HLA SYSTEM **2** *noun* person; *most animals are afraid of humans*

humeroulnar joint [hjuːmərəʊˈʌlnə ˈdʒɔɪnt] *noun* part of the elbow joint, where the trochlea of the humerus and the trochlear notch of the ulna articulate

humerus [ˈhjuːmərəs] *noun* top bone in the arm, running from the shoulder to the elbow; *see illustration at* SHOULDER (NOTE: plural is **humeri)**

humid [ˈhjuːmɪd] *adjective* which is damp, which contains moisture vapour

humidity [hjuːˈmɪdəti] *noun* measurement of how much water vapour is contained in the air

humour *US* **humor** [ˈhjuːmə] *noun* fluid in the body; **aqueous humour** = fluid in the eye between the lens and the cornea; **vitreous**

humour = jelly behind the lens in the eye; *see illustration at* EYE

hunchback ['hʌnʃbæk] *noun* (i) excessive curvature of the spine; (ii) person suffering from excessive curvature of the spine

hunger ['hʌŋgə] *noun* feeling a need to eat; **hunger pains** = pains in the abdomen when a person feels hungry (sometimes a sign of a duodenal ulcer); **air hunger** = *see* AIR

hungry ['hʌŋgri] *adjective* wanting to eat; *I'm hungry*; *are you hungry?*; *you must be hungry after that long walk*; *the patient will not be hungry after the operation*; *I'm not very hungry - I had a big breakfast* (NOTE: **hungry - hungrier - hungriest**)

Huntington's chorea ['hʌntɪŋtənz kəʊ'rɪə] *see* CHOREA

Hurler's syndrome ['hɜːləz 'sɪndrəum] = GARGOYLISM

hurry ['hʌri] **1** *noun* rush; *get out of the way - we're in a hurry!*; **he's always in a hurry** = he is always rushing about *or* doing things very fast; **what's the hurry?** = why are you going so fast? **2** *verb* to go or do something fast; to make someone go faster; *she hurried along the passage*; *you'll have to hurry if you want to see the doctor, he's just leaving the hospital*; *don't hurry - we've got plenty of time*; *don't hurry me, I'm working as fast as I can*

hurt [hɜːt] **1** *noun (used by children)* painful area; *she has a hurt on her knee* **2** *verb* (i) to have pain; (ii) to give pain; *he's hurt his hand*; *where does your foot hurt?*; *his arm is hurting so much he can't write*; *she fell down and hurt herself*; *are you hurt?*; *is he badly hurt?*; *my foot hurts*; *he was slightly hurt in the car crash*; *two players got hurt in the football game* (NOTE: **hurting - hurt - has hurt**)

husky ['hʌski] *adjective* slightly hoarse; *husky voice*

Hutchinson-Gilford syndrome ['hʌtʃɪnsən'gɪlfəd 'sɪndrəum] *noun* progeria, premature senility

Hutchinson's tooth ['hʌtʃɪnsənz 'tuːθ] *noun* narrow upper incisor tooth, with notches along the cutting edge, a symptom of congenital syphilis but also occurring naturally

hyal- ['haɪəl] *prefix* like glass

hyalin ['haɪəlɪn] *noun* transparent substance produced from collagen and deposited around blood vessels and scars when certain tissues degenerate

hyaline ['haɪəlɪn] *adjective* nearly transparent like glass; **hyaline cartilage** = type of cartilage found in the nose, larynx and joints; *see illustration at* JOINTS; **hyaline membrane disease** = respiratory distress syndrome, condition of newborn babies, where the lungs do not expand properly

hyalitis [haɪə'laɪtɪs] *noun* inflammation of the vitreous humour or the hyaloid membrane in the eye

hyaloid membrane ['haɪəlɔɪd 'membreɪn] *noun* transparent membrane round the vitreous humour in the eye

hyaluronic acid [haɪəlu'rɒnɪk 'æsɪd] *noun* substance which binds connective tissue and is found in the eyes

hyaluronidase [haɪəlu'rɒnɪdeɪz] *noun* enzyme which destroys hyaluronic acid

hybrid ['haɪbrɪd] *adjective & noun* cross between two species of plant or animal; **hybrid vigour** = increase in size, rate of growth, fertility or resistance to disease found in offspring of a cross between two species

hydatid (cyst) ['haɪdətɪd 'sɪst] *noun* cyst which covers the larvae of the tapeworm *Taenia solium*

hydatid disease *or* **hydatidosis** ['haɪdətɪd dɪ'ziːz *or* haɪdətɪ'dəusɪs] *noun* disease caused by hydatid cysts in the lung or brain

hydatidiform mole [haɪdə'tɪdɪfɔːm 'məul] *noun* growth in the uterus, which looks like a hydatid cyst, and is formed of villous sacs swollen with fluid

hydr- [haɪdr] *prefix* referring to water

hydraemia [haɪ'driːmɪə] *noun* excess of water in the blood

hydragogue ['haɪdrəgɒg] *noun* laxative, substance which produces watery faeces

hydrarthrosis [haɪdrɑː'θrəusɪs] *noun* swelling caused by excess synovial liquid at a joint

hydro- ['haɪdrəu] *prefix* referring to water

hydroa [haɪ'drəuə] *noun* eruption of small itchy blisters (as those caused by sunlight)

hydrocele ['haɪdrəusiːl] *noun* collection of watery liquid found in a cavity such as the scrotum

hydrocephalus [haɪdrəʊˈsefələs] *noun* excessive quantity of cerebrospinal fluid in the brain

hydrochloric acid (HCl) [haɪdrəʊˈklɒrɪk ˈæsɪd] *noun* acid found in the gastric juices which helps the maceration of food

hydrocolpos [haɪdrəʊˈkɒlpəs] *noun* cyst in the vagina containing clear fluid

hydrocortisone [haɪdrəʊˈkɔːtɪzəʊn] *noun* steroid hormone secreted by the adrenal cortex; used to treat rheumatism and inflammatory and allergic conditions

hydrocyanic acid (HCN) [haɪdrəʊsaɪˈænɪk ˈæsɪd] *noun* acid which forms cyanide

hydrogen [ˈhaɪdrədʒn] *noun* chemical element, a gas which combines with oxygen to form water, and with other elements to form acids, and is present in all animal tissue (NOTE: chemical symbol is **H**)

hydrogen peroxide (H₂O₂) [ˈhaɪdrədʒn pəˈrɒksaɪd] *noun* solution used as a disinfectant

hydrometer [haɪˈdrɒmɪtə] *noun* instrument which measures the density of a liquid

hydromyelia [haɪdrəʊmaɪˈiːliə] *noun* condition where fluid swells the central canal of the spinal cord

hydronephrosis [haɪdrəʊnəˈfrəʊsɪs] *noun* swelling of the pelvis of a kidney caused by accumulation of water due to infection or a kidney stone blocking the ureter

hydropericarditis *or* **hydropericardium** [haɪdrəʊperikɑːˈdaɪtɪs or haɪdrəʊperiˈkɑːdiəm] *noun* accumulation of liquid round the heart

hydrophobia [haɪdrəʊˈfəʊbiə] *noun* rabies, frequently fatal virus disease transmitted by infected animals

> COMMENT: hydrophobia affects the mental balance, and the symptoms include difficulty in breathing or swallowing and a horror of water

hydrorrhoea [haɪdrəʊˈriːə] *noun* discharge of watery fluid

hydrotherapy [haɪdrəʊˈθerəpi] *noun* type of physiotherapy, the treatment of patients with water, where the patients are put in hot baths or are encouraged to swim

hydrothorax [haɪdrəʊˈθɔːræks] *noun* collection of liquid in the pleural cavity

hydroxide [haɪˈdrɒksaɪd] *noun* chemical compound containing a hydroxyl group; **aluminium hydroxide** *US* **aluminum hydroxide (Al(OH)₃** *or* **Al₂O₃3H₂0)** = chemical substance used as an antacid

hydroxyproline [haɪdrɒksiˈprəʊliːn] *noun* amino acid present in some proteins, especially in collagen

5-hydroxy-tryptamine [ˈfaɪv haɪˈdrɒksiˈtrɪptəmiːn] *noun* serotonin, compound which exists in blood platelets and is released after tissue is injured, and is a neurotransmitter important in sleep, mood and vasoconstriction

hygiene [ˈhaɪdʒiːn] *noun* (i) being clean and keeping healthy conditions; (ii) science of health; *nurses have to maintain a strict personal hygiene*; **dental hygiene** = keeping the teeth clean and healthy; **oral hygiene** = keeping the mouth clean by gargling and mouthwashes

hygienic [haɪˈdʒiːnɪk] *adjective* (i) clean; (ii) which produces healthy conditions; *don't touch the food with dirty hands - it isn't hygienic*

hygienist [haɪˈdʒiːnɪst] *noun* person who specializes in hygiene and its application; **dental hygienist** = person who works in a dentist's surgery, cleaning teeth and gums, removing plaque from teeth and giving fluoride treatment

hymen [ˈhaɪmen] *noun* membrane which partially covers the vaginal passage in a virgin

hymenectomy [haɪməˈnektəmi] *noun* surgical removal of the hymen, operation to increase the size of the opening of the hymen; surgical removal of any membrane

hymenotomy [haɪməˈnɒtəmi] *noun* incision of the hymen during surgery

hyoglossus [haɪəʊˈglɒsəs] *noun* muscle which is attached to the hyoid bone and depresses the tongue

hyoid bone [ˈhaɪɔɪd ˈbəʊn] *noun* small U-shaped bone at the base of the tongue

hyoscine [ˈhaɪəʊsiːn] *noun* drug used as a sedative, in particular for treatment of motion sickness

hyp- *or* **hypo-** [haɪp or hɪp or ˈhaɪpəʊ] *prefix* meaning less, too little or too small; *opposite is* HYPER-

hypaemia [haɪˈpiːmiə] *noun* insufficient amount of blood in the body

hypalgesia [haɪpælˈdʒiːziə] *noun* low sensitivity to pain

hyper- [ˈhaɪpə] *prefix* meaning higher or too much; *opposite is* HYP- *or* HYPO-

hyperacidity [haɪpərəˈsɪdəti] *noun* increase in acid in the stomach

hyperactive [haɪpərˈæktɪv] *adjective* being very active

hyperactivity [haɪpəræktˈɪvəti] *noun* condition where something (a gland or a child) is too active; **attention deficit hyperactivity disorder (ADHD)** = condition where a child has an inability to concentrate and shows disruptive behaviour

hyperacusis *or* **hyperacousia** [haɪpərəˈkjuːsɪs or haɪpərəˈkjuːziə] *noun* being very sensitive to sounds

hyperaemia [haɪpərˈiːmiə] *noun* excess blood in any part of the body

hyperaesthesia [haɪpəriːsˈθiːziə] *noun* extremely high sensitivity in the skin

hyperalgesia [haɪpərælˈdʒiːziə] *noun* increased sensitivity to pain

hyperbaric [haɪpəˈbeərɪk] *adjective* (treatment) where a patient is given oxygen at high pressure, used to treat carbon monoxide poisoning

hypercalcaemia [haɪpəkælˈsiːmiə] *noun* excess of calcium in the blood

hyperchlorhydria [haɪpəklɔːˈhaɪdriə] *noun* excess of hydrochloric acid in the stomach

hyperdactylism [haɪpəˈdæktɪlɪzm] *noun* polydactylism, having more than the normal number of fingers or toes

hyperemesis gravidarum [haɪpərˈemɪsɪs grævɪˈdeərəm] *noun* uncontrollable vomiting in pregnancy

hyperglycaemia [haɪpəglaɪˈsiːmiə] *noun* excess of glucose in the blood

hyperinsulinism [haɪpərˈɪnsjʊlɪnɪzm] *noun* reaction of a diabetic to an excessive dose of insulin or to hypoglycaemia

hyperkinesia [haɪpəkɪˈniːziə] *noun* condition where there is abnormally great strength or movement; **essential hyperkinesia** = condition of children where their movements are excessive and repeated

hyperkinetic syndrome [haɪpəkɪˈnetɪk ˈsɪndrəʊm] *noun* effort syndrome, a condition where the patient experiences fatigue, shortness of breath, pain under the heart and palpitation

hyperlipidaemia [haɪpəlɪpɪˈdiːmiə] *noun* pathological increase of the amount of lipids (or fat) in the blood

hypermenorrhoea [haɪpəmenəˈriːə] *noun* menstruation in which the flow is excessive

hypermetropia *or* **hyperopia** [haɪpəmɪˈtrəʊpiə or haɪpəˈrəʊpiə] *noun* longsightedness, a condition where the patient sees more clearly objects which are a long way away, but cannot see objects which are close; *compare* MYOPIA

hypernephroma [haɪpənəˈfrəʊmə] = GRAWITZ TUMOUR

hyperopia [haɪpəˈrəʊpiə] *noun* = HYPERMETROPIA

hyperostosis [haɪpərɒˈstəʊsɪs] *noun* excessive overgrowth on the outside surface of a bone, especially the frontal bone

hyperpiesis [haɪpəpaɪˈiːsɪs] *noun* abnormally high pressure, especially of the blood

hyperpituitarism [haɪpəˈpɪtjuːətərɪzm] *noun* condition where the pituitary gland is overactive; *see also* PITUITARY

hyperplasia [haɪpəˈpleɪziə] *noun* condition in which there is an increase in the number of cells in an organ

hyperpyrexia [haɪpəpaɪˈreksiə] *noun* high body temperature (above 41.1°C)

hypersensitive [haɪpəˈsensətɪv] *adjective* (person) who reacts more strongly than normal to an antigen

hypersensitivity [haɪpəsensəˈtɪvəti] *noun* condition where the patient reacts very strongly to something (such as an allergic substance); *her hypersensitivity to dust*; *anaphylactic shock shows hypersensitivity to an injection*

hypertension [haɪpəˈtenʃn] *noun* high blood pressure, condition where the pressure of the blood in the arteries is higher than 160/95 for adults without heart disease or diabetes; **portal hypertension** = high pressure in the portal vein, caused by cirrhosis of the liver or a clot in the vein and causing internal bleeding; **pulmonary hypertension** = high blood pressure in the blood vessels supplying the lungs

COMMENT: high blood pressure can have many causes: the arteries are too narrow, causing the heart to strain; kidney disease;

Cushing's syndrome, etc. High blood pressure is treated with drugs such as beta blockers, ACE inhibitors, diuretics and calcium channel blockers

hypertensive [haɪpə'tensɪv] *adjective* referring to high blood pressure; **hypertensive headache** = headache caused by high blood pressure

hyperthermia [haɪpə'θɜːmiə] *noun* very high body temperature

hyperthyroidism [haɪpə'θaɪrɔɪdɪzm] *noun* condition where the thyroid gland is too active and swells, as in Graves' disease

hypertonia [haɪpə'təʊniə] *noun* increased rigidity and spasticity of the muscles

hypertrichosis [haɪpətraɪ'kəʊsɪs] *noun* condition where the patient has excessive growth of hair on the body or on part of the body

hypertrophic [haɪpə'trɒfɪk] *adjective* associated with hypertrophy; **hypertrophic rhinitis** = condition where the mucous membranes in the nose become thicker

hypertrophy [haɪ'pɜːtrəfi] *noun* increase in the number or size of cells in a tissue

hypertropia [haɪpə'trəʊpiə] *noun* US = HYPERMETROPIA

hyperventilate [haɪpə'ventɪleɪt] *verb* to breathe very fast; *we all hyperventilate as an expression of fear or excitement*

hyperventilation [haɪpəventɪ'leɪʃn] *noun* very fast breathing which can be accompanied by dizziness or tetany

hypervitaminosis [haɪpəvɪtəmɪ'nəʊsɪs] *noun* condition caused by taking too many synthetic vitamins, especially Vitamins A and D

hyphaema [haɪ'fiːmiə] *noun* bleeding into the front chamber of the eye

hypn- [hɪpn] *prefix* referring to sleep

hypnosis [hɪp'nəʊsɪs] *noun* state like sleep, but caused artificially, where the patient can remember forgotten events in the past, will do whatever the hypnotist tells him to do

hypnotherapist [hɪpnəʊ'θerəpɪst] *noun* person who practises hypnotherapy

hypnotherapy [hɪpnəʊ'θerəpi] *noun* treatment by hypnosis, used in treating some addictions

hypnotic [hɪp'nɒtɪk] *adjective* referring to hypnotism; (drug) which causes sleep;

(state) which is like sleep but which is caused artificially

hypnotism ['hɪpnətɪzm] *noun* inducing hypnosis

hypnotist ['hɪpnətɪst] *noun* person who hypnotizes other people; *the hypnotist passed his hand in front of her eyes and she went immediately to sleep*

hypnotize ['hɪpnətaɪz] *verb* to make someone go into a state where he appears to be asleep, and will do whatever the hypnotist suggests; *he hypnotizes his patients, and then persuades them to reveal their hidden problems*

hypo ['haɪpəʊ] *(informal)* = HYPODERMIC SYRINGE

hypo- ['haɪpəʊ] *prefix* meaning less, too little or beneath

hypoaesthesia [haɪpəʊiːs'θiːziə] *noun* condition where the patient has a diminished sense of touch

hypocalcaemia [haɪpəʊkæl'siːmiə] *noun* abnormally low amount of calcium in the blood, which can cause tetany

hypochondria [haɪpəʊ'kɒndriə] *noun* condition where a person is too worried about his health and believes he is ill

hypochondriac [haɪpəʊ'kɒndriæk] **1** *noun* person who worries about his health too much **2** *adjective* **hypochondriac regions** = two parts of the upper abdomen, on either side of the epigastrium below the floating ribs

hypochondrium [haɪpə'kɒndriəm] *noun* one of the hypochondriac regions in the upper part of the abdomen

hypochromic anaemia [haɪpəʊ'krəʊmɪk ə'niːmiə] *noun* anaemia where haemoglobin is reduced in proportion to the number of red blood cells, which then appear very pale

hypodermic [haɪpə'dɜːmɪk] **1** *adjective* beneath the skin; **hypodermic syringe** *or* a **hypodermic** = syringe which injects liquid under the skin; **hypodermic needle** = needle for injecting liquid under the skin **2** *noun* *(informal)* hypodermic syringe, needle or injection

hypogastrium [haɪpə'gæstriəm] *noun* part of the abdomen beneath the stomach

hypoglossal nerve [haɪpə'glɒsl 'nɜːv] *noun* twelfth cranial nerve which governs the muscles of the tongue

hypoglycaemia [haɪpəglaɪ'siːmiə] *noun* low concentration of glucose in the blood

COMMENT: hypoglycaemia affects diabetics who feel weak from lack of sugar. A hypoglycaemic attack can be prevented by eating glucose or a lump of sugar when feeling faint

hypoglycaemic [haɪpəglaɪˈsiːmɪk] *adjective* suffering from hypoglycaemia; **hypoglycaemic coma** = state of unconsciousness affecting diabetics after taking an overdose of insulin

hypohidrosis *or* **hypoidrosis** [haɪpəhaɪˈdrəʊsɪs *or* haɪpɔɪˈdrəʊsɪs] *noun* producing too little sweat

hypokalaemia [haɪpəkæˈliːmɪə] *noun* deficiency of potassium in the blood

hypomenorrhoea [haɪpəmenəˈriːə] *noun* production of too little blood at menstruation

hyponatraemia [haɪpənæˈtriːmɪə] *noun* lack of sodium in the body

hypophyseal [haɪpəˈfɪzɪəl] *adjective* referring to the hypophysis or pituitary gland; **hypophyseal stalk** = stalk which attaches the pituitary gland to the hypothalamus

hypophysis cerebri [haɪˈpɒfəsɪs ˈserəbri] *see* PITUITARY GLAND

hypopituitarism [haɪpəˈpɪtjʊətərɪzm] *noun* condition where the pituitary gland is underactive; *see* PITUITARY

hypoplasia [haɪpəˈpleɪzɪə] *noun* lack of development, defective formation of tissue or an organ

hypopyon [haɪpəˈpaɪən] *noun* pus in the aqueous humour in the front chamber of the eye

hyposensitive [haɪpəˈsensətɪv] *adjective* being less sensitive than normal

hypospadias [haɪpəˈspeɪdɪəs] *noun* congenital defect of the wall of the male urethra or the vagina, so that the opening occurs on the under side of the penis or in the vagina; *compare* EPISPADIAS

hypostasis [haɪˈpɒstəsɪs] *noun* condition where fluid accumulates in part of the body because of poor circulation

hypostatic [haɪpəˈstætɪk] *adjective* referring to hypostasis; **hypostatic eczema** = eczema which develops on the legs, caused by bad circulation; **hypostatic pneumonia** = pneumonia caused by fluid accumulating in the lungs of a bedridden patient with a weak heart

hypotension [haɪpəˈtenʃn] *noun* low blood pressure

hypotensive [haɪpəˈtensɪv] *adjective* suffering from low blood pressure

hypothalamic [haɪpəʊθəˈlæmɪk] *adjective* referring to the hypothalamus; **hypothalamic hormones** = releasing hormones, hormones secreted by the hypothalamus which make the pituitary gland release certain hormones

hypothalamus [haɪpəʊˈθæləməs] *noun* part of the brain above the pituitary gland, which controls the production of hormones by the pituitary gland and regulates important bodily functions such as hunger, thirst and sleep; *see illustration at* BRAIN

hypothenar [haɪˈpɒθenə] *adjective* referring to the soft fat part of the palm beneath the little finger; **hypothenar eminence** = lump on the palm beneath the little finger; *compare* THENAR

hypothermia [haɪpəˈθɜːmɪə] *noun* reduction in body temperature below normal, for official purposes taken to be below 35°C

inadvertent hypothermia can readily occur in patients undergoing surgery when there is reduced heat production and a greater potential for heat loss to the environment
British Journal of Nursing

hypothermic [haɪpəˈθɜːmɪk] *adjective* suffering from hypothermia; *examination revealed that she was hypothermic, with a rectal temperature of only 29.4°C*

hypothyroidism [haɪpəˈθaɪrɔɪdɪzm] *noun* underactivity of the thyroid gland

hypotonia [haɪpəˈtəʊnɪə] *noun* reduced tension in any part of the body

hypotonic [haɪpəˈtɒnɪk] *adjective* **(a)** with reduced tension **(b)** (solution) with lower osmotic pressure than plasma

hypotropia [haɪpəˈtrəʊpɪə] *noun* form of squint where one eye looks downwards

hypoventilation [haɪpəventɪˈleɪʃn] *noun* very slow breathing

hypovitaminosis [haɪpəvɪtəmɪˈnəʊsɪs] *noun* lack of vitamins

hypoxaemia [haɪpɒˈksiːmɪə] *noun* inadequate supply of oxygen in arterial blood

hypoxia [haɪˈpɒksɪə] *noun* **(a)** inadequate supply of oxygen to tissue as a result of a lack of oxygen in arterial blood **(b)** = HYPOXAEMIA

hyster- ['hɪstə] *prefix* referring to the uterus

hysteralgia [hɪstər'ældʒə] *noun* pain in the uterus

hysterectomy [hɪstə'rektəmi] *noun* surgical removal of the uterus, either to treat cancer or because of the presence of fibroids; **subtotal hysterectomy** = removal of the uterus, but not the cervix; **total hysterectomy** = removal of the whole uterus

hysteria [hɪ'stɪərɪə] *noun* neurotic state, where the patient is unstable, and may scream and wave the arms about, but also is repressed, and may be slow to react to outside stimuli

hysterical [hɪ'sterɪkl] *adjective* (reaction) of hysteria; *he burst into hysterical crying*; **hysterical personality** = mental condition of a person who is unstable, lacks normal feelings and is dependent on others

hysterically [hɪ'sterɪkli] *adverb* in a hysterical way; *she was laughing hysterically*

hysterics [hɪ'sterɪks] *noun* attack of hysteria; *she had an attack or a fit of hysterics or she went into hysterics*

hystericus [hɪ'sterɪkəs] *see* GLOBUS

hystero- ['hɪstərəʊ] *prefix* referring to the uterus

hysterocele ['hɪstərəʊsi:l] *noun* hernia of the uterus

hysteroptosis [hɪstərɒp'təʊsɪs] *noun* prolapse of the uterus

hysterosalpingography [hɪstərəʊsælpɪŋ'gɒgrəfi] *noun* uterosalpingography, X-ray examination of the uterus and Fallopian tubes following injection of radio-opaque material

hysteroscope ['hɪstərəskəʊp] *noun* tube for inspecting the inside of the uterus

hysteroscopy [hɪstə'rɒskəpi] *noun* examination of the uterine cavity using a hysteroscope or fibrescope

hysterotomy [hɪstə'rɒtəmi] *noun* surgical incision into the uterus (as in Caesarean section or for some types of abortion)

Ii

I *chemical symbol for* iodine

-iasis ['aɪəsɪs] *suffix* meaning disease caused by something; **amoebiasis** = disease caused by an amoeba

iatrogenic [aɪætrə'dʒenɪk] *adjective* condition which is caused by a doctor's treatment for another disease or condition

> COMMENT: can be caused by a drug (a side effect), by infection from the doctor, or simply by worry about possible treatment

I band ['aɪ 'bænd] *noun* part of the pattern in muscle tissue, seen through a microscope as a light-coloured band

ice [aɪs] *noun* (a) frozen water (b) dry ice = solid carbon dioxide

icebag *or* **ice pack** ['aɪsbæg *or* 'aɪs 'pæk] *noun* cold compress made of lumps of ice wrapped in a cloth or put in a special bag, applied to a bruise or swelling to reduce the pain

ice cream ['aɪs 'kriːm] *noun* frozen sweet made from cream, water and flavouring; *after a tonsillectomy, children can be allowed ice cream*

ichor ['aɪkɔː] *noun* watery liquid which comes from a wound or suppurating sore

ichthyosis [ɪkθɪ'əʊsɪs] *noun* hereditary condition where the skin is dry and covered with scales

ICRC ['aɪ 'siː 'ɑː 'siː] = INTERNATIONAL COMMITTEE OF THE RED CROSS

ICSH ['aɪ 'siː 'es 'eɪtʃ] = INTERSTITIAL CELL STIMULATING HORMONE

icteric [ɪk'terɪk] *adjective* (patient) with jaundice

icterus ['ɪktərəs] = JAUNDICE; **icterus gravis neonatorum** = jaundice associated with erythroblastosis fetalis

ictus ['ɪktəs] *noun* stroke or fit

ICU ['aɪ 'siː 'juː] = INTENSIVE CARE UNIT

id [ɪd] *noun* (in psychology) basic unconscious drives which exist in hidden forms in a person

ideal [aɪ'dɪəl] *adjective* very suitable or perfect; referring to an idea; *this is an ideal place for a new hospital*

identical [aɪ'dentɪkl] *adjective* exactly the same; **identical twins** = monozygotic twins, two children born at the same time and from the same ovum, and therefore of the same sex and exactly the same in appearance; *compare* FRATERNAL

identifiable [aɪdentɪ'faɪəbl] *adjective* which can be identified; *cot deaths often have no identifiable cause*

identification [aɪdentɪfɪ'keɪʃn] *noun* act of identifying; **identification with someone** = taking on some characteristics of an older person (such as a parent or teacher)

identifier [aɪ'dentɪfaɪə] *noun* **patient identifier** = code of letters and digits attached to the patient's medical records by which all information concerning the patient can be traced, for example, cause of death

identify [aɪ'dentɪfaɪ] *verb* to determine the identity of something or someone; *the next of kin were asked to identify the body*; *doctors have identified the cause of the outbreak of dysentery*

identity [aɪ'dentətɪ] *noun* who a person is; **identity bracelet** *or* **label** = label attached to the wrist of a newborn baby or patient in hospital, so that he or she can be identified

idio- ['ɪdiəʊ] *prefix* referring to one particular person

idiocy ['ɪdiəsi] *noun* severe mental subnormality (IQ below 20)

idiopathic [ɪdiə'pæθɪk] *adjective* (i) referring to idiopathy; (ii) (disease) with no obvious cause; **idiopathic epilepsy** =

epilepsy not caused by a brain disorder, beginning during childhood or adolescence

idiopathy [ɪdɪˈɒpəθɪ] *noun* condition which develops without any known cause

idiosyncrasy [ɪdɪəˈsɪŋkrəsi] *noun* (i) way of behaving which is particular to one person; (ii) one person's strong reaction to treatment or to a drug

idiot [ˈɪdɪət] *noun* person suffering from severe mental subnormality; **idiot savant** = person with mental subnormality who also possesses a single particular mental ability (such as the ability to play music by ear, to draw remembered objects, to do mental calculations) (NOTE: the term idiot is no longer used by the medical profession)

idioventricular rhythm [ɪdɪəvenˈtrɪkjʊlə ˈrɪðm] *noun* slow natural rhythm in the ventricles of the heart, but not in the atria

IDK [ˈaɪ ˈdiː ˈkeɪ] = INTERNAL DERANGEMENT OF THE KNEE

Ig [ˈaɪ ˈdʒiː] = IMMUNOGLOBULIN

IgA antiendomysial antibody (EmA) [ˈaɪ ˈdʒiː ˈeɪ] *noun* serological screening test for coeliac disease

IHD [ˈaɪ ˈeɪtʃ ˈdiː] = ISCHAEMIC HEART DISEASE

IL-1, IL-2 [ˈaɪ ˈel ˈwʌn] = INTERLEUKIN-1, INTERLEUKIN-2

ile(o)- [ˈɪli or ˈɪliəʊ] *prefix* referring to the ileum

ileal [ˈɪliəl] *adjective* referring to the ileum; **ileal bladder** *or* **ileal conduit** = artificial tube formed when the ureters are linked to part of the ileum, and that part is linked to an opening in the abdominal wall

ileectomy [ɪliˈektəmi] *noun* surgical removal of all or part of the ileum

ileitis [ɪliˈaɪtɪs] *noun* inflammation of the ileum; **regional ileitis** = inflammation of part of the intestine (usually the ileum) resulting in pain, diarrhoea and loss of weight (NOTE: also called **regional enteritis** or **Crohn's disease**); *compare* ULCERATIVE COLITIS

COMMENT: no certain cause has been found for Crohn's disease, where only one section of the intestine becomes inflamed and can be blocked

ileocaecal [ɪliəʊˈsiːkl] *adjective* referring to the ileum and the caecum; **ileocaecal**

orifice = point where the small intestine joins the large intestine

ileocolic [ɪliəʊˈkɒlɪk] *adjective* referring to both the ileum and the colon; **ileocolic artery** = branch of the superior mesenteric artery

ileocolitis [ɪliəʊkəˈlaɪtɪs] *noun* inflammation of both the ileum and the colon

ileocolostomy [ɪliəʊkəˈlɒstəmi] *noun* surgical operation to make a link directly between the ileum and the colon

ileoproctostomy [ɪliəʊprɒkˈtɒstəmi] *noun* surgical operation to create a link between the ileum and the rectum

ileorectal [ɪliəʊˈrektl] *adjective* referring to both the ileum and the rectum

ileosigmoidostomy [ɪliəʊsɪgmɔɪˈdɒstəmi] *noun* surgical operation to create a link between the ileum and the sigmoid colon

ileostomy [ɪliˈɒstəmi] *noun* surgical operation to make an opening between the ileum and the abdominal wall to act as an artificial opening for excretion of faeces; **ileostomy bag** = bag attached to the opening made by an ileostomy, to collect faeces as they are passed out of the body

ileum [ˈɪliəm] *noun* lower part of the small intestine, between the jejunum and the caecum; *compare* ILIUM; *see illustration at* DIGESTIVE SYSTEM

COMMENT: the ileum is the longest section of the small intestine, being about 2.5 metres long

ileus [ˈɪliəs] *noun* obstruction in the intestine, but usually distension caused by loss of muscular action in the bowel (paralytic or adynamic ileus)

ili(o)- [ˈɪli or ˈɪliəʊ] *prefix* referring to the ilium

iliac [ˈɪliæk] *adjective* referring to the ilium; **common iliac artery** = one of two arteries which branch from the aorta in the abdomen and in turn divide into the internal iliac artery (leading to the pelvis) and the external iliac artery (leading to the leg); **common iliac veins** = two veins draining the legs, pelvis and abdomen, which join to form the inferior vena cava; **external iliac artery** = artery which branches from the aorta in the abdomen and leads to the leg; **internal iliac artery** = artery which branches from the aorta in the abdomen and leads to the pelvis; **iliac crest** = curved top edge of the ilium; *see illustration at* PELVIS; **iliac fossa** = depression on the inner side of the hip bone; **iliac regions** = two regions of the lower abdomen, on either side of the hypogastrium; **iliac spine** = projection at the posterior end of the iliac crest

iliacus [ɪliˈækəs] *noun* muscle in the groin which flexes the thigh

iliococcygeal [ɪliəʊkɒkˈsɪdʒl] *adjective* referring to both the ilium and the coccyx

iliolumbar [ɪliəʊˈlʌmbə] *adjective* referring to the iliac and lumbar regions

iliopectineal *or* **iliopubic** [ɪliəʊpekˈtɪniəl *or* ɪliəʊˈpjuːbɪk] *adjective* referring to both the ilium and the pubis; **iliopectineal** *or* **iliopubic eminence** = raised area on the inner surface of the innominate bone

iliopsoas [ɪliəʊˈsəʊəs] *noun* muscle formed from the iliacus and psoas muscles

iliotibial tract [ɪliəʊˈtɪbiəl ˈtrækt] *noun* thick fascia which runs from the ilium to the tibia

ilium [ˈɪliəm] *noun* top part of each of the hip bones, which form the pelvis; *compare* ILEUM; *see illustration at* PELVIS

ill [ɪl] *adjective* not well, sick; *eating green apples will make you ill; if you feel ill you ought to see a doctor; he's not as ill as he was last week* (NOTE: **ill - worse - worst**)

illegal [ɪˈliːgl] *adjective* not done according to the law; *she had an illegal abortion*

ill health [ˈɪl ˈhelθ] *noun* not being well; *he has been in ill health for some time; she has a history of ill health; he had to retire early for reasons of ill health*

illness [ˈɪlnəs] *noun* **(a)** state of being ill, of not being well; *his illness makes him very tired; most of the children stayed away from school because of illness* **(b)** type of disease; *he is in hospital with an infectious tropical illness; scarlet fever is no longer considered to be a very serious illness*

illusion [ɪˈluːʒn] *noun* condition where a person has a wrong perception of external objects; **optical illusion** = something which is seen wrongly, usually when it is moving, so that it appears to be something else

i.m. *or* **IM** [ˈaɪ ˈem] = INTRAMUSCULAR

image [ˈɪmɪdʒ] *noun* sensation (such as smell, sight or taste) which is remembered clearly

imagery [ˈɪmɪdʒri] *noun* producing visual sensations clearly in the mind

imaginary [ɪˈmædʒɪnri] *adjective* which does not exist but which is imagined; **imaginary playmates** = friends who do not exist but who are imagined by a small child to exist

imagination [ɪmædʒɪˈneɪʃn] *noun* being able to see things in your mind; *in his imagination he saw himself sitting on a beach in the sun*

imagine [ɪˈmædʒɪn] *verb* to see, hear or feel something in your mind; *imagine yourself sitting on the beach in the sun; I thought I heard someone shout, but I must have imagined it because there is no one there*; **to imagine things** = to have delusions; *she keeps imagining things; sometimes he imagines he is swimming in the sea*

imaging [ˈɪmɪdʒɪŋ] *noun* technique for creating pictures of sections of the body, using scanners attached to computers; **magnetic resonance imaging (MRI)** = scanning technique, using magnetic fields and radio waves, for examining soft tissue and cells; **X-ray imaging** = showing X-ray pictures of the inside of part of the body on a screen

imbalance [ɪmˈbæləns] *noun* wrong proportions of substances as, for example, in the diet

imbecile [ˈɪmbəsiːl] *noun* person who is mentally subnormal

imbecility [ɪmbəˈsɪləti] *noun* mental subnormality (where the IQ is below 50) (NOTE: these terms are no longer used by the medical profession)

imitate [ˈɪmɪteɪt] *verb* to do what someone else does; *when he walks he imitates his father; she is very good at imitating the English teacher; children learn by imitating adults or older children*

immature [ɪməˈtjʊə] *adjective* not mature; **an immature cell** = cell which is still developing

immaturity [ɪməˈtʃʊrəti] *noun* behaviour which is lacking in maturity; *(in psychology)* **emotional immaturity** = lacking in emotional development

immediate [ɪˈmiːdjət] *adjective* which happens now, without waiting; *his condition needs immediate treatment*

immediately [ɪˈmiːdjətli] *adverb* just after; *he became ill immediately after he came back from holiday; she will phone the doctor immediately (after) her father regains* *consciousness*; *if the child's temperature rises, you must call the doctor immediately*

immersion foot [ɪˈmɜːʃn ˈfʊt] *noun* trench foot, condition, caused by exposure to cold and damp, where the skin of the foot becomes red and blistered and in severe cases turns black when gangrene sets in. (The condition was common among soldiers serving in the trenches during the First World War)

immiscible [ɪˈmɪsəbl] *adjective; (of liquids)* which cannot be mixed

immobile [ɪˈməʊbaɪl] *adjective* not moving, which cannot move

immobilization [ɪməʊbɪlaɪˈzeɪʃn] *noun* being kept still, without moving

immobilize [ɪˈməʊbɪlaɪz] *verb* to make someone keep still and not move; to attach a splint to a joint to prevent the bones moving

immovable [ɪˈmuːvəbl] *adjective* (joint) which cannot be moved

immune [ɪˈmjuːn] *adjective* protected against an infection or allergic disease; *she seems to be immune to colds*; *the injection should make you immune to yellow fever*; **immune deficiency** = lack of immunity to a disease; *see also* AIDS; **immune reaction** *or* **immune response** = reaction of a body to an antigen; **immune system** = complex network of cells and cell products which protects the body from disease; it includes the thymus, spleen, lymph nodes, white blood cells and antibodies

the reason for this susceptibility is a profound abnormality of the immune system in children with sickle-cell disease

Lancet

the AIDS virus attacks a person's immune system and damages his or her ability to fight other diseases

Journal of the American Medical Association

immunity [ɪˈmjuːnəti] *noun* ability to resist attacks of a disease because antibodies are produced; *the vaccine gives immunity to tuberculosis*; **acquired immunity** = immunity which a body acquires (from having caught a disease or from immunization), not one which is congenital; **active immunity** = immunity which is acquired by catching and surviving an infectious disease or by vaccination with a

weakened form of the disease which makes the body form antibodies; **natural immunity** = immunity which a body acquires in the uterus or from the mother's milk; **passive immunity** = immunity which is acquired by a baby in the uterus or by a patient through an injection with an antitoxin

immunization [ɪmjunaɪˈzeɪʃn] *noun* making a person immune to an infection, either by injecting an antiserum (passive immunization) or by giving the body the disease in such a small dose that the body does not develop the disease, but produces antibodies to counteract it; *see also* VACCINATION

vaccination is the most effective way to prevent children getting the disease. Children up to 6 years old can be vaccinated if they missed earlier immunization

Health Visitor

immunize [ˈɪmjunaɪz] *verb* to give someone immunity from an infection; *see also* VACCINATE (NOTE: you immunize someone **against** a disease)

COMMENT: in the UK, infants are immunized against diphtheria, pertussis, polio, tetanus, Hib, mumps, measles and rubella, unless there are contra-indications or the parents object

immunoassay [ɪmjunəʊæˈseɪ] *noun* test for the presence and strength of antibodies

immunocompetent [ɪmjunəʊˈkɒmpɪtənt] *adjective* able to participate in the process of immunization

immunocompromised
[ɪmjunəʊˈkɒmprəmaɪzd] *adjective* not able to offer resistance to infection

immunodeficiency [ɪmjunəʊdɪˈfɪʃnsi] *noun* lack of immunity to a disease; **immunodeficiency virus** = retrovirus which attacks the immune system; **acquired immunodeficiency syndrome (AIDS)** = viral infection which breaks down the body's immune system (NOTE: also called **acquired immune deficiency syndrome**); *see also* HIV

immunodeficient [ɪmjunəʊdɪˈfɪʃnt] *adjective* lacking immunity to a disease; *this form of meningitis occurs in persons who are immunodeficient*

immunoelectrophoresis
[ɪmjunəʊɪletrəʊfəˈriːsɪs] *noun* method of

identifying antigens in a laboratory, using electrophoresis

immunoglobulin (Ig) [ɪmjunəʊˈglɒbjʊlɪn] *noun* antibody, a protein produced in blood plasma as protection against infection (the commonest is gamma globulin) (NOTE: the 5 main classes are called: **immunoglobulin G, A, D, E and M** *or* **IgG, IgA, IgD, IgE and IgM**)

immunological [ɪmjunəˈlɒdʒɪkl] *adjective* referring to immunology; **immunological tolerance** = tolerance of the lymphoid tissues to an antigen

immunologist [ɪmjuˈnɒlədʒɪst] *noun* specialist in immunology

immunology [ɪmjuˈnɒlədʒi] *noun* study of immunity and immunization

immunosuppressant [ɪmjunəʊsəˈpresənt] *noun* drug used to counteract the response of the immune system to reject a transplanted organ

immunosuppression [ɪmjunəʊsəˈpreʃn] *noun* suppressing the body's natural immune system so that it will not reject a transplanted organ

immunosuppressive [ɪmjunəʊsəˈpresɪv] *adjective & noun* (drug) used to counteract the response of the immune system to reject a transplanted organ

immunotherapy [ɪmjunəʊˈθerəpi] *see* ADOPTIVE

immunotransfusion [ɪmjunəʊtrænsˈfjuːʒn] *noun* transfusion of blood, serum or plasma containing immune bodies

impacted [ɪmˈpæktɪd] *adjective* tightly pressed or firmly lodged against something; **impacted fracture** = fracture where the broken parts of the bones are driven against each other; **impacted tooth** = tooth which is held against another tooth and so cannot grow normally; **impacted ureteric calculus** = stone which is lodged in a ureter

impaction [ɪmˈpækʃn] *noun* condition where two things are impacted; **dental impaction** = condition where a tooth is impacted in the jaw; **faecal impaction** = condition where a hardened mass of faeces stays in the rectum

impair [ɪmˈpeə] *verb* to harm (a sense or function) so that it does not work properly; **impaired hearing** = hearing which is not acute; **impaired vision** = eyesight which is not fully clear; **visually impaired person** = person whose eyesight is not clear

impairment [ɪmˈpeəmənt] *noun* condition where a sense or function is harmed so that it does not work properly; *his hearing impairment does not affect his work*; *the impairment was progressive, but she did not notice that her eyesight was getting worse*

```
impairment - any loss or
abnormality of psychological,
physical or anatomical
structure or function
                              WHO
```

impalpable [ɪmˈpælpəbl] *adjective* which cannot be felt when touched

impediment [ɪmˈpedɪmənt] *noun* obstruction; **speech impediment** = condition where a person cannot speak properly because of a deformed mouth

imperfecta [ɪmpəˈfektə] *see* OSTEOGENESIS

imperforate [ɪmˈpɜːfrət] *adjective* without an opening; **imperforate anus** = condition where the anus does not have an opening; **imperforate hymen** = membrane in the vagina which has no opening for the menstrual fluid

impetigo [ɪmpɪˈtaɪgəʊ] *noun* irritating and very contagious skin disease caused by staphylococci, which spreads rapidly and is easily passed from one child to another, but can be treated with antibiotics

implant 1 [ˈɪmplɑːnt] *noun* tissue, drug, inert material or device (such as a pacemaker) grafted or inserted into a patient; **lens implant** = artificial lens implanted in the eye when the natural lens is removed as is the case of cataract; **implant material** = substance grafted or inserted into a patient; **implant site** = place in or on the body where the implant is positioned **2** [ɪmˈplɑːnt] *verb* to become fixed; to graft or insert (tissue, drug, inert material or device); *the ovum implants in the wall of the uterus*; *the site was implanted with the biomaterial*

implantation [ɪmplɑːnˈteɪʃn] *noun* **(a)** grafting or inserting of a drug, tissue, inert material or device into a patient; introduction of one tissue into another surgically **(b)** place in or on the body where an implant is positioned **(c)** point in the development of an embryo when the fertilized ovum reaches the uterus and becomes fixed in the wall of the uterus; *see also* NIDATION

impotence [ˈɪmpətəns] *noun* inability in a male to have an erection or to ejaculate, and so have sexual intercourse

impotent ['ɪmpətənt] *adjective (of a man)* unable to have sexual intercourse

impregnate ['ɪmpregneɪt] *verb* **(a)** to make (a female) pregnant **(b)** to soak (a cloth) with a liquid; *a cloth impregnated with antiseptic*

impregnation [ɪmpreg'neɪʃn] *noun* action of impregnating

impression [ɪm'preʃn] *noun* **(a)** mould of a patient's jaw made by a dentist before making a denture **(b)** depression on an organ or structure into which another organ or structure fits; **cardiac impression** = (i) concave area near the centre of the upper surface of the liver under the heart; (ii) depression on the mediastinal part of the lungs where they touch the pericardium

improve [ɪm'pruːv] *verb* to get better; to make better; *he was very ill, but he is improving now*

improvement [ɪm'pruːvmənt] *noun* getting better; *the patient's condition has shown a slight improvement*; *doctors have not detected any improvement in her asthma*

impulse ['ɪmpʌls] *noun* **(a)** message transmitted by a nerve **(b)** sudden feeling that you want to act in a certain way

impure [ɪm'pjuə] *adjective* not pure

impurities [ɪm'pjuərətiz] *plural noun* substances which are not pure or clean; *the kidneys filter impurities out of the blood*

inability [ɪnə'bɪləti] *noun* being unable to do something; *he suffered from a temporary inability to pass water*

inactive [ɪn'æktɪv] *adjective* **(a)** not being active, not moving; *patients must not be allowed to become inactive* **(b)** which does not work; *the serum makes the poison inactive*

inactivity [ɪnæk'tɪvəti] *noun* lack of activity; *he has periods of complete inactivity*

inadequate [ɪn'ædɪkwət] *adjective* not sufficient; *the hospital has inadequate staff to deal with a major accident*

inanition [ɪnə'nɪʃn] *noun* state of exhaustion caused by starvation

in articulo mortis [ɪn ɑː'tɪkjuləu 'mɔːtɪs] *Latin phrase meaning* 'at the onset of death'

inborn [ɪn'bɔːn] *adjective* congenital, which is in the body from birth; *a body has an inborn tendency to reject transplanted organs*

inbred [ɪn'bred] *adjective* suffering from inbreeding

inbreeding ['ɪnbriːdɪŋ] *noun* breeding between a closely related male and female, who have the same parents or grandparents, so making congenital defects spread

incapable [ɪn'keɪpəbl] *adjective* not able to do something; *she was incapable of feeding herself*

incapacitated [ɪnkə'pæsɪteɪtɪd] *adjective* not able to act; *he was incapacitated for three weeks by his accident*

incarcerated [ɪn'kɑːsəreɪtɪd] *adjective* (hernia) which cannot be corrected by physical manipulation

inception rate [ɪn'sepʃn 'reɪt] *noun* number of new cases of a disease during a period of time, per thousand of population

incest ['ɪnsest] *noun* crime of having sexual intercourse with a close relative (daughter, son, mother, father)

incestuous [ɪn'sestjuəs] *adjective* referring to incest; *they had an incestuous relationship*

incidence ['ɪnsɪdəns] *noun* number of times something happens in a certain population over a period of time; *the incidence of drug-related deaths*; *men have a higher incidence of stroke than women*; **incidence rate** = number of new cases of a disease during a given period, per thousand of population

incipient [ɪn'sɪpiənt] *adjective* which is just beginning, which is in its early stages; *he has an incipient appendicitis*; *the tests detected incipient diabetes mellitus*

incise [ɪn'saɪz] *verb* to cut; **incised wound** = wound with clean edges, caused by a sharp knife or razor

incision [ɪn'sɪʒn] *noun* cut in a patient's body made by a surgeon using a scalpel; any cut made with a sharp knife or razor; *the first incision is made two millimetres below the second rib; compare* EXCISION

incisional [ɪn'sɪʒənl] *adjective* referring to an incision; **incisional hernia** = hernia which breaks through the abdominal wall at a place where a surgical incision was made during an operation

incisor (tooth) [ɪn'saɪzə 'tuːθ] *noun* one of the front teeth (four each in the upper and lower jaws) which are used to cut off pieces of food; *see illustration at* TEETH

include [ɪn'kluːd] *verb* to count something or someone with others; *does the number of cases include the figures for outpatients? the dentist will be on holiday up to and* including next Tuesday

inclusion [ɪn'kluːʒn] *noun* something enclosed inside something else; **inclusion bodies** = very small particles found in cells infected by virus

incoherent [ɪnkə'hɪərənt] *adjective* not able to speak in a way which makes sense

incompatibility [ɪnkəmpætə'bɪləti] *noun* being incompatible; *the incompatibility of the donor's blood with that of the patient*

incompatible [ɪnkəm'pætəbl] *adjective* which does not go together with something else; (drugs) which must not be used together because they undergo chemical change and the therapeutic effect is lost or changed to something undesirable; (tissue) which is genetically different from other tissue, making it impossible to transplant into that tissue; **incompatible blood** = blood from a donor that does not match the blood of the patient receiving the transfusion

incompetence [ɪn'kɒmpətns] *noun* (i) not being able to do a certain act; (ii) *(of valves)* not closing properly; **aortic incompetence** = condition where the aortic valve does not close properly, causing regurgitation; *(of the cervix)* **cervical incompetence** = dysfunction of the cervix of the uterus which is often the cause of spontaneous abortions and premature births and can be remedied by pursestring stitch (Shirodkar's operation); **mitral incompetence** = situation where the mitral valve does not close completely so that blood flows back into the atrium

incompetent [ɪn'kɒmpətnt] *adjective* **(a)** (part of the body) which is unable to function; *an incompetent mitral valve*; **incompetent cervix** = dysfunctional cervix of the uterus which is often the cause of spontaneous abortions and premature births and can be remedied by pursestring stitch (Shirodkar's operation) **(b)** (person) who is mentally deficient

incomplete [ɪnkəm'pliːt] *adjective* which is not complete; **incomplete abortion** = *see* ABORTION

incontinence [ɪn'kɒntɪnəns] *noun* inability to control the discharge of urine (or faeces); **faecal incontinence** = encopresis, inability to control the bowel movements; **urinary incontinence** = involuntary emission of urine; **stress incontinence** = condition in women where the sufferer is incapable of retaining urine when the intra-abdominal pressure is raised by coughing or laughing; **incontinence pad** = pad of material to absorb urine

incontinent [ɪn'kɒntɪnənt] *adjective* unable to control the discharge of urine or faeces

incoordination [ɪnkəʊɔːdɪ'neɪʃn] *noun* situation where the muscles in various parts of the body do not act together, making it impossible to do certain actions

incorrect [ɪnkə'rekt] *adjective* not correct; *the doctor made an incorrect diagnosis*; *the dosage prescribed was incorrect*

increase 1 ['ɪŋkriːs] *noun* getting larger or higher; *an increase in heart rate* **2** [ɪn'kriːs] *verb* to get larger or higher; *his pulse rate increased by 10 per cent*

incubation period [ɪŋkju'beɪʃn 'pɪəriəd] *noun* (i) time during which a virus or bacterium develops in the body after contamination or infection, before the appearance of the symptoms of the disease; (ii) time during which a bacterial sample grows in a laboratory culture

incubator ['ɪŋkjubeɪtə] *noun* **(a)** apparatus for growing bacterial cultures **(b)** specially controlled container in which a premature baby can be kept in ideal conditions

incurable [ɪn'kjʊərəbl] *noun & adjective* (patient) who will never be cured, (illness) which cannot be cured; *he is suffering from an incurable disease of the blood*; *she has been admitted to a hospital for incurables*

incus ['ɪŋkəs] *noun* one of the three ossicles in the middle ear, shaped like an anvil; *see illustration at* EAR

COMMENT: the incus is the central one of the three bones: the malleus articulates with it, and the incus articulates with the stapes

independent [ɪndɪ'pendənt] *adjective* free, not controlled by someone or something else

independently [ɪndɪ'pendəntli] *adverb* not being controlled by anyone or anything; *the autonomic nervous system functions independently of the conscious will*

index finger ['ɪndeks 'fɪŋgə] *noun* first finger next to the thumb

Indian hemp ['ɪndiən 'hemp] *noun* tropical plant from whose leaves or flowers cannabis (marijuana or hashish) is produced

indican ['ɪndɪkæn] *noun* potassium salt

indicate ['ɪndɪkeɪt] *verb* (a) to show; *the skin reaction indicates a highly allergenic state* (b) to suggest that a certain type of treatment should be given; *a course of antibiotics is indicated*; *therapeutic intervention was indicated in nine of the patients tested*

indication [ɪndɪ'keɪʃn] *noun* situation or sign which suggests that a certain type of treatment should be given or that a condition has a particular cause; *sulpha drugs have been replaced by antibiotics in many indications*; *see also* CONTRAINDICATION

indicator ['ɪndɪkeɪtə] *noun* substance which shows something, especially a substance secreted in body fluids which shows which blood group a person belongs to

indigestion [ɪndɪ'dʒestʃn] *noun* dyspepsia, disturbance of the normal process of digestion, where the patient experiences pain or discomfort in the stomach; *he is taking tablets to relieve his indigestion or he is taking indigestion tablets*

indirect [ɪndə'rekt or ɪndaɪ'rekt] *adjective* not direct; **indirect contact** = catching a disease by inhaling bacteria or by being in contact with a vector, but not in direct contact with an infected person

indisposed [ɪndɪ'spəʊzd] *adjective* slightly ill; *my mother is indisposed and cannot see any visitors*

indisposition [ɪndɪspə'zɪʃn] *noun* slight illness

individual [ɪndɪ'vɪdjul] *noun & adjective* (for) one particular person; single

indolence ['ɪndələns] *noun* lack of activity

indolent ['ɪndələnt] *adjective* causing little pain; (ulcer) which develops slowly and does not heal

indrawing [ɪn'drɔːɪŋ] *noun* pulling towards the inside

indrawn [ɪn'drɔːn] *adjective* which is pulled inside

induce [ɪn'djuːs] *verb* to make something happen; **to induce labour** = to make a woman go into labour; **induced abortion** = abortion which is produced by drugs or by surgery

induction of labour [ɪn'dʌkʃn əf 'leɪbə] *noun* action of starting childbirth artificially

induration [ɪndjʊə'reɪʃn] *noun* hardening of tissue or of an artery because of pathological change

induratum [ɪndjʊə'reɪtəm] *see* ERYTHEMA

industrial [ɪn'dʌstrɪəl] *adjective* referring to industries or factories; **industrial disease** = disease which is caused by the type of work done by a worker (such as by dust produced or chemicals used in the factory)

indwelling catheter [ɪn'dwelɪŋ 'kæθɪtə] *noun* catheter left in place for a period of time after its introduction

inebriation [ɪniːbrɪ'eɪʃn] *noun* state where a person is habitually drunk

inert [ɪ'nɜːt] *adjective* (a) *(of person)* not moving; lifeless (b) *(of chemical, etc.)* which is not active; which will not produce a chemical reaction

inertia [ɪ'nɜːʃə] *noun* complete lack of activity, condition of indolence of the body or mind

in extremis ['ɪn ɪks'triːmɪs] *Latin phrase* meaning 'at the moment of death'

infant ['ɪnfənt] *noun* small child under two years of age; **infant mortality rate** = number of infants who die per thousand births

infantile ['ɪnfəntaɪl] *adjective* (i) referring to small children; (ii) (disease) which affects children; **infantile convulsions** *or* **spasms** = convulsions, minor epileptic fits in small children; **infantile paralysis** = POLIOMYELITIS

infantilism [ɪn'fæntɪlɪzm] *noun* condition where a person keeps some characteristics of an infant when he or she becomes an adult

infarct ['ɪnfɑːkt] *noun* area of tissue which is killed when the blood supply is cut off by the blockage of an artery

infarction [ɪn'fɑːkʃn] *noun* killing of tissue by cutting off the blood supply; **cardiac** *or* **myocardial infarction** = death of part of the heart muscle after coronary thrombosis; **cerebral infarction** = death of brain tissue as a result of reduction in the blood supply to the brain

cerebral infarction accounts for about 80% of first-ever strokes

British Journal of Hospital Medicine

infect [ɪn'fekt] *verb* to contaminate with disease-producing microorganisms or toxins; to transmit infection; *the disease infected his* *liver*; *the whole arm soon became infected*; **infected wound** = wound which has become poisoned by bacteria

infection [ɪnˈfekʃn] *noun* entry of microbes into the body, which then multiply in the body; *as a carrier he was spreading infection to other people in the office*; *she is susceptible to minor infections*

infectious [ɪnˈfekʃəs] *adjective* (disease) which is caused by microbes and can be transmitted to other persons by direct means; *this strain of flu is highly infectious*; *her measles is at the infectious stage*; **infectious hepatitis** = hepatitis A, hepatitis transmitted by a carrier through food or drink; **infectious mononucleosis** = glandular fever, infectious disease where the body has an excessive number of white blood cells

COMMENT: the symptoms include sore throat, fever and swelling of the lymph glands in the neck. The disease is probably caused by the Epstein-Barr virus

infective [ɪnˈfektɪv] *adjective* (disease) caused by a microbe, which can be caught from another person but which cannot always be directly transmitted; **(subacute) infective endocarditis** = infection of the endocardium (the membrane covering the inner surfaces of the heart) by bacteria; **infective enteritis** = enteritis caused by bacteria; **infective hepatitis** = hepatitis A, hepatitis transmitted by a carrier through food or drink

infectivity [ɪnfekˈtɪvəti] *noun* being infective; *the patient's infectivity can last about a week*

inferior [ɪnˈfɪəriə] *adjective* lower (part of the body); **inferior aspect** = view of the body from below; **inferior vena cava** = main vein carrying blood from the lower part of the body to the heart

inferiority [ɪnfɪəriˈɒrəti] *noun* being lower, less important or less intelligent than others; **inferiority complex** = mental state where the patient feels very inferior to others and compensates for this by behaving violently towards them (NOTE: the opposite is **superior**, **superiority**)

infertile [ɪnˈfɜːtaɪl] *adjective* not fertile, not able to reproduce

infertility [ɪnfəˈtɪləti] *noun* not being fertile, able to reproduce

infest [ɪnˈfest] *verb* (*of parasites*) to be present in large numbers; *the child's hair was infested with lice*

infestation [ɪnfesˈteɪʃn] *noun* having large numbers of parasites; invasion of the body by parasites; *the condition is caused by infestation of the hair with lice*

infiltrate [ˈɪnfɪltreɪt] **1** *verb* (*of liquid or waste*) to pass from one part of the body to another through a wall or membrane and be deposited in the other part **2** *noun* substance which has infiltrated part of the body

the chest roentgenogram often discloses interstitial pulmonary infiltrates, but may occasionally be normal
Southern Medical Journal

infiltration [ɪnfɪlˈtreɪʃn] *noun* passing of a liquid through the walls of one part of the body into another part; condition where waste is brought to and deposited round cells

the lacrimal and salivary glands become infiltrated with lymphocytes and plasma cells. The infiltration reduces lacrimal and salivary secretions which in turn leads to dry eyes and dry mouth
American Journal of Nursing

infirm [ɪnˈfɜːm] *adjective* old and weak; *my grandfather is quite infirm now*

infirmary [ɪnˈfɜːməri] *noun* **(a)** room in a school or factory where people can go if they are ill **(b)** old name for a hospital (NOTE: **infirmary** is still used in names of hospitals: **the Glasgow Royal Infirmary**)

infirmity [ɪnˈfɜːməti] *noun* (i) being old and weak; (ii) illness; *in spite of his infirmities he still reads all the newspapers*

inflame [ɪnˈfleɪm] *verb* to make an organ or a tissue react to an infection, an irritation or a blow by becoming sore, red and swollen; *the skin has become inflamed around the sore*

inflammation [ɪnfləˈmeɪʃn] *noun* being inflamed, having become sore, red and swollen as a reaction to an infection or an irritation or a blow; *she has an inflammation of the bladder or a bladder inflammation*; *the body's reaction to infection took the form of an inflammation of the eyelid*

inflammatory [ɪnˈflæmətri] *adjective* which makes an organ or a tissue become sore, red and swollen; **inflammatory bowel disease** = any condition (such as Crohn's disease, colitis or ileitis) where the bowel becomes inflamed; **inflammatory response** *or* **reaction** = any condition where an organ or a tissue reacts to an external stimulus by becoming inflamed; *she showed an inflammatory response to the ointment*

inflatable [ɪnˈfleɪtəbl] *adjective* which can be inflated

inflate [ɪnˈfleɪt] *verb* to fill with air; *the abdomen is inflated with air before a coelioscopy*; *in valvuloplasty, a balloon is introduced into the valve and inflated*

influence [ˈɪnfluəns] **1** *noun* being able to have an effect on someone or something **2** *verb* to have an effect on someone or something; *the development of the serum has been influenced by research carried out in the USA*

influenza [ɪnfluˈenzə] *noun* infectious disease of the upper respiratory tract with fever, malaise and muscular aches, transmitted by a virus, which occurs in epidemics; *she is in bed with influenza*; *half the staff in the office are off work with influenza*; *the influenza epidemic has killed several people*

COMMENT: influenza virus is spread by droplets of moisture in the air, so the disease can be spread by coughing or sneezing. Influenza can be quite mild, but virulent strains occur from time to time (Spanish influenza, Hong Kong flu) and can weaken the patient so much that he becomes susceptible to pneumonia and other more serious infections

inform [ɪnˈfɔːm] *verb* to tell someone; *have you informed the police that the drugs have been stolen?*

informal [ɪnˈfɔːml] *adjective* not official; **informal patient** = patient who has admitted himself to a hospital, without being referred by a doctor

information [ɪnfəˈmeɪʃn] *noun* facts about something; *have you any information about the treatment of sunburn?*; *the police won't give us any information about how the accident happened*; *you haven't given me enough information about when your symptoms started*; *that's a very useful piece or bit of information* (NOTE: no plural: **some information; a piece of information)**

informed [ɪnˈfɔːmd] *adjective* having the latest information; **informed consent** = agreement given by a patient or the guardians of a patient after they have been given all the necessary information, that an operation can be carried out

infra- [ˈɪnfrə] *prefix* meaning below

infraorbital nerve [ɪnfrəˈɔːbɪtl ˈnɜːv] *noun* continuation of the maxillary nerve below the orbit of the eye; **infraorbital vein** = vessel draining the face through the infraorbital canal to the pterygoid plexus

infrared rays *or* **infrared radiation** [ɪnfrəˈred ˈreɪz *or* ɪnfrəˈred reɪdiˈeɪʃn] *noun* long invisible rays, below the visible red end of the colour spectrum, used to produce heat in body tissues in the treatment of traumatic and inflammatory conditions; *she was advised to take a course of infrared ray treatment*; *see also* LIGHT THERAPY

infundibulum [ɪnfʌnˈdɪbjʊləm] *noun* any part of the body shaped like a funnel, especially the stem which attaches the pituitary gland to the hypothalamus

infusion [ɪnˈfjuːʒn] *noun* (i) drink made by pouring boiling water on a dry substance (such as herb tea or a powdered drug); (ii) putting liquid into a body, using a drip

ingestion [ɪnˈdʒestʃn] *noun* **(a)** taking in food, drink or medicine by the mouth **(b)** process by which a foreign body (such as a bacillus) is surrounded by a cell

ingredient [ɪnˈgriːdiənt] *noun* substance which is used with others to make something (food to eat, lotion to put on the skin, etc.); **active ingredient** = *see* ACTIVE

ingrowing toenail [ɪnˈgrəʊɪŋ ˈtəʊneɪl] *noun* condition where the nail cuts into the tissue at the side of it, and creates inflammation; sepsis and ulceration can also occur; *if the nail is slightly ingrown, it can be treated by cutting at the sides*

ingrown toenail [ɪnˈgrəʊn ˈtəʊneɪl] = INGROWING TOENAIL

inguinal [ˈɪŋgwɪnl] *adjective* referring to the groin; **inguinal canal** = passage in the lower abdominal wall, carrying the spermatic cord in the male and the round ligament of the uterus in the female; **inguinal hernia** = hernia where the intestine bulges through the muscles in the groin, especially through the inguinal canal; **inguinal ligament** = Poupart's ligament, a ligament in the groin, running from the spine to the pubis; **inguinal region** = groin, the part of the body where the lower abdomen joins the top of the thigh

inguinale [ɪŋgwɪˈneɪli] *see* GRANULOMA

inhalant [ɪnˈheɪlənt] *noun* medicinal substance which is breathed in

inhalation [ɪnhəˈleɪʃn] *noun* **(a)** action of breathing in; **smoke inhalation** = breathing in smoke (as in a fire) **(b)** action of breathing in a medicinal substance as part of treatment; medicinal substance which is breathed in; **steam inhalation** = treatment of respiratory disease by breathing in steam with medicinal substances in it

inhale [ɪnˈheɪl] *verb* to breathe in; *he inhaled some toxic gas fumes and was rushed to hospital; even smoking cigars can be bad for you if you inhale the smoke* (NOTE: the opposite is **exhale**)

inhaler [ɪnˈheɪlə] *noun* small device for administering medicinal substances into the mouth or nose so that they can be breathed in (NOTE: the opposite is **exhalation**)

inherent [ɪnˈhɪərnt] *adjective* thing which is part of the essential character of a person, a permanent characteristic of an organism

inherit [ɪnˈherɪt] *verb* to receive characteristics from a parent's genes; *she inherited her father's red hair; haemophilia is a condition which is inherited through the mother's genes*

inhibit [ɪnˈhɪbɪt] *verb* to block, to prevent an action happening; to stop a functional process; *aspirin inhibits the clotting of blood*; **to have an inhibiting effect on something** = to block something, to stop something happening

inhibition [ɪnhɪˈbɪʃn] *noun* **(a)** action of blocking or preventing something happening, especially preventing a muscle or organ from functioning properly **(b)** *(in psychology)* suppressing a thought which is associated to a sense of guilt; blocking of a normal spontaneous action by some mental influence

inhibitor [ɪnˈhɪbɪtə] *noun* substance which inhibits

inhibitory nerve [ɪnˈhɪbɪtəri ˈnɜːv] *noun* nerve which stops a function taking place; *the vagus nerve is an inhibitory nerve which slows down the action of the heart*

inject [ɪnˈdʒekt] *verb* to put a liquid into a patient's body under pressure, by using a hollow needle inserted into the tissues; *he was injected with morphine; she injected herself with a drug*

injection [ɪnˈdʒekʃn] *noun* **(a)** act of injecting a liquid into the body; **intracutaneous injection** = injection of a liquid between the layers of skin (as for a test for an allergy); **intramuscular injection** = injection of liquid into a muscle (as for a slow release of a drug); **intravenous injection** = injection of liquid into a vein (as for fast release of a drug); **hypodermic injection** = injection of a liquid beneath the skin (as for pain-killing drugs) (NOTE: also **subcutaneous injection**) **(b)** liquid introduced into the body; *he had a penicillin injection*

injure [ˈɪndʒə] *verb* to hurt; *six people were injured in the accident*

injured [ˈɪndʒəd] **1** *adjective* (person) who has been hurt **2** *noun* **the injured** = people who have been injured; *all the injured were taken to the nearest hospital*

injury [ˈɪndʒəri] *noun* damage or wound caused to a person's body; *his injuries required hospital treatment; she never recovered from her injuries; he received severe facial injuries in the accident*; **accidental injury** = injury sustained in an accident; **internal injury** = damage to one of the internal organs; **non-accidental injury** = injury which is not caused accidentally

ink [ɪŋk] *noun* coloured liquid which is used for writing; **ink blot test** = RORSCHACH TEST

inlay [ˈɪnleɪ] *noun* *(in dentistry)* type of filling for teeth

inlet [ˈɪnlet] *noun* passage or opening through which a cavity can be entered; **thoracic inlet** = upper bony margin of the thorax

innate [ɪˈneɪt] *adjective* inherited, which is present in a body from birth

inner [ˈɪnə] *adjective* (part) which is inside; **inner ear** = part of the ear inside the head, behind the eardrum, containing the semicircular canals, the vestibule and the cochlea; **inner pleura** = membrane attached to the surface of a lung (NOTE: the opposite is **outer**)

innermost [ˈɪnəməʊst] *adjective* furthest inside

innervation [ɪnɜːˈveɪʃn] *noun* nerve supply to an organ (both motor nerves and sensory nerves)

innocent [ˈɪnəsənt] *adjective* (growth) which is benign, not malignant

innominate [ɪˈnɒmɪnət] *adjective* with no name; **innominate artery** = brachiocephalic artery, the largest branch of the arch of the aorta, which continues as the right common carotid and right subclavian arteries; **innominate bone** = HIPBONE; **innominate veins** = brachiocephalic veins, the two veins which continue the subclavian and jugular veins to the superior vena cava

inoculate [ɪ'nɒkjuleɪt] *verb* to introduce vaccine into a person's body in order to make the body create antibodies, so making the person immune to the disease; *the baby was inoculated against diphtheria* (NOTE: you inoculate someone **against** a disease)

inoculation [ɪnɒkju'leɪʃn] *noun* action of inoculating someone; *has the baby had a diphtheria inoculation?*

inoculum [ɪ'nɒkjuləm] *noun* substance (such as a vaccine) used for inoculation

inoperable [ɪn'ɒpərəbl] *adjective* (condition) which cannot be operated on; *the surgeon decided that the cancer was inoperable*

inorganic [ɪnɔː'gænɪk] *adjective* (substance) which is not made from animal or vegetable sources

inotropic [ɪnəʊ'trɒpɪk] *adjective* which affects the way muscles contract, especially those of the heart

inpatient ['ɪnpeɪʃənt] *noun* patient living in a hospital for treatment or observation; *compare* OUTPATIENT

inquest ['ɪnkwest] *noun* inquiry (by a coroner) into the cause of a death

COMMENT: an inquest has to take place where death is violent or not expected, where death could be murder, or where a prisoner dies and when police are involved

inquire [ɪn'kwaɪə] *verb* to ask questions about something; *he inquired if anything was wrong; she inquired about the success rate of that type of operation; the committee is inquiring into the administration of the District Health Authority*

inquiry [ɪn'kwaɪri] *noun* official investigation; *there has been a government inquiry into the outbreak of legionnaires' disease*

insane [ɪn'seɪn] *adjective* mad, suffering from a mental disorder

insanitary [ɪn'sænətri] *adjective* not sanitary or unhygienic; *cholera spread rapidly because of the insanitary conditions in the town*

insanity [ɪn'sænəti] *noun* psychotic mental disorder or illness

COMMENT: insanity is the legal term used to describe patients whose mental condition is so unstable that they need to be placed in a hospital to prevent them doing actions which could harm themselves or other people, although some are cared for in the community

insect ['ɪnsekt] *noun* small animal with six legs and a body in three parts; *insects were flying round the lamp*; *he was stung by an insect*; **insect bites** = stings caused by insects which puncture the skin to suck blood, and in so doing introduce irritants

COMMENT: most insect bites are simply irritating, but some patients can be extremely sensitive to certain types of insect (such as bee stings). Other insect bites can be more serious, as insects can carry the organisms which produce typhus, sleeping sickness, malaria, filariasis, etc.

insecticide [ɪn'sektɪsaɪd] *noun* substance which kills insects

insemination [ɪnsemɪ'neɪʃn] *noun* (i) fertilization of an ovum by a sperm; (ii) introduction of sperm into the vagina; **artificial insemination** = introduction of semen into a woman's uterus by artificial means; **artificial insemination by donor (AID)** *or* **donor insemination (DI)** = artificial insemination using the sperm of an anonymous donor; **artificial insemination by husband (AIH)** = artificial insemination using the semen of the husband

insert [ɪn'sɜːt] *verb* to put something into something; *the catheter is inserted into the passage*

insertion [ɪn'sɜːʃn] *noun* **(a)** (i) point of attachment of a muscle to a bone; (ii) point where an organ is attached to its support **(b)** action of putting something into something **(c)** change in the structure of a chromosome, where a segment of the chromosome is introduced into another member of the complement

insides ['ɪnsaɪdz] *plural noun (informal)* internal organs, especially the stomach and intestines; *he says he has a pain in his insides*; *you ought to see the doctor if you think there is something wrong with your insides*

insidious [ɪn'sɪdiəs] *adjective* causing harm without showing any obvious signs; **insidious disease** = disease which causes damage before being detected; *this disorder is insidious and may develop for some time before being detected*

insight ['ɪnsaɪt] *noun* ability of a patient to realise that he is ill or has particular problems or characteristics

insipidus [ɪnˈsɪpɪdəs] *see* DIABETES

in situ [ˈɪn ˈsɪtjuː] *adjective* in place

insoluble [ɪnˈsɒljʊbl] *adjective* which cannot be dissolved in liquid; **insoluble fibre** = fibre in bread and cereals, which is not digested, but which swells inside the intestine

insomnia [ɪnˈsɒmniə] *noun* inability to sleep, sleeplessness; *she suffers from insomnia*; *what does the doctor give you for your insomnia?*

insomniac [ɪnˈsɒmniæk] *noun* person who suffers from insomnia

inspect [ɪnˈspekt] *verb* to examine, to look at something carefully; *the doctor inspected the boy's throat*; *he used a bronchoscope to inspect the inside of the lungs*

inspection [ɪnˈspekʃn] *noun* act of examining something; *the officials have carried out an inspection of the hospital kitchens*

inspector [ɪnˈspektə] *noun* person who inspects; **Government Health Inspector** = government official who examines offices or factories to see if they are clean and healthy

inspiration [ɪnspəˈreɪʃn] *noun* breathing in, taking air into the lungs (NOTE: the opposite is expiration)

COMMENT: inspiration takes place when the muscles of the diaphragm contract, allowing the lungs to expand

inspissated [ɪnˈspɪseɪtɪd] *adjective* (liquid) which is thickened by removing water from it

inspissation [ɪnspɪˈseɪʃn] *noun* removing water from a solution to make it thicker

instability [ɪnstəˈbɪləti] *noun* not being stable or steady

instep [ˈɪnstep] *noun* arched top part of the foot

instil *or* **instill** [ɪnˈstɪl] *verb* to put a liquid in drop by drop; *instil four drops in each nostril twice a day*

instillation [ɪnstɪˈleɪʃn] *noun* (a) putting a liquid in drop by drop (b) liquid put in drop by drop

instinct [ˈɪnstɪŋkt] *noun* tendency or ability which the body has from birth, and does not need to learn; *the body has a natural instinct to protect itself from danger*

instinctive [ɪnˈstɪŋktɪv] *adjective* referring to instinct; *everyone has an instinctive reaction to move away from fire*

institution [ɪnstɪˈtjuːʃn] *noun* hospital or clinic, especially a psychiatric hospital or children's home; *he has lived all his life in institutions*

institutionalization *or* **institutional neurosis** [ɪnstɪˈtjuːʃənalaɪˈzeɪʃn *or* ɪnstɪˈtjuːʃnl njuˈrəʊsɪs] *noun* condition where a patient has become so adapted to life in an institution that it is impossible for him to live outside it

institutionalize [ɪnstɪˈtjuːʃənalaɪz] *verb* to put a person into an institution

instruction [ɪnˈstrʌkʃn] *noun* teaching how to do something; *the students are given instruction in dealing with emergency cases*; **instructions** = words which explain how something is used or how to do something; *the instructions are written on the medicine bottle*; *we can't use this machine because we have lost the book of instructions*; *she gave the taxi driver instructions how to get to the hospital*

instrument [ˈɪnstrəmənt] *noun* piece of equipment; tool; *the doctor had a box of surgical instruments*

instrumental [ɪnstrəˈmentl] *adjective* (a) using an instrument; **instrumental delivery** = childbirth where the doctor uses forceps to help the baby out of the mother's uterus (b) **instrumental in** = helping to do something; *she was instrumental in developing the new technique*

insufficiency [ɪnsəˈfɪʃənsi] *noun* (i) not being enough to perform normal functions; (ii) incompetence of an organ; *the patient is suffering from a renal insufficiency*

insufflation [ɪnsəˈfleɪʃn] *noun* blowing something, such as air or a powder, into a cavity in the body

insula [ˈɪnsjʊlə] *noun* part of the cerebral cortex which is covered by the folds of the sulcus

insulin [ˈɪnsjʊlɪn] *noun* hormone produced by the islets of Langerhans in the pancreas; **insulin dependence** = being dependent on insulin; **insulin-dependent** = *see* DIABETES; **insulin resistant** = condition in which the muscle and other tissue cells respond inadequately to insulin, common in Type2 diabetes

COMMENT: insulin controls the way in which the body converts sugar into energy and regulates the level of sugar in the blood; a lack of insulin caused by diabetes mellitus makes the level of glucose in the blood rise. Insulin injections are regularly used to treat diabetes mellitus, but care has to be taken not to exceed the dose as this will cause hyperinsulinism and hypoglycaemia

insulinase ['ɪnsjʊlɪneɪz] *noun* enzyme which breaks down insulin

insulinoma *or* **insuloma** [ɪnsjʊlɪ'nəʊmə or ɪnsjʊ'ləʊmə] *noun* tumour in the islets of Langerhans

insurance [ɪn'ʃʊərəns] *noun* agreement with a company that they will pay you money if something is lost or damaged; **accident insurance** = insurance which pays out money when an accident happens; **life insurance** = insurance which pays out money when someone dies; **medical insurance** = insurance which pays for private medical treatment; **National Insurance** = weekly payment from a person's wages (with a supplement from the employer) which pays for state assistance, medical treatment, etc.

insure [ɪn'ʃʊə] *verb* to agree with a company that they will pay you money if something is lost or damaged; *is your car insured?*

intake ['ɪnteɪk] *noun* amount of a substance taken in; taking in (of a substance); *a high intake of alcohol*; *she was advised to reduce her intake of sugar*; **suggested daily intake** = amount of a substance which it is recommended to take in each day

integration [ɪntɪ'greɪʃn] *noun* process where a whole is made into a single unit by the functional combination of the parts

COMMENT: there are two modes of integration: nervous and hormonal

integument [ɪn'tegjumənt] *noun* covering layer, such as the skin

intelligence [ɪn'telɪdʒəns] *noun* ability to learn and understand quickly; **intelligence quotient (IQ)** = ratio of the mental age as given by an intelligence test, to the actual age of the person; **intelligence test** = test to see how intelligent someone is, giving a mental age, as opposed to the chronological age of the person

COMMENT: the average IQ is between 90 and 110

intelligent [ɪn'telɪdʒənt] *adjective* clever, able to learn quickly; *he's the most intelligent boy in the class*

intense [ɪn'tens] *adjective* very strong (pain); *she is suffering from intense post herpetic neuralgia*

intensity [ɪn'tensəti] *noun* strength (of pain)

intensive care [ɪn'tensɪv 'keə] *noun* continual supervision and treatment of a patient in a special section of a hospital; *the patient was put in intensive care*; *he came out of intensive care and was moved to the general ward*; **intensive care unit (ICU)** = special section of a hospital which supervises seriously ill patients who need constant supervision

intention [ɪn'tenʃn] *noun* **(a)** healing process; **healing by first intention** = healing of a clean wound where the tissue reforms quickly; **healing by second intention** = healing of an infected wound or ulcer, which takes place slowly and may leave a permanent scar **(b)** aiming to do something; **intention tremor** = trembling of the hands when a person makes a voluntary movement to try to touch something

inter- ['ɪntə] *prefix* meaning between

interaction [ɪntər'ækʃn] *noun* effect which two or more substances (such as drugs) have on each other

interatrial septum [ɪntər'eɪtriəl 'septəm] *noun* membrane between the right and left atria in the heart

interbreed [ɪntə'briːd] *verb* to reproduce with another member of the same species

intercalated [ɪntəkə'leɪtɪd or ɪn'tɜːkələɪtɪd] *adjective* inserted between other tissues; **intercalated disc** = closely applied cell membranes at the end of adjacent cells in cardiac muscle, seen as transverse lines

intercellular [ɪntə'seljʊlə] *adjective* between the cells in tissue

intercostal [ɪntə'kɒstl] *adjective* between the ribs; **intercostal muscles** *or* **the intercostals** = muscles between the ribs

COMMENT: the intercostal muscles expand and contract the thorax, so changing the pressure in the thorax and making the person breathe in or out. There are three layers of intercostal muscle: external, internal and innermost or intercostalis intimis

intercourse ['ɪntəkɔːs] *noun* **(sexual) intercourse** = action of inserting the man's penis into the woman's vagina, releasing spermatozoa from the penis by ejaculation, which may fertilize an ovum from the woman's ovaries

intercurrent [ɪntə'kʌrənt] *noun* **intercurrent disease** *or* **infection** = disease or infection which affects someone who is suffering from another disease

interdigital [ɪntə'dɪdʒɪtl] *adjective* referring to the space between the fingers or toes

interest ['ɪntrəst] **1** *noun* **(a)** special attention; *the consultant takes a lot of interest in his students; she has no interest in what goes on in the ward around her; why doesn't he take more interest in physiotherapy?* **(b)** something which attracts you particularly; *her main interest is the treatment of cardiac patients; do you have any special interests apart from your work?* **2** *verb* to attract someone's attention; *he's specially interested in the work of the physiotherapy department; nothing seems to interest her very much*

interesting ['ɪntrəstɪŋ] *adjective* which attracts your attention; *there's an interesting article on the treatment of drug addiction in the magazine*

interfere [ɪntə'fɪə] *verb* to get involved, to stop or hinder a function

interference [ɪntə'fɪərəns] *noun* act of interfering

interferon [ɪntə'fɪərɒn] *noun* protein produced by cells, usually in response to a virus and which then reduces the spread of viruses

COMMENT: although it is now possible to synthesize interferon outside the body, large-scale production is extremely expensive and the substance has not proved as successful at combating viruses as had been hoped, though it is used in multiple sclerosis with some success

interior [ɪn'tɪərɪə] *adjective & noun* (part) which is inside; *the interior of the intestine is lined with millions of villi*

interleukin [ɪntə'luːkɪn] *noun* protein produced by the body's immune system; **interleukin-1 (IL-1)** = protein which causes high temperature; **interleukin-2 (IL-2)** = protein which stimulates T-cell production, used in the treatment of cancer

interlobar [ɪntə'ləʊbə] *adjective* between lobes; **interlobar artery** = artery running

towards the cortex on each side of a renal pyramid

interlobular [ɪntə'lɒbjʊlə] *adjective* between lobules; **interlobular arteries** = arteries running to the glomeruli of the kidneys

intermediate [ɪntə'miːdɪət] *adjective* which is in the middle between two things

intermedius [ɪntə'miːdɪəs] *see* VASTUS

intermenstrual [ɪntə'menstrul] *adjective* between the menstrual periods

intermittent [ɪntə'mɪtənt] *adjective* occurring at intervals; **intermittent claudication** = condition of the arteries causing severe pain in the legs which makes the patient limp after having walked a short distance (the symptoms increase with more walking, but stop after a short rest, and recur when the patient walks again); **intermittent fever** = fever which rises and falls, like malaria

intern ['ɪntɜːn] *noun* US medical school graduate who is working in a hospital while at the same time continuing his studies (NOTE: the GB English is **houseman, house officer**)

interna [ɪn'tɜːnə] *see* OTITIS

internal [ɪn'tɜːnl] *adjective* **(a)** inside the body; **the drug is for internal use only** = it should not be used on the outside of the body; **internal auditory meatus** = channel which takes the auditory nerve through the temporal bone; **internal bleeding** = loss of blood from an injury inside the body; **internal capsule** = broad band of fibres passing to and from the cerebral cortex; **internal carotid** = artery in the neck, behind the external carotid, which gives off the ophthalmic artery and ends by dividing into the anterior and middle cerebral arteries; **internal derangement of the knee (IDK)** = condition where the knee cannot function properly because of a torn meniscus; **internal ear** = the part of the ear inside the head, behind the eardrum, containing the semicircular canals, the vestibule and the cochlea; **internal haemorrhage** = haemorrhage which takes place inside the body; **internal injury** = damage to one of the internal organs; **internal jugular** = largest jugular vein in the neck, leading to the brachiocephalic veins; US **internal medicine** = treatment of diseases of the internal organs by specialists; **internal oblique** = middle layer of muscle covering the abdomen, beneath the external oblique;

internal organs = organs situated inside the body; *compare* EXTERNAL **(b) internal market** = system within the NHS, where hospitals are considered as suppliers of health care services and health authorities and GPs are considered as purchasers of services, the aim being to improve the efficiency of the system by introducing a more commercial approach to its organization

internally [ɪnˈtɜːnəli] *adverb* inside the body; *he was bleeding internally*

international unit (IU) [ɪntəˈnæʃnl ˈjuːnɪt] *noun* internationally agreed standard used in pharmacy as a measure of a substance such as drug or hormone

interneurone [ɪntəˈnjuːrəʊn] *noun* neurone with short processes which is a link between two other neurones in sensory or motor pathways

internist [ɪnˈtɜːnɪst] *noun* specialist who treats diseases of the internal organs by non-surgical means

internodal [ɪntəˈnəʊdl] *adjective* between two nodes

internship [ɪnˈtɜːnʃɪp] *noun US* position of an intern in a hospital

internuncial neurone [ɪntəˈnʌnʃl ˈnjuːrəʊn] *noun* neurone which links two other nerve cells

internus [ɪnˈtɜːnəs] *noun* medial rectus muscle in the orbit of the eye

interoceptor [ɪntərəʊˈseptə] *noun* nerve cell which reacts to a change taking place inside the body; *see also* CHEMORECEPTOR, EXTEROCEPTOR, PROPRIOCEPTOR, RECEPTOR, VISCEROCEPTOR

interosseous [ɪntərˈɒsɪəs] *adjective* between bones

interpeduncular cistern
[ɪntəpəˈdʌŋkjʊlər ˈsɪstən] *noun* subarachnoid space between the two cerebral hemispheres beneath the midbrain and the hypothalamus

interphalangeal joint (IP joint)
[ɪntəfəˈlændʒɪəl ˈdʒɔɪnt] *noun* joint between the phalanges; **distal interphalangeal joint (DIP)** = joint nearest the end of the finger or toe; **proximal interphalangeal joint (PIP)** = joint nearest the point of attachment of a finger or toe

interphase [ˈɪntəfeɪz] *noun* stage of a cell between divisions

interpret [ɪnˈtɜːprɪt] *verb* to examine and decide what something means; *to interpret an X-ray*

interpubic joint [ɪntəˈpjuːbɪk ˈdʒɔɪnt] *noun* pubic symphysis, piece of cartilage which joins the two sections of the pubic bone

interruptus [ɪntəˈrʌptəs] *see* COITUS

intersexuality [ɪntəsekʃuˈæləti] *noun* condition where a baby has both male and female characteristics, as in Klinefelter's syndrome and Turner's syndrome

interstices [ɪnˈtɜːstɪsɪz] *plural noun* small spaces between parts of the body or between cells

interstitial [ɪntəˈstɪʃl] *adjective* (tissue, etc.) in the spaces between parts of something, especially the tissue between the active tissue in an organ; **interstitial cells** = Leydig cells, the testosterone-producing cells between the tubules in the testes; **interstitial cell stimulating hormone (ICSH)** = hormone produced by the pituitary gland which stimulates the formation of corpus luteum in females and testosterone in males (NOTE: also called luteinizing hormone orLH)

intertrigo [ɪntəˈtraɪgəʊ] *noun* irritation which occurs when two skin surfaces rub against each other (as in the armpit or between the buttocks)

intertubercular plane [ɪntətjuˈbɜːkjʊlə ˈpleɪn] *noun* imaginary horizontal line drawn across the lower abdomen at the level of the projecting parts of the iliac bones

interval [ˈɪntəvəl] *noun* period of time between two points; *there will be an interval of about two months between treatments*; **at intervals** = from time to time; **at regular intervals** = quite often but regularly - such as every two months; *the test must be repeated at regular intervals*; **in the interval** = in the meantime; *I will see you in two weeks time, in the interval continue to take the medicine twice a day*

intervention [ɪntəˈvenʃn] *noun* treatment; **medical intervention** *or* **surgical intervention** = treatment of illness by drugs or by surgery; **nursing intervention** = treatment of illness by nursing care, without surgery

interventricular [ɪntəvenˈtrɪkjʊlə] *adjective* between ventricles (in the heart or brain); **interventricular septum** = wall in the lower part of the heart, separating the ventricles; **interventricular foramen** = opening in the brain between the lateral ventricle and the third ventricle, through which the cerebrospinal fluid passes

intervertebral [ɪntə'vɜːtɪbrl] *adjective* between vertebrae; **intervertebral disc** = thick piece of cartilage which lies between two vertebrae; **intervertebral foramen** = hole between two vertebrae; *see also* VERTEBRAL; *see illustrations at* JOINTS, VERTEBRAL COLUMN

intestinal [ɪn'testɪnl] *adjective* referring to the intestine; **intestinal anastomosis** = surgical operation to join one part of the intestine to another (after a section has been removed); **intestinal flora** = bacteria which are always present in the intestine; **intestinal glands** = glands of Lieberkuhn, tubular glands found in the mucous membrane of the small and large intestine, especially those between the bases of the villi in the small intestine; **intestinal infection** = infection in the intestines; **intestinal juice** = colourless fluid secreted by the small intestine which contains enzymes that help digestion; **intestinal obstruction** = blocking of the intestine; **intestinal wall** = layers of tissue which form the intestine (NOTE: for other terms referring to the intestine, see words beginning with **entero-**)

intestine [ɪn'testɪn] *noun* **the intestines** = the bowel or gut, the tract which passes from the stomach to the anus in which food is digested as it passes through; **small intestine** = section of the intestine from the stomach to the caecum, consisting of the duodenum, the jejunum and the ileum; **large intestine** = the colon, the section of the intestine from the caecum to the rectum, consisting of the caecum, the ascending, transverse, descending and sigmoid colons and the rectum

COMMENT: absorption of substances in partly digested food is the main function of the small intestine. This is carried out by the little villi in the walls of the intestine which absorb nutrients into the bloodstream. The large intestine absorbs water from the food after it has passed through the small intestine, and the remaining material passes out of the body through the anus as faeces

intima ['ɪntɪmə] *noun & adjective;* **(tunica) intima** = inner layer of the wall of an artery or vein

intolerance [ɪn'tɒlərəns] *noun* (i) being unable to endure something, such as pain; (ii) being unable to take certain drugs because of the body's reaction to them; *he developed an intolerance to penicillin*

intoxicant [ɪn'tɒksɪkənt] *noun* substance, such as an alcoholic drink, which induces a state of intoxication or poisoning

intoxicate [ɪn'tɒksɪkeɪt] *verb* to make a person drunk, to make a person incapable of controlling his actions, because of the influence of alcohol on his nervous system; *he drank six glasses of whisky and became completely intoxicated*

intoxication [ɪntɒksɪ'keɪʃn] *noun* condition which results from the absorption and diffusion in the body of a poison, such as alcohol; *she was driving a bus in a state of intoxication*

intra- ['ɪntrə] *prefix* meaning inside

intra-abdominal [ɪntrəæb'dɒmɪnl] *adjective* inside the abdomen

intra-articular [ɪntrəɑː'tɪkjʊlə] *adjective* inside a joint

intracellular [ɪntrə'seljʊlə] *adjective* inside a cell

intracerebral haematoma [ɪntrə'serəbrl hiːmə'təʊmə] *noun* blood clot inside a cerebral hemisphere

intracranial [ɪntrə'kreɪniəl] *adjective* inside the skull

intractable [ɪn'træktəbl] *adjective* which cannot be treated; *an operation to relieve intractable pain*

intracutaneous *or* **intradermal** [ɪntrəkju'teɪniəs *or* ɪntrə'dɜːml] *adjective* inside layers of skin tissue; **intradermal test** = allergy or other test (such as Mantoux test) requiring an injection into the thickness of the skin

intradural [ɪntrə'djʊərl] *adjective* inside the dura mater

intramedullary [ɪntrəme'dʌləri] *adjective* inside the bone marrow or spinal cord

intramural [ɪntrə'mjʊərl] *adjective* inside the wall of an organ

intramuscular [ɪntrə'mʌskjʊlə] *adjective* inside a muscle; **intramuscular injection** = injection made into a muscle

intraocular [ɪntrə'ɒkjʊlə] *adjective* inside the eye; **intraocular lens (IOL)** = artificial lens implanted inside the eye; **intraocular**

pressure = pressure inside the eyeball (if too high, it gives glaucoma)

intrathecal [ɪntrə'θiːkl] *adjective* inside a sheath, inside the intradural or subarachnoid space

intratubercular plane [ɪntrətjuː'bɜːkjʊlə 'pleɪn] *noun* plane at right angles to the sagittal plane, passing through the tubercles of the iliac crests

intrauterine [ɪntrə'juːtəraɪn] *adjective* inside the uterus; **intrauterine device (IUD)** = plastic coil placed inside the uterus to prevent conception

intravenous (IV) [ɪntrə'viːnəs] *adjective* into a vein; **intravenous feeding** = giving liquid food to a patient by means of a tube inserted into a vein; *see also* DRIP; **intravenous injection** = injection into a vein for fast release of a drug; **intravenous pyelogram (IVP)** = series of X-ray photographs of the kidneys using pyelography; **intravenous pyelography** = X-ray examination of the kidneys after an opaque substance is injected intravenously into the body, and is carried by the blood into the kidneys

intravenously [ɪntrə'viːnəsli] *adverb* into a vein; *a fluid given intravenously*

intra vitam ['ɪntrə 'vaɪtəm] *Latin phrase meaning* 'during life'

intrinsic [ɪn'trɪnsɪk] *adjective* referring to the essential nature of an organism, included inside an organ or part; **intrinsic factor** = protein produced in the gastric glands which reacts with the extrinsic factor, and which, if lacking, causes pernicious anaemia; **intrinsic ligament** = ligament which forms part of the capsule surrounding a joint; **intrinsic muscle** = muscle lying completely inside the part or segment, especially of a limb which it moves

introduce [ɪntrə'djuːs] *verb* **(a)** to put something into something; *he used a syringe to introduce a medicinal substance into the body*; *the nurse introduced the catheter into the vein* **(b)** to present two people to one another when they have never met before; *can I introduce my new assistant?* **(c)** to start a new way of doing something; *the hospital has introduced a new screening process for cervical cancer*

introduction [ɪntrə'dʌkʃn] *noun* **(a)** putting something inside; *the introduction of semen into the woman's uterus*; *the introduction of an endotracheal tube into*

the patient's mouth **(b)** starting a new process

introitus [ɪn'trəuitəs] *noun* opening into any hollow organ or canal

introversion [ɪntrə'vɜːʃn] *noun* condition where a person is excessively interested in himself and his own mental state

introvert ['ɪntrəvɜːt] *noun* person who thinks only about himself and his own mental state; *compare* EXTROVERT, EXTROVERSION

introverted [ɪntrə'vɜːtɪd] *adjective* (person) who thinks only about himself

intubate ['ɪntjubeit] *verb* to catheterize, to insert a tube into any organ or part of the body

intubation [ɪntju'beɪʃn] *noun* catheterization, therapeutic insertion of a tube into the larynx through the glottis to allow passage of air

intumescence [ɪntju'mesəns] *noun* swelling of an organ

intussusception [ɪntəsə'sepʃn] *noun* condition where part of the gastrointestinal tract telescopes into the part beneath it, causing an obstruction and strangulation of the part which has telescoped

invagination [ɪnvædʒə'neɪʃn] *noun* **(a)** intussusception **(b)** surgical treatment of hernia, in which a sheath of tissue is made to cover the opening

invalid ['ɪnvəliːd] *noun & adjective* (person) who has had an illness and has not fully recovered from it; (person) who is disabled; *he has been an invalid since he had the accident six years ago*; *she is looking after her invalid parents*; **invalid carriage** = small car, specially made for use by an invalid; **invalid chair** = wheelchair, a chair with wheels in which an invalid can sit and move about; *she manages to do all her shopping using her invalid chair*; *some buildings have special entrances for invalid chairs*

invalidity [ɪnvə'lɪdəti] *noun* being disabled; **invalidity benefit** = money paid by the government to someone who is permanently disabled

invasion [ɪn'veɪʒn] *noun* entry of bacteria into a body, first attack of a disease

invasive [ɪn'veɪzɪv] *adjective* **(a)** (cancer) which tends to spread throughout the body **(b)** (inspection or treatment) which involves entering the body by making an incision; *see also* NON-INVASIVE

invent [ɪnˈvent] *verb* (**a**) to make something which has never been made before; *he invented a new type of catheter* (**b**) to make up, using your imagination; *he invented the whole story*; *small children often invent imaginary friends*

invention [ɪnˈvenʃn] *noun* thing which someone has invented; *we have seen his latest invention, a brain scanner*

inversion [ɪnˈvɜːʃn] *noun* being turned towards the inside, turning of part of the body (such as the foot) towards the inside; **inversion of the uterus** = condition where the top part of the uterus touches the cervix, as if it were inside out (which may happen after childbirth)

invertase [ɪnˈvɜːteɪz] *noun* enzyme in the intestine which splits sucrose

investigate [ɪnˈvestɪgeɪt] *verb* to examine something to try to find out what caused it; *health inspectors are investigating the outbreak of legionnaires' disease*

investigation [ɪnvestɪˈgeɪʃn] *noun* examination to find out the cause of something which has happened; *the Health Authority ordered an investigation into how the drugs were stolen*

investigative surgery [ɪnˈvestɪgeɪtɪv ˈsɜːdʒəri] *noun* surgery to investigate the cause of a condition

invisible [ɪnˈvɪzəbl] *adjective* which cannot be seen; *the microbes are invisible to the naked eye, but can be clearly seen under a microscope*

in vitro [ˈɪn ˈviːtrəʊ] *Latin phrase meaning* 'in a glass'; **in vitro activity** *or* **in vitro experiment** = experiment which takes place in the laboratory; **in vitro fertilization (IVF)** = fertilization of an ovum in the laboratory; *see also* TEST-TUBE BABY

in vivo [ˈɪn ˈviːvəʊ] *Latin phrase meaning* 'in living tissue'; **in vivo experiment** = experiment on a living body (such as an animal)

involucrum [ɪnvəˈluːkrəm] *noun* covering of new bone which forms over diseased bone

involuntary [ɪnˈvɒləntəri] *adjective* independent of the will, done without any mental processes being involved; *patients are advised not to eat or drink, to reduce the risk of involuntary vomiting while on the* operating table; **involuntary action** = action where a patient does not use his will power; **involuntary muscle** = muscle supplied by

the autonomic nervous system, and therefore not under voluntary control (such as the muscle which activates a vital organ like the heart)

involution [ɪnvəˈluːʃn] *noun* (**a**) return of an organ to normal size, such as the return of the uterus to normal size after childbirth (**b**) period of decline of organs which sets in after middle age

involutional [ɪnvəˈluːʃənl] *adjective* referring to involution; **involutional melancholia** = depression which occurs in people (mainly women) after middle age, probably caused by a change of endocrine secretions

involve [ɪnˈvɒlv] *verb* to concern, to have to do with; *the operation involves removing part of the duodenum and attaching the stomach directly to the jejunum*

iodaemia [aɪəʊˈdiːmiə] *noun* (high) level of iodine in the blood

iodine [ˈaɪədiːn] *noun* chemical element which is essential to the body, especially to the functioning of the thyroid gland; **tincture of iodine** = weak solution of iodine in alcohol, used as an antiseptic (NOTE: chemical symbol is I)

COMMENT: lack of iodine in the diet can cause goitre

IOL [ˈaɪ ˈəʊ ˈel] = INTRAOCULAR LENS

ion [ˈaɪən] *noun* atom which has an electric charge (ions with a positive charge are called cations and those with a negative charge are anions)

ionize [ˈaɪənaɪz] *verb* to give an atom an electric charge

ionizer [ˈaɪənaɪzə] *noun* negative ion generator, a machine that increases the amount of negative ions in the atmosphere of a room, so counteracting the effect of positive ions

COMMENT: it is believed that living organisms, including human beings, react to the presence of ionized particles in the atmosphere. Hot dry winds contain a higher proportion of positive ions than normal and these winds cause headaches and other illnesses. If negative ionized air is introduced into an air-conditioning system, the incidence of headaches and nausea among people working in the building may be reduced

ionotherapy [aɪɒnə'θerəpi] *noun* treatment by ions introduced into the body via an electric current

IP ['aɪ 'piː] = INTERPHALANGEAL JOINT

ipecacuanha *US* **ipecac** [ɪpɪkækju'ænə or 'ɪpɪkæk] *noun* drug made from the root of an American plant, used as treatment for coughs, and also as an emetic

ipsilateral [ɪpsɪ'lætərl] *adjective* on the same side of the body

IQ ['aɪ 'kjuː] = INTELLIGENCE QUOTIENT

irid- ['ɪrɪd] *prefix* referring to the iris

iridectomy [ɪrɪ'dektəmi] *noun* surgical removal of part of the iris

iridencleisis [ɪrɪden'klaɪsɪs] *noun* operation to treat glaucoma, where part of the iris is used as a drainage channel through a hole in the conjunctiva

iridocyclitis [ɪrɪdəʊsɪ'klaɪtɪs] *noun* inflammation of the iris and the tissues which surround it

iridodialysis [ɪrɪdəʊdaɪ'æləsɪs] *noun* separation of the iris from its insertion

iridoplegia [ɪrɪdəʊ'pliːdʒə] *noun* paralysis of the iris

iridotomy [ɪrɪ'dɒtəmi] *noun* surgical incision into the iris

iris ['aɪrɪs] *noun* coloured ring in the eye, with at its centre the pupil; *see illustration at* EYE

COMMENT: the iris acts like the aperture in a camera shutter, opening and closing to allow more or less light through the pupil into the eye

iritis [aɪ'raɪtɪs] *noun* inflammation of the iris

iron ['aɪən] *noun* **(a)** chemical element essential to the body, found in liver, eggs, etc. (NOTE: chemical symbol is Fe) **(b)** common grey metal

COMMENT: iron is an essential part of the red pigment in red blood cells. Lack of iron in haemoglobin results in iron-deficiency anaemia. Storage of too much iron in the body results in haemochromatosis

iron lung ['aɪən 'lʌŋ] = DRINKER RESPIRATOR

irradiation [ɪreɪdi'eɪʃn] *noun* **(a)** spread from a centre, as nerve impulses **(b)** use of rays to treat patients or to kill bacteria in food; **total body irradiation** = treating the whole body with radiation

irreducible [ɪrɪ'djuːsəbl] *adjective* (hernia) where the organ cannot be returned to its original position without an operation

irregular [ɪ'regjulə] *adjective* not regular, abnormal; *the patient's breathing was irregular*; *the nurse noted that the patient had developed an irregular pulse*; *he has irregular bowel movements*

irrigate ['ɪrɪgeɪt] *verb* to wash out a cavity in the body

irrigation [ɪrɪ'geɪʃn] *noun* washing out of a cavity in the body; **colonic irrigation** = washing out the large intestine

irritability [ɪrɪtə'bɪləti] *noun* state of being irritable

irritable ['ɪrɪtəbl] *adjective* which can be easily excited; **irritable colon** *or* **irritable bowel syndrome** = MUCOUS COLITIS

irritant ['ɪrɪtənt] *noun* substance which can irritate; **irritant dermatitis** = contact dermatitis, a skin inflammation caused by touching

irritate ['ɪrɪteɪt] *verb* to make something painful, itchy or sore; *some types of wool can irritate the skin*

irritation [ɪrɪ'teɪʃn] *noun* action of irritating; *an irritation caused by the ointment*

isch- [ɪsk] *prefix* meaning reduction, too little

ischaemia [ɪ'skiːmiə] *noun* deficient blood supply to part of the body; **cerebral ischaemia** = failure in the blood supply to the brain

ischaemic [ɪ'skiːmɪk] *adjective* lacking in blood; **ischaemic heart disease (IHD)** = disease of the heart caused by a failure in the blood supply (as in coronary thrombosis); **transient ischaemic attack (TIA)** = mild stroke caused by a brief stoppage of blood supply to the brain

changes in life style factors have been related to the decline in total mortality from IHD. In many studies a sedentary life style has been reported as a risk factor for IHD

Journal of the American Medical Association

the term stroke does not refer to a single pathological entity. Stroke may be haemorrhagic or ischaemic: the latter is usually caused by thrombosis or embolism

British Journal of Hospital Medicine

ischial ['ɪskɪəl] *adjective* referring to the ischium or hip joint; **ischial tuberosity** = lump of bone forming the ring of the ischium

ischiocavernosus muscle [ˌɪskɪəʊkævə'nəʊsəs 'mʌsl] *noun* muscle along one side of the perineum

ischiorectal [ˌɪskɪəʊ'rektl] *adjective* referring to both the ischium and the rectum; **ischiorectal abscess** = abscess which forms in fat cells between the anus and the ischium; **ischiorectal fossa** = space on either side of the lower end of the rectum and anal canal

ischium ['ɪskɪəm] *noun* lower part of the hip bone in the pelvis; *see illustration at* PELVIS

ischuria [ɪ'skjʊərɪə] *noun* retention or suppression of urine

Ishihara test [ɪʃɪ'hærə 'test] *noun* test for colour blindness where the patient is asked to identify letters or numbers among a mass of coloured dots

islets of Langerhans *or* **islands of Langerhans** *or* **islet cells** ['aɪləts or 'aɪlɒnz əv 'læŋəhæns or 'aɪlət 'selz] *plural noun* groups of cells in the pancreas which secrete the hormones glucagon and insulin

iso- ['aɪsəʊ] *prefix* meaning equal

isoantibody [ˌaɪsəʊ'æntɪbɒdɪ] *noun* antibody which forms in one person as a reaction to antigens from another person

isograft ['aɪsəʊgrɑːft] *noun* syngraft, graft of tissue from an identical twin

isoimmunization [ˌaɪsəʊɪmjʊnaɪ'zeɪʃn] *noun* immunization of a person with antigens derived from another person

isolate ['aɪsəleɪt] *verb* **(a)** to keep one patient apart from others (because he has a dangerous infectious disease) **(b)** to identify a single virus or bacteria among many; *scientists have been able to isolate the virus which causes legionnaires' disease; candida is easily isolated from the mouths of healthy adults*

isolation [ˌaɪsə'leɪʃn] *noun* separation of a patient, especially one with an infectious disease, from other patients; **isolation hospital** *or* **isolation ward** = special hospital or special ward in a hospital where patients suffering from infectious dangerous diseases can be isolated

isoleucine [ˌaɪsəʊ'luːsɪn] *noun* essential amino acid

isometric exercises [ˌaɪsəʊ'metrɪk 'eksəsaɪzɪz] *noun* exercises which strengthen the muscles, where the muscles contract but do not shorten

isotonic [ˌaɪsə'tɒnɪk] *adjective* (solution, such as a saline drip) which has the same osmotic pressure as blood and which can therefore be passed directly into the body

isotonicity [ˌaɪsətɒ'nɪsətɪ] *noun* equal osmotic pressure of two or more solutions

isotope ['aɪsətəʊp] *noun* form of a chemical element which has the same chemical properties as other forms, but different atomic mass; **radioactive isotope** = isotope which sends out radiation, used in radiotherapy and scanning

isthmus ['ɪsməs] *noun* (i) short narrow canal or cavity; (ii) narrow band of tissue joining two larger masses of similar tissue (such as the section in the centre of the thyroid gland, which joins the two lobes)

itch [ɪtʃ] **1** *noun* any irritated place on the skin, which makes a person want to scratch; **the itch** = scabies, an infection of the skin caused by a mite, producing violent irritation **2** *verb* to produce an irritating sensation, making a person want to scratch; *the cream made his skin itch more*

itching ['ɪtʃɪŋ] *noun* pruritus, irritation of the skin which makes a person want to scratch

itchy ['ɪtʃɪ] *adjective* which makes a person want to scratch; *the main symptom of the disease is an itchy red rash*

-itis ['aɪtɪs] *suffix* meaning inflammation; **otitis** = inflammation of the ear; **rhinitis** = inflammation of the nasal passages

IU ['aɪ 'juː] = INTERNATIONAL UNIT

IUD ['aɪ 'juː 'diː] = INTRAUTERINE DEVICE

IV ['aɪ 'viː] = INTRAVENOUS

IVF ['aɪ 'viː 'ef] = IN VITRO FERTILIZATION

IVP ['aɪ 'viː 'piː] = INTRAVENOUS PYELOGRAM

Jj

J [dʒeɪ] = JOULE

jab [dʒæb] *noun (informal)* injection, inoculation; *he has had a tetanus jab; go to the doctor to get a cholera jab*

jacket ['dʒækɪt] *noun* short coat; *the dentist was wearing a white jacket*; **bed jacket** = short warm jacket which a patient can wear when sitting in bed

Jacksonian epilepsy [dʒæk'səʊniən 'epɪlepsɪ] *see* EPILEPSY

Jakob ['dʒækɒb] *see* CREUTZFELDT

Jacquemier's sign ['dʒækəmɪəz 'saɪn] *noun* sign of early pregnancy, when the vaginal mucosa becomes bluish in colour due to an increased amount of blood in the arteries

jar [dʒɑː] **1** *noun* pot (usually glass) for keeping liquids or food in; *specimens of diseased organs can be kept in glass jars* **2** *verb* to give a shock with a blow; *the patient fell awkwardly and jarred his spine*

jaundice ['dʒɔːndɪs] *noun* icterus, a condition where there is an excess of bile pigment in the blood, and where the pigment is deposited in the skin and the whites of the eyes which have a yellow colour; **haemolytic jaundice** *or* **prehepatic jaundice** = jaundice caused by haemolysis of the red blood cells; **hepatocellular jaundice** = jaundice caused by injury to or disease of the liver cells; **infective jaundice** = jaundice caused by a viral disease such as hepatitis; **obstructive jaundice** *or* **posthepatic jaundice** = jaundice caused by an obstruction of the bile ducts; *see also* ACHOLURIC, ICTERUS NEONATORUM

COMMENT: jaundice can have many causes, usually relating to the liver: the most common are blockage of the bile ducts by gallstones or by disease of the liver and Weil's disease

jaw [dʒɔː] *noun* bones in the face which hold the teeth and form the mouth; **upper jaw and lower jaw** = the two parts of the jaw, the upper (the maxillae) being fixed parts of the skull, and the lower (the mandible) being attached to the skull with a hinge so that it can move up and down; *teeth are fixed in both the upper and lower jaw; he fell down and broke his jaw; the punch on his mouth broke his lower jaw*

jawbone ['dʒɔːbəʊn] *noun* one of the bones (the maxillae and the mandible) which form the jaw (NOTE: **jawbone** usually refers to the lower jaw or mandible)

jejun(o)- [dʒiːdʒun] *prefix* referring to the jejunum

jejunal [dʒɪ'dʒuːnl] *adjective* referring to the jejunum; **jejunal ulcer** = ulcer in the jejunum

jejunectomy [dʒiːdʒuː'nektəmi] *noun* surgical removal of all or part of the jejunum

jejunoileostomy [dʒɪdʒuːnəʊɪli'ɒstəmi] *noun* surgical operation to make an artificial link between the jejunum and the ileum

jejunostomy [dʒiːdʒu'nɒstəmi] *noun* surgical operation to make an artificial passage to the jejunum through the wall of the abdomen

jejunotomy [dʒiːdʒu'nɒtəmi] *noun* surgical operation to cut into the jejunum

jejunum [dʒiː'dʒuːnəm] *noun* part of the small intestine between the duodenum and the ileum; *see illustration at* DIGESTIVE SYSTEM

COMMENT: the jejunum is about 2 metres long

jelly ['dʒeli] *noun* semi-solid substance; **lubricating jelly** = jelly used to make a surface slippery

jerk [dʒɜːk] **1** *noun* sudden movement of part of the body which indicates that the local reflex arc is intact; **ankle jerk** = jerk as a reflex action of the foot when the back of the ankle is tapped; **knee jerk** = jerk made as a reflex action by the knee, when the legs are crossed and the patellar tendon is tapped sharply **2** *verb* to make sudden movements; *some forms of epilepsy are accompanied by jerking of the limbs*

jerky ['dʒɜːki] *adjective* with sudden movement; *the patient made jerky movements with his hand*

jet lag ['dʒet læg] *noun* condition suffered by people who travel long distances in planes, caused by rapid changes in time zones which affect sleep patterns and meal times and thus interfere with the body's metabolism (NOTE: does not take **the** or **a: she is suffering from jet lag; he took several days to get over his jet lag**)

jigger ['dʒɪgə] = SANDFLEA

join [dʒɔɪn] *verb* to put things together; to come together; *the bones are joined together by a cartilage*; *the inflammation started at the point where the ileum joins the caecum*

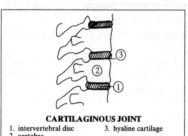

CARTILAGINOUS JOINT
1. intervertebral disc   3. hyaline cartilage
2. vertebra

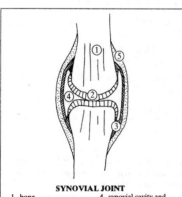

SYNOVIAL JOINT
1. bone   4. synovial cavity and
2. articular cartilage   fluid
3. synovial membrane   5. joint capsule (ligament)

joint [dʒɔɪnt] *noun* junction of two or more bones, especially one which allows movement of the bones; *the elbow is a joint in the arm*; *arthritis is accompanied by stiffness in the joints*; **hip joint** = place where the hip is joined to the upper leg; **wrist joint** = place where the wrist joins the arm; **ball and socket joint** = joint (like the shoulder) where the rounded end of a long bone fits into a socket on another bone; **primary cartilaginous joint** = temporary joint where the intervening cartilage is converted into adult bone; **secondary cartilaginous joint** = joint where the surfaces of the two bones are connected by a piece of cartilage so that they cannot move (such as the pubic symphysis); **fibrous joint** = joint where two bones are fixed together by fibrous tissue, so that they can move only slightly (as in the bones of the skull); **hinge joint** = joint (like the knee) which allows the two bones to move in one plane only; **locking joints** = joints (such as the knee or elbow) which can be locked in an extended position; **pivot joint** *or* **trochoid joint** = joint where a bone can rotate easily; **synovial joint** = joint where the two bones are separated by a space filled with synovial fluid which nourishes and lubricates the surfaces of the bones; **joint capsule** = white fibrous tissue which surrounds and holds a joint together; **joint mice** = loose pieces of bone or cartilage in the knee joint, making the joint lock; *see also* CHARCOT'S JOINT (NOTE: for other terms referring to joints, see words beginning with **arthr-, articul-**)

joint-breaker fever ['dʒɔɪntbreɪkə 'fiːvə] = O'NYONG-NYONG FEVER

jointed ['dʒɔɪntɪd] *adjective* linked with joints

joule [dʒuːl] *noun* SI unit of measurement of energy (NOTE: usually written **J** with figures: **25J**)

COMMENT: one joule is the amount of energy used to move one kilogram the distance of one metre, using the force of one newton. 4.184 joules equals one calorie

jugular ['dʒʌgjʊlə] *adjective* referring to the throat or neck; **jugular nerve** = one of the nerves in the neck; **jugular trunk** = terminal lymph vessel in the neck, draining into the subclavian vein; **jugular vein** *or* **jugular** = one of the veins which pass down either side of the neck

COMMENT: there are three jugular veins on each side: the internal jugular is large and leads to the brachiocephalic vein, the external jugular is smaller and leads to the subclavian vein and the anterior jugular is the smallest

juice [dʒuːs] *noun* **(a)** liquid from a fruit or vegtable; fluid secretion of an animal or plant; *a glass of orange juice or tomato juice*; *a tin of grapefruit juice* **(b)** gastric juice = acid liquid secreted by the stomach which helps digest food; **intestinal juice** = alkaline liquid secreted by the small intestine which helps digest food

junction [ˈdʒʌŋkʃn] *noun* joining point

juvenile [ˈdʒuːvənaɪl] *adjective* referring to children or adolescents; *the area has six new cases of juvenile diabetes mellitus*

juxta- [ˈdʒʌkstə] *prefix* meaning beside or near

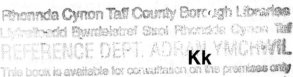
Kk

K [keɪ] **1** *chemical symbol for* potassium **2** *noun* **Vitamin K** = vitamin found in green vegetables like spinach and cabbage, and which helps the clotting of blood and is needed to activate prothrombin

k *symbol for* kilo-

Kahn test ['kɑːn 'test] *noun* test of blood serum to diagnose syphilis

kala-azar ['kæləə'zɑː] *noun* severe infection, occurring in tropical countries

> COMMENT: kala-azar is a form of leishmaniasis, caused by the infection of the intestines and internal organs by a parasite *Leishmania* pread by flies. Symptoms are fever, anaemia, general wasting of the body and swelling of the spleen and liver

kalium ['keɪliəm] = POTASSIUM

kaolin ['keɪəlɪn] *noun* white powder, the natural form of aluminium silicate or china clay

> COMMENT: kaolin is used internally in liquid form to reduce diarrhoea and can also be used externally as a talc or as a poultice

Kaposi's sarcoma [kə'pəʊzɪz sɑː'kəʊmə] *noun* cancer which takes the form of many haemorrhagic nodes affecting the skin, especially on the extremities

> COMMENT: formerly a relatively rare disease, found mainly in tropical countries; now more common as it is one of the sequelae of AIDS

karyotype ['kærɪəʊtaɪp] *noun* the chromosome complement of a cell, shown as a diagram or as a set of letters and numbers

Kayser-Fleischer ring ['kaɪzə'flaɪʃə 'rɪŋ] *noun* brown ring on the outer edge of the cornea, which is a diagnostic sign of hepatolenticular degeneration

kcal = KILOCALORIE

keen [kiːn] *adjective* **(a)** eager or willing; *he's keen to go to medical school*; *she is not at all keen on prescribing placebos* **(b)** *(of senses)* which can notice differences very well; *he has a keen sense of smell*; *she has keen eyesight* (NOTE: **keen - keener - keenest**)

keep [kiːp] *verb* **(a)** to have for a very long time or for ever; *the hospital keeps its medical records for ten years* **(b)** to continue to do something; *the pump has to be kept going twenty-four hours a day*; *keep taking the tablets for ten days* **(c)** to make someone stay in a state; *the patient must be kept warm and quiet*; *dangerous medicines should be kept locked in a cupboard* (NOTE: **keeping - kept - has kept**)

keep down ['kiːp 'daʊn] *verb* to take food and retain it in the stomach; *he managed to keep down some soup*; *she could not even keep a glass of orange juice down*

keep on ['kiːp 'ɒn] *verb* to continue to do something; *the patient kept on calling out in his sleep*; *you should keep on doing the exercises at home for several weeks*

Keller's operation ['kɛləz ɒpə'reɪʃn] *noun* operation on the big toe, to remove a bunion or to correct an ankylosed joint

keloid ['kiːlɔɪd] *noun* excessive amount of scar tissue at the site of a skin injury

kerat(o)- ['kerət or 'kerətəʊ] *prefix* referring to horn, horny tissue or the cornea

keratalgia [kerə'tældʒiə] *noun* pain felt in the cornea

keratectasia [kerətek'teɪziə] *noun* condition where the cornea bulges

keratectomy [kerə'tektəmi] *noun* surgical removal of the whole or part of the cornea

keratin ['kerətɪn] *noun* protein found in horny tissue (such as fingernails, hair or the outer surface of the skin)

keratinization [kerətɪnaɪˈzeɪʃn] *noun* cornification, the appearance of horny characteristics in tissue

keratinize [ˈkerətɪnaɪz] *verb* to convert into keratin, into horny tissue; *the cells are gradually keratinized*

keratinocyte [ˈkerətɪnəʊsaɪt] *noun* cell which produces keratin

keratitis [kerəˈtaɪtɪs] *noun* inflammation of the cornea

keratoacanthoma [kerətəʊækənˈθəʊmə] *noun* type of benign skin tumour, which disappears after a few months

keratoconjunctivitis [kerətəʊkəndʒʌntɪˈvaɪtɪs] *noun* inflammation of the cornea with conjunctivitis

keratoconus [kerətəʊˈkəʊnəs] *noun* cone-shaped lump on the cornea

keratoglobus [kerətəʊˈgləʊbəs] *noun* swelling of the eyeball

keratoma [kerəˈtəʊmə] *noun* hard thickened growth due to hypertrophy of the horny zone of the skin (NOTE: plural is **keratomata**)

keratomalacia [kerətəʊməˈleɪʃə] *noun* (i) softening of the cornea frequently caused by Vitamin A deficiency; (ii) softening of the horny layer of the skin

keratome [ˈkerətəʊm] *noun* surgical knife used for operations on the cornea

keratometer [kerəˈtɒmɪtə] *noun* instrument for measuring the curvature of the cornea

keratometry [kerəˈtɒmɪtri] *noun* process of measuring the curvature of the cornea

keratoplasty [ˈkerətəplæsti] *noun* corneal graft, grafting corneal tissue from a donor in place of diseased tissue

keratoscope [ˈkerətəskəʊp] *noun* Placido's disc, an instrument for examining the cornea to see if it has an abnormal curvature

keratosis [kerəˈtəʊsɪs] *noun* hard lesion covering the skin

keratotomy [kerəˈtɒtəmi] *noun* surgical operation to make a cut in the cornea, the first step in many intraocular operations

kerion [ˈkɪərɪɒn] *noun* painful soft mass, usually on the scalp, caused by ringworm

kernicterus [kəˈnɪktərəs] *noun* yellow pigmentation of the basal ganglia and other nerve cells in the spinal cord and brain, found in children with icterus

> COMMENT: the symptoms are convulsions, anorexia and drowsiness. In babies the disease can be fatal, and where it is not fatal, spasticity and mental defects appear

Kernig's sign [ˈkɜːnɪgz ˈsaɪn] *noun* symptom of meningitis, when the knee cannot be straightened if the patient is lying down with the thigh brought up against the abdomen

ketoacidosis [kiːtəʊæsɪˈdəʊsɪs] *noun* accumulation of ketone bodies in tissue in diabetes, causing acidosis

ketogenesis [kiːtəʊˈdʒenəsɪs] *noun* production of ketone bodies

ketogenic diet [kiːtəʊˈdʒenɪk ˈdaɪət] *noun* diet with a high fat content, producing ketosis

ketonaemia [kiːtəʊˈniːmiə] *noun* morbid state where ketone bodies exist in the blood

ketone [ˈkiːtəʊn] *noun* chemical compound containing the group CO attached to two alkyl groups; **ketone bodies** = ketone compounds formed from fatty acids

ketonuria [kiːtəʊˈnjʊəriə] *noun* state where ketone bodies are excreted in the urine

ketosis [kiːˈtəʊsɪs] *noun* state where ketone bodies (such as acetone and acetic acid) accumulate in the tissues, a late complication of juvenile diabetes mellitus; *see also* ACETONE, ACETONURIA

key [kiː] **1** *noun* **(a)** piece of shaped metal used to open a lock; *she has a set of keys to the laboratory*; *he signed for the key to the medicine cupboard* **(b)** part of a piano, a typewriter or a computer which you push down with your fingers **(c)** answer to a problem, explanation; *the key to successful treatment of arthritis is movement* **2** *adjective* most important; *he has the key position in the laboratory*; *penicillin is the key factor in the treatment of gangrene*

keyhole surgery [ˈkiːhəʊl ˈsɜːdʒəri] *noun* (*informal*) laparoscopic surgery involving inserting tiny surgical instruments through an endoscope

kg = KILOGRAM

kick [kɪk] **1** *noun* hitting with your foot; *she could feel the baby give a kick* **2** *verb* to hit something with your foot; *she could feel the baby kicking*

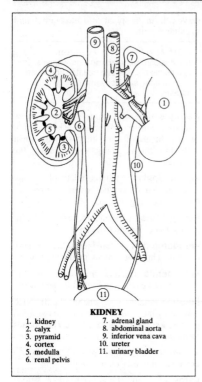

KIDNEY

1. kidney
2. calyx
3. pyramid
4. cortex
5. medulla
6. renal pelvis
7. adrenal gland
8. abdominal aorta
9. inferior vena cava
10. ureter
11. urinary bladder

kidney ['kɪdni] *noun* one of two organs situated in the lower part of the back on either side of the spine behind the abdomen, whose function is to maintain normal concentrations of the main constituents of blood, passing the waste matter into the urine; *he has a kidney infection*; *the kidneys have begun to malfunction*; *she is being treated for kidney trouble*; **kidney dialysis** = removing waste matter from the blood of a patient by passing it through a kidney machine; **kidney failure** = situation where a patient's kidneys do not function properly; **kidney machine** = apparatus through which a patient's blood is passed to be cleaned by dialysis if the patient's kidneys have failed; **kidney stone** = hard mass of calcium like a little piece of stone, which forms in the kidney; **floating kidney** = NEPHROPTOSIS; **horseshoe kidney** = congenital defect of the kidney, where sometimes the upper but usually the lower parts of both kidneys are joined together (NOTE: for other terms referring to the kidney, see words beginning with **nephr-, ren-, reno-**)

COMMENT: a kidney is formed of an outer cortex and an inner medulla. The nephrons which run from the cortex into the medulla filter the blood and form urine. The urine is passed through the ureters into the bladder. Sudden sharp pain in back of the abdomen, going downwards, is an indication of a kidney stone passing into the ureter

kill [kɪl] *verb* to make someone or something die; *she was given the kidney of a person killed in a car crash*; *heart attacks kill more people every year*; *antibodies are created to kill bacteria*

killer ['kɪlə] *noun* person or disease which kills; *virulent typhoid fever can be a killer disease*; *in the winter, bronchitis is the killer of hundreds of old people*; *see also* PAINKILLER

Killian's operation ['kɪliənz ɒpə'reɪʃn] *noun* clearing of the frontal sinus by curetting

COMMENT: in Killian's operation the incision is made in the eyebrow

kilo ['kɪləʊ] *abbreviation for* KILOGRAM

kilo- ['kɪləʊ] *prefix* meaning one thousand (10^3 (NOTE: symbol is **k**)

kilocalorie ['kɪləʊkæləri] *noun* SI unit of measurement of heat (= 1,000 calories) (NOTE: with figures usually written **kcal**. Note also that it is now more usual to use the term **joule**)

kilogram *or* **kilo** ['kɪləgræm *or* 'kiːləʊ] *noun* base SI unit of measurement of weight (= 1,000 grams); *two kilos of sugar*; *he weighs 62 kilos (62 kg)* (NOTE: with figures usually written **kg**)

kilojoule ['kɪləʊdʒuːl] *noun* SI unit of measurement of energy or heat (= 1,000 joules) (NOTE: with figures usually written **kJ**)

kilopascal ['kɪləʊpæskəl] *noun* SI unit of measurement of pressure (= 1,000 pascals) (NOTE: with figures usually written **kPa**)

Kimmelstiel-Wilson disease *or* **syndrome** ['kɪməlstiːl'wɪlsən dɪ'ziːz *or* 'sɪndrəʊm] *noun* form of nephrosclerosis found in diabetics

kin [kɪn] *noun* relatives or close members of the family; **next of kin** = person or persons who are most closely related to someone; *the hospital has notified the next of kin of the death of the accident victim*

kin- *or* **kine-** [kɪn *or* 'kɪni] *prefix* meaning movement

kinaesthesia [kɪniːsˈθiːziə] *noun* being aware of the movement and position of parts of the body

> COMMENT: kinaesthesia is the result of information from muscles and ligaments which is passed to the brain and which allows the brain to recognize movements, touch and weight

kinanaesthesia [kɪnæniːsˈθiːziə] *noun* not being able to sense the movement and position of parts of the body

kinematics [kɪnɪˈmætɪks] *noun* science of movement, especially of body movements (NOTE: also spelled **cinematics**)

kineplasty [ˈkɪnəplæsti] *noun* amputation where the muscles of the stump of the amputated limb are used to operate an artificial limb (NOTE: also spelled **cineplasty**)

kinesiology [kaɪniːsiˈɒlədʒi] *noun* study of human movements, referring particularly to their use in treatment (NOTE: also spelled **cinesiology**)

kinesitherapy [kɪniːsiˈθerəpi] *noun* therapy involving movement of parts of the body

kinetochore [kaɪˈniːtəkɔː] = CENTROMERE

Kirschner wire [ˈkɜːʃnəz ˈwaɪə] *noun* wire attached to a bone and tightened to provide traction to a fracture

kissing disease [ˈkɪsɪŋ diˈziːz] *(informal)* = GLANDULAR FEVER

kiss of life [ˈkɪs əv ˈlaɪf] *noun* method of artificial respiration where the aider breathes into the patient's lungs (either through the mouth or through the nose); *he was given the kiss of life*

kit [kɪt] *noun* equipment put together in a container; **first-aid kit** = box with bandages and dressings kept ready to be used in an emergency

kJ = KILOJOULE

Klebsiella [klebsiˈelə] *noun* form of Gram negative bacteria, one of which, *Klebsiella pneumoniae*, can cause pneumonia

Klebs-Loeffler bacillus [ˈklebzˈlɜːflə bəˈsɪləs] *noun* diphtheria bacillus

kleptomania [kleptəˈmeɪniə] *noun* form of mental disorder where the patient has a compulsive desire to steal things (even things of little value)

kleptomaniac [kleptəˈmeɪniæk] *noun* person who suffers from a compulsive desire to steal

Klinefelter's syndrome [ˈklaɪnfeltəz ˈsɪndrəʊm] *noun* genetic disorder where a male has an extra female chromosome (making an XXY set), giving sterility and partial female characteristics

Klumpke's paralysis [ˈkluːmpkəz pəˈræləsɪs] *noun* form of paralysis due to an injury during birth, affecting the forearm and hand (NOTE: also called **Déjerine-Klumpke's syndrome**)

knee [niː] *noun* joint in the middle of the leg, joining the femur and the tibia; **water on the knee** = condition where synovial fluid accumulates in the knee joint; **knee jerk** = PATELLAR REFLEX; **knee joint** = joint where the femur and the tibia are joined, covered by the kneecap

kneecap [ˈniːkæp] *noun* the patella, a small bone in front of the knee joint (NOTE: for other terms referring to the knee see words beginning with **genu-**)

knit [nɪt] *verb* **(a)** to make something out of wool, using two long needles **(b)** *(of broken bones)* to join together again; *broken bones take longer to knit in old people than in children* (NOTE: **knitting - has knitted** *or* **has knit**)

knock [nɒk] **1** *noun* **(a)** sound made by hitting something **(b)** hitting of something; *he was concussed after having had a knock on the head* **2** *verb* to hit something; *he knocked his head on the floor as he fell*

knock down [ˈnɒk ˈdaʊn] *verb* to make something fall down by hitting it hard; *he was knocked down by a car*

knock knee [ˈnɒk ˈniː] *noun* genu valgum, a state where the knees touch and the ankles are apart when a person is standing straight; *compare* BOW LEGS

knock-kneed [ˈnɒkˈniːd] *adjective* (person) whose knees touch when he stands straight with feet slightly apart

knock out [ˈnɒk ˈaʊt] *verb* to hit someone so hard that he is no longer conscious; *he was knocked out by a blow on the head*

knot [nɒt] **1** *noun* place where two pieces of string or gut are tied together; *he tied a knot at the end of the piece of string* **2** *verb* to attach with a knot; *the nurse knotted the two bandages* (NOTE: **knotting - knotted**)

knuckle ['nʌkl] *noun* the back of each joint on a person's hand

Koch's bacillus ['kəʊks bə'sıləs] *noun* bacillus, *Mycobacterium tuberculosis,* which causes tuberculosis

Koch-Weeks bacillus ['kəʊk'wiːks bə'sıləs] *noun* bacillus which causes conjunctivitis

Köhler's disease ['kɜːləz dı'siːz] *noun* scaphoiditis, degeneration of the navicular bone in children

koilonychia [kɔıləʊ'nıkıə] *noun* spoon nail, state where the fingernails are brittle and concave, caused by iron-deficiency anaemia

Koplik's spots ['kɒplıks 'spɒts] *plural noun* small bluish-white spots surrounded by red areola, found in the mouth in the early stages of measles

Korsakoff's syndrome ['kɔːsəkɒfs 'sındrəʊm] *noun* condition where the patient's memory fails and he invents things which have not happened and is confused, caused usually by chronic alcoholism or disorders in which there is a deficiency of vitamin B

kraurosis [krɔː'rəʊsıs] *noun* dryness and shrivelling of a part; **kraurosis penis** = state where the foreskin becomes dry and shrivelled; **kraurosis vulvae** = condition where the vulva becomes thin and dry due to lack of oestrogen (found usually in elderly women)

Krause corpuscles ['krauzə 'kɔːpʌslz] *see* CORPUSCLE; *see illustration at* SKIN AND SENSORY RECEPTORS

Krebs cycle ['krebz 'saıkl] = CITRIC ACID CYCLE

Krukenberg tumour ['kruːkənbɜːg 'tjuːmə] *noun* malignant tumour in the ovary secondary to a tumour in the stomach

Kuntscher nail *or* **Küntscher nail** ['kʌntʃə 'neıl] *noun* long steel nail used to pin fractures of long bones through the bone marrow

Kupffer's cells ['kupfəz 'selz] *noun* large specialized liver cells which break down haemoglobin into bile

Kveim test ['kvaım 'test] *noun* skin test to confirm the presence of sarcoidosis

kwashiorkor [kwɒʃi'ɔːkɔː] *noun* malnutrition of small children, mostly in tropical countries, causing anaemia, wasting of the body and swollen liver

kyphos ['kaıfəs] *noun* lump on the back in kyphosis

kyphoscoliosis [kaıfəʊskɒli'əʊsıs] *noun* condition where the patient has both backward and lateral curvature of the spine

kyphosis [kaı'fəʊsıs] *noun* hunchback, excessive backward curvature of the top part of the spine; *see also* LORDOSIS

kyphotic [kaı'fɒtık] *adjective* referring to kyphosis

LI

l = LITRE

lab [læb] *noun* *(informal)* = LABORATORY; *we'll send the specimens away for a lab test*; *the lab report is negative*; *the samples have been returned by the lab*

lab- [leɪb] *prefix* referring to the lips or to labia

label ['leɪbl] **1** *noun* piece of paper or card attached to an object or person to identify them; **identity label** = label attached to the wrist of a newborn baby or a patient in hospital, so that he can be identified easily **2** *verb* to write on a label, to attach a label to an object; *the bottle is labelled 'poison'*

labia ['leɪbiə] *see* LABIUM

labial ['leɪbiəl] *adjective* referring to the lips or to labia

labile ['leɪbaɪl] *adjective* (drug) which is unstable and likely to change if heated or cooled

labio- ['leɪbiəʊ] *prefix* referring to lips or to labia

labioplasty ['leɪbiəʊplæsti] *noun* surgical operation to repair damaged or deformed lips

labium ['leɪbiəm] *noun* (i) lip; (ii) structure which looks like a lip; **labia majora** = two large fleshy folds at the outside edge of the vulva; **labia minora** = nymphae, two small fleshy folds on the inside edge of the vulva; *see illustration at* UROGENITAL SYSTEM (female) (NOTE: plural is **labia**)

labor ['leɪbə] *see* LABOUR

laboratory [ləˈbɒrətri] *noun* special room(s) where scientists can do research, can test chemical substances, can grow tissues in culture, etc.; *the new drug has passed its laboratory tests*; *the samples of water from the hospital have been sent to the laboratory for testing*; **laboratory officer** = qualified person in charge of a laboratory; **laboratory techniques** = methods or skills needed to perform experiments in a laboratory; **laboratory technician** = person who does practical work in a laboratory and has particular care of equipment

labour *US* **labor** ['leɪbə] *noun* childbirth, especially the contractions in the uterus which take place during childbirth; **woman in labour** = experiencing the physical changes, contractions in the uterus, pains, etc., which precede the birth of a child; **to go into labour** = to start to experience the contractions which indicate the birth of a child is imminent; *she was in labour for 14 hours*; *she went into labour at 6 o'clock*; *see also* INDUCE, PREMATURE

COMMENT: labour usually starts about nine months (or 266 days) after conception. The cervix expands and the muscles in the uterus contract, causing the amnion to burst. The muscles continue to contract regularly, pushing the baby into, and then through, the vagina

labyrinth ['læbərɪnθ] *noun* interconnecting tubes, especially those in the inside of the ear; **bony labyrinth** *or* **osseous labyrinth** = hard part of the temporal bone surrounding the membranous labyrinth in the inner ear; **membranous labyrinth** = series of ducts and canals formed of membrane inside the osseous labyrinth

COMMENT: the labyrinth of the inner ear is in three parts: the three semicircular canals, the vestibule and the cochlea. The osseous labyrinth is filled with a fluid (perilymph) and the membranous labyrinth is a series of ducts and canals inside the osseous labyrinth. The membranous labyrinth contains a fluid (endolymph). As the endolymph moves about in the membranous labyrinth it stimulates the vestibular nerve which communicates the sense of movement of the head to the brain. If a person turns round and round and then stops, the endolymph continues to move and creates the sensation of giddiness

labyrinthitis [ˌlæbərɪnˈθaɪtɪs] *noun* otitis interna, inflammation of the labyrinth

lacerated [ˈlæsəreɪtɪd] *adjective* torn, with a rough edge; **lacerated wound** = wound where the skin is torn, as by a rough surface or barbed wire

laceration [ˌlæsəˈreɪʃn] *noun* act of tearing tissue; wound which has been cut or torn with rough edges, and not the result of stabbing or pricking

lachrymal [ˈlækrɪml] *see* LACRIMAL

lack [læk] **1** *noun* not having something; *the children are dying because of lack of food*; *the hospital had to close two wards because of lack of money* **2** *verb* not to have enough of something; *the children lack winter clothing*; *their diet lacks essential proteins*; **he lacks the strength to feed himself** = he isn't strong enough to feed himself

lacrimal *or* **lacrymal** *or* **lachrymal** [ˈlækrɪml] *adjective* referring to tears, tear ducts or tear glands; **lacrimal apparatus** *or* **system** = arrangement of glands and ducts which produce and drain tears; **lacrimal bones** = two little bones which join with others to form the orbits; **lacrimal canaliculus** = small canal draining tears into the lacrimal sac; **lacrimal caruncle** = small red point at the inner corner of each eye; **lacrimal duct** = tear duct, small duct leading from the lacrimal gland; **lacrimal gland** = tear gland, gland beneath the upper eyelid which secretes tears; **lacrimal puncta** = small openings of the lacrimal canaliculus at the corners of the eyes through which tears drain into the nose; **lacrimal sac** = sac at the upper end of the nasolacrimal duct, linking it with the lacrimal canaliculus; *see also* NASOLACRIMAL

lacrimation [ˌlækrɪˈmeɪʃn] *noun* crying, the production of tears

lacrimator [ˈlækrɪmeɪtə] *noun* substance which irritates the eyes and makes tears flow

lact- [lækt] *prefix* referring to milk

lactase [ˈlækteɪz] *noun* enzyme, secreted in the small intestine, which converts milk sugar into glucose and galactose

lactate [ˈlækteɪt] *verb* to produce milk

lactation [lækˈteɪʃn] *noun* (i) production of milk; (ii) period during which a mother is breast feeding a baby

COMMENT: lactation is stimulated by the production of the hormone prolactin by the pituitary gland. It starts about three days after childbirth, during which period the breasts secrete colostrum

lacteal [ˈlæktɪəl] **1** *adjective* referring to milk **2** *noun* lymph vessel in a villus, which helps the digestive process in the small intestine by absorbing fat

lactic acid [ˈlæktɪk ˈæsɪd] *noun* sugar which forms in cells and tissue, also in sour milk, cheese and yoghurt

COMMENT: lactic acid is produced as the body uses up sugar during exercise. Excessive amounts of lactic acid in the body can produce muscle cramp

lactiferous [lækˈtɪfərəs] *adjective* which produces or secretes or carries milk; **lactiferous duct** = duct in the breast which carries milk; **lactiferous sinus** = dilatation of the lactiferous duct at the base of the nipple

Lactobacillus [ˌlæktəʊbəˈsɪləs] *noun* genus of Gram-positive bacteria which can produce lactic acid from glucose and may be found in the digestive tract and the vagina

lactogenic hormone [ˌlæktəʊˈdʒenɪk ˈhɔːməʊn] = PROLACTIN

lactose [ˈlæktəʊz] *noun* milk sugar, sugar found in milk; **lactose intolerance** = condition where a person cannot digest lactose because lactase is absent in the intestine, or because of an allergy to milk, causing diarrhoea

lactosuria [ˌlæktəʊˈsjʊərɪə] *noun* excretion of lactose in the urine

lactovegetarian [ˌlæktəʊvedʒɪˈteərɪən] *noun* & *adjective* (person) who does not eat meat, but eats vegetables, fruit, dairy produce and eggs and sometimes fish; *he has been on a lactovegetarian diet for twenty years*; *compare* VEGAN, VEGETARIAN

lacuna [ləˈkjuːnə] *noun* small hollow or cavity (NOTE: the plural is **lacunae**)

Laennec's cirrhosis [ˈleɪəneks səˈrəʊsɪs] *noun* commonest form of alcoholic cirrhosis of the liver

laevocardia [ˌliːvəʊˈkɑːdɪə] *noun* normal position of the apex of the heart towards the left side of the body; *compare* DEXTROCARDIA

lambda [ˈlæmdə] *noun* point at the back of the skull where the sagittal suture and lambdoidal suture meet

lambdoid(al) suture [ˈlæmdɔɪdəl ˈsuːtʃə] *noun* horizontal joint across the back of the skull between the parietal and occipital bones; *see illustration at* SKULL

lamblia [ˈlæmbliə] *see* GIARDIA

lambliasis [læmˈblaɪəsɪs] *see* GIARDIASIS

lame [leɪm] *adjective* not able to walk normally because of pain, stiffness or deformity in a leg or foot; *he has been lame since his accident*

lamella [ləˈmelə] *noun* (i) thin sheet of tissue; (ii) thin disc placed under the eyelid to apply a drug to the eye (NOTE: the plural is **lamellae**)

lameness [ˈleɪmnəs] *noun* limping, the inability to walk normally because of pain, stiffness or deformity in a leg or foot

lamina [ˈlæmɪnə] *noun* (i) thin membrane; (ii) side part of the posterior arch in a vertebra; **lamina propria** = connective tissue of mucous membrane containing blood vessels, lymphatics, etc. (NOTE: plural is **laminae**)

laminectomy [læmɪˈnektəmi] *noun* rachiotomy, surgical operation to cut through the lamina of a vertebra in the spine to get to the spinal cord

lamp [læmp] *noun* electric device which makes light; *an electric lamp*; *an endoscope can have a small lamp at the end of it*; *the ear specialist shone his lamp into the patient's ear*; *she lay for thirty minutes under an ultraviolet lamp*

lance [lɑːns] *verb* to make a cut in a boil or abscess to remove the pus

lancet [ˈlɑːnsɪt] *noun* sharp two-edged pointed knife formerly used in surgery

lancinate [ˈlænsɪneɪt] *verb* to lacerate or cut

lancinating [ˈlænsɪneɪtɪŋ] *adjective* (pain) which is sharp and cutting

Landry's paralysis [ˈlændrɪz pəˈræləsɪs] *see* GUILLAIN-BARRÉ SYNDROME

Langerhans [ˈlæŋəhæns] *noun* **islets** *or* **islands of Langerhans** = groups of cells in the pancreas which secrete the hormones glucagon, insulin and gastrin; **Langerhans' cells** = cells on the outer layers of the skin

Lange test [ˈlæŋgə ˈtest] *noun* method of detecting globulin in the cerebrospinal fluid

lanolin [ˈlænəlɪn] *noun* grease (from sheep's wool) which absorbs water, and is used to rub on dried skin, or in the preparation of cosmetics

lanugo [ləˈnjuːgəʊ] *noun* soft hair on the body of a fetus or newborn baby; soft hair on the body of an adult (except on the palms of the hands, the soles of the feet, and the parts where long hair grows)

laparo- [ˈlæpərəʊ] *prefix* referring to the lower abdomen

laparoscope [ˈlæpərəskəʊp] *noun* peritoneoscope, a surgical instrument which is inserted through a hole in the abdominal wall to allow a surgeon to examine the inside of the abdominal cavity

laparoscopic [læpərəˈskɒpɪk] *adjective* using a laparoscope; **laparoscopic surgery** = surgery involving inserting tiny surgical instruments through an endoscope

laparoscopy [læpəˈrɒskəpi] *noun* peritoneoscopy, using a laparoscope to examine the inside of the abdominal cavity

laparotomy [læpəˈrɒtəmi] *noun* surgical operation to cut open the abdominal cavity

large [lɑːdʒ] *adjective* very big; *he has a large tumour on the right cerebrum* (NOTE: **large - larger - largest**)

large intestine [ˈlɑːdʒ ɪnˈtestɪn] *noun* section of the digestive system from the caecum to the rectum

larva [ˈlɑːvə] *noun* stage in the development of an insect or tapeworm, after the egg has hatched but before the animal becomes adult (NOTE: the plural is **larvae**)

laryng- *or* **laryngo-** [ləˈrɪndʒ or ləˈrɪŋgəʊ] *prefix* referring to the larynx

laryngeal [ləˈrɪndʒɪəl] *adjective* referring to the larynx; **laryngeal inlet** = entrance from the laryngopharynx leading through the vocal cords to the trachea; **laryngeal prominence** = Adam's apple; **laryngeal reflex** = cough

laryngectomy [lærɪnˈdʒektəmi] *noun* surgical removal of the larynx, usually as treatment for throat cancer

laryngismus (stridulus) [lærɪnˈdʒɪzməs ˈstrɪdjuləs] *noun* spasm of the throat muscles with a sharp intake of breath which occurs when the larynx is irritated, as in children suffering from croup

laryngitis [lærɪnˈdʒaɪtɪs] *noun* inflammation of the larynx

laryngofissure [lərɪŋgəʊˈfɪʃə] *noun* surgical operation to make an opening into the larynx through the thyroid cartilage

laryngologist [lærɪn'gɒlədʒɪst] *noun* doctor who specializes in diseases of the larynx, throat and vocal cords

laryngology [lærɪn'gɒlədʒi] *noun* study of diseases of the larynx, throat and vocal cords

laryngopharyngeal [lærɪŋgəʊfə'rɪndʒiəl] *adjective* referring to the larynx and pharynx

laryngopharynx [lærɪŋgəʊ'færɪŋks] *noun* part of the pharynx below the hyoid bone

laryngoscope [lə'rɪŋgəskəʊp] *noun* instrument for examining the inside of the larynx, using a light and mirrors

laryngoscopy [lærɪŋ'gɒskəpi] *noun* examination of the larynx with a laryngoscope

laryngospasm ['lærɪŋgəspæzm] *noun* muscular spasm which suddenly closes the larynx

laryngostenosis [lærɪŋgəstə'nəʊsɪs] *noun* narrowing of the lumen of the larynx

laryngotomy [lærɪŋ'gɒtəmi] *noun* surgical operation to make an opening in the larynx through the membrane (especially in an emergency, when the throat is blocked)

laryngotracheobronchitis [lərɪŋgəʊtræɪkiəʊbrɒŋ'kaɪtɪs] *noun* inflammation of the larynx, trachea and bronchi, as in croup

larynx ['lærɪŋks] *noun* the voice box, the organ in the throat which produces sounds; *see illustration at* THROAT

COMMENT: the larynx is a hollow passage made of cartilage, containing the vocal cords, situated behind the Adam's apple. It is closed by the epiglottis when swallowing or before coughing

laser ['leɪzə] *noun* instrument which produces a highly concentrated beam of light, which can be used to cut or attach tissue, as in operations for detached retina; **argon laser** = laser which uses argon as its medium; **endometrial laser ablation** = gynaecological surgical procedure using a laser to treat fibroids or other causes of thickening of the lining of the uterus; **tunable dye laser** = laser used to coagulate fine blood vessels to blanch port wine stains; **laser probe** = metal probe which is inserted into the body and through which a laser beam can be passed to remove a blockage in an artery; **laser surgery** = surgery using lasers (such as removal of tumours, sealing blood vessels, etc.)

Lassa fever ['læsə 'fiːvə] *noun* highly infectious virus disease found in Central and West Africa

COMMENT: the symptoms are high fever, pains, and ulcers in the mouth. It is often fatal

Lassar's paste ['læsəz 'peɪst] *noun* ointment made of zinc oxide, used to treat eczema

lassitude ['læsɪtjuːd] *noun* state where a person does not want to do anything, sometimes because he is depressed

lata ['lætə] *see* FASCIA

latent ['leɪtənt] *adjective* (disease) which is present in the body, but does not show any signs; *the children were tested for latent viral infection*

lateral ['lætrəl] *adjective* (i) further away from the midline of the body; (ii) referring to one side of the body; **lateral aspect** *or* **view** = view of the side of part of the body; **lateral malleolus** = prominence on the outer surface of the ankle joint; *compare* MEDIAL

lateralis [lætə'reɪlɪs] *see* VASTUS

laterally ['lætrəli] *adverb* towards or on the side of the body

lateroversion [lætrəʊ'vɜːʃn] *noun* turning (of an organ) to one side

latissimus dorsi [lə'tɪsɪməs 'dɔːsi] *noun* large flat triangular muscle covering the lumbar region and the lower part of the chest

laugh [lɑːf] **1** *noun* sound made by the throat when a person is amused; *he said it with a laugh*; *she gave a hysterical laugh* **2** *verb* to make a sound which shows amusement; *he started to laugh hysterically*

laughing gas ['lɑːfɪŋ gæs] *noun* nitrous oxide (N_2O), colourless gas with a sweet smell, used in combination with other gases as an anaesthetic in dentistry and surgery

laundry ['lɔːndri] *noun* (a) place where clothes, etc., are washed; *the bedclothes will be sent to the hospital laundry to be sterilized* (b) clothes, etc., which need to be washed or which have been washed; *the report criticized the piles of dirty laundry left lying in the wards*

lavage ['lævɪdʒ or 'lævɑːʒ] *noun* washing out or irrigating an organ, such as the stomach; **gastric lavage** = stomach washout, usually to remove a poisonous substance which has been absorbed

lavatory ['lævətri] *noun* toilet, a place or room where one can get rid of water or solid waste from the body; *the ladies' lavatory is to the right*; *there are three lavatories for the ward of ten people*

laxative ['læksətɪv] *noun & adjective* (medicine) which causes a bowel movement, such as bisacodyl which stimulates intestinal motility, or lactulose which alters fluid retention in the bowel

COMMENT: laxatives are very commonly used without prescription to treat constipation, although they should only be used as a short term solution. Change of diet and regular exercise are better ways of treating most types of constipation

layer ['leɪə] *noun* flat area, sheet of a substance under or over another area; *they put three layers of cotton wadding over his eye*

lazy ['leɪzi] *adjective* not wanting to do any work; **lazy eye** = eye which does not focus properly

lb *see* POUND

LD ['el 'diː] = LETHAL DOSE

LDL ['el 'diː 'el] = LOW DENSITY LIPOPROTEIN

l.e. *or* **LE** ['el 'iː] *abbreviation for* LUPUS ERYTHEMATOSUS; **LE cells** = white blood cells which show that a patient has lupus erythematosus

lead [led] *noun* very heavy soft metallic element, which is poisonous in compounds; **lead line** = blue line seen on the gums in cases of lead poisoning (NOTE: chemical symbol is **Pb**)

lead-free ['led'friː] *adjective* with no lead in it; *lead-free paint*; *lead-free petrol*

lead poisoning ['led 'pɔɪzənɪŋ] *noun* plumbism or saturnism, poisoning caused by taking in lead salts

COMMENT: lead salts are used externally to treat bruises or eczema, but if taken internally produce lead poisoning, which can also be caused by paint (children's toys must be painted in lead-free paint) or by lead fumes from car engines (which can be avoided by using lead-free petrol)

leak [liːk] *verb (of liquids)* to flow out by accident or by mistake; *blood leaked into the subcutaneous layers*

learning ['lɜːnɪŋ] *noun* gaining knowledge of something or of how to do something;

person with learning difficulties *or* **learning disabilities** = person who has low to average intelligence and finds it difficult to learn a skill; *school for children with learning disabilities*

lecithins ['lesɪθɪnz] *noun* constituents of all animal and plant cells, involved with the transport and absorption of fats

leech [liːtʃ] *noun* type of parasitic worm which lives in water and sucks the blood of animals by attaching itself to the skin; **medicinal leech** = leech which is raised specially for use in medicine

COMMENT: leeches were formerly commonly used in medicine to remove blood from a patient. Today they are used in special cases, where it is necessary to make sure that blood does not build up in part of the body (as in a severed finger which has been sewn back on)

left [left] *adverb, adjective & noun* referring to the side of the body which usually has the weaker hand; *he can't write with his left hand*; *the heart is on the left side of the body*

left-hand ['left'hænd] *adjective* on the left side; *look in the left-hand drawer of the desk*; *the tablets are on the top left-hand shelf in the cupboard*

left-handed ['left'hændɪd] *adjective* using the left hand more often than the right, such as for writing; *she's left-handed*; *left-handed people need special scissors*; *about five per cent of the population is left-handed*

left-handedness [left'hændɪdnəs] *noun* condition of a person who is left-handed

leg [leg] *noun* part of the body with which a person or animal walks and stands; *she made him stand on one leg and lift the other leg up*; *he is limping from a leg injury which he received playing football*; *his left leg is slightly shorter than the right*; *she complained of pains in her right leg*; *she fell off the wall and broke her leg*

COMMENT: the leg is formed of the thigh (with the thighbone or femur), the knee (with the kneecap or patella), and the lower leg (with two bones - the tibia and fibula)

legal ['liːgl] *adjective* which is allowed by law; **legal abortion** = abortion carried out according to the law

Legg-Calvé-Perthes disease
['leg'kælveɪ'pɜːtɪz dɪ'ziːz] *noun* degeneration of the upper end of the thighbone in young

boys, which prevents the bone growing properly and can result in a permanent limp

legionnaires' disease [liːdʒəˈneəz dɪˈziːz] *noun* bacterial disease similar to pneumonia

> COMMENT: the disease is thought to be transmitted in droplets of moisture in the air, and so the bacterium is found in central air-conditioning systems. It can be fatal to old or sick people, and so is especially dangerous if present in a hospital

leiomyoma [laɪəʊmaɪˈəʊmə] *noun* tumour of smooth muscle, especially the smooth muscle coating the uterus

leiomyosarcoma [laɪəʊmaɪəʊsɑːˈkəʊmə] *noun* sarcoma in which large bundles of smooth muscle are found

Leishmania [liːʃˈmeɪniə] *noun* tropical parasite which is passed to humans by the bites of sandflies

leishmaniasis [liːʃməˈnaɪəsɪs] *noun* any of several diseases (such as Delhi boil or kala-azar) caused by the parasite *Leishmania*, one form giving disfiguring ulcers, another attacking the liver and bone marrow; **mucocutaneous leishmaniasis** = disorder affecting the skin and mucous membrane

Lembert's suture [ˈlɑːmbeəz ˈsuːtʃə] *noun* suture used to close a wound in the intestine which includes all the coats of the intestine

Lempert operation [ˈlempət ɒpəˈreɪʃn] *noun* fenestration, a surgical operation to relieve deafness by making a small opening in the inner ear

length [leŋθ] *noun* measurement of how long something is; *the small intestine is about 5 metres in length*

lens [lenz] *noun* **(a)** part of the eye behind the iris and pupil, which focuses light coming from the cornea onto the retina; *see illustration at* EYE **(b)** piece of shaped glass or plastic which forms part of a pair of spectacles or microscope; **contact lens** = tiny glass or plastic lens which fits over the eyeball and is worn instead of spectacles

> COMMENT: the lens in the eye is elastic, and can change its shape under the influence of the ciliary muscle, to allow the eye to focus on objects at different distances

lenticular [lenˈtɪkjʊlə] *adjective* referring to a lens, like a lens

lentigo [lenˈtaɪɡəʊ] *noun* freckle, a small brown spot on the skin often caused by exposure to sunlight

leper [ˈlepə] *noun* person suffering from leprosy; *he works in a leper hospital*

lepidosis [lepɪˈdəʊsɪs] *noun* skin eruption, where pieces of skin fall off in flakes

leproma [leˈprəʊmə] *noun* lesion of the skin caused by leprosy

leprosy [ˈleprəsi] *noun* infectious bacterial disease of skin and peripheral nerve tracts caused by *Mycobacterium leprae,* which destroys the tissues and can cripple the patient if left untreated (NOTE: also called **Hansen's disease**)

> COMMENT: Leprosy attacks the nerves in the skin, and finally the patient loses all feeling in a limb, and parts, such as fingers or toes, can drop off

lepto- [ˈleptəʊ] *prefix* meaning thin

leptocyte [ˈleptəsaɪt] *noun* thin red blood cell found in anaemia

leptomeninges [leptəmeˈnɪndʒiːz] *noun* two inner meninges (pia mater and arachnoid)

leptomeningitis [leptəmenɪnˈdʒaɪtɪs] *noun* inflammation of the leptomeninges

leptospirosis [leptəspaɪˈrəʊsɪs] *noun* infectious disease caused by the spirochaete *Leptospira* transmitted to humans from rat urine, giving jaundice and kidney damage (NOTE: also called **Weil's disease**)

leresis [ləˈriːsɪs] *noun* uncoordinated speech, a sign of dementia

lesbian [ˈlezbiən] *noun & adjective* woman who experiences sexual attraction towards other women

lesbianism [ˈlezbiənɪzm] *noun* sexual attraction in one woman for another; *compare* HOMOSEXUAL

lesion [ˈliːʒn] *noun* wound, sore or damage to the body (NOTE: lesion is used to refer to any damage to the body, from the fracture of a bone to a cut on the skin)

lessen [ˈlesn] *verb* to make less strong; *the injection will lessen the pain*; *modern antibiotics lessen the chance of a patient getting gangrene*

lesser [ˈlesə] *adjective* smaller; **lesser trochanter** = projection on the femur which is the insertion of the psoas major muscle

lethal ['li:θl] *adjective* which can kill; *she took a lethal dose of aspirin*; *these fumes are lethal if inhaled*; **lethal gene** = gene which can kill the person who inherits it

lethargic [lə'θɑ:dʒɪk] *adjective* showing lethargy; **lethargic encephalitis** *or* **encephalitis lethargica** = a common type of virus encephalitis occurring in epidemics in the 1920s

lethargy ['leθədʒi] *noun* mental torpor or tired feeling, when the patient has slow movements and is almost inactive

leucine ['lu:si:n] *noun* essential amino acid

leuco- *or* **leuko-** ['lu:kəʊ] *prefix* meaning white

leucocyte *or* **leukocyte** ['lu:kəsaɪt] *noun* white blood cell which contains a nucleus but has no haemoglobin

COMMENT: in normal conditions the blood contains far fewer leucocytes than erythrocytes (red blood cells), but their numbers increase rapidly when infection is present in the body. Leucocytes are either granular (with granules in the cytoplasm) or nongranular. The main types of leucocyte are: lymphocytes and monocytes which are nongranular, and neutrophils, eosinophils and basophils which are granular (granulocytes). Granular leucocytes are produced by the bone marrow, and their main function is to remove foreign particles from the blood and fight infection by forming antibodies

leucocytolysis *or* **leukocytolysis** [lu:kəsaɪ'tɒləsɪs] *noun* destruction of leucocytes

leucocytosis *or* **leukocytosis** [lu:kəsaɪ'təʊsɪs] *noun* increase in numbers of leucocytes in the blood above the normal upper limit (in order to fight an infection)

leucodeplete [lu:kəʊdɪ'pli:t] *verb* to remove white cells from the blood

leucoderma [lu:kə'dɜ:mə] *noun* vitiligo, condition where white patches appear on the skin

leucolysin [lu:kəʊ'laɪsɪn] *noun* protein which destroys white blood cells

leucoma [lu'kəʊmə] *noun* white scar of the cornea

leuconychia [lu:kə'nɪkiə] *noun* white marks on the fingernails

leucopenia [lu:kə'pi:niə] *noun* reduction in the number of leucocytes in the blood, usually as a result of a disease

leucoplakia [lu:kə'plækiə] *noun* condition where white patches form on mucous membranes (such as on the tongue or inside of the mouth)

leucopoiesis [lu:kəʊpɔɪ'i:sɪs] *noun* production of leucocytes

leucorrhoea [lu:kə'ri:ə] *noun* excessive discharge of white mucus from the vagina (NOTE: also informally called **whites**)

leucotomy [lu'kɒtəmi] *noun* **prefrontal leucotomy** = operation to divide some of the white matter in the prefrontal lobe, formerly used as a treatment for schizophrenia

leukaemia [lu'ki:miə] *noun* any of several malignant diseases where an abnormal number of leucocytes form in the blood

COMMENT: apart from the increase in the number of leucocytes, the symptoms include swelling of the spleen and the lymph glands. There are several forms of leukaemia: the commonest is acute lymphoblastic leukaemia which occurs in children and can be treated by radiotherapy

levator [lə'veɪtə] *noun* **(a)** surgical instrument for lifting pieces of fractured bone **(b)** muscle which lifts a limb or a part of the body

level ['levl] **1** *adjective* flat, horizontal or not rising and falling; *her temperature has remained level for the last hour* **2** *noun* amount; *he has a very high level of cholesterol in his blood*

levodopa [li:və'dəʊpə] *noun; see* DRUGS TABLE IN SUPPLEMENT

Lewy body ['lu:wi 'bɒdi] *noun* deposit of protein in the brain caused by neurodegeneration; **Lewy body dementia** = disease which affects the mental processes, similar to Alzheimer's disease, but with the presence of Lewy bodies in the brain and patients are more prone to hallucinations and delusions

Leydig cells ['laɪdɪg 'selz] *noun* interstitial cells, testosterone-producing cells between the tubules in the testes

l.g.v. ['el 'dʒi: 'vi:] = LYMPHOGRANULOMA VENEREUM

LH ['el 'eɪtʃ] = LUTEINIZING HORMONE

liable to ['laɪəbl 'tʊ] *adjective* likely to; *people in sedentary occupations are liable to have digestive disorders*

libido [lɪ'bi:dəʊ] *noun* **(a)** sexual urge; **loss of libido** = loss of sexual urge **(b)** *(in* *psychology*) force which drives the unconscious mind, used especially referring to the sexual urge

lice [laɪs] *see* LOUSE

licence *US* **license** ['laɪsəns] *noun* official document which allows someone to do something (such as allowing a doctor to practise, a pharmacist to make and sell drugs or, in the USA, allowing a nurse to practise); *he was practising as a doctor without a licence*; *she is sitting her registered nurse license examination*

license ['laɪsəns] *verb* to give someone a licence to do something; *he is licensed to sell dangerous drugs*

licensure ['laɪsənʃə] *noun US* act of licensing a nurse to practise nursing

licentiate [laɪ'senʃiət] *noun* person who has been given a licence to practise as a doctor

lichen ['laɪkn or 'lɪtʃn] *noun* type of skin disease with thick skin and small lesions; **lichen planus** = skin disease where itchy purple spots appear on the arms and thighs

lichenification [laɪkenɪfɪ'keɪʃn] *noun* thickening of the skin at the site of a lesion

lichenoid ['laɪkənɔɪd] *adjective* like a lichen

lick [lɪk] *verb* to make the tongue move over something to taste it or to wet it

lid [lɪd] *noun* top which covers a container; *put the lid back on the jar*; *a medicine bottle with a child-proof lid*

lie [laɪ] **1** *noun* way in which a fetus is present in the uterus; **longitudinal lie** = normal position of the fetus lying along the axis of the mother's body; **transverse lie** = position of the fetus across the body of the mother **2** *verb* to be in a flat position; *the accident victim was lying on the pavement*; *make sure the patient lies still and does not move* (NOTE: **lies - lying - lay - has lain**)

Lieberkühn's glands *or* **crypts of Lieberkühn** ['liːbəkuːnz 'glændz or 'krɪpts əv 'liːbəkuːn] *noun* tubular glands found in the mucous membrane of the small and large intestine, especially those between the bases of the villi in the small intestine

lie down ['laɪ 'daʊn] *verb* to put yourself in a flat position; *she lay down on the floor or on the bed*; *the doctor asked him to lie down on the couch*; *when I was lying down he asked me to lift my legs in the air*

lientery *or* **lienteric diarrhoea** ['laɪəntri or laɪən'terɪk daɪə'riːə] *noun* form of diarrhoea where the food passes through the intestine rapidly without being digested

life [laɪf] *noun* being alive, not being dead; *the surgeons saved the patient's life*; *his life is in danger because the drugs are not available*; *the victim showed no sign of life*; **life expectancy** = number of years a person of a certain age is likely to live; **life insurance** = insurance against death; **life-threatening disease** = disease which may kill the patient

lifebelt ['laɪfbelt] *noun* large ring which helps a person to float in water

life-saving equipment ['laɪf'seɪvɪŋ ɪ'kwɪpmənt] *noun* equipment (such as boats, stretchers and first-aid kit) kept ready in case of an emergency

lift [lɪft] **1** *noun* **(a)** machine which takes people from one floor to another in a tall building **(b)** way of carrying an injured person; **fireman's lift** = way of carrying an unconscious person on the shoulders of one carrier with the carrier's right arm passing between or around the patient's legs and holding the patient's right hand, allowing the carrier's left hand to remain free; **shoulder lift** = way of carrying a heavy person, where the upper part of his body rests on the shoulders of two carriers **2** *verb* to raise to a higher position; to pick something up; *this box is so heavy he can't lift it off the floor*; *she hurt her back lifting a box down from the shelf*

ligament ['lɪgəmənt] *noun* thick band of fibrous tissue which connects the bones at a joint and forms the joint capsule; *see also* BROAD, EXTRINSIC, INTRINSIC, ROUND, SACRO-UTERINE

ligate ['laɪgeɪt] *verb* to tie with a ligature, as to tie a blood vessel to stop bleeding, or to tie the Fallopian tubes as a sterilization procedure

ligation [laɪ'geɪʃn] *noun* surgical operation to tie up a blood vessel; **tubal ligation** = surgical operation to tie up the Fallopian tubes as a sterilization procedure

ligature ['lɪgətʃə] **1** *noun* thread used to tie vessels or a lumen, such as a blood vessel to stop bleeding **2** *verb* = LIGATE

light [laɪt] **1** *adjective* **(a)** not heavy; *she can carry this box easily - it's quite light*; *he's not fit, so he can only do light work* **(b)** bright so that one can see well; *at six o'clock* *in the morning it was just getting light* **(c)** (hair or skin) which is nearer white in colour rather than dark; *she has a very light complexion*; *he has light coloured hair* (NOTE: light - lighter - lightest) **2** *noun* **(a)** brightness, something which shines and helps you to see; *the light of the sun makes plants green*; *there's not enough light in here to take a photo*; **light adaptation** = changes in the eye to adapt to an abnormally bright or dim light or to adapt to normal light after being in darkness; **light reflex** = reflex of the pupil of the eye which contracts when exposed to bright light; **light therapy** *or* **light treatment** = treatment of a disorder by exposing the patient to light (sunlight, infrared light, etc.); **light waves** = waves travelling in all directions from a source of light which stimulate the retina and are visible **(b)** object (usually a glass bulb) which gives out light; *switch on the lights - it's getting dark*; *the car was travelling with no lights*; *the endoscope has a small light at the end*

lightening ['laɪtənɪŋ] *noun* late stage in pregnancy where the fetus goes down into the pelvic cavity

lighting ['laɪtɪŋ] *noun* way of giving light; *the lighting in the operating theatre has to be very good*

lightly ['laɪtli] *adverb* without using much pressure; *the doctor pressed lightly round the swollen area with the tips of his fingers*

lightning pains ['laɪtnɪŋ 'peɪnz] *plural noun* sharp pains in the legs in a patient suffering from locomotor ataxia

lignocaine *US* **lidocaine** ['lɪgnəkeɪn or 'laɪdəkeɪn] *noun; see* DRUGS TABLE IN SUPPLEMENT

limb [lɪm] *noun* one of the legs or arms; **lower limbs** = legs; **upper limbs** = arms; **limb lead** = electrode attached to an arm or leg when taking an electrocardiogram

limbic system ['lɪmbɪk 'sɪstəm] *noun* system of nerves in the brain, including the hippocampus, the amygdala and the hypothalamus, which are associated with emotions such as fear and anger

limbless ['lɪmləs] *adjective* lacking one or more limbs; *a limbless ex-soldier*

limbus ['lɪmbəs] *noun* edge, especially the edge of the cornea where it joins the sclera (NOTE: plural is **limbi**)

liminal ['lɪmɪnl] *adjective* (stimulus) at the lowest level which can be sensed

limit ['lɪmɪt] **1** *noun* furthest point or place beyond which you cannot go; *there is a speed limit of 30 miles per hour in towns*; **there is no age limit for joining the club** = people of all ages can join **2** *verb* to set a limit to something; *you must limit your intake of coffee to two cups a day*

limp [lɪmp] **1** *noun* way of walking awkwardly because of pain, stiffness or deformity in a leg or foot; *he walks with a limp*; *the operation has left him with a limp* **2** *verb* to walk awkwardly because of pain, stiffness or deformity in a leg or foot; *he was still limping three weeks after the accident*

linctus ['lɪŋktəs] *noun* sweet cough medicine

line [laɪn] **1** *noun* ridge or mark which connects two points **2** *verb* to provide an inner coat to something; *the intestine is lined with mucus*; *the inner ear is lined with fine hairs*

linea ['lɪniə] *noun* thin line; **linea alba** = tendon running from the breastbone to the pubic area, to which abdominal muscles are attached; **linea nigra** = dark line on the skin from the navel to the pubis which appears during the later months of pregnancy

lingual ['lɪŋgwəl] *adjective* referring to the tongue; **lingual artery** = artery which supplies blood to the tongue; **lingual tonsil** = lymphoid tissue on the top surface of the back of the tongue; *see illustration at* TONGUE; **lingual vein** = vein which takes blood from the tongue

liniment ['lɪnəmənt] *noun* embrocation or oily liquid rubbed on the skin, which eases the pain or stiffness of a sprain or bruise by acting as a vasodilator or counterirritant

lining ['laɪnɪŋ] *noun* substance or tissue on the inside of an organ; *the thick lining of the aorta*

link [lɪŋk] *verb* to join things together; *the ankle bone links the bones of the lower leg to the calcaneus*

linkage ['lɪŋkɪdʒ] *noun (of genes)* being close together on a chromosome, and therefore likely to be inherited together

linoleic acid [lɪnəʊ'liːɪk 'æsɪd] *noun* one of the essential fatty acids which cannot be synthesized and has to be taken into the body from food (such as vegetable oil)

linolenic acid [lɪnəʊ'lenɪk 'æsɪd] *noun* one of the essential fatty acids

lint [lɪnt] *noun* thick flat cotton wadding, used as a surgical dressing; *she put some lint on the wound before bandaging it*

liothyronine [laɪəʊ'θaɪrəʊniːn] *noun* hormone produced by the thyroid gland which can be artificially synthesized for use as a rapid-acting treatment for hypothyroidism

lip [lɪp] *noun* (i) one of two fleshy muscular parts round the edge of the mouth; (ii) flesh round the edge of an opening; *her lips were cracked from the cold*; *lips of a wound or of an incision* = the two sides of a wound, which need to be sutured, etc., to heal (NOTE: for terms referring to lips, see words beginning with **cheil-, lab-, labi-**)

lipaemia [lɪ'piːmiə] *noun* excessive amount of fat (such as cholesterol) in the blood

lipase ['lɪpeɪz] *noun* enzyme which breaks down fats in the intestine

lipid ['lɪpɪd] *noun* fat or fatlike substance which exists in human tissue and forms an important part of the human diet; **lipid metabolism** = chemical changes where lipids are broken down into fatty acids

COMMENT: lipids are not water soluble. They float in the blood and can attach themselves to the walls of arteries causing atherosclerosis

lipid-lowering drug ['lɪpɪd'ləʊərɪŋ 'drʌg] *noun* drug which lowers serum triglycerides and low density lipoprotein cholesterol and raises high density lipoprotein cholesterol to reduce the progression of coronary artherosclerosis, used in patients with, or at high risk of developing coronary heart disease (NOTE: lipid-lowering drugs have names ending in **-fibrate: bezafibrate**)

lipidosis [lɪpɪ'dəʊsɪs] *noun* disorder of lipid metabolism, where subcutaneous fat is not present in some parts of the body

lipochondrodystrophy [lɪpəʊkɒndrəʊ'dɪstrəfi] *noun* congenital disorder of the lipid metabolism, the bones and main organs, causing mental deficiency and physical deformity

lipodystrophy [lɪpəʊ'dɪstrəfi] *noun* disorder of lipid metabolism

lipogenesis [lɪpəʊ'dʒenəsɪs] *noun* production or making deposits of fat

lipoid ['lɪpɔɪd] *noun & adjective* compound lipid or fatty substance (such as cholesterol) which is like a lipid

lipoidosis [lɪpɔɪ'dəʊsɪs] *noun* group of diseases with reticuloendothelial hyperplasia and abnormal deposits of lipoids in the cells

lipolysis [lɪ'pɒləsɪs] *noun* process of breaking down fat by lipase

lipolytic enzyme [lɪpə'lɪtɪk 'enzaɪm] = LIPASE

lipoma [lɪ'pəʊmə] *noun* benign tumour formed of fatty tissue

lipomatosis [lɪpəʊmə'təʊsɪs] *noun* excessive deposit of fat in the tissues in tumour-like masses

lipoprotein [lɪpəʊ'prəʊtiːn] *noun* protein which combines with lipids and carries them in the bloodstream and lymph system; lipoproteins are classified according to the percentage of protein which they carry; **high-density lipoproteins (HDLs)** = lipoproteins with a lower percentage of cholesterol; **low-density lipoproteins (LDLs)** = lipoproteins with a large percentage of cholesterol which deposit fats in muscles and arteries; **very low density lipoprotein (VLDL)** = fat produced by the liver after food has been absorbed and before it becomes low density lipoprotein

liposarcoma [lɪpəʊsɑː'kəʊmə] *noun* lipoma and sarcoma

liposuction [lɪpəʊ'sʌkʃn] *noun* surgical removal of fatty tissue for cosmetic reasons

lipotrophic [lɪpəʊ'trɒfik] *adjective* (substance) which increases the amount of fat present in the tissues

Lippes loop ['lɪpəz 'luːp] *noun* type of intrauterine device

lipping ['lɪpɪŋ] *noun* condition where bone tissue grows over other bones

lipuria [lɪ'pjʊəriə] *noun* presence of fat or oily emulsion in the urine

liquid ['lɪkwɪd] *adjective & noun* matter (like water) which is not solid and is not a gas; *sick patients need a lot of liquids*; *he was put on a liquid diet*; **liquid paraffin** = oil used as a laxative

liquor ['lɪkə] *noun (in pharmacy)* solution, usually aqueous, of a pure substance

lisp [lɪsp] **1** *noun* speech defect where the patient has difficulty in pronouncing 's' sounds and replaces them with 'th' **2** *verb* to talk with a lisp

list [lɪst] **1** *noun* number of things written down one after the other; *there is a list of names in alphabetical order*; *the names of* *duty nurses are on the list in the office*; **he's on the danger list** = he is critically ill; **she's off the danger list** = she is no longer critically ill **2** *verb* to write something in the form of a list; *the drugs are listed at the back of the book*; *the telephone numbers of the emergency services are listed in the Yellow Pages*

listen ['lɪsn] *verb* to pay attention to something heard; *the doctor listened to the patient's chest*

Listeria [lɪ'stɪərɪə] *noun* genus of bacteria found on domestic animals and in unpasteurized milk products, which can cause uterine infection or meningitis

listeriosis [lɪstərɪ'əʊsɪs] *noun* infectious disease transmitted from animals to humans by the bacteria Listeria

listless ['lɪstləs] *adjective* weak and tired

listlessness ['lɪstləsnəs] *noun* being generally weak and tired

lith- [lɪθ] *prefix* meaning stone

lithaemia [lɪ'θiːmɪə] *noun* uricacidaemia, abnormal amount of uric acid in the blood

lithiasis [lɪ'θaɪəsɪs] *noun* forming of stones in an organ

litholapaxy *or* **lithotrity** ['lɪθɒləpæksi *or* lɪ'θɒtrɪti] *noun* evacuation of pieces of a stone in the bladder after crushing it with a lithotrite

lithonephrotomy [lɪθəʊnə'frɒtəmi] *noun* surgical removal of a stone in the kidney

lithotomy [lɪ'θɒtəmi] *noun* surgical removal of a stone from the bladder; **lithotomy position** = position of a patient for some medical examinations, where the patient lies on his back with his legs flexed and his thighs on his abdomen

lithotrite ['lɪθəʊtraɪt] *noun* surgical instrument which crushes a stone in the bladder

lithotrity [lɪ'θɒtrɪti] = LITHOLAPAXY

lithuresis [lɪθju'riːsɪs] *noun* passage of small stones from the bladder during urination

lithuria [lɪ'θjʊərɪə] *noun* presence of excessive amounts of uric acid or urates in the urine

litmus ['lɪtməs] *noun* substance which turns red in acid and blue in alkali; **litmus paper** = small piece of paper impregnated with litmus, used to test for acidity or alkalinity

litre *US* **liter** ['liːtə] *noun* unit of measurement of liquids (= 1.76 pints) (NOTE: with figures usually written **l: 2.5l** but it can be written in full to avoid confusion with the numeral **1**)

little ['lɪtl] *adjective* **(a)** small, not big; **little finger** *or* **little toe** = smallest finger on the hand, smallest toe on the foot; *he has a ring on his little finger*; *her little toe was crushed by the door* **(b)** not much; *she eats very little bread*

Little's area ['lɪtlz 'eərɪə] *noun* area of blood vessels in the nasal septum

Little's disease ['lɪtlz dɪ'ziːz] = SPASTIC DIPLEGIA

live 1 [laɪv] *adjective* **(a)** living, not dead; *graft using live tissue*; *see also* BIRTH **(b)** carrying electricity; *he was killed when he touched a live wire* **2** [lɪv] *verb* to be alive; *he is very ill, and the doctor doesn't think he will live much longer*

livedo [lɪ'viːdəʊ] *noun* discoloured spots on the skin

liver ['lɪvə] *noun* large gland in the upper part of the abdomen; *she has been suffering from liver trouble*; *he has been having treatment for a liver infection*; **liver extract** = food made from animal livers, used as an injection to treat anaemia; **liver fluke** = parasitic flatworm which can infest the liver; **liver spot** = little brown spot on the skin; *see illustration at* DIGESTIVE SYSTEM (NOTE: for other terms referring to the liver, see words beginning with **hepat-**)

COMMENT: the liver is situated in the top part of the abdomen on the right side of the body next to the stomach. It is the largest gland in the body, weighing almost 2 kg. Blood carrying nutrients from the intestines enters the liver by the hepatic portal vein; the nutrients are removed and the blood returned to the heart through the hepatic vein. The liver is the major detoxicating organ in the body; it destroys harmful organisms in the blood, produces clotting agents, secretes bile, stores glycogen and metabolizes proteins, carbohydrates and fats. Diseases affecting the liver include hepatitis and cirrhosis; the symptom of liver disease is often jaundice

livid ['lɪvɪd] *adjective* (skin) with a blue colour because of being bruised or because of asphyxiation

LMC = LOCAL MEDICAL COMMITTEE

Loa loa ['ləʊə 'ləʊə] *noun* tropical threadworm which digs under the skin, especially around and into the eye, causing loa loa and loiasis

loa loa [ˈləʊə ˈləʊə] *noun* tropical disease of the eye caused when the threadworm *Loa loa* enters the eye or the skin around the eye

lobar [ˈləʊbə] *adjective* referring to a lobe; **lobar bronchi** = secondary bronchi, air passages supplying a lobe of a lung; **lobar pneumonia** = infection in one or more lobes of the lung

lobe [ləʊb] *noun* (i) rounded section of an organ, such as the brain, lung or liver; (ii) soft fleshy part at the bottom of the ear; (iii) cusp on the crown of a tooth; **caudate lobe** = lobe at the back of the liver, behind the right and left lobes; **frontal lobe** = front lobe of each cerebral hemisphere; **occipital lobe** = lobe at the back of each cerebral hemisphere; **parietal lobe** = lobe at the side and to the top of each cerebral hemisphere; **prefrontal lobe** = part of the brain in the front part of each hemisphere, in front of the frontal lobe, which is concerned with memory and learning; **temporal lobe** = lobe above the ear in each cerebral hemisphere; *see illustration at* LUNGS

lobectomy [ləʊˈbektəmi] *noun* surgical removal of one of the lobes of an organ such as the lung

lobotomy [ləˈbɒtəmi] *noun* formerly, surgical operation to treat mental disease by cutting into a lobe of the brain to cut the nerve fibres; *see* LEUCOTOMY

lobule [ˈlɒbjuːl] *noun* small section of a lobe in the lung, formed of acini

local [ˈləʊkl] *adjective* referring to a separate place; confined to one part; **local anaesthesia** = loss of feeling in a single part of the body; **local anaesthetic** *or* **a local** = anaesthetic which removes the feeling in a certain part of the body only, such as lignocaine; *he had a local for the operation for an ingrowing toenail*; *the surgeon removed the growth under local anaesthetic*; **Local Medical Committee (LMC)** = committee responsible for monitoring the interests of providers of primary care (GPs, dentists, pharmacists) in a district

> few parts of the body are inaccessible to modern catheter techniques, which are all performed under local anaesthesia
>
> *British Medical Journal*

localize [ˈləʊkəlaɪz] *verb* to locate something, to find where something is; to restrict the spread of something to a particular area

> these patients may be candidates for embolization of their bleeding point, particularly as angiography will often be necessary to localize that point
>
> *British Medical Journal*

localized [ˈləʊkəlaɪzd] *adjective* (infection) which occurs in one part of the body only (NOTE: the opposite is **generalized**)

locate [ləˈkeɪt] *verb* (i) to find where something is; (ii) to situate, to be situated in a place

> ultrasonography is helpful in determining sites of incompetence and in locating the course of veins in more obese patients
>
> *British Journal of Hospital Medicine*

> the target cells for adult myeloid leukaemia are located in the bone marrow, and there is now evidence that childhood leukaemias also arise in the bone marrow
>
> *British Medical Journal*

lochia [ˈləʊkiə] *noun* discharge from the vagina after childbirth or abortion

lochial [ˈləʊkiəl] *adjective* referring to lochia

lock [lɒk] *verb* **(a)** to close a door, box, etc., so that it has to be opened with a key; *the drugs have to be kept in a locked cupboard* **(b)** to fix in a position; **locked knee** = displaced piece of cartilage of the knee, condition where a piece of the cartilage in the knee slips (the symptom is a sharp pain, and the knee remains permanently bent); **locking of the knee** = condition where the knee joint suddenly becomes rigid

lockjaw [ˈlɒkdʒɔː] = TETANUS

locomotion [ləʊkəˈməʊʃn] *noun* being able to move

locomotor ataxia [ləʊkəʊˈməʊtər əˈtæksiə] = TABES DORSALIS

loculus [ˈlɒkjʊləs] *noun* small space (in an organ)

locum (tenens) ['ləʊkəm 'tenəns] *noun* doctor who takes the place of another doctor for a time

locus ['ləʊkəs] *noun* area or point (of infection or disease); position on a chromosome where a gene is present

lodge [lɒdʒ] *verb* to stay or to stick; *the piece of bone lodged in her throat*; *the larvae of the tapeworm lodge in the walls of the intestine*

logrolling ['lɒgrəʊlɪŋ] *noun* method of moving a patient who is lying down into another position

loiasis [ləʊ'aɪəsɪs] *noun* tropical disease of the eye caused when the threadworm *Loa loa* enters the eye or the skin around the eye

loin [lɔɪn] *noun* lower back part of the body above the buttocks

long-acting ['lɒŋ'æktɪŋ] *adjective* (drug or treatment) which has an effect that lasts a long time

longitudinal [lɒndʒɪ'tjuːdɪnl] *adjective* lengthwise, in the direction of the long axis of the body; **longitudinal arch** = part of the sole of the foot which curves upwards, running along the length of the foot from the heel to the ball of the foot

longsighted [lɒŋ'saɪtɪd] *adjective* able to see clearly things which are far away, but not things which are close

longsightedness [lɒŋ'saɪtɪdnəs] = HYPERMETROPIA

long-stay ['lɒŋ'steɪ] *adjective* staying a long time in hospital; *patients in long-stay units or long-stay patients*

longus ['lɒŋgəs] *see* MUSCLE

look after ['lʊk 'ɑːftə] *verb* to take care of or to attend to the needs of (a patient); *the nurses looked after him very well or he was very well looked after in hospital*; *she is off work looking after her children who have mumps*; *some patients need a lot of looking after* = they need continual attention

loop [luːp] *noun* **(a)** curve or bend in a line, especially one of the particular curves in a fingerprint; **loop of Henle** = curved tube which forms the main part of a nephron in the kidney; *(of the small intestine)* **blind loop syndrome** *or* **stagnant loop syndrome** = condition which occurs in cases of diverticulosis or of Crohn's disease, with steatorrhoea, abdominal pain and megaloblastic anaemia **(b)** curved piece of

wire placed in the uterus to prevent contraception

loose [luːs] *adjective* not fixed, not attached, not tight; *one of my molars has come loose* (NOTE: **loose - looser - loosest**)

loosely ['luːsli] *adverb* not tightly; *the bandage was loosely tied round her wrist*

loosen ['luːsən] *verb* to make loose; *loosen the tie round the victim's neck*

lordosis [lɔː'dəʊsɪs] *noun* excessive forward curvature of the lower part of the spine; *see also* KYPHOSIS

lordotic [lɔː'dɒtɪk] *adjective* referring to lordosis

lose [luːz] *verb* not to have something any longer; *he lost the ability to walk*; *when you have a cold you can easily lose all sense of smell and taste*; *she has lost weight since last summer* = she has got thinner (NOTE: **losing - lost - has lost**)

loss [lɒs] *noun* not having something any more; **loss of appetite** = not having as much appetite as before; **loss of sensation** = not being able to feel the limbs any more; **loss of weight** *or* **weight loss** = not weighing as much as before; *see also* HEARING

lotion ['ləʊʃn] *noun* medicinal liquid used to rub on the skin or to use on the body; *he bathed his eyes in a mild antiseptic lotion*; *use this lotion on your eczema*

louse [laʊs] *noun* small insect of the *Pediculus* genus, which sucks blood and lives on the skin as a parasite on animals and humans (NOTE: plural is **lice**)

COMMENT: there are several forms of louse: the commonest are the body louse, the crab louse and the head louse and some diseases can be transmitted by lice

low [ləʊ] *adjective & adverb* near the bottom or towards the bottom; not high; *he hit his head on the low ceiling*; *the temperature is too low here for oranges to grow*; **low blood pressure** = hypotension, condition where the pressure of the blood is abnormally low; **low-calorie diet** = diet with few calories (to help a person to lose weight); **low-fat diet** = diet with little animal fat which can help reduce the risk of heart disease and alleviate some skin conditions; **low-risk patient** = patient not likely to catch or develop a certain disease; **low-salt diet** = diet with little salt which has been shown to help reduce high blood pressure; *see also* NEURONE (NOTE:

low - lower - lowest. Note also that the opposite of **low** is **high**)

lower ['ləʊə] **1** *adjective* further down; **lower jaw** = bottom jaw; **lower limbs** = legs (NOTE: the opposite of **lower** is **upper**) **2** *verb* to make something go down; to reduce; *they covered the patient with wet cloth to try to lower his body temperature*

lozenge ['lɒzɪndʒ] *noun* sweet medicinal tablet; *she was sucking a cough lozenge*

LPN ['el 'pi: 'en] *US* = LICENSED PRACTICAL NURSE

LRCP ['el 'ɑ: 'si: 'pi:] = LICENTIATE OF THE ROYAL COLLEGE OF PHYSICIANS

LSD ['el 'es 'di:] *noun* = LYSERGIC ACID DIETHYLAMIDE powerful hallucinogenic drug

lubb-dupp [lʌb'dʌb] *noun* two sounds made by the heart, which represent each cardiac cycle when heard through a stethoscope

lubricant ['lu:brɪkənt] *noun* fluid which lubricates

lubricate ['lu:brɪkeɪt] *verb* to make smooth with oil or liquid

lucid ['lu:sɪd] *adjective* with a clearly working mind; *in spite of the pain, he was still lucid*

lucidum ['lu:sɪdəm] *see* STRATUM

Ludwig's angina ['lu:dvɪgz æn'dʒaɪnə] *noun* cellulitis of the mouth and some parts of the neck which causes the neck to swell and may obstruct the airway

lues ['lu:i:z] *noun* former name for syphilis or the plague

lumbago [lʌm'beɪgəʊ] *noun* pain in the lower back; *she has been suffering from lumbago for years*; *he has had an attack of lumbago*

COMMENT: mainly due to rheumatism, but can be brought on by straining the back muscles, lesions of the intervertebral discs or bad posture

lumbar ['lʌmbə] *adjective* referring to the lower part of the back; **lumbar arteries** = five arteries altogether, which supply blood to the back muscles and skin; **lumbar cistern** = subarachnoid space in the spinal cord, where the dura mater ends, filled with cerebrospinal fluid; **lumbar enlargement** = wider part of the spinal cord in the lower spine, where the nerves of the lower limbs are attached; **lumbar plexus** = point where several nerves which supply the thighs and abdomen join together, lying in the upper psoas muscle; **lumbar puncture** = *see* PUNCTURE; **lumbar region** = two parts of the abdomen on either side of the umbilical region; **lumbar vertebrae** = five vertebrae between the thoracic vertebrae and the sacrum

lumbosacral [lʌmbəʊ'seɪkrl] *adjective* referring to the lumbar vertebrae and the sacrum; **lumbosacral joint** = joint at the bottom of the back between the lumbar vertebrae and the sacrum

lumbricus [lʌm'braɪkəs] *noun* earthworm

lumen ['lu:mɪn] *noun* **(a)** SI unit of light emitted per second **(b)** (i) space inside a passage in the body or an instrument (such as an endoscope); (ii) hole at the end of a passage in the body or an instrument (such as an endoscope)

lump [lʌmp] *noun* mass of hard tissue which rises on the surface or under the surface of the skin; *he has a lump where he hit his head on the low door*; *she noticed a lump in her right breast and went to see the doctor*

lumpectomy [lʌm'pektəmi] *noun* surgical removal of a hard mass or lump, as in the case of some cancers

lunate (bone) ['lu:neɪt 'bəʊn] *noun* one of the eight small carpal bones in the wrist; *see illustration at* HAND

lung [lʌŋ] *noun* one of two organs of respiration in the body into which air is sucked when a person breathes; *the doctor listened to his chest to see if his lungs were all right*; **lung cancer** = cancer in the lung; **lung trouble** = disorder in the lung, such as bronchitis or pneumonia, etc.; **artificial lung** = machine through which the patient's deoxygenated blood is passed to absorb oxygen to take back to the bloodstream; **farmer's lung** = type of asthma caused by an allergy to rotting hay; **shock lung** = serious condition after a blow, where the patient's lungs fail to work (NOTE: for other terms referring to the lungs, see words beginning with **bronch-**, **pneumo-**, **pneumon-**, **pulmo-**, **pulmon-**)

COMMENT: the two lungs are situated in the chest cavity, protected by the ribcage. The heart lies between the lungs. The right lung has three lobes, the left lung only two. Air goes down into the lungs through the trachea and bronchi. It passes to the alveoli where its oxygen is deposited in the blood in exchange for waste carbon dioxide which is exhaled (gas exchange). Lung cancer can be caused by smoking tobacco, and is commonest in people who are heavy smokers

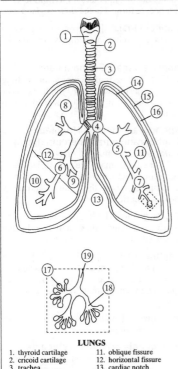

LUNGS

1. thyroid cartilage	11. oblique fissure
2. cricoid cartilage	12. horizontal fissure
3. trachea	13. cardiac notch
4. main bronchus	14. visceral pleura
5. superior lobe bronchus	15. parietal pleura
6. middle lobe bronchus	16. pleural cavity
7. inferior lobe bronchus	17. alveolus
8. superior lobe	18. alveolar duct
9. middle lobe	19. bronchiole
10. inferior lobe	

lunula [ˈluːnjʊlə] *noun* curved white mark at the base of a fingernail

lupus [ˈluːpəs] *noun* type of chronic skin disease; **lupus erythematosus acutus (LE)** = one of several collagen diseases, a form of lupus, involving the heart and blood vessels; **lupus vulgaris** = form of tuberculosis of the skin, where red spots appear on the face and become infected; *see also* DISSEMINATED, SYSTEMIC

lutein [ˈluːtiːn] *noun* yellow pigment in the corpus luteum

luteinizing hormone (LH) [ˈluːtiːnaɪzɪŋ ˈhɔːməʊn] *noun* interstitial cell stimulating hormone, a hormone produced by the pituitary gland, which stimulates the formation of the corpus luteum in females and of testosterone in males

luteum [ˈluːtiəm] *noun* **corpus luteum** = *see* CORPUS, MACULA LUTEA

lux [lʌks] *noun* SI unit of brightness of light shining on a surface

luxation [lʌkˈseɪʃn] *noun* dislocation, a condition where a bone is displaced from its normal position

Lyme disease [ˈlaɪm dɪˈziːz] *noun* viral disease transmitted by bites from deer ticks *(Borrelia burgdorferi)*. It causes rashes, nervous pains, paralysis and, in extreme cases, death

lymph- *or* **lympho-** [lɪmf *or* ˈlɪmfəʊ] *prefix meaning* lymph

lymph (fluid) [ˈlɪmf ˈfluːɪd] *noun* colourless liquid containing white blood cells, which circulates in the lymph system from all body tissues, carrying waste matter away from tissues to the veins; **lymph duct** = any channel carrying lymph; **lymph nodes** *or* **lymph glands** = collections of lymphoid tissue situated in various points of the lymphatic system (especially under the armpits and in the groin) through which lymph passes and in which lymphocytes are produced; **lymph vessels** = tubes which carry lymph round the body from the tissues to the veins

COMMENT: lymph drains from the tissues through capillaries into lymph vessels. It is formed of water, protein and white blood cells (lymphocytes). Waste matter (such as infection) in the lymph is filtered out and destroyed as it passes through the lymph nodes, which then add further lymphocytes to the lymph before it continues into the system. It eventually drains into the brachiocephalic (innominate) veins, and joins the venous bloodstream. Lymph is not pumped round the body like blood but moves by muscle pressure on the lymph vessels and by the negative pressure of the large veins into which the vessels empty. Lymph is an essential part of the body's defence against infection

lymphadenectomy [lɪmfædəˈnektəmi] *noun* surgical removal of a lymph node

lymphadenitis [lımfædə'naıtıs] *noun* inflammation of the lymph nodes

lymphadenoma [lımfædə'nəumə] *noun* hypertrophy of a lymph node

lymphadenopathy [lımfædə'nɒpəθi] *noun* any condition of the lymph nodes

lymphangiectasis [lımfændʒi'ektəsıs] *noun* swelling of the smaller lymph vessels as a result of obstructions in larger vessels

lymphangiography [lımfændʒi'ɒgrəfi] *noun* X-ray examination of the lymph vessels following introduction of radio-opaque material

lymphangioma [lımfændʒi'əumə] *noun* tumour formed of lymph tissues

lymphangioplasty [lımfændʒi'ɒplæsti] *noun* surgical operation to make artificial lymph channels

lymphangiosarcoma
[lımfændʒiəusɑː'kəumə] *noun* malignant tumour of the endothelial cells lining the lymph vessels

lymphangitis [lımfæn'dʒaıtıs] *noun* inflammation of the lymph vessels

lymphatic [lım'fætık] **1** *adjective* referring to lymph; **lymphatic capillaries** = capillaries which lead from tissue and join lymphatic vessels; **lymphatic duct** = main channel for carrying lymph; **right lymphatic duct** = one of the main terminal channels for carrying lymph, draining the right side of the head and neck and entering the junction of the right subclavian and internal jugular veins. It is the smaller of the two main discharge points of the lymphatic system into the venous system, the larger being the thoracic duct; **lymphatic nodes** *or* **lymphatic glands** = glands situated in various points of the lymphatic system, especially under the armpits and in the groin where they produce lymphocytes; **lymphatic nodule** = small lymph node found in clusters in tissues; **lymphatic system** = series of vessels which transport lymph from the tissues through the lymph nodes and into the bloodstream; **lymphatic vessel** = tube which carries lymph round the body from the tissue to the veins **2** *noun* **the lymphatics** = lymph vessels

lymphoblast ['lımfəublæst] *noun* abnormal cell which forms in acute lymphatic leukaemia, a cell formed by the change which takes place in a lymphocyte on contact with an antigen

lymphoblastic [lımfəu'blæstık] *adjective* referring to lymphoblasts, forming lymphocytes

lymphocyte ['lımfəusaıt] *noun* type of mature leucocyte or white blood cell formed by the lymph nodes, and concerned with the production of antibodies; **T-lymphocyte** = lymphocyte formed in the thymus gland

lymphocytosis [lımfəusaı'təusıs] *noun* increased number of lymphocytes in the blood

lymphoedema *US* **lymphedema** [lımfəuı'diːmə *or* lımfı'diːmə] *noun* swelling caused by obstruction of the lymph vessels or abnormalities in the development of lymph vessels

lymphogranuloma inguinale *or* **lymphogranuloma venereum (l.g.v.)** [lımfəugrænju'ləumə 'ıngwıneıli *or* lımfəugrænju'ləumə ve'nıəriəm] *noun* venereal disease which causes a swelling of the lymph glands in the groin, occurring in tropical countries

lymphography [lım'fɒgrəfi] *noun* making images of the lymphatic system, after having introduced a radio-opaque substance

lymphoid tissue ['lımfɔıd 'tıʃuː] *noun* tissue in the lymph nodes, the tonsils and the spleen where masses of lymphocytes are supported by a network of reticular fibres and cells

lymphoma [lım'fəumə] *noun* tumour arising from lymphoid tissue

lymphopenia *or* **lymphocytopenia** [lımfəu'piːniə *or* lımfəusaıtəu'piːniə] *noun* reduction in the number of lymphocytes in the blood

lymphopoiesis [lımfəupɔı'iːsıs] *noun* production of lymphocytes or lymphoid tissue

lymphorrhagia *or* **lymphorrhoea** [lımfə'reıdʒə *or* lımfə'rıə] *noun* escape of lymph from ruptured or severed lymphatic vessels

lymphosarcoma [lımfəusɑː'kəumə] *noun* malignant growth arising from lymphocytes and their cells of origin in the lymph nodes

lymphuria [lım'fjuəriə] *noun* presence of lymph in the urine

lyophilization [laıɒfılaı'zeıʃn] *noun* preserving tissue, plasma, serum, etc., by freeze-drying in a vacuum

lyophilize [laɪˈɒfɪlaɪz] *verb* to preserve tissue, plasma, serum, etc., by freeze-drying in a vacuum

lysergic acid diethylamide (LSD) [laɪˈsɜːdʒɪk ˈæsɪd daɪˈeθɪləmaɪd] *noun* powerful hallucinogenic drug, which can cause psychosis

lysin [ˈlaɪsɪn] *noun* protein in the blood which destroys the cell against which it is directed, toxin which causes the lysis of cells; *see also* BACTERIOLYSIN, HAEMOLYSIN, LEUCOLYSIN

lysine [ˈlaɪsiːn] *noun* essential amino acid

lysis [ˈlaɪsɪs] *noun* **(a)** destruction of a cell by a lysin, where the membrane of the cell is destroyed **(b)** reduction in a fever or disease over a period of time

> COMMENT: in diseases such as typhoid fever, the patient's condition only improves gradually. The opposite where a patient gets rapidly better or worse, is called crisis

lysol [ˈlaɪsɒl] *noun* strong disinfectant, made of cresol and soap

lysosome [ˈlaɪsəsəʊm] *noun* particle in a cell which contains enzymes which break down substances (such as bacteria) which enter the cell

lysozyme [ˈlaɪsəzaɪm] *noun* enzyme found in whites of eggs and in tears, and which destroys certain bacteria

Mm

M *symbol for* mega-

m (a) = METRE **(b)** *symbol for* milli-

MAAG = MEDICAL AUDIT ADVISORY GROUP

macerate ['mæsəreɪt] *verb* to make something soft by letting it lie in a liquid for a time

maceration [mæsə'reɪʃn] *noun* softening of a solid by letting it lie in a liquid so that the soluble matter dissolves; **neonatal maceration** = softening or rotting of fetal tissue after the fetus has died in the uterus and has remained in the amniotic fluid

Macmillan nurse [mək'mɪlən 'nɜːs] *noun* nurse who specializes in cancer care, employed by the organization Macmillan Cancer Relief

macro- ['mækrəʊ] *prefix* meaning large (NOTE: opposite is **micro-**)

macrobiotic [mækrəʊbaɪ'ɒtɪk] *adjective* (food) which is healthy, which has been produced naturally without artificial additives or preservatives

> COMMENT: macrobiotic diets are usually vegetarian and are prepared in a special way; they consist of beans, coarse flour, fruit and vegetables. They may not contain enough protein or trace elements, especially to satisfy the needs of children

macrocephaly [mækrəʊ'sefəli] *noun* having an abnormally large head

macrocheilia [mækrəʊ'kaɪliə] *noun* having large lips

macrocyte ['mækrəʊsaɪt] *noun* abnormally large red blood cell found in patients suffering from pernicious anaemia

macrocytic [mækrəʊ'sɪtɪk] *adjective* referring to macrocytes; **macrocytic anaemia** = anaemia where the patient has abnormally large red blood cells

macrocytosis *or* **macrocythaemia** [mækrəʊsaɪ'təʊsɪs *or* mækrəʊsaɪ'θiːmiə] *noun* having macrocytes in the blood

macrodactyly [mækrəʊ'dæktəli] *noun* hypertrophy of the fingers or toes

macrogenitosoma [mækrəʊdʒenɪtə'səʊmə] *noun* premature development of the body with the genitals being of an abnormally large size

macroglobulin [mækrəʊ'glɒbjʊlɪn] *noun* immunoglobulin, a globulin protein of high molecular weight, which serves as an antibody

macroglossia [mækrəʊ'glɒsiə] *noun* having an abnormally large tongue

macrognathia [mækrəʊ'neɪθiə] *noun* condition in which the jaw is larger than normal

macrolide drug ['mækrəlaɪd 'drʌg] *noun* drug used in the treatment of bacterial infection, often in place of penicillin in patients sensitive to penicillin (NOTE: macrolide drugs have names ending in **-omycin: erythromycin**)

macromastia [mækrəʊ'mæstiə] *noun* overdevelopment of breasts

macromelia [mækrəʊ'miːliə] *noun* having abnormally large limbs

macrophage ['mækrəʊfeɪdʒ] *noun* any of several large cells, which destroy inflammatory tissue, found in connective tissue, wounds, lymph nodes and other parts

macropsia [mæ'krɒpsiə] *noun* seeing objects larger than they really are, caused by a defect in the retina

macroscopic [mækrəʊ'skɒpɪk] *adjective* which can be seen with the naked eye

macula ['mækjʊlə] *noun* **(a)** change in the colour of a small part of the body without changing the surface (as in freckles); **macula lutea** = yellow spot on the retina, surrounding the fovea, the part of the eye which sees most clearly (NOTE: plural is **maculae**) **(b)** area of hair cells inside the utricle and saccule of the ear

macular ['mækjʊlə] *adjective* referring to a macula; **macular degeneration** = eye disorder in elderly patients, where fluid leaks into the retina and destroys cones and rods, reducing central vision; **macular oedema** = disorder of the eye where fluid gathers in the fovea

macule ['mækjuːl] *noun* small flat coloured spot on the skin (NOTE: a spot which is raised above the surface of the skin is a **papule**)

maculopapular [mækjʊləʊ'pæpjʊlə] *adjective* (rash) made up of macules and papules

mad [mæd] *adjective* (person) who is suffering from a mental disorder (NOTE: not a medical term)

maduromycosis *or* **Madura foot** *or* **maduromycetoma** [mədjʊərəʊmaɪ'kəʊsɪs or mə'djʊərə 'fʊt or mədjʊərəʊmaɪsə'təʊmə] *noun* tropical fungus infection in the feet, which can destroy tissue and infect bones

Magendie's foramen [mə'dʒendɪz fə'reɪmen] *noun* opening in the fourth ventricle of the brain which allows cerebrospinal fluid to flow

magna ['mægnə] *see* CISTERNA

Magnesia [mæg'niːzɪə] *see* MILK

magnesium [mæg'niːzɪəm] *noun* chemical element found in green vegetables, which is essential especially for the correct functioning of muscles; **magnesium sulphate** = Epsom salts, magnesium salt used as a laxative; **magnesium trisilicate** = magnesium compound used to treat peptic ulcers (NOTE: chemical symbol is **Mg**)

magnetic [mæg'netɪk] *adjective* having the attraction of a magnet; **magnetic field** = area round a body which is under the influence of its attraction; **magnetic resonance imaging (MRI)** = scanning technique for examining soft body tissue and cells; *see also* NUCLEAR MAGNETIC RESONANCE

Magnetic Resonance Imaging scans produce more sensitive images than X-rays, so they are more useful in determining pathophysiology. Although MRI scans are similar to CT scans, they work differently

Nursing 87

magnum ['mægnəm] *see* FORAMEN

maidenhead ['meɪdənhed] *noun* hymen, the membrane which partially covers the vaginal passage in a virgin

maim [meɪm] *verb* to incapacitate someone with a major injury; *the car crash maimed him for life*

maintain [meɪn'teɪn] *verb* to keep up; *the heart beats regularly to maintain the supply of oxygen to the tissues*

major ['meɪdʒə] *adjective* greater, important, serious; *he had to undergo major surgery on his heart*; *the operation was a major one*; **labia majora** = two large fleshy folds at the edge of the vulva; *see illustration at* UROGENITAL SYSTEM (female) (NOTE: the opposite is **minor**)

mal [mæl] *noun* illness or disease; **grand mal** = commonest form of epilepsy, where the patient loses consciousness and falls to the ground with convulsions; urinary incontinence is common; **petit mal** = less severe form of epilepsy, where loss of consciousness happens suddenly but lasts a few seconds only and the patient does not fall or urinate

mal- [mæl] *prefix* meaning bad or abnormal

malabsorption [mæləb'sɔːpʃn] *noun* defective absorption by the intestines of fluids and nutrients in food; **malabsorption syndrome** = group of symptoms and signs resulting from steatorrhoea and malabsorption of vitamins, protein, carbohydrates and water, including malnutrition, anaemia, oedema, dermatitis

malacia [mə'leɪʃə] *noun* & *suffix* pathological softening of an organ or tissue

maladjusted [mælə'dʒʌstɪd] *adjective* (child) who has difficulty fitting into society or family

maladjustment [mælə'dʒʌstmənt] *noun* difficulty experienced in fitting into society or family

malaise [mə'leɪz] *noun* feeling of discomfort

malaligned [mə'laɪnd] *adjective* (bone) which is not correctly aligned

malar ['meɪlə] *adjective* referring to the cheek; **malar bone** = zygoma or zygomatic bone, the cheekbone which forms the prominent part of the cheek and the lower part of the eye socket

malaria [mə'leəriə] *noun* paludism, a mainly tropical disease caused by a parasite *Plasmodium* which enters the body after a bite from the female anopheles mosquito

COMMENT: malaria is a recurrent disease; it produces headaches, shivering, vomiting, sweating and sometimes hallucinations which are caused by toxins coming from the waste of the plasmodium in the blood.

malarial [mə'leəriəl] *adjective* referring to malaria; **malarial parasite** = parasite transmitted into the human bloodstream by the bite of the female anopheles mosquito

malarious [mə'leəriəs] *adjective* (region) where malaria is endemic

male [meɪl] *noun & adjective* referring to a man, of the same sex as a man; **male sex hormone** = testosterone, the hormone produced by the testes, which causes physical changes to take place in males as they become sexually mature; **male sex organs** = the testes, epididymis, vasa deferentia, seminal vesicles, ejaculatory ducts and penis

malformation [mælfɔː'meɪʃn] *noun* abnormal development of a structure; **congenital malformation** = malformation (such as cleft palate) which is present at birth

malformed [mæl'fɔːmd] *adjective* (part of the body) which has been badly formed

malfunction [mæl'fʌŋkʃn] **1** *noun* abnormal working of an organ; *his loss of consciousness was due to a malfunction of the kidneys or to a kidney malfunction* **2** *verb* to work badly; *during the operation his heart began to malfunction*

malignancy [mə'lɪgnənsi] *noun* state of being malignant; *the tests confirmed the malignancy of the growth*

without a functioning immune system to ward off germs, the patient now becomes vulnerable to becoming infected by bacteria, protozoa, fungi and other viruses and malignancies which may cause life-threatening illness
Journal of the American Medical Association

malignant [mə'lɪgnənt] *adjective* threatening life, tending to cause death, virulent (tumour); **malignant hypertension** = dangerously high blood pressure; **malignant melanoma** = dark tumour which develops on the skin from a mole, caused by

exposure to strong sunlight; **malignant tumour** = cancer, a tumour which is cancerous and can reappear or spread into other tissue, even if removed surgically (NOTE: the opposite is **benign** or **non-malignant**)

malingerer [mə'lɪŋɡərə] *noun* person who pretends to be ill

malingering [mə'lɪŋɡərɪŋ] *adjective* pretending to be ill

malleolar [mə'liːələ] *adjective* referring to a malleolus

malleolus [mə'liːələs] *noun* one of two bony prominences at each side of the ankle; **lateral malleolus** = part of the end of the fibula which protrudes on the outside of the ankle; **medial malleolus** = part of the end of the tibia which protrudes on the inside of the ankle (NOTE: plural is **malleoli**)

mallet finger ['mælɪt 'fɪŋɡə] *noun* finger which cannot be straightened because the tendon attaching the top joint has been torn

malleus ['mæliəs] *noun* largest of the three ossicles in the middle ear, shaped like a hammer; *see illustration at* EAR

Mallory's stain ['mæləriz 'steɪn] *noun* trichrome stain, used in histology to distinguish collagen, cytoplasm and nuclei

Mallory-Weiss tears ['mæləri'vaɪs 'teəz] *plural noun* tearing of the mucous membrane at the junction of the oesophagus and the stomach

malnourished [mæl'nʌrɪʃt] *adjective* (person) who does not have enough to eat

malnutrition [mælnju'trɪʃn] *noun* (i) bad nutrition, as a result of starvation, wrong diet or bad absorption of food; (ii) not having enough to eat

malocclusion [mælə'kluːʒn] *noun* condition where the teeth in the upper and lower jaws do not meet properly when the patient's mouth is closed; *see also* OCCLUSION

malodorous [mæl'əudərəs] *adjective* with a strong unpleasant smell

Malpighian body *or* **Malpighian corpuscle** [mæl'pɪɡiən 'bɒdi or mæl'pɪɡiən 'kɔːpʌsl] *see* CORPUSCLE (NOTE: also called **renal corpuscle**)

Malpighian glomerulus [mæl'pɪɡiən gləu'merjuləs] *noun* expanded end of a renal tubule, surrounding a glomerular tuft in the kidney, which filters plasma in order to reabsorb useful foodstuffs and eliminate waste (NOTE: also called **Bowman's capsule**)

Malpighian layer [mæl'pɪgɪən 'leɪə] *noun* deepest layer of the epidermis

malposition [mælpə'zɪʃn] *noun* wrong position (as of the fetus in the uterus or of fractured bones)

malpractice [mæl'præktɪs] *noun* (i) acting in an unprofessional or illegal way; (ii) wrong treatment of a patient (by a doctor, surgeon, dentist, etc.) for which the doctor may be tried in court; *the surgeon was found guilty of malpractice*

malpresentation [mælprezn'teɪʃn] *noun* abnormal presentation of the fetus in the uterus

Malta fever ['mɔːltə 'fiːvə] = BRUCELLOSIS

maltase ['mɔːlteɪz] *noun* enzyme in the small intestine which converts maltose into glucose

maltose [mɔːl'təʊz] *noun* sugar formed by digesting starch or glycogen

malunion [mæl'juːnɪən] *noun* incorrect union of pieces of a broken bone

mamilla *see* MAMMILLA

mamillary *see* MAMMILLARY

mamma ['mæmə] *noun* the breast, one of two glands on the chest of a woman which secrete milk

mammal ['mæml] *noun* type of animal (such as the human being) which gives birth to live young, secretes milk to feed them, keeps a constant body temperature and is covered with hair

mammary ['mæməri] *adjective* referring to the breast; **mammary gland** = gland in females which produces milk

mammilla *or* **mamilla** [mə'mɪlə] *noun* nipple, protruding part in the centre of the breast, containing the milk ducts through which the milk flows

mammillary *or* **mamillary** ['mæmɪlri] *adjective* referring to the nipple; **mamillary bodies** = two little projections on the base of the hypothalamus

mammogram ['mæməgræm] *noun* picture of a breast made using soft-tissue radiography

mammography [mæ'mɒgrəfi] *noun* examination of the breast, using a special X-ray technique

mammography is the most effective technique available for the detection of occult (non-palpable) breast cancer. It has been estimated that mammography can detect a carcinoma two years before it becomes palpable
Southern Medical Journal

mammoplasty ['mæməplæsti] *noun* plastic surgery to reduce the size of the breasts

mammothermography [mæməʊθɜ'mɒgrəfi] *noun* thermography of a breast

manage ['mænɪdʒ] *verb* **(a)** to control; to be in charge of; *she manages the ward very efficiently*; *we want to appoint someone to manage the group of hospitals*; *bleeding can usually be managed, but sometimes an operation may be necessary* **(b)** to be able to do something; to succeed in doing something; *did you manage to phone the doctor?*; *can she manage at home all by herself?*; *how are we going to manage without the nursing staff?*; *I managed to get him back into bed*

management ['mænɪdʒmənt] *noun* (i) organization or running (of a hospital, clinic, health authority, etc.); (ii) organization of a series of different treatments for a patient

manager ['mænɪdʒə] *noun* person in charge of a department in the health service, person in charge of a group of hospitals; **nurse manager** = nurse who has administrative duties in a hospital or the health service

mandible ['mændɪbl] *noun* lower bone in the jaw; *compare* MAXILLA; *see illustration at* SKULL

COMMENT: the jaw is formed of two bones, the mandible which is attached to the skull with a hinge joint and can move up and down, and the maxillae which are fixed parts of the skull

mandibular [mæn'dɪbjʊlə] *adjective* referring to the lower jaw; **mandibular fossae** = sockets in the skull into which the ends of the lower jaw fit; **mandibular nerve** = sensory nerve which supplies the teeth in the lower jaw, the temple, the floor of the mouth and the back part of the tongue

mane ['meɪni] *Latin word meaning* 'during the daytime': used on prescriptions (NOTE: the opposite is **nocte**)

he was diagnosed as having diabetes mellitus at age 14, and

was successfully controlled on insulin 15 units mane and 10 units nocte

British Journal of Hospital Medicine

manganese [ˈmæŋgəniːz] *noun* metallic trace element (NOTE: chemical symbol is **Mn**)

mania [ˈmeɪniə] *noun* state of manic-depressive psychosis where the patient is in a state of excitement, very sure of his own abilities and has increased energy

-mania [ˈmeɪniə] *suffix* obsession with something; **dipsomania** = addiction to alcohol; **kleptomania** = obsessive stealing of objects

maniac [ˈmeɪniæk] *noun* person suffering from an obsession

manic [ˈmænɪk] *adjective* referring to mania; **manic depression** = MANIC-DEPRESSIVE ILLNESS

manic-depressive [mænɪkdɪˈpresɪv] *adjective* (person) suffering from manic depression; **manic-depressive illness** *or* **manic-depressive psychosis** = bipolar disorder, a psychological condition where a patient moves between mania and depression and experiences delusion

manifestation [mænɪfesˈteɪʃn] *noun* sign, indication or symptom (of a disease)

the reason for this susceptibility is a profound abnormality of the immune system in children with sickle cell disease. The major manifestations of pneumococcal infection in SCD are septicaemia, meningitis and pneumonia

Lancet

manipulate [məˈnɪpjuleɪt] *verb* to rub or to move parts of the body with the hands to treat a joint, a slipped disc or a hernia

manipulation [mənɪpjuˈleɪʃn] *noun* moving or rubbing parts of the body with the hands to treat a disorder of a joint or a hernia

manner [ˈmænə] *noun* way of doing something, way of behaving; *he was behaving in a strange manner*; **doctor with a good bedside manner** = doctor who comforts and reassures patients when he examines them in hospital

mannitol [ˈmænɪtɒl] *noun see* DRUGS TABLE IN SUPPLEMENT

manometer [məˈnɒmɪtə] *noun* instrument for comparing pressures

Mantoux test [mænˈtuː ˈtest] *noun* test for tuberculosis, where the patient is given an intracutaneous injection of tuberculin; *compare* PATCH TEST

manual [ˈmænjuəl] *adjective* done by hand

manubrium (sterni) [məˈnuːbriəm ˈstɜːnaɪ] *noun* top part of the breastbone

MAO [ˈem ˈaɪ ˈəʊ] = MONOAMINE OXIDASE; **MAO inhibitor** = drug used to treat depression by inhibiting the action of MAO, causing an accumulation of catecholamine neurotransmitters but which can cause high blood pressure

MAOI [ˈem ˈaɪ ˈəʊ ˈaɪ] = MONOAMINE OXIDASE INHIBITOR

mapping [ˈmæpɪŋ] *noun* **chromosome mapping** = procedure by which the position of genes on a chromosome is established

map out [ˈmæp ˈaʊt] *verb* to show clearly in a diagram; *to map out the extent of a tumour*

marasmus [məˈræzməs] *noun* wasting disease which affects small children who have difficulty in absorbing nutrients or who are suffering from malnutrition (NOTE: also called **failure to thrive**)

marble bone disease [ˈmɑːbl ˈbəʊn dɪˈziːz] = OSTEOPETROSIS

Marburg virus disease [ˈmɑːbɜːg ˈvaɪrəs dɪˈziːz] *noun* green monkey disease, virus disease of green monkeys which is transmitted to humans

COMMENT: because monkeys are used in laboratory experiments, the disease mainly affects laboratory workers. Symptoms include headaches and bleeding from mucous membranes; the disease is often fatal

march fracture [ˈmɑːtʃ ˈfræktʃə] *noun* fracture of one of the metatarsal bones in the foot, caused by excessive exercise to which the body is not accustomed

Marfan's syndrome [ˈmɑːfænz ˈsɪndrəʊm] *noun* hereditary condition where the patient has extremely long fingers and toes, with abnormalities of the heart, aorta and eyes

margarine [mɑːdʒəˈriːn] *noun* vegetable fat which looks like butter and is used instead of butter

marijuana [mærɪˈwɑːnə] *noun* cannabis, (i) addictive drug made from the leaves or flowers of the Indian hemp plant; (ii) tropical plant from whose leaves or flowers an addictive drug is produced

mark [mɑːk] **1** *noun* spot, small area of a different colour; *there's a red mark where you hit your head*; *the rash has left marks on the chest and back* **2** *verb* to make a mark; **the tin is marked 'dangerous'** = it has the word 'dangerous' written on it

marked [mɑːkt] *adjective* obvious or noticeable; *there has been a marked improvement in his condition*

marker ['mɑːkə] *noun* (i) label, thing which marks a place; (ii) substance which is part of a chromosome and gives it a genetic mark which can be used as a point of reference; (iii) substance introduced into the body to make internal structures clearer to X-rays

market *see* INTERNAL

marrow *or* **bone marrow** ['mærəʊ or 'bəʊn 'mærəʊ] *noun* soft tissue in cancellous bone; **bone marrow transplant** = transplant of marrow from a donor to a recipient; *see illustration at* BONE STRUCTURE (NOTE: for other terms referring to bone marrow, see words beginning with **myel-, myelo-**)

COMMENT: two types of bone marrow are to be found: red bone marrow or myeloid tissue, which forms red blood cells and is found in cancellous bone in the vertebrae, in the ends of long bones, and in the sternum and other flat bones; as a person gets older, fatty yellow bone marrow develops in the central cavity of long bones

masculinization [mæskjʊlɪnaɪ'zeɪʃn] *noun* development of male characteristics (such as body hair and a deep voice) in a woman, caused by hormone deficiency or by treatment with male hormones

mask [mɑːsk] *noun* (i) metal and rubber frame that fits over the patient's nose and mouth and is used to administer an anaesthetic; (ii) piece of gauze which fits over the mouth and nose to prevent droplet infection; (iii) cover which fits over the face of a person who has been disfigured in an accident

masochism ['mæsəkɪzm] *noun* abnormal sexual condition where a person takes pleasure in being hurt or badly treated

masochist ['mæsəkɪst] *noun* person suffering from masochism

masochistic [mæsə'kɪstɪk] *adjective* referring to masochism; *compare* SADISM, SADIST, SADISTIC

mass [mæs] *noun* **(a)** (i) body of matter; (ii) mixture for making pills; (iii) main solid part of bone **(b)** large quantity, such as a large number of people; *the patient's back was covered with a mass of red spots*; **mass radiography** = taking X-ray photographs of large numbers of people to check for tuberculosis; **mass screening** = testing large numbers of people for the presence of a disease

massage ['mæsɑːʒ] **1** *noun* treatment of muscular conditions which involves rubbing, stroking or pressing a patient's body with the hands; **external cardiac massage** = method of making a patient's heart start beating again by rhythmic pressing on the breastbone; **internal cardiac massage** = method of making a patient's heart start beating again by pressing on the heart itself (NOTE: no plural, but **a massage** is used to refer to a single treatment: **he had a hot bath and a massage**) **2** *verb* to rub, stroke or press a patient's body with the hands

masseter (muscle) [mæ'siːtə 'mʌsl] *noun* muscle which clenches the lower jaw making it move up

massive ['mæsɪv] *adjective* very large; *he was given a massive injection of penicillin*; *she had a massive heart attack*

mast- [mæst] *prefix* referring to a breast

mastalgia [mæ'stældʒə] *noun* pain in the mammary gland

mastatrophy [mæ'stætrəfi] *noun* atrophy of the mammary gland

mast cell ['mɑːst 'sel] *noun* large cell in connective tissue, which carries histamine and reacts to allergens

mastectomy [mæ'stektəmi] *noun* surgical removal of a breast; **radical mastectomy** = removal of the breast, and also the associated lymph nodes and muscles

masticate ['mæstɪkeɪt] *verb* to chew food

mastication [mæstɪ'keɪʃn] *noun* chewing food

mastitis [mæs'taɪtɪs] *noun* inflammation of the breast

mastoid ['mæstɔɪd] *adjective & noun* (i) shaped like a nipple; (ii) belonging to the mastoid part of the temporal bone; **mastoid antrum** = *see* ANTRUM; **mastoid (air) cells** = air cells in the mastoid process; **mastoid**

process or **mastoid** = part of the temporal bone which protrudes at the side of the head behind the ear; *see illustration at* SKULL

mastoidectomy [mæstɔɪ'dektəmi] *noun* surgical operation to remove part of the mastoid process, as a treatment for mastoiditis

mastoiditis [mæstɔɪ'daɪtɪs] *noun* inflammation of the mastoid process and air cells

COMMENT: symptoms are fever, and pain in the ears. The mastoid process can be infected by infection from the middle ear through the mastoid antrum. Mastoiditis can cause deafness and can affect the meninges if not treated

mastoidotomy [mæstɔɪ'dɒtəmi] *noun* surgical operation to make a cut into the mastoid process to treat infection

masturbate ['mæstəbeɪt] *verb* to excite one's own genitals so as to produce an orgasm

masturbation [mæstə'beɪʃn] *noun* stimulation of one's own genitals to produce an orgasm

match [mætʃ] *verb* (a) to examine two things to see if they are similar, to see if they fit together; *they are trying to match the donor to the recipient* (b) to fit together in a certain way; *the two samples don't match*

bone marrow from donors has to be carefully matched with the recipient or graft-versus-host disease will ensue

Hospital Update

mater ['meɪtə] *see* ARACHNOID, DURA MATER, PIA MATER

material [mə'tɪəriəl] *noun* (a) matter which can be used to make something (b) cloth; *the wound should be covered with gauze or other light material* (c) all that is necessary in surgery

materia medica [mə'tɪəriə 'medɪkə] *Latin words meaning* 'medical substance': study of drugs or dosages as used in treatment

maternal [mə'tɜːnl] *adjective* referring to a mother; **maternal death** = death of a mother during pregnancy, childbirth or up to twelve months after childbirth; **maternal deprivation** = *see* DEPRIVATION; **maternal instincts** = instinctive feelings in a woman to look after and protect her child

maternity [mə'tɜːnəti] *noun* childbirth, becoming a mother; **maternity case** = woman who is about to give birth; **maternity clinic** = clinic where expectant mothers are taught how to look after babies, do exercises and have medical checkups; **maternity hospital** or **maternity ward** or **maternity unit** = hospital, ward or unit which deals only with women giving birth

matrix ['meɪtrɪks] *noun* ground substance, amorphous mass of cells forming the basis of connective tissue

matron ['meɪtrn] *noun* woman in charge of the nurses in a hospital; *she has been made matron of the maternity hospital*; *such cases should be reported to (the) matron* (NOTE: **matron** can be used with names: **Matron Jones**; the official title is '**Nursing officer**')

matter ['mætə] *noun* (a) substance; **grey matter** = nerve tissue which is of a dark grey colour and forms part of the central nervous system; **white matter** = nerve tissue in the central nervous system which contains more myelin than grey matter (b) (**infected**) **matter** = pus

mattress ['mætrəs] *noun* thick soft part of a bed which you lie on; **mattress suture** = suture made with a loop on each side of the incision

maturation [mætʃu'reɪʃn] *noun* becoming mature or fully developed

mature [mə'tʃʊə] *adjective* fully developed; **mature follicle** = Graafian follicle just before ovulation

maturing [mə'tʃʊərɪŋ] *adjective* becoming mature; **maturing egg** or **ovum** = ovum contained by a Graafian follicle

maturity [mə'tʃʊərəti] *noun* (a) being fully developed (b) (*in psychology*) being a responsible adult

maxilla (bone) [mæk'sɪlə 'bəʊn] *noun* upper jaw bone; *see illustration at* SKULL (NOTE: plural is **maxillae**. It is more correct to refer to the upper jaw as the **maxillae** as it is in fact formed of two bones which are fused together)

maxillary [mæk'sɪlri] *adjective* referring to the maxilla; **maxillary air sinus** or **maxillary antrum** = one of two sinuses behind the cheekbones in the upper jaw (NOTE: also called **antrum of Highmore**)

maxillo-facial [mæk'sɪləʊ'feɪʃəl] *adjective* referring to the maxillary bone and the face; *maxillo-facial surgery*

MB ['em 'bi:] = BACHELOR OF MEDICINE

McBurney's point [mək'bɜ:nız 'pɔɪnt] *noun* point which indicates the normal position of the appendix on the right side of the abdomen, between the hip bone and the navel, which is extremely painful if pressed when the patient has appendicitis

MCP ['em 'si: 'pi:] = METACARPOPHALANGEAL

MD ['em 'di:] = DOCTOR OF MEDICINE

ME ['em 'i:] = MYALGIC ENCEPHALOMYELITIS

meal [mi:l] *noun* eating food at a particular time; *we have three meals a day - breakfast, lunch and dinner*; *you should only have a light meal in the evening*; **barium meal** = liquid solution containing barium sulphate which a patient drinks so that an X-ray can be taken of his stomach

measles ['mi:zlz] *noun* morbilli or rubeola, infectious disease of children, where the body is covered with a red rash; *she's in bed with measles*; *have you had measles?*; *he's got measles*; *they caught measles from their friend at school*; *see also* GERMAN MEASLES, KOPLIK'S SPOTS

COMMENT: measles can be a serious disease as it weakens the body's resistance to other diseases, especially bronchitis and ear infections; it can be prevented by immunization. If caught by an adult it can be very serious

measure ['meʒə] **1** *noun* **(a)** unit of size, quantity or degree; *a metre is a measure of length* **(b) tape measure** = long tape with centimetres, inches, etc., marked on it **2** *verb* to find out the size of something; to be a certain size; *the room measures 3 metres by 2 metres*; *a thermometer measures temperature*

measurement ['meʒəmənt] *noun* size, length, etc., of something which has been measured

meat [mi:t] *noun* animal flesh which is eaten (NOTE: no plural: **some meat, a piece** *or* **a slice of meat; he refuses to eat meat**)

meatus [mɪ'eɪtəs] *noun* opening leading to an internal passage in the body, such as the urethra or the nasal cavity; **external auditory meatus** = tube in the skull leading from the outer ear to the eardrum; **internal auditory meatus** = channel which takes the

auditory nerve through the temporal bone; *see illustrations at* EAR, SKULL

mechanism ['mekənɪzm] *noun* physical or chemical changes by which a function is carried out, system in the body which functions in a particular way; *the inner ear is the body's mechanism for the sense of balance*

Meckel's diverticulum ['mekəlz daɪvə'tɪkjʊləm] *see* DIVERTICULUM

meconium [mɪ'kəʊnɪəm] *noun* first dark green faeces produced by a newborn baby

media ['mi:dɪə] *noun* tunica media, the middle layer of the wall of an artery or vein

medial ['mi:dɪəl] *adjective* nearer to the central midline of the body or to the centre of an organ; **medial arcuate ligament** = fibrous arch to which the diaphragm is attached; **medial malleolus** = bone at the end of the tibia which protrudes at the inside of the ankle; **medial rectus** = muscle arising from the medial part of the common tendinous ring and inserted into the sclera anterior of the eyeball; *compare* LATERAL

medialis [mi:dɪ'eɪlɪs] *see* VASTUS

medially ['mi:dɪəli] *adverb* towards or on the sagittal plane of the body

median ['mi:dɪən] *adjective* towards the central midline of the body, placed in the middle; **median nerve** = one of the main nerves of the forearm and hand; **median plane** = midline at right angles to the coronal plane and dividing the body into right and left parts

mediastinal [mi:dɪə'staɪnl] *adjective* referring to the mediastinum; *the mediastinal surface of pleura or of the lungs*

mediastinitis [mi:dɪæstə'naɪtɪs] *noun* inflammation of the mediastinum

mediastinum [mi:dɪə'staɪnəm] *noun* section of the chest between the lungs, where the heart, oesophagus, and phrenic and vagus nerves are situated

medical ['medɪkl] **1** *adjective* (i) referring to the study of diseases; (ii) referring to treatment of disease which does not involve surgery; (iii) (treatment) given by a doctor (as opposed to a surgeon) in a hospital or in his surgery; *a medical student*; *medical help was provided by the Red Cross*; **medical assistance** = help provided by a nurse, by an ambulanceman or by a member of the Red Cross, etc.; **medical audit** = systematic critical analysis of the quality of medical care including the procedures used for diagnosis and treatment, the use of resources and the resulting outcome and quality of life for the patient; **medical audit advisory group (MAAG)** = body with the responsibility of advising on medical audit in primary care; **medical certificate** = official document signed by a doctor, giving a patient permission to be away from work or not to do certain types of work; **medical committee** = committee of doctors in a hospital who advise the management on medical matters; **medical doctor (MD)** = doctor who practises medicine, but not usually a surgeon; **medical examination** = examination of a patient by a doctor; **medical history** = details of a patient's medical records over a period of time; **chief medical officer** = government official responsible for all aspects of public health; **Medical Officer of Health (MOH)** = formerly, local government official in charge of the health service in a certain district; **medical practitioner** = person qualified in medicine (a doctor or surgeon); **Medical Research Council (MRC)** = government body which organizes and pays for medical research; **medical secretary** = qualified secretary who specializes in medical documentation, either in a hospital or in a doctor's surgery; **medical social worker** = person who helps patients with their family problems or problems related to their work, which may have an effect on their response to treatment; **medical ward** = ward for patients who do not have to undergo surgical operations **2** *noun* official examination of a person by a doctor; *he wanted to join the army, but failed his medical; you will have to have a medical if you take out an insurance policy*

Medic-Alert bracelet ['medɪkə'lɜːt 'breɪslət] *noun* bracelet worn by a person to show that he suffers from a certain condition (such as diabetes or an allergy)

Medicare ['medɪkeə] *noun* system of public health insurance in the USA

medicated ['medɪkeɪtɪd] *adjective* (talcum powder, cough sweet, etc.) which contains a medicinal drug; **medicated shampoo** = shampoo containing a chemical which is supposed to prevent dandruff

medication [medɪ'keɪʃn] *noun* (i) method of treatment by giving drugs to a patient; (ii) medicine or drug taken by a patient; *he was given medication by the ambulancemen; what sort of medication has she been taking?; 80% of elderly patients admitted to*

geriatric units are on medication; *see also* PREMEDICATION

medicinal [mə'dɪsənl] *adjective* referring to medicine; (substance) with healing properties; *he has a drink of whisky before he goes to bed for medicinal purposes;* **medicinal drug** = drug used to treat a disease as opposed to hallucinatory or addictive drugs

medicinally [mə'dɪsənli] *adverb* (used) as a medicine; *the herb can be used medicinally*

medicine ['medsɪn] *noun* **(a)** drug, preparation taken to treat a disease or condition; *take some cough medicine if your cough is bad; you should take the medicine three times a day;* **medicine bottle** = special bottle which contains medicine; **medicine cabinet** *or* **medicine chest** = cupboard where medicines, bandages, thermometers, etc., can be left locked up, but ready for use in an emergency **(b)** (i) study of diseases and how to cure or prevent them; (ii) study and treatment of diseases which does not involve surgery; *he is studying medicine because he wants to be a doctor;* **clinical medicine** = study and treatment of patients in a hospital ward or in the doctor's surgery (as opposed to the operating theatre or laboratory) (NOTE: no plural in this meaning)

medico ['medɪkəu] *noun (informal)* doctor; *my medico said I was perfectly fit*

medico- ['medɪkəu] *prefix* referring to medicine or to doctors

medicochirurgical [medɪkəukaɪ'rɜːdʒɪkl] *adjective* referring to both medicine and surgery

medicolegal [medɪkəu'liːgəl] *adjective* referring to both medicine and the law

medium ['miːdiəm] **1** *adjective* average, in the middle or at the halfway point **2** *noun* substance through which something acts; **contrast medium** = radio-opaque dye introduced into an organ or part of the body so that soft tissue will show clearly on an X-ray photograph; **culture medium** = jelly (such as agar) in which a bacterial culture is grown in a laboratory

medulla [me'dʌlə] *noun* (i) soft inner part of an organ (as opposed to the outer cortex); (ii) bone marrow; (iii) any structure similar to bone marrow; **medulla oblongata** = continuation of the spinal cord going through the foramen magnum into the brain; **renal medulla** = inner part of a kidney containing no glomeruli; *see illustration at* KIDNEY;

adrenal medulla *or* suprarenal medulla = inner part of the adrenal gland which secretes adrenaline and noradrenaline

medullary [me'dʌləri] *adjective* (i) similar to marrow; (ii) referring to a medulla; **medullary cavity** = hollow centre of a long bone, containing bone marrow; *see illustration at* BONE STRUCTURE; **medullary cord** = epithelial fibre found near the hilum of the fetal ovary

medullated nerve ['medəleɪtɪd 'nɜːv] *noun* nerve surrounded by a myelin sheath

medulloblastoma [medʌləublæ'stəumə] *noun* tumour which develops in the medulla oblongata and the fourth ventricle of the brain in children

mega- *or* **megalo-** ['megə *or* 'megələu] *prefix* **(a)** meaning large (NOTE: the opposite is **micro-) (b)** meaning one million (10^6); **megajoule** = unit of measurement of energy (= one million joules) (NOTE: symbol is **M**)

megacolon [megə'kəulən] *noun* condition where the lower colon is very much larger than normal, because part of the colon above is constricted, making bowel movements impossible

megakaryocyte [megə'kæriəsaɪt] *noun* bone marrow cell which produces blood platelets

megaloblast ['megələublæst] *noun* abnormally large blood cell found in the bone marrow of patients suffering from certain types of anaemia caused by vitamin B_{12} deficiency

megaloblastic [megələu'blæstɪk] *adjective* referring to megaloblasts; **megaloblastic anaemia** = anaemia caused by vitamin B_{12} deficiency

megalocephaly [megələu'sefəli] *noun* having an abnormally large head

megalocyte ['megələusaɪt] *noun* abnormally large red blood cell, found in pernicious anaemia

-megaly ['megəli] *suffix meaning* enlargement

meibomian cyst [maɪ'bəumiən 'sɪst] *noun* chalazion, swelling of a sebaceous gland in the eyelid

meibomian gland [maɪ'bəumiən 'glænd] *noun* tarsal gland, a sebaceous gland on the edge of the eyelid which secretes a liquid to lubricate the eyelid

meiosis *US* **miosis** [maɪ'əusɪs] *noun* process of cell division which results in two pairs of haploid cells (cells with only one set of chromosomes); *compare* MITOSIS

Meissner's corpuscle ['maɪsnəz 'kɔːpʌsl] *noun* receptor cell in the skin which is thought to be sensitive to touch; *see illustration at* SKIN & SENSORY RECEPTORS

Meissner's plexus ['maɪsnəz 'pleksəs] *noun* network of nerve fibres in the wall of the alimentary canal

melaena *or* **melena** [mə'liːnə] *noun* black faeces where the colour is caused by bleeding in the intestine

melancholia [melən'kəuliə] *noun* (i) severe depressive illness occurring usually between the ages of 45 and 65; (ii) clinical syndrome with tendency to delusion, fixed personality, and agitated movements; **involutional melancholia** = depression which occurs in people (mainly women) after middle age, probably caused by a change of endocrine secretions

melanin ['melənɪn] *noun* dark pigment which gives colour to skin and hair, also found in the choroid of the eye and in certain tumours

melanism *or* **melanosis** ['melənɪzm *or* melə'nəusɪs] *noun* (i) abnormally depositing of dark pigment; (ii) staining of all body tissue with melanin in a form of carcinoma

melanocyte ['melənəsaɪt] *noun* any cell which carries pigment

melanocyte-stimulating hormone (MSH) ['melənəsaɪt 'stɪmjuleɪtɪŋ 'hɔːməum] *noun* hormone produced by the pituitary gland which causes darkening in the colour of the skin

melanoderma [melənə'dɜːmə] *noun* (i) abnormally large amount of melanin in the skin; (ii) discoloration of patches of the skin

melanoma [melə'nəumə] *noun* tumour formed of dark pigmented cells; **malignant melanoma** = dark tumour which develops on the skin from a mole, often caused by exposure to strong sunlight

COMMENT: ABCD is the key to remember if you want to know if there is a risk of developing a melanoma: A = ASSYMMETRY, ie. the two sides are not quite the same, and the mole does not have a perfect shape; B = BORDER, the edge becomes irregular; C = COLOUR , there may be a change in colour, with the mole becoming darker; D = DIAMETER, any change in diameter should be considered an important factor. Among other features, pain is rarely an important feature but itching could be one

melanophore ['melənəfɔː] *noun* cell which contains melanin

melanoplakia ['melənəpleɪkiə] *noun* areas of pigment in the mucous membrane inside the mouth

melanosis [melə'nəʊsɪs] *see* MELANISM

melanuria [melə'njʊəriə] *noun* (i) presence of dark colouring in the urine; (ii) condition where the urine turns black after being allowed to stand (as in cases of malignant melanoma)

melasma [mə'læzmə] *noun* presence of little brown, yellow or black spots on the skin

melatonin [melə'təʊnɪn] *noun* hormone produced by the pineal gland during the hours of darkness, which makes animals sleep during the winter months; it is thought to control the body's rhythms and is taken as a drug to prevent jet lag

COMMENT: bright light hitting the eye has the effect of stopping the production of melatonin

melena [mə'liːnə] = MELAENA

mellitus ['melɪtəs] *see* DIABETES

membrane ['membreɪn] *noun* thin layer of tissue which lines or covers an organ; **membrane bone** = bone which develops from tissue and not from cartilage; **basement membrane** = membrane at the base of an epithelium; **mucous membrane** = membrane which lines internal passages in the body (such as nose or mouth) and secretes mucus; **serous membrane** = membrane which lines an internal cavity which does not come into contact with air (such as the peritoneum or pericardium); **synovial membrane** = smooth membrane which forms the inner lining of the capsule covering a joint, and secretes the fluid which lubricates the joint; **tectorial membrane** = spiral membrane in the inner ear above the organ of Corti, which contains the hair cells which transmit impulses to the auditory nerve; **tympanic membrane** = eardrum; *see illustration at* EAR

membranous ['membrənəs] *adjective* referring to membrane; **membranous labyrinth** = canals round the cochlea

memory ['memri] *noun* ability to remember; *he has a very good memory for dates*; *I have no memory for names*; *he said the whole list from memory*; **loss of memory** = not being able to remember anything; *she was found wandering in the street suffering from loss of memory*; *he lost his memory after the accident*

menarche [mə'nɑːki] *noun* start of menstrual periods

mend [mend] *verb* to repair; to make something perfect which has a fault in it; *the surgeons are trying to mend the defective heart valves*

Mendel's laws ['mendəlz 'lɔːz] *noun* laws of heredity

Mendelson's syndrome ['mendəlsənz 'sɪndrəʊm] *noun* sometimes fatal condition where acid fluid from the stomach is brought up into the windpipe and passes into the lungs, occurring mainly in obstetric patients

Ménière's disease *or* **syndrome** [meni'eəz dɪ'ziːz or 'sɪndrəʊm] *noun* disease of the middle ear, where the patient becomes dizzy, hears ringing in the ears and may vomit and becomes progressively deaf

COMMENT: the causes are not certain, but may include infections or allergies, which increase the fluid contents of the labyrinth in the middle ear

mening- *or* **meningo-** [me'nɪndʒ or mə'nɪŋgəʊ] *prefix* referring to the meninges

meningeal [me'nɪndʒiəl] *adjective* referring to the meninges; **meningeal haemorrhage** = haemorrhage from a meningeal artery; **meningeal sarcoma** = malignant tumour in the meninges

meninges [me'nɪndʒiːz] *plural noun* membranes which surround the brain and spinal cord (NOTE: the singular is **meninx**)

COMMENT: the meninges are divided into three layers: the tough outer layer (dura mater) which protects the brain and spinal cord, the middle layer (arachnoid mater) and the delicate inner layer (pia mater) which contains the blood vessels. The cerebrospinal fluid flows in the space (subarachnoid space) between the arachnoid mater and pia mater

meningioma [menɪndʒi'əʊmə] *noun* benign tumour in the meninges

meningism [me'nɪndʒɪzm] *noun* condition where there are signs of meningeal irritation suggesting meningitis, but where there is no pathological change in the cerebrospinal fluid

meningitis [menɪn'dʒaɪtɪs] *noun* inflammation of the meninges, where the patient has violent headaches, fever, and stiff neck muscles, and can become delirious; **aseptic meningitis** = relatively mild viral form of meningitis; *see also* HIB, MENINGOCOCCAL

COMMENT: meningitis is a serious viral or bacterial disease which can cause brain damage and even death. The bacterial form can be treated with antibiotics. The most common forms of bacterial meningitis are Hib and meningococcal

meningocele [mə'nɪŋgəʊsiːl] *noun* condition where the meninges protrude through the vertebral column or skull

meningococcal [mənɪŋgəʊ'kɒkl] *adjective* referring to meningococcus; **meningococcal disease** = disease caused by a meningococcus; **meningococcal meningitis** = cerebrospinal fever, cerebrospinal meningitis or spotted fever, the commonest epidemic form of meningitis, caused by a bacterium *Neisseria meningitidis,* where the meninges become inflamed causing headaches and fever

meningococcus [mənɪŋgəʊ'kɒkəs] *noun* bacterium *Neisseria meningitidis* which causes meningococcal meningitis (NOTE: plural is **meningococci**)

meningoencephalitis [mənɪŋgəʊensefə'laɪtɪs] *noun* inflammation of the meninges and the brain

meningoencephalocele [mənɪŋgəʊen'sefələʊsiːl] *noun* condition where part of the meninges and the brain push through a gap in the skull

meningomyelocele [mənɪŋgəʊ'maɪələʊsiːl] *noun* hernia of part of the meninges and the spinal cord

meningovascular [mənɪŋgəʊ'væskjʊlə] *adjective* referring to the meningeal blood vessels

meniscectomy [menɪ'sektəmi] *noun* surgical removal of a cartilage from the knee

meniscus [mə'nɪskəs] *noun* semilunar cartilage, one of two pads of cartilage (lateral meniscus and medial meniscus) between the femur and tibia in a knee joint (NOTE: the plural is **menisci**)

meno- ['menəʊ] *prefix* referring to menstruation

menopausal [menə'pɔːzl] *adjective* referring to the menopause

menopause ['menəpɔːz] *noun* period (usually between 45 and 55 years of age) when a woman stops menstruating and can no longer bear children; **male menopause** = non-medical term given to a period in a man's life in middle age (NOTE: also called **climacteric** *or* **change of life**)

menorrhagia [menə'reɪdʒiə] *noun* very heavy bleeding during menstruation

menses ['mensiːz] *plural noun* = MENSTRUATION

menstrual ['menstrʊəl] *adjective* referring to menstruation; **menstrual cramp** = cramp in the muscles round the uterus during menstruation; **menstrual cycle** = period (usually 28 days) during which a woman ovulates, then the walls of the uterus swell and bleeding takes place if the ovum has not been fertilized; **menstrual flow** = discharge of blood from the uterus during menstruation

menstruate ['menstrueɪt] *verb* to bleed from the uterus during menstruation

menstruation [menstru'eɪʃn] *noun* bleeding from the uterus which occurs in a woman each month when the lining of the uterus is shed because no fertilized egg is present

menstruum ['menstruːəm] *noun* liquid used in the extract of active principles from an unrefined drug

mental ['mentl] *adjective* **(a)** referring to the mind; **mental age** = age of a person's mental development, measured by intelligence tests; *she has a mental age of three*; **mental block** = temporary inability to remember something, caused by the effect of nervous stress on the mental processes; **mental deficiency** *or* **defect** *or* **disorder** *or* **handicap** *or* **retardation** *or* **subnormality** = condition where a person's mind has not developed as fully as the body, so that he is not so mentally advanced as others of the same age; **mental development** = development of the mind; *although physically handicapped her mental development is higher than normal for her age*; **mental hospital** = special hospital for the treatment of mentally ill patients; **mental illness** = any disorder which affects the mind; **mental patient** = patient suffering from a mental illness **(b)** referring to the chin; **mental nerve** = nerve which supplies the chin

mentalis muscle [men'teɪlɪs 'mʌsl] *noun* muscle attached to the front of the lower jaw and the skin of the chin

mentally ['mentli] *adverb* in the mind, referring to the mind; *mentally, she is very advanced for her age*; **mentally defective** *or* **mentally retarded** = (person) with a mental ability which is less than normal for his age; *by the age of four he was showing signs of being mentally retarded*; **the mentally ill** = people suffering from mental illness

menthol ['menθɒl] *noun* strongly scented compound, produced from peppermint oil, used in cough medicines and in the treatment of neuralgia

mentholated ['menθəleɪtɪd] *adjective* impregnated with menthol

mentum ['mentəm] *noun* chin

meralgia (paraesthetica) [mə'rældʒə pæres'θetɪkə] *noun* pain in the top of the thigh (caused by a pinched nerve)

mercurialism [mə'kjʊəriəlɪzm] *noun* mercury poisoning

mercurochrome [mə'kjʊərəʊkrəʊm] *noun* red antiseptic solution

mercury ['mɜːkjʊri] *noun* poisonous liquid metal, used in thermometers; **mercury poisoning** = poisoning by drinking mercury, mercury compounds or by inhaling mercury vapour (NOTE: the chemical symbol is **Hg**)

mercy killing ['mɜːsi 'kɪlɪŋ] *noun* euthanasia, the killing of a sick person to put an end to his or her suffering

Merkel's cells *or* **discs** ['mɜːkelz 'selz *or* 'dɪsks] *noun* epithelial cells in the deeper part of the dermis which form touch receptors

merocrine ['merəʊkraɪn] *adjective* (gland, especially a sweat gland) which does not disintegrate and remains intact during secretion (NOTE: also called **eccrine**)

mes- *or* **meso-** [mes *or* 'mesəʊ] *prefix* meaning middle

mesaortitis [meseɪɔː'taɪtɪs] *noun* inflammation of the media of the aorta

mesarteritis [mesɑːtə'raɪtɪs] *noun* inflammation of the media of an artery

mesencephalon [mesen'sefəlɒn] *noun* the midbrain, a small section of the brain stem, above the pons, between the hindbrain and the cerebrum

mesenteric [mesen'terɪk] *adjective* referring to the mesentery; **superior mesenteric arteries** = arteries which supply the small intestine; **inferior mesenteric arteries** = arteries which supply the transverse colon and rectum; **mesenteric vein** = vein in the portal system running from the intestine to the portal vein

mesenterica [mesen'terɪkə] *see* TABES

mesentery ['mesentri] *noun* double layer peritoneum which attaches the small intestine and other abdominal organs to the abdominal wall

mesoappendix [mesəʊə'pendɪks] *noun* fold of peritoneum which links the appendix and the ileum

mesocolon [mesəʊ'kəʊlən] *noun* fold of peritoneum which supports the colon (in an adult it supports the transverse and sigmoid sections only)

mesoderm *or* **embryonic mesoderm** ['mesəʊdɜːm *or* embri'ɒnɪk 'mesəʊdɜːm] *noun* middle layer of an embryo, which develops into muscles, bones, blood, kidneys, cartilages, urinary ducts, and the cardiovascular and lymphatic systems

mesodermal [mesəʊ'dɜːml] *adjective* referring to the mesoderm

mesometrium [mesəʊ'miːtriəm] *noun* muscle layer of the uterus

mesomorph ['mesəʊmɔːf] *noun* type of person of average height but strong build

mesomorphic [mesəʊ'mɔːfɪk] *adjective* like a mesomorph; *see also* ECTOMORPH, ENDOMORPH

mesonephros [mesəʊ'nefrɒs] *noun* Wolffian body, kidney tissue which exists in a human embryo

mesosalpinx [mesəʊ'sælpɪŋks] *noun* upper part of the broad ligament around the Fallopian tubes

mesotendon [mesəʊ'tendən] *noun* synovial membrane connecting the lining of the fibrous sheath to that of a tendon

mesothelioma [mesəʊθeli'əʊmə] *noun* tumour of the serous membrane, which can be benign or malignant; **pleural mesothelioma** = tumour of the pleura, due to inhaling asbestos dust

mesothelium [mesəʊ'θiːliəm] *noun* layer of cells lining a serous membrane; *see also* EPITHELIUM, ENDOTHELIUM

mesovarium [mesəʊ'veəriəm] *noun* fold of peritoneum around the ovaries

messenger ['mesəndʒə] *noun* person who brings a message; **messenger RNA (mRNA)** = type of ribonucleic acid which transmits the genetic code from the DNA to the ribosomes which form the proteins coded on the DNA

meta- ['metə] *prefix* which changes

meta analysis ['metə ə'næləsɪs] *noun* statistical procedure to combine the results from many studies to give a single estimate, giving weight to large studies

metabolic [metə'bɒlɪk] *adjective* referring to metabolism; **basal metabolic rate (BMR)** = amount of energy used by a body in exchanging oxygen and carbon dioxide when at rest, i.e. energy needed to keep the body functioning and the temperature normal (formerly used as a way of testing the thyroid gland); *see also* ACIDOSIS, ALKALOSIS

metabolism [mə'tæbəlɪzm] *noun* chemical processes which are continually taking place in the human body and which are essential to life; **basal metabolism** = minimum amount of energy needed to keep the body functioning and the temperature normal when at rest

COMMENT: metabolism covers all changes which take place in the body: the building of tissue (anabolism); the breaking down of tissue (catabolism); the conversion of nutrients into tissue; the elimination of waste matter; the action of hormones, etc.

metabolite [mə'tæbəlaɪt] *noun* substance produced by metabolism, substance taken into the body in food and then metabolized

metabolize [mə'tæbəlaɪz] *verb* to change the nature of something by metabolism; *the liver metabolizes proteins and carbohydrates*

metacarpal [metə'kɑːpl] *noun & adjective;* **metacarpal bone** *or* **metacarpal** = one of the five bones in the metacarpus

metacarpophalangeal joint (MCP *or* **MP joint)** [metəkɑːpəfə'lændʒiəl 'dʒɔɪnt] *noun* joint between a metacarpal bone and a finger

replacement of the MCP joint is usually undertaken to relieve pain, deformity and immobility due to rheumatoid arthritis
Nursing Times

metacarpus [metə'kɑːpəs] *noun* the five bones in the hand between the fingers and the wrist; *see illustration at* HAND

metal ['metl] *noun* material (either an element or a compound) which can carry heat and electricity (some metals are essential for life)

metallic [me'tælɪk] *adjective* like a metal, referring to a metal; **metallic element** = chemical element which is a metal

metamorphopsia [metəmɔː'fɒpsiə] *noun* condition where the patient sees objects in distorted form, usually due to inflammation of the choroid

metaphase ['metəfeɪz] *noun* one of the stages in mitosis or meiosis

metaphysis [me'tæfəsɪs] *noun* end of the central section of a long bone, where the bone grows and where it joins the epiphysis

metaplasia [metə'pleɪziə] *noun* change of one tissue to another

metastasis [me'tæstəsɪs] *noun* spreading of a malignant disease from one part of the body to another through the bloodstream or the lymph system (NOTE: plural is **metastases**)

he suddenly developed problems with his balance and a solitary brain metastasis was diagnosed
British Journal of Nursing

metastasize [me'tæstəsaɪz] *noun* to spread by metastasis

metastatic [metə'stætɪk] *adjective* referring to metastasis; *metastatic growths developed in the liver*

metatarsal [metə'tɑːsl] *noun & adjective* one of the five bones in the metatarsus; **metatarsal arch** = arched part of the sole of the foot, running across the sole of the foot from side to side

metatarsalgia [metətɑː'sældʒə] *noun* pain in the heads of the metatarsal bones

metatarsophalangeal joint [metətɑːsəfə'lændʒiəl 'dʒɔɪnt] *noun* joint between a metatarsal bone and a toe

metatarsus [metə'tɑːsəs] *noun* the five long bones in the foot between the toes and the tarsus (NOTE: plural is **metatarsi**)

meteorism ['miːtiərɪzm] *noun* tympanites, condition where gas is present in the stomach or intestines, causing dilatation and pain

methaemoglobin [met'hiːməʊgləʊbɪn] *noun* dark brown substance formed from haemoglobin which develops during illness, following treatment with certain drugs

COMMENT: methaemoglobin cannot transport oxygen round the body, and so causes cyanosis

methaemoglobinaemia [methiːməʊgləʊbɪˈniːmɪə] *noun* presence of methaemoglobin in the blood

methionine [meˈθaɪəniːn] *noun* essential amino acid

method [ˈmeθəd] *noun* way of doing something

methycillin-resistant staphylococcus aureus (MRSA) [meθɪˈsɪlɪn rɪˈzɪstənt stæfɪləˈkɒkəs ˈɔːriəs] *noun* bacterium resistant to almost all antibiotics, so which can cause life-threatening infection in patients recovering from surgery

methyl alcohol [ˈmeθl ˈælkəhɒl] *noun* wood alcohol (a poisonous alcohol used as fuel)

methylated spirits [meθəleɪtɪd ˈspɪrɪts] *noun* almost pure alcohol, with wood alcohol and colouring added

methylene blue [ˈmeθəliːn ˈbluː] *noun* blue dye, formerly used as a mild urinary antiseptic, now used to treat drug-induced methaemoglobinaemia

metr- *or* **metro-** [metr *or* ˈmetrəʊ] *prefix* referring to the uterus

metralgia [meˈtrældʒə] *noun* pain in the uterus

metre *US* **meter** [ˈmiːtə] *noun* SI unit of length; *the room is four metres by three* (NOTE: **metre** is usually written **m** with figures: **the colon is 1.3 m long**)

metritis [meˈtraɪtɪs] *noun* inflammation of the myometrium

metrocolpocele [metrəˈkɒlpəʊsiːl] *noun* condition where the uterus protrudes into the vagina

metropathia haemorrhagica [metrəˈpæθɪə heməˈreɪdʒɪkə] *noun* essential uterine haemorrhage, abnormal condition of the uterus, where the lining swells and there is heavy menstrual bleeding

metroptosis [metrɒˈptəʊsɪs] *noun* prolapsed uterus or prolapse of the uterus, condition where the uterus has moved downwards out of its normal position

metrorrhagia [miːtrəʊˈreɪdʒɪə] *noun* abnormal bleeding from the vagina between the menstrual periods

metrostaxis [miːtrəʊˈstæksɪs] *noun* continual light bleeding from the uterus

Mg *chemical symbol for* magnesium

mg = MILLIGRAM

MI [ˈem ˈaɪ] = MITRAL INCOMPETENCE

micelle [maɪˈsel] *noun* tiny particle formed by the digestion of fat in the small intestine

Michel's clips [mɪˈʃels ˈklɪps] *see* CLIP

micro- [ˈmaɪkrəʊ] *prefix* **(a)** meaning very small (NOTE: the opposite is **macro-** or **mega-** or **megalo-**) **(b)** meaning one millionth (10^{-6}); **microgram** = unit of measurement of weight (= one millionth of a gram); **micromole** = unit of measurement of the amount of substance (= one millionth of a mole) (NOTE: symbol is μ)

microaneurysm [maɪkrəʊˈænjərɪzm] *noun* tiny swelling in the wall of a capillary in the retina

microangiopathy [maɪkrəʊændʒɪˈɒpəθi] *noun* any disease of the capillaries

microbe [ˈmaɪkrəʊb] *noun* microorganism, such as a bacterium, which may cause disease and which can only be seen with a microscope

microbial [maɪˈkrəʊbiəl] *adjective* referring to microbes; **microbial disease** = disease caused by a microbe; **microbial ecology** = study of the way in which microbes develop in nature

microbiological [maɪkrəʊbaɪəˈlɒdʒɪkl] *adjective* referring to microbiology

microbiologist [maɪkrəʊbaɪˈɒlədʒɪst] *noun* scientist who specializes in the study of microorganisms

microbiology [maɪkrəʊbaɪˈɒlədʒi] *noun* scientific study of microorganisms

microcephalic [maɪkrəʊseˈfælɪk] *adjective* suffering from microcephaly

microcephaly [maɪkrəʊˈsefəli] *noun* condition where a person has an abnormally small head

COMMENT: microcephaly in a baby can be caused by the mother having had German measles during pregnancy

microcheilia [maɪkrəʊˈkaɪliə] *noun* having abnormally small lips

Micrococcus [maɪkrəʊ'kɒkəs] *noun* genus of bacterium, some species of which cause arthritis, endocarditis and meningitis

microcyte ['maɪkrəʊsaɪt] *noun* abnormally small red blood cell

microcytic [maɪkrə'sɪtɪk] *adjective* referring to microcytes

microcytosis *or* **microcythaemia** [maɪkrəʊsaɪ'təʊsɪs *or* maɪkrəʊsaɪ'θiːmiə] *noun* presence of excess microcytes in the blood

microdactylia [maɪkrəʊdæk'tɪliə] *noun* having abnormally small or short fingers or toes

microdontism *or* **microdontia** [maɪkrəʊ'dɒntɪzm *or* maɪkrəʊ'dɒntiə] *noun* having abnormally small teeth

microglia [maɪkrəʊ'gliːə] *noun* tiny cells in the central nervous system which destroy other cells

microglossia [maɪkrəʊ'glɒsiə] *noun* having an abnormally small tongue

micrognathia [maɪkrəʊ'neɪθiə] *noun* condition where one jaw is abnormally smaller than the other

micromastia [maɪkrəʊ'mæstiə] *noun* having abnormally small breasts

micromelia [maɪkrəʊ'miːliə] *noun* having abnormally small arms or legs

micrometer [maɪ'krɒmɪtə] *noun* **(a)** instrument for taking very small measurements, such as measuring the width or thickness of very thin pieces of tissue **(b)** *US* = MICROMETRE

micrometre *or* **micron** [maɪ'krɒmɪtə *or* 'maɪkrɒn] unit of measurement of thickness (= one millionth of a metre) (NOTE: with figures usually written **µm**)

microorganism [maɪkrəʊ'ɔːgənɪzm] *noun* very small organism which may cause disease and which can only be seen under a microscope

COMMENT: viruses, bacteria, protozoa and fungi are all forms of microorganism

micropsia [maɪ'krɒpsiə] *noun* seeing objects smaller than they really are, caused by a defect in the retina

microscope ['maɪkrəskəʊp] *noun* scientific instrument with lenses, which makes very small objects appear larger; *the tissue was examined under the microscope*; *under the microscope it was possible to see*

the cancer cells; **electron microscope (EM)** = microscope which uses a beam of electrons instead of light

COMMENT: in an ordinary or light microscope the image is magnified by lenses. In an electron microscope the lenses are electromagnets and a beam of electrons is used instead of light, thereby achieving much greater magnifications

microscopic [maɪkrə'skɒpɪk] *noun* so small that it can only be seen through a microscope

microscopy [maɪ'krɒskəpi] *noun* science of the use of microscopes

microsecond ['maɪkrəʊsekənd] *noun* unit of measurement of time (= one millionth of a second) (NOTE: with figures usually written **µs**)

Microsporum [maɪkrəʊ'spɔːrəm] *noun* type of fungus which causes ringworm of the hair, skin and sometimes nails

microsurgery [maɪkrəʊ'sɜːdʒəri] *noun* surgery on very small parts of the body, using tiny instruments and a microscope

COMMENT: microsurgery is used in operations on eyes and ears, and also to connect severed nerves and blood vessels

microvillus [maɪkrəʊ'vɪləs] *noun* very small process found on the surface of many cells, especially the epithelial cells in the intestine (NOTE: plural is **microvilli**)

micturate ['mɪktjʊreɪt] *verb* to urinate, to pass urine from the body

micturition [mɪktju'rɪʃn] *noun* urination, passing of urine from the body

mid- [mɪd] *prefix* meaning middle

midbrain ['mɪdbreɪn] *noun* the mesencephalon, the small section of the brain stem, above the pons, between the cerebrum and the hindbrain

midcarpal [mɪd'kɑːpl] *adjective* between the two rows of carpal bones

middle ['mɪdl] *noun* **(a)** centre or central point of something **(b)** waist; *the water came up to my middle*

middle-aged ['mɪdl'eɪdʒd] *adjective* not very young and not very old; *a disease which affects middle-aged women*

middle ear ['mɪdl 'ɪə] *noun* section of the ear between the eardrum and the inner ear; **middle ear infection** = otitis media, infection of the middle ear, usually accompanied by headaches and fever

COMMENT: the middle ear contains the three ossicles which receive vibrations from the eardrum and transmit them to the cochlea. The middle ear is connected to the throat by the Eustachian tube

middle finger ['mɪdl 'fɪŋgə] *noun* finger between the forefinger and the ring finger, usually the longest of the five fingers

midgut ['mɪdgʌt] *noun* middle part of the gut in an embryo, which develops into the small intestine

mid-life crisis ['mɪdlaɪf 'kraɪsɪs] = MENOPAUSE

midline ['mɪdlaɪn] *noun* imaginary line drawn down the middle of the body from the head through the navel to the point between the feet

patients admitted with acute abdominal pains were referred for study. Abdominal puncture was carried out in the midline immediately above or below the umbilicus

Lancet

midriff ['mɪdrɪf] *noun* the diaphragm

midstream specimen *or* **midstream urine** [mɪd'striːm 'spesəmɪn *or* mɪd'striːm 'juərɪn] *noun* urine sample taken in the middle of a flow of urine

midtarsal [mɪd'tɑːsəl] *adjective* between the tarsal bones

midwife ['mɪdwaɪf] *noun* professional person who helps a woman give birth to a child (often at home); **community midwife** = midwife who works in a community as part of a primary health care team (NOTE: plural is **midwives**)

COMMENT: to become a Registered Midwife (RM), a Registered General Nurse has to take a further 18 month course, or alternatively can follow a full 3 year course

midwifery [mɪd'wɪfri] *noun* (i) profession of a midwife; (ii) study of practical aspects of obstetrics; **midwifery course** = training course to teach nurses the techniques of being a midwife

migraine ['miːgreɪn *or* 'maɪgreɪn] *noun* sharp severe recurrent headache, often associated with vomiting and visual disturbances; *he had an attack of migraine and could not come to work*; *her migraine attacks seem to be worse in the summer*

COMMENT: the cause of migraine is not known. Attacks are often preceded by an 'aura', where the patient sees flashing lights or the eyesight becomes blurred. The pain is normally intense and affects one side of the head only

migrainous ['mɪgreɪnəs] *adjective* (person) who is subject to migraine attacks

mild [maɪld] *adjective* not severe, not cold, gentle; *we had a very mild winter*; *she's had a mild attack of measles*; *he was off work with a mild throat infection* (NOTE: **mild - milder - mildest**)

mildly ['maɪldli] *adverb* slightly, not strongly; *a mildly infectious disease*; *a mildly antiseptic solution*

milia ['mɪliə] *see* MILIUM

miliaria [mɪli'eəriə] *noun* prickly heat or heat rash, itchy red spots which develop on the chest, under the armpits and between the thighs in hot countries, caused by blocked sweat glands

miliary ['mɪliəri] *adjective* small in size, like a seed; **miliary tuberculosis** = tuberculosis which occurs as little nodes in various parts of the body including the meninges of the brain and spinal cord

milium ['mɪliəm] *noun* (i) white pinhead-sized tumour on the face in adults; (ii) retention cyst in infants; (iii) cyst on the skin (NOTE: plural is **milia**)

milk [mɪlk] *noun* (a) white liquid produced by female mammals to feed their young; *can I have a glass of milk, please?*; *have you enough milk?*; *the patient can only drink warm milk* (b) (*breast milk*) milk produced by a woman; *the milk will start to flow a few days after childbirth* (NOTE: no plural **some milk, a bottle of milk** *or* **a glass of milk**)

milk leg ['mɪlk 'leg] *noun* white leg or phlegmasia alba dolens, acute oedema of the leg, a condition which affects women after childbirth, where a leg becomes pale and inflamed as a result of lymphatic obstruction

milk sugar ['mɪlk 'ʃugə] = LACTOSE

milk teeth ['mɪlk 'tiːθ] *noun* deciduous teeth, a child's first twenty teeth, which are gradually replaced by permanent teeth

milky ['mɪlki] *adjective* (liquid) which is white like milk (NOTE: for other terms referring to milk, see words beginning with **galact-, lact-**)

milli- ['mɪli] *prefix* meaning one thousandth (10^{-3}) (NOTE: symbol is **m**)

milligram ['mɪlɪgræm] *noun* unit of measurement of weight (= one thousandth of a gram) (NOTE: with figures usually written **mg**)

millilitre *US* **milliliter** ['mɪlili:tə] *noun* unit of measurement of liquid (= one thousandth of a litre) (NOTE: with figures usually written **ml**)

millimetre *US* **millimeter** ['mɪlimi:tə] *noun* unit of measurement of length (= one thousandth of a metre) (NOTE: with figures usually written **mm**)

millimole ['mɪlimoʊl] *noun* unit of measurement of the amount of substance (= one thousandth of a mole) (NOTE: with figures usually written **mmol**)

millisievert ['mɪlisi:vət] *noun* unit of measurement of radiation; **millisievert/year** **(mSv/year)** = number of millisieverts per year (NOTE: with figures usually written **mSv**)

radiation limits for workers should be cut from 50 to 5 millisieverts, and those for members of the public from 5 to 0.25

Guardian

Milroy's disease ['mɪlrɔɪz dɪ'zi:z] *noun* hereditary condition where the lymph vessels are blocked and the legs swell

Minamata disease ['mɪnəmɑːtə dɪ'zi:z] *noun* form of mercury poisoning from eating polluted fish, found first in Japan

mind [maɪnd] *noun* part of the brain which controls memory, consciousness or reasoning; **he's got something on his mind** = he's worrying about something; **let's try to take her mind off her exams** = try to stop her worrying about them; **state of mind** = general feeling; *he's in a very miserable state of mind* (NOTE: for terms referring to mind, see **mental**, and words beginning with **psych-**)

miner ['maɪnə] *noun* person who works in a coal mine; **miner's elbow** = inflammation of the elbow caused by pressure

mineral ['mɪnərl] *noun* inorganic substance; **mineral water** = water taken out of the ground and sold in bottles

COMMENT: the most important minerals required by the body are: calcium (found in cheese, milk and green vegetables) which helps the growth of bones and encourages blood clotting; iron (found in bread and liver) which helps produce red blood cells; phosphorus (found in bread and fish) which helps in the growth of bones and the

metabolism of fats; iodine (found in fish) is essential to the functioning of the thyroid gland

minim ['mɪnɪm] *noun* liquid measure used in pharmacy (one sixtieth of a drachm)

minimal ['mɪnɪməl] *adjective* very small

mini mental state examination ['mɪni 'mentl 'steɪt ɪgzæmɪ'neɪʃn] *noun* test performed mainly by psychiatrists to determine the mental ability of the patient, used in the diagnosis of dementia

minimum ['mɪnɪmʌm] **1** *adjective* smallest possible **2** *noun* smallest possible amount (NOTE: plural is **minimums** or **minima**)

minor ['maɪnə] *adjective* not important; **minor illness** = illness which is not serious; **minor surgery** = surgery which can be undertaken even when there are no hospital facilities; **labia minora** = two small fleshy folds at the edge of the vulva (NOTE: the opposite is **major**)

practice nurses play a major role in the care of patients with chronic disease and they undertake many preventive procedures. They also deal with a substantial amount of minor trauma

Nursing Times

minute 1 [maɪ'njuːt] *adjective* very small; *a minute piece of dust got in my eye* **2** ['mɪnɪt] *noun* unit of time equal to 60 seconds

miosis or **myosis** [maɪ'oʊsɪs] *noun* **(a)** contraction of the pupil of the eye (as in bright light) **(b)** *US* = MEIOSIS

miotic [maɪ'ɒtɪk] *noun* drug which makes the pupil of the eye become smaller

mis- [mɪs] *prefix* meaning wrong

miscarriage [mɪs'kærɪdʒ] *noun* spontaneous abortion, situation where an unborn baby leaves the uterus before the end of the pregnancy, especially during the first seven months of pregnancy; *she had two miscarriages before having her first child*

miscarry [mɪs'kæri] *verb* to have a miscarriage; *the accident made her miscarry*; *she miscarried after catching the infection*

misconduct [mɪs'kɒndʌkt] *noun* wrong action by a professional person, such as a doctor; **professional misconduct** = actions which are considered to be wrong by the body which regulates a profession (such as an action by a doctor which is considered wrong by the Professional Conduct Committee of the General Medical Council)

misdiagnose [mɪsdaɪəgˈnəʊz] *verb* to make an incorrect diagnosis

mismatch [mɪsˈmætʃ] *verb* to match tissues wrongly

finding donors of correct histocompatible type is difficult but necessary because results using mismatched bone marrow are disappointing
Hospital Update

mist. *or* **mistura** [mɪst *or* mɪsˈtjʊərə] *see* RE. MIST.

misuse 1 [mɪsˈjuːs] *noun* wrong use; *he was arrested for misuse of drugs* **2** [mɪsˈjuːz] *verb* to use (a drug) wrongly

mite [maɪt] *noun* very small parasite, which causes dermatitis; **harvest mite** = chigger, a tiny parasite which enters the skin near a hair follicle and travels under the skin, causing intense irritation

mitochondrial [maɪtəˈkɒndriəl] *adjective* referring to mitochondria

mitochondrion [maɪtəˈkɒndriən] *noun* tiny rod-shaped part of a cell's cytoplasm responsible for cell respiration (NOTE: plural is **mitochondria)**

mitosis [maɪˈtəʊsɪs] *noun* process of cell division, where the mother cell divides into two identical daughter cells; *compare* MEIOSIS

mitral [ˈmaɪtrl] *adjective* referring to the mitral valve; **mitral incompetence (MI)** = situation where the mitral valve does not close completely so that blood goes back into the atrium; **mitral stenosis** = condition where the opening in the mitral valve is made smaller because the cusps have stuck together; **mitral valve** = bicuspid valve, a valve in the heart which allows blood to flow from the left atrium to the left ventricle but not in the opposite direction; **mitral valvotomy** = surgical operation to detach the cusps of the mitral valve in mitral stenosis

mittelschmerz [mɪtelˈʃmeəts] *noun* pain felt by women in the lower abdomen at ovulation

mix [mɪks] *verb* to put things together; *the pharmacist mixed the chemicals in a bottle*

mixture [ˈmɪkstʃə] *noun* chemical substances mixed together; *the doctor gave me an unpleasant mixture to drink*; *take one spoonful of the mixture every three hours*; **cough mixture** = medicine taken to stop you coughing

ml = MILLILITRE

mm = MILLIMETRE

mmol = MILLIMOLE

MMR [ˈem ˈem ˈɑː] = MEASLES, MUMPS AND RUBELLA

Mn *chemical symbol for* manganese

Mo *chemical symbol for* molybdenum

MO [ˈem ˈəʊ] = MEDICAL OFFICER

mobile [ˈməʊbaɪl] *adjective* able to move about; *it is important for elderly patients to remain mobile*

mobility [məˈbɪləti] *noun (of patients)* being able to move about; **mobility allowance** = government benefit to help disabled people pay for transport

mobilization [məʊbəlaɪˈzeɪʃn] *noun* making something mobile; **stapedial mobilization** = operation to relieve deafness by detaching the stapes from the fenestra ovalis

moderate [ˈmɒdrət] *adjective* not high or low

moderately [ˈmɒdrətli] *adverb* not at one or other extreme; *the patient had a moderately comfortable night*

modiolus [məʊˈdiːələs] *noun* central stalk in the cochlea

MOH [ˈem ˈəʊ ˈeɪtʃ] = MEDICAL OFFICER OF HEALTH

moist [mɔɪst] *adjective* slightly wet or damp; *the compress should be kept moist*; **moist gangrene** = condition where dead tissue decays and swells with fluid because of infection

moisten [ˈmɔɪsn] *verb* to make something damp

moisture [ˈmɔɪstʃə] *noun* water or other liquid; *moisture can collect in the scar tissue*; *there is moisture in the air on a humid day*; **moisture content** = amount of water or other liquid which a substance contains

mol = MOLE (b)

molar [ˈməʊlə] **1** *adjective* **(a)** referring to the large back teeth **(b)** referring to the mole, the SI unit of amount of a substance **2** *noun* one of the large back teeth, used for grinding food; **third molar** = wisdom tooth, one of the four molars at the back of the jaw, which only appears at about the age of 20 and sometimes does not appear at all; *see illustration at* TEETH

COMMENT: in milk teeth there are eight molars and in permanent teeth there are twelve

molarity [məʊˈlærəti] *noun* strength of a solution shown as the number of moles of a substance per litre of solution

molasses [məˈlæsɪz] *noun* dark sweet substance made of sugar before it has been refined

mole [məʊl] *noun* (a) dark raised spot on the skin; *she has a large mole on her chin*; *see also* MELANOMA (b) SI unit of measurement of the amount of substance (NOTE: with figures usually written **mol**)

molecular [məˈlekjʊlə] *adjective* referring to a molecule; **molecular biology** = study of the molecules of living matter; **molecular weight** = weight of one molecule of a substance

molecule [ˈmɒlɪkjuːl] *noun* smallest independent mass of a substance

molluscum [məˈlʌskəm] *noun* soft round skin tumour; **molluscum contagiosum** = contagious viral skin infection which gives a small soft sore; **molluscum fibrosum** = skin tumours of neurofibromatosis; **molluscum sebaceum** = benign skin tumour which disappears after a short time

molybdenum [mɒˈlɪbdənəm] *noun* metallic trace element (NOTE: the chemical symbol is **Mo**)

monaural [mɒnˈɔːrəl] *adjective* referring to the use of one ear only

Mönckeberg's arteriosclerosis
[ˈmʌnkəbeəgz ɑːtiːriəʊskleˈrəʊsɪs] *noun* condition of old people, where the media of the arteries in the legs harden, causing limping

mongol [ˈmɒŋgəl] *noun* former word for a person suffering from Down's syndrome

mongolism [ˈmɒŋgəlɪzm] *noun* former name for Down's syndrome

Monilia [məʊˈnɪliə] = CANDIDA

moniliasis [mɒniˈlaɪəsɪs] = CANDIDIASIS

monitor [ˈmɒnɪtə] **1** *noun* screen (like a TV screen) on a computer; **cardiac monitor** = instrument which checks the functioning of the heart in an intensive care unit; **fetal monitor** = electronic device which monitors the fetus in the uterus **2** *verb* to check, to examine how a patient is progressing

monitoring [ˈmɒnɪtrɪŋ] *noun* regular examination and recording of a patient's temperature, weight, blood pressure, etc.

mono- [ˈmɒnəʊ] *prefix* meaning single or one

monoamine oxidase (MAO)
[mɒnəʊˈæmiːn ˈɒksɪdeɪz] *noun* enzyme which breaks down the catecholamines to their inactive forms

monoamine oxidase inhibitor (MAO inhibitor or MAOI) [mɒnəʊˈæmiːn ˈɒksɪdeɪz ɪnˈhɪbɪtə] *noun* drug (such as phenelzine) which inhibits monoamine oxidase (used to treat depression, it can also cause high blood pressure)

COMMENT: use is limited, because of the potential for drug and dietary interactions and the necessity for slow withdrawal

monoblast [ˈmɒnəʊblæst] *noun* cell which produces a monocyte

monochromat [mɒnəʊˈkrəʊmæt] *noun* colour-blind person

monocular [mɒˈnɒkjʊlə] *adjective* referring to one eye; **monocular vision** = seeing with one eye only, so that the sense of distance is impaired; *compare* BINOCULAR

monocyte [ˈmɒnəʊsaɪt] *noun* type of nongranular leucocyte, a white blood cell with a nucleus shaped like a kidney, which destroys bacterial cells

monocytosis or mononucleosis
[mɒnəʊsaɪˈtəʊsɪs or mɒnəʊnjuːkliˈəʊsɪs] *noun* glandular fever, condition in which there is an abnormally high number of monocytes in the blood

COMMENT: symptoms include sore throat, swelling of the lymph nodes and fever; it is probably caused by the Epstein-Barr virus

monodactylism [mɒnəʊˈdæktɪlɪzm] *noun* congenital condition in which only one finger or toe is present on the hand or foot

monomania [mɒnəʊˈmeɪnjə] *noun* deranged state where a person concentrates attention on one idea

mononeuritis [mɒnəʊnjuːˈraɪtɪs] *noun* neuritis which affects one nerve

mononuclear [mɒnəʊ'njuːkliə] *adjective* (cell, such as a monocyte) which has one nucleus

mononucleosis [mɒnəʊnjuːkli'əʊsɪs] *see* MONOCYTOSIS

monoplegia ['mɒnəʊpliːdʒə] *noun* paralysis of one part of the body only (i.e. one muscle, one limb)

monorchism ['mɒnɔːkɪzm] *noun* condition in which only one testis is visible

monosodium glutamate [mɒnə'səʊdiəm 'gluːtəmeɪt] *noun* a salt, often used to make food taste better; *see also* CHINESE RESTAURANT SYNDROME

monosomy ['mɒnəʊsəʊmi] *noun* condition where a person has a chromosome missing from one or more pairs

monosynaptic [mɒnəʊsɪ'næptɪk] *adjective* (nervous pathway) with only one synapse

monovalent [mɒnəʊ'veɪlənt] *adjective* having a valency of one

monoxide [mə'nɒksaɪd] *see* CARBON

monozygotic twins [mɒnəzaɪ'gɒtɪk 'twɪnz] = IDENTICAL TWINS

mons pubis *or* **mons veneris** ['mɒnz 'pjuːbɪs *or* 'mɒnz və'nɪərɪs] *noun* cushion of fat covering the pubis

monster ['mɒnstə] *noun* deformed fetus which cannot live

Montezuma's revenge [mɒntɪ'zuːməz rɪ'vendʒ] *noun (informal)* diarrhoea which affects people travelling in foreign countries, eating unwashed fruit or drinking water which has not been boiled

Montgomery's glands [mənt'gʌməriz 'glændz] *noun* sebaceous glands around the nipple which become more marked in pregnancy

mood [muːd] *noun* a person's mental state (of excitement, depression, euphoria, etc.)

Mooren's ulcer ['muːrənz 'ʌlsə] *noun* chronic ulcer of the cornea, found in elderly patients

morbid ['mɔːbɪd] *adjective* (i) showing symptoms of being diseased; (ii) referring to disease; (iii) unhealthy (mental faculty); *the X-ray showed a morbid condition of the kidneys*; **morbid anatomy** *or* **pathology** = visual study of a diseased body and the changes which the disease has caused to the body

morbidity [mɔː'bɪdəti] *noun* being diseased or sick; **morbidity rate** = number of cases of a disease per hundred thousand of population

> apart from death, coronary heart disease causes considerable morbidity in the form of heart attack, angina and a number of related diseases
>
> *Health Education Journal*

morbilli [mɔː'bɪli] = MEASLES

morbilliform [mɔː'bɪlifɔːm] *adjective* (rash) similar to measles

moribund ['mɒrɪbʌnd] *noun & adjective* dying (person)

morning ['mɔːnɪŋ] *noun* first part of the day before 12 o'clock noon; **morning sickness** = illness (including nausea and vomiting) experienced by women in the early stages of pregnancy when they get up in the morning; *(informal)* **morning-after feeling** = HANGOVER; **morning-after pill** = contraceptive pill which is effective if taken after sexual intercourse

Moro reflex ['mɔːrəʊ 'riːfleks] *noun* reflex of a newborn baby when it hears a loud noise (the baby is laid on a table and raises its arms if the table is struck)

morphea *or* **morphoea** [mɔː'fiə] *noun* form of scleroderma, a disease where the skin is replaced by thick connective tissue

morphine ['mɔːfiːn] *noun; see* DRUGS TABLE IN SUPPLEMENT

morphology [mɔː'fɒlədʒi] *noun* study of the structure and shape of living organisms

mortality (rate) [mɔː'tæləti 'reɪt] *noun* number of deaths per year, shown per hundred thousand of population

mortis ['mɔːtɪs] *see* RIGOR

mortuary ['mɔːtjʊəri] *noun* room in a hospital where dead bodies are kept until removed by an undertaker for burial

morula ['mɒrʊlə] *noun* early stage in the development of an embryo, where the cleavage of the ovum creates a mass of cells

mosquito [məs'kiːtəʊ] *noun* insect which sucks human blood, some species of which can pass viruses or parasites into the bloodstream

COMMENT: in northern countries a mosquito bite merely produces an itchy spot; in tropical countries dengue, filariasis, malaria and yellow fever are transmitted in this way. Mosquitoes breed in water and they spread rapidly in lakes or canals created by dams and other irrigation schemes. Because irrigation is more widely practised in tropical countries, mosquitoes are increasing and diseases such as malaria are spreading

mother ['mʌðə] *noun* female parent; **mother cell** = original cell which splits into daughter cells by mitosis; **mother-fixation** = condition where a patient's development has been stopped at a stage where the adult remains like a child, dependent on the mother

motile ['məʊtaɪl] *adjective* (cell or microbe) which can move spontaneously; *sperm cells are extremely motile*

motility [məʊ'tɪləti] *noun* (a) *(of cells or microbes)* being able to move about (b) *(of gut)* action of peristalsis

motion ['məʊʃn] *noun* (a) faeces, the matter which is evacuated in a bowel movement; *he passed blood with his motions* (b) movement; **motion sickness** = illness and nausea felt when travelling (NOTE: also called **travel sickness**)

COMMENT: the movement of liquid inside the labyrinth of the middle ear causes motion sickness, which is particularly noticeable in vehicles which are closed, such as planes, coaches, hovercraft

motionless ['məʊʃnləs] *noun* not moving; *catatonic patients can sit motionless for hours*

motor ['məʊtə] *adjective* referring to movement, which produces movement; **motor area** or **motor cortex** = part of the cortex in the brain which controls voluntary muscle movement by sending impulses to the motor nerves (NOTE: also called **pyramidal area**); **motor end plate** = end of a motor nerve where it joins muscle fibre; **motor nerve** = nerve which carries impulses from the brain to muscles and causes voluntary movement; **motor neurone** = neurone which forms part of a motor nerve pathway leading from the brain to a muscle; **motor neurone disease** = disease of the nerve cells which control the movement of the muscles; **motor pathway** = series of motor neurones leading from the motor cortex to a muscle

COMMENT: motor neurone disease has three forms: progressive muscular atrophy

(PMA), which affects movements of the hands, lateral sclerosis, which is a form of spasticity, and bulbar palsy, which affects the mouth and throat

mottled ['mɒtld] *adjective* (skin) with patches of different colours

mountain fever ['maʊntɪn 'fiːvə] = BRUCELLOSIS

mountain sickness ['maʊntɪn 'sɪknəs] *noun* altitude sickness, condition where a person suffers from oxygen deficiency from being at a high altitude (as on a mountain) where the level of oxygen in the air is low

mouth [maʊθ] *noun* opening at the head of the alimentary canal, through which food and drink are taken in, and through which a person speaks and can breathe; *she was sleeping with her mouth open*; **roof of the mouth** = the palate, the top part of the inside of the mouth, which is divided into a hard front part and soft back part; **mouth-to-mouth breathing** or **ventilation** or **resuscitation** = method of making a patient start to breathe again, by blowing air through his mouth into his lungs (NOTE: for terms referring to the mouth, see **oral,** and words beginning with **stomat-**)

mouthful ['maʊθfʊl] *noun* amount which you can hold in your mouth; *he had a mouthful of soup*

mouthwash ['maʊθwɒʃ] *noun* antiseptic solution used to treat infection in the mouth

move [muːv] *verb* to change from one place to another; *try to move your arm*; *he found he was unable to move*

movement ['muːvmənt] *noun* (a) act of moving; **active movement** = movement made by a patient using his own will (b) **bowel movement** = defecation, evacuation of solid waste matter from the bowel through the anus; *the patient had a bowel movement this morning*

moxybustion [mɒksɪ'bʌstʃn] *noun* treatment used in the Far East, where dried herbs are placed on the skin and set on fire

MP ['em 'piː] = METACARPOPHALANGEAL (JOINT)

MPS ['em 'piː 'es] = MEMBER OF THE PHARMACEUTICAL SOCIETY

MRC ['em 'aː 'siː] = MEDICAL RESEARCH COUNCIL

MRCGP ['em 'ɑ: 'si: 'dʒi: 'pi:] = MEMBER OF THE ROYAL COLLEGE OF GENERAL PRACTITIONERS

MRCP ['em 'ɑ: 'si: 'pi:] = MEMBER OF THE ROYAL COLLEGE OF PHYSICIANS

MRCS ['em 'ɑ: 'si: 'es] = MEMBER OF THE ROYAL COLLEGE OF SURGEONS

MRI ['em 'ɑ: 'aɪ] = MAGNETIC RESONANCE IMAGING

---

during a MRI scan, the patient lies within a strong magnetic field as selected sections of his body are stimulated with radio frequency waves. Resulting energy changes are measured and used by the MRI computer to generate images

Nursing 87

---

mRNA = MESSENGER RNA

MRSA = METHYCILLIN-RESISTANT STAPHYLOCOCCUS AUREUS

MS ['em 'es] = MULTIPLE SCLEROSIS, MITRAL STENOSIS

MSH ['em 'es 'eɪtʃ] = MELANOCYTE-STIMULATING HORMONE

mSv = MILLISIEVERT

mucin ['mjuːsɪn] *noun* compound of sugars and protein which is the main substance in mucus

muco- ['mjuːkəʊ] *prefix* referring to mucus

mucocele ['mjuːkəʊsiːl] *noun* cavity containing an accumulation of mucus

mucocutaneous [mjuːkəʊkjuˈteɪniəs] *adjective* referring to mucous membrane and the skin

mucoid ['mjukɔɪd] *adjective* similar to mucus

mucolytic [mjukəʊˈlɪtɪk] *noun* substance which dissolves mucus

mucomembranous colitis [mjuːkəʊˈmembrənəs kəˈlaɪtɪs] = MUCOUS COLITIS

mucoprotein [mjuːkəʊˈprəʊtiːn] *noun* form of protein found in blood plasma

mucopurulent [mjuːkəʊˈpjʊərʊlənt] *adjective* consisting of a mixture of mucus and pus

mucopus [mjuːkəʊˈpʌs] *noun* mixture of mucus and pus

mucormycosis [mjuːkɔːmaɪˈkəʊsɪs] *noun* disease of the ear and throat caused by the fungus *Mucor*

mucosa [mjuˈkəʊzə] *noun* mucous membrane

mucosal [mjuˈkəʊzl] *adjective* referring to a mucous membrane

mucous ['mjuːkəs] *adjective* referring to mucus, covered in mucus; **mucous cell** = cell which contains mucinogen which secretes mucin; **mucous colitis** = inflammation of the mucous membrane in the intestine, where the patient suffers pain caused by spasms in the muscles of the walls of the colon (NOTE: also called **irritable bowel syndrome** *or* **irritable colon** *or* **spastic colon**); **mucous membrane** *or* **mucosa** = wet membrane which lines internal passages in the body (such as the nose, mouth, stomach and throat) and secretes mucus; **mucous plug** = plug of mucus which blocks the cervical canal during pregnancy

mucoviscidosis [mjuːkəʊvɪsiˈdəʊsɪs] *noun* cystic fibrosis, hereditary disease in which there is malfunction of the exocrine glands, such as the pancreas, in particular those which secrete mucus

mucus ['mjuːkəs] *noun* slippery liquid secreted by mucous membranes inside the body, which protects those membranes (NOTE: for other terms referring to mucus, see words beginning with **blenno-**)

muddled ['mʌdld] *adjective* (person) whose thought processes are confused

Müllerian duct [mʌˈlɪəriən 'dʌkt] = PARAMESONEPHRIC DUCT

multi- ['mʌlti] *prefix* meaning many

multicentric [mʌltiˈsentrɪk] *adjective* in several centres; **multicentric trial** *or* **testing** = trials carried out in several centres at the same time

multifocal lens [mʌltiˈfəʊkl 'lenz] *noun* lens in spectacles whose focus changes from top to bottom so that the person wearing the spectacles can see objects clearly at different distances; *compare* BIFOCAL

multiforme ['mʌltifɔːm] *see* ERYTHEMA

multigravida [mʌltiˈgrævɪdə] *noun* pregnant woman who has been pregnant two or more times before

multi-infarct dementia [ˈmʌltiˈɪnfɑːkt dɪˈmenʃə] *noun* dementia caused by a number of small strokes, when the dementia is not progressive as in Alzheimer's disease but increases in steps as new strokes occur

multinucleated [mʌltiˈnjuːklieɪtɪd] *adjective* (cell) with several nuclei, such as a megakaryocyte

multipara [mʌlˈtɪpərə] *noun* woman who has given birth to two or more live children (mainly used for a woman in labour for the second time); **gravides multiparae =** women who have had a least four live births (NOTE: plural is **multiparae**)

multiple [ˈmʌltɪpl] *adjective* which occurs several times or in several places; **multiple birth =** giving birth to more than one child at the same time; **multiple fracture =** condition where a bone is broken in several places; **multiple myeloma =** malignant tumour in bone marrow, most often affecting flat bones; **multiple pregnancy =** pregnancy where the mother is going to produce more than one baby (i.e. twins, triplets, etc.); **multiple sclerosis (MS) =** disease of the central nervous system which gets progressively worse, where patches of fibres lose their myelin, causing numbness in the limbs, progressive weakness and paralysis (NOTE: also called **disseminated sclerosis**)

multipolar [mʌltiˈpəʊlə] *adjective* (neurone) with several processes; *see also* BIPOLAR, UNIPOLAR

multiresistant [mʌltirɪˈzɪstnt] *adjective* (disease) which is resistant against several types of antibiotic

mumps [mʌmps] *plural noun* infectious parotitis, an infectious disease of children, with fever and swellings in the salivary glands, caused by a paramyxovirus; *he caught mumps from the children next door*; *she's in bed with mumps*; *he can't go to school - he's got mumps*

COMMENT: mumps is a relatively mild disease in children; in adult males it can have serious complications and cause inflammation of the testicles (mumps orchitis)

Münchhausen's syndrome [ˈmʌntʃhaʊzənz ˈsɪndrəʊm] *noun* condition where the patient pretends to be ill in order to be admitted to hospital

murder [ˈmɜːdə] **1** *noun* **(a)** killing someone illegally and intentionally; *he was charged with murder* or *he was found guilty of murder; the murder rate has fallen over the last year* **(b)** an act of killing someone illegally and intentionally; *three murders have been committed during the last week; the police are looking for the knife used in the murder* **2** *verb* to kill someone illegally and intentionally

murmur [ˈmɜːmə] *noun* sound (usually the sound of the heart), heard through a stethoscope; **friction murmur =** sound of two serous membranes rubbing together, heard with a stethoscope in patients suffering from pericarditis, pleurisy

Murphy's sign [ˈmɜːfiz ˈsaɪn] *noun* sign of an inflamed gall bladder, where the patient will experience pain if the abdomen is pressed while he inhales

muscae volitantes [ˈmʌskaɪ vɒliˈtænteɪz] *noun* cellular or blood debris present in the vitreous of the eye, common in old age, but a sudden event can be a symptom of retinal haemorrhage (NOTE: also called **floaters**)

muscarine [ˈmʌskəriːn] *noun* poison found in fungi

muscarinic [mʌskəˈrɪnɪk] *adjective* (neurone or receptor) stimulated by acetylcholine and muscarine

COMMENT: acetylcholine receptors are of two types, muscarinic, found in parasympathetic post-ganglionic nerve junctions, and nicotinic, found at neuromuscular junctions and in autonomic ganglia. Acetylcholine acts on both types of receptors, but other drugs act on one or the other

muscle [ˈmʌsl] *noun* organ in the body, which contracts to make part of the body move; *if you do a lot of exercises you develop strong muscles; the muscles in his legs were still weak after he had spent two months in bed; he had muscle cramp after going into the cold water*; **muscle fatigue =** tiredness in the muscles after strenuous exercise; **muscle fibre =** component fibre of muscles (there are two types of fibre which form striated and smooth muscles); **muscle relaxant =** drug (such as baclofen) which reduces contractions in the muscles; **muscle spasm =** sudden sharp contraction of a muscle; **muscle spindles =** sensory receptors which lie along striated muscle fibres; **muscle tissue =** tissue which forms the muscles and which is able to expand and contract; **muscle wasting =** condition where the muscles lose weight and become thin; **cardiac muscle =** muscle in the heart which makes the heart beat; **skeletal**

muscle = muscle attached to a bone, which makes a limb move; **smooth muscle** or **unstriated muscle** = type of muscle found in involuntary muscles; **striated muscle** or **striped muscle** = type of muscle found in skeletal muscles whose movements are controlled by the central nervous system; **visceral muscle** = muscle in the walls of the intestines which makes the intestine contract (NOTE: for other terms referring to muscles, see words beginning with **my-, myo-**)

COMMENT: there are two types of muscle: voluntary (striated) muscles, which are attached to bones and move parts of the body when made to do so by the brain, and involuntary (smooth) muscles which move essential organs such as the intestines and bladder automatically. The heart muscle also works automatically

muscular ['mʌskjʊlə] *adjective* referring to muscle; **muscular branch** = branch of a nerve to a muscle carrying efferent impulses to produce contraction; **muscular defence** = rigidity of muscles associated with inflammation such as peritonitis; **muscular disorders** = disorders (such as cramp or strain) which affect the muscles; **muscular dystrophy** = type of muscle disease where some muscles become weak and are replaced with fatty tissue; *see also* DUCHENNE; **muscular relaxant** = drug which relaxes the muscles; **muscular rheumatism** = pains in the back or neck, usually caused by fibrositis or inflammation of the muscles; **muscular system** = the muscles in the body, usually applied only to striated muscles; **muscular tissue** = tissue which forms the muscles and which is able to expand and contract

muscularis [mʌskjʊ'leərɪs] *noun* muscular layer of an internal organ

musculocutaneous ['mʌskjʊləʊkju'temɪəs] *noun* referring to muscle and skin; **musculocutaneous nerve (in the upper limb)** = nerve in the brachial plexus which supplies the muscles in the arm

musculoskeletal [mʌskjʊləʊ'skelɪtl] *adjective* referring to muscles and bone

musculotendinous [mʌskjʊləʊ'tendɪnəs] *adjective* referring to both muscular and tendinous tissue

mutant ['mju:tənt] *noun & adjective* (i) (gene) in which mutation has occurred; (ii) (organism) carrying a mutant gene; **mutant gene** = gene which has undergone mutation

mutate [mju'teɪt] *verb* to undergo a genetic change; *bacteria can mutate suddenly, and become increasingly able to infect*

mutation [mju'teɪʃn] *noun* change in the DNA which changes the physiological effect of the DNA on the cell

COMMENT: a mutation in the gene for amyloid precursor protein (APP) in some families causes early-onset Alzheimer's disease, when abnormal deposits of beta amyloid are formed and dementia occurs

mutism ['mju:tɪzm] *noun* dumbness, being unable to speak

MW = MOLECULAR WEIGHT

my- or **myo-** [maɪ or 'maɪəʊ] *prefix* referring to muscle

myalgia [maɪ'ældʒə] *noun* muscle pain

myalgic encephalomyelitis (ME) [maɪ'ældʒɪk ensefələʊmaɪə'laɪtɪs] postviral fatigue syndrome, a long-term condition affecting the nervous system, where the patient feels tired and depressed and has pain and weakness in the muscles

myasthenia (gravis) [maɪəs'θi:nɪə 'grɑ:vɪs] *noun* general weakness and dysfunction of the muscles, caused by defective conduction at the motor end plates

myc- [maɪk or maɪs] *prefix* referring to fungus

mycelium [maɪ'si:lɪəm] *noun* mass of threads which forms the main part of a fungus

mycetoma [maɪsi'təʊmə] = MADUROMYCOSIS

Mycobacterium [maɪkəʊbæk'tɪərɪəm] *noun* one of a group of bacteria, including those which cause leprosy and tuberculosis

mycology [maɪ'kɒlədʒi] *noun* study of fungi

Mycoplasma [maɪkəʊ'plæzmə] *noun* type of microorganism similar to a bacterium, associated with diseases such as pneumonia and urethritis

mycosis [maɪ'kəʊsɪs] *noun* any disease (such as athlete's foot) caused by a fungus; **mycosis fungoides** = form of skin cancer, with irritating nodules

mydriasis [maɪ'draɪəsɪs] *noun* enlargement of the pupil of the eye

mydriatic [mɪdri'ætɪk] *noun* drug which makes the pupil of the eye become larger

myectomy [maɪˈektəmi] *noun* surgical removal of part or all of a muscle

myel- *or* **myelo-** [ˈmaɪəl *or* ˈmaɪələu] *prefix* referring (i) to bone marrow; (ii) to the spinal cord

myelin [ˈmaɪəlɪn] *noun* protective white substance which is formed into a covering (myelin sheath) round nerve fibres by Schwann cells which speeds nerve impulse conduction; *see illustration at* NEURONE

myelinated [ˈmaɪəlɪneɪtɪd] *adjective* (nerve fibre) covered by a myelin sheath

myelination [maɪəliˈneɪʃn] *noun* process by which a myelin sheath forms round nerve fibres

myelitis [maɪəˈlaɪtɪs] *noun* (i) inflammation of the spinal cord; (ii) inflammation of bone marrow

myeloblast [ˈmaɪələblæst] *noun* precursor of a granulocyte

myelocele [ˈmaɪələsiːl] *noun* form of spina bifida where part of the spinal cord passes through a gap in the vertebrae

myelocyte [ˈmaɪələsaɪt] *noun* cell in bone marrow which develops into a granulocyte

myelofibrosis [maɪələfaɪˈbrəusɪs] *noun* fibrosis of bone marrow, associated with anaemia

myelogram [ˈmaɪələgræm] *noun* record of the spinal cord taken by myelography

myelography [maɪəˈlɒgrəfi] *noun* X-ray examination of the spinal cord and subarachnoid space after a radio-opaque substance has been injected

myeloid [ˈmaɪələɪd] *adjective* referring to bone marrow, to the spinal cord; produced by bone marrow; **myeloid leukaemia** = acute form of leukaemia in adults; **myeloid tissue** = red bone marrow

myeloma [maɪəˈləumə] *noun* malignant tumour in bone marrow, at the ends of long bones or in the jaw

myelomalacia [maɪələuməˈleɪʃə] *noun* softening of tissue in the spinal cord

myelomatosis [maɪələuməˈtəusɪs] *noun* disease where malignant tumours infiltrate the bone marrow

myelopathy [maɪəˈlɒpəθi] *noun* any disorder of the spinal cord or bone marrow

myenteron [maɪˈentərɒn] *noun* layer of muscles in the small intestine, which produces peristalsis

myiasis [ˈmaɪəsɪs] *noun* infestation by larvae of flies

mylohyoid [maɪləˈhaɪɔɪd] *noun & adjective* referring to the molar teeth in the lower jaw and the hyoid bone; **mylohyoid line** = line running along the outside of the lower jawbone, dividing the upper part of the bone which forms part of the mouth from the lower part which is part of the neck

myo- [ˈmaɪəu] *prefix* meaning muscle

myoblast [ˈmaɪəblæst] *noun* embryonic cell which develops into muscle

myoblastic [maɪəuˈblæstɪk] *adjective* referring to myoblast

myocardial [maɪəuˈkɑːdɪəl] *adjective* referring to the myocardium; **myocardial infarction** = death of part of the heart muscle after coronary thrombosis

myocarditis [maɪəukɑːˈdaɪtɪs] *noun* inflammation of the heart muscle

myocardium [maɪəuˈkɑːdɪəm] *noun* middle layer of the wall of the heart, formed of heart muscle; *see illustration at* HEART

myocele [ˈmaɪəsiːl] *noun* condition where a muscle pushes through a gap in the surrounding membrane

myoclonic [maɪəuˈklɒnɪk] *adjective* referring to myoclonus; **myoclonic epilepsy** = form of epilepsy where the limbs jerk frequently

myoclonus [maɪəuˈklɒnəs] *noun* muscle spasm which makes a limb give an involuntary jerk

myodynia [maɪəuˈdɪnɪə] *noun* pain in muscles

myofibril [maɪəuˈfaɪbrɪl] *noun* long thread of striated muscle fibre

myofibrosis [maɪəufaɪˈbrəusɪs] *noun* condition where muscle tissue is replaced by fibrous tissue

myogenic [maɪəuˈdʒenɪk] *adjective* (movement) which comes from an involuntary muscle

myoglobin [maɪəuˈgləubɪn] *noun* muscle haemoglobin, which takes oxygen from blood and passes it to the muscle

myoglobinuria [maɪəugləubɪˈnjuərɪə] *noun* presence of myoglobin in the urine

myogram [ˈmaɪəugræm] *noun* record showing how a muscle is functioning

myograph ['maɪəʊɡrɑːf] *noun* instrument which records the degree and strength of a muscle contraction

myography [maɪ'ɒɡrəfi] *noun* recording the degree and strength of a muscle contraction with a myograph

myokymia [maɪəʊ'kaɪmɪə] *noun* twitching of a certain muscle

myology [maɪ'ɒlədʒi] *noun* study of muscles and their associated structures and diseases

myoma [maɪ'əʊmə] *noun* benign tumour in a smooth muscle

myomectomy [maɪəʊ'mektəmi] *noun* (i) surgical removal of a benign growth from a muscle, especially removal of a fibroid from the uterus; (ii) myectomy

myometritis [maɪəʊmə'traɪtɪs] *noun* inflammation of the myometrium

myometrium [maɪəʊ'miːtriəm] *noun* muscular tissue in the uterus

myoneural junction [maɪəʊ'njʊərl 'dʒʌŋkʃn] = NEUROMUSCULAR JUNCTION

myopathy [maɪ'ɒpəθi] *noun* disease of a muscle, especially where the muscle wastes away; **focal myopathy** = destruction of muscle tissue caused by the substance injected; **needle myopathy** = destruction of muscle tissue caused by using a large needle in intramuscular injections

myopia [maɪ'əʊpiə] *noun* shortsightedness or nearsightedness, condition where a patient can see clearly objects which are close, but not ones which are further away

myopic [maɪ'ɒpɪk] *adjective* shortsighted or nearsighted, able to see close objects clearly, but not objects which are further away (NOTE: the opposite is **longsightedness** or **hypermetropia**)

myoplasm ['maɪəʊplæzm] *noun* sarcoplasm, cytoplasm of muscle cells

myoplasty ['maɪəʊplæsti] *noun* plastic surgery to repair a muscle

myosarcoma [maɪəʊsɑː'kəʊmə] *noun* (i) malignant tumour containing unstriated muscle; (ii) combined myoma and sarcoma

myosin ['maɪəʊsɪn] *noun* protein in the A bands of muscle fibre which makes muscles elastic

myosis, myotic [maɪ'əʊsɪs or maɪ'ɒtɪk] *see* MIOSIS, MIOTIC

myositis [maɪəʊ'saɪtɪs] *noun* inflammation and degeneration of a muscle

myotatic [maɪəʊ'tætɪk] *adjective* referring to the sense of touch in a muscle; **myotatic reflex** = reflex action in a muscle which contracts after being stretched

myotomy [maɪ'ɒtəmi] *noun* surgical operation to cut a muscle

myotonia [maɪəʊ'təʊniə] *noun* difficulty in relaxing a muscle after exercise

myotonic [maɪəʊ'tɒnɪk] *adjective* referring to tone in a muscle; **myotonic dystrophy** *or* **dystrophia myotonica** = hereditary disease with muscle stiffness leading to atrophy of the muscles of the face and neck

myotonus [maɪ'ɒtənəs] *noun* muscle tone

myringa [mɪ'rɪŋɡə] *noun* the eardrum, membrane at the end of the external auditory meatus leading from the outer ear, which vibrates with sound and passes the vibrations on to the ossicles in the middle ear

myringitis [mɪrɪn'dʒaɪtɪs] *noun* inflammation of the eardrum

myringoplasty [mɪ'rɪŋɡəʊplæsti] *noun* plastic surgery to correct a defect in the eardrum

myringotome [mɪ'rɪŋɡəʊtəʊm] *noun* sharp knife used in myringotomy

myringotomy [mɪrɪn'ɡɒtəmi] *noun* surgical operation to make an opening in the eardrum

myxoedema *US* **myxedema** [mɪksə'diːmə] *noun* condition caused when the thyroid gland does not produce enough thyroid hormone

COMMENT: the patient (usually a middle-aged woman) becomes fat, moves slowly and develops coarse skin; the condition can be treated with thyroxine

myxoedematous [mɪksə'demətəs] *adjective* referring to myxoedema

myxoma [mɪk'səʊmə] *noun* benign tumour of mucous tissue, usually found in subcutaneous tissue of the limbs and neck

myxosarcoma [mɪksəʊsɑː'kəʊmə] *noun* malignant tumour of mucous tissue

myxovirus [mɪksəʊ'vaɪrəs] *noun* any virus which has an affinity for the mucoprotein receptors in red blood cells (one of which causes influenza)

Nn

N (a) *chemical symbol for* nitrogen **(b)** = NEWTON

n *symbol for* nano-

Na *chemical symbol for* sodium

nabothian cyst *or* **nabothian follicle** *or* **nabothian gland** [nə'bəuθiən 'sɪst or 'fɒlɪkl or 'glænd] *noun* cyst which forms in the cervix of the uterus when the ducts in the cervical glands are blocked

naevus ['niːvəs] *noun* birthmark, a mark on the skin which a baby has at birth and which cannot be removed; *see also* HAEMANGIOMA, PORT WINE STAIN, STRAWBERRY (NOTE: plural is **naevi**)

Naga sore ['nɑːgə 'sɔː] *noun* tropical ulcer, large area of infection which forms round a wound in tropical countries

nagging pain ['nægɪŋ 'peɪn] *noun* dull, continuous throbbing pain

nail [neɪl] *noun* unguis, hard growth, formed of keratin, which forms on the top surface at the end of each finger and toe; **nail bed** = part of the finger which is just under the nail and on which the nail rests; **nail biting** = obsessive chewing of the fingernails, usually a sign of stress; **nail matrix** = the internal structure of the nail, the part of the finger from which the nail grows; **nail scissors** = special curved scissors for cutting nails; *see also* FINGERNAIL, TOENAIL (NOTE: for terms referring to nail, see words beginning with **onych-**)

nano- ['nænəu] *prefix meaning* one thousand millionth (10^{-9}) (NOTE: symbol is **n**)

nanometre *US* **nanometer** ['nænəumiːtə] *noun* unit of measurement of length (= one thousand millionth of a metre) (NOTE: with figures usually written **nm**)

nanomole ['nænəuməul] *noun* unit of measurement of the amount of substance (= one thousand millionth of a mole) (NOTE: with figures usually written **nmol**)

nanosecond ['nænəusekənd] *noun* unit of measurement of time (= one thousand millionth of a second) (NOTE: with figures usually written **ns**)

nape [neɪp] *noun* nucha, the back of the neck

napkin ['næpkɪn] *noun* soft cloth, used for wiping or absorbing; **sanitary napkin** = sanitary towel, a wad of absorbent cotton material attached by a woman over the vulva to absorb the menstrual flow; **napkin rash** = NAPPY RASH

nappy ['næpi] *noun* cloth used to wrap round a baby's bottom and groin to keep clothing clean and dry; **disposable nappy** = paper nappy which is thrown away when dirty, and not washed and used again; **nappy rash** = sore red skin on a baby's buttocks and groin, caused by reaction to long contact with ammonia in a wet nappy (NOTE: the American English is **diaper**)

narco- ['nɑːkəu] *prefix* meaning sleep or stupor

narcoanalysis [nɑːkəuə'næləsɪs] *noun* use of narcotics to induce a comatose state in a patient about to undergo psychoanalysis which may be emotionally disturbing

narcolepsy ['nɑːkəlepsi] *noun* condition where the patient has an uncontrollable tendency to fall asleep at any time

narcoleptic [nɑːkə'leptɪk] *noun & adjective* (substance) which causes narcolepsy; (patient) suffering from narcolepsy

narcosis [nɑː'kəusɪs] *noun* state of lowered consciousness induced by a drug; **basal narcosis** = making a patient completely unconscious by administering a narcotic before a general anaesthetic; **nitrogen narcosis** = loss of consciousness due to the formation of nitrogen in the tissues, caused by pressure change

narcotic [nɑː'kɒtɪk] *noun & adjective* (pain-relieving drug) which makes a patient sleep or become unconscious; *the doctor put*

her to sleep with a powerful narcotic; the
narcotic side-effects of an antihistamine

COMMENT: although narcotics are used
medicinally as pain-killers, they are highly
addictive. The main narcotics are
barbiturates, cocaine, and opium and
drugs derived from opium, such as
morphine, codeine and heroin. Addictive
narcotics are widely used for the relief of
pain in terminally ill patients

nares ['neəriːz] *plural noun* nostrils, two
passages in the nose through which air is
breathed in or out; **anterior nares** *or*
external nares = the two nostrils; **internal
nares** *or* **posterior nares** = choanae, the two
openings shaped like funnels leading from
the nasal cavity to the pharynx (NOTE: singular
is **naris**)

narrow ['nærəʊ] **1** *adjective* not wide; *the
blood vessel is a narrow channel which
takes blood to the tissues; the surgeon
inserted a narrow tube into the vein* (NOTE:
narrow - narrower - narrowest. Note also the
opposite is **broad**) **2** *verb* to become narrow;
*the bronchial tubes are narrowed causing
asthma*

nasal ['neɪzl] *adjective* referring to the nose;
nasal apertures = choanae, two openings
shaped like funnels leading from the nasal
cavity to the pharynx; **nasal bones** = two
small bones which form the bridge at the top
of the nose; *see illustration at* SKULL; **nasal
cavity** = cavity behind the nose between the
cribriform plates above and the hard palate
below, divided in two by the nasal septum
and leading to the nasopharynx; *see
illustration at* THROAT; **nasal cartilage** =
two cartilages in the nose (the upper is
attached to the nasal bone and the front of the
maxilla, the lower is thinner and curls round
each nostril to the septum); **nasal conchae** =
turbinate bones, three ridges of bone
(superior, middle and inferior conchae)
which project into the nasal cavity from the
side walls; **nasal congestion** = condition
where the nose is blocked by inflamed and
congested mucous membrane and mucus;
nasal drops = drops of liquid inserted into
the nose; **nasal septum** = division between
the two parts of the nasal cavity, formed of
the vomer and the nasal cartilage; **nasal
spray** = spray of liquid into the nose

naso- ['neɪzəʊ] *prefix* referring to the nose

nasogastric [neɪzəʊ'gæstrɪk] *adjective*
referring to the nose and stomach;

nasogastric tube = tube passed through the
nose into the stomach

nasogastrically [neɪzəʊ'gæstrɪkli] *adverb*
(to feed a patient) via a tube passed through
the nose into the stomach

all patients requiring
nutrition are fed enterally,
whether nasogastrically or
directly into the small
intestine

nasolacrimal [neɪzəʊ'lækrɪml] *adjective*
referring to the nose and the tear glands;
nasolacrimal duct = duct which drains tears
from the lacrimal sac into the nose

nasopharyngeal [neɪzəʊfə'rɪndʒɪəl]
adjective referring to the nasopharynx

nasopharyngitis [neɪzəʊfærɪn'dʒaɪtɪs]
noun inflammation of the mucous membrane
of the nasal part of the pharynx

nasopharynx [neɪzəʊ'færɪŋks] *noun* top
part of the pharynx which connects with the
nose

nasty ['nɑːsti] *adjective* unpleasant; *this
medicine has a nasty taste; drink some
orange juice to take away the nasty taste;
this new drug has some nasty side-effects*
(NOTE: **nasty - nastier - nastiest**)

nates ['neɪtiːz] *plural noun* buttocks

National Health Service (NHS) ['næʃənl
'helθ 'sɜːvɪs] *noun* government service in the
UK which provides medical services free of
charge at the point of delivery, or at reduced
cost, to the whole population; the service is
paid for out of tax revenue; **a NHS doctor** = a
doctor who works in the National Health
Service; **NHS glasses** = cheap spectacles
provided by the National Health Service; **on
the NHS** = free, paid for by the NHS; *he had
his operation on the NHS; she went to see a
specialist on the NHS* (NOTE: the opposite of
'on the NHS' is 'privately')

figures reveal that 5% more
employees in the professional
and technical category were
working in the NHS compared
with three years before

**National Institute for Clinical
Excellence (NICE)** ['næʃənl 'ɪnstɪtjuːt fə
'klɪnɪkl 'eksələns] *noun* British government
organization which produces
recommendations for treatments based on
clinical evidence and cost-effectiveness

natural ['nætʃrl] *adjective* **(a)** normal, not surprising; *his behaviour was quite natural*; *it's natural for old people to go deaf*; **natural childbirth** = childbirth where the mother is not given pain-killing drugs but is encouraged to give birth to the baby with as little medical assistance as possible; **natural immunity** = immunity from disease a newborn baby has from birth, which is inherited, acquired in the uterus or from the mother's milk **(b)** not made by men; (thing) which comes from nature; **natural gas** = gas which is found in the earth and not made in a factory; **natural history** = study of nature

nature ['neɪtʃə] *noun* **(a)** (i) essential quality of something; (ii) kind or sort **(b)** genetic makeup which affects personality, behaviour or risk of disease; *see also* NURTURE **(c) human nature** = general behavioural characteristics of human beings **(d)** plants and animals; **nature study** = learning about plant and animal life at school

naturopathy [neɪtʃə'rɒpəθi] *noun* treatment of diseases and disorders which does not use medical or surgical means, but natural forces such as light, heat, massage, eating natural foods and using herbal remedies

nausea ['nɔːsɪə] *noun* feeling sick, feeling that you want to vomit; *she suffered from nausea in the morning*; *he felt slight nausea in getting onto the boat*

COMMENT: nausea can be caused by eating habits, such as eating too much rich food or drinking too much alcohol; it can also be caused by sensations such as unpleasant smells or motion sickness. Other causes include stomach disorders, such as gastritis, ulcers and liver infections. Nausea is commonly experienced by women in the early stages of pregnancy, and is called 'morning sickness'

nauseated *US* **nauseous** ['nɔːsieitid or 'nɔːsiəs] *adjective* feeling sick, feeling about to vomit; *the casualty may feel nauseated*

navel ['neivl] *noun* umbilicus, scar with a depression in the middle of the abdomen where the umbilical cord was detached after birth (NOTE: for terms referring to the navel, see words beginning with **omphal-**)

navicular bone [nə'vikjulə 'bəun] *noun* one of the tarsal bones in the foot; *see illustration at* FOOT

nearsighted [nɪə'saitid] = MYOPIC

nearsightedness [nɪə'saitidnəs] = MYOPIA

nebula ['nebjulə] *noun* (i) slightly cloudy spot on the cornea; (ii) spray of medicinal solution, applied to the nose or throat using a nebulizer

nebulizer ['nebjulaizə] = ATOMIZER

Necator [ne'keitə] *noun* genus of hookworm which infests the small intestine

necatoriasis [nekeitə'raiəsis] *noun* infestation of the small intestine by the parasite Necator

neck [nek] *noun* **(a)** part of the body which joins the head to the body; *he is suffering from pains in the neck*; *the front of the neck is swollen with goitre*; *the jugular veins run down the side of the neck*; **stiff neck** = condition where moving the neck is painful, usually caused by a strained muscle or by sitting in a cold draught; **neck collar** = special strong collar to support the head of a patient with neck injuries or a condition such as cervical spondylosis **(b)** narrow part (of a bone or organ); **neck of the femur** *or* **femoral neck** = the narrow part between the head and the diaphysis of the femur; **neck of tooth** = point where a tooth narrows slightly, between the crown and the root; **neck of the uterus** = CERVIX (NOTE: for terms referring to the neck, see **cervical**)

COMMENT: the neck is formed of the seven cervical vertebrae, and is held vertical by strong muscles. Many organs pass through the neck, including the oesophagus, the larynx and the arteries and veins which connect the brain to the bloodstream. The front of the neck is usually referred to as the throat

necro- ['nekrəu] *prefix* meaning death

necrobiosis [nekrəubai'əusis] *noun* (i) death of cells surrounded by living tissue; (ii) gradual localized death of a part or tissue

necrology [ne'krɒlədʒi] *noun* scientific study of mortality statistics

necrophilia *or* **necrophilism** [nekrə'filiə or ne'krɒfilizm] *noun* (i) abnormal pleasure in corpses; (ii) sexual attraction to dead bodies

necropsy ['nekrɒpsi] = POST MORTEM

necrosed ['nekrəuzd] *adjective* dead (tissue or bone)

necrosis [ne'krəusis] *noun* death of a part of the body, such as a bone, tissue or an organ; *gangrene is a form of necrosis*

necrospermia [nekrəʊ'spɜːmiə] *noun* condition where dead sperm exist in the semen

necrotic [ne'krɒtɪk] *adjective* referring to necrosis; dead (tissue)

necrotomy [ne'krɒtəmi] *noun* dissection of a dead body; **osteoplastic necrotomy** = surgical removal of a piece of necrosed bone tissue

needle ['niːdl] *noun* (i) thin metal instrument with a hole at one end for attaching a thread, and a sharp point at the other end, used for sewing up surgical incisions; (ii) thin hollow metal instrument with a point at one end, attached to a hypodermic syringe and used for giving injections; *it is important that needles used for injections should be sterilized; AIDS can be transmitted by using non-sterile needles*; **stop needle** = needle with a ring round it, so that it can only be pushed a certain distance into the body; **surgical needle** = needle for sewing up surgical incisions; **needle myopathy** = destruction of muscle tissue caused by using a large needle for intramuscular injections

needlestick ['niːdlstɪk] *noun* accidental pricking of one's own skin by a needle (as by a nurse picking up a used syringe)

needling ['niːdlɪŋ] *noun* puncture of a cataract with a needle

needs assessment ['niːdz ə'sesmənt] *noun* the investigation of the (health and social care) needs of a particular group of people, in order to match services to need

negative ['negətɪv] *adjective & noun* showing 'no'; **the answer is in the negative** = the answer is 'no'; **the test was negative** = the test showed that the patient did not have the disease; **negative feedback** = situation where the result of a process represses the process which caused it

negativism ['negətɪvɪzm] *noun* attitude of a patient who opposes what someone says

COMMENT: there are two types of negativism: active, where the patient does the opposite of what a doctor tells him, and passive, where the patient does not do what he has been asked to do

negra ['niːgrə] *see* LINEA

Negri bodies ['neɪgri 'bɒdɪz] *plural noun* particles found in the cerebral cells of patients suffering from rabies

Neil Robertson stretcher ['niːl 'rɒbətsən 'stretʃə] *see* STRETCHER

Neisseria [naɪ'sɪəriə] *noun* genus of bacteria, including gonococcus which causes gonorrhoea, and meningococcus which causes meningitis

nematode ['nemətəʊd] *noun* type of parasitic roundworm, such as hookworms, pinworms and threadworms

neo- ['niːəʊ] *prefix* meaning new

neocerebellum [niːəʊserə'beləm] *noun* middle part of the cerebellum

neomycin [niːəʊ'maɪsɪn] *noun; see* DRUGS TABLE IN SUPPLEMENT

neonatal [niːəʊ'neɪtl] *adjective* referring to the first few weeks after birth; **neonatal death rate** = number of newborn babies who die, shown per thousand babies born

one of the most common routes of neonatal poisoning is percutaneous absorption following topical administration

Southern Medical Journal

neonate ['niːəʊneɪt] *noun* newborn baby, less than four weeks old

neonatologist [niːənə'tɒlədʒɪst] *noun* specialist who looks after small babies during the first few weeks, also one who looks after premature babies and babies with some congenital disorders

neonatology [niːənə'tɒlədʒi] *noun* branch of medicine dealing with newborn babies

neonatorum [niːəʊneɪ'tɔːrəm] *see* ASPHYXIA

neoplasm ['niːəʊplæzm] *noun* any new and morbid formation of tissue

testicular cancer comprises only 1% of all malignant neoplasms in the male, but it is one of the most frequently occurring types of tumours in late adolescence

Journal of American College Health

nephr- [nefr] *prefix* referring to the kidney

nephralgia [nɪ'frældʒə] *noun* pain in the kidney

nephrectomy [nɪ'frektɒmi] *noun* surgical removal of the whole kidney

nephritis [nɪ'fraɪtɪs] *noun* inflammation of the kidney

COMMENT: acute nephritis can be caused by a streptococcal infection. Symptoms can include headaches, swollen ankles, and fever

nephroblastoma [nefrəublæ'stəumə] *noun* Wilms' tumour, malignant tumour in the kidneys in young children, usually under the age of 10, leading to swelling of the abdomen, which is treated by removal of the affected kidney

nephrocalcinosis [nefrəukælsɪ'nəusɪs] *noun* condition where calcium deposits are found in the kidney

nephrocapsulectomy [nefrəukæpsju'lektəmi] *noun* surgical removal of the capsule round a kidney

nephrolithiasis [nefrəulɪ'θaɪəsɪs] *noun* condition where stones form in the kidney

nephrolithotomy [nefrəulɪ'θɒtəmi] *noun* surgical removal of a stone in the kidney

nephrologist [nɪ'frɒlədʒɪst] *noun* doctor who specializes in the study of the kidney and its diseases

nephrology [nɪ'frɒlədʒi] *noun* study of the kidney and its diseases

nephroma [nɪ'frəumə] *noun* tumour in the kidney, tumour derived from renal substances

nephron ['nefrɒn] *noun* tiny structure in the kidney, through which fluid is filtered

COMMENT: a nephron is formed of a series of tubules, the loop of Henle, Bowman's capsule and a glomerulus. Blood enters the nephron from the renal artery, and waste materials are filtered out by the Bowman's capsule. Some substances return to the bloodstream by reabsorption in the tubules. Urine is collected in the ducts leading from the tubules to the ureters

nephropexy ['nefrəupeksi] *noun* surgical operation to attach a mobile kidney

nephroptosis [nefrɒp'təusɪs] *noun* floating kidney, condition where the kidney is mobile

nephrosclerosis [nefrəusklə'rəusɪs] *noun* kidney disease due to vascular change

nephrosis [nɪ'frəusɪs] *noun* degeneration of the tissue of a kidney

nephrostomy [nɪ'frɒstəmi] *noun* surgical operation to make a permanent opening into the pelvis of the kidney from the surface

nephrotic syndrome [nɪ'frɒtɪk 'sɪndrəum] *noun* increasing oedema, albuminuria and raised blood pressure

nephrotomy [nɪ'frɒtəmi] *noun* surgical operation to cut into a kidney

nephroureterectomy [nefrəujuərɪtə'rektəmi] *noun* ureteronephrectomy, surgical removal of all or part of a kidney and the ureter attached to it

nerve [nɜːv] *noun* **(a)** bundle of fibres in a body which take impulses from one part of the body to another (each fibre being the axon of a nerve cell); **cranial nerves** = twelve pairs of nerves which are connected directly to the brain, and govern mainly the structures of the head and neck; *see also the list at* CRANIAL; **spinal nerves** = thirty-one pairs of nerves which lead from the spinal cord, and govern mainly the trunk and limbs; **motor nerve** *or* **efferent nerve** = nerve which carries impulses from the brain and spinal cord to muscles and causes movements; **peripheral nerves** = parts of motor and sensory nerves which branch from the brain and spinal cord; **sensory nerve** *or* **afferent nerve** = nerve which registers a sensation, such as heat, taste, smell, etc., and carries impulses to the brain and spinal cord; **vasomotor nerve** = nerve whose impulses make the arterioles become narrower **(b)** *(names of nerves)* **abducent nerve** = sixth cranial nerve which controls the muscle which makes the eyeball turn; **accessory nerve** = eleventh cranial nerve which supplies the muscles in the neck and shoulders; **acoustic nerve** *or* **auditory nerve** *or* **vestibulocochlear nerve** = eighth cranial nerve which governs hearing and balance; **circumflex nerve** = sensory and motor nerve in the upper arm; **cochlear nerve** = division of the auditory nerve; **facial nerve** = seventh cranial nerve which governs the muscles of the face, the taste buds on the front of the tongue and the salivary and lacrimal glands; **femoral nerve** = nerve which governs the muscle at the front of the thigh; **glossopharyngeal nerve** = ninth cranial nerve which controls the pharynx, the salivary glands and part of the tongue; **hypoglossal nerve** = twelfth cranial nerve which governs the muscles of the tongue; **oculomotor nerve** = third cranial nerve which controls the eyeballs and eyelids; **olfactory nerve** = first cranial nerve which controls the sense of smell; **optic nerve** = second cranial nerve which takes sensation of sight from the eye to the brain; **phrenic nerve** = nerve which controls the muscles in the diaphragm; **pneumogastric nerve** *or* **vagus nerve** = tenth cranial nerve which controls swallowing and nerve fibres in the heart and chest; **radial nerve** = main motor nerve of the arm; **sacral nerves** = nerves which branch from the spinal cord in the sacrum and govern the legs, the arms and the genital area; **trigeminal nerve** = fifth cranial nerve which controls the sensory nerves in the forehead and face and the muscles in the jaw; **trochlear nerve** = fourth cranial nerve which controls the muscles of the eyeball; **ulnar nerve** = nerve running from the neck to the elbow, which controls the muscles in the forearm and fingers; **vestibulocochlear nerve** = eighth cranial nerve which governs hearing and balance **(c) nerve block** = stopping the function of a nerve by injecting an anaesthetic; **nerve cell** = neurone, cell in the nervous system, consisting of a cell body, axon(s) and dendrites, which transmits nerve impulses; **nerve centre** = point at which nerves come together; **nerve ending** = terminal at the end of a nerve fibre, where a nerve cell connects with another nerve or with a muscle; **nerve fibre** = axon, a thread-like structure which is part of a nerve cell and carries nerve impulses; **nerve gas** = gas which attacks the nervous system; **nerve impulse** = electrochemical impulse which is transmitted by nerve cells; **nerve root** = first part of a nerve as it leaves or joins the spinal column (the dorsal nerve root is the entry for a sensory nerve, and the ventral nerve root is the exit for a motor nerve); **nerve tissue** = tissue which forms nerves, and which is able to transmit the nerve impulses (NOTE: for other terms referring to nerves, see words beginning with **neur-**)

COMMENT: nerves are the fibres along which impulses are carried. Motor nerves or efferent nerves take messages between the central nervous system and muscles, making the muscles move. Sensory nerves or afferent nerves transmit impulses (such as sight or pain) from the sense organs to the brain

nervosa [nəˈvəusə] *see* ANOREXIA

nervous [ˈnɜːvəs] *adjective* **(a)** referring to nerves; **nervous breakdown** = non-medical term for a sudden mental illness, where a patient becomes so depressed and worried that he is incapable of doing anything; **nervous system** = nervous tissues of the body, including the peripheral nerves, spinal cord, ganglia and nerve centres; **autonomic nervous system** = nervous system which

regulates the automatic functioning of the structures of the body, such as the heart and lungs; **central nervous system (CNS)** = brain and spinal cord which link together all the nerves; **peripheral nervous system (PNS)** = nervous tissue outside the central nervous system; *see also* PARASYMPATHETIC, SYMPATHETIC **(b)** very easily worried; *she's nervous about her exams*; *don't be nervous - the operation is a very simple one*

nervousness [ˈnɜːvəsnəs] *noun* state of being nervous

nervy [ˈnɜːvi] *adjective (informal)* worried and nervous

nettle rash [ˈnetl ˈræʃ] *noun* urticaria, affection of the skin, with white or red weals which sting or itch, caused by an allergic reaction (often to plants)

network [ˈnetwɜːk] *noun* interconnecting system of lines and spaces, like a net; *a network of fine blood vessels*

neur- *or* **neuro-** [ˈnjʊər or ˈnjʊərəu] *prefix* referring to a nerve or the nervous system

neural [ˈnjʊərl] *adjective* referring to a nerve or the nervous system; **neural arch** = curved part of a vertebra, which forms the space through which the spinal cord passes; **neural crest** = ridge of cells in an embryo which forms nerve cells of the sensory and autonomic ganglia; **neural groove** = groove on the back of an embryo, formed as the neural plate closes to form the neural tube; **neural plate** = thickening of an embryonic disc which folds over to form the neural tube; **neural tube** = tube lined with ectodermal cells running the length of an embryo, which develops into the brain and spinal cord; **neural tube defect** = congenital defect (such as spina bifida) which occurs when the edges of the neural tube do not close up properly

neuralgia [njuˈrældʒə] *noun* spasm of pain which runs along a nerve; **trigeminal neuralgia** = pain in the trigeminal nerve, which sends intense pains shooting across the face

neurapraxia [njuərəˈpræksiə] *noun* lesion of a nerve which leads to paralysis for a very short time, giving a tingling feeling and loss of function

neurasthenia [njuərəsˈθiːnjə] *noun* type of neurosis where the patient is mentally and physically irritable and extremely fatigued

neurasthenic [njʊərəs'θenɪk] *noun & adjective* (person) suffering from neurasthenia

neurectasis [njʊ'rektəsɪs] *noun* surgical operation to stretch a peripheral nerve

neurectomy [njʊ'rektəmi] *noun* surgical removal of all or part of a nerve

neurilemma *or* **neurolemma** [njʊəri'lemə *or* njʊərəʊ'lemə] *noun* outer sheath formed of Schwann cells, which covers the myelin sheath covering a nerve fibre

neurilemmoma *or* **neurinoma** [njʊərile'məʊmə *or* njʊəri'nəʊmə] *noun* benign tumour of a nerve, formed from the neurilemma

neuritis [njʊ'raɪtɪs] *noun* inflammation of a nerve, giving a constant pain

neuroanatomy [njʊərəʊə'nætəmi] *noun* scientific study of the structure of the nervous system

neuroblast ['njʊərəʊblæst] *noun* cell in the embryonic spinal cord which forms a nerve cell

neuroblastoma [njʊərəʊblæ'stəʊmə] *noun* malignant tumour formed from the neural crest, found mainly in young children

neurocranium [njʊərəʊ'kreɪniəm] *noun* part of the skull which encloses and protects the brain

neurodermatitis [njʊərəʊdɜːmə'taɪtɪs] *noun* inflammation of the skin caused by psychological factors

neurodermatosis [njʊərəʊdɜːmə'təʊsɪs] *noun* nervous condition involving the skin

neuroendocrine system [njʊərəʊ'endəkraɪn 'sɪstəm] *noun* system in which the CNS and hormonal systems interact to control the function of organs and tissues

neuroepithelial [njʊərəʊepi'θiːliəl] *adjective* referring to the neuroepithelium

neuroepithelioma [njʊərəʊepiθiːli'əʊmə] *noun* malignant tumour in the retina

neuroepithelium [njʊərəʊepi'θiːliəm] *noun* epithelial cells forming part of the lining of the mucosa of the nose or the labyrinth of the middle ear

neurofibril [njʊərəʊ'faɪbrɪl] *noun* fine thread in the cytoplasm of a neurone

neurofibroma [njʊərəʊfaɪ'brəʊmə] *noun* benign tumour of a nerve, formed from the neurilemma; **acoustic neurofibroma** = tumour in the sheath of the auditory nerve

neurofibromatosis (NF) [njʊərəʊfaɪbrəʊmə'təʊsɪs] *noun* hereditary condition where the patient has neurofibromata on the nerve trunks, limb plexuses or spinal roots, and pale brown spots appear on the skin (NOTE: also called **molluscum fibrosum** *or* **von Recklinghausen's disease**)

neurogenesis [njʊərəʊ'dʒenəsɪs] *noun* development and growth of nerves and nervous tissue

neurogenic [njʊərəʊ'dʒenɪk] *adjective* (i) coming from the nervous system; (ii) referring to neurogenesis; **neurogenic bladder** = any disturbance of the bladder function caused by lesions in the nerve supply to the bladder

neuroglandular junction [njʊərəʊ'glændjʊlə 'dʒʌŋkʃn] *noun* point where a nerve joins the gland which it controls

neuroglia [nju'rɒgliə] *noun* supporting cells of the spinal cord and brain

neurohormone [njʊərəʊ'hɔːməʊn] *noun* hormone produced in some nerve cells and secreted from the nerve endings

neurohypophysis [njʊərəʊhaɪ'pɒfəsɪs] *noun* lobe at the back of the pituitary gland, which secretes oxytocin and vasopressin

neurolemma [njʊərəʊ'lemə] *noun* = NEURILEMMA

neuroleptic [njʊərəʊ'leptɪk] *noun* anti-psychotic drug (such as chlorpromazine hydrochloride) which calms a patient and stops him or her worrying

neurological [njʊərə'lɒdʒɪkl] *adjective* referring to neurology

neurologist [nju'rɒlədʒɪst] *noun* doctor who specializes in the study of the nervous system and the treatment of its diseases

neurology [nju'rɒlədʒi] *noun* scientific study of the nervous system and its diseases

neuroma [nju'rəʊmə] *noun* benign tumour formed of nerve cells and nerve fibres; **acoustic neuroma** = tumour in the sheath of the auditory nerve

neuromuscular [njʊərəʊ'mʌskjʊlə] *adjective* referring to nerves and muscles; **neuromuscular junction** = myoneural junction, the point where a motor nerve joins muscle fibre

neuromyelitis optica [njuərəumaɪə'laɪtɪs 'ɒptɪkə] *noun* Devic's disease, condition similar to multiple sclerosis, where the patient has acute myelitis and the optic nerve is also affected

neurone *or* **neuron** ['njuərəun or 'njuərɒn] *noun* nerve cell, a cell in the nervous system which transmits nerve impulses; **bipolar neurone** = neurone with two processes (found in the retina); **motor neurone** = neurone which is part of a nerve pathway transmitting impulses from the brain to a muscle or gland; **upper motor neurone** = neurone which takes impulses from the cerebral cortex; **lower motor neurone** = linked neurones which carry motor impulses from the spinal cord to the muscles; **multipolar neurone** = neurone with several processes; **sensory neurone** = neurone which receives its stimulus directly from the receptor, and passes the impulse to the sensory cortex; **unipolar neurone** = neurone with a single process

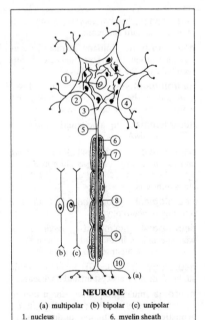

NEURONE

(a) multipolar (b) bipolar (c) unipolar

1. nucleus	6. myelin sheath
2. Nissl granules	7. Schwann cell nucleus
3. neurofibrilla	8. node of Ranvier
4. dendrite	9. neurilemma
5. axon	10. terminal branch

neuropathology [njuərəupə'θɒlədʒi] *noun* study of diseases of the nervous system

neuropathy [njuə'rɒpəθi] *noun* disease involving destruction of the tissues of the nervous system

neurophysiologist [njuərəufɪzɪ'ɒlədʒɪst] *noun* scientist who studies the physiology of the nervous system

neurophysiology [njuərəufɪzɪ'ɒlədʒi] *noun* study of the physiology of nerves

neuroplasty ['njuərəuplæsti] *noun* surgery to repair damaged nerves

neuropsychiatric [njuərəusaɪki'ætrɪk] *adjective* referring to neuropsychiatry

neuropsychiatrist [njuərəusaɪ'kaɪətrɪst] *noun* doctor who specializes in the study and treatment of mental and nervous disorders

neuropsychiatry [njuərəusaɪ'kaɪətri] *noun* study of mental and nervous disorders

neurorrhaphy [nju'rɔːrəfi] *noun* surgical operation to join by suture a nerve which has been cut

neurosarcoma [njuərəusɑː'kəumə] *noun* malignant neuroma

neuroscientist [njuərəu'saɪəntɪst] *noun* scientist who studies the nervous system

neurosecretion [njuərəusɪ'kriːʃn] *noun* (i) substance secreted by a nerve cell; (ii) secretion of active substance by nerve cells

neurosis [nju'rəusɪs] *noun* illness of the personality, in which a patient becomes obsessed with something and experiences strong emotions towards it, such as fear of empty spaces, jealousy of a sibling, etc.; **anxiety neurosis** = neurotic condition where the patient is anxious and has morbid fears (NOTE: plural is **neuroses**)

neurosurgeon [njuərəu'sɜːdʒn] *noun* surgeon who operates on the nervous system, including the brain

neurosurgery [njuərəu'sɜːdʒri] *noun* surgery on the nervous system, including the brain and spinal cord

neurosyphilis [njuərəu'sɪfəlɪs] *noun* syphilis which attacks the nervous system

neurotic [nju'rɒtɪk] *noun & adjective* (i) (person) who suffers from neurosis; (ii) (any person) who is worried or obsessed with something

neurotically [nju'rɒtɪkli] *adverb* in a neurotic way; *she is neurotically obsessed with keeping herself clean*

neurotmesis [njuːrɒt'miːsɪs] *noun* cutting a nerve completely

neurotomy [njʊˈrɒtəmi] *noun* surgical operation to cut a nerve

neurotoxic [njʊərəʊˈtɒksɪk] *adjective* (substance) which can harm or be poisonous to nerve cells

neurotransmitter [njʊərəʊtrænsˈmɪtə] *noun* chemical substance which transmits nerve impulses from one neurone to another

> COMMENT: the main neurotransmitters are the catecholamines (adrenaline, noradrenaline, 5-hydroxytryptamine) and acetylcholine. Other neurotransmitters such as gamma aminobutyric acid, glutamine and substance P are less common

neurotripsy [ˈnjʊərəʊtrɪpsi] *noun* surgical bruising or crushing of a nerve

neurotropic [njʊərəʊˈtrɒpɪk] *adjective* (bacterium) which is attracted to and attacks nerves

neuter [ˈnjuːtə] *adjective* neither male nor female

neutral [ˈnjuːtrl] *adjective* neither acid nor alkali; *a pH factor of 7 is neutral*

neutralize [ˈnjuːtrəlaɪz] *verb* to counteract the effect of something; *(in bacteriology)* to make a toxin harmless by combining it with the correct amount of antitoxin; *alkali poisoning can be neutralized by applying acid solution*

neutropenia [njuːtrəˈpiːniə] *noun* condition where there are fewer neutrophils than normal in the blood

neutrophil [ˈnjuːtrəfɪl] *adjective* polymorph, type of white blood cell with an irregular nucleus, which can attack and destroy bacteria

nevus [ˈniːvəs] *US* = NAEVUS

newborn [ˈnjuːbɔːn] *adjective & noun* (baby) which has been born recently

newton [ˈnjuːtn] *noun* SI unit of measurement of force (NOTE: usually written N with figures: **the muscle exerted a force of 5N**)

> COMMENT: 1 newton is the force required to move 1 kilogram at the speed of 1 metre per second

nexus [ˈneksəs] *noun* link, point where two organs or tissues join

NF [ˈen ˈef] = NEUROFIBROMATOSIS

NHS [ˈen ˈeɪtʃ ˈes] = NATIONAL HEALTH SERVICE

niacin ($C_6H_5NO_2$) [ˈnaɪəsɪn] *noun* nicotinic acid, a vitamin of the vitamin B complex found in milk, meat, liver, kidney, yeast, beans, peas and bread (lack of niacin can cause mental disorders and pellagra)

NICE [naɪs] = NATIONAL INSTITUTE FOR CLINICAL EXCELLENCE

nick [nɪk] **1** *noun* little cut; *he had a nick in his ear lobe which bled* **2** *verb* to make a little cut; *he nicked his chin while shaving*

nicotine ($C_{10}H_{14}N_2$) [ˈnɪkətiːn] *noun* main alkaloid substance found in tobacco; **nicotine addiction** = addiction to nicotine, derived from smoking tobacco; **nicotine patch** = patch containing nicotine which is released slowly into the bloodstream, as a method of curing nicotine addiction; **nicotine poisoning** *or* **nicotinism** = poisoning of the autonomic nervous system with large quantities of nicotine; **nicotine receptor** = cholinergic receptor found at the neuromuscular junction on skeletal muscle and in the autonomic ganglia, which responds to nicotine and nicotine-like drugs

nicotinic [nɪkəˈtɪnɪk] **nicotinic acid** = NIACIN; **nicotinic receptor** = NICOTINE RECEPTOR

nictation *or* **nictitation** [nɪkˈteɪʃn *or* nɪktɪˈteɪʃn] *noun* act of winking

nidation [naɪˈdeɪʃn] *noun* **(a)** building of the endometrial layers of the uterus between menstrual periods **(b)** implantation, the point in the development of an embryo, when the fertilized ovum reaches the uterus and implants in the wall of the uterus

nidus [ˈnaɪdəs] *noun* centre of infection, site where bacteria can settle and breed

Nielsen [ˈniːlsn] *see* HOLGER

night [naɪt] *noun* period between sunset and sunrise, part of the day when it is dark; *I don't like going out alone late at night*; *there are two nurses on duty each night*; **night blindness** = NYCTALOPIA; **night duty** = being on duty at night; **night nurse** = nurse who is on duty at night; **night sweat** = heavy sweating when asleep at night; **night terror** = disturbed sleep, which a child does not remember

nightmare [ˈnaɪtmeə] *noun* dream which frightens; *the little girl had a nightmare and woke up screaming*

nightshade [ˈnaɪtʃeɪd] *see* BELLADONNA

nigra [ˈnaɪgrə] *see* LINEA

ninety-nine (99) ['namti'nam] *number* number which a doctor asks someone to say, so that he can inspect the back of the throat; *the doctor told him to open his mouth wide and say ninety-nine*

nipple ['nɪpl] *noun* **(a)** mammilla, protruding darker part in the centre of the breast, containing the milk ducts through which the milk passes **(b)** *US* rubber teat on a baby's feeding bottle

Nissl granules *or* **Nissl bodies** ['nɪsl 'grænjuːlz *or* 'bɒdiz] *noun* coarse granules surrounding the nucleus in the cytoplasm of nerve cells; *see illustration at* NEURONE

nit [nɪt] *noun* egg or larva of a louse

nitrate ['naɪtreɪt] *noun* drug (such as glyceryl trinitrate taken under the tongue) which dilates the vessels to the heart muscle and lowers cardiac work by reducing venous return to the heart, for rapid relief of angina and in heart failure (NOTE: nitrate drugs have names ending in -nitrate: glyceryl trinitrate)

COMMENT: patients can develop tolerance to these drugs

-nitrate ['naɪtreɪt] *suffix* used in names of nitrate drugs; *glyceryl trinitrate*

nitrogen ['naɪtrədʒn] *noun* chemical element, a gas which is the main component of air and is an essential part of protein (NOTE: chemical symbol is N)

COMMENT: nitrogen is taken into the body by digesting protein-rich foods; excess nitrogen is excreted in urine. When the intake of nitrogen and the excretion rate are equal, the body is in nitrogen balance or protein balance

nitrous oxide (N_2O) ['naɪtrəs 'ɒksaɪd] *noun* laughing gas, colourless gas with a sweet smell, used in combination with other gases as an anaesthetic in dentistry and surgery

nm = NANOMETRE

nmol = NANOMOLE

NMR ['en 'em 'aː] = NUCLEAR MAGNETIC RESONANCE

Nocardia [nəʊ'kaːdɪə] *noun* genus of bacteria found in soil, some species of which cause nocardiosis and Madura foot

nocardiosis *or* **nocardiasis** [nəʊkaːdi'əʊsɪs *or* nəʊkaː'daɪəsɪs] *noun* lung infection which may metastasize to other tissue, caused by *Nocardia*

nociceptive [nəʊsi'septɪv] *adjective* (nerves) which carry pain to the brain

nociceptor [nəʊsi'septə] *noun* sensory nerve which carries pain to the brain

nocte ['nɒkti] *Latin word meaning* 'at night' (written on prescriptions) (NOTE: opposite is **mane**)

nocturia [nɒk'tjʊərɪə] *noun* passing abnormally large quantity of urine during the night

nocturnal [nɒk'tɜːnl] *adjective* at night; **nocturnal enuresis** = bedwetting, passing urine when asleep in bed at night (especially used of children)

nod [nɒd] **1** *noun* moving the head forward (as to show agreement); *when the nurse asked him if he wanted a drink, he gave a nod* **2** *verb* **(a)** to move the head forward (as to show agreement); *when she asked if anyone wanted an ice cream, all the children nodded* **(b)** *(informal)* **to nod off** = to begin to go to sleep (with the head falling forward); *he nodded off in his chair*

nodal ['nəʊdl] *adjective* referring to nodes; **nodal tachycardia** = sudden attack of rapid heartbeats

node [nəʊd] *noun* (i) small mass of tissue; (ii) group of nerve cells; **atrioventricular node** *or* **AV node** = mass of conducting tissue in the right atrium of the heart, which continues as the bundle of His and passes impulses from the atria to the ventricles; **axillary nodes** = part of the lymphatic system in the arm; **cervical nodes** = lymph nodes in the neck; **Heberden's node** = small bony lump which develops on the terminal phalanges of fingers in osteoarthritis; **lymph nodes** = glands of lymphoid tissue situated at various points of the lymphatic system (especially under the armpits and in the groin), through which lymph passes and in which lymphocytes are produced; **Osler's nodes** = tender swellings at the ends of fingers and toes in patients suffering from subacute bacterial endocarditis; **node of Ranvier** = one of a series of points along the length of a nerve, where the myelin sheath round the nerve fibre ends and connective tissue touches the axon through which the axon is depolarized

nodosa [nəʊ'dəʊsə] *see* PERIARTERITIS

nodosum [nəʊ'dəʊsəm] *see* ERYTHEMA

nodular ['nɒdjʊlə] *adjective* formed of nodules

nodule ['nɒdjuːl] *noun* small node or group of cells; anterior part of the inferior vermis; *see also* BOHN

noma ['nəʊmə] *noun* cancrum oris, severe ulcers in the mouth, leading to gangrene

nomen proprium ['nəʊmən 'prəʊpriəm] *see* N.P.

non- ['nɒn] *prefix* meaning not; **non-absorbable suture** = suture made of a substance which cannot be absorbed into the body, and which eventually has to be removed; **non-allergenic** = (cosmetic, etc.) which will not aggravate an allergy; **non-contagious** = not contagious; **non-emergency surgery** *or* **non-urgent surgery** = operation, such as a joint replacement, for a condition which is not life-threatening and which, therefore, does not need to be performed immediately; **non-nucleated** = (cell) with no nucleus; **non-smoker** = person who does not smoke; **non-venereal disease** = disease which is not a venereal disease

non compos mentis ['nɒn 'kɒmpəs 'mentɪs] *Latin phrase meaning* 'not of sound mind': (person) who is mentally incapable of managing his own affairs

nongranular leucocytes [nɒn'grænjʊlə 'luːkəʊsaɪts] *noun* leucocytes (such as lymphocytes or monocytes) which have no granules

non-invasive ['nɒnɪn'veɪzɪv] *adjective* (inspection or treatment) which does not involve entering the body by making an incision; *see also* INVASIVE

non-malignant [nɒnmə'lɪgnənt] *adjective* not malignant; *a non-malignant growth*

non-medical ['nɒn'medɪkl] *adjective* (word) which is not used in specialized medical speech; *'nervous breakdown' is a non-medical term for a type of sudden mental illness*

non-secretor [nɒnsɪ'kriːtə] *noun* person who does not secrete indicators of blood grouping into body fluids

non-specific [nɒnspe'sɪfɪk] *adjective* (condition) which is not caused by any single identifiable cause; **non-specific urethritis (NSU)** = formerly, sexually transmitted inflammation of the urethra not caused by gonorrhea

non-sterile [nɒn'steraɪl] *adjective* (dressing) which is not sterile, (instrument) which has not been sterilized

non-steroidal ['nɒn'stɪərɔɪdəl] *adjective* not containing steroids (NOTE: the opposite is **steroidal**)

non-steroidal anti-inflammatory drug (NSAID) ['nɒn'stɪərɔɪdəl 'æntiɪn'flæmətri 'drʌg] *noun* drug used in the treatment of pain associated with inflammation, including rheumatic disease, post-operative analgesia and dysmenorrhoea, by inhibiting the release of prostaglandins (NOTE: non-steroidal anti-inflammatory drugs have names ending in **-fen: ibuprofen**)

> COMMENT: serious gastro-intestinal side effects can occur, especially in the elderly. Asthma can worsen

non-union [nɒn'juːniən] *noun* condition where the two parts of a fractured bone do not join together and do not heal

noradrenaline *US* **norepinephrine** [nɔːrə'drenəlɪn *or* nɔːrepi'nefrɪn] *noun* hormone secreted by the medulla of the adrenal glands which acts as a vasoconstrictor and is used to maintain blood pressure in shock or haemorrhage or hypotension

norma ['nɔːmə] *noun* in anatomy, the skull as seen from a certain angle

normal ['nɔːml] *adjective* usual, ordinary, according to a standard; *after taking the tablets, his blood pressure went back to normal; her temperature is two degrees above normal; he had an above normal pulse rate; it is normal for a person with myopia to suffer from headaches*

normally ['nɔːmli] *adverb* in a normal or ordinary way; *the patients are normally worried before the operation; he was breathing normally*

normoblast ['nɔːməʊblæst] *noun* early form of a red blood cell, normally found only in bone marrow but found in the blood in certain types of leukaemia and anaemia

normocyte ['nɔːməʊsaɪt] *noun* normal red blood cell

normocytic [nɔːməʊ'saɪtɪk] *adjective* referring to a normocyte

normocytosis [nɔːməʊsaɪ'təʊsɪs] *noun* having the normal number of red blood cells in the peripheral blood

normotension [nɔːməʊ'tenʃn] *noun* normal blood pressure

normotensive [nɔːməʊ'tensɪv] *adjective* (blood pressure) at normal level

nose [nəʊz] *noun* organ through which a person breathes and smells; **she must have a cold - her nose is running** = liquid mucus is dripping from her nose; **he blew his nose** = he blew air through his nose into a handkerchief to get rid of mucus in his nose; **to speak through your nose** = to speak as if your nose is blocked, so that you say 'b' instead of 'm' and 'd' instead of 'n' (NOTE: for other terms referring to the nose, see **nasal** and words beginning with **naso-, rhin-, rhino-**)

COMMENT: the nose is formed of cartilage and small bones making the bridge at the top. It leads into two passages (the nostrils) which in turn lead to the nasal cavity, divided in two by the septum. The nasal passages connect with the sinuses, with the ears through the Eustachian tubes, and with the pharynx. The receptors which detect smell are in the top of the nasal passage.

nosebleed ['nəʊzbliːd] *noun* epistaxis, bleeding from the nose, usually caused by a blow or by sneezing, by blowing the nose hard or by high blood pressure; *she had a headache, followed by a violent nosebleed*

noso- ['nɒsəʊ] *prefix* referring to diseases

nosocomial [nɒsəʊ'kəʊmiəl] *adjective* referring to hospitals; **nosocomial infection** = infection which is passed on to someone in a hospital

nosology [nɒ'sɒlədʒi] *noun* classification of diseases

nostril ['nɒstrl] *noun* naris, one of the two passages in the nose through which air is breathed in or out; *his right nostril is blocked*

notch [nɒtʃ] *noun* depression on a surface, usually on a bone, but sometimes on an organ; **cardiac notch** = (i) point in the left lung, where the right inside wall is bent; (ii) notch at the point where the oesophagus joins the greater curvature of the stomach; **occipital notch** = point on the lower edge of the cerebral hemisphere, where the surface has a notch

notice ['nəʊtɪs] **1** *noun* **(a)** piece of writing giving information, usually put in a place where everyone can see it; *he pinned up a notice about the meeting; notices warning the public about the dangers of rabies are posted at every port and airport* **(b)** warning; *they had to leave with ten minutes' notice*; **it had to be done at short notice** = with very little warning time **(c)** attention; **take no notice of what he says** = pay no attention to it, don't worry about it; *she took no notice of what the doctor suggested* **2** *verb* to see, to take note of; *nobody noticed that the patient was sweating*; *did you notice the development of any new symptoms?*

noticeable ['nəʊtɪsəbl] *adjective* which can be noticed; *the disease has no easily noticeable symptoms*

noticeboard ['nəʊtɪsbɔːd] *noun* flat piece of wood, etc., on a wall, on which notices can be pinned

notifiable disease ['nəʊtɪfaɪəbl dɪ'ziːz] *noun* serious infectious disease which in Great Britain has to be reported by a doctor to the Department of Health so that steps can be taken to stop it spreading

COMMENT: the following are notifiable diseases: cholera, diphtheria, dysentery, encephalitis, food poisoning, jaundice, malaria, measles, meningitis, ophthalmia neonatorum, paratyphoid, plague, poliomyelitis, relapsing fever, scarlet fever, smallpox, tuberculosis, typhoid, typhus, whooping cough, yellow fever

notify ['nəʊtɪfaɪ] *verb* to inform someone officially; *the local doctor notified the Health Service of the case of cholera* (NOTE: you notify someone of something)

nourish ['nʌrɪʃ] *verb* to give food or nutrients to (someone); **nourishing food** = food (such as liver or brown bread) which supplies nourishment

nourishment ['nʌrɪʃmənt] *noun* (i) act of supplying nutrients; (ii) nutrients (such as proteins, fats or vitamins)

noxious ['nɒkʃəs] *adjective* harmful (drug or gas)

n.p. ['en 'piː] *abbreviation for the Latin phrase* 'nomen proprium': the name of the drug (written on the label of the container)

NPO ['en 'piː 'əʊ] *abbreviation for the Latin phrase* 'nil per oram': nothing by the mouth (used to refer to patients being kept without food); *the patient should be kept NPO for five hours before the operation*

NSAID = NON-STEROIDAL ANTI-INFLAMMATORY DRUG

NSU ['en 'es 'juː] = NON-SPECIFIC URETHRITIS

nucha ['njuːkə] *noun* nape, the back of the neck

nuchal ['njuːkl] *adjective* referring to the nape

nuclear ['njuːklɪə] *adjective* referring to nuclei; **nuclear magnetic resonance (NMR)** = scanning technique, using magnetic fields and radio waves, which reveals abnormalities in soft tissue, body fluids, etc.; *see also* MAGNETIC RESONANCE IMAGING; **nuclear medicine** = use of radioactive substances for detecting and treating disorders; **nuclear radiation**; *see* RADIATION

nuclease ['njuːklɪeɪz] *noun* enzyme which breaks down the nucleic acids

nucleic acids [njuː'kliːɪk 'æsɪdz] *noun* organic acids combined with proteins (DNA or RNA) which exist in the nucleus and protoplasm of all cells

nucleolus [njuː'kliːələs] *noun* structure inside a cell nucleus, containing RNA

nucleoprotein [njuːklɪəu'prəutiːn] *noun* compound of protein and nucleic acid, such as chromosomes or ribosomes

nucleus ['njuːklɪəs] *noun* **(a)** central body in a cell, containing DNA and RNA, and controlling the function and characteristics of the cell **(b)** group of nerve cells in the brain or spinal cord; **basal nuclei** = masses of grey matter at the bottom of each cerebral hemisphere; **nucleus pulposus** = soft central part of an intervertebral disc which disappears in old age; *see illustration at* NEURONE (NOTE: the plural is **nuclei**)

nullipara [nʌ'lɪpərə] *noun & adjective* (woman) who has never had a child

numb [nʌm] *adjective* (limb) which has no feeling; *her fingers were numb with cold*; *the tips of his ears went numb or became numb*

numbness ['nʌmnəs] *noun* loss of feeling

nurse [nɜːs] **1** *noun* person (usually a woman) who looks after sick people in a hospital or helps a doctor in his surgery; *she works as a nurse in the local hospital*; *she's training to be a nurse*; **charge nurse** = nurse who is in charge of a group of patients, a ward or a department in a hospital; **district nurse** *or* **home nurse** = nurse who visits and treats patients in their homes; **escort nurse** = nurse who goes with a patient to the operating theatre and back to the ward; **practice nurse** *or* **nurse practitioner** = nurse employed by a clinic or doctor's practice who can give advice to patients; **staff nurse** = nurse who is on the permanent staff of a hospital; **theatre nurse** = nurse who is specially trained to assist a surgeon

during an operation; **ward nurse** = nurse who works in a hospital ward; **nurse manager** = nurse who has administrative duties in the health service or in a hospital; *see also* ENROLLED NURSE (NOTE: although the term nurse applies to both men and women, in popular speech it is used more frequently to refer to women, and **male nurse** is used for men. Nurse can be used as a title before a name: **Nurse Jones**) **2** *verb* to look after sick people; *when he was ill his mother nursed him until he was better*

COMMENT: in the UK qualified nurses are either ENs (Enrolled Nurses) or RNs (Registered Nurses). Registered nurses follow a three year course and have to pass the ENB examinations before becoming RGN, RMN or RNMH. RSCNs have a further 6 months or 4 term course before they qualify. Enrolled nurses follow 2 year courses

nursery school ['nɜːsəri 'skuːl] *noun* school for little children; **day nursery** = place where small children can be looked after during the daytime, and go home in the evenings

nursing ['nɜːsɪŋ] **1** *noun* work or profession of being a nurse; *she enjoys nursing*; *he is taking a nursing course*; *he has chosen nursing as his career*; **nursing home** = house where convalescents or old people can live under medical supervision by a qualified nurse; **nursing practice** = treatment given by nurses; **nursing process** = standard method of treatment carried out by nurses and its documentation **2** *adjective* providing care as a nurse; **nursing mother** = mother who breast-feeds her baby; **nursing officer** = nurse who has administrative duties in the National Health Service

few would now dispute the need for clear, concise nursing plans to guide nursing practice, provide educational tools and give an accurate legal record

Nursing Times

all relevant sections of the nurses' care plan and nursing process records had been left blank

Nursing Times

nurture ['nɜːtʃə] **1** *noun* sociological factors from the environment affecting personality, behaviour or risk of disease; *see also*

NATURE **2** *verb* to bring up and care for (children)

nutans ['njuːtns] *see* SPASMUS

nutation [njuːˈteɪʃn] *noun* involuntary nodding of the head

nutrient ['njuːtriənt] *noun* substance (such as protein, fat or vitamin) in food which is necessary to provide energy or to help the body grow

nutrition [njuˈtrɪʃn] *noun* (i) study of the supply of nutrients to the body from digesting food; (ii) nourishment or food

nutritional [njuˈtrɪʃnl] *adjective* referring to nutrition; **nutritional anaemia** = anaemia caused by an imbalance in the diet; **nutritional disorder** = disorder (such as obesity) related to food and nutrients

nutritionist [njuˈtrɪʃənɪst] *noun* dietitian, person who specializes in the study of nutrition and advises on diets

nyctalopia [nɪktəˈləʊpiə] *noun* night blindness, being unable to see in bad light

nyctophobia [nɪktəˈfəʊbiə] *noun* fear of the dark

nymphae ['nɪmfiː] *noun* the labia minora, two small fleshy folds at the edge of the vulva

nymphomania [nɪmfəˈmeɪniə] *noun* obsessive sexual urge in a woman (NOTE: in a man, called **satyriasis**)

nymphomaniac [nɪmfəˈmeɪniæk] *noun* woman who has an abnormally obsessive sexual urge

nystagmus [nɪˈstægməs] *noun* rapid, involuntary movement of the eyes up and down or from side to side

COMMENT: nystagmus can be horizontal, vertical, torsional or rotary; it can be congenital, but is also a symptom of multiple sclerosis and Ménière's disease

Oo

O *chemical symbol for* oxygen

oat cell carcinoma [ˈəʊt ˈsel kɑːsɪˈnəʊmə] *noun* type of cancer of the bronchi, with distinctive small cells

OB = OBSTETRICS

obese [əʊˈbiːs] **1** *adjective* (person who is) too fat or too heavy **2** *plural noun* **the obese** = overweight people

obesity [əʊˈbiːsəti] *noun* being overweight

> COMMENT: obesity is caused by excess fat accumulating under the skin and around organs in the body. It is sometimes due to glandular disorders, but it is usually caused by eating or drinking too much. A tendency to obesity can be hereditary

obey [əˈbeɪ] *verb* to do what someone or a rule says you should do; *you ought to obey the doctor's instructions and go to bed*; *patients must obey the hospital rules*

obligate [ˈɒblɪgeɪt] *adjective* (organism) which exists and develops in only one way (as viruses which are parasites only inside cells)

oblique [əˈbliːk] *noun & adjective* (muscle) which lies at an angle; **oblique fissure** = groove between the lobes of the lungs; **oblique fracture** = fracture where the bone is not broken directly across its axis; **oblique muscle** = (i) muscle which controls the eyeball; (ii) muscle which controls the abdominal wall; **external oblique** = outer abdominal muscle; **internal oblique** = muscle covering the abdomen beneath the external oblique

> there are four recti muscles and two oblique muscles in each eye, which coordinate the movement of the eyes and enable them to work as a pair
>
> *Nursing Times*

obliterans [əˈblɪtərns] *see* ENDARTERITIS

obliterate [əˈblɪtəreɪt] *verb* to block a cavity completely

obliteration [əblɪtəˈreɪʃn] *noun* complete blocking (of a cavity, etc.)

oblongata [ɒblɒŋˈgeɪtə] *see* MEDULLA

observation [ɒbzəˈveɪʃn] *noun* examining something over a period of time; *he was admitted to hospital for observation*

observe [əbˈzɜːv] *verb* to notice, to see something and understand it; *the nurses observed signs of improvement in the patient's condition*; *the girl's mother observed symptoms of anorexia and reported them to her doctor*

obsessed [əbˈsest] *adjective* suffering from an obsession; *he is obsessed with the idea that his wife is trying to kill him*

obsession [əbˈseʃn] *noun* mental disorder where the patient has a fixed idea or emotion which he cannot get rid of, even if he knows it is wrong or unpleasant; *she has an obsession about cats*

obsessional [əbˈseʃənl] *adjective* referring to an obsession; *he is suffering from an obsessional disorder*

obsessive [əbˈsesɪv] *adjective* showing an obsession; *he has an obsessive desire to steal little objects*; **obsessive action** = repeated actions (such as washing) which indicate a mental disorder; **obsessive compulsion disorder** = neurotic illness characterized by the need to perform repeated ritual acts, such as checking or cleaning, treated with psychotherapy and antidepressants

obstetric(al) [əbˈstetrɪk *or* əbˈstetrɪkəl] *adjective* referring to obstetrics; **obstetrical forceps** = type of large forceps used to hold a baby's head during childbirth; **obstetric patient** = woman who is being treated by an obstetrician

obstetrician [ɒbstəˈtrɪʃn] *noun* doctor who specializes in obstetrics

obstetrics (OB) [əb'stetrɪks] *noun* branch of medicine and surgery dealing with pregnancy, childbirth and the period immediately after childbirth

obstruct [əb'strʌkt] *verb* to block; *the artery was obstructed by a blood clot*

obstruction [əb'strʌkʃn] *noun* (i) something which blocks (a passage or a blood vessel); (ii) blocking of a passage or blood vessel; **intestinal obstruction** *or* **obstruction of the bowels** = blockage of the intestine; **urinary obstruction** = blockage of the urethra, which prevents urine being passed

obstructive [əb'strʌktɪv] *adjective* caused by an obstruction; **obstructive jaundice** = jaundice caused by an obstruction in the bile ducts; **obstructive lung disease** = bronchitis and emphysema

obtain [əb'teɪn] *verb* to get; *some amino acids are obtained from food; where did he obtain the drugs?*

obtrusive [ɒb'truːsɪv] *adjective* (scar) which is very noticeable

obturator ['ɒbtjʊreɪtə] *noun* (i) one of two muscles in the pelvis which govern the movement of the hip and thigh; (ii) device which closes an opening, such as a dental prosthesis which covers a cleft palate; (iii) metal bulb which fits into a bronchoscope or sigmoidoscope; **obturator foramen** = opening in the hip bone near the acetabulum

obtusion [əb'tjuːʒn] *noun* condition where perception and feelings become dulled

OC = ORAL CONTRACEPTIVE

OCD ['əʊ; 'siː; 'diː] = OBSESSIVE COMPULSION DISORDER

occipital [ɒk'sɪpɪtl] *adjective* referring to the back of the head; **occipital bone** *or* **occipital** = one of the bones in the skull, the bone at the back of the head; **occipital condyle** = round part of the occipital bone which joins it to the atlas; **occipital lobe** = lobe at the back of each cerebral hemisphere; **occipital notch** = point on the lower edge of the cerebral hemisphere where the surface has a notch

occipito-anterior [ɒk'sɪpɪtəʊæn'tɪərɪə] *adjective* (position of a baby at birth) where the baby faces the mother's back

occipito-posterior [ɒk'sɪpɪtəʊpɒ'stɪərɪə] *adjective* (position of a baby at birth) where the baby faces the front

occiput ['ɒksɪpʌt] *noun* lower part of the back of the head or skull

occluded [ə'kluːdɪd] *adjective* closed or blocked

occlusion [ə'kluːʒn] *noun* **(a)** blockage, thing which blocks a passage or which closes an opening; **coronary occlusion** = blood clot in the coronary arteries leading to heart failure **(b)** the way in which the teeth in the upper and lower jaws fit together when the jaws are closed (NOTE: a bad fit between the teeth is a **malocclusion**)

occlusive [ə'kluːsɪv] *adjective* referring to occlusion or to blocking; **occlusive stroke** = stroke caused by a blood clot; **occlusive therapy** = treatment of a squint where the good eye is covered up in order to encourage the squinting eye to become straight

occult [ə'kʌlt] *adjective* (i) not easy to see with the naked eye; (ii) (symptom or sign) which is hidden; **occult blood** = very small quantities of blood in the faeces, which can only be detected by tests (NOTE: the opposite is **overt**)

occulta [ə'kʌltə] *see* SPINA BIFIDA

occupancy rate ['ɒkjʊpənsi 'reɪt] *noun* number of beds occupied in a hospital, shown as a percentage of all the beds

occupation [ɒkjʊ'peɪʃn] *noun* job or work; *what is his occupation?; people in sedentary occupations are liable to digestive disorders*

occupational [ɒkjʊ'peɪʃənl] *adjective* referring to work; **occupational asthma** *or* **occupational dermatitis** = asthma or dermatitis caused by materials with which one comes into contact at work; **occupational disease** = disease which is caused by the type of work or the conditions in which someone works (such as disease caused by dust or chemicals in a factory); **occupational hazard** = dangerous situation related to the working environment; **occupational health (OH) nurse** = nurse who deals with health problems of people at work; **occupational medicine** = part of medicine which looks after accidents and diseases connected with work; **occupational therapist** = qualified therapist who treats people with mental or physical handicaps by using activities such as light work, hobbies, etc.; **occupational therapy** = light work or hobbies used as a means of treatment to promote independence, especially for handicapped or mentally ill patients and during the recovery period after an illness or operation

occur [ə'kɜ:] *verb* to happen, to take place; to be found; *thrombosis occurred in the artery*; *a form of glaucoma which occurs in infants*; *one of the most frequently occurring types of tumour*

occurrence [ə'kʌrəns] *noun* taking place, happening; *neuralgia is a common occurrence after shingles*

ochronosis [ɒkrəu'nəusɪs] *noun* condition where cartilage, ligaments and other fibrous tissue become dark as a result of a metabolic disorder, and also the urine turns black on exposure to air

ocular ['ɒkjulə] *adjective* referring to the eye; *opticians are trained to detect all kinds of ocular imbalance*

oculi ['ɒkjulaɪ] *see* ALBUGINEA, ORBICULARIS

oculist ['ɒkjulɪst] *noun* qualified physician or surgeon who specializes in the treatment of eye disorders

oculo- ['ɒkjuləu] *prefix meaning* eye

oculogyric [ɒkjuləu'dʒɪrɪk] *adjective* which causes eye movements

oculomotor [ɒkjuləu'məutə] *adjective* referring to movements of the eyeball; **oculomotor nerve** = third cranial nerve which controls the eyeball and upper eyelid

oculonasal [ɒkjuləu'neɪzl] *adjective* referring to the eye and the nose

o.d. ['əu 'di:] **(a)** *abbreviation for the Latin phrase* 'omni die': every day (written on a prescription) **(b)** *abbreviation for* overdose

ODA ['əu 'di: 'eɪ] = OPERATING DEPARTMENT ASSISTANT

odont(o)- [ɒdɒnt] *prefix meaning* teeth

odontalgia [ɒdɒn'tældʒə] *noun* toothache

odontitis [ɒdɒn'taɪtɪs] *noun* inflammation of the pulpy interior of a tooth

odontoid process [ɒ'dɒntɔɪd 'prəuses] *noun* projecting part of a vertebra, shaped like a tooth

odontology [ɒdɒn'tɒlədʒi] *noun* study of teeth and associated structures, and their disorders

odontoma *or* **odontome** [ɒdɒn'təumə *or* 'ɒdɒntəum] *noun* **(a)** structure like a tooth which has an abnormal arrangement of its component tissues **(b)** solid or cystic tumour

derived from cells concerned with the development of a tooth

odour *US* **odor** ['əudə] *noun* smell; **body odour** = unpleasant smell caused by perspiration

odourless ['əudələs] *adjective* (liquid, etc.) with no smell

odynophagia [ɒdɪnə'feɪdʒə] *noun* condition where pain occurs when food is swallowed

oe- [i:] (NOTE: words beginning with oe- are written e- in American English)

oedema *US* **edema** [ɪ'di:mə] *noun* dropsy, swelling of part of the body caused by accumulation of fluid in the intercellular tissue spaces; *her main problem is oedema of the feet*; **macular oedema** = disorder of the eye where fluid gathers in the fovea; **pulmonary oedema** = collection of fluid in the lungs as in left-sided heart failure; **subcutaneous oedema** = fluid collecting under the skin, usually at the ankles

oedematous [ɪ'dɪmətəs] *adjective* referring to oedema

Oedipus complex ['i:dɪpəs 'kɒmpleks] *noun; (in psychology)* condition where a boy feels sexually attracted to his mother and sees his father as an obstacle

oesophageal [i:sɒfə'dʒi:əl] *adjective* referring to the oesophagus; **oesophageal hiatus** = opening in the diaphragm through which the oesophagus passes; **oesophageal spasm** = spasm in the oesophagus; **oesophageal ulcer** = ulcer in the oesophagus; **oesophageal varices** = varicose veins in the oesophagus

oesophagectomy [i:sɒfə'dʒektəmi] *noun* surgical removal of part of the oesophagus

oesophagitis [i:sɒfə'dʒaɪtɪs] *noun* inflammation of the oesophagus (caused by acid juices from the stomach or by infection)

oesophagocele [i:'sɒfəgəusi:l] *noun* condition where the mucous membrane lining the oesophagus protrudes through the wall

oesophagoscope [i:'sɒfəgəuskəup] *noun* thin tube with a light at the end, which is passed down the oesophagus to examine it

oesophagoscopy [i:sɒfə'gɒskəpi] *noun* examination of the oesophagus with an oesophagoscope

oesophagostomy [i:sɒfə'gɒstəmi] *noun* surgical operation to make an opening in the oesophagus to allow the patient to be fed, usually after an operation on the pharynx

oesophagotomy [iːsɒfəˈgɒtəmi] *noun* surgical operation to make an opening in the oesophagus to remove something which is blocking it

oesophagus *US* **esophagus** [iˈsɒfəgəs] *noun* tube down which food passes from the pharynx to the stomach; *see illustrations at* STOMACH, THROAT

oestradiol [iːstrəˈdaɪɒl] *noun* type of oestrogen secreted by an ovarian follicle, which stimulates the development of secondary sexual characteristics in females at puberty (a synthetic form is given as treatment for oestrogen deficiency)

oestriol [ˈiːstrɪɒl] *noun* placental hormone with oestrogenic properties, found in the urine of pregnant women

oestrogen [ˈiːstrədʒn] *noun* any substance with the physiological activity of oestradiol

COMMENT: synthetic oestrogens form most oral contraceptives, and are also used in the treatment of menstrual and menopausal disorders

oestrogenic hormone [iːstrəˈdʒenɪk ˈhɔːməʊn] *noun* oestrogen used to treat conditions which develop during menopause

oestrone [ˈiːstrəʊn] *noun* type of oestrogen

official [əˈfɪʃl] *adjective* (i) accepted by an authority; (ii) (drug) which is permitted by an authority

officially [əˈfɪʃli] *adverb* (accepted or permitted) by an authority; *the drug has been officially listed as a dangerous drug*

OH [ˈəʊ ˈeɪtʃ] = OCCUPATIONAL HEALTH; *an OH nurse*

oil [ɔɪl] *noun* liquid which cannot be mixed with water (there are three types: fixed vegetable or animal oils; volatile oils; mineral oils); **cod liver oil** = oil from the liver of the cod fish, which is rich in calories and in vitamins A and D; **essential oils** = oils from scented plants used in cosmetics and as antiseptics; **fixed oil** = oil which is liquid at 20°C

oily [ˈɔɪli] *adjective* containing oil

ointment [ˈɔɪntmənt] *noun* smooth oily medicinal preparation which can be spread on the skin to soothe or to protect; **eye ointment** = ointment in a special tube to be used in eye treatment

oleaginous [əʊlɪˈædʒɪnəs] *adjective* oily; *see also* OLEIC; OLEUM

olecranon (process) [əʊˈlekrənɒn ˈprəʊsəs] *noun* curved process at the end of the ulna (NOTE: called also **funny bone**)

oleic [ˈəʊliːɪk] *adjective* referring to oil; **oleic acid** = one of the fatty acids, present in most oils

oleum [ˈəʊliəm] *noun* (*term used in pharmacy*) oil

olfaction [ɒlˈfækʃn] *noun* (i) sense of smell; (ii) way in which a person's sensory organs detect smells

olfactory [ɒlˈfæktəri] *adjective* referring to the sense of smell; **olfactory area** = part of the brain that registers smell; **olfactory bulb** = end of the olfactory tract, where the processes of the sensory cells in the nose are linked to the fibres of the olfactory nerve; **olfactory nerve** = first cranial nerve which controls the sense of smell; **olfactory tract** = nerve tract which takes the olfactory nerve from the nose to the brain

olig- *or* **oligo-** [ˈɒlɪg *or* ˈɒlɪgəʊ] *prefix* meaning few or little

oligaemia [ɒlɪˈgiːmiə] *noun* condition where the patient has too little blood in his circulatory system

oligodactylism [ɒlɪgəʊˈdæktɪlɪzm] *noun* congenital condition where a baby is born without some fingers or toes

oligodipsia [ɒlɪgəʊˈdɪpsiə] *noun* condition where a patient does not want to drink

oligodontia [ɒlɪgəʊˈdɒnʃə] *noun* state in which most of the teeth are lacking

oligohydramnios [ɒlɪgəʊhaɪˈdræmniəs] *noun* condition where the amnion surrounding the fetus contains too little amniotic fluid

oligomenorrhoea [ɒlɪgəʊmenəˈriːə] *noun* condition where the patient menstruates infrequently

oligospermia [ɒlɪgəʊˈspɜːmiə] *noun* condition where there are too few spermatozoa in the semen

oliguria [ɒlɪˈgjʊəriə] *noun* condition where the patient does not produce enough urine

olive [ˈɒlɪv] *noun* (**a**) fruit of a tree, which gives an edible oil (**b**) swelling containing grey matter, on the side of the pyramid of the medulla oblongata

-olol [ˈɒlɒl] *suffix* used for beta blockers; *atenolol*; *propranolol hydrochloride*

o.m. ['əʊ 'em] *abbreviation for the Latin phrase* 'omni mane': every morning (written on a prescription)

-oma ['əʊmə] *suffix* meaning tumour (NOTE: plural is **-omata**)

Ombudsman ['ɒmbʊdzmən] *see* HEALTH SERVICE COMMISSIONER

oment- [əʊ'ment] *prefix* referring to the omentum

omental [əʊ'mentl] *adjective* referring to the omentum

omentectomy [əʊmen'tektəmi] *noun* surgical removal of part of the omentum

omentopexy [əʊ'mentəpeksi] *noun* surgical operation to attach the omentum to the abdominal wall

omentum [əʊ'mentəm] *noun* epiploon, double fold of peritoneum hanging down over the intestines (NOTE: the plural is **omenta**. Note that for other terms referring to the omentum see words beginning with **epiplo-**)

COMMENT: the omentum is in two sections: the greater omentum which covers the intestines, and the lesser omentum which hangs between the liver and the stomach and the liver and the duodenum

omphal- ['ɒmfəl] *prefix* referring to the navel

omphalitis [ɒmfə'laɪtɪs] *noun* inflammation of the navel

omphalocele ['ɒmfələsi:l] *noun* hernia where part of the intestine protrudes through the abdominal wall near the navel

omphalus ['ɒmfələs] *noun* navel or umbilicus, scar with a depression in the middle of the abdomen where the umbilical cord was detached after birth

-omycin [əʊ'maɪsɪn] *suffix* used in names of macrolide drugs; *erythromycin*

o.n. ['əʊ 'en] *abbreviation for the Latin phrase* 'omni nocte': every night (written on a prescription)

onanism ['əʊnənɪzm] *noun* masturbation

Onchocerca [ɒŋkəʊ'sɜːkə] *noun* genus of tropical parasitic threadworm

onchocerciasis [ɒŋkəʊsɜː'kaɪəsɪs] *noun* infestation with *Onchocerca* where the larvae can move into the eye, causing river blindness

onco- ['ɒŋkəʊ] *prefix* referring to tumours

oncogene ['ɒŋkədʒiːn] *noun* part of the genetic system which causes malignant tumours to develop

all cancers may be reduced to fundamental mechanisms based on cancer risk genes or oncogenes within ourselves. An oncogene is a gene that encodes a protein that contributes to the malignant phenotype of the cell
British Medical Journal

oncogenesis [ɒŋkə'dʒenəsɪs] *noun* origin and development of a tumour

oncogenic [ɒŋkə'dʒenɪk] *adjective* (substance or virus) which causes tumours to develop

oncologist [ɒŋ'kɒlədʒɪst] *noun* doctor who specializes in oncology, especially cancer

oncology [ɒŋ'kɒlədʒi] *noun* scientific study of new growths

oncolysis [ɒŋ'kɒlɪsɪs] *noun* destruction of a tumour or of tumour cells

oncotic [ɒŋ'kɒtɪk] *adjective* referring to a tumour

onset ['ɒnset] *noun* beginning; *the onset of the illness is marked by sudden high temperature*

a follow-up study of 84 patients with early onset pre-eclampsia (before 37 weeks' gestation) showed a high prevalence of renal disease
British Medical Journal

ontogeny [ɒn'tɒdʒəni] *noun* origin and development of an individual organism

onych- [ɒnɪk] *prefix* referring to nails

onychauxis [ɒnɪ'kɔːksɪs] *noun* overgrowth of the nails of the fingers or toes

onychia [ɒ'nɪkiə] *noun* abnormality of the nails, caused by inflammation of the matrix

onychogryphosis [ɒnɪkəʊgrɪ'fəʊsɪs] *noun* condition where the nails are bent or curved over the ends of the fingers or toes

onycholysis [ɒnɪ'kɒləsɪs] *noun* condition where a nail becomes separated from its bed, without falling out

onychomadesis [ɒnɪkəʊmə'diːsɪs] *noun* condition where the nails fall out

onychomycosis [ɒnɪkəʊmaɪ'kəʊsɪs] *noun* infection of the nail with a fungus

onychosis [ɒnɪ'kəʊsɪs] *noun* any disease of the nails

o'nyong-nyong fever [əʊniˈɒŋniɒŋ ˈfiːvə] *noun* infectious virus disease prevalent in East Africa, spread by mosquitoes (NOTE: also called **joint-breaker fever**)

COMMENT: the symptoms are high fever, inflammation of the lymph nodes and excruciating pains in the joints

oo- [ˈəʊə] *prefix* referring to an ovum or to an embryo

oocyesis [əʊəsaɪˈiːsɪs] *noun* pregnancy which develops in the ovary

oocyte [ˈəʊəsaɪt] *noun* cell which forms from an oogonium and becomes an ovum by meiosis

oogenesis [əʊəˈdʒenəsɪs] *noun* formation and development of ova

oogenetic [əʊədʒəˈnetɪk] *adjective* referring to oogenesis

oogonium [əʊəˈgəʊniəm] *noun* cell produced at the beginning of the development of an ovum (NOTE: the plural is **oogonia**)

COMMENT: in oogenesis, an oogonium produces an oocyte which develops through several stages to produce a mature ovum. Polar bodies are also formed which do not develop into ova

oopho- or **oophoro-** [ˈəʊəfəʊ or əʊˈɒfərəʊ] *prefix* referring to the ovaries

oophoralgia [əʊəfəˈrældʒə] *noun* pain in the ovaries

oophorectomy [əʊəfəˈrektəmi] *noun* ovariectomy, the surgical removal of an ovary

oophoritis [əʊəfəˈraɪtɪs] *noun* ovaritis, inflammation in an ovary, which can be caused by mumps

oophoroma [əʊəfəˈrəʊmə] *noun* rare ovarian tumour, occurring in middle age

oophoron [əʊˈɒfərɒn] *noun* an ovary, one of two organs in a woman which produce ova or egg cells and secrete the female hormone oestrogen

oophoropexy [əʊˈɒfərəpeksi] *noun* surgical operation to attach an ovary

oophorosalpingectomy [əʊɒfərəsælpɪnˈdʒektəmi] *noun* surgical removal of an ovary and the Fallopian tube attached to it

ooze [uːz] *verb* (*of pus or blood*) to flow slowly

OP [ˈəʊ ˈpiː] = OUTPATIENT

opacification [əˈpæsɪfɪkeɪʃn] *noun* becoming opaque (such as the lens in a case of cataract)

opacity [əʊˈpæsəti] *noun* (i) not allowing light to pass through; (ii) area in the eye which is not clear

opaque [əʊˈpeɪk] *adjective* not transparent; **radio-opaque dye** = liquid which appears on an X-ray, and which is introduced into soft organs (such as the kidney) so that they show up clearly on an X-ray photograph

open [ˈəʊpən] *adjective* not closed; **open fracture** = compound fracture, fracture where the skin surface is damaged or where the broken bone penetrates the surface of the skin; **open-heart surgery** = surgery to repair part of the heart or one of the coronary arteries, performed while the heart has been bypassed and the blood is circulated by a pump; **open visiting** = arrangement in a hospital where visitors can enter the wards at any time

opening [ˈəʊpnɪŋ] *noun* place where something opens

operable [ˈɒpərəbl] *adjective* (condition) which can be treated by an operation; *the cancer is still operable*

operate [ˈɒpəreɪt] *verb* (a) to operate on a patient = to treat a patient's condition by cutting open his body and removing a part which is diseased or repairing a part which is not functioning correctly; *the patient was operated on yesterday*; *the surgeons decided to operate as the only way of saving the baby's life*

operating [ˈɒpəreɪtɪŋ] *adjective & noun* (a) **operating department assistant (ODA)** = nurse working in the operating department; **operating microscope** = special microscope with two eyepieces and a light, used in very delicate surgery; **operating table** = special table on which the patient is placed to undergo a surgical operation; **operating theatre**, *US* **operating room (OR)** = special room in a hospital where surgeons carry out operations (b) **operating gene** = the gene in an operon which regulates the functions of the others

operation [ɒpəˈreɪʃn] *noun* (i) way in which a drug acts; (ii) surgical intervention, act of cutting open a patient's body to treat a disease or disorder; *she's had an operation on her foot*; *the operation to remove the cataract was successful*; *a team of surgeons* *performed the operation*; *heart operations are always difficult* (NOTE: a surgeon **performs** an operation **on** a patient)

operative ['ɒpərətɪv] *adjective* peroperative, taking place during a surgical operation; *see also* POSTOPERATIVE, PREOPERATIVE

operator ['ɒpəreɪtə] *noun* surgeon who operates; **operator gene** = OPERATING GENE

operculum [ə'pɜːkjʊləm] *noun* (i) part of the cerebral hemisphere which overlaps the insula; (ii) plug of mucus which can block the cervical canal during pregnancy

operon ['ɒpərɒn] *noun* group of genes which controls the production of enzymes

ophth- [ɒfθ or ɒpθ] *prefix* referring to the eye

ophthalmectomy [ɒfθæl'mektəmi] *noun* surgical removal of an eye

ophthalmia [ɒf'θælmiə] *noun* inflammation of the eye; **ophthalmia neonatorum** = conjunctivitis of a newborn baby, beginning 21 days after birth, caused by infection in the birth canal; **Egyptian ophthalmia** = trachoma, virus disease of the eyes, common in tropical countries

ophthalmic [ɒf'θælmɪk] *adjective* referring to the eye; **ophthalmic practitioner** = optician, qualified person who specializes in testing eyes and prescribing lenses; **ophthalmic surgeon** = surgeon who specializes in surgery to treat eye disorders; **ophthalmic nerve** = branch of the trigeminal nerve, supplying the eyeball, the upper eyelid, the brow and one side of the scalp

ophthalmitis [ɒfθæl'maɪtɪs] *noun* inflammation of the eye

ophthalmological [ɒfθælmə'lɒdʒɪkl] *adjective* referring to ophthalmology

ophthalmologist [ɒfθæl'mɒlədʒɪst] *noun* doctor who specializes in the study of the eye and its diseases

ophthalmology [ɒfθæl'mɒlədʒi] *noun* study of the eye and its diseases

ophthalmoplegia [ɒfθælmə'pliːdʒə] *noun* paralysis of the muscles of the eye

ophthalmoscope [ɒf'θælməskəʊp] *noun* instrument containing a bright light and small lenses, used by a doctor to examine the inside of an eye

ophthalmoscopy [ɒfθæl'mɒskəpi] *noun* examination of the inside of an eye using an ophthalmoscope

ophthalmotomy [ɒfθæl'mɒtəmi] *noun* surgical operation to make a cut in the eyeball

ophthalmotonometer [ɒfθælmətə'nɒmɪtə] *noun* tonometer, instrument which measures pressure inside the eye

-opia ['əʊpiə] *suffix* referring to a defect in the eye; **myopia** = being shortsighted

opiate ['əʊpiət] *noun* sedative which is prepared from opium, such as morphine or codeine

opinion [ə'pɪnjən] *noun* what someone thinks about something; *what's the surgeon's opinion of the case?*; *the doctor asked the consultant for his opinion as to the best method of treatment*; *she has a very high or very low opinion of her doctor* = she thinks he is very good or very bad; **to ask for a second opinion** = to ask another doctor or consultant to examine a patient and give his opinion on diagnosis or treatment

opioid ['əʊpiɔɪd] *adjective* based on opium; *codeine is an opioid analgesic*

opium ['əʊpiəm] *noun* substance made from poppies, used in the preparation of codeine and heroin

opponens [ə'pəʊnəns] *noun* muscles of the fingers which tend to draw these fingers opposite to other fingers; *see* OPPOSITION

opportunist(ic) [ɒpə'tjuːnɪst or ɒpətjuː'nɪstɪk] *adjective* (parasite or microbe) which takes advantage of the host's weakened state to cause infection

opposition [ɒpə'zɪʃn] *noun* movement of the hand muscles where the tip of the thumb is made to touch the tip of another finger so as to hold something

opsonic index [ɒp'sɒnɪk 'ɪndeks] *noun* number which gives the strength of an individual's serum reaction to bacteria

opsonin ['ɒpsənɪn] *noun* substance, usually an antibody, in blood which sticks to the surface of bacteria and helps to destroy them

optic ['ɒptɪk] *adjective* referring to the eye or to sight; **optic chiasma** = structure where some of the optic nerves from each eye partially cross each other in the hypothalamus; **optic disc** *or* **optic papilla** = point on the retina where the optic nerve starts; **optic nerve** = second cranial nerve which transmits the sensation of sight from the eye to the brain; *see illustration at* EYE; **optic neuritis** = inflammation of the optic nerve, which makes objects appear blurred; **optic radiations** = nerve tracts which take the optic impulses from the optic tracts to the visual cortex; **optic tracts** = nerve tracts which take the optic nerves from the optic chiasma to the optic radiations

optical [ˈɒptɪkl] *adjective* referring to optics; **optical illusion** = something which is seen wrongly so that it appears to be something else

optician [ɒpˈtɪʃn] *noun* **dispensing optician** = person who fits and sells glasses but does not test eyes; **ophthalmic optician** = qualified person who specializes in making glasses and in testing eyes and prescribing lenses (NOTE: in American English an **optician** is a technician who makes lenses and fits glasses, but cannot test patient's eyesight)

COMMENT: in the UK qualified ophthalmic opticians must be registered by the General Optical Council before they can practise

optics [ˈɒptɪks] *noun* study of light rays and sight; **fibre optics** = *see* FIBRE

optometer [ɒpˈtɒmɪtə] = REFRACTOMETER

optometrist [ɒpˈtɒmətrɪst] *noun mainly US* person who specializes in testing eyes and prescribing lenses

optometry [ɒpˈtɒmətri] *noun* testing of eyes and prescribing of lenses to correct defects in sight

-oquine [ɒkwɪn] *suffix* used for antimalarial drugs; *chloroquine*

OR [ˈəʊ ˈɑː] *US* = OPERATING ROOM; *an OR nurse*

oral [ˈɔːrəl] *adjective* referring to the mouth; **oral cavity** = the mouth; **oral contraceptive** = contraceptive pill which is swallowed; **oral hygiene** = keeping the mouth clean by gargling and mouthwashes; **oral medication** = medicine which is taken by swallowing; **oral thermometer** = thermometer which is put into the mouth to take a patient's temperature

orally [ˈɔːrəli] *adverb* (medicine taken) by the mouth; *the lotion cannot be taken orally*; *compare* PARENTERAL

orbicularis [ɔːbɪkjuˈleərɪs] *adjective* circular muscle in the face; **orbicularis oculi** = muscle which opens and closes the eye;

orbicularis oris = muscle which closes the lips tight

orbit [ˈɔːbɪt] *noun* eye socket, the hollow bony depression in the front of the skull in which each eye and lacrimal gland are situated; *see illustration at* SKULL

orbital [ˈɔːbɪtl] *adjective* referring to the orbit

orchi- [ˈɔːkɪ] *prefix* referring to the testes

orchidalgia [ɔːkɪˈdældʒə] *noun* neuralgic-type pain in a testis

orchidectomy [ɔːkɪˈdektəmi] *noun* surgical removal of a testis

orchidopexy *or* **orchiopexy** [ˈɔːkɪdəʊpeksi or ɔːkiəʊˈpeksi] *noun* surgical operation to place an undescended testis in the scrotum

orchidotomy [ɔːkɪˈdɒtəmi] *noun* surgical operation to make a cut into a testis

orchis [ˈɔːkɪs] *noun* testis

orchitis [ɔːˈkaɪtɪs] *noun* inflammation of the testes, characterized by hypertrophy, pain and a sensation of weight

orderly [ˈɔːdəli] *noun* person who does general work; **hospital orderly** = person who does heavy work in a hospital, such as wheeling patients into the operating theatre, moving equipment about, etc.

organ [ˈɔːgən] *noun* part of the body which is distinct from other parts and has a particular function (such as the liver, an eye, the ovaries, etc.); **organ of Corti** *or* **spiral organ** = membrane in the cochlea which takes sounds and converts them into impulses sent to the brain along the auditory nerve; **organ transplant** = transplanting of an organ from one person to another

organic [ɔːˈgænɪk] *adjective* **(a)** referring to organs in the body; **organic disorder** = disorder caused by changes in body tissue or in an organ **(b)** (i) (substance) which comes from an animal or plant; (ii) (food) which has been cultivated naturally, without any chemical fertilizers or pesticides

organically [ɔːˈgænɪkli] *adverb* (food) grown using natural fertilizers and not chemicals

organism [ˈɔːgənɪzm] *noun* any single living plant, animal, bacterium or fungus

organotherapy [ɔːgənəʊˈθerəpi] *noun* treatment of a disease by using an extract from the organ of an animal (such as using liver extract to treat anaemia)

orgasm ['ɔːgæzm] *noun* climax of the sexual act, when a person experiences a moment of great excitement

oriental sore [ɔːri'entl 'sɔː] *noun* Leishmaniasis, skin disease of tropical countries caused by the parasite *Leishmania*

orifice ['ɒrəfis] *noun* opening; **cardiac orifice** = opening where the oesophagus joins the stomach; **ileocaecal orifice** = opening where the small intestine joins the large intestine; **pyloric orifice** = opening where the stomach joins the duodenum

origin ['ɒridʒin] *noun* place where a muscle is attached, where the branch of a nerve or blood vessel begins

original [ə'ridʒənl] *adjective* as in the first place; *the surgeon was able to move the organ back to its original position*

originate [ə'ridʒəneit] *verb* to start (in a place); to begin, to make something begin; *the treatment originated in China; drugs which originated in the tropics*

oris ['ɔːris] *see* CANCRUM ORIS, ORBICULARIS ORIS

ornithine ['ɔːniθain] *noun* amino acid produced by the liver

ornithosis [ɔːni'θəusis] *noun* disease of birds which can be passed to humans as a form of pneumonia; *see also* PSITTACOSIS

oropharynx ['ɔːrəufærɪŋks] *noun* part of the pharynx below the soft palate at the back of the mouth

ortho- ['ɔːθəu] *prefix* meaning correct or straight

orthodiagraph [ɔːθəu'daiəgrɑːf] *noun* X-ray photograph of an organ taken using only a thin stream of X-rays which allows accurate measurements of the organ to be made

orthodontic [ɔːθəu'dɒntik] *adjective* which corrects badly formed or placed teeth; referring to orthodontics; *he had to undergo a course of orthodontic treatment*

orthodontics *US* **orthodontia** [ɔːθə'dɒntiks or ɔːθə'dɒnʃə] *noun* branch of dentistry which deals with correcting badly placed teeth

orthodontist [ɔːθə'dɒntist] *noun* dental surgeon who specializes in correcting badly placed teeth

orthopaedic [ɔːθə'piːdik] *adjective* which corrects badly formed or damaged bones or joints; referring to or used in orthopaedics; **orthopaedic collar** = special strong collar to support the head of a patient with neck injuries or a condition such as cervical spondylosis; **orthopaedic hospital** = hospital which specializes in operations to correct badly formed joints or bones; **orthopaedic surgeon** = surgeon who specializes in orthopaedics

orthopaedics [ɔːθə'piːdiks] *noun* branch of surgery dealing with abnormalities, diseases and injuries of the locomotor system

orthopaedist [ɔːθə'piːdist] *noun* surgeon who specializes in orthopaedics

orthopnoea [ɔːθəp'niə] *noun* condition where the patient has great difficulty in breathing while lying down; *see also* DYSPNOEA

orthopnoeic [ɔːθəp'niːik] *adjective* referring to orthopnoea

orthopsychiatry [ɔːθəusai'kaiətri] *noun* science and treatment of behavioural and personality disorders

orthoptics [ɔː'θɒptiks] *noun* methods used to treat squints

orthoptist [ɔː'θɒptist] *noun* eye specialist working in an eye hospital, who treats squints and other disorders of eye movement

orthosis [ɔː'θəusis] *noun* device which is fitted to the outside of the body to support a weakness or correct a deformity (such as a surgical collar, leg braces, etc.) (NOTE: plural is **orthoses**)

orthostatic [ɔːθə'stætik] *adjective* referring to the position of the body when standing up straight; **orthostatic hypotension** = common condition where the blood pressure drops when someone stands up suddenly, causing dizziness

orthotist ['ɔːθətist] *noun* qualified person who fits orthoses

Ortolani's sign [ɔːtə'lɑːniz 'sain] *noun* test for congenital dislocation of the hip, where the hip makes a clicking noise if the joint is rotated

os [ɒs] *Latin noun* **(a)** bone (NOTE: plural is **ossa**) **(b)** mouth (NOTE: plural is **ora**)

osculum ['ɒskjuləm] *noun* small opening or pore

-osis ['əusis] *suffix* referring to disease

Osler's nodes ['ɒsləz 'nəudz] *noun* tender swellings at the ends of fingers and toes in patients suffering from subacute bacterial endocarditis

osmoreceptor [ɒzməʊrɪ'septə] *noun* cell in the hypothalamus which checks the level of osmotic pressure in the blood by altering the secretion of ADH and regulates the amount of water in the blood

osmosis [ɒz'məʊsɪs] *noun* movement of solvent from one part of the body through a semipermeable membrane to another part where there is a higher concentration of molecules

osmotic pressure [ɒz'mɒtɪk 'preʃə] *noun* pressure required to stop the flow of the solvent through a membrane

osseous ['ɒsiəs] *adjective* bony, referring to bones; **osseous labyrinth** = hard part of the temporal bone surrounding the inner ear

ossicle ['ɒsɪkl] *noun* small bone; **auditory ossicles** = three little bones (the malleus, the incus and the stapes) in the middle ear

COMMENT: the auditory ossicles pick up the vibrations from the eardrum and transmit them through the oval window to the cochlea in the inner ear. The three bones are articulated together; the stapes is attached to the membrane of the oval window, and the malleus to the eardrum, and the incus lies between the other two

ossification [ɒsɪfɪ'keɪʃn] *noun* osteogenesis, formation of bone

ossium ['ɒsiəm] *see* FRAGILITAS

ost- *or* **osteo-** [ɒst *or* 'ɒstiəʊ] *prefix* referring to bone

osteitis [ɒsti'aɪtɪs] *noun* inflammation of a bone due to injury or infection; **osteitis deformans** = Paget's disease, a disease which gradually softens bones in the spine, legs and skull, so that they become curved; **osteitis fibrosis cystica** = generalized weakness of bones, associated with formation of cysts, where bone tissue is replaced by fibrous tissue, caused by excessive activity of the thyroid gland (the localized form is osteitis fibrosis localista)

osteoarthritis *or* **osteoarthrosis** [ɒstiəʊɑː'θraɪtɪs *or* ɒstiəʊɑː'θrəʊsɪs] *noun* chronic degenerative arthritic disease of middle-aged and elderly people, where the joints are inflamed and become stiff and painful

osteoarthropathy [ɒstiəʊɑː'θrɒpəθi] *noun* disease of the bone and cartilage at a joint, particularly the ankles, knees or wrists, associated with carcinoma of the bronchi

osteoarthrosis [ɒstiəʊɑː'θrəʊsɪs] *noun* = OSTEOARTHRITIS

osteoarthrotomy [ɒstiəʊɑː'θrɒtəmi] *noun* surgical removal of the articular end of a bone

osteoblast ['ɒstiəʊblæst] *noun* cell in an embryo which forms bone

osteochondritis [ɒstiəʊkɒn'draɪtɪs] *noun* degeneration of epiphyses; **osteochondritis dissecans** = painful condition where pieces of articular cartilage become detached from the joint surface

osteochondroma [ɒstiəʊkɒn'drəʊmə] *noun* tumour containing both bony and cartilaginous cells

osteoclasia *or* **osteoclasis** [ɒstiəʊ'kleɪziə *or* ɒsti'ɒkləsɪs] *noun* (i) destruction of bone tissue by osteoclasts; (ii) surgical operation to fracture or refracture bone to correct a deformity

osteoclast ['ɒstiəʊklæst] *noun* **(a)** cell which destroys bone **(b)** surgical instrument for breaking bones

osteoclastoma [ɒstiəʊklæ'stəʊmə] *noun* usually benign tumour occurring at the ends of long bones

osteocyte ['ɒstiəʊsaɪt] *noun* bone cell

osteodystrophia *or* **osteodystrophy** [ɒstiəʊdɪ'strəʊfiə *or* ɒstiəʊ'dɪstrəfi] *noun* bone disease, especially one caused by disorder of the metabolism

osteogenesis [ɒstiəʊ'dʒenəsɪs] *noun* formation of bone; **osteogenesis imperfecta** = congenital condition where bones are brittle and break easily due to abnormal bone formation (NOTE: also called **fragilitas ossium**)

osteogenic [ɒstiəʊ'dʒenɪk] *adjective* made of bone tissue, starting from bone tissue

osteology [ɒsti'ɒlədʒi] *noun* study of bones and their structure

osteolysis [ɒsti'ɒlɪsɪs] *noun* (i) destruction of bone tissue by osteoclasts; (ii) removal of bone calcium

osteolytic [ɒstiəʊ'lɪtɪk] *adjective* referring to osteolysis

osteoma [ɒsti'əʊmə] *noun* benign tumour in a bone

osteomalacia [ɒstiəʊmə'leɪʃiə] *noun* condition in adults, where the bones become soft because of lack of calcium and vitamin D, or limited exposure to sunlight

osteomyelitis [ɒstɪəʊmaɪəˈlaɪtɪs] *noun* inflammation of the interior of bone, especially the marrow spaces

osteon [ˈɒstɪɒn] *noun* = HAVERSIAN SYSTEM

osteopath [ˈɒstɪəpæθ] *noun* person who practises osteopathy

osteopathy [ɒstɪˈɒpəθi] *noun* (i) way of treating diseases and disorders by massage and manipulation of bones and joints; (ii) any disease of bone

osteopetrosis [ɒstɪəʊpəˈtrəʊsɪs] *noun* marble bone disease, disease where bones become condensed

osteophony [ɒstɪˈɒfəni] *see* CONDUCTION

osteophyte [ˈɒstɪəʊfaɪt] *noun* bony growth

osteoplasty [ˈɒstɪəʊplæsti] *noun* plastic surgery on bones

osteoporosis [ɒstɪəʊpɔːˈrəʊsɪs] *noun* condition where the bones become thin, porous and brittle, due to low levels of oestrogen, lack of calcium and lack of physical exercise

COMMENT: osteoporosis mainly affects post-menopausal women, increasing the risk of fractures; hormone replacement therapy is the most effective method of preventing osteoporosis

osteosarcoma [ɔːstɪəʊsɑːˈkəʊmə] *noun* malignant tumour of bone cells

osteosclerosis [ɒstɪəʊskləˈrəʊsɪs] *noun* condition where the bony spaces become hardened as a result of chronic inflammation

osteotome [ˈɒstɪəʊtəʊm] *noun* type of chisel used by surgeons to cut bone

osteotomy [ɒstɪˈɒtəmi] *noun* surgical operation to cut a bone, especially to relieve pain in a joint

ostium [ˈɒstɪəm] *noun* opening into a passage

-ostomy [ˈɒstəmi] *suffix* referring to an operation to make an opening

ostomy [ˈɒstəmi] *noun* (*informal*) colostomy or ileostomy

OT [ˈəʊ ˈtiː] = OCCUPATIONAL THERAPIST

ot- *or* **oto-** [əʊt *or* ˈəʊtəʊ] *prefix* referring to the ear

otalgia [əʊˈtældʒə] *noun* earache, pain in the ear

OTC [ˈəʊ ˈtiː ˈsiː] *abbreviation* 'over the counter': (drug) which can be bought freely at the chemist's shop, and does not need a prescription

otic [ˈəʊtɪk] *adjective* referring to the ear

otitis [əʊˈtaɪtɪs] *noun* inflammation of the ear; **otitis externa** *or* **external otitis** = any inflammation of the external auditory meatus to the eardrum; **otitis interna** = labyrinthitis, inflammation of the inner ear; **otitis media** = tympanitis, inflammation of the middle ear; **secretory otitis media** = glue ear, a condition where fluid forms behind the eardrum and causes deafness; *see also* PANOTITIS

otolaryngologist [əʊtəlærɪŋˈgɒlədʒɪst] *noun* doctor who specializes in treatment of diseases of the ear and throat

otolaryngology [əʊtəlærɪŋˈgɒlədʒi] *noun* study of diseases of the ear and throat

otolith [ˈəʊtəlɪθ] *noun* (i) stone which forms in the inner ear; (ii) tiny piece of calcium carbonate attached to the hair cells in the saccule and utricle of the inner ear; **otolith organs** = two pairs of sensory organs (the saccule and the utricle) in the inner ear which pass information to the brain about the position of the head

otologist [əʊˈtɒlədʒɪst] *noun* doctor who specializes in the study of the ear

otology [əʊˈtɒlədʒi] *noun* scientific study of the ear and its diseases

otomycosis [əʊtəmaɪˈkəʊsɪs] *noun* infection of the external auditory meatus by a fungus

otoplasty [ˈəʊtəplæsti] *noun* plastic surgery of the external ear to repair damage or deformity

otorhinolaryngologist [əʊtəraɪnəʊlærɪŋˈgɒlədʒɪst] *noun* ENT specialist, doctor who specializes in the study of the ear, nose and throat

otorhinolaryngology (ENT) [əʊtəraɪnəʊlærɪŋˈgɒlədʒi] *noun* study of the ear, nose and throat

otorrhagia [əʊtəˈreɪdʒə] *noun* bleeding from the external ear

otorrhoea [əʊtəˈriːə] *noun* discharge of pus from the ear

otosclerosis [əʊtəskləˈrəʊsɪs] *noun* condition where the ossicles in the middle ear become thicker, the stapes becomes fixed to the oval window, and the patient becomes deaf

otoscope ['əutəskəup] = AURISCOPE

outbreak ['autbreik] *noun* series of cases of a disease which start suddenly; *there is an outbreak of typhoid fever or a typhoid outbreak in the town*

outcome ['autkʌm] *noun* a measure of the result of an intervention or treatment, such as the mortality rate following different methods of surgery

outer ['autə] *adjective* (part) which is outside; **outer ear** = pinna, the part of the ear on the outside of the head, with a channel leading to the eardrum; **outer pleura** = membrane attached to the diaphragm and covering the chest cavity (NOTE: opposite is **inner**)

outlet ['autlet] *noun* opening or channel through which something can go out; **thoracic outlet** = large opening at the base of the thorax

out of hours ['aut əv 'auəz] *adverb* not during the normal opening hours of a doctor's surgery; *there is a special telephone number if you need to call the doctor out of hours*

outpatient ['autpeiʃənt] *noun* patient living at home, who comes to the hospital for treatment; *she goes for treatment as an outpatient*; **outpatient department** *or* **outpatients' department** *or* **clinic** = department of a hospital which deals with outpatients; *he cut his hand badly in the accident and the police took him to the outpatients' department to have it* dressed; *25 patients were selected from the outpatient department for testing*; *see also* INPATIENT

outreach ['autriːtʃ] *noun* services provided for patients or the public in general, outside a hospital, clinic or local government department

ov- *or* **ovar-** ['əuv *or* 'əuvər] *prefix* referring to the ovaries

ova ['əuvə] *see* OVUM

oval window ['əuvəl 'windəu] *noun* the fenestra ovalis, oval opening between the middle ear and the inner ear; *see illustration at* EAR

ovaralgia *or* **ovarialgia** [əuvə'rældʒə *or* əuveəri'ældʒə] *noun* pain in the ovaries

ovarian [əu'veəriən] *adjective* referring to the ovaries; **ovarian cyst** = cyst which develops in the ovaries; **ovarian follicle** = cell which contains an ovum (NOTE: also called **Graafian follicle**)

ovariectomy [əuveəri'ektəmi] *noun* oophorectomy, surgical removal of an ovary

ovariocele [əu'veəriəusiːl] *noun* hernia of an ovary

ovariotomy [əuveəri'ɒtəmi] *noun* surgical removal of an ovary or a tumour in an ovary

ovaritis [əuvə'raitis] *noun* oophoritis, inflammation of an ovary or both ovaries

ovary ['əuvəri] *noun* one of two organs in a woman, which produce ova or egg cells and secrete the female hormone oestrogen; *see illustration at* UROGENITAL SYSTEM (female) (NOTE: for other terms referring to ovaries, see words beginning with **oophor-**)

over- ['əuvə] *prefix* too much

overbite ['əuvəbait] *noun* normal formation of the teeth, where the top incisors come down over and in front of the bottom incisors when the jaws are closed

overcome [əuvə'kʌm] *verb* **(a)** to fight something and win; *she overcame her disabilities and now leads a normal life* **(b)** to make someone lose consciousness; *two people were overcome by smoke in the fire* (NOTE: **overcoming - overcame - has overcome**)

overcompensate [əuvə'kɒmpənseit] *verb* to try to cover the effects of a handicap by making too strenuous efforts

overdo [əuvə'duː] *verb* (*informal*) **to overdo it** *or* **to overdo things** = to work too hard, to do too much exercise; *she overdid it, working until 9 o'clock every evening*; *he has been overdoing things and has to rest* (NOTE: **overdoing - overdid - has overdone**)

overdose ['əuvədəus] *noun* dose (of a drug) which is larger than normal; *she went into a coma after an overdose of heroin or after a heroin overdose*

overeating [əuvə'riːtiŋ] *noun* eating too much food

overexertion [əuvərig'zɜːʃn] *noun* doing too much physical work, taking too much exercise

overgrow [əuvə'grəu] *verb* to grow over a tissue

overgrowth ['əuvəgrəuθ] *noun* growth of tissue over another tissue

overjet [ˈəʊvədʒet] *noun* space which separates the top incisors from the bottom incisors when the jaws are closed

overlap [əʊvəˈlæp] *verb (of bandages, etc.)* to lie partly on top of another

overprescribe [əʊvəprɪˈskraɪb] *verb* to issue too many prescriptions; *some doctors seriously overprescribe tranquillizers*

overproduction [əʊvəprəˈdʌkʃn] *noun* producing too much; *the condition is caused by overproduction of thyroxine by the thyroid gland*

oversew [ˈəʊvəsəʊ] *verb* to sew a patch of tissue over a perforation (NOTE: **oversewing - oversewed - has oversewn**)

overweight [ˈəʊvəweɪt] *adjective* too fat and heavy; *he is several kilos overweight for his age and height*

overwork [əʊvəˈwɜːk] **1** *noun* doing too much work; *he collapsed from overwork* **2** *verb* to work too much, to make something work too much; *he has been overworking his heart*

overwrought [əʊvəˈrɔːt] *adjective* very tense and nervous; *he is rather overwrought because of troubles at work*

overt [ɒˈvɜːt] *adjective* easily seen with the naked eye (NOTE: the opposite is **occult**)

oviduct [ˈəʊvɪdʌkt] = FALLOPIAN TUBE

ovulate [ˈɒvjuleɪt] *verb* to release a mature ovum into a Fallopian tube

ovulation [ɒvjuˈleɪʃn] *noun* release of an ovum from the mature ovarian follicle into the Fallopian tube

ovum [ˈəʊvəm] *noun* female egg cell which, when fertilized by a spermatozoon, begins to develop into an embryo (NOTE: the plural is **ova**. Note that for other terms referring to ova, see words beginning with **oo-**)

-oxacin [ˈɒksəsɪn] *suffix* used in names of quinolone drugs; *ciprofloxacin*

oxidase [ˈɒksɪdeɪz] *noun* enzyme which encourages oxidation by removing hydrogen; *see also* MONOAMINE

oxidation [ɒksɪˈdeɪʃn] *noun* action of making oxides by combining with oxygen or removing hydrogen

COMMENT: carbon compounds form oxides when metabolised with oxygen in the body, producing carbon dioxide

oxide [ˈɒksaɪd] *noun* compound formed with oxygen; **zinc oxide (ZnO)** = compound of zinc and oxygen, which forms a soft white soothing powder used in creams and lotions

oximetry [ɒkˈsɪmətri] *noun* **pulse oximetry** = method of measuring the oxygen content of arterial blood

oxycephalic [ɒksɪsəˈfælɪk] *adjective* referring to oxycephaly

oxycephaly [ɒksɪˈsefəli] *noun* turricephaly, condition where the skull is deformed into a point, with exophthalmos and defective sight

oxygen [ˈɒksɪdʒn] *noun* chemical element, a common colourless gas which is present in the air and essential to human life; **oxygen cylinder** = heavy metal tube which contains oxygen and is connected to a patient's oxygen mask; **oxygen mask** = mask connected to a supply of oxygen, which can be put over the face to help a patient with breathing difficulties; **oxygen tent** = type of cover put over a patient so that he can breathe in oxygen; **oxygen therapy** = any treatment involving the administering of oxygen, as in an oxygen tent, in emergency treatment for heart failure, etc. (NOTE: chemical symbol is **O**)

COMMENT: oxygen is absorbed into the bloodstream through the lungs and is carried to the tissues along the arteries; it is essential to normal metabolism and given to patients with breathing difficulties

oxygenate [ˈɒksɪdʒəneɪt] *verb* to treat (blood) with oxygen; **oxygenated blood** = arterial blood, blood which has received oxygen in the lungs and is being carried to the tissues along the arteries (it is brighter red than venous deoxygenated blood)

oxygenation [ɒksɪdʒəˈneɪʃn] *noun* becoming filled with oxygen; *blood is carried along the pulmonary artery to the lungs for oxygenation*

oxygenator [ɒksɪdʒəˈneɪtə] *noun* machine which puts oxygen into the blood, used as an artificial lung in surgery

oxyhaemoglobin [ɒksɪhiːməˈɡləʊbɪn] *noun* compound of haemoglobin and oxygen, which is the way oxygen is carried in arterial blood from the lungs to the tissues; *see also* HAEMOGLOBIN

oxyntic cell [ɒkˈsɪntɪk ˈsel] *noun* parietal cell, cell in the gastric gland which secretes hydrochloric acid

oxytocin [ɒksɪˈtəʊsɪn] *noun* hormone secreted by the posterior pituitary gland, which controls the contractions of the uterus and encourages the flow of milk

COMMENT: an extract of oxytocin is used as an injection to start contractions of the uterus and to assist in the third stage of labour

oxyuriasis [ɒksɪjuˈraɪəsɪs] = ENTEROBIASIS

Oxyuris [ɒksɪˈjuərɪs] = ENTEROBIUS

ozaena [əʊˈziːnə] *noun* (i) disease of the nose, where the nasal passage is blocked and mucus forms, giving off an unpleasant smell; (ii) any unpleasant discharge from the nose

ozone [ˈəʊzəʊn] *noun* gas present in the atmosphere in small quantities, which is harmful at high levels of concentration; **ozone sickness** = condition suffered by jet travellers, due to levels of ozone in aircraft (NOTE: chemical symbol O_3)

COMMENT: The maximum amount of ozone which is considered safe for humans to breathe is 80 parts per billion. Even in lower concentrations it irritates the throat, makes people cough and gives headaches and asthma attacks similar to hay fever. Ozone is created in the stratosphere by the effect of ultraviolet radiation from the sun on oxygen. Ozone is destroyed by reaction with nitric oxide (created by burning fossil fuel) or water or chlorine compounds (from chlorofluorocarbons used in aerosols and packaging). The reduction of ozone in the stratosphere by any of these reactions creates a thin area or 'hole' in the ozone layer. The ozone layer in the stratosphere acts as a protection against the harmful effects of the sun's radiation, and the destruction or reduction of the layer has the effect of allowing more radiation to pass through the atmosphere with harmful effects (such as skin cancer) on humans

Pp

P 1 *chemical symbol for* phosphorus **2** *see* SUBSTANCE P

Pa = PASCAL

pacemaker ['peɪsmeɪkə] *noun* **(a)** sinoatrial node or SA node, node in the heart which regulates the heartbeat; **ectopic pacemaker** = abnormal focus of the heart muscle which takes the place of the SA node **(b) (cardiac) pacemaker** = electronic device implanted on a patient's heart or which a patient wears attached to his chest, which stimulates and regulates the heartbeat; *the patient was fitted with a pacemaker*; **endocardial pacemaker** = pacemaker attached to the lining of the heart; **epicardial pacemaker** = pacemaker attached to the surface of the ventricle

COMMENT: an electrode is usually attached to the epicardium and linked to the device which can be implanted in various positions in the chest

pachy- ['pæki] *prefix* meaning thickening

pachydactyly [pæki'dæktɪli] *noun* condition where the fingers and toes become thicker than normal

pachydermia *or* **pachyderma** [pæki'dɜːmiə or pɜːki'dɜːmə] *noun* condition where the skin becomes thicker than normal

pachymeningitis [pækimenɪn'dʒaɪtɪs] *noun* inflammation of the dura mater

pachymeninx [pæki'miːnɪŋks] *noun* the dura mater, thicker outer layer covering the brain and spinal cord

pachysomia [pæki'səʊmiə] *noun* condition where soft tissues of the body become abnormally thick

pacifier ['pæsɪfaɪə] *noun US* rubber teat given to a baby to suck, to prevent it crying (NOTE: British English is **dummy**)

pacing [peɪsɪŋ] *noun* surgical operation to implant or attach a cardiac pacemaker

Pacinian corpuscle [pə'sɪniən 'kɔːpʌsl] *see* CORPUSCLE

pack [pæk] **1** *noun* **(a)** (i) tampon of gauze or cotton wool, used to fill an orifice such as the nose; (ii) wet material folded tightly, used to press on the body; (iii) treatment where a blanket or sheet is used to wrap round the patient's body; **cold pack** *or* **hot pack** = cold or hot wet cloth put on a patient's body to reduce or increase his body temperature; **ice pack** = cold compress made of lumps of ice wrapped in a cloth, or put in a special bag, and pressed on a swelling or bruise to reduce the pain **(b)** box or bag of goods for sale; *a pack of sticking plaster*; *she bought a sterile dressing pack*; *the cough tablets are sold in packs of fifty* **2** *verb* **(a)** to fill an orifice with a tampon (of cotton wool); *the ear was packed with cotton wool to absorb the discharge* **(b)** to put things in cases or boxes; *the transplant organ arrived at the hospital packed in ice*; **packed cell volume (haematocrit)** = volume of red blood cells in a patient's blood shown against the total volume of blood

packing ['pækɪŋ] *noun* absorbent material put into a wound or part of the body to absorb fluids

pack up ['pæk 'ʌp] *verb* (*informal*) to stop working; *his heart simply packed up under the strain*

PACT = PRESCRIBING, ANALYSES AND COST

pad [pæd] *noun* (i) soft absorbent material, placed on part of the body to protect it; (ii) thickening of part of the skin; *she wrapped a pad of soft cotton wool round the sore*

paed- *or* **paedo-** ['ped or 'piːd or 'piːdəʊ] *prefix* referring to children (NOTE: words beginning with the prefix **paed-** *or* **paedo-** are written **ped-** *or* **pedo-** in US English)

paediatric [piːdi'ætrɪk] *adjective* referring to the treatment of the diseases of children; *a* *new paediatric hospital has been opened; parents can visit children in the paediatric wards at any time*

```
Paediatric    day    surgery
minimizes   the   length   of
hospital stay and therefore is
less traumatic for both child
and parents
```
British Journal of Nursing

---

paediatrician [piːdɪə'trɪʃn] *noun* doctor who specializes in the treatment of diseases of children

paediatrics [piːdɪ'ætrɪks] *noun* study of children, their development and diseases; *compare* GERIATRICS

Paget's disease ['pædʒəts dɪ'ziːz] *noun* **(a)** osteitis deformans, a disease which gradually softens and thickens the bones in the spine, skull and legs, so that they become curved **(b)** form of breast cancer which starts as an itchy rash round the nipple

pain [peɪn] *noun* feeling which a person has when hurt; *she had pains in her legs after playing tennis*; *the doctor gave him an injection to relieve the pain*; *she is suffering from back pain*; **to be in great pain** = to have very sharp pains which are difficult to bear; **abdominal pain** = pain in the abdomen, caused by indigestion or serious disorder; **burning pain** = sensation as if of being burnt; **chest pains** = pains in the chest which may be caused by heart disease; **labour pains** = pains felt at regular intervals by a woman as the muscles of the uterus contract during childbirth; **lightning pain** = quick, sharp pain which is very painful but goes rapidly; **nagging pain** = dull, continuous throbbing pain; **stabbing pain** = pain which comes in a series of short sharp stabs, as if being jabbed with the point of a knife; **throbbing pain** = pain which continues in repeated short attacks; **referred pain** = SYNALGIA; **pain pathway** = series of linking nerve fibres and neurones which carry impulses of pain from the site to the sensory cortex; **pain receptor** = nerve ending which is sensitive to pain; **pain relief** = easing pain by using analgesics; **pain threshold** = point at which a person finds it impossible to bear pain without crying (NOTE: pain can be used in the plural to show that it recurs: **she has pains in her left leg)**

COMMENT: pain is carried by the sensory nerves to the central nervous system; from the site it travels up the spinal column to the

---

medulla and through a series of neurones which use Substance P as the neurotransmitter to the sensory cortex. Pain is the method by which a person knows that part of the body is damaged or infected, though the pain is not always felt in the affected part (see synalgia)

---

painful ['peɪnfʊl] *adjective* which hurts; *she has a painful skin disease*; *his foot is so painful he can hardly walk*; *your eye looks very red - is it very painful?*

painkiller *or* **painkilling drug** *or* **pain-relieving drug** ['peɪnkɪlə *or* 'peɪnkɪlɪŋ 'drʌg *or* 'peɪnrɪ'liːvɪŋ 'drʌg] *noun* analgesic, a drug (such as paracetamol) which stops a patient feeling pain

painless ['peɪnləs] *adjective* which does not hurt, which gives no pain; *a painless method of removing warts*

paint [peɪnt] **1** *noun* coloured antiseptic, analgesic or astringent liquid which is put on the surface of the body **2** *verb* to cover (a wound) with an antiseptic, analgesic or astringent liquid or lotion; *she painted the rash with calamine*

painter's colic ['peɪntəz 'kɒlɪk] *noun* form of lead poisoning caused by working with paint

palate ['pælət] *noun* roof of the mouth and floor of the nasal cavity (formed of the hard and soft palates); **hard palate** = front part of the palate between the upper teeth, made of the horizontal parts of the palatine bone and processes of the maxillae; **soft palate** = back part of the palate leading to the uvula; *see illustration at* THROAT; *see also* CLEFT PALATE

palatine ['pælətaɪn] *adjective* referring to the palate; **palatine arches** = folds of tissue between the soft palate and the pharynx; **palate bones** *or* **palatine bones** = two bones which form part of the hard palate, the orbits of the eyes and the cavity behind the nose; **palatine tonsil** = tonsil, lymphoid tissue at the back of the throat, between the soft palate, the tongue and the pharynx

palato- ['pælətəʊ] *prefix* referring to the palate

palatoglossal arch [pælətəʊ'glɒsl 'ɑːtʃ] *noun* fold between the soft palate and the tongue, anterior to the tonsil

palatopharyngeal arch [pælətəfærɪn'dʒɪəl 'ɑːtʃ] *noun* fold between the soft palate and the pharynx, posterior to the tonsil

palatoplasty ['pælətəplæsti] *noun* plastic surgery of the roof of the mouth, such as to repair a cleft palate

palatoplegia [pælətə'pli:dʒə] *noun* paralysis of the soft palate

palatorrhaphy [pælə'tɔːrəfi] *noun* surgical operation to suture and close a cleft palate (NOTE: also called **staphylorrhaphy** or **uraniscorrhaphy**)

pale [peɪl] *adjective* light coloured or white; *after her illness she looked pale and tired; with his pale complexion and dark rings round his eyes, he did not look at all well*; **to turn pale** = to become white in the face, because the flow of blood is reduced; *some people turn pale at the sight of blood*

paleness *or* **pallor** ['peɪlnəs *or* 'pælə] *noun* being pale

pali- *or* **palin-** ['pæli *or* 'pælin] *prefix* which repeats

palilalia [pæli'leɪliə] *noun* speech defect where the patient repeats words

palindromic [pælin'drəumik] *adjective* (disease) which recurs

palliative ['pæliətiv] *noun & adjective* treatment or drug which relieves the symptoms, but does nothing to cure the disease which causes the symptoms (a pain killer can reduce the pain in a tooth, but will not cure the caries which causes the pain)

```
coronary    artery    bypass
grafting   is   a   palliative
procedure  aimed  at  the  relief
of persistent angina pectoris
```
British Journal of Hospital Medicine

pallor ['pælə] *noun* paleness, being pale

palm [pɑːm] *noun* soft inside part of the hand

palmar ['pælmə] *adjective* referring to the palm; **palmar arch** = one of two arches in the palm formed by two arteries which link together; **palmar interosseus** = deep muscle between the bones in the hand; **palmar region** = area of skin around the palm (NOTE: in the hand **palmar** is the opposite of **dorsal**)

palpable ['pælpəbl] *adjective* which can be felt when touched; which can be examined with the hand

```
mammography  is  the  most
effective  technique  available
for  the  detection  of  occult
(non-palpable) breast cancer.
It  has  been  estimated  that
```

```
mammography   can   detect   a
carcinoma  two  years  before  it
becomes palpable
```
Southern Medical Journal

palpate [pæl'peɪt] *verb* to examine part of the body by feeling it with the hand

palpation [pæl'peɪʃn] *noun* examination of part of the body by feeling it with the hand; **breast palpation** = feeling a breast to see if a lump is present which might indicate breast cancer; **digital palpation** = pressing part of the body with the fingers

palpebra ['pælpɪbrə] *noun* eyelid (NOTE: plural is **palpebrae**)

palpebral ['pælpɪbrəl] *adjective* referring to the eyelids

palpitate ['pælpɪteɪt] *verb* to beat rapidly, to throb, to flutter

palpitation [pælpɪ'teɪʃn] *noun* awareness that the heart is beating abnormally, caused by stress or by a disease

palsied ['pɔːlzid] *adjective* suffering from palsy; *cerebral palsied children*

palsy ['pɔːlzi] *noun* paralysis; **cerebral palsy** = disorder of the brain, mainly due to brain damage occurring before birth, or due to lack of oxygen during birth; **Erb's palsy** = condition where an arm is paralysed because of birth injuries to the brachial plexus; *see also* BELL'S PALSY

COMMENT: cerebral palsy is the disorder affecting spastics. The patient may have bad coordination of muscular movements, impaired speech, hearing and sight, and sometimes mental retardation

paludism ['pæljudɪzm] = MALARIA

pan- *or* **pant-** *or* **panto-** [pæn *or* 'pænt *or* 'pæntəu] *prefix* meaning generalized, affecting everything

panacea [pænə'sɪə] *noun* medicine which is supposed to cure everything

panarthritis [pænɑː'θraɪtɪs] *noun* inflammation of all the tissues of a joint or of all the joints in the body

pancarditis [pænkɑːdaɪtɪs] *noun* inflammation of all the tissues in the heart, i.e. the heart muscle, the endocardium and the pericardium

pancreas ['pæŋkrɪəs] *noun* gland which lies across the back of the body between the kidneys

COMMENT: the pancreas has two functions: the first is to secrete the pancreatic juice which goes into the duodenum and digests proteins and carbohydrates; the second function is to produce the hormone insulin which regulates the use of sugar by the body. This hormone is secreted into the bloodstream by the islets of Langerhans which are in the pancreas

pancreatectomy [pæŋkriə'tektəmi] *noun* surgical removal of all or part of the pancreas; **partial pancreatectomy** = removal of part of the pancreas; **subtotal pancreatectomy** = removal of most of the pancreas; **total pancreatectomy** = removal of the whole pancreas together with part of the duodenum (NOTE: also called **Whipple's operation**)

pancreatic [pæŋkri'ætɪk] *adjective* referring to the pancreas; **benign pancreatic disease** = chronic pancreatitis; **pancreatic duct** = duct leading through the pancreas to the duodenum; **pancreatic fibrosis** = CYSTIC FIBROSIS; **pancreatic juice** *or* **pancreatic secretion** = digestive juice formed of enzymes produced by the pancreas which digests fats and carbohydrates

pancreatin ['pæŋkriətɪn] *noun* substance made from enzymes secreted by the pancreas and used to treat a patient whose pancreas does not produce pancreatic enzymes

pancreatitis [pæŋkriə'taɪtɪs] *noun* inflammation of the pancreas; **acute pancreatitis** = inflammation after pancreatic enzymes have escaped into the pancreas, causing symptoms of acute abdominal pain; **chronic pancreatitis** = chronic inflammation, after repeated attacks of acute pancreatitis, where the gland becomes calcified; **relapsing pancreatitis** = form of pancreatitis where the symptoms recur, but in a less painful form

pancreatomy *or* **pancreatotomy** [pæŋkri'ætəmi *or* pæŋkriə'tɒtəmi] *noun* surgical operation to open the pancreatic duct

pancytopenia [pænsaɪtə'piːniə] *noun* condition where the numbers of red and white blood cells and blood platelets are all reduced together

pandemic [pæn'demɪk] *noun & adjective* (epidemic disease) which affects many parts of the world; *compare* ENDEMIC, EPIDEMIC

pang [pæŋ] *noun* sudden sharp pain (especially in the intestine); *after not eating for a day, he suffered pangs of hunger*

panhysterectomy [pænhɪstə'rektmi] *noun* surgical removal of all the uterus and the cervix

panic ['pænɪk] **1** *noun* sudden great fear which cannot be stopped and which sometimes results in irrational behaviour; *he was in a panic as he sat in the consultant's waiting room*; **panic attack** = sudden attack of panic **2** *verb* to be suddenly afraid; *he panicked when the surgeon told him he might have to have an operation*

panniculitis [pənɪkju'laɪtɪs] *noun* inflammation of the panniculus adiposus, producing tender swellings on the thighs and breasts

panniculus [pə'nɪkjuləs] *noun* layer of membranous tissue; **panniculus adiposus** = fatty layer of tissue underneath the skin

pannus ['pænəs] *noun* growth on the cornea containing tiny blood vessels

panophthalmia *or* **panophthalmitis** [pænɒf'θælmiə *or* pænɒfθæl'maɪtɪs] *noun* inflammation of the whole of the eye

panosteitis *or* **panostitis** [pænɒsti'aɪtɪs *or* pænɒ'staɪtɪs] *noun* inflammation of all of a bone

panotitis [pænəʊ'taɪtɪs] *noun* inflammation affecting all of the ear, but especially the middle ear

panproctocolectomy [pænprɒktəkə'lektəmi] *noun* surgical removal of the whole of the rectum and the colon

pant [pænt] *verb* to take short breaths because of overexertion, to gasp for breath; *he was panting when he reached the top of the stairs*

pantothenic acid [pæntə'θenɪk 'æsɪd] *noun* vitamin of the vitamin B complex, found in liver, yeast and eggs

pantotropic *or* **pantropic** [pæntə'trɒpɪk *or* pæn'trɒpɪk] *adjective* (virus) which attacks many different parts of the body

Papanicolaou test *or* **Pap test** *or* **Pap smear** ['pæpənɪkə'leɪu 'test *or* 'pæp 'test *or* 'pæp 'smɪə] *noun* method of staining smears from various body secretions to test for malignancy, such as testing a cervical smear sample to see if cancer is present

papilla [pə'pɪlə] *noun* small swelling which protrudes above the normal surface level; *the upper surface of the tongue is covered with papillae*; **hair papilla** = part of the skin containing capillaries which feed blood to the hair; **optic papilla** = optic disc, the point on the retina where the optic nerve starts; *see illustration at* TONGUE; *see also* CIRCUMVALLATE, FILIFORM, FUNGIFORM, VALLATE (NOTE: plural is **papillae**)

papillary [pə'pɪləri] *adjective* referring to papillae

papillitis [pæpɪ'laɪtɪs] *noun* inflammation of the optic disc at the back of the eye

papilloedema [pæpɪləʊ'diːmə] *noun* oedema of the optic disc at the back of the eye

papilloma [pæpɪ'ləʊmə] *noun* benign tumour on the skin or mucous membrane

papillomatosis [pæpɪləʊmə'təʊsɪs] *noun* (i) being affected with papillomata; (ii) formation of papillomata

papovavirus [pə'pəʊvəvaɪrəs] *noun* family of viruses which start tumours, some of which are malignant, and some of which, like warts, are benign

Pap test *or* **Pap smear** ['pæp 'test *or* 'pæp 'smɪə] *see* PAPANICOLAOU TEST

papular ['pæpjʊlə] *adjective* referring to a papule

papule ['pæpjuːl] *noun* small coloured spot raised above the surface of the skin as part of a rash (NOTE: a flat spot is a **macule**)

papulopustular [pæpjʊlə'pʌstjʊlə] *adjective* (rash) with both papules and pustules

papulosquamous [pæpjʊlə'skweɪməs] *adjective* (rash) with papules and a scaly skin

para- ['pærə] *prefix* meaning (i) similar to or near; (ii) changed or beyond

paracentesis [pærəsen'tiːsɪs] *noun* draining of fluid from a cavity inside the body, using a hollow needle, either for diagnostic purposes or because the fluid is harmful

paracetamol [pærə'siːtəmɒl] *noun see* DRUGS TABLE IN SUPPLEMENT

paracolpitis [pærəkɒl'paɪtɪs] = PERICOLPITIS

paracusis *or* **paracousia** [pærə'kjuːsɪs *or* pærə'kuːsɪə] *noun* disorder of hearing

paradoxical breathing *or* **respiration** [pærə'dɒksɪkl 'briːðɪŋ *or* respə'reɪʃn] *noun* condition of a patient with broken ribs, where the chest appears to move in when the patient breathes in, and appears to move out when he breathes out

paradoxus [pærə'dɒksəs] *see* PULSUS

paraesthesia [pæriːs'θiːzɪə] *noun* numbness and tingling feeling, like pins and needles (NOTE: plural is **paraesthesiae**)

> the sensory symptoms are paraesthesiae which may spread up the arm over the course of about 20 minutes
> *British Journal of Hospital Medicine*

paraffin ['pærəfɪn] *noun* oil produced from petroleum, forming the base of some ointments, and also used for heating and light; **liquid paraffin** = oil used as a laxative; **paraffin gauze** = gauze covered with solid paraffin, used as a dressing

parageusia [pærə'gjuːsɪə] *noun* (i) disorder of the sense of taste; (ii) unpleasant taste in the mouth

paragonimiasis [pærəgɒnə'maɪəsɪs] *noun* endemic haemoptysis, tropical disease where the patient's lungs are infested with a fluke and he coughs up blood

paraguard stretcher ['pærəgɑːd 'stretʃə] *see* STRETCHER

para-influenza virus [pærəɪnflu'enzə 'vaɪrəs] *noun* virus which causes upper respiratory tract infection (in its structure it is identical to paramyxoviruses and the measles virus)

paralyse *US* **paralyze** ['pærəlaɪz] *verb* to weaken (muscles) so that they cannot function; *his arm was paralysed after the stroke*; *she is paralysed from the waist down*

paralysis [pə'ræləsɪs] *noun* condition where the muscles of part of the body become weak and cannot be moved because the motor nerves have been damaged; *the condition causes paralysis of the lower limbs*; *he suffered temporary paralysis of the right arm*; **bulbar paralysis** = form of motor neurone disease which affects the muscles of the mouth, jaw and throat; **facial paralysis** = BELL'S PALSY; **infantile paralysis** = POLIOMYELITIS; **paralysis agitans** = PARKINSON'S DISEASE; **general paralysis of the insane (GPI)** = old term for tertiary syphilis when the brain is affected; **spastic paralysis** = cerebral palsy, disorder of the brain affecting spastics, caused by brain damage before birth or lack of oxygen at birth; *see also* DIPLEGIA, HEMIPLEGIA, MONOPLEGIA, PARAPLEGIA, QUADRIPLEGIA

COMMENT: paralysis can have many causes: the commonest are injuries to or diseases of the brain or the spinal column

paralytic [pærə'lɪtɪk] *adjective* referring to paralysis; (person) who is paralysed; **paralytic ileus** = obstruction in the ileum caused by paralysis of the muscles of the intestine

paralytica [pærə'lɪtɪkə] *see* DEMENTIA PARALYTICA

paramedian [pærə'miːdiən] *adjective* near the midline of the body; **paramedian plane** = plane near the midline of the body, parallel to the sagittal plane and at right angles to the coronal plane

paramedic [pærə'medɪk] *noun* person in a profession linked to that of nurse, doctor or surgeon (NOTE: paramedic is used to refer to all types of services and staff, from therapists and hygienists, to ambulancemen and radiographers, but does not include doctors, nurses or midwives)

paramedical [pærə'medɪkl] *adjective* referring to services linked to those given by nurses, doctors and surgeons

paramesonephric duct [pærəmesə'nefrɪk 'dʌkt] *noun* Müllerian duct, one of the two ducts in an embryo which develop into the uterus and Fallopian tubes

parameter [pə'ræmɪtə] *noun* measurement of something (such as blood pressure) which may be an important factor in treating the condition which the patient is suffering from

parametritis [pærəmɪ'traɪtɪs] *noun* inflammation of the parametrium

parametrium [pærə'miːtriəm] *noun* connective tissue around the uterus

paramnesia [pæræm'niːziə] *noun* disorder of the memory where the patient remembers events which have not happened

paramyxovirus [pærəmɪksəʊ'vaɪrəs] *noun* one of a group of viruses, which cause mumps, measles and other infectious diseases

paranasal [pærə'neɪzl] *adjective* by the side of the nose; **paranasal air sinus** = one of the four sinuses in the skull near the nose

COMMENT: the four pairs of paranasal sinuses are the frontal, maxillary, ethmoidal, and sphenoidal

paranoia [pærə'nɔɪə] *noun* mental disorder where the patient has fixed delusions, usually that he is being persecuted or attacked

paranoiac [pærə'nɔɪæk] *noun* person suffering from paranoia

paranoid ['pærənɔɪd] *adjective* suffering from a fixed delusion; **paranoid schizophrenia** = form of schizophrenia where the patient believes he is being persecuted

paraparesis [pærəpə'riːsɪs] *noun* incomplete paralysis of the legs

paraphasia [pærə'feɪziə] *noun* speech defect where the patient uses a wrong sound in the place of the correct word or phrase

paraphimosis [pærəfaɪ'məʊsɪs] *noun* condition where the foreskin is tight and has to be removed by circumcision

paraphrenia [pærə'friːniə] *noun* paranoid psychosis, where the patient has delusions and the personality disintegrates

paraplegia [pærə'pliːdʒə] *noun* paralysis which affects the lower part of the body and the legs, usually caused by an injury to the spinal cord; **spastic paraplegia** = paraplegia caused by disturbed nutrition of the cortex in elderly people

paraplegic [pærə'pliːdʒɪk] *noun* & *adjective* (person) suffering from paraplegia

parapsoriasis [pærəsə'raɪəsɪs] *noun* group of skin diseases with scales, similar to psoriasis

parasagittal [pærə'sædʒɪtl] *adjective* near the midline of the body; **parasagittal plane** = plane near the midline of the body, parallel to the sagittal plane and at right angles to the coronal plane

parasitaemia [pærəsɪ'tiːmiə] *noun* presence of parasites in the blood

parasite ['pærəsaɪt] *noun* plant or animal which lives on or inside another organism and draws nourishment from that organism

COMMENT: the commonest parasites affecting humans are lice on the skin, and various types of worms in the intestines. Many diseases (such as malaria and amoebic dysentery) are caused by infestation with parasites

parasitic [pærə'sɪtɪk] *adjective* referring to parasites; **parasitic cyst** = cyst produced by a parasite, usually in the liver

parasiticide [pærə'saɪtəsaɪd] *noun & adjective* (substance) which kills parasites

parasitology [pærəsɪ'tɒlədʒi] *noun* scientific study of parasites

parasuicide [pærə'suːɪsaɪd] *noun* act where the patient tries to kill himself, but without really intending to do so, rather as a way of drawing attention to his psychological condition

parasympathetic nervous system [pærəsɪmpə'θetɪk 'nɜːvəs 'sɪstəm] *noun* one of two systems in the autonomic nervous system; *see also* SYMPATHETIC

> COMMENT: the parasympathetic nervous system originates in some of the cranial and sacral nerves. It acts in opposition to the sympathetic nervous system, slowing down the action of the heart, reducing blood pressure, and increasing the rate of digestion

parathormone [pærə'θɔːməʊn] *noun* parathyroid hormone, the hormone secreted by the parathryoid glands which regulates the level of calcium in blood plasma

parathyroid [pærə'θaɪrɔɪd] *noun & adjective;* **parathyroid (gland)** = one of four glands in the neck, near the thyroid gland, which secrete parathyroid hormones; **parathyroid hormone** = hormone secreted by the parathyroid gland which regulates the level of calcium in blood plasma

parathyroidectomy [pærəθaɪrɔɪ'dektəmi] *noun* surgical removal of a parathyroid gland

paratyphoid [pærə'taɪfɔɪd] *noun & adjective;* **paratyphoid (fever)** = infectious disease which has similar symptoms to typhoid and is caused by bacteria transmitted by humans or animals

> COMMENT: there are three forms of paratyphoid fever, known by the letters A, B, and C. They are caused by three types of bacterium, *Salmonella paratyphi* A, B, and C. TAB injections give immunity against paratyphoid A and B, but not against C

paravertebral [pærə'vɜːtɪbrl] *adjective* near the vertebrae, beside the spinal column; **paravertebral injection** = injection of local anaesthetic into the back near the vertebrae

parenchyma [pə'reŋkɪmə] *noun* tissues which contain the working cells of an organ as opposed to the stoma or supporting tissue

parent ['peərənt] *noun* mother or father; **single parent family** = family which consists of a child or children and only one parent (because of death, divorce or separation); **parent cell** *or* **mother cell** = original cell which splits into daughter cells by mitosis

> in most paediatric wards today open visiting is the norm, with parent care much in evidence. Parents who are resident in the hospital also need time spent with them
>
> *Nursing Times*

parenteral [pæ'rentərl] *adjective* (drug) which is not given orally and so not by way of the digestive tract, but given in the form of injections or suppositories; **parenteral nutrition** *or* **feeding** = feeding of a patient by means other than by way of the digestive tract, especially giving injections of glucose to a critically ill patient; *compare* ENTERAL

parenthood ['peərənthʊd] *noun* state of being a parent; **planned parenthood** = situation where two people plan to have a certain number of children and take contraceptives to limit the number of children in the family

paresis [pə'riːsɪs] *noun* partial paralysis

paresthesia [pæriːs'θiːziə] = PARAESTHESIA

paries ['peəriːz] *noun* (i) superficial parts of a structure of organ; (ii) wall of a cavity (NOTE: plural is **parietes**)

parietal [pə'raɪətl] *adjective* referring to the wall of a cavity or any organ; **parietal bones** *or* **parietals** = two bones which form the sides of the skull; **parietal cell** = OXYNTIC CELL; **parietal lobe** = middle lobe of the cerebral hemisphere, which is associated with language and other mental processes, and also contains the postcentral gyrus; **parietal pericardium** = outer layer of the serous pericardium not in direct contact with the heart muscle, which lies inside and is attached to the fibrous pericardium; **parietal peritoneum** = part of the peritoneum which lines the abdominal cavity and covers the abdominal viscera; **parietal pleura** = membrane attached to the diaphragm, and covering the chest cavity and lungs

-parin ['pærɪn] *suffix* used for anticoagulants; *heparin*

Paris ['pærɪs] *see* PLASTER

parkinsonian [pɑːkɪn'səʊnɪən] *adjective* referring to Parkinson's disease; *parkinsonian tremor*

Parkinsonism *or* **Parkinson's disease** ['pɑːkɪnsənɪzm *or* 'pɑːkɪnsənz dɪ'ziːz] *noun* slow progressive disorder affecting elderly people

COMMENT: Parkinson's disease affects the basal ganglia of brain which control movement, due to destruction of dopaminergic neurones. The symptoms include trembling of the limbs, a shuffling walk and difficulty in speaking. Some cases can be improved by treatment with levodopa, which is the precursor of the missing neurotransmitter dopamine, or by drugs which inhibit the breakdown of dopamine

paronychia [pærə'nɪkiə] *noun* inflammation near the nail which forms pus, caused by an infection in the fleshy part of the tip of a finger; *see also* WHITLOW

parosmia [pə'rɒzmiə] *noun* disorder of the sense of smell

parotid [pə'rɒtɪd] *adjective & noun* near the ear; **parotid glands** *or* **parotids** = glands which produce saliva, situated in the neck behind the joint of the jaw and ear; *see illustration at* THROAT

parotitis [pærə'taɪtɪs] *noun* inflammation of the parotid glands

COMMENT: mumps is the commonest form of parotitis, where the parotid gland becomes swollen and the sides of the face become fat

parous ['peərəs] *adjective* (woman) who has given birth to one or more children

paroxysm ['pærəksɪzm] *noun* (i) sudden movement of the muscles; (ii) sudden appearance of symptoms of the disease; (iii) sudden attack of coughing or sneezing; *he suffered paroxysms of coughing during the night*

paroxysmal [pærək'sɪzml] *adjective* referring to a paroxysm; similar to a paroxysm; **paroxysmal dyspnoea** = attack of breathlessness at night, caused by heart failure; **paroxysmal tachycardia** = sudden attack of rapid heartbeats

parrot disease ['pærət dɪ'ziːz] = PSITTACOSIS

pars [pɑːz] *Latin word meaning* part

part [pɑːt] *noun* piece, one of the sections which make up a whole organ or body; **spare part surgery** = surgery where parts of the body (such as bones or joints) are replaced by artificial pieces

partial ['pɑːʃl] *adjective* not complete, affecting only part of something; *he only made a partial recovery*; **partial amnesia** = being unable to remember certain facts, such as the names of people; **partial deafness** = being able to hear some sounds but not all; **partial gastrectomy** *or* **partial mastectomy** = operations to remove part of the stomach or part of a breast; **partial vision** = being able to see only a part of the total field of vision, not being able to see anything very clearly

partially ['pɑːʃəli] *adverb* not completely; *he is partially paralysed in his right side*; **the partially sighted** = people who have only partial vision

particle ['pɑːtɪkl] *noun* very small piece of matter

particulate [pɑː'tɪkjʊlət] *adjective* (i) referring to particles; (ii) made up of separate particles; **particulate matter (PM10, PM2.5, PM1)** = particles of less than a specified size, usually of carbon, which are used as a measure of air pollution and can affect asthma

partly ['pɑːtli] *adverb* not completely; *she is partly paralysed*

parturient [pɑː'tjʊəriənt] *adjective & noun* (i) referring to childbirth; (ii) (woman) who is in labour

parturition [pɑːtju'rɪʃn] *noun* childbirth

pascal ['pæskəl] *noun* SI unit of measurement of pressure (NOTE: with figures usually written **Pa**)

COMMENT: 1 pascal is the pressure exerted on an area of 1 square metre by a force of 1 newton

Paschen bodies ['pæʃken 'bɒdɪz] *plural noun* particles which occur in the skin lesions of smallpox patients

pass [pɑːs] *verb* to allow (faeces or urine) to come out of the body; *he passed blood in his bowel movement*; *she had pains when she passed water*; *he passed a small stone in his urine*

passage ['pæsɪdʒ] *noun* (i) long narrow channel inside the body; (ii) moving from one place to another; (iii) evacuation of the bowels; (iv) introduction of an instrument into a cavity; **air passage** = tube which takes air to the lungs; **anal passage** or **back passage** = the anus; **front passage** = (i) the urethra; (ii) the vagina

pass away ['pɑːs ə'weɪ] *verb* to die; *see also* PASS ON (b); *mother passed away during the night*

passive ['pæsɪv] *adjective* not active; **passive immunity** = immunity which is acquired by a baby in the uterus or by a patient through an injection with an antitoxin; **passive movement** = movement of a joint by a doctor or therapist, not by the patient himself; **passive smoking** = breathing in smoke from other people's cigarettes when you do not smoke yourself

pass on ['pɑːs 'ɒn] *verb* **(a)** to give (a disease) to someone; *haemophilia is passed on by a woman to her sons; the disease was quickly passed on by carriers to the rest of the population* **(b)** to die; *my father passed on two years ago; see also* PASS AWAY

pass out ['pɑːs 'aʊt] *verb* to faint; *when we told her her father was ill, she passed out*

past [pɑːst] *adjective* (time) which has passed; **past history** = records of earlier illnesses; *he has no past history of renal disease*

paste [peɪst] *noun* medicinal ointment which is quite solid and is spread or rubbed onto the skin

Pasteurella [pæstə'relə] *noun* genus of parasitic bacteria, one of which causes the plague

pasteurization [pæstəraɪ'zeɪʃn] *noun* heating of food or food products to destroy bacteria

COMMENT: Pasteurization is carried out by heating food for a short time at a lower temperature than that used for sterilization: the two methods used are heating to 72ºC for fifteen seconds (the high temperature short time method) or to 65º for half an hour, and then cooling rapidly. This has the effect of killing tuberculosis bacteria

pasteurize ['pæstəraɪz] *verb* to kill bacteria in food by heating it; *the government is telling people to drink only pasteurized milk*

pastille ['pæstl] *noun* (i) sweet jelly with medication in it, which can be sucked to relieve a sore throat; (ii) small paper disc

covered with barium platinocyanide, which changes colour when exposed to radiation

pat [pæt] *verb* to hit lightly; *she patted the baby on the back to make it burp*

patch ['pætʃ] *noun* piece of plaster with a substance on it, which is stuck to the skin of a patient to allow the substance to be gradually absorbed into the system through the skin (as in HRT); **nicotine patch** = patch containing nicotine which is released slowly into the bloodstream, as a method of curing nicotine addiction; **patch test** = test for allergies or tuberculosis, where a piece of plaster containing an allergic substance or tuberculin is stuck to the skin to see if there is a reaction; *compare* MANTOUX TEST

COMMENT: Patches are available on prescription for various treatments, especially for administering hormone replacement therapy. They are also used for treating nicotine addiction and in this case can be bought without a prescription

patella [pə'telə] *noun* kneecap, the small bone in front of the knee joint

patellar [pə'telə] *noun* referring to the kneecap; **patellar reflex** = knee jerk, the jerk made as a reflex action by the knee, when the legs are crossed and the patellar tendon is tapped sharply; **patellar tendon** = tendon just below the kneecap

patellectomy [pætə'lektəmi] *noun* surgical operation to remove the kneecap

patency ['peɪtənsi] *noun* being open; *they carried out an examination to determine the patency of the Fallopian tubes; a salpingostomy was performed to restore the patency of the Fallopian tube*

patent ['peɪtənt] *adjective* **(a)** open; exposed; *the presence of a pulse shows that the main blood vessels from the heart to the site of the pulse are patent;* **patent ductus arteriosus** = congenital condition where the ductus arteriosus does not close, allowing blood into the circulation without having passed through the lungs **(b) patent medicine** = medicinal preparation with special ingredients which is made and sold under a trade name

paternity [pə'tɜːnəti] *noun* **(a)** being a father; **paternity leave (b)** the identity of a father; *the court had first to establish the child's paternity;* **paternity test** = test (such as blood grouping) which allows to determine the identity of the father of a child (DNA fingerprinting may be required in order to identify a man who might be the father according to his blood group and that of the child, but is not in fact the father) (NOTE: compare **maternity**)

path- *or* **patho-** ['pæθ or 'pæθə] *prefix* referring to disease

pathogen ['pæθədʒn] *noun* microbe which causes a disease

pathogenesis [pæθə'dʒenəsɪs] *noun* origin, production, development of a morbid or diseased condition

pathogenetic [pæθədʒə'netɪk] *adjective* referring to pathogenesis

pathogenic [pæθə'dʒenɪk] *adjective* which can cause or produce a disease

pathogenicity [pæθədʒə'nɪsəti] *noun* ability of a pathogen to cause a disease

pathognomonic [pæθəgnəu'mɒnɪk] *adjective* (symptom) which is typical and characteristic, and which indicates that a patient has a particular disease

pathological *or* **pathologic** [pæθə'lɒdʒɪkl or pə'θɒlədʒɪk] *adjective* referring to a disease, which is caused by a disease; which indicates a disease; **pathological fracture** = fracture of a diseased bone

pathologist [pə'θɒlədʒɪst] *noun* **(a)** doctor who specializes in the study of diseases and the changes in the body caused by disease; he examines tissue specimens from patients and reports on the presence or absence of disease in them **(b)** doctor who examines dead bodies to find out the cause of death

pathology [pə'θɒlədʒi] *noun* study of diseases and the changes in structure and function which diseases cause in the body; **clinical pathology** = study of disease as applied to treatment of patients; **pathology report** = report on tests carried out to find the cause of a disease

pathophysiology [pæθəfɪzi'ɒlədʒi] *noun* study of abnormal or diseased organs

pathway ['pɑːθweɪ] *noun* series of linked neurones along which nerve impulses travel; **final common pathway** = linked neurones which take all impulses from the central nervous system to a muscle; **motor pathway** = series of motor neurones leading from the brain to the muscles

-pathy [pəθi] *suffix* (i) diseased; (ii) treatment of a disease

patient ['peɪʃənt] **1** *adjective* being able to wait a long time without getting annoyed; *you will have to be patient if you are waiting for treatment - the doctor is late with his appointments* **2** *noun* person who is in hospital or who is being treated by a doctor; *the patients are all asleep in their beds*; *the doctor is taking the patient's temperature*; **patient identifier** = code of letters and digits attached to the patient's medical records by which all information concerning the patient can be traced, for example, cause of death; **private patient** = patient who is paying for treatment, and who is not being treated under the National Health Service

patiently ['peɪʃəntli] *adverb* without getting annoyed; *they waited patiently for two hours before the consultant could see them*

patulous ['pætjʊləs] *adjective* stretched open, patent

Paul-Bunnell reaction *or* **Paul-Bunnell test** ['pɔːlbʌ'nel rɪ'ækʃn or 'test] *noun* blood test to see if a patient has glandular fever, where the patient's blood is tested against a solution containing glandular fever bacilli

Paul's tube ['pɔːlz 'tjuːb] *noun* glass tube used to remove the contents of the bowel after an opening has been made between the intestine and the abdominal wall

pavement epithelium ['peɪvmənt epɪ'θiːliəm] *noun* squamous epithelium, a simple type of epithelium with flattened cells like scales, forming the lining of the serous membrane of the pericardium, the peritoneum and the pleura

pay bed ['peɪ 'bed] *noun* bed (usually in a separate room) in a National Health Service hospital for which a patient pays separately

Pb *chemical symbol for* lead

PBI test ['piː 'biː 'aɪ 'test] = PROTEIN-BOUND IODINE TEST

p.c. ['piː 'siː] *abbreviation for the Latin phrase* 'post cibum': after food (written on prescriptions)

PCC ['piː 'siː 'siː] = PROFESSIONAL CONDUCT COMMITTEE

PCG ['piː 'siː 'dʒiː] = PRIMARY CARE GROUP

PCR ['piː 'siː 'ɑː] = POLYMERASE CHAIN REACTION

PCT ['piː 'siː 'tiː] = PRIMARY CARE TRUST

peak [pi:k] *noun* the highest point; **peak period** = time of the day, days of the month or months of the year, during which something (such as fever, tiredness, infectious diseases, colds) reaches its highest point

pearl [pɜ:l] *see* BOHN

Pearson bed ['pɪəsən 'bed] *noun* type of bed with a Balkan frame, used for patients with fractures

peau d'orange ['pəu dɒ'rɑ:nʒ] *French phrase meaning* 'orange peel': thickened skin with many little depressions caused by lymphoedema which forms over a breast tumour or in elephantiasis

pecten ['pektɪn] *noun* (i) middle section of the wall of the anal passage; (ii) hard ridge on the pubis

pectineal [pek'tɪnɪəl] *adjective* (i) referring to the pecten of the pubis; (ii) (structure) with ridges like a comb

pectoral ['pektərəl] **1** *noun* **(a)** therapeutic substance which has a good effect on respiratory disease **(b)** = PECTORAL MUSCLE **2** *adjective* referring to the chest; **pectoral girdle** = shoulder girdle, the shoulder bones (the scapulae and clavicles) to which the upper arm bones are attached; **pectoral muscle** = chest muscle, one of two muscles which lie across the chest and control movements of the shoulder and arm

pectoralis [pektə'reɪlɪs] *noun* chest muscle; **pectoralis major** = large chest muscle which pulls the arm forward or rotates it; **pectoralis minor** = small chest muscle which allows the shoulder to be depressed

pectoris ['pektərɪs] *see* ANGINA

pectus ['pektəs] *noun* anterior part of the chest; **pectus excavatum** = FUNNEL CHEST

ped- *or* **pedo-** ['ped *or* 'pi:d *or* 'pi:dəu] *US*; *see* PAED-

pediatrics, pediatrician [pi:di'ætrɪks *or* pi:diə'trɪʃn] *US*; *see* PAEDIATRICS, PAEDIATRICIAN

pedicle ['pedɪkl] *noun* (i) long thin piece of skin which attaches a skin graft to the place where it was growing originally; (ii) piece of tissue which connects a tumour to healthy tissue; (iii) bridge which connects the lamina of a vertebra to the body

pediculosis [pɪdɪkju'ləusɪs] *noun* skin disease caused by being infested with lice

Pediculus [pɪ'dɪkjuləs] *noun* louse, little insect which lives on humans and sucks blood; **Pediculus capitis** = head louse; **Pediculus corporis** = body louse; **Pediculus pubis** = pubic louse (NOTE: plural is **Pediculi**)

pediodontia [pidiə'dɒnʃə] *noun* study of children's teeth

pediodontist [pi:diə'dɒntɪst] *noun* dentist who specializes in the treatment of children's teeth

peduncle [pɪ'dʌŋkl] *noun* stem or stalk; **cerebellar peduncle** = band of nerve tissue connecting parts of the cerebellum; **cerebral peduncle** = mass of nerve fibres connecting the cerebral hemispheres to the midbrain; *see illustration at* BRAIN

pedunculate [pɪ'dʌŋkjuleɪt] *adjective* having a stem or stalk (NOTE: the opposite is **sessile**)

peel [pi:l] *verb* to take the skin off a fruit or vegetable; *(of skin)* to come off in pieces; *after getting sunburnt his skin began to peel*

PEEP ['pi: 'i: 'i: 'pi:] = POSITIVE END-EXPIRATORY PRESSURE

Pel-Ebstein fever ['pel'ebstaɪn 'fi:və] *noun* fever (associated with Hodgkin's disease) which recurs regularly

pellagra [pə'lægrə] *noun* disease caused by deficiency of nicotinic acid, riboflavine and pyridoxine from the vitamin B complex, where patches of skin become inflamed, and the patient has anorexia, nausea and diarrhoea

COMMENT: in some cases the patient's mental faculties can be affected, with depression, headaches and numbness of the extremities. Treatment is by improving the patient's diet

Pellegrini-Stieda's disease [pelə'gri:ni'sti:dəz dɪ'zi:z] *noun* disease where an injury to a knee causes the ligament to become calcified

pellet ['pelɪt] *noun* (i) pill of steroid hormone, usually either oestrogen or testosterone; (ii) solid sediment at base of container after centrifuging

pellicle ['pelɪkl] *noun* thin layer of skin tissue

pellucida [pɪ'lu:sɪdə] *see* ZONA

pelvic ['pelvɪk] *adjective* referring to the pelvis; **pelvic brim** = line on the ilium which separates the false pelvis from the true pelvis; **pelvic cavity** = space below the abdominal cavity above the pelvis; **pelvic floor** = lower part of the space beneath the pelvic girdle formed of muscle; **pelvic fracture** = fracture of the pelvis; **pelvic girdle** = hip girdle, the ring formed by the two hip bones to which the thigh bones are attached; **pelvic outlet** = opening at the base of the pelvis

pelvimeter [pel'vɪmɪtə] *noun* instrument to measure the diameter and capacity of the pelvis

pelvimetry [pel'vɪmətri] *noun* measuring the pelvis, especially to see if the internal ring is wide enough for a baby to pass through in childbirth

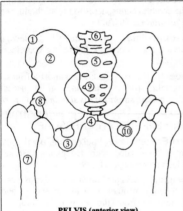

PELVIS (anterior view)

1. iliac crest
2. ilium
3. ischium
4. pubis
5. sacrum
6. vertebral column
7. femur
8. hip joint
9. sacral foramen
10. obturator foramen

pelvis ['pelvɪs] *noun* **(a)** (i) group of bones and cartilage which form a ring and connect the thigh bones to the spine; (ii) the internal space inside the pelvic girdle **(b) renal pelvis** *or* **pelvis of the kidney** = main central tube leading into the kidney from where the ureter joins it; *see illustration at* KIDNEY (NOTE: the plural is **pelves** *or* **pelvises**. Note also that for terms referring to the renal pelvis, see words beginning with **pyel-** or **pyelo-**)

COMMENT: the pelvis is a bowl-shaped ring, formed of the two hip bones, with the sacrum and the coccyx at the back. The hip bones are each in three sections: the ilium, the ischium and the pubis and are linked in front by the pubic symphysis. The pelvic girdle is shaped in a different way in men and women, the internal space being wider

in women. The top part of the pelvis, which does not form a complete ring, is called the 'false pelvis'; the lower part is the 'true pelvis'.

pemphigoid ['pemfɪgɔɪd] *adjective & noun* (skin disease) which is similar to pemphigus

pemphigus ['pemfɪgəs] *noun* rare disease where large blisters form inside the skin

penetrate ['penətreɪt] *verb* to go through something, to go into something; *the end of the broken bone has penetrated the liver; the ulcer burst, penetrating the wall of the duodenum*

penetration [penə'treɪʃn] *noun* act of penetrating; *the penetration of the vagina by the penis; penetration of an ovum by a spermatozoon*

-penia [piːniə] *suffix* meaning lack, not enough of something; **cytopenia** = lack of cellular elements in the blood

penicillin [penə'sɪlɪn] *noun* common antibiotic produced from a fungus (NOTE: penicillin drugs have names ending in **-cillin: amoxycillin**)

COMMENT: penicillin is effective against many microbial diseases, but some people can be allergic to it, and this fact should be noted on medical record cards

Penicillium [penə'sɪliəm] *noun* fungus from which penicillin is derived

penile ['piːnaɪl] *adjective* referring to the penis; **penile urethra** = tube in the penis through which urine and semen pass

penis ['piːnɪs] *noun* male genital organ, which also passes urine; *see illustration at* UROGENITAL SYSTEM (male); *see also* KRAUROSIS

COMMENT: the penis is a mass of tissue containing the urethra. When stimulated the tissue of the penis fills with blood and becomes erect

pentose ['pentəuz] *noun* sugar containing five carbon atoms

pentosuria [pentə'ʃuəriə] *noun* abnormal condition where pentose is present in the urine

pep [pep] *verb (informal)* to give (someone) a feeling of well-being; *these pills will pep you up*

pep pill ['pep 'pɪl] = AMPHETAMINE

pepsin ['pepsɪn] *noun* enzyme in the stomach which breaks down the proteins in food into peptones

pepsinogen [pep'sɪnədʒn] *noun* secretion from the gastric gland which is the inactive form of pepsin

peptic ['peptɪk] *adjective* referring to digestion or to the digestive system; **peptic ulcer** = benign ulcer in the duodenum or in the stomach

peptidase ['peptɪdeɪz] *noun* enzyme which breaks down proteins in the intestine into amino acids

peptide ['peptaɪd] *noun* compound formed of two or more amino acids

peptone ['peptəʊn] *noun* substance produced by the action of pepsins on proteins in food

peptonuria [peptə'njʊərɪə] *noun* abnormal condition where peptones are present in the urine

per [pɜː or pə] *preposition* out of, for each; **ten per thousand** = ten out of every thousand; *the number of cases of cervical cancer per thousand patients tested*

per cent [pə'sent] *adverb & noun* in or for every hundred; *fifty per cent (50%) of the tests were positive*; *seventy-five per cent (75%) of hospital cases remain in hospital for less than four days*; **there has been a five per cent increase in applications** = the number of applications has gone up by five in every hundred (NOTE: usually written % with figures: **we need to increase output by 5%**)

percentage [pə'sentɪdʒ] *noun* proportion rate in every hundred or for every hundred; *what is the percentage of long-stay patients in the hospital?*

perception [pə'sepʃn] *noun* impression formed in the brain as a result of information about the outside world which is passed back by the senses

perceptive deafness [pe'septɪv 'defnəs] *noun* deafness caused by a disorder of the auditory nerves or the brain centres which receive nerve impulses

percussion [pə'kʌʃn] *noun* test (usually on the heart and lungs) in which the doctor taps part of the patient's body and listens to the sound produced

percutaneous [pɜːkju'teɪnɪəs] *adjective* through the skin

per diem ['pɜː 'diːem] *Latin phrase meaning* 'per day' (written on prescriptions)

perennial [pə'renɪəl] *adjective* which continues all the time, for a period of years; *she suffers from perennial bronchial asthma*

perforate ['pɜːfəreɪt] *verb* to make a hole through something; *the ulcer perforated the duodenum*; **perforated eardrum** = eardrum with a hole in it; **perforated ulcer** = ulcer which has made a hole in the wall of the intestine

perforation [pɜːfə'reɪʃn] *noun* hole through the whole thickness of a tissue or membrane (such as a hole in the intestine or in the eardrum)

perform [pə'fɔːm] *verb* **(a)** to do (an operation); *a team of three surgeons performed the heart transplant operation* **(b)** to work; *the new heart has performed very well*; *the kidneys are not performing as well as they should*

performance [pə'fɔːməns] *noun* way in which something works; *the doctors are not satisfied with the performance of the transplanted heart*

perfusion [pə'fjuːʒn] *noun* passing of a liquid through vessels, an organ or tissue, especially the flow of blood into lung tissue; **hypothermic perfusion** = method of preserving donor organs by introducing a preserving solution and the storing the organ at a low temperature

peri- ['peri] *prefix* meaning near, around or enclosing

periadenitis [perɪədɪ'naɪtɪs] *noun* inflammation of tissue round a gland

perianal [perɪ'eɪnl] *adjective* around the anus; **perianal haematoma** = small painful swelling outside the anus caused by forcing a bowel movement

periarteritis [perɪɑːtə'raɪtɪs] *noun* inflammation of the outer coat of an artery and the tissue round it; **periarteritis nodosa** = collagen disease, where the walls of the arteries become inflamed, causing asthma, high blood pressure and kidney failure (NOTE: also called **polyarteritis nodosa**)

periarthritis [perɪɑː'θraɪtɪs] *noun* inflammation of the tissue round a joint; **chronic periarthritis** = inflammation of tissues round the shoulder joint (NOTE: also called **scapulohumeral arthritis**)

pericard- [peri'kɑːd] *prefix* referring to the pericardium

pericardectomy *or* **pericardiectomy** [perikɑː'dektəmi *or* perikɑːdi'ektəmi] *noun* surgical removal of the pericardium

pericardial [peri'kɑːdiəl] *adjective* referring to the pericardium; **pericardial effusion** = fluid which forms in the pericardial sac during pericarditis; **pericardial friction** = rubbing together of the two parts of the pericardium in pericarditis; **pericardial sac** *or* **serous pericardium** = the inner part of the pericardium forming a sac which contains fluid to prevent the two parts of the pericardium rubbing together

pericardiocentesis [perikɑːdiəusen'tiːsɪs] *noun* puncture of the pericardium to remove fluid

pericardiorrhaphy [perikɑːdi'ɔːrəfi] *noun* surgical operation to repair a wound in the pericardium

pericardiostomy [perikɑːdi'ɒstəmi] *noun* surgical operation to open the pericardium through the thoracic wall to drain off fluid

pericarditis [perikɑː'daɪtɪs] *noun* inflammation of the pericardium; **acute pericarditis** = sudden attack of fever and pains in the chest, caused by the two parts of the pericardium rubbing together; **chronic pericarditis** *or* **constrictive pericarditis** = condition where the pericardium becomes thickened and prevents the heart from functioning normally

pericardium [peri'kɑːdiəm] *noun* membrane which surrounds and supports the heart; **fibrous pericardium** = outer part of the pericardium which surrounds the heart and is attached to the main blood vessels; **parietal pericardium** = outer layer of serous pericardium attached to the fibrous pericardium; **serous pericardium** *or* **pericardial sac** = the inner part of the pericardium, forming a double sac which contains fluid to prevent the two parts of the pericardium from rubbing together; **visceral pericardium** = inner layer of serous pericardium, attached to the wall of the heart

pericardotomy *or* **pericardiotomy** [perikɑː'dɒtəmi *or* perikɑːdi'ɒtəmi] *noun* surgical operation to open the pericardium

perichondritis [perikɒn'draɪtɪs] *noun* inflammation of cartilage, especially in the outer ear

perichondrium [peri'kɒndriəm] *noun* fibrous connective tissue which covers cartilage

pericolpitis *or* **paracolpitis** [perikɒl'paɪtɪs *or* pærəkɒl'paɪtɪs] *noun* inflammation of the connective tissue round the vagina

pericranium [peri'kreɪniəm] *noun* connective tissue which covers the surface of the skull

pericystitis [perisi'staɪtɪs] *noun* inflammation of the structures round the bladder, usually caused by infection in the uterus

perifolliculitis [perifəlɪkju'laɪtɪs] *noun* inflammation of the skin round hair follicles

perihepatitis [perihepə'taɪtɪs] *noun* inflammation of the membrane round the liver

perilymph ['perilɪmf] *noun* fluid found in the labyrinth of the inner ear

perimeter [pə'rɪmɪtə] *noun* **(a)** instrument to measure the field of vision **(b)** length of the outside line around an enclosed area

perimetritis [perimə'traɪtɪs] *noun* inflammation of the perimetrium

perimetrium [peri'miːtriəm] *noun* membrane round the uterus

perimetry [pə'rɪmətri] *noun* measurement of the field of vision

perimysium [peri'maɪsiəm] *noun* sheath which surrounds a bundle of muscle fibres

perinatal [peri'neɪtl] *adjective* referring to the period just before and after childbirth; **perinatal mortality rate** = number of babies born dead or who die during the period immediately after childbirth, shown per thousand babies born; **perinatal period** = period of time before and after childbirth (from the 28th week after conception to the first week after delivery)

perinatology [perinə'tɒlədʒi] *noun* branch of medicine which studies and treats physiological and pathological conditions affecting the mother and/or infant just before and just after the birth of a baby

perineal [peri'niːəl] *adjective* referring to the perineum; **perineal body** = mass of muscle and fibres between the anus and the vagina or prostate; **perineal muscles** = muscles which lie in the perineum

perineoplasty [peri'niːəplæsti] *noun* surgical operation to repair the perineum by grafting tissue

perineorrhaphy [perini'ɔːrəfi] *noun* surgical operation to stitch up a perineum which has torn during childbirth

perinephric [peri'nefrɪk] *adjective* around the kidney

perinephritis [perinɪ'fraɪtɪs] *noun* inflammation of tissue round the kidney, which spreads from an infected kidney

perineum [perɪ'niːəm] *noun* skin and tissue between the opening of the urethra and the anus

perineurium [peri'njʊəriəm] *noun* connective tissue which surrounds bundles of nerve fibres

period ['pɪəriəd] *noun* **(a)** length of time; *the patient regained consciousness after a short period of time*; *she is allowed out of bed for two periods each day*; **safe period** = time during the menstrual cycle when conception is not likely to occur (used as a method of contraception); *see also* RHYTHM METHOD **(b)** menstruation or the menses, bleeding from the uterus which occurs in a woman each month when the lining of the uterus is shed because no fertilized egg is present; *she always has heavy periods*; *some women experience abdominal pain during their periods*; *she has bleeding between periods*

periodic [pɪəri'ɒdɪk] *adjective* which occurs from time to time; *he has periodic attacks of migraine*; *she has to go to the clinic for periodic checkups*; **periodic fever** = disease of the kidneys, common in Mediterranean countries; **periodic paralysis** = recurrent attacks of weakness where the level of potassium in the blood is low

periodicity [pɪəriə'dɪsəti] *noun* timing of recurrent attacks of a disease

periodontal *or* **periodontic** [periəʊ'dɒntl *or* periəʊ'dɒntɪk] *adjective* referring to the area around the teeth; **periodontal disease** = PERIODONTITIS; **periodontal membrane** *or* **periodontal ligament** = membrane which attaches a tooth to the bone of the jaw; *see illustration at* TOOTH

periodontics *or* **periodontia** [periəʊ'dɒntɪks *or* periəʊ'dɒnʃə] *noun* study of diseases of the periodontal membrane

periodontist [periəʊ'dɒntɪst] *noun* dentist who specializes in the treatment of gum diseases

periodontitis [periəʊdɒn'taɪtɪs] *noun* infection of the periodontal membrane leading to pyorrhoea, and resulting in the teeth falling out if untreated

periodontium [periəʊ'dɒnʃiəm] *noun* periodontal membrane, but also used to refer to the gums and bone around a tooth

perionychia *or* **perionyxis** [periəʊ'nɪkiə *or* periəʊ'nɪksɪs] *noun* painful swelling round a fingernail

perioperative [peri'ɒpərətɪv] *adjective* before and after a surgical operation

During the perioperative period little attention is given to thermoregulation

British Journal of Nursing

periosteal [peri'ɒstiəl] *adjective* referring to the periosteum; attached to the periosteum

periosteotome [peri'ɒstiəutəʊm] *noun* surgical instrument used to cut the periosteum

periosteum [peri'ɒstiəm] *noun* dense layer of connective tissue around a bone; *see illustration at* BONE STRUCTURE

periostitis [periɒ'staɪtɪs] *noun* inflammation of the periosteum

peripheral [pə'rɪfərl] *adjective* at the edge; **peripheral nerves** = pairs of motor and sensory nerves which branch out from the brain and spinal cord; **peripheral nervous system (PNS)** = all the nerves in different parts of the body which are linked and governed by the central nervous system; **peripheral vasodilator** = chemical substance which acts to widen the blood vessels in the arms and legs and so improves bad circulation; **peripheral vascular disease** = disease affecting the blood vessels which supply the arms and legs

periphlebitis [perɪflə'baɪtɪs] *noun* (i) inflammation of the outer coat of a vein; (ii) inflammation of the connective tissue round a vein

perisalpingitis [perisælpɪn'dʒaɪtɪs] *noun* inflammation of the peritoneum and other parts round a Fallopian tube

perisplenitis [perisplə'naɪtɪs] *noun* inflammation of the peritoneum and other parts round the spleen

peristalsis [peri'stælsɪs] *noun* movement (like waves) produced by alternate contraction and relaxation of muscles along an organ such as the intestine or oesophagus, which pushes the contents of the organ along it automatically; *compare* ANTIPERISTALSIS

peristaltic [perɪˈstæltɪk] *adjective* occurring in waves, as in peristalsis

peritendinitis [peritendiˈnaɪtɪs] *noun* painful inflammation of the sheath round a tendon

peritomy [pəˈrɪtəmi] *noun* (a) surgical operation on the eye, where the conjunctiva is cut in a circle round the cornea (b) circumcision

peritoneal [peritəˈnɪəl] *adjective* referring to the peritoneum; belonging to the peritoneum; **peritoneal cavity** = space between the layers of the peritoneum, containing the major organs of the abdomen; **peritoneal dialysis** = removing waste matter from a patient's blood by introducing fluid into the peritoneum which then acts as a filter (as opposed to haemodialysis)

peritoneoscope [periˈtəuniəskəup] = LAPAROSCOPE

peritoneoscopy [peritəuniˈɒskəpi] = LAPAROSCOPY

peritoneum [peritəuˈniːəm] *noun* membrane which lines the abdominal cavity and covers the organs in it; **parietal peritoneum** = part of the peritoneum which lines the inner abdominal wall; **visceral peritoneum** = part of the peritoneum which covers the organs in the abdominal cavity

peritonitis [peritəuˈnaɪtɪs] *noun* inflammation of the peritoneum as a result of bacterial infection; **primary peritonitis** = peritonitis caused by direct infection from the blood or the lymph; **secondary peritonitis** = peritonitis caused by infection from an adjoining tissue, such as the rupturing of the appendix

COMMENT: peritonitis is a serious condition and can have many causes. One of its effects is to stop the peristalsis of the intestine so making it impossible for the patient to eat and digest

peritonsillar [periˈtɒnsɪlə] *adjective* around the tonsils; **peritonsillar abscess** = QUINSY

peritrichous [pərɪˈtraɪkəs] *adjective* (bacteria) where the surface of the cell is covered with flagella

periumbilical [periʌmˈbɪlɪkl] *adjective* around the navel

periureteritis [perijuərɪtəˈraɪtɪs] *noun* inflammation of the tissue round a ureter, usually caused by inflammation of the ureter itself

periurethral [perijuˈriːθrəl] *adjective* around the urethra

perlèche [pəˈleʃ] *noun* (a) cracks in dry skin at the corners of the mouth, often caused by riboflavine deficiency (b) candidiasis

permanent [ˈpɜːmənənt] *adjective* which exists always; *the accident left him with a permanent disability*; **permanent teeth** = teeth in an adult, which replace the child's milk teeth during late childhood

COMMENT: the permanent teeth consist of eight incisors, four canines, eight premolars and twelve molars, the last four molars (one on each side of the upper and lower jaw) being called the wisdom teeth

permanently [ˈpɜːmənəntli] *adverb* always, for ever; *he was permanently disabled in the accident*

permeability [pɜːmiəˈbɪləti] *noun* (of a membrane) ability to allow certain substances in a fluid to pass through

permeable membrane [ˈpɜːmiəbl ˈmembreɪn] *noun* membrane which allows certain substances in a fluid to pass through it

pernicious [pəˈnɪʃəs] *adjective* harmful or dangerous (disease), abnormally severe (disease) which is likely to end in death; **pernicious anaemia** = disease where an inability to absorb vitamin B_{12} prevents the production of red blood cells and damages the spinal cord (NOTE: also called **Addison's anaemia**)

pernio [ˈpɜːniəu] *noun* **erythema pernio** = chilblain, the condition where the skin of the fingers, toes, nose or ears reacts to cold by becoming red, swollen and itchy

perniosis [pɜːniˈəusɪs] *noun* any condition caused by cold which affects blood vessels in the skin

pero- [ˈperəu] *prefix* meaning deformed or defective

peromelia [perəuˈmiːliə] *noun* congenital deformity of the limbs

peroneal [perəuˈniːəl] *adjective* referring to the outside of the leg; **peroneal muscle** *or* **peroneus** = one of three muscles (brevis, longus, tertius) on the outside of the lower leg which make the leg turn outwards

peroperative [pə'rɒpərətɪv] *adjective* taking place during a surgical operation

peroral [pər'ɔːrəl] *adjective* through the mouth

persecute ['pɜːsɪkjuːt] *verb* to treat someone badly, to make someone suffer all the time; *in paranoia, the patient feels he is being persecuted*

persecution [pɜːsɪ'kjuːʃn] *noun* being treated badly, being made to suffer; *he suffers from persecution mania*

perseveration [pəsəvə'reɪʃn] *noun* repeating actions or words without any stimulus

persist [pə'sɪst] *verb* to continue for some time; *the weakness in the right arm persisted for two weeks*

persistent [pə'sɪstənt] *adjective* which continues for some time; *she suffered from a persistent cough*; *treatment aimed at the relief of persistent angina*; *see also* VEGETATIVE

person ['pɜːsən] *noun* man or woman

personal ['pɜːsənl] *adjective* (i) referring to a person; (ii) belonging to a person; *only certain senior members of staff can consult the personal records of the patients*

personality [pɜːsə'næləti] *noun* way in which one person is mentally different from another; **personality disorder** = disorder which affects the way a person behaves, especially in relation to other people

> Alzheimer's disease is a progressive disorder which sees a gradual decline in intellectual functioning and deterioration of personality and physical coordination and activity
>
> *Nursing Times*

personnel [pɜːsə'nel] *noun* members of staff; *all hospital personnel must be immunized against hepatitis*; *only senior personnel can inspect the patients' medical records* (NOTE: **personnel** is plural)

perspiration [pɜːspə'reɪʃn] *noun* (i) action of sweating, of producing moisture through the sweat glands; (ii) sweat, moisture produced by the sweat glands; *perspiration broke out on his forehead*; **sensible perspiration** = drops of sweat which can be seen on the skin, secreted by the sweat glands

> COMMENT: perspiration is formed in the sweat glands under the epidermis and cools the body as the moisture evaporates from the skin. Sweat contains salt, and in hot countries it may be necessary to take salt tablets to replace the salt lost through perspiration

perspire [pə'spaɪə] *verb* to sweat, to produce moisture through the sweat glands; *after the game of tennis he was perspiring*

Perthes' disease *or* **Perthes' hip** ['pɜːtiːz dɪ'ziːz *or* 'pɜːtiːz 'hɪp] *noun* disease (found in young boys) where the upper end of the femur degenerates and does not develop normally, sometimes resulting in a permanent limp

pertussis [pə'tʌsɪs] = WHOOPING COUGH

perversion [pə'vɜːʃn] *noun* any abnormal behaviour; *he is suffering from a form of sexual perversion*

pes [pes] *noun* foot; **pes cavus** = CLAW FOOT; **pes planus** = FLAT FOOT

pessary ['pesəri] *noun* **(a)** vaginal suppository, drug in soluble material which is pushed into the vagina and absorbed into the blood there **(b)** contraceptive device worn inside the vagina to prevent spermatozoa entering **(c)** device like a ring, which is put into the vagina as treatment for prolapse of the uterus

pest [pest] *noun* animal which carries disease, attacks plants and animals and harms or kills them; *a spray to remove insect pests*

pesticide ['pestɪsaɪd] *noun* substance which kills pests

petechia [pe'tiːkɪə] *noun* small red spot, where blood has entered the skin (NOTE: the plural is **petechiae**)

petit mal ['pəti 'mæl] *noun* less severe form of epilepsy, where loss of consciousness attacks last only a few seconds and the patient appears simply to be thinking deeply

petri dish ['peɪtri 'dɪʃ] *noun* small round and shallow glass or plastic dish, sometimes with a lid, in which a culture is grown

petrosal [pə'trəʊsl] *adjective* referring to the petrous part of the temporal bone

petrositis [petrəʊ'saɪtɪs] *noun* inflammation of the petrous part of the temporal bone

petrous ['petrəs] *adjective* (i) like stone; (ii) petrosal; **petrous bone** = part of the temporal bone which forms the base of the skull and the inner and middle ears

-pexy [peksi] *suffix* referring to fixation of an organ by surgery

Peyer's patches ['paɪəz 'pætʃɪz] *noun* patches of lymphoid tissue on the mucous membrane of the small intestine

Peyronie's disease ['peɪrəni:z dɪ'zi:z] *noun* condition where hard fibre develops in the penis which becomes painful when erect (associated with Dupuytren's contracture)

PGEA = POSTGRADUATE EDUCATION ALLOWANCE

pH ['pi: 'eɪtʃ] *noun* concentration of hydrogen ions in a solution, which determines its acidity; **pH factor** = factor which indicates acidity or alkalinity; **pH test** = test to see how acid or alkaline a solution is

COMMENT: the pH factor is shown as a number; pH 7 is neutral; pH 8 and above show that the solution is alkaline and pH 6 and below show that the solution is acid

phaco- *or* **phako-** ['fækəʊ] *prefix* referring to the lens of the eye

phaeochromocytoma [fi:əʊkrəʊməʊsaɪ'təʊmə] *noun* tumour of the adrenal glands which affects the secretion of hormones such as adrenaline, which in turn results in hypertension and hyperglycaemia

phag- *or* **phago-** [fæg or 'fægəʊ] *prefix* referring to eating

-phage [feɪdʒ] *suffix* which eats

-phagia ['feɪdʒə] *suffix* referring to eating

phagocyte ['fægəsaɪt] *noun* cell, especially a white blood cell, which can surround and destroy other cells, such as bacteria cells

phagocytic [fægə'saɪtɪk] *adjective* (i) referring to phagocytes; (ii) which destroys cells; *monocytes become phagocytic during infection*

phagocytosis [fægəsaɪ'təʊsɪs] *noun* destruction of bacteria cells and foreign bodies by phagocytes

phako- *or* **phaco-** ['fækəʊ] *prefix* referring to the lens of the eye

phakic ['fækɪk] *adjective* (eye) which has its natural lens

phalangeal [fə'lændʒɪəl] *adjective* referring to the phalanges

phalanges [fə'lændʒi:z] *plural of* PHALANX

phalangitis [fælən'dʒaɪtɪs] *noun* inflammation of the fingers or toes caused by infection of tissue

phalanx ['fælæŋks] *noun* bone in a finger or toe; *see illustrations at* HAND, FOOT

COMMENT: the fingers and toes have three phalanges each, except the thumb and big toe, which have only two

phalloplasty ['fæləplæsti] *noun* surgical operation to repair a damaged or deformed penis

phallus ['fæləs] *noun* penis, male genital organ

phantom ['fæntəm] *noun* **(a)** model of the whole body or part of the body, used to practise or demonstrate surgical operations **(b)** ghost, something which is not there but seems to be there; **phantom limb** = condition where a patient seems to feel sensations in a limb which has been amputated; **phantom pregnancy** = PSEUDOCYESIS; **phantom tumour** = condition where a swelling occurs which imitates a swelling caused by a tumour

pharmaceutical [fɑːmə'su:tɪkl] **1** *adjective* referring to pharmacy or drugs; **the Pharmaceutical Society** = professional association for pharmacists in Great Britain **2** *noun* **pharmaceuticals** = drugs

pharmacist ['fɑːməsɪst] *noun* trained person who is qualified to prepare medicines according to the instructions on a doctor's prescription; **community pharmacist** *or* **retail pharmacist** = person who makes medicines and sells them in a chemist's shop

COMMENT: qualified pharmacists must be registered by the Pharmaceutical Society of Great Britain before they can practise

pharmaco- ['fɑːməkəʊ] *prefix* referring to drugs

pharmacodynamic [fɑːməkəʊdaɪ'næmɪk] *adjective* (property of a drug) which affects the part where it is applied

pharmacokinetic [fɑːməkəʊkaɪ'netɪk] *adjective* (property of a drug) which has an effect over a period of time

pharmacological [fɑːmækə'lɒdʒɪkl] *adjective* referring to pharmacology

pharmacologist [fɑːmə'kɒlədʒɪst] *noun* scientist who specializes in the study of drugs

pharmacology [fɑːmə'kɒlədʒi] *noun* study of drugs or medicines, and their actions, properties and characteristics

pharmacopoeia [fɑːməkəˈpiːə] *noun* official list of drugs, their methods of preparation, dosages and the ways in which they should be used

COMMENT: the British Pharmocopoeia is the official list of drugs used in the United Kingdom. The drugs listed in it have the letters BP after their name. In the USA the official list is the United States Pharmacopeia or USP

pharmacy [ˈfɑːməsi] *noun* **(a)** study of making and dispensing of drugs; *the six pharmacy students are taking their diploma examinations this year*; *he has a qualification in pharmacy* **(b)** shop or department in a hospital where drugs are prepared

Pharmacy Act [ˈfɑːməsi ˈækt] *noun* one of several Acts of the British Parliament (Pharmacy and Poisons Act 1933, Misuse of Drugs Act 1971, Poisons Act 1972) which regulate the making, prescribing and selling of drugs

pharyng- *or* **pharyngo-** [ˈfærɪndʒ or fəˈrɪŋgəʊ] *prefix* referring to the pharynx

pharyngeal [færɪnˈdʒiːəl] *adjective* referring to the pharynx; **pharyngeal pouch** = visceral pouch, one of the pouches in the side of the throat of an embryo; **pharyngeal tonsil** = adenoidal tonsil, lymphoid tissue at the back of the throat where the passages from the nose join the pharynx

pharyngectomy [færɪnˈdʒektəmi] *noun* surgical removal of part of the pharynx, especially in cases of cancer of the pharynx

pharyngismus *or* **pharyngism** [færɪnˈdʒɪzməs or ˈfærɪndʒɪzm] *noun* spasm which contracts the muscles of the pharynx

pharyngitis [færɪnˈdʒaɪtɪs] *noun* inflammation of the pharynx

pharyngocele [fəˈrɪŋgəʊsiːl] *noun* (i) cyst which opens off the pharynx; (ii) hernia of part of the pharynx

pharyngolaryngeal [fəˈrɪŋgəʊləˈrɪndʒl] *adjective* referring to the pharynx and the larynx

pharyngoscope [fəˈrɪŋgəʊskəʊp] *noun* instrument with a light attached, used by a doctor to examine the pharynx

pharyngotympanic tube [fərɪŋgəʊtɪmˈpænɪk ˈtjuːb] *noun* Eustachian tube, one of two tubes which connect the back of the throat to the middle ear

pharynx [ˈfærɪŋks] *noun* muscular passage leading from the back of the mouth to the oesophagus

COMMENT: the nasal cavity (or nasopharynx) leads to the back of the mouth (or oropharynx) and then into the pharynx proper, which in turn becomes the oesophagus when it reaches the sixth cervical vertebra. The pharynx is the channel both for air and food; the trachea (or windpipe) leads off it before it joins the oesophagus. The upper part of the pharynx (the nasopharynx) connects with the middle ear through the Eustachian tubes. When air pressure in the middle ear is not equal to that outside (as when going up or down in a plane), the tube becomes blocked and pressure can be reduced by swallowing

phase [feɪz] *noun* stage or period of development; *if the cancer is diagnosed in its early phase, the chances of complete cure are much greater*

phenol [ˈfiːnɒl] *noun* carbolic acid, strong disinfectant used for external use

phenotype [ˈfiːnəʊtaɪp] *noun* the particular characteristics of an organism; *compare* GENOTYPE

all cancers may be reduced to fundamental mechanisms based on cancer risk genes or oncogenes within ourselves. An oncogene is a gene that encodes a protein that contributes to the malignant phenotype of the cell
British Medical Journal

phenylalanine [fiːnɪˈlæləniːn] *noun* essential amino acid

phenylketonuria [fiːnɪlkiːtəʊˈnjʊəriə] *noun* hereditary defect which affects the way in which the body breaks down phenylalanine, which in turn concentrates toxic metabolites in the nervous system causing brain damage

COMMENT: to have phenylketonuria, a child has to inherit the gene from both parents. The condition can be treated by giving the child a special diet but early diagnosis is essential to avoid brain damage

phial [ˈfaɪəl] *noun* small medicine bottle

-philia [ˈfɪliə] *suffix* meaning attraction or liking for something

philtrum [ˈfɪltrəm] *noun* **(a)** groove in the centre of the top lip **(b)** drug believed to stimulate sexual desire

phimosis [faɪ'məʊsɪs] *noun* condition where the foreskin is tight and has to be removed by circumcision

phleb- *or* **phlebo-** ['fleb or 'flɪb or 'fliːbəʊ or 'flebəʊ] *prefix* referring to a vein

phlebectomy [flɪ'bektəmi] *noun* surgical removal of a vein or part of a vein

phlebitis [flɪ'baɪtɪs] *noun* inflammation of a vein

phlebogram ['flebəgræm] *noun* venogram, an X-ray picture of a vein or system of veins

phlebography [flɪ'bɒgrəfi] *noun* venography, X-ray examination of a vein using a radio-opaque dye so that the vein will show up on the film

phlebolith ['flebəlɪθ] *noun* stone which forms in a vein as a result of an old thrombus becoming calcified

phlebothrombosis [flebəʊθrɒm'bəʊsɪs] *noun* blood clot in a deep vein in the legs or pelvis, which can easily detach and form an embolus in a lung

phlebotomy [flɪ'bɒtəmi] *noun* operation where a vein or an artery is cut so that blood can be removed (as when taking blood from a donor)

phlegm [flem] *noun* sputum, mucus found in an inflamed nose, throat or lung and coughed up by the patient; *she was coughing up phlegm into her handkerchief*

phlegmasia alba dolens [fleg'meɪziə 'ælbə 'dəʊləns] *noun* milk leg or white leg, acute oedema of the leg, a condition which affects women after childbirth, where a leg becomes pale and inflamed as a result of lymphatic obstruction

phlyctenule [flɪk'tenjuːl] *noun* (i) tiny blister on the cornea or conjunctiva; (ii) any small blister

phobia ['fəʊbiə] *noun* abnormal fear; *he has a phobia about or of dogs*; *fear of snakes is one of the commonest phobias*

-phobia ['fəʊbiə] *suffix* meaning neurotic fear of something; **agoraphobia** = fear of open spaces; **claustrophobia** = fear of enclosed spaces

phobic ['fəʊbɪk] *adjective* referring to a phobia; **phobic anxiety** = state of worry caused by a phobia

-phobic ['fəʊbɪk] *suffix* person who has a phobia of something; **agoraphobic** = person who is afraid of open spaces

phocomelia *or* **phocomely** [fəʊkə'miːliə or fəʊ'kɒməli] *noun* (i) congenital condition where the upper part of the limbs do not develop, leaving the hands or feet directly attached to the body; (ii) congenital condition in which the legs develop normally, but the arms are absent or underdeveloped

phon- *or* **phono-** ['fəʊn or 'fəʊnəʊ] *prefix* referring to sound or voice

phonocardiogram [fəʊnəʊ'kɑːdiəgræm] *noun* chart of the sounds made by the heart

phonocardiography [fəʊnəʊkɑːdi'ɒgrəfi] *noun* recording the sounds made by the heart

phosphataemia [fɒsfə'tiːmiə] *noun* presence of excess phosphates (such as calcium or sodium) in the blood

phosphatase ['fɒsfəteɪz] *noun* group of enzymes which are important in the cycle of muscle contraction and in the calcification of bones

phosphate ['fɒsfeɪt] *noun* salt of phosphoric acid, used in tonics

phosphaturia [fɒsfə'tjʊəriə] *noun* condition where excess phosphates are present in the urine

COMMENT: the urine becomes cloudy, which can indicate stones in the bladder or kidney

phospholipid [fɒsfə'lɪpɪd] *noun* compound with fatty acids, which is one of the main components of membranous tissue

phosphonecrosis [fɒsfəne'krəʊsɪs] *noun* necrotic condition affecting the kidneys, liver and bones, usually seen in people who work with phosphorus

phosphorescent [fɒsfə'resənt] *adjective* which shines without producing heat

phosphoric acid [fɒs'fɒrɪk 'æsɪd] *noun* acid which forms phosphates

phosphorus ['fɒsfərəs] *noun* toxic chemical element which is present in minute quantities in bones and nerve tissue; it causes burns if it touches the skin, and can poison if swallowed (NOTE: chemical symbol is **P**)

phossy jaw ['fɒsi 'dʒɔː] *noun* type of phosphonecrosis resulting in disintegration of the bones of the lower jaw, caused by inhaling phosphorus fumes (the disease was once common among workers in match factories)

phot- *or* **photo-** [fɒt or fəʊt or 'fəʊtəʊ] *prefix* referring to light

photalgia [fəʊˈtældʒə] *noun* (i) pain in the eye caused by bright light; (ii) severe photophobia

photocoagulation [fəʊtəʊkəʊægjuˈleɪʃn] *noun* process where tissue coagulates from the heat caused by light

COMMENT: photocoagulation is used to treat a detached retina

photodermatosis [fəʊtəʊdɜːməˈtəʊsɪs] *noun* lesion of the skin after exposure to bright light

photogenic [fəʊtəʊˈdʒenɪk] *adjective* (i) which is produced by the action of light; (ii) which produces light

photograph [ˈfəʊtəɡrɑːf] **1** *noun* picture taken with a camera, which uses the chemical action of light on sensitive film; **X-ray photograph** = picture produced by exposing sensitive film to X-rays; *he was examining the X-ray photographs of the patient's chest* **2** *verb* to take a picture with a camera

photography [fəˈtɒɡrəfi] *noun* taking pictures with a camera; *the development of X-ray photography has meant that internal disorders can be more easily diagnosed*

photophobia [fəʊtəʊˈfəʊbɪə] *noun* (i) condition where the eyes become sensitive to light and conjunctivitis may be caused (it can be associated with measles and some other infectious diseases); (ii) morbid fear of light

photophthalmia [fəʊtəfˈθælmɪə] *noun* inflammation of the eye caused by bright light, as in snow blindness

photopic vision [fəʊˈtɒpɪk ˈvɪʒn] *noun* vision which is adapted to bright light (as in daylight) by using the cones in the retina instead of the rods, as in scotopic vision; *see also* LIGHT ADAPTATION

photoreceptor neurone [fəʊtəʊrɪˈseptə ˈnjʊərəʊn] *noun* rod or cone in the retina, which is sensitive to light or colour

photoretinitis [fəʊtəʊretiˈnaɪtɪs] *noun* sun blindness, damaged retina caused by looking at the sun

photosensitive [fəʊtəʊˈsensətɪv] *adjective* (skin or lens) which is sensitive to light, which is stimulated by light

photosensitivity [fəʊtəʊsensəˈtɪvəti] *noun* being sensitive to light

phototherapy [fəʊtəʊˈθerəpi] *noun* treatment of jaundice and vitamin D deficiency, which involves exposing a patient to rays of ultraviolet light

phototoxicity [fəʊtəʊtɒkˈsɪsəti] *noun* cause of damage to the retina of the eye due to exposure to too much ultraviolet light or radiation (UVR); *children's retinas are more likely to suffer damage as a result of phototoxicity from excess ultraviolet light than those of adults; see also* RETINOPATHY

photuria [fəʊˈtjʊərɪə] *noun* phosphorescent urine

phren- *or* **phreno-** [ˈfren *or* ˈfrenəʊ] *prefix* referring to (i) the brain; (ii) the phrenic nerve

phrenemphraxis [frenemˈfræksɪs] *noun* surgical operation to crush the phrenic nerve in order to paralyse the diaphragm

-phrenia [ˈfriːnɪə] *suffix* meaning disorder of the mind

phrenic [ˈfrenɪk] *adjective* **(a)** referring to the diaphragm; **phrenic nerve** = pair of nerves which controls the muscles in the diaphragm; **phrenic avulsion** = *see* AVULSION **(b)** referring to the mind or intellect

phrenicectomy [frenɪˈsektəmi] *noun* surgical removal of all or part of the phrenic nerve

phreniclasia [frenɪˈkleɪzɪə] *noun* operation to clamp the phrenic nerve

phrenicotomy [frenɪˈkɒtəmi] *noun* operation to divide the phrenic nerve

phthiriasis [θəˈraɪəsɪs] *noun* infestation with the crab louse

Phthirius pubis [ˈθaɪərəs ˈpjuːbɪs] pubic louse or crab louse, louse which infests the pubic region

phthisis [ˈθaɪsɪs] *noun* old term for tuberculosis

phycomycosis [faɪkəʊmaɪˈkəʊsɪs] *noun* acute infection of the lungs, central nervous system and other organs by a fungus

physi- *or* **physio-** [ˈfɪzi *or* ˈfɪzɪəʊ] *prefix* referring to (i) physiology; (ii) physical

physic [ˈfɪzɪk] *noun* old term for medicine

physical [ˈfɪzɪkl] **1** *adjective* referring to the body, as opposed to the mind; **physical dependence** = state where a person is addicted to a drug such as heroin and suffers physical effects if he stops taking the drug; **physical education** = teaching of sports and exercises in school; **physical examination** =

examination of a patient's body to see if he is healthy; **physical medicine** = branch of medicine which deals with physical disabilities or with treatment of disorders after they have been diagnosed; **physical sign** = symptom which can be seen on the patient's body or which can be produced by percussion and palpitation; **physical therapy** = treatment of disorders by heat, by massage, by exercise and other physical means **2** *noun* physical examination; *he has to pass a physical before being accepted by the police force*

physically ['fızıklı] *adverb* referring to the body; *physically he is very weak, but his mind is still alert*

physician [fı'zıʃn] *noun* registered doctor who is not a surgeon (NOTE: in British English, physician refers to a specialist doctor, though not usually a surgeon, while in American English it is used for any qualified doctor)

physio ['fızıəu] *noun (informal)* **(a)** session of physiotherapy treatment **(b)** physiotherapist

physiological [fızıə'lɒdʒıkl] *adjective* referring to physiology, to the normal functions of the body; **physiological saline** *or* **solution** = any solution used to keep cells or tissue alive

physiologist [fızı'ɒlədʒıst] *noun* scientist who specializes in the study of the functions of living organisms

physiology [fızı'ɒlədʒi] *noun* study of living organisms and their normal functions

physiotherapist [fızıə'θerəpıst] *noun* trained specialist who gives physiotherapy

physiotherapy [fızıə'θerəpi] *noun* treatment of a disorder or condition by exercise, massage, heat treatment, infrared lamps, etc., to restore strength, to restore function after a disease or injury, to correct a deformity; **physiotherapy clinic** = clinic where patients can have physiotherapy

phyt- *or* **phyto-** ['faɪt *or* 'faɪtəu] *prefix* referring to plants, coming from plants

phytooestrogen [faɪtəu'iːstrədʒən] *noun* substance obtained from cereals, legumes and seeds which has a similar effect on the body as oestrogen, used increasingly as an alternative to hormone replacement therapy

phyto-photo dermatitis ['faɪtəu'fəutəu dɜːmə'taɪtıs] *noun* acute skin reaction due to the combination of plant irritation and sunlight

pia mater ['paɪə 'meɪtə] *noun* delicate inner layer of the meninges, the membrane which covers the brain and spinal cord

pian [piː'ɑːn] = YAWS

pica ['paɪkə] *noun* desire to eat things (such as wood or paper) which are not food, often found in pregnant women and small children

pick [pık] *verb* to take away small pieces of something with the fingers or with a tool; *she picked the pieces of glass out of the wound with tweezers*; **to pick one's nose** = to take pieces of mucus out of the nostrils; **to pick one's teeth with a pin** = to take away pieces of food which are stuck between the teeth

Pick's disease ['pıks dı'ziːz] *noun* **(a)** rare condition, a form of presenile dementia, where a disorder of the lipoid metabolism causes retarded mental development, anaemia, loss of weight and swelling of the spleen and liver **(b)** constrictive pericarditis

pick up ['pık 'ʌp] *verb (informal)* **(a)** to catch a disease; *he must have picked up the disease when he was travelling in Africa* **(b)** to get stronger or better; *he was ill for months, but he's picking up now*

pico- ['piːkəu] *prefix* meaning one million millionth (10^{-12}) (NOTE: symbol is **p**)

picomole ['piːkəuməul] *noun* unit of measurement of the amount of substance (= one million millionth of a mole) (NOTE: with figures usually written **pmol**)

picornavirus [piːkɔːnə'vaɪrəs] *noun* virus containing RNA, such as enteroviruses and rhinoviruses

PID ['piː 'aɪ 'diː] = PROLAPSED INTERVERTEBRAL DISC

pigeon chest ['pıdʒən 'tʃest] *noun* deformity of the chest, where the breastbone sticks out

pigeon toes ['pıdʒən 'təuz] *noun* condition where the feet turn towards the inside when a person is standing upright

pigment ['pıgmənt] *noun* (i) substance which gives colour to part of the body such as blood, the skin or hair; (ii) *(in pharmacy)* a paint; **bile pigment** = yellow colouring matter in bile; **blood pigment** = HAEMOGLOBIN; **respiratory pigment** = blood pigment which can carry oxygen collected in the lungs and release it in tissues

COMMENT: the body contains several substances which control colour: melanin gives dark colour to the skin and hair;

bilirubin gives yellow colour to bile and urine; haemoglobin in the blood gives the skin a pink colour; carotene can give a reddish-yellow colour to the skin if the patient eats too many tomatoes or carrots. Some pigment cells can carry oxygen and are called 'respiratory pigments'

pigmentation [pɪgmen'teɪʃn] *noun* colouring of the body, especially that produced by deposits of pigment

pigmented [pɪg'mentɪd] *adjective* coloured, showing an abnormal colour; **pigmented epithelium** *or* **pigmented layer** = coloured tissue at the back of the retina

piles [paɪlz] = HAEMORRHOIDS

pill [pɪl] *noun* small hard round ball of drug which is to be swallowed whole; *he has to take the pills twice a day*; *the doctor put her on a course of vitamin pills*; **the pill** = oral contraceptive; **she's on the pill** = she is taking a regular course of contraceptive pills; **morning-after pill** *or* **next-day pill** = contraceptive pill taken after intercourse

pillow ['pɪləʊ] *noun* soft cushion on a bed which the head lies on when the patient is lying down; *the nurse gave her an extra pillow to keep her head raised*

pill-rolling ['pɪl'rəʊlɪŋ] *noun* nervous action of the fingers, in which the patient seems to be rolling a very small object, associated with Parkinson's disease

pilo- ['paɪlə] *prefix* referring to hair

pilomotor nerve [paɪlə'məʊtə 'nɜ:v] *noun* nerve which supplies the arrector pili muscles attached to hair follicles

pilomotor reflex [paɪlə'məʊtə 'ri:fleks] *noun* reaction of the dermal papillae of the skin to cold, fear, etc., which causes the hairs on the skin to become erect

pilonidal cyst [paɪlə'naɪdl 'sɪst] *noun* cyst containing hair, usually found at the bottom of the spine near the buttocks

pilonidal sinus [paɪlə'naɪdl 'saɪnəs] *noun* small depression with hairs at the base of the spine

pilosebaceous [paɪləsə'beɪʃəs] *adjective* referring to the hair follicles and the glands attached to them

pilosis *or* **pilosism** [paɪ'ləʊsɪs *or* 'paɪləsɪzm] *noun* condition where someone has an abnormal amount of hair or where hair is present in an abnormal place

pilus ['paɪləs] *noun* (i) one hair; (ii) hair-like process on the surface of a bacterium; *see also* ARRECTOR PILI

pimple ['pɪmpl] *noun* papule or pustule (small swelling on the skin, containing pus); *he had pimples on his neck*; *is that red pimple painful?*; **goose pimples** = reaction of the skin to being cold or frightened, where the skin is raised into many little bumps by the action of the erector pili muscles

pimply ['pɪmpli] *adjective* covered with pimples

pin [pɪn] **1** *noun* **(a)** small sharp piece of metal for attaching things together; *the nurse fastened the bandage with a pin*; **safety pin** = special type of bent pin with a guard which protects the point, used for attaching nappies or bandages **(b)** metal nail used to attach broken bones; *he has had a pin inserted in his hip* **2** *verb* to attach with a pin; *she pinned the bandages carefully to stop them slipping*; *the bone had fractured in several places and needed pinning*

pinch [pɪnʃ] **1** *noun* (i) squeezing the thumb and first finger together; (ii) quantity of something which can be held between the thumb and first finger; *she put a pinch of salt into the water* **2** *verb* **(a)** to squeeze something tightly between the thumb and first finger **(b)** to squeeze; *she developed a sore on her ankle where her shoe pinched*

pineal (body) *or* **pineal gland** ['pɪniəl 'bɒdi *or* 'pɪniəl 'glænd] *noun* small cone-shaped gland situated below the corpus callosum in the brain, which produces melatonin and is believed to be associated with the circadian rhythm; *see illustration at* BRAIN

pinguecula *or* **pinguicula** [pɪŋ'gwekjʊlə *or* pɪŋ'gwɪkjʊlə] *noun* condition affecting old people, where the conjunctiva in the eyes has small yellow growths near the edge of the cornea, usually on the nasal side

pink [pɪŋk] *adjective* of a colour like very pale red; **pink disease** = erythroedema or acrodynia, children's disease where the child's hands, feet and face swell and become pink, with a fever and loss of appetite, caused by an allergy to mercury; **pink eye** = inflammation of the conjunctiva, where the eyelids become swollen and sticky and discharge pus, common in schools and other institutions, caused by the Koch-Weeks bacillus (NOTE: also called **epidemic conjunctivitis**)

pinna ['pɪnə] *noun* the outer ear, the part of the ear which is outside the head, connected by a passage to the eardrum; *see illustration at* EAR

pinnaplasty ['pɪnəplæsti] *noun* cosmetic surgical procedure to correct the shape of the ear

pinocytosis [paɪnəʊsaɪ'təʊsɪs] *noun* process by which a cell surrounds and takes in fluid

pins and needles ['pɪnz ən 'niːdlz] *noun* non-medical term for paraesthesia, an unpleasant tingling feeling, caused when a nerve is irritated, as when a limb has become numb after the circulation has been blocked for a short time

pint [paɪnt] *noun* unit of measurement of liquids (= about 0.56 of a litre); *he was given six pints of blood in blood transfusions during the operation*

pinta ['pɪntə] *noun* skin disease of the tropical regions of America, caused by a spirochaete *Treponema*

COMMENT: the skin on the hands and feet swells and loses its colour

pinworm ['pɪnwɜːm] *noun US* threadworm, thin nematode worm *Enterobius vermicularis* which infests the large intestine

PIP ['piː 'aː 'piː] = PROXIMAL INTERPHALANGEAL JOINT

pipette [pɪ'pet] *noun* thin glass tube used in the laboratory for taking or measuring samples of liquid

piriform fossae ['pɪrɪfɔːm 'fɒsiː] *plural noun* two hollows at the sides of the upper end of the larynx

pisiform (bone) ['pɪsɪfɔːm 'bəʊn] *noun* one of the eight small carpal bones in the wrist; *see illustration at* HAND

pit [pɪt] *noun* hollow place on a surface; **the pit of the stomach** = the epigastrium, the part of the upper abdomen between the ribcage above the navel; *see also* ARMPIT

pitcher's elbow ['pɪtʃəz 'elbəʊ] *US* = TENNIS ELBOW

pithiatism [pɪ'θaɪətɪzm] *noun* way of influencing the patient's mind by persuading him of something, as when the doctor treats a condition by telling the patient that he is in fact well

pitted ['pɪtɪd] *adjective* covered with small hollows; *his skin was pitted by acne*

pitting ['pɪtɪŋ] *noun* formation of hollows in the skin

pituitary body *or* **pituitary gland** [pɪ'tjuːɪtri 'bɒdi *or* 'glænd] *noun* hypophysis cerebri, the main endocrine gland in the body; *see illustration at* BRAIN; **pituitary fossa** = hollow in the upper surface of the sphenoid bone in which the pituitary gland sits (NOTE: also called **sella turcica**)

COMMENT: the pituitary gland is about the size of a pea and hangs down from the base of the brain, inside the sphenoid bone, on a stalk which attaches it to the hypothalamus. The front lobe of the gland (the adenohypophysis) secretes several hormones (TSH, ACTH) which stimulate the adrenal and thyroid glands, or which stimulate the production of sex hormones, melanin and milk. The posterior lobe of the pituitary gland (the neurohypophysis) secretes the antidiuretic hormone (ADH) and oxytocin. The pituitary gland is the most important gland in the body because the hormones it secretes control the functioning of the other glands

pituitrin [pɪ'tjuːɪtrɪn] *noun* hormone secreted by the pituitary gland

pityriasis [pɪtɪ'raɪəsɪs] *noun* any skin disease where the skin develops thin scales; **pityriasis alba** = disease of children with flat white patches on the cheeks; **pityriasis capitis** = dandruff, a condition where pieces of dead skin form on the scalp and fall out when the hair is combed; **pityriasis rosea** = mild irritating rash affecting young people, which appears especially in the early part of the year and has no known cause; **pityriasis rubra** = serious, sometimes fatal, skin disease, a type of exfoliative dermatitis, where the skin turns dark red and is covered with white scales

pivot ['pɪvət] **1** *noun* stem used to attach an artificial crown to the root of a tooth **2** *verb* to rest and turn on a point; *the atlas bone pivots on the second vertebra*; **pivot joint** = joint where a bone can rotate freely (NOTE: also called **trochoid joint**)

placebo [plə'siːbəʊ] *noun* tablet which appears to be a drug, but has no medicinal substance in it; **placebo effect** = apparently beneficial effect of telling a patient that he is having a treatment, even if this is not true, caused by the patient's hope that the treatment will be effective

COMMENT: placebos may be given to patients who have imaginary illnesses;

placebos can also help in treating real disorders by stimulating the patient's psychological will to be cured. Placebos are also used on control groups in tests of new drugs (a placebo-controlled study)

placenta [plə'sentə] *noun* tissue which grows inside the uterus during pregnancy and links the baby to the mother; **placenta praevia** = condition where the fertilized egg becomes implanted in the lower part of the uterus, which means that the placenta lies across the cervix and may become detached during childbirth and cause brain damage to the baby; **battledore placenta** = placenta where the umbilical cord is attached to the edge and not the centre

COMMENT: the vascular system of the fetus is not directly connected to that of the mother. The placenta allows an exchange of oxygen and nutrients to be passed from the mother to the fetus to which she is linked by the umbilical cord. It stops functioning when the baby breathes for the first time and is then passed out of the uterus as the afterbirth

placental [plə'sentl] *adjective* referring to the placenta; **placental insufficiency** = condition where the placenta does not provide the fetus with the necessary oxygen and nutrients; *see also* BARRIER

placentography [plæsən'tɒgrəfi] *noun* X-ray examination of the placenta of a pregnant woman after a radio-opaque dye has been injected

Placido's disc [plæsɪdəʊz 'dɪsk] *noun* keratoscope, an instrument for examining the cornea to see if it has an abnormal curvature

plagiocephaly [pleɪdʒɪə'sefəli] *noun* condition where a person has a distorted head

plague [pleɪg] *noun* infectious disease which occurs in epidemics where many people are killed; **bubonic plague** = fatal disease caused by *Yersinia pestis* in the lymph system transmitted to humans by fleas from rats; **pneumonic plague** = form of bubonic plague where mainly the lungs are affected; **septicaemic plague** = form of bubonic plague where the symptoms are generalized; *the hospitals cannot cope with all the plague victims; thousands of people are dying of plague*

COMMENT: bubonic plague was the Black Death of the Middle Ages; its symptoms are fever, delirium, prostration, rigor and swellings on the lymph nodes

plan [plæn] **1** *noun* arrangement of how something should be done; **care plan** = plan drawn up by the nursing staff for the treatment of an individual patient **2** *verb* to arrange how something is going to be done; **they are planning to have a family** = they expect to have children and so are not taking contraceptives

one issue has arisen - the amount of time and effort which nurses need to put into the writing of detailed care plans. Few would now dispute the need for clear, concise nursing plans to guide nursing practice, provide educational tools and give an accurate legal record

Nursing Times

plane [pleɪn] *noun* flat surface, especially that of the body seen from a certain angle; *see* CORONAL, MEDIAN, SAGITTAL

planned parenthood ['plænd 'peərənthʊd] *noun* situation where two people plan to have a certain number of children, and take contraceptives to control the number of children in the family

planning ['plænɪŋ] *noun* arranging how something should be done; **family planning** = using contraceptives to control the number of children in a family; **family planning clinic** = clinic which gives advice on contraception

planta ['plæntə] *noun* the sole of the foot

plantar ['plæntə] *adjective* referring to the sole of the foot; **plantar arch** = curved part of the sole of the foot running along the length of the foot; **deep plantar arch** = curved artery crossing the sole of the foot; **plantar flexion** = bending of the toes downwards; **plantar reflex** *or* **plantar response** = normal downward movement of the toes when the sole of the foot is stroked in Babinski test; **plantar region** = the sole of the foot; **plantar surface** = the skin of the sole of the foot; **plantar wart** = wart on the sole of the foot

planus ['pleɪnəs] *see* LICHEN, PES

plaque [plæk] *noun* flat area; **bacterial plaque** = hard smooth bacterial deposit on teeth; **atherosclerotic plaque** = deposit on the walls of arteries; **senile plaque** = spherical deposit of beta amyloid in brain areas in Alzheimer's disease

-plasia ['pleɪziə] *suffix* which develops or grows

plasm- *or* **plasmo-** ['plæzm *or* 'plæzməʊ] *prefix* referring to blood plasma

plasma ['plæzmə] *noun* (i) yellow watery liquid which makes up the main part of blood; (ii) lymph with no corpuscles; (iii) cytoplasm; *the accident victim was given plasma*; **plasma cell** = lymphocyte which produces a certain type of antibody; **plasma protein** = protein in plasma (such as albumin, gamma globulin and fibrinogen)

COMMENT: if blood does not clot it separates into blood corpuscles and plasma, which is formed of water and proteins, including the clotting agent fibrinogen. If blood clots, the corpuscles separate from serum, which is a watery liquid similar to plasma, but not containing fibrinogen. Dried plasma can be kept for a long time, and is used, after water has been added, for transfusions

plasmacytoma [plæzməsaɪ'təʊmə] *noun* malignant tumour of plasma cells, normally found in lymph nodes or bone marrow

plasmapheresis [plæzməfə'riːsɪs] *noun* operation to take blood from a patient, then to separate the red blood cells from the plasma, and to return the red blood cells suspended in a saline solution to the patient through a transfusion

plasmin ['plæzmɪn] *noun* fibrinolysin, enzyme which digests fibrin

plasminogen [plæz'mɪnədʒn] *noun* substance in blood plasma which becomes activated and forms plasmin

Plasmodium [plæz'məʊdiəm] *noun* type of parasite which infests red blood cells and causes malaria

plasmolysis [plæz'mɒlɪsɪs] *noun* contraction of a cell protoplasm by dehydration, where the surrounding cell wall becomes smaller

plaster ['plɑːstə] *noun* (a) white powder which is mixed with water and used to make a solid support to cover a broken limb; *after his accident he had his leg in plaster for two months*; **plaster of Paris** = fine white plaster used to make plaster casts; **frog plaster** = plaster cast made to keep the legs in the correct position after an operation to correct a dislocated hip; **plaster cast** = hard support

made of bandage soaked in liquid plaster of Paris, which is allowed to harden after being wrapped round a broken limb and which prevents the limb moving while the bone heals **(b) sticking plaster** = adhesive plaster, sticky tape used to cover a small wound or to attach a pad of dressing to the skin; *put a plaster on your cut*

plastic ['plæstɪk] **1** *noun* artificial material made from petroleum, and used to make many objects, including replacement organs **2** *adjective* which can be made in different shapes; **plastic lymph** = inflammatory lymph, yellow liquid produced by an inflamed wound and which helps the healing process; **plastic surgery** = surgery which repairs defective or deformed parts of the body; **plastic surgeon** = surgeon who specializes in plastic surgery

COMMENT: plastic surgery is especially important in treating accident victims or people who have suffered burns. It is also used to correct congenital deformities such as a cleft palate. When the object is simply to improve the patient's appearance, it is usually referred to as 'cosmetic surgery'

-plasty ['plæsti] *suffix* referring to plastic surgery

plate [pleɪt] *noun* **(a)** flat round piece of china for putting food on; *the nurses brought round sandwiches on a plate for lunch; pass your dirty plates to the person at the end of the table* **(b)** (i) flat sheet of metal, bone, etc.; (ii) flat piece of metal attached to a fractured bone to hold the broken parts together; *the surgeon inserted a plate in her skull*; **cribriform plate** = top part of the ethmoid bone which forms the roof of the nasal cavity and part of the top of the eye sockets; **dental plate** = prosthesis made to the shape of the mouth, which holds artificial teeth

platelet ['pleɪtlɪt] *noun* thrombocyte, a small blood cell which releases thromboplastin and which multiplies rapidly after an injury, encouraging the coagulation of blood; **platelet count** = test to count the number of platelets in a certain quantity of blood

platy- ['plæti] *prefix* meaning flat

platysma [plə'tɪzmə] *noun* flat muscle running from the collarbone to the lower jaw

-plegia ['pliːdʒə] *suffix* meaning paralysis

pleio- *or* **pleo-** ['plaɪəʊ *or* 'pliːəʊ] *prefix* meaning too many

pleocytosis [pliːəʊsaɪ'təʊsɪs] *noun* condition where there are an abnormal number of leucocytes in the cerebrospinal fluid

pleoptics [pliːˈɒptɪks] *noun* treatment to help the partially sighted

plessor [ˈplesə] *noun* little hammer with a rubber tip, used by doctors to tap tendons to test for reflexes or for percussion of the chest

plethora [ˈpleθərə] *noun* old term meaning too much blood in the body

plethoric [pleˈθɒrɪk] *adjective* (appearance) due to dilatation of superficial blood vessels

plethysmography [pleθɪzˈmɒɡrəfi] *noun* method of recording the changes in the volume of organs, mainly used to measure blood flow in the limbs

pleur- *or* **pleuro-** [ˈpluər *or* ˈpluərəu] *prefix* referring to the pleura

pleura [ˈpluərə] *noun* one of two membranes lining the chest cavity and covering each lung; **parietal pleura** *or* **outer pleura** = membrane attached to the diaphragm and covering the chest cavity; **visceral pleura** *or* **inner pleura** = membrane attached to the surface of the lung; *see illustration at* LUNGS (NOTE: plural is **pleurae**)

pleuracentesis [pluərəsenˈtiːsɪs] *see* PLEUROCENTESIS

pleural [ˈpluərl] *adjective* referring to the pleura; **pleural cavity** = space between the inner and outer pleura; **pleural effusion** = excess fluid formed in the pleural sac; **pleural fluid** = fluid which forms between the layers of the pleura in pleurisy; **pleural membrane** = PLEURA

pleurectomy [pluəˈrektəmi] *noun* surgical removal of part of the pleura which has been thickened or made stiff by chronic empyema

pleurisy [ˈpluərɪsi] *noun* inflammation of the pleura, usually caused by pneumonia; **diaphragmatic pleurisy** = inflammation of the outer pleura only

COMMENT: the symptoms of pleurisy are coughing, fever, and sharp pains when breathing, caused by the two layers of pleura rubbing together

pleuritis [pluəˈraɪtɪs] = PLEURISY

pleurocele [ˈpluərəusiːl] *noun* (i) condition where part of the lung or pleura is herniated; (ii) fluid in the pleural cavity

pleurocentesis *or* **pleuracentesis** [pluərəusenˈtiːsɪs *or* pluərəsenˈtiːsɪs] *noun* operation where a hollow needle is put into the pleura to drain liquid

pleurodesis [pluərəˈdiːsɪs] *noun* treatment for a collapsed lung, where the inner and outer pleura are stuck together

pleurodynia [pluərəˈdɪniə] *noun* pain in the muscles between the ribs, due to rheumatic inflammation; **epidemic pleurodynia** = virus disease affecting the intestinal muscles, with symptoms like influenza, (fever, headaches and pains in the chest) (NOTE: also called **Bornholm disease**)

pleuropneumonia [pluərənjuˈməuniə] *noun* acute lobar pneumonia (the classic type of pneumonia)

plexor [ˈpleksə] *see* PLESSOR

plexus [ˈpleksəs] *noun* network of nerves, blood vessels or lymphatics; **Auerbach's plexus** = group of nerve fibres in the intestine; **brachial plexus** = group of nerves at the armpit and base of the neck which lead to the nerves in the arms and hands; injury to the brachial plexus at birth leads to Erb's palsy; **cervical plexus** = group of nerves in front of the vertebrae in the neck, which lead to nerves supplying the skin and muscles of the neck, and also the phrenic nerve which controls the diaphragm; **choroid plexus (of the lateral ventricle)** = part of the pia mater, a network of small blood vessels in the ventricles of the brain which produce cerebrospinal fluid; **lumbar plexus** = point near the spine above the pelvis where several nerves supplying the thigh and abdomen are joined together; **sacral plexus** = group of nerves inside the pelvis near the sacrum which lead to nerves in the buttocks, back of the thigh and lower leg and foot; **solar plexus** *or* **coeliac plexus** = network of nerves in the abdomen, behind the stomach

pliable [ˈplaɪəbl] *adjective* which can bend easily

plica [ˈplaɪkə] *noun* fold

plicate [ˈplaɪkeɪt] *adjective* folded

plication [plaɪˈkeɪʃn] *noun* (i) surgical operation to reduce the size of a muscle or a hollow organ by making folds in its walls and attaching them; (ii) the action of folding; (iii) a fold

plombage [plɒmˈbɑːʒ] *noun* (i) packing bone cavities with antiseptic material; (ii) packing of the lung or pleural cavities with inert material

plumbism ['plʌmbɪzm] *noun* lead poisoning

Plummer-Vinson syndrome ['plʌmə'vɪnsən 'sɪndrəum] *noun* type of iron-deficiency anaemia, where the tongue and mouth become inflamed and the patient cannot swallow

plunger ['plʌnʒə] *noun* part of a hypodermic syringe which slides up and down inside the tube, either sucking liquid into the syringe or forcing the contents out

PM ['pi: 'em] **(a)** = POST MORTEM; *what are the results of the PM?* **(b)** = PARTICULATE MATTER

PMA ['pi: 'em 'eɪ] = PROGRESSIVE MUSCULAR ATROPHY

pmol = PICOMOLE

PMS ['pi: 'em 'es] = PREMENSTRUAL SYNDROME

PMT ['pi: 'em 'ti:] = PREMENSTRUAL TENSION; *she is being treated for PMT; the hospital has a special clinic for PMT sufferers*

-pnea *or* **-pnoea** [pni:ə] *suffix* referring to breathing

pneum- *or* **pneumo-** ['nju:m or 'nju:məu] *prefix* referring to air, to the lungs or to breathing

pneumatocele [nju'mætəusi:l] *noun* (i) sac or tumour filled with gas; (ii) herniation of the lung

pneumaturia [nju:mə'tjuəriə] *noun* passing air or gas in the urine

pneumocephalus [nju:məu'sefələs] *noun* presence of air or gas in the brain

pneumococcal [nju:məu'kɒkl] *adjective* referring to pneumococci

pneumococcus [nju:məu'kɒkəs] *noun* genus of bacteria which causes respiratory tract infections, including pneumonia (NOTE: plural is **pneumococci**)

pneumoconiosis [nju:məkəuni'əusɪs] *noun* lung disease where fibrous tissue forms in the lungs because the patient has inhaled particles of stone or dust over a long period of time

pneumoencephalography [nju:məuensefə'lɒgrəfi] *noun* X-ray examination of the ventricles and spaces of the brain taken after air has been injected into the cerebrospinal fluid by lumbar puncture

COMMENT: the air takes the place of the cerebrospinal fluid and makes it easier to photograph the ventricles clearly. This technique has been superseded by CAT and MRI

pneumogastric [nju:məu'gæstrɪk] *adjective* referring to the lungs and the stomach; **pneumogastric nerve** = vagus nerve, tenth cranial nerve, which controls swallowing and nerve fibres in the heart and chest

pneumograph ['nju:məgrɑ:f] *noun* instrument which records chest movements during breathing

pneumohaemothorax [nju:məuhi:məu'θɔ:ræks] *noun* blood or air in the pleural cavity (NOTE: also called **haemopneumothorax**)

pneumomycosis [nju:məumaɪ'kəusɪs] *noun* infection of the lungs caused by a fungus

pneumon- *or* **pneumono-** ['nju:mən or 'nju:mənəu] *prefix* referring to the lungs

pneumonectomy [nju:mə'nektəmi] *noun* surgical removal of all or part of a lung

pneumonia [nju'məuniə] *noun* inflammation of a lung, where the tiny alveoli of the lung become filled with fluid; *he developed pneumonia and had to be hospitalized*; *she died of pneumonia*; **bacterial pneumonia** = form of pneumonia caused by pneumococcus; *see also* BRONCHOPNEUMONIA; **double pneumonia** *or* **bilateral pneumonia** = pneumonia affecting both lungs; **hypostatic pneumonia** = pneumonia caused by fluid which accumulates in the posterior bases of the lungs of a bedridden patient; **lobar pneumonia** = pneumonia which affects one or more lobes of the lung; **viral** *or* **virus pneumonia** = type of inflammation of the lungs caused by a virus; *see also* ASPIRATION

COMMENT: the symptoms of pneumonia are shivering, pains in the chest, high temperature and sputum brought up by coughing

pneumonic plague [nju'mɒnɪk 'pleɪg] *noun* form of bubonic plague which mainly affects the lungs

pneumonitis [nju:məu'naɪtɪs] *noun* inflammation of the lungs

pneumoperitoneum
[nju:məuperitə'ni:əm] *noun* air in the peritoneal cavity

pneumoradiography
[nju:məureidi'ɒgrəfi] *noun* X-ray examination of part of the body after air or a gas has been inserted to make the organs show more clearly

pneumothorax [nju:məu'θɔ:ræks] *noun* collapsed lung, condition where air or gas is in the thorax; **artificial pneumothorax** = former method of treating tuberculosis, where air was introduced between the layers of the pleura to make the lung collapse; **spontaneous pneumothorax** = pneumothorax caused by a rupture of an abnormal condition on the surface of the pleura; **tension pneumothorax** = pneumothorax where rupture of the pleura forms an opening like a valve, through which air is forced during coughing but cannot escape; **traumatic pneumothorax** = pneumothorax which results from damage to the lung surface or the wall of the chest, which allows air to leak into the space between the pleurae

-pnoea [pni:ə] *suffix* referring to breathing

PNS ['pi: 'en 'es] = PERIPHERAL NERVOUS SYSTEM

pock [pɒk] *noun* (i) localized lesion on the skin, due to smallpox or chickenpox; (ii) infective focus on the membrane of a fertile egg, caused by a virus

pocket ['pɒkit] *noun* (i) small bag attached to the inside to a coat, etc. in which money, handkerchief, keys, etc., can be kept; (ii) cavity in the body; **pocket of infection** = place where an infection remains

pockmark ['pɒkmɑ:k] *noun* scar left by a pustule, as in smallpox

pockmarked ['pɒkmɑ:kt] *adjective* (face) with scars from smallpox

pod- [pɒd] *prefix* referring to the foot

podagra [pɒ'dægrə] = GOUT

podalic version [pəu'dælik 'vɜ:ʃn] *noun* turning of the fetus in the uterus by the feet

podiatrist [pəu'daiətrist] *noun US* person who specializes in the care of the foot and its diseases

podiatry [pəu'daiətri] *noun US* study of minor diseases and disorders of the feet

-poiesis [pɔi'i:sis] *suffix* which forms

poikilo- ['pɔikiləu] *prefix* meaning irregular or varied

poikilocyte ['pɔikiləusait] *noun* abnormally large red blood cell with an irregular shape

poikilocytosis [pɔikiləusai'təusis] *noun* condition where poikilocytes exist in the blood

poikilothermic [pɔikiləu'θɜ:mik] *adjective* (animal) with cold blood, cold-blooded (animal); *compare* HOMOIOTHERMIC

COMMENT: the body temperature of cold-blooded animals changes with the outside temperature

point [pɔint] *noun* **(a)** sharp end; *surgical needles have to have very sharp points* **(b)** dot used to show the division between whole numbers and parts of numbers (NOTE: **3.256**: say 'three point two five six'; **his temperature was 38.7**: say 'thirty-eight point seven') **(c)** mark in a series of numbers; *what's the freezing point of water?*

pointed ['pɔintid] *adjective* with a sharp point; *a pointed rod*

poison ['pɔizən] **1** *noun* substance which can kill or harm body tissues if eaten or drunk; *he died after someone put poison in his coffee*; *poisons must be kept locked up*; **poison ivy** *or* **poison oak** = American plants whose leaves can cause a painful rash if touched **2** *verb* to give someone a poison or a substance which can harm or kill; *the workers were poisoned by toxic fumes*; *the wound was poisoned by bacterial infection*

COMMENT: The commonest poisons, of which even a small amount can kill, are arsenic, cyanide and strychnine. Many common foods and drugs can be poisonous if taken in large doses. Common household materials such as bleach, glue and insecticides can also be poisonous. Some types of poisoning, such as Salmonella, can be passed to other people through lack of hygienic conditions

poisoning ['pɔizənɪŋ] *noun* condition where a person is made ill or is killed by a poisonous substance; **blood poisoning** = condition where bacteria are present in blood and cause illness; **Salmonella poisoning** = poisoning by Salmonellae which develop in the intestines; **staphylococcal poisoning** = poisoning by staphylococci in food

poisonous ['pɔizənəs] *adjective* (substance) which is full of poison or which can kill or harm; *some mushrooms are good to eat and some are poisonous*; **poisonous**

gas = gas which can kill, which can make someone ill

Poisons Act ['pɔɪzənəs 'ækt] *noun* one of several Acts of the British Parliament (Pharmacy and Poisons Act 1933, Misuse of Drugs Act 1971, Poisons Act 1972) which regulate the making, prescribing and selling of drugs

polar ['pəulə] *adjective* with a pole; **polar body** = small cell which is produced from an oocyte but does not develop into an ovum

pole [pəul] *noun* (i) end of an axis; (ii) end of a rounded organ, such as the end of a lobe in the cerebral hemisphere

poli- *or* **polio-** ['pɒlɪ *or* 'pəuliəu] *prefix* referring to grey matter in the nervous system

polio ['pəuliəu] *(informal) see* POLIOMYELITIS

polioencephalitis [pəuliəuensefə'laɪtɪs] *noun* type of viral encephalitis, an inflammation of the grey matter in the brain caused by the same virus as poliomyelitis

polioencephalomyelitis [pəuliəuensefələumaɪə'laɪtɪs] *noun* polioencephalitis which also affects the spinal cord

poliomyelitis *or* **polio** [pəuliəumaɪə'laɪtɪs *or* 'pəuliəu] *noun* infantile paralysis, an infection of the anterior horn cells of the spinal cord caused by a virus which attacks the motor neurones and can lead to paralysis; **abortive poliomyelitis** = mild form of poliomyelitis which only affects the throat and intestines; **bulbar poliomyelitis** = type of polio affecting the brain stem, which makes it difficult for a patient to swallow or breathe; **nonparalytic poliomyelitis** = form of poliomyelitis similar to the abortive form but which also affects the muscles to a certain degree; **paralytic poliomyelitis** = poliomyelitis which affects the patient's muscles

COMMENT: symptoms of poliomyelitis are paralysis of the limbs, fever and stiffness in the neck. The bulbar form may start with difficulty in swallowing. Poliomyelitis can be prevented by immunization and two vaccines are used: the Sabin vaccine is formed of live polio virus and is taken orally on a piece of sugar; Salk vaccine is given as an injection of dead virus

poliovirus [pəuliəu'vaɪrəs] *noun* virus which causes poliomyelitis

Politzer's bag ['pɒlɪtsəz 'bæg] *noun* rubber bag which is used to blow air into the middle ear to unblock a Eustachian tube

pollen ['pɒlən] *noun* male gamete from plants (produced by the flower stamens) which floats in the air in spring and summer, and which causes hay fever; **pollen count** = figure which shows the amount of pollen in a sample of air

pollex ['pɒleks] *noun* thumb (NOTE: the plural is **pollices**)

pollinosis [pɒlə'nəusɪs] = HAY FEVER

pollutant [pə'lu:tnt] *noun* substance which pollutes

pollute [pə'lu:t] *verb* to make the air, a river or the sea, etc., dirty, especially with industrial waste

pollution [pə'lu:ʃn] *noun* making dirty; **atmospheric pollution** = pollution of the air

poly- ['pɒli] *prefix* meaning many or much, touching many organs

polyarteritis nodosa [pɒliɑ:tə'raɪtɪs nə'dəusə] *noun* collagen disease where the walls of the arteries in various parts of the body become inflamed, leading to asthma, high blood pressure and kidney failure (NOTE: also called **periarteritis nodosa**)

polyarthritis [pɒliɑ:'θraɪtɪs] *noun* inflammation of several joints, such as rheumatoid arthritis

polycystic ovaries [pɒli'sɪstɪk 'əuvəriz] *noun* condition where the ovaries produce cysts, causing anovulation which results in infertility

polycystitis [pɒlɪsɪ'staɪtɪs] *noun* congenital disease where several cysts form in the kidney at the same time

polycythaemia [pɒlɪsaɪ'θi:miə] *noun* blood disease where the number of red blood cells increases, often due to difficulties which the patient has in breathing; **polycythaemia vera** = erythraemia, a blood disease where the number of red blood cells increases, together with an increase in the number of white blood cells, making the blood thicker and slowing its flow

polydactylism [pɒli'dæktɪlɪzm] *noun* hyperdactylism, condition where a person has more than five fingers or toes

polydipsia [pɒli'dɪpsiə] *noun* condition (often caused by diabetes insipidus) where the patient is abnormally thirsty

polygraph ['pɒligrɑːf] *noun* instrument which records the pulse in several parts of the body at the same time

polymenorrhoea [pɒlimenə'riːə] *noun* abnormally frequent menstruations

polymerase chain reaction (PCR) ['pɒliməreɪz 'tʃeɪn ri'ækʃn] *noun* the technique used to amplify genetic material in order to analyse it for genetic defects, such as material from a single cell in an embryo

polymorph ['pɒlimɔːf] *noun* neutrophil, type of leucocyte or white blood cell with an irregular nucleus

polymyalgia rheumatica [pɒlimaɪ'æ1dʒə ruː'mætɪkə] *noun* disease of elderly people where the patient has pain and stiffness in the shoulder and hip muscles making them weak and sensitive

polyneuritis [pɒlinjuː'raɪtɪs] *noun* inflammation of many nerves

polyneuropathy [pɒlinjuː'rɒpəθi] *noun* any disease which affects several nerves

polyopia *or* **polyopsia** *or* **polyopy** [pɒli'əupiə *or* pɒli'ɒpsiə *or* 'pɒliəupi] *noun* condition where the patient sees several images of one object at the same time; *compare* DIPLOPIA

polyp *or* **polypus** ['pɒlɪp *or* 'pɒlɪpəs] *noun* tumour, growing on a stalk in mucous membrane, which can be cauterized, often found in the nose, mouth or throat (NOTE: plural of **polypus** is **polypi**)

polypeptide [pɒli'peptaɪd] *noun* type of protein formed of linked amino acids

polyphagia [pɒli'feɪdʒə] *noun* (i) condition where a patient eats too much; (ii) morbid desire for every kind of food

polypharmacy [pɒli'fɑːməsi] *noun* prescribing several drugs to be taken at the same time

polyploid ['pɒliplɔɪd] *adjective* (cell) where there are more than three sets of the haploid number of chromosomes; *compare* DIPLOID, HAPLOID

polyposis [pɒli'pəusɪs] *noun* condition where many polyps form in the mucous membrane of the colon; *see also* FAMILIAL ADENOMATOUS POLYPOSIS

polypus ['pɒlɪpəs] = POLYP

polyradiculitis [pɒlirædɪkju'laɪtɪs] *noun* disease of the nervous system which affects the roots of the nerves

polysaccharide [pɒli'sækəraɪd] *noun* type of carbohydrate

polyserositis [pɒlisɪərəu'saɪtɪs] *noun* inflammation of the membranes lining the abdomen, chest and joints and exudation of serous fluid

polyspermia *or* **polyspermism** *or* **polyspermy** [pɒli'spɜːmiə *or* pɒli'spɜːmɪzm *or* pɒli'spɜːmi] *noun* (i) excessive seminal secretion; (ii) fertilization of one ovum by several spermatozoa

polyunsaturated fat [pɒliʌn'sætʃəreɪtɪd 'fæt] *noun* fatty acid capable of absorbing more hydrogen (typical of vegetable and fish oils)

polyuria [pɒli'juəriə] *noun* condition where a patient passes a large quantity of urine, usually as a result of diabetes insipidus

polyvalent [pɒlɪ'veɪlənt] *adjective* having more than one valency

pompholyx ['pɒmfɒlɪks] *noun* (i) type of eczema with many irritating little blisters on the hands and feet; (ii) morbid skin condition with bulbous swellings

pons [pɒnz] *noun* (a) bridge of tissue joining parts of an organ (b) **pons (Varolii)** = part of the hindbrain, formed of fibres which continue the medulla oblongata; *see illustration at* BRAIN (NOTE: plural is **pontes**)

pontine ['pɒntaɪn] *noun* referring to a pons; **pontine cistern** = subarachnoid space in front of the pons, containing the basilar artery

poor [puə] *adjective* not very good; *he's in poor health*; *she suffers from poor circulation*

poorly ['puəli] *adjective (informal)* not very well; *her mother has been quite poorly recently*; *he felt poorly and stayed in bed*

POP ['piː 'əu 'piː] = PROGESTERONE ONLY PILL

popeyes ['pɒpaɪz] *plural noun* US protruding eyes

popliteal [pɒp'lɪtiəl] *adjective* referring to the back of the knee; **popliteal artery** = artery which branches from the femoral artery behind the knee and leads into the tibial arteries; **popliteal fossa** *or* **popliteal space** = space behind the knee between the hamstring and the calf muscle

popliteus *or* **popliteal muscle** [pɒp'lɪtiəs *or* pɒp'lɪtiəl 'mʌsl] *noun* muscle at the back of the knee

population [pɒpju'leɪʃn] *noun* **(a)** number of people living in a country or town; *population statistics show that the birth rate is slowing down*; *the government has decided to screen the whole population of the area* **(b)** number of patients in hospital; *the hospital population in the area has fallen below ten thousand*

pore [pɔː] *noun* (i) tiny hole in the skin through which the sweat passes; (ii) small communicating passage between cavities; *see illustration at* SKIN & SENSORY RECEPTORS

porencephaly *or* **porencephalia** *or* **porencephalus** [pɔːren'sefəli *or* pɔːrensə'feɪliə *or* pɔːren'sefələs] *noun* abnormal cysts in the cerebral cortex, as a result of defective development

porous ['pɔːrəs] *adjective* (i) containing pores; (ii) (tissue) which allows fluid to pass through; *porous bone surrounds the Eustachian tubes*

porphyria [pɔː'fɪriə] *noun* hereditary disease affecting the metabolism of porphyrin pigments

COMMENT: porphyria causes abdominal pains and attacks of mental confusion. The skin becomes sensitive to light and the urine becomes coloured and turns dark brown when exposed to the light

porphyrin ['pɔːfərɪn] *noun* family of biological pigments (the commonest is protoporphyrin IX)

porphyrinuria [pɔːfɪrɪ'njuəriə] *noun* presence of excess porphyrins in the urine, a sign of porphyria or of metal poisoning

porta ['pɔːtə] *noun* opening which allows blood vessels to pass into an organ; **porta hepatis** = opening in the liver through which the hepatic artery, hepatic duct and portal vein pass

portable ['pɔːtəbl] *adjective* which can be carried; *he keeps a portable first aid kit in his car*; *the ambulance team carried a portable blood testing unit*

portal ['pɔːtl] *adjective* referring to a porta, especially the portal system or the portal vein; **portal hypertension** = high pressure in the portal vein, caused by cirrhosis of the liver or a clot in the vein, causing internal bleeding; *see also* BANTI'S SYNDROME; **portal pyaemia** = infection of the portal vein in the liver, giving abscesses; **portal system** = group of veins which have capillaries at both ends and do not go to the heart, such as the portal vein; **portal vein** = vein which takes blood from the stomach, pancreas, gall bladder, intestines and spleen to the liver

porter ['pɔːtə] *noun* person who does general work in a hospital, such as wheeling a patient's trolley into the operating theatre, moving heavy equipment, etc.

portocaval [pɔːtəu'keɪvl] *adjective* linking the portal vein to the inferior vena cava; **portocaval anastomosis** = surgical operation to join the portal vein to the inferior vena cava; **portocaval shunt** = artificial passage made between the portal vein and the inferior vena cava to relieve portal hypertension

porto-systemic encephalopathy ['pɔːtəusɪs'tiːmɪk ensefə'lɒpəθi] *noun* mental disorder and coma caused by liver disorder due to portal hypertension (NOTE: for terms referring to the portal vein, see words beginning with **pyl-** or **pyle-**)

port wine stain ['pɔːt 'waɪn 'steɪn] *noun* naevus, purple birthmark

position [pə'zɪʃn] **1** *noun* **(a)** place (where something is); *the exact position of the tumour is located by an X-ray* **(b)** the way a patient stands, sits or lies; **genupectoral position** = kneeling with the chest on the floor; **lithotomy position** = lying on the back with the hips and knees bent; **recovery position** *or* **semiprone position** = lying face downwards, with one knee and one arm bent forwards and the face turned to one side; *see also* TRENDELENBURG'S **2** *verb* to place in a certain position; *the fetus is correctly positioned in the uterus*

positive ['pɒzətɪv] *adjective* which indicates the answer 'yes' or which shows the presence of something; *her cervical smear was positive or she gave a positive test for cervical cancer*; **positive end-expiratory pressure (PEEP)** = forcing the patient to breathe through a mask in cases where fluid has collected in the lungs; **positive feedback** = situation where the result of a process stimulates the process which caused it; **positive pressure ventilation (PPV)** = forcing air into the lungs to encourage the lungs to expand; **positive pressure respirator** = machine which forces air into a patient's lungs through a tube inserted in the mouth

positively ['pɒzətɪvli] *adverb* in a positive way; *she reacted positively to the test*

posology [pə'sɒlədʒi] *noun* study of doses of medicine

posseting ['pɒsɪtɪŋ] *noun (in babies)* bringing up small quantities of curdled milk into the mouth after feeding

Possum ['pɒsəm] *noun* device using electronic switches which helps a severely paralysed patient to work a machine such as a telephone or typewriter (NOTE: the name is derived from the first letters of **Patient-Operated Selector Mechanism**)

post- [pəʊst] *prefix* meaning after or later

postcentral gyrus [pəʊst'sentrl 'dʒaɪrəs] *noun* sensory area of the cerebral cortex, which receives impulses from receptor cells and senses pain, heat, touch, etc.

post-cibal [pəʊst'saɪbl] *adjective* after having eaten food

post-coital [pəʊst'kɔɪtl] *adjective* after having sexual intercourse

postconcussional [pəʊstkən'kʌʃnl] *adjective* (symptoms) which follow after a patient has had concussion

post-epileptic [pəʊstepɪ'leptɪk] *adjective* after an epileptic fit

posterior [pɒ'stɪəriə] *adjective* at the back; *the cerebellum is posterior to the medulla oblongata*; **posterior approach** = (operation) carried out from the back; **posterior aspect** = view of the back of the body or of part of the body; **posterior chamber (of the eye)** = part of the aqueous chamber which is behind the iris; **posterior synechia** = condition of the eye where the iris sticks to the anterior surface of the lens (NOTE: the opposite is **anterior**)

posteriorly [pɒ'stɪəriəli] *adverb* behind; *an artery leads to a posteriorly placed organ*; *rectal biopsy specimens are best taken posteriorly* (NOTE: the opposite is **anteriorly**)

postganglionic [pəʊstgæŋli'ɒnɪk] *adjective* placed after a ganglion; **postganglionic fibre** = axon of a nerve cell which starts in a ganglion and extends beyond the ganglion; **postganglionic neurone** = neurone which starts in a ganglion and ends in a gland or unstriated muscle

postgraduate education allowance (PGEA) ['pəʊst'grædjʊət edjʊ'keɪʃn ə'laʊəns] *noun* payment made to GPs to reward continued education

posthepatic [pəʊsthɪ'pætɪk] *adjective* after the liver; **posthepatic bilirubin** = bilirubin which enters the plasma after being treated by the liver; **posthepatic jaundice** = obstructive jaundice, jaundice caused by an obstruction in the bile ducts

post herpetic neuralgia ['pəʊst hə'petɪk njuː'rældʒə] *noun* pains felt after an attack of shingles

posthitis [pɒs'θaɪtɪs] *noun* inflammation of the foreskin

posthumous ['pɒstjʊməs] *adjective* after death; **posthumous birth** = (i) birth of a baby after the death of the father; (ii) birth of a baby by Caesarean section after the mother has died

post-irradiation ['pəʊstɪrɪdi'eɪʃn] *adjective* (pain or disorder) caused by X-rays

postmature baby [pəʊstmə'tʃʊə 'beɪbi] *noun* baby born more than nine months after conception

postmaturity [pəʊstmə'tʃʊərəti] *noun* pregnancy which lasts longer than nine months

postmenopausal [pəʊstmenəʊ'pɔːzl] *adjective* after the menopause; *she experienced some postmenopausal bleeding*; **postmenopausal woman** = woman whose menopause is over

post mortem (PM) ['pəʊst 'mɔːtəm] *noun* examination of a dead body by a pathologist to find out the cause of death; *the post mortem (examination) showed that he had been poisoned*

postnasal [pəʊst'neɪzl] *noun* behind the nose; **postnasal drip** = condition where mucus from the nose runs down into the throat and is swallowed

postnatal [pəʊst'neɪtl] *adjective* after the birth of a child; **postnatal depression** = depression which sometimes affects a woman after childbirth

postnecrotic cirrhosis [pəʊstne'krɒtɪk sə'rəʊsɪs] *noun* cirrhosis of the liver caused by viral hepatitis

post-op ['pəʊst'ɒp] *(informal)* = POSTOPERATIVE, POSTOPERATIVELY

postoperative [pəʊst'ɒprətɪv] *adjective* after a surgical operation; *the patient has suffered postoperative nausea and vomiting*; *occlusion may appear as postoperative angina pectoris*; **the second postoperative day** = the second day after an operation;

postoperative pain = pain felt by a patient after an operation

---

the nurse will help ensure that the parent is physically fit to cope with the postoperative child

British Journal of Nursing

---

postoperatively [pəʊstˈɒprətɪvli] *adverb* after a surgical operation; **at twelve months post-op** *or* **postoperatively** = twelve months after the operation

postpartum [pəʊstˈpɑːtəm] *adjective* postnatal, after the birth of a child; **postpartum haemorrhage (PPH)** = heavy bleeding after childbirth

postprandial [pəʊstˈprændɪəl] *adjective* after eating a meal

post-primary tuberculosis [pəʊstˈpraɪməri tjubɜːkjuˈləʊsɪs] *noun* reappearance of tuberculosis in a patient who has been infected with it before

postsynaptic [pəʊstsɪˈnæptɪk] *adjective* after a synapse; **postsynaptic axon** = nerve leaving one side of a synapse

post-traumatic [pəʊsttrɔːˈmætɪk] *adjective* after a trauma (such as an accident, rape, fire, etc.); **post-traumatic amnesia** = amnesia which follows a trauma; **post-traumatic disorder** = mental disorder which follows a trauma

postural [ˈpɒstʃrl] *adjective* referring to posture; *a study of postural disorders*; **postural drainage** = removing matter from infected lungs by making the patient lie down with his head lower than his feet, so that he can cough more easily; **postural hypotension** = low blood pressure when standing up suddenly, causing dizziness

posture [ˈpɒstʃə] *noun* way of standing or sitting; *bad posture can cause pain in the back*; *she has to do exercises to correct her bad posture* *or* *she has to do posture exercises*

postviral [pəʊstˈvaɪrl] *adjective* after a virus; **postviral fatigue syndrome** = myalgic encephalomyelitis, a long-term condition affecting the nervous system, where the patient feels tired and depressed and has pain and weakness in the muscles

potassium [pəˈtæsɪəm] *noun* metallic element (NOTE: chemical symbol is **K**)

potassium permanganate (KMnO₄) [pəˈtæsɪəm pəˈmæŋgəneɪt] *noun*

purple-coloured poisonous salt, used as a disinfectant

Pott's disease *or* **Pott's caries** [ˈpɒts dɪˈziːz *or* ˈpɒts ˈkeəriz] *noun* tuberculosis of the spine, causing paralysis

Pott's fracture [ˈpɒts ˈfræktʃə] *noun* fracture of the lower end of the fibula together with displacement of the ankle and foot outwards

pouch [paʊtʃ] *noun* small sac or pocket attached to an organ; **branchial pouch** = pouch on the side of the neck of an embryo

poultice [ˈpəʊltɪs] *noun* fomentation, compress made of hot water and flour paste or other substances which is pressed on to an infected part to draw out pus, to relieve pain or to encourage the circulation

pound [paʊnd] *noun* measure of weight (about 450 grams); *the baby weighed only four pounds at birth* (NOTE: with numbers **pound** is usually written **lb; the baby weighs 6lb**)

Poupart's ligament [puˈpɑːts ˈlɪgəmənt] *noun* inguinal ligament, ligament in the groin, running from the spine to the pubis

powder [ˈpaʊdə] *noun* medicine like fine dry dust made from particles of drugs; *he took a powder to help his indigestion* *or* *he took an indigestion powder*

powdered [ˈpaʊdəd] *adjective* crushed so that it forms a fine dry dust; *the medicine is available in tablets or in powdered form*

pox [pɒks] *noun* (i) old name for syphilis; (ii) disease with eruption of vesicles or pustules

poxvirus [pɒksˈvaɪrəs] *noun* any of a group of viruses, such as those which cause cowpox and smallpox

---

Molluscum contagiosum is a harmless skin infection caused by a poxvirus that affects mainly children and young adults

British Medical Journal

PPD [ˈpiː ˈpiː ˈdiː] = PURIFIED PROTEIN DERIVATIVE

PPH [ˈpiː ˈpiː ˈeɪtʃ] = POSTPARTUM HAEMORRHAGE

PPV [ˈpiː ˈpiː ˈviː] = POSITIVE PRESSURE VENTILATION

p.r. [ˈpiː ˈɑː] *abbreviation for the Latin phrase* 'per rectum': examination by way of the rectum

practice ['præktɪs] *noun* **(a)** patients of a doctor or dentist; work of a doctor or dentist; *he has been in practice for six years*; *after qualifying he joined his father's practice*; **general practice** = doctor's practice where patients from an area are treated for all types of disease; *he left the hospital and went into general practice*; *she is in general practice in the North of London or she has a general practice in North London*; **group practice** = medical practice where several doctors or dentists share the same office building and support services; **practice leaflet** = leaflet produced by the doctors in a practice, giving details of the telephone numbers, hours when the surgery is open, etc.; **practice nurse** = nurse employed by a clinic or doctor's practice who can take blood samples, give help and advice to patients, etc. **(b)** when actually done; *it's a good idea, but will it work in practice?*

practice nurses play a major role in the care of patients with chronic disease and they undertake many preventive procedures

Nursing Times

patients presenting with symptoms of urinary tract infection were recruited in a general practice survey
Journal of the Royal College of General Practitioners

practise ['præktɪs] *verb* to work as a doctor; *he practises in North London*; *she practises homeopathy*; *a doctor must be registered before he can practise*

practitioner [præk'tɪʃnə] *noun* doctor, a qualified person who practises; **general practitioner (GP)** = doctor who treats many patients in an area for all types of illness and does not specialize; **nurse practitioner** = (i) nurse employed by a clinic or doctor's practice who can take blood samples, give advice to patients, etc.; (ii) *US* trained nurse who has not been licensed; **ophthalmic practitioner** = qualified person who specializes in testing eyes and prescribing lenses; *see also* FAMILY

praecox ['priːkɒks] *see* DEMENTIA, EJACULATIO

praevia ['priːviə] *see* PLACENTA

pre- [priː] *prefix* meaning before or in front of; **preadmission information** = information given to a patient before he is admitted to hospital; **pre-anaesthetic round** = examination of patients by the surgeon before they are anaesthetized

precancer [priː'kænsə] *noun* growth or cell which is not malignant but which may become cancerous

precancerous [priː'kænsrəs] *adjective* (growth) which is not malignant now, but which can become cancerous later

precaution [prɪ'kɔːʃn] *noun* action taken before something happens; *she took the tablets as a precaution against seasickness*; **to take safety precautions** = to do things which will make yourself safe

precede [prɪ'siːd] *verb* to happen before or earlier; *the attack was preceded by a sudden rise in body temperature*

precentral gyrus [priː'sentrl 'dʒaɪrəs] *noun* motor area of the cerebral cortex

precipitate 1 [prɪ'sɪpɪtət] *noun* substance which is precipitated during a chemical reaction **2** *verb* [prɪ'sɪpɪteɪt] **(a)** to make a substance separate from a chemical compound and fall to the bottom of a liquid during a chemical reaction; *casein is precipitated when milk comes into contact with an acid* **(b)** to make something start suddenly

it has been established that myocardial infarction and sudden coronary death are precipitated in the majority of patients by thrombus formation in the coronary arteries
British Journal of Hospital Medicine

precipitation [prɪsɪpɪ'teɪʃn] *noun* action of forming a precipitate

precipitin [prɪ'sɪpɪtɪn] *noun* antibody which reacts to an antigen and forms a precipitate, used in many diagnostic tests

precise [prɪ'saɪs] *adjective* very exact or correct; *the instrument can give precise measurements of changes in heartbeat*

preclinical [priː'klɪnɪkl] *adjective* **(a)** before diagnosis; *the preclinical stage of an infection* **(b)** first part of a medical course, before the students are allowed to examine real patients; *a preclinical student*

precocious [prɪ'kəʊʃəs] *adjective* more physically or mentally developed than is normal for a certain age

precocity [prɪ'kɒsəti] *noun* being precocious

precordial [priː'kɔːdiəl] *adjective* referring to the precordium

precordium [priː'kɔːdiəm] *noun* part of the thorax over the heart

precursor [prɪ'kɜːsə] *noun* substance or cell from which another substance or cell is developed, such as dopa, the precursor for dopamine, which is converted to dopamine by the enzyme dopa decarboxylase

predict [prɪ'dɪkt] *verb* to say what will happen in the future; *doctors are predicting a rise in cases of whooping cough*

prediction [prɪ'dɪkʃn] *noun* saying what you expect will happen in the future; *the Health Ministry's prediction of a rise in cases of hepatitis B*

predictive [prɪ'dɪktɪv] *adjective* which predicts; **the predictive value of a test** = the accuracy of the test in predicting a medical condition

predigested food [priːdaɪ'dʒestɪd 'fuːd] *noun* food which has undergone predigestion

predigestion [priːdaɪ'dʒestʃn] *noun* artificial starting of the digestive process before food is eaten

predisposed to [priːdɪ'spəʊzd tʊ] *adjective* with a tendency to; *all the members of the family are predisposed to vascular diseases*

predisposition [priːdɪspə'zɪʃn] *noun* tendency; *she has a predisposition to obesity*

predominant [prɪ'dɒmɪnənt] *adjective* which is more powerful than others

pre-eclampsia [priːɪ'klæmpsiə] *noun* condition of pregnant women towards the end of the pregnancy, which may lead to eclampsia; **early onset pre-eclampsia** = pre-eclampsia which appears before 37 weeks' gestation

COMMENT: symptoms are high blood pressure, oedema and protein in the urine

preemie ['priːmi] *noun US (informal)* premature infant

prefrontal [priː'frʌntl] *adjective* in the front part of the frontal lobe; **prefrontal leucotomy** = operation to divide some of the white matter in the prefrontal lobe, formerly used as a treatment for schizophrenia; **prefrontal lobe** = part of the brain in the front part of each hemisphere, in front of the frontal lobe, which is concerned with memory and learning

preganglionic [priːgæŋglɪ'ɒnɪk] *adjective* near to and in front of a ganglion; **preganglionic fibre** = nerve fibre which ends in a ganglion where it is linked in a synapse to a postganglionic fibre; **preganglionic neurone** = neurone which ends in a ganglion

pregnancy ['pregnənsi] *noun* (i) time between conception and childbirth when a woman is carrying the unborn child in her uterus; (ii) condition of being pregnant; **extrauterine** *or* **ectopic pregnancy** = pregnancy where the embryo develops outside the uterus, usually in one of the Fallopian tubes; **multiple pregnancy** = pregnancy a woman is pregnant with more than one child; **phantom pregnancy** = pseudocyesis, psychological condition where a woman has all the symptoms of pregnancy without being pregnant; **tubal pregnancy** = the most common form of ectopic pregnancy, where the fetus develops in a Fallopian tube instead of the uterus; **unwanted pregnancy** = condition where a woman becomes pregnant without wanting to have a child; **pregnancy-associated hypertension** = high blood pressure which is associated with pregnancy; **pregnancy test** = test to see if a woman is pregnant or not

pregnant ['pregnənt] *adjective* (woman) with an unborn child in her uterus; *she is six months pregnant*

prehepatic [priːhɪ'pætɪk] *adjective* before the liver; **prehepatic bilirubin** = bilirubin in plasma before it passes through the liver; **prehepatic jaundice** = jaundice which occurs because of haemolysis before the blood reaches the liver

premature ['premətʃʊə] *adjective* early, before the normal time; *the baby was born five weeks premature*; **premature baby** = baby born earlier than 37 weeks from conception, or weighing less than 2.5 kilos, but capable of independent life; **premature beat** = ectopic beat, abnormal extra beat of the heart which can be caused by caffeine or other stimulants; **premature birth** = birth of a baby earlier than 37 weeks from conception; **premature ejaculation** = situation where a man ejaculates too early during sexual intercourse; **premature labour** = starting to give birth earlier than 37 weeks from conception; *after the accident she went into premature labour*

COMMENT: babies can survive even if born several weeks premature. Even babies weighing less than one kilo at birth can survive in an incubator, and develop normally

prematurely ['prematʃʊəli] *adverb* early, before the normal time; *the baby was born two weeks prematurely*; *a large number of people die prematurely from ischaemic heart disease*

prematurity [premə'tʃʊərəti] *noun* situation where something occurs early, before the normal time

premed [pri:'med] *noun* (*informal*) stage of being given premedication; *the patient is in premed*

premedication *or* **premedicant drug** [pri:medɪ'keɪʃn] *noun* drug (such as a sedative) given to a patient before an operation begins in order to block the parasympathetic nervous system and prevent vomiting during the operation

premenstrual [pri:'menstrʊl] *adjective* before menstruation; **premenstrual syndrome (PMS)** *or* **premenstrual tension (PMT)** = nervous stress experienced by a woman for one or two weeks before a menstrual period starts

premolar [pri:'məʊlə] *noun* tooth with two points, situated between the canines and the first proper molar; *see illustration at* TEETH

prenatal [pri:'neɪtl] *adjective* during the period between conception and childbirth; **prenatal diagnosis** = antenatal diagnosis, medical examination of a pregnant woman to see if the fetus is developing normally

pre-op ['pri:'ɒp] (*informal*) = PREOPERATIVE

preoperative [pri:'ɒprətɪv] *adjective* before a surgical operation; **preoperative medication** = drug (such as a sedative) given to a patient before an operation begins

preoperatively [pri:'ɒprətɪvli] *adverb* before a surgical operation

prep [prep] (*informal*) **1** *noun* preparing, getting a patient ready for an operation; *the prep is finished, so the patient can be taken to the operating theatre* **2** *verb* to prepare or get a patient ready for an operation; *has the patient been prepped?*

preparation [prepə'reɪʃn] *noun* (**a**) act of preparing a patient before an operation (**b**) medicine or liquid containing a drug; *he was given a preparation containing an antihistamine*

prepare [prɪ'peə] *verb* to get something ready; to make something; *he prepared a soothing linctus*; *six rooms in the hospital were prepared for the accident victims*; *the nurses were preparing the patient for the operation*

prepatellar bursitis [pri:pə'telə bə'saɪtɪs] *noun* housemaid's knee, condition where the fluid sac at the knee becomes inflamed, caused by kneeling on hard surfaces

prepubertal [pri:'pju:bətl] *adjective* referring to the period before puberty

prepuberty [pri:'pju:bəti] *noun* period before puberty

prepuce ['pri:pju:s] *noun* foreskin, skin covering the top of the penis, which can be removed by circumcision

presby- *or* **presbyo-** ['prezbi *or* 'prezbiəʊ] *prefix* referring to old age

presbyacusis [prezbiə'ku:sɪs] *noun* condition where an old person's hearing fails gradually, due to degeneration of the internal ear

presbyopia [prezbi'əʊpiə] *noun* condition where an old person's sight fails gradually, due to hardening of the lens

prescribe [prɪs'kraɪb] *verb* to give instructions for a patient to get a certain dosage of a drug or a certain form of therapeutic treatment; *the doctor prescribed a course of antibiotics*; **prescribing analyses and cost (PACT)** = data on the prescribing of drugs in primary care

prescription [prɪ'skrɪpʃn] *noun* order written by a doctor to a pharmacist asking for a drug to be prepared and given or sold to a patient

presence ['prezns] *noun* being there; *tests showed the presence of sugar in the urine*

presenile [pri:'si:naɪl] *adjective* (i) prematurely old; (ii) (condition) which affects people of early or middle age, but has characteristics of old age; **presenile dementia** = old term used to describe a form of mental degeneration affecting adults before old age (as in Alzheimer's disease)

COMMENT: patients used to be diagnosed with presenile dementia if they showed symptoms of dementia and were under the age of 65, and senile dementia if over 65. However, the terms are no longer often used and instead the type of dementia is used for diagnostic purposes (Alzheimer's disease, multi-infarct, vascular etc.)

presenility [priːsəˈnɪləti] *noun* ageing of the body or brain before the normal time, with the patient showing symptoms which are normally associated with old people

present 1 [prɪˈzent] *verb* **(a)** to show, to be present; *the patient presented with severe chest pains*; *the doctors' first task is to relieve the presenting symptoms*; *the condition may also present in a baby* **(b)** *(in obstetrics)* to appear (in the vaginal channel); **the presenting part** = the part of the fetus which appears first **2** [ˈpreznt] *adjective* which is there; *all the symptoms of the disease are present*

chlamydia in the male commonly presents a urethritis characterized by dysuria
Journal of American College Health

26 patients were selected from the outpatient department on grounds of disabling breathlessness present for at least five years
Lancet

sickle cell chest syndrome is a common complication of sickle cell disease, presenting with chest pain, fever and leucocytosis
British Medical Journal

a 24 year-old woman presents with an influenza-like illness of five days' duration
British Journal of Hospital Medicine

the presenting symptoms of Crohn's disease may be extremely variable
New Zealand Medical Journal

presentation [prezənˈteɪʃn] *noun* way in which a baby will be born, i.e. the part of the baby's body which will appear first in the vaginal channel; **breech presentation** = position of the baby in the uterus, where the buttocks will appear first; **cephalic presentation** = normal presentation, where the baby's head will appear first; **face presentation** = position of the baby in the uterus, where the face will appear first; **shoulder presentation** = position of the baby in the uterus, where the shoulder will appear first; **transverse presentation** = position of the baby in the uterus, where the baby's side will appear first, normally requiring urgent manipulation or Caesarean section to prevent complications

preservation [prezəˈveɪʃn] *noun* keeping of tissue sample or donor organ in good condition

preserve [prɪˈzɜːv] *verb* to keep or to stop (tissue sample) from rotting

press [pres] *verb* to push or to squeeze; *the tumour is pressing against a nerve*

pressor [ˈpresə] *adjective* (nerve) which increases the action of part of the body; (substance) which raises blood pressure

pressure [ˈpreʃə] *noun* **(a)** (i) action of squeezing or of forcing (ii) force of something on its surroundings; **blood pressure** = *see* BLOOD; **diastolic pressure** = low point of blood pressure during the diastole; **osmotic pressure** = pressure by which certain molecules in a fluid go through a membrane into another part of the body; **pulse pressure** = difference between the diastolic and systolic pressure; **systolic pressure** = high point of blood pressure during the systole; **pressure area** = area of the body where a bone is near the surface of the skin, so that if the skin is pressed the circulation will be cut off; **pressure point** = place where an artery crosses over a bone, so that the blood can be cut off by pressing with the finger; **pressure sore** = ulcer which forms on the skin at a pressure area or where something presses on it **(b)** mental or physical stress caused by external events;

presynaptic [priːsɪˈnæptɪk] *adjective* before a synapse; **presynaptic axon** = nerve leading to one side of a synapse

presystole [priːˈsɪstəli] *noun* period before systole in the cycle of heartbeats

preterm [priːˈtɜːm] *adjective* (birth of a child) taking place before the normal time

prevalence [ˈprevləns] *noun* percentage, number of cases of a disease in a certain place at a certain time; *the prevalence of malaria in some tropical countries*; *the prevalence of cases of malnutrition in large towns*; *a high prevalence of renal disease*

prevalent [ˈprevlənt] *adjective* common (in comparison to something); *the disease is prevalent in some African countries*; *a condition which is more prevalent in the cold winter months*

prevent [prɪˈvent] *verb* to stop something happening; *the treatment is given to prevent the patient's condition from getting worse*; *doctors are trying to prevent the spread of the outbreak of legionnaires' disease* (NOTE:

you prevent something **from** happening or simply **prevent something happening**)

prevention [prɪ'venʃn] *noun* stopping something happening; **accident prevention** = taking steps to prevent accidents happening

preventive [prɪ'ventɪv] *adjective* which prevents; **preventive medicine** = medical action to prevent a disease from occurring; **preventive measure** = step taken to prevent a disease from occurring

> COMMENT: preventive measures include immunization, vaccination, sterilization, quarantine and improving standards of housing and sanitation. Health education also has an important role to play in the prevention of disease

prevertebral [priː'vɜːtɪbrl] *adjective* in front of the spinal column or a vertebra

priapism ['praɪəpɪzm] *noun* erection of the penis without sexual stimulus, caused by a blood clot in the tissue of the penis, injury to the spinal cord or stone in the urinary bladder

prick [prɪk] *verb* to make a small hole with a sharp point; *the nurse pricked the patient's finger to take a blood sample*; *she pricked her finger on the needle and the spot became infected*

prickle cell ['prɪkl 'sel] *noun* cell with many processes connecting it to other cells, found in the inner layer of the epidermis

prickly heat ['prɪkli 'hiːt] = MILIARIA

-pril [prɪl] *suffix* for ACE inhibitors; *Captopril*

primary ['praɪməri] *adjective* **(a)** (condition) which is first, and leads to another (the secondary condition); **primary complex** = first lymph node to be infected by tuberculosis; **primary haemorrhage** = bleeding which occurs immediately after an injury has been suffered; **primary tubercle** = first infected spot where tuberculosis starts in a lung; **primary tumour** = site of original malignant growth from which the cancer spreads; **primary tuberculosis** = infection of a patient with tuberculosis for the first time; *see also* AMENORRHOEA **(b)** which is most important; **primary health care** *or* **primary medical care** = treatment provided by a general practitioner; **primary care group (PCG)** = organization responsible for overseeing the provision of primary healthcare and the commissioning of secondary care in a district; key members

include GPs, community nurses, social services and lay members; **primary care trust (PCT)** = the top level of the primary care group with extra responsibilities such as direct employment of community staff ; *compare* SECONDARY

---

among primary health care services, 1.5% of all GP consultations are due to coronary heart disease
Health Services Journal

---

primary care is largely concerned with clinical management of individual patients, while community medicine tends to view the whole population as its patient
Journal of the Royal College of General Practitioners

---

primigravida *or* **primigravid patient** [praɪmɪ'grævɪdə or 'praɪmɪgrævɪd 'peɪʃnt] *noun* woman who is pregnant for the first time

primipara [praɪ'mɪpərə] *noun* woman who has given birth to one child (NOTE: also called **unipara**)

primordial [praɪ'mɔːdiəl] *adjective* in the very first stage of development; **primordial follicle** = first stage of development of an ovarian follicle

principle ['prɪnsəpl] *noun* rule or theory; **active principle** = main ingredient of a drug which makes it have the required effect on a patient

prioritize [praɪ'ɒrɪtaɪz] *verb* to give priority to something; *the hospital prioritized respiratory cases during the flu epidemic*

priority [praɪ'ɒrəti] *noun* right to be first; *urgent surgical cases must be given top priority*

private ['praɪvət] *adjective* **(i)** belonging to one person, not to the public; **(ii)** which is paid for by a person; *he runs a private clinic for alcoholics*; *she is in private practice as an orthopaedic consultant*; **private patient** = patient who is paying for his treatment, not having it done through the National Health Service; **private practice** = services of a doctor, surgeon or dentist which are paid for by the patients themselves (or by a medical insurance), but not by the National Health Service

privately ['praɪvətli] *adverb* paid by the patient, not by the National Health Service;

she decided to have the operation done privately (NOTE: the opposite is **'on the National Health'**)

p.r.n. ['piː 'ɑː 'en] *abbreviation for the Latin phrase* 'pro re nata': as and when required (written on a prescription)

pro- [prəʊ] *prefix* meaning before or in front of

probang ['prəʊbæŋ] *noun* surgical instrument, like a long rod with a brush at one end, formerly used to test and find strictures in the oesophagus and to push foreign bodies into the stomach

probe [prəʊb] **1** *noun* (i) instrument used to explore inside a cavity or wound; (ii) device inserted into a medium to obtain information; **laser probe** = metal probe which is inserted into the body and through which a laser beam can be passed to remove a blockage in an artery; **ultrasonic** *or* **ultrasound probe** = instrument which locates organs or tissues inside the body, using ultrasound **2** *verb* to investigate the inside of something; *the surgeon probed the wound with a scalpel*

problem ['prɒbləm] *noun* **(a)** something which is difficult to find an answer to; *scientists are trying to find a solution to the problem of drug-related disease*; **problem child** = child who is difficult to control **(b)** medical disorder, usually an addiction; **he has an alcohol problem** *or* **a drugs problem** = he is addicted to alcohol or drugs; **problem drinking** = alcoholism which has a bad effect on a person's behaviour or work

procedure [prə'siːdʒə] *noun* (i) type of treatment; (ii) treatment given at one time; *the hospital has developed some new procedures for treating Parkinson's disease; we are hoping to increase the number of procedures carried out per day*; **surgical procedure** = one surgical operation

disposable items now available for medical and nursing procedures range from cheap syringes to expensive cardiac pacemakers

Nursing Times

the electromyograms and CT scans were done as outpatient procedures

Southern Medical Journal

process ['prəʊses] **1** *noun* **(a)** projecting part of the body; **articular process** = piece of bone which sticks out of the neural arch in a vertebra and articulates with the next vertebra; **ciliary processes** = series of ridges behind the iris to which the lens of the eye is attached; *see illustration at* EYE; **mastoid process** = part of the temporal bone which protrudes at the side of the head behind the ear; *see illustration at* SKULL; **transverse process** = part of a vertebra which protrudes at the side; **xiphoid process** = bottom part of the breastbone which is originally cartilage but becomes bone by middle age **(b)** technical or scientific action; *a new process for testing serum samples has been developed in the research laboratory* **(c)** **nursing process** = standard method of treatment carried out by nurses, and the documents which go with it **2** *verb* to examine or to test samples; *the blood samples are being processed by the laboratory*

the nursing process serves to divide overall patient care into that part performed by nurses and that performed by the other professions

Nursing Times

all relevant sections of the nurses' care plan and nursing process records had been left blank

Nursing Times

procidentia [prəʊsɪ'denʃə] *noun* movement of an organ downwards; **uterine procidentia** = condition where the uterus has passed through the vagina

proct- *or* **procto-** ['prɒkt or 'prɒktəʊ] *prefix* referring to the anus or rectum

proctalgia [prɒk'tældʒə] *noun* pain in the lower rectum or anus, caused by neuralgia; **proctalgia fugax** = condition where the patient suffers sudden pains in the rectum during the night, usually relieved by eating or drinking

proctatresia [prɒktə'triːzɪə] *noun* imperforate anus, condition where the anus does not have an opening

proctectasia [prɒktek'teɪzɪə] *noun* condition where the rectum or anus is dilated because of continued constipation

proctectomy [prɒk'tektəmi] *noun* surgical removal of the rectum

proctitis [prɒk'taɪtɪs] *noun* inflammation of the rectum

proctocele ['prɒktəsiːl] *noun* **vaginal proctocele** = condition associated with prolapse of the uterus, where the rectum protrudes into the vagina

proctoclysis [prɒkˈtɒkləsɪs] *noun* introduction of a lot of fluid into the rectum slowly

proctocolectomy [prɒktəʊkɒˈlektəmi] *noun* surgical removal of the rectum and the colon

proctocolitis [prɒktəkəˈlaɪtɪs] *noun* inflammation of the rectum and part of the colon

proctodynia [prɒktəˈdɪniə] *noun* sensation of pain in the anus

proctologist [prɒkˈtɒlədʒɪst] *noun* specialist in proctology

proctology [prɒkˈtɒlədʒi] *noun* scientific study of the rectum and anus and their associated diseases

proctorrhaphy [prɒkˈtɔːrəfi] *noun* surgical operation to stitch up a tear in the rectum or anus

proctoscope [ˈprɒktəskəʊp] *noun* surgical instrument consisting of a long tube with a light in the end, used to examine the rectum

proctoscopy [prɒkˈtɒskəpi] *noun* examination of the rectum using a proctoscope

proctosigmoiditis [prɒktəʊsɪgmɔɪˈdaɪtɪs] *noun* inflammation of the rectum and the sigmoid colon

proctotomy [prɒkˈtɒtəmi] *noun* (i) surgical operation to divide a structure of the rectum or anus; (ii) opening of an imperforate anus

prodromal [prəʊˈdrəʊml] *adjective* (time) between when the first symptoms of a disease appear, and the appearance of the major effect, such as a fever or rash; **prodromal rash** = early rash, rash which appears as a symptom of a disease before the major rash

prodrome *or* **prodroma** [ˈprəʊdrəʊm *or* prəʊˈdrəʊmə] *noun* early symptom of an attack of a disease

in classic migraine a prodrome is followed by an aura, then a headache, and finally a recovery phase. The prodrome may not be recognised
British Journal of Hospital Medicine

produce [prəˈdjuːs] *verb* to make; *the drug produces a sensation of dizziness*; *doctors*

are worried by the side-effects produced by the new painkiller

product [ˈprɒdʌkt] *noun* (i) thing which is produced; (ii) result or effect of a process; **pharmaceutical products** = medicines, pills, lozenges or creams which are sold in chemists' shops

proenzyme [prəʊˈenzaɪm] *noun* zymogen, first mature form of an enzyme, before it develops into an active enzyme

profession [prəˈfeʃn] *noun* (i) type of job for which special training is needed; (ii) all people working in a specialized type of employment for which they have been trained; **the medical profession** = all doctors; **he's a doctor by profession** = his job is being a doctor

professional [prəˈfeʃnl] *adjective* referring to a profession; **professional body** = organization which acts for all the members of a profession; **Professional Conduct Committee (PCC)** = committee of the General Medical Council which decides on cases of professional misconduct; **professional misconduct** = action which is thought to be wrong by the body which regulates a profession (such as an action by a doctor which is considered wrong by the General Medical Council)

profound [prəˈfaʊnd] *adjective* serious; *a profound abnormality of the immune system*

profunda [prəˈfʌndə] *adjective* (blood vessels) which lie deep in tissues

profuse [prəˈfjuːs] *adjective* very large quantity; *fever accompanied by profuse sweating*; *pains with profuse internal bleeding*

progeria [prəʊˈdʒɪəriə] *noun* premature senility (NOTE: also called **Hutchinson-Gilford syndrome**)

progesterone [prəˈdʒestərəʊn] *noun* hormone produced in the second part of the menstrual cycle by the corpus luteum and which stimulates the formation of the placenta if an ovum is fertilized (it is also produced by the placenta itself)

progestogen [prəˈdʒestədʒn] *noun* any substance which has the same effect as progesterone

COMMENT: because natural progesterones prevent ovulation during pregnancy, synthetically produced progestogens are used to make contraceptive pills

prognathic jaw [prɒgˈnæθɪk ˈdʒɔː] *noun* jaw which protrudes further than the other

prognathism [ˈprɒgnəθɪzm] *noun* condition where one jaw (especially the lower) or both jaws protrude

prognosis [prɒgˈnəʊsɪs] *noun* opinion of how a disease or disorder will develop; **this cancer has a prognosis of about two years** = the patient will die within two years unless this cancer is eradicated; *compare* DIAGNOSIS

prognostic [prɒgˈnɒstɪk] *adjective* referring to prognosis; **prognostic test** = test to decide how a disease will develop, how long a patient will survive an operation

programme [ˈprəʊgræm] *noun* series of medical treatments given in a set way at set times; *the doctor prescribed a programme of injections*; *she took a programme of steroid treatment*

progress 1 [ˈprəʊgres] *noun* development, way in which a person is becoming well; *the doctors seem pleased that she has made such good progress since her operation* **2** [prəˈgres] *verb* to develop or to continue to do well; *the patient is progressing well*; *the doctor asked how the patient was progressing*

progression [prəˈgreʃn] *noun* development; **progression of a disease** = way in which a disease develops

progressive [prəˈgresɪv] *adjective* which develops all the time; *Alzheimer's disease is a progressive disorder which sees a gradual decline in intellectual functioning*; **progressive deafness** = condition where the patient becomes more and more deaf; **progressive muscular atrophy** = any form of muscular dystrophy, with progressive weakening of the muscles, particularly in the pelvic and shoulder girdles

progressively [prəˈgresɪvli] *adverb* more and more; *he became progressively more disabled*

proinsulin [prəʊˈɪnsjʊlɪn] *noun* substance produced by the pancreas, then converted to insulin

project [prəˈdʒekt] *verb* to protrude or to stick out

projection [prəˈdʒekʃn] *noun* **(a)** piece of a part which protrudes; **projection tract** =

fibres connecting the cerebral cortex with the lower parts of the brain and spinal cord **(b)** *(in psychology)* mental action, where the patient blames another person for his own faults

prolactin [prəʊˈlæktɪn] *noun* lactogenic hormone, a hormone secreted by the pituitary gland which stimulates the production of milk

prolapse [ˈprəʊlæps] *noun* condition where an organ has moved downwards out of its normal position; **rectal prolapse** *or* **prolapse of the rectum** = condition where mucous membrane of the rectum moves downwards and passes through the anus; **prolapsed intervertebral disc (PID)** = slipped disc, a condition where an intervertebral disc becomes displaced or where the soft centre of a disc passes through the hard cartilage of the exterior and presses onto a nerve; **prolapsed uterus** *or* **prolapse of the uterus** = UTERINE PROLAPSE

proliferate [prəˈlɪfəreɪt] *verb* to produce many similar cells or parts, and so grow

proliferation [prəlɪfəˈreɪʃn] *noun* process of proliferating

proliferative [prəˈlɪfərətɪv] *adjective* which multiplies; **proliferative phase** = period when a disease is spreading fast

proline [ˈprəʊlɪn] *noun* amino acid found in proteins, especially in collagen

prolong [prəˈlɒŋ] *verb* to make longer; *the treatment prolonged her life by three years*

prolonged [prəˈlɒŋd] *adjective* very long; *she had to undergo a prolonged course of radiation treatment*

prominence [ˈprɒmɪnəns] *noun* projection, part of the body which stands out; **the laryngeal prominence** = the Adam's apple

prominent [ˈprɒmɪnənt] *adjective* which stands out, which is very visible; *she had a prominent scar on her neck which she wanted to have removed*

promontory [ˈprɒməntri] *noun* projection, section of an organ (especially the middle ear and sacrum) which stands out above the rest

promote [prəˈməʊt] *verb* to help something take place; *the drug is used to promote blood clotting*

pronate [ˈprəʊneɪt] *verb* (i) to lie face downwards; (ii) to turn the hand so that palm faces downwards

pronation [prəʊ'neɪʃn] *noun* turning the hand round so that the palm faces downwards

pronator [prəʊ'neɪtə] *noun* muscle which makes the hand turn face downwards

prone [prəʊn] *adjective* (i) lying face downwards; (ii) (arm) with the palm facing downwards (NOTE: the opposite is **supination, supine**)

pronounced [prə'naʊnst] *adjective* very obvious or marked; *she has a pronounced limp*

propagate ['prɒpəgeɪt] *verb* to multiply

propagation [prɒpə'geɪʃn] *noun* increasing, causing something to spread

properdin ['prəʊpədɪn] *noun* protein in blood plasma which can destroy Gram-negative bacteria and neutralize viruses when acting together with magnesium

prophase ['prəʊfeɪz] *noun* first stage of mitosis when the chromosomes are visible as long thin double threads

prophylactic [prɒfə'læktɪk] *noun* & *adjective* (substance) which helps to prevent the development of a disease

prophylaxis [prɒfə'læksɪs] *noun* (i) prevention of disease; (ii) preventive treatment

proportion [prə'pɔːʃn] *noun* quantity of something, especially as compared to the whole; *a high proportion of cancers can be treated by surgery*; *the proportion of outpatients to inpatients is increasing*

the target cells for adult myeloid leukaemia are located in the bone marrow, and there is now evidence that a substantial proportion of childhood leukaemias also arise in the bone marrow
British Medical Journal

proprietary [prə'praɪətri] *adjective* which belongs to a commercial company; **proprietary medicine** *or* **proprietary drug** = patent medicine, drug which is sold under a trade name; **proprietary name** = trade name for a drug; *compare* GENERIC

proprioception [prəʊprɪə'sepʃn] *noun* reaction of nerves to body movements and relation of information about movements to the brain

proprioceptive [prəʊprɪə'septɪv] *adjective* referring to sensory impulses from the joints, muscles and tendons, which relate information about body movements to the brain

proprioceptor [prəʊprɪə'septə] *noun* end of a sensory nerve which reacts to stimuli from muscles and tendons as they move

proptosis [prɒp'təʊsɪs] *noun* forward displacement of the eyeball

prop up ['prɒp 'ʌp] *verb* to support a patient (as with pillows)

prosop- *or* **prosopo-** ['prɒsəp or 'prɒsəpəʊ] *prefix* referring to the face

prospective [prə'spektɪv] *adjective* (study) applying to the future, following what happens to selected patients; *see also* RETROSPECTIVE

prostaglandins [prɒstə'glændɪnz] *noun* fatty acids present in many parts of the body, which are associated with the sensation of pain and have an effect on the nervous system, blood pressure and in particular the uterus at menstruation

prostate ['prɒsteɪt] *noun;* **prostate (gland)** = gland in men which produces a secretion in which sperm cells float; **he has prostate trouble** = he is suffering from prostatitis, he has an enlarged prostate gland; *see illustration at* UROGENITAL SYSTEM (MALE)

COMMENT: the prostate gland lies under the bladder and surrounds the urethra (the tube leading from the bladder to the penis). It secretes a fluid containing enzymes. As a man grows older, the prostate gland tends to enlarge and constrict the point at which the urethra leaves the bladder, making it difficult to pass urine

prostatectomy [prɒstə'tektəmi] *noun* surgical removal of all or part of the prostate gland; **retropubic prostatectomy** = prostatectomy where the operation is performed through the membrane surrounding the prostate gland; **transurethral prostatectomy** = prostatectomy where the operation is performed through the urethra (NOTE: also called **transurethral resection**); **transvesical prostatectomy** = prostatectomy where the operation is performed through the bladder; *see also* HARRIS'S OPERATION

prostatic [prɒ'stætɪk] *adjective* referring to the prostate gland; belonging to the prostate gland; **prostatic hypertrophy** = enlargement of the prostate gland; **prostatic massage** = removing fluid from the prostate gland through the rectum; **prostatic urethra** = section of the urethra which passes through the prostate; **prostatic utricle** = sac branching from the prostatic urethra

prostatitis [prɒstə'taɪtɪs] *noun* inflammation of the prostate gland

prostatocystitis [prɒsteɪtəʊsɪ'staɪtɪs] *noun* inflammation of the prostatic part of the urethra and the bladder

prostatorrhoea [prɒstətə'rɪə] *noun* discharge of fluid from the prostate gland

prosthesis [prɒs'θiːsɪs] *noun* device which is attached to the body to take the place of a part which is missing (such as an artificial leg, glass eye, etc.); **dental prosthesis** = one or more false teeth; **ocular prosthesis** = artificial or glass eye (NOTE: plural is **prostheses**)

prosthetic [prɒs'θetɪk] *adjective* (artificial limb) which replaces a part of the body which has been amputated or removed; *he was fitted with a prosthetic hand*

prosthetics [prɒs'θetɪks] *noun* study and making of prostheses

prosthetist ['prɒsθətɪst] *noun* qualified person who fits prostheses

The average life span of a joint prosthesis is 10-15 years
                    British Journal of Nursing

prostration [prɒs'treɪʃn] *noun* extreme tiredness of body or mind

protamine ['prəʊtəmiːn] *noun* simple protein found in fish, used with insulin to slow down the insulin absorption rate

protanopia [prəʊtə'nəʊpɪə] = DALTONISM

protease ['prəʊtɪeɪz] *noun* proteolytic enzyme, digestive enzyme which breaks down protein in food by splitting the peptide link

protect [prə'tekt] *verb* to keep something safe from harm; *the population must be protected against the spread of the virus*

protection [prə'tekʃn] *noun* thing which protects; *children are vaccinated as a protection against disease*

protective [prə'tektɪv] *adjective* which protects; **protective cap** = condom, a rubber sheath put over the penis before intercourse as a contraceptive or as a protection against venereal disease

protein ['prəʊtiːn] *noun* nitrogen compound which is present in and is an essential part of all living cells in the body, formed by the condensation of amino acids; **protein balance** = situation when the nitrogen intake in protein is equal to the excretion rate (in the urine); **protein deficiency** = lack of enough proteins in the diet

COMMENT: proteins are necessary for growth and repair of the body's tissue; they are mainly formed of carbon, nitrogen and oxygen in various combinations as amino acids. Certain foods (such as beans, meat, eggs, fish and milk) are rich in protein

protein-bound iodine ['prəʊtiːn'baʊnd 'aɪədiːn] *noun* compound of thyroxine and iodine; **protein-bound iodine test (PBI test)** = test to measure if the thyroid gland is producing adequate quantities of thyroxine

proteinuria [prəʊti'njʊərɪə] *noun* proteins in the urine

proteolysis [prəʊti'ɒləsɪs] *noun* breaking down of proteins in food by proteolytic enzymes

proteolytic [prəʊtiɒ'lɪtɪk] *adjective* referring to proteolysis; **proteolytic enzyme** = PROTEASE

Proteus ['prəʊtjuːs] *noun* genus of bacteria commonly found in the intestines

prothrombin [prəʊ'θrɒmbɪn] *noun* Factor II, a protein in blood which helps blood to coagulate and which needs vitamin K to be effective; **prothrombin time** = time taken (in Quick's test) for clotting to take place

proto- ['prəʊtəʊ] *prefix* meaning first, at the beginning

protocol ['prəʊtəkɒl] *noun* instructions for the clinical management of a particular condition, including tests, surgery and drug treatments

protopathic [prəʊtəʊ'pæθɪk] *adjective* (i) referring to nerves which are able to sense only strong sensations; (ii) referring to a first symptom or lesion; (iii) referring to the first sign of partially restored function in an injured nerve; *see also* EPICRITIC

protoplasm ['prəʊtəʊplæzm] *noun* substance like a jelly which makes up the largest part of each cell

protoplasmic [prəʊtəʊ'plæzmɪk] *adjective* referring to protoplasm

protoporphyrin IX [prəʊtəʊˈpɔːfərɪn ˈnaɪn] *noun* commonest form of porphyrin, found in haemoglobin and chlorophyll

Protozoa [prəʊtəʊˈzəʊə] *plural noun* tiny simple organisms with a single cell (NOTE: the singular is **protozoon**)

COMMENT: parasitic Protozoa can cause several diseases, such as amoebiasis, malaria and other tropical diseases

protozoan [prəʊtəˈzəʊən] *adjective* referring to the Protozoa

protrude [prəˈtruːd] *verb* to stick out; *she wears a brace to correct her protruding teeth*; *protruding eyes are associated with some forms of goitre*

protuberance [prəˈtjuːbərns] *noun* rounded part of the body which projects above the rest

proud flesh [ˈpraʊd ˈfleʃ] *noun* new vessels and young fibrous tissue which form when a wound, incision or lesion is healing

provide [prəˈvaɪd] *verb* to supply or to give; *a balanced diet should provide the necessary proteins required by the body*; *a dentist's surgery should provide adequate room for patients to wait in*; *the hospital provides an ambulance service to the whole area*

provider [prəˈvaɪdə] *noun* hospital which provides secondary care which is paid for by another body such as PCG or social services; *see also* PURCHASER

provision [prəˈvɪʒn] *noun* act of providing; *the provision of aftercare facilities for patients recently discharged from hospital*

provisional [prəˈvɪʒnl] *adjective* temporary, which may be changed; *the hospital has given me a provisional date for the operation*; *the paramedical team attached sticks to the broken leg to act as provisional splints*

provisionally [prəˈvɪʒnli] *adverb* in a temporary way, not certainly; *she has provisionally accepted the offer of a bed in the hospital*

provoke [prəˈvəʊk] *verb* to stimulate, make something happen; *the medication provoked a sudden rise in body temperature*; *the fit was provoked by the shock of the accident*

proximal [ˈprɒksɪml] *adjective* near the midline, the central part of the body; **proximal convoluted tubule** = part of the kidney filtering system, between the loop of

Henle and the glomerulus; **proximal interphalangeal joint (PIP)** = joint nearest the point of attachment of a finger or toe

proximally [ˈprɒksɪmli] *adverb* placed further towards the centre or point of attachment (NOTE: the opposite is **distal, distally**)

prurigo [pruˈraɪgəʊ] *noun* itchy eruption of papules; **Besnier's prurigo** = irritating form of prurigo on the backs of the knees and the insides of the elbows

pruritus [pruˈraɪtəs] *noun* irritation of the skin which makes a patient want to scratch; **pruritus ani** = itching round the anal orifice; **pruritus vulvae** = itching round the vulva

prussic acid [ˈprʌsɪk ˈæsɪd] = CYANIDE

pseud- *or* **pseudo-** [ˈsjuːd *or* ˈsjuːdəʊ] *prefix* meaning false, similar to something, but not the same

pseudarthrosis [sjuːdɑːˈθrəʊsɪs] *noun* false joint, as when the two broken ends of a fractured bone do not bind together but heal separately

pseudoangina [sjuːdəʊænˈdʒaɪnə] *noun* pain in the chest, caused by worry but not indicating heart disease

pseudocoxalgia [sjuːdəʊkɒkˈsældʒə] *noun* Legg-Calvé-Perthes disease, degeneration of the upper end of the femur (in young boys) which prevents the femur from growing properly and can result in a permanent limp

pseudocrisis [sjuːdəʊˈkraɪsɪs] *noun* sudden fall in the temperature of the patient with fever, but which does not mark the end of the fever

pseudocroup [sjuːdəʊˈkruːp] *noun* (i) laryngismus stridulus; (ii) form of asthma, where contractions take place in the larynx

pseudocyesis [sjuːdəʊsaɪˈiːsɪs] *noun* phantom pregnancy, condition where a woman has the physical symptoms of pregnancy, but is not pregnant

pseudocyst [ˈsjuːdəʊsɪst] *noun* (i) false cyst; (ii) space which fills with fluid in an organ, but without the walls which would form a cyst, as a result of softening or necrosis of the tissue

pseudodementia [sjuːdəʊdɪˈmenʃə] *noun* condition of extreme apathy found in hysterical people (where their behaviour corresponds to what they imagine to be insanity, though they show no signs of true dementia)

pseudohypertrophic muscular dystrophy [sjuːdəʊhaɪpəˈtrɒfik ˈmʌskjʊlə ˈdɪstrəfi] *noun* Duchenne muscular dystrophy, a hereditary disease affecting the muscles, which swell and become weak, beginning in early childhood

pseudohypertrophy [sjuːdəʊhaɪˈpɜːtrəfi] *noun* overgrowth of fatty or fibrous tissue in a part or organ, which results in the part or organ being enlarged

pseudomyxoma [sjuːdəʊmɪkˈsəʊmə] *noun* tumour rich in mucus

pseudoplegia *or* **pseudoparalysis** [sjuːdəʊˈpliːdʒə *or* sjuːdəʊpəˈræləsɪs] *noun* (i) loss of muscular power in the limbs, but without true paralysis; (ii) paralysis caused by hysteria

pseudopolyposis [sjuːdəʊpɒliˈpəʊsɪs] *noun* condition where polyps are found in many places in the intestine, usually resulting from an earlier infection

psilosis [saɪˈləʊsɪs] *noun* sprue, disease of the small intestine, which prevents the patient from absorbing food properly

COMMENT: the condition is often found in the tropics, and results in diarrhoea and loss of weight

psittacosis [sɪtəˈkəʊsɪs] *noun* parrot disease, disease of parrots which can be transmitted to humans

COMMENT: the disease is similar to typhoid fever, but atypical pneumonia is present; symptoms include fever, diarrhoea and distension of the abdomen

psoas major [ˈsəʊæs ˈmeɪdʒə] *noun* muscle in the groin which flexes the hip; **psoas minor** = small muscle, similar to the psoas major, but which is not always present

psoriasis [səˈraɪəsɪs] *noun* common inflammatory skin disease where red patches of skin are covered with white scales

psoriatic [sɔːriˈætɪk] *adjective* referring to psoriasis; **psoriatic arthritis** = form of psoriasis which is associated with arthritis

psych- *or* **psycho-** [ˈsaɪk *or* ˈsaɪkəʊ] *prefix* referring to the mind

psychasthenia [saɪkæsˈθiːniə] *noun* (i) any psychoneurosis, except hysteria; (ii) psychoneurosis characterized by fears and phobias

psyche [ˈsaɪki] *noun* the mind

psychedelic [saɪkəˈdelɪk] *adjective* (drug, such as LSD) which expands a person's consciousness

psychiatric [saɪkiˈætrɪk] *adjective* referring to psychiatry; *he is undergoing psychiatric treatment*; **psychiatric hospital** = hospital which specializes in the treatment of patients with mental disorders

psychiatrist [saɪˈkaɪətrɪst] *noun* doctor who specializes in the diagnosis and treatment of mental disorders and behaviour

psychiatry [saɪˈkaɪətri] *noun* branch of medicine concerned with diagnosis and treatment of mental disorders and behaviour

psychoanalysis [saɪkəʊəˈnæləsɪs] *noun* treatment of mental disorder, where a specialist talks to the patient and analyses with him his condition and the past events which have caused it

psychoanalyst [saɪkəʊˈænəlɪst] *noun* doctor who is trained in psychoanalysis

psychogenic *or* **psychogenetic** *or* **psychogenous** [saɪkəˈdʒenɪk *or* saɪkədʒəˈnetɪk *or* saɪˈkɒdʒənəs] *adjective* (illness) which starts in the mind, rather than in a physical cause

psychogeriatrics [saɪkəʊdʒeriˈætrɪks] *adjective* study of the mental disorders of old people

psychological [saɪkəˈlɒdʒɪkl] *adjective* referring to psychology; caused by a mental state; **psychological dependence** = state where a person is addicted to a drug (such as cannabis) but does not suffer physical effects if he stops taking it

psychologically [saɪkəˈlɒdʒɪkli] *adverb* in a way which is caused by a mental state; *she is psychologically incapable of making decisions*; *he is psychologically addicted to tobacco*

psychologist [saɪˈkɒlədʒɪst] *noun* person who specializes in the study of the mind and mental processes; **clinical psychologist** = psychologist who studies and treats sick patients in hospital; **educational psychologist** = psychologist who studies the problems of education

psychology [saɪˈkɒlədʒi] *noun* study of the mind and mental processes

psychometrics [saɪkəˈmetrɪks] *noun* way of measuring intelligence and personality where the result is shown as a number on a scale

psychomotor [saɪkə'məutə] *adjective* referring to muscle movements caused by mental activity; **psychomotor disturbance** = muscles movements (such as twitching) caused by mental disorder; **psychomotor epilepsy** = epilepsy in which fits are characterized by blurring of consciousness and accompanied by coordinated but wrong movements; **psychomotor retardation** = slowing of thought and action

psychoneurosis [saɪkənju'rəusɪs] *noun* neurosis, any of a group of mental disorders in which a patient has a faulty response to the stresses of life

psychopath ['saɪkəpæθ] *noun* person whose behaviour is abnormal and may be violent and antisocial

psychopathic [saɪkə'pæθɪk] *adjective* referring to psychopathy

psychopathological
[saɪkəupæθə'lɒdʒɪkl] *adjective* referring to psychopathology

psychopathology [saɪkəpə'θɒlədʒi] *noun* branch of medicine concerned with the pathology of mental disorders and diseases

psychopathy [saɪ'kɒpəθi] *noun* any disease of the mind

psychopharmacology
[saɪkəufɑːmə'kɒlədʒi] *noun* study of the actions and applications of drugs which have a powerful effect on the mind and behaviour

psychophysiological
[saɪkəufɪziə'lɒdʒɪkl] *adjective* referring to psychophysiology

psychophysiology [saɪkəufɪzi'ɒlədʒi] *noun* physiology of the mind and its functions

psychosis [saɪ'kəusɪs] *noun* general term for any serious mental disorder where the patient shows lack of insight

psychosocial [saɪkəu'səuʃl] *adjective* concerning the interaction of psychological and social factors

recent efforts to redefine nursing have moved away from the traditional medically dominated approach towards psychosocial care and forming relationships with patients
British Journal of Nursing

psychosomatic [saɪkəsə'mætɪk] *adjective* referring to the relationship between body and mind

COMMENT: many physical disorders, such as duodenal ulcers or high blood pressure, can be caused by mental conditions like worry or stress, and are then termed psychosomatic in order to distinguish them from the same conditions having physical or hereditary causes

psychosurgery [saɪkəu'sɜːdʒri] *noun* brain surgery, used as a treatment for psychological disorders

psychosurgical [saɪkəu'sɜːdʒikl] *adjective* referring to psychosurgery

psychotherapeutic [saɪkəθerə'pjuːtɪk] *adjective* referring to psychotherapy

psychotherapist [saɪkə'θerəpɪst] *noun* person trained to give psychotherapy

psychotherapy [saɪkə'θerəpi] *noun* treatment of mental disorders by psychological methods, as when a psychotherapist talks to the patient and encourages him to talk about his problems; *see also* THERAPY

psychotic [saɪ'kɒtɪk] *adjective* (i) referring to psychosis; (ii) characterized by mental disorder

psychotropic [saɪkə'trɒpɪk] *adjective* (drug) which affects a patient's mood (such as a stimulant or a sedative)

pt = PINT

pterion ['tɪərɪɒn] *noun* point on the side of the skull where the frontal, temporal parietal and sphenoid bones meet

pterygium [tə'rɪdʒɪəm] *noun* degenerative condition where a triangular growth of conjunctiva covers part of the cornea, with its apex towards the pupil

pterygo- ['terɪgəu] *suffix* referring to the pterygoid process

pterygoid process ['terɪgɔɪd 'prəuses] *noun* one of two projecting parts on the sphenoid bone; **pterygoid plate** = small flat bony projection on the pterygoid process; **pterygoid plexus** = group of veins and sinuses which join together behind the cheek

pterygomandibular [terɪgəmæn'dɪbjulə] *adjective* referring to the pterygoid process and the mandible

pterygopalatine fossa [terɪgə'pælətɪn 'fɒsə] *noun* space between the pterygoid process and the upper jaw

ptomaine ['təumeɪn] *noun* group of nitrogenous substances produced in rotting food, which gives the food a special smell

(NOTE: **ptomaine poisoning** was the term formerly used to refer to any form of food poisoning)

ptosis ['təʊsɪs] *noun* (i) prolapse of an organ; (ii) drooping of the upper eyelid, which makes the eye stay half closed

-ptosis ['təʊsɪs] *suffix* meaning prolapse, fallen position of an organ

ptyal- *or* **ptyalo-** ['taɪəl or 'taɪələʊ] *prefix* referring to the saliva

ptyalin ['taɪəlɪn] *noun* enzyme in saliva which cleanses the mouth and converts starch into sugar

ptyalism ['taɪəlɪzm] *noun* production of an excessive amount of saliva

ptyalith ['taɪəlɪθ] *noun* sialolith, a stone in the salivary gland

ptyalography [taɪə'lɒgrəfi] *noun* sialography, the X-ray examination of the ducts of the salivary gland

pubertal *or* **puberal** ['pjuːbətl or 'pjuːbərl] *adjective* referring to puberty

puberty ['pjuːbəti] *noun* physical and psychological changes which take place when childhood ends and adolescence and sexual maturity begin and the sex glands become active

COMMENT: puberty starts at about the age of 10 in girls, and slightly later in boys

pubes ['pjuːbiːz] *noun* part of the body just above the groin, where the pubic bones are found

pubic ['pjuːbɪk] *adjective* referring to the area near the genitals; **pubic bone** = pubis, the bone in front of the pelvis; **pubic hair** = tough hair growing in the genital region; **pubic louse** = *Phthirius,* louse which infests the pubic regions; **pubic symphysis** = piece of cartilage which joins the two sections of the pubic bone

COMMENT: in a pregnant woman, the pubic symphysis stretches to allow the pelvic girdle to expand so that there is room for the baby to pass through

pubis ['pjuːbɪs] *noun* bone forming the front part of the pelvis (NOTE: the plural is **pubes**)

public health ['pʌblɪk 'helθ] *noun* the study of illness, health and disease in the community; *see also* COMMUNITY MEDICINE

pudendal [pjuː'dendl] *adjective* referring to the pudendum; **pudendal block** = operation

to anaesthetize the pudendum during childbirth

pudendum [pjuː'dendəm] *noun* external genital organ of a woman (NOTE: the plural is **pudenda)**

puerpera [pjuː'ɜːprə] *noun* woman who has recently given birth, is giving birth, and whose uterus is still distended

puerperal *or* **puerperous** [pjuː'ɜːprl or pjuː'ɜːprəs] *adjective* (i) referring to the puerperium; (ii) referring to childbirth; (iii) which occurs after childbirth; **puerperal fever** = form of septicaemia, which was formerly common in mothers immediately after childbirth and caused many deaths

puerperalism [pjuː'ɜːprəlɪzm] *noun* illness of a baby or its mother resulting from or associated with childbirth

puerperium [pjuːə'pɪəriəm] *noun* period of about six weeks which follows immediately after the birth of a child, during which the mother's sexual organs recover from childbirth

puke [pjuːk] *verb (informal)* to vomit, to be sick

Pulex ['pjuːleks] *noun* genus of human fleas

pull [pʊl] *verb* to strain, to make a muscle move in a wrong direction; *he pulled a muscle in his back*

pulley ['pʊli] *noun* device with wheels over or under which wires or cords pass, used in traction to make wires tense

pull through ['pʊl 'θruː] *verb (informal)* to recover from a serious illness; *the doctor says she is strong and should pull through*

pull together ['pʊl tə'geðə] *verb* **to pull yourself together** = to become calmer; *although he was very angry he soon pulled himself together*

pulmo- *or* **pulmon-** *or* **pulmono-** ['pʌlməʊ or 'pʌlmən or 'pʌlmənəʊ] *prefix* referring to the lungs

pulmonale [pʌlmə'neɪli] *see* COR PULMONALE

pulmonary ['pʌlmənəri] *adjective* referring to the lungs; **pulmonary arteries** = arteries which take deoxygenated blood from the heart to the lungs for oxygenation; *see illustration at* HEART; **pulmonary circulation** = circulation of blood from the heart through the pulmonary arteries to the lungs for oxygenation and back to the heart through the pulmonary veins; **pulmonary**

embolism = blockage of a pulmonary artery by a blood clot; **pulmonary hypertension** = high blood pressure in the blood vessels supplying blood to the lungs; **pulmonary insufficiency** *or* **incompetence** = dilatation of the main pulmonary artery and stretching of the valve ring, due to pulmonary hypertension; **pulmonary oedema** = collection of fluid in the lungs, as occurs in left-sided heart failure; **pulmonary stenosis** = condition where the opening of the right ventricle becomes narrow; **pulmonary valve** = valve at the opening of the pulmonary artery; **pulmonary vein** = vein which takes oxygenated blood from the lungs to the left atrium of the heart (it is the only vein which carries oxygenated blood)

pulmonectomy [pʌlmə'nektəmi] *noun* pneumonectomy, surgical removal of a lung or part of a lung

pulp [pʌlp] *noun* soft tissue, especially when surrounded by hard tissue such as the inside of a tooth; **pulp cavity** = centre of a tooth containing soft tissue; *see illustration at* TOOTH

pulpy ['pʌlpi] *adjective* made of pulp; *the pulpy tissue inside a tooth*

pulsation [pʌl'seɪʃn] *noun* action of beating regularly, such as the visible pulse which can be seen under the skin in some parts of the body

pulse [pʌls] *noun* **(a)** (i) any regular recurring variation in quantity; (ii) pressure wave which can be felt in an artery each time the heart beats to pump blood; **to take** *or* **to feel someone's pulse** = to place fingers on an artery to feel the pulse and count the number of beats per minute; *has the patient's pulse been taken?*; *her pulse is very irregular*; **carotid pulse** = pulse in the carotid artery at the side of the neck; **femoral pulse** = pulse taken in the groin; **radial pulse** = main pulse in the wrist, taken near the outer edge of the forearm, just above the wrist; **ulnar pulse** = secondary pulse in the wrist, taken near the inner edge of the forearm; **pulse oximetry** = method of measuring the oxygen content of arterial blood; **pulse point** = place on the body where the pulse can be taken; **pulse pressure** = difference between the diastolic and systolic pressure; *see also* CORRIGAN **(b)** *(food)* **pulses** = beans and peas; *pulses provide a large amount of protein*

COMMENT: the normal, adult pulse is about 72 beats per minute, but it is higher in children. The pulse is normally taken by placing the fingers on the patient's wrist, at the point where the radial artery passes through the depression just below the thumb

pulseless ['pʌlsləs] *adjective* (patient) who has no pulse because the heart is beating very weakly

pulsus ['pʌlsəs] *noun* the pulse; **pulsus alternans** = pulse with a beat which is alternately strong and weak; **pulsus bigeminus** = double pulse, with an extra ectopic beat; **pulsus paradoxus** = condition where there is a sharp fall in the pulse when a patient breathes in

pulvis ['pʌlvɪs] *noun* powder

pump [pʌmp] **1** *noun* machine which forces liquids or air into or out of something; **stomach pump** = instrument for sucking out the contents of a patient's stomach, especially if he has just swallowed a poison **2** *verb* to force liquid or air along a tube; *the heart pumps blood round the body*; *the nurses tried to pump the poison out of the stomach*

punch drunk syndrome ['pʌnʃ 'drʌŋk 'sɪndrəʊm] *noun* condition of a patient (usually a boxer) who has been hit on the head many times, and develops impaired mental faculties, trembling limbs and speech disorders

punctum ['pʌŋktəm] *noun* point; **puncta lacrimalia** = small openings at the corners of the eyes through which tears drain into the nose (NOTE: plural is **puncta**)

puncture ['pʌŋktʃə] **1** *noun* (i) neat hole made by a sharp instrument; (ii) making a hole in an organ or swelling to take a sample of the contents or to remove fluid; **lumbar puncture** *or* **spinal puncture** = surgical operation to remove a sample of cerebrospinal fluid by inserting a hollow needle into the lower part of the spinal canal (NOTE: US English is also **spinal tap**); **sternal puncture** = surgical operation to remove a sample of bone marrow from the breastbone for testing; **puncture wound** = wound made by a sharp instrument which makes a hole in the tissue **2** *verb* to make a hole in tissue with a sharp instrument

pupil ['pjuːpl] *noun* central opening in the iris of the eye, through which light enters the eye; *see illustration at* EYE

pupillary [pjuː'pɪləri] *adjective* referring to the pupil; **pupillary reaction** = light reflex, the reflex where the pupil changes size according to the amount of light going into the eye

purchaser ['pɜːtʃəsə] *noun* body (usually a PCG) which commissions healthcare and manages the budget to pay for the service; *see also* PROVIDER

pure [pjʊə] *adjective* very clean, not mixed with other substances; **pure alcohol** = alcohol BP, alcohol with 5% water

purgation [pɜː'geɪʃn] *noun* using a drug to make a bowel movement

purgative ['pɜːgətɪv] *noun* & *adjective* laxative; (medicine) which causes evacuation of the bowels

purge [pɜːdʒ] *verb* to induce evacuation of a patient's bowels

purify ['pjʊərɪfaɪ] *verb* to make pure; **purified protein derivative (PPD)** = pure form of tuberculin, used in tuberculin tests

Purkinje cells [pə'kɪndʒi 'selz] *noun* neurones in the cerebellar cortex

Purkinje fibres [pə'kɪndʒi 'faɪbəz] *noun* bundle of fibres which form the atrioventricular bundle and pass from the AV node to the septum

Purkinje shift [pə'kɪndʒi 'ʃɪft] *noun* change in colour sensitivity which takes place in the eye in low light when the eye starts using the rods in the retina because the light is too weak to stimulate the cones

purpura ['pɜːpjʊrə] *noun* purple colouring on the skin, similar to a bruise, caused by blood disease and not by trauma; **Henoch's purpura** = blood disorder of children, where the skin becomes purple and bleeding takes place in the intestine; **Schönlein's purpura** = blood disorder of children, where the skin becomes purple and the joints are swollen and painful

pursestring ['pɜːsstrɪŋ] *see* SHIRODKAR

purulent ['pjʊərʊlənt] *adjective* suppurating, containing or producing pus

pus [pʌs] *noun* yellow liquid composed of blood serum, pieces of dead tissue, white blood cells and the remains of bacteria, formed by the body in reaction to infection (NOTE: for terms referring to pus, see words beginning with **py-** or **pyo-**)

pustular ['pʌstjʊlə] *adjective* (i) covered with or composed of pustules; (ii) referring to pustules

pustule ['pʌstjuːl] *noun* small pimple filled with pus

putrefaction [pjuːtrɪ'fækʃn] *noun* decompositon of organic substances by bacteria, making an unpleasant smell

putrefy ['pjuːtrɪfaɪ] *verb* to rot or to decompose

put up ['pʊt 'ʌp] *verb* to arrange (a drip for a patient)

p.v. ['piː 'viː] *abbreviation for the Latin phrase* 'per vaginam': by way of the vagina

PVS ['piː 'viː 'es] = PERSISTENT VEGETATIVE STATE

PWA ['piː 'dʌbljuː 'eɪ] *noun* person with AIDS

py- *or* **pyo-** ['paɪ *or* 'paɪəʊ] *prefix* referring to pus

pyaemia [paɪ'iːmiə] *noun* invasion of blood with bacteria, which then multiply and form many little abscesses in various parts of the body

pyarthrosis [paɪɑː'θrəʊsɪs] *noun* acute suppurative arthritis, a condition where a joint becomes infected with pyogenic organisms and fills with pus

pyel- *or* **pyelo-** ['paɪəl *or* 'paɪələʊ] *prefix* referring to the pelvis of the kidney, renal pelvis

pyelitis [paɪə'laɪtɪs] *noun* inflammation of the central part of the kidney

pyelocystitis [paɪələsɪ'staɪtɪs] *noun* inflammation of the pelvis of the kidney and the urinary bladder

pyelogram ['paɪələgræm] *noun* X-ray photograph of a kidney and the urinary tract; **intravenous pyelogram** = X-ray photograph of a kidney using intravenous pyelography

pyelography [paɪə'lɒgrəfi] *noun* X-ray examination of a kidney after introduction of a contrast medium; **intravenous pyelography** = X-ray examination of a kidney after opaque liquid has been injected intravenously into the body and taken by the blood into the kidneys; **retrograde pyelography** = X-ray examination of the kidney where a catheter is passed into the kidney and the opaque liquid is injected directly into it

pyelolithotomy [paɪələlɪ'θɒtəmi] *noun* surgical removal of a stone from the pelvis of the kidney

pyelonephritis [paɪələʊnɪ'fraɪtɪs] *noun* inflammation of the kidney and the pelvis of the kidney

pyeloplasty ['paɪələplæsti] *noun* any surgical operation on the pelvis of the kidney

pyelotomy [paɪə'lɒtəmi] *noun* surgical operation to make an opening in the pelvis of the kidney

pyemia [paɪ'iːmiə] = PYAEMIA

pyknolepsy [pɪknə'lepsi] *noun* former name for a type of frequent attack of petit mal epilepsy, affecting children

pyl- *or* **pyle-** ['paɪl or 'paɪli] *prefix* referring to the portal vein

pylephlebitis [paɪliflə'baɪtɪs] *noun* thrombosis of the portal vein

pylethrombosis [paɪliθrɒm'bəʊsɪs] *noun* condition where blood clots are present in the portal vein or any of its branches

pylor- *or* **pyloro-** [paɪ'lɔːr or paɪ'lɔːrəʊ] *prefix* referring to the pylorus

pylorectomy [paɪlə'rektəmi] *noun* surgical removal of the pylorus and the antrum of the stomach

pyloric [paɪ'lɒrɪk] *adjective* referring to the pylorus; **pyloric antrum** = space at the bottom of the stomach before the pyloric sphincter; **pyloric orifice** = opening where the stomach joins the duodenum; **pyloric sphincter** = muscle which surrounds the pylorus, makes it contract and separates it from the duodenum; **pyloric stenosis** = blockage of the pylorus, which prevents food from passing from the stomach into the duodenum

pyloroplasty [paɪ'lɔːrəplæsti] *noun* surgical operation to make the pylorus larger, sometimes combined with treatment for peptic ulcers

pylorospasm [paɪ'lɔːrəspæzm] *noun* muscle spasm which closes the pylorus so that food cannot pass through into the duodenum

pylorotomy [paɪlə'rɒtəmi] *noun* Ramstedt's operation, surgical operation to cut into the muscle surrounding the pylorus to relieve pyloric stenosis

pylorus [paɪ'lɔːrəs] *noun* opening at the bottom of the stomach leading into the duodenum

pyo- ['paɪəʊ] *prefix* referring to pus

pyocele ['paɪəsiːl] *noun* enlargement of a tube or cavity due to accumulation of pus

pyocolpos [paɪə'kɒlpəs] *noun* accumulation of pus in the vagina

pyoderma [paɪə'dɜːmə] *noun* eruption of pus in the skin

pyogenic [paɪə'dʒenɪk] *adjective* which produces or forms pus

pyometra [paɪə'miːtrə] *noun* accumulation of pus in the uterus

pyomyositis [paɪəmaɪə'saɪtɪs] *noun* inflammation of a muscle caused by staphylococci or streptococci

pyonephrosis [paɪənɪ'frəʊsɪs] *noun* distension of the kidney with pus

pyopericarditis [paɪəperɪkɑː'daɪtɪs] *noun* bacterial pericarditis, an inflammation of the pericardium due to infection with staphylococci, streptococci or pneumococci

pyorrhoea [paɪə'rɪə] *noun* discharge of pus; **pyorrhoea alveolaris** = suppuration from the supporting tissues round the teeth

pyosalpinx [paɪə'sælpɪŋks] *noun* inflammation and formation of pus in a Fallopian tube

pyosis [paɪ'əʊsɪs] *noun* formation of pus, suppuration

pyothorax [paɪə'θɔːræks] = EMPYEMA

pyr- *or* **pyro-** [paɪr or 'paɪrəʊ] *prefix* referring to burning or fever

pyramid ['pɪrəmɪd] *noun* cone-shaped part of the body, especially a cone-shaped projection on the surface of the medulla oblongata or in the medulla of the kidney; *see illustration at* KIDNEY

pyramidal [pɪ'ræmɪdl] *adjective* referring to a pyramid; **pyramidal cell** = cone-shaped cell in the cerebral cortex; **pyramidal tracts** = tracts in the brain and spinal cord which carry the motor neurone fibres from the cerebral cortex

pyrexia [paɪ'reksiə] *noun* fever, a rise in body temperature, or a sickness when the temperature of the body is higher than normal

pyrexic [paɪ'reksɪk] *adjective* with fever

pyridoxine [pɪri'dɒksɪn] = VITAMIN B$_6$

pyrogen ['paɪrədʒen] *noun* substance which causes a fever

pyrogenic [paɪrə'dʒenɪk] *adjective* which causes a fever

pyrosis [paɪ'rəusɪs] = HEARTBURN

pyruvic acid [paɪ'ruːvɪk 'æsɪd] *noun* substance formed from muscle glycogen when it is broken down to release energy

pyuria [paɪ'juəriə] *noun* pus in the urine

Qq

q.d.s. *or* **q.i.d.** ['kju: 'di: 'es *or* 'kju: 'aɪ 'di:] *abbreviation for the Latin phrase* 'quater in die sumendus': four times a day (written on prescriptions)

Q fever ['kju: 'fi:və] *noun* infectious rickettsial disease of sheep and cows caused by *Coxiella burnetti* transmitted to humans

COMMENT: Q fever mainly affects farm workers and workers in the meat industry. The symptoms are fever, cough and headaches

q.s. ['kju: 'es] *abbreviation for the Latin phrase* 'quantum sufficiat': as much as necessary (written on prescriptions)

quad [kwɒd] = QUADRUPLET

quadrant ['kwɒdrənt] *noun* quarter of a circle; sector of the body; *tenderness in the right lower quadrant of the abdomen*

quadrantanopia [kwɒdrɒntə'nəʊpɪə] *noun* blindness in a quarter of the field of vision

quadrate lobe ['kwɒdreɪt 'ləʊb] *noun* lobe on the lower side of the liver

quadratus [kwɒ'dreɪtəs] *noun* any muscle with four sides; **quadratus femoris** = muscle at the top of the femur, that rotates the thigh

quadri- ['kwɒdri] *prefix* referring to four

quadriceps femoris ['kwɒdrɪseps 'femɒrɪs] *noun* large muscle in the front of the thigh, which extends to the leg

COMMENT: the quadriceps femoris is divided into four parts: the rectus femoris, vastus lateralis, vastus medialis, and the vastus intermedius. It is the sensory receptors in the quadriceps which react to give a knee jerk when the patellar tendon is tapped

quadriplegia [kwɒdrɪ'pli:dʒə] *noun* paralysis of all four limbs: both arms and both legs

quadriplegic [kwɒdri'pli:dʒɪk] *noun & adjective* (person) paralysed in all four limbs: both arms and legs

quadruple ['kwɒdrʊpl] *adjective* four times, in four parts; **quadruple vaccine** = vaccine which immunizes against four diseases: diphtheria, whooping cough, poliomyelitis, and tetanus

quadruplet *or* **quad** ['kwɒdrʊplət *or* kwɒd] *noun* one of four babies born to a mother at the same time; *she had quadruplets or quads*; *see also* QUINTUPLET, SEXTUPLET, TRIPLET, TWIN

quadrupod ['kwɒdrʊpɒd] *noun* walking stick which ends in four little legs

qualification [kwɒlɪfɪ'keɪʃn] *noun* being qualified; *she has a qualification in pharmacy*; *are his qualifications recognized in Great Britain?*

qualify ['kwɒlɪfaɪ] *verb* to pass a course of study and be accepted as being able to practise; *he qualified as a doctor two years ago*

qualitative ['kwɒlɪtətɪv] *adjective* (study) in which descriptive information is collected; *compare* QUANTITATIVE

quantitative ['kwɒnɪtətɪv] *adjective* (study) in which numerical information is collected; *compare* QUALITATIVE

quarantine ['kwɒrənti:n] **1** *noun* period (originally forty days) when an animal, person or ship just arrived in a country has to be kept separate in case a serious disease may be carried, to allow the disease time to develop; *the animals were put in quarantine on arrival at the port*; *a ship in quarantine shows a yellow flag called the quarantine flag* **2** *verb* to put a person or animal in quarantine

COMMENT: animals coming into Great Britain are quarantined for six months because of the danger of rabies. People who are suspected of having an infectious disease can be kept in quarantine for a period which varies according to the incubation period of the disease. The main diseases concerned are cholera, yellow fever and typhus

quartan fever ['kwɔːtn 'fiːvə] *noun* infectious disease, a form of malaria caused by *Plasmodium malariae* where the fever returns every four days; *see also* TERTIAN

Queckenstedt test ['kwekənsted 'test] *noun* test done during a lumbar puncture where pressure is applied to the jugular veins, to see if the cerebrospinal fluid is flowing correctly

quickening ['kwɪknɪŋ] *noun* first sign of life in an unborn baby, usually after about four months of pregnancy, when the mother can feel it moving in her uterus

Quick test ['kwɪk 'test] *noun* test to identify the clotting factors in a blood sample

quiescent [kwɪ'esnt] *adjective* inactive; (disease) with symptoms reduced either by treatment or in the normal course of the disease

quin [kwɪn] = QUINTUPLET

quinine [kwɪ'niːn] *noun* alkaloid drug made from the bark of a South American tree (the cinchona); **quinine poisoning** = illness caused by taking too much quinine

COMMENT: quinine was formerly used to treat the fever symptoms of malaria, but is not often used now because of its side-effects. Symptoms of quinine poisoning are dizziness and noises in the

head. Small amounts of quinine have a tonic effect and are used in tonic water

quininism *or* **quinism** ['kwɪniːnɪzm *or* 'kwɪnɪzm] *noun* quinine poisoning

quinolone antibiotic [kwɪnə'ləʊn antibaɪ'ɒtik] *noun* drug used to treat Gram-negative and Gram-positive bacterial infections of the respiratory and urinary tracts and of the gastro-intestinal system (NOTE: quinolone drugs have names ending in **-oxacin: ciprofloxacin**)

COMMENT: contra-indications include use in pregnancy, renal disease and for use in children

quinsy ['kwɪnzi] *noun* peritonsillar abscess, acute throat inflammation with an abscess round a tonsil

quintuplet *or* **quin** ['kwɪntjʊplət *or* kwɪn] *noun* one of five babies born to a mother at the same time; *see also* QUADRUPLET, SEXTUPLET, TRIPLET, TWIN

quotidian [kwə'tɪdiən] *adjective* recurring daily; **quotidian fever** = violent form of malaria where the fever returns at daily or even shorter intervals

quotient ['kwəʊʃnt] *noun* result when one number is divided by another; **intelligence quotient (IQ)** = ratio of the result of an intelligence test shown as a relationship of the mental age to the actual age of the person tested (the average being 100); **respiratory quotient** = ratio of the amount of carbon dioxide passed from the blood into the lungs to the amount of oxygen absorbed into the blood from the air

Rr

R = ROENTGEN

R/ *abbreviation for the Latin word* 'recipe': prescription

R & D ['aː n 'diː] = RESEARCH AND DEVELOPMENT

Ra *chemical symbol for* radium

rabbit fever ['ræbɪt 'fiːvə] = TULARAEMIA

rabid ['ræbɪd or 'reɪbɪd] *adjective* referring to rabies, suffering from rabies; *he was bitten by a rabid dog*; **rabid encephalitis** = fatal encephalitis resulting from the bite of a rabid animal

rabies ['reɪbiːz] *noun* hydrophobia, frequently fatal viral disease transmitted to humans by infected animals; *the hospital ordered a batch of rabies vaccine*

COMMENT: rabies affects the mental balance, and the symptoms include difficulty in breathing or swallowing and an intense fear of water (hydrophobia) to the point of causing convulsions at the sight of water

rachi- *or* **rachio-** ['reɪki or 'reɪkiəʊ] *prefix* referring to the spine

rachianaesthesia [reɪkiænəs'θiːziə] = SPINAL ANAESTHESIA

rachiotomy [reɪki'ɒtəmi] *noun* laminectomy, surgical operation to cut through a vertebra in the spine to reach the spinal cord

rachis ['reɪkɪs] = BACKBONE

rachischisis [reɪ'kɪskɪsɪs] = SPINA BIFIDA

rachitic [rə'kɪtɪk] *adjective* (child) with rickets

rachitis [rə'kaɪtɪs] = RICKETS

rad [ræd] *noun* unit of measurement of absorbed radiation dose; *see also* BECQUEREL, GRAY (NOTE: **gray** is now used to mean one hundred rads)

radial ['reɪdiəl] *adjective* (i) referring to something which branches; (ii) referring to the radius, one of the bones in the forearm; **radial artery** = artery which branches from the brachial artery, running near the radius, from the elbow to the palm of the hand; **radial nerve** = main motor nerve in the arm, running down the back of the upper arm and the outer side of the forearm; **radial pulse** = main pulse in the wrist, taken near the outer edge of the forearm, just above the wrist; **radial recurrent** = artery in the arm which forms a loop beside the brachial artery; **radial reflex** = jerk made by the forearm when the insertion in the radius of one of the muscles (the brachioradialis) is hit

radiate ['reɪdɪeɪt] *verb* **(a)** to spread out in all directions from a central point; *the pain radiates from the site of the infection* **(b)** to send out rays; *heat radiates from the body*

radiation [reɪdi'eɪʃn] *noun* waves of energy which are given off by certain substances, especially radioactive substances; **radiation burn** = burning of the skin caused by exposure to large amounts of radiation; **radiation enteritis** = enteritis caused by X-rays; **radiation sickness** = illness caused by exposure to radiation from radioactive substances; **radiation treatment** = RADIOTHERAPY; *see also* OPTIC RADIATION, SENSORY RADIATION

COMMENT: prolonged exposure to many types of radiation can be harmful. Nuclear radiation is the most obvious, but exposure to X-rays (either as a patient being treated, or as a radiographer) can cause radiation sickness. First symptoms of the sickness are diarrhoea and vomiting, but radiation can also be followed by skins burns and loss of hair. Massive exposure to radiation can kill quickly, and any person exposed to radiation is more likely to develop certain types of cancer than other members of the population

radical ['rædɪkl] *adjective* (i) very serious, which deals with the root of a problem; (ii) (operation) which removes the whole of a part or of an organ, together with its lymph system and other tissue; **radical mastectomy** = surgical removal of a breast and the lymph nodes and muscles associated with it; **radical mastoidectomy** = operation to remove all of the mastoid process; **radical treatment** = treatment which aims at complete eradication of a disease

radicle ['rædɪkl] *noun* (i) a small root or vein; (ii) tiny fibre which forms the root of a nerve

radicular [rə'dɪkjulə] *adjective* referring to a radicle

radiculitis [rədɪkju'laɪtɪs] *noun* inflammation of a radicle of a cranial or spinal nerve; *see also* POLYRADICULITIS

radio- ['reɪdiəu] *prefix* referring to (i) radiation; (ii) radioactive substances; (iii) the radius in the arm

radioactive [reɪdiəu'æktɪv] *adjective* (substance) whose nucleus disintegrates and gives off energy in the form of radiation which can pass through other substances; **radioactive isotope** = *see* RADIOISOTOPE

COMMENT: the commonest naturally radioactive substances are radium and uranium. Other substances can be made radioactive for medical purposes by making their nuclei unstable, so forming radioactive isotopes. Radioactive iodine is used to treat conditions such as thyrotoxicosis. Radioactive isotopes of various chemicals are used to check the functioning of or disease in internal organs

radioactivity [reɪdiəuæk'tɪvəti] *noun* energy in the form of radiation emitted by a radioactive substance

radiobiologist [reɪdiəubaɪ'ɒlədʒɪst] *noun* doctor who specializes in radiobiology

radiobiology [reɪdiəubaɪ'ɒlədʒi] *noun* scientific study of radiation and its effects on living things

radiocarpal joint [reɪdiəu'kɑːpl 'dʒɔɪnt] *noun* wrist joint, the joint where the radius articulates with the scaphoid (one of the carpal bones)

radiodermatitis [reɪdiəudɜːmə'taɪtɪs] *noun* inflammation of the skin caused by exposure to radiation

radiodiagnosis [reɪdiəudaɪəg'nəusɪs] *noun* X-ray diagnosis

radiographer [reɪdi'ɒgrəfə] *noun* (i) person specially trained to operate a machine to take X-ray photographs or radiographs (diagnostic radiographer); (ii) person specially trained to use X-rays or radioactive isotopes in treatment of patients (therapeutic radiographer)

radiography [reɪdi'ɒgrəfi] *noun* examining the internal parts of a patient by taking X-ray photographs

radioimmunoassay [reɪdiəuɪmjuːnəu'æseɪ] *noun* use of radioactive tracers to investigate the presence of antibodies in blood samples, in order to measure the antibodies themselves or the amount of particular substances in the blood such as hormones

radioisotope [reɪdiəu'aɪsətəup] *noun* isotope of a chemical element which is radioactive

COMMENT: radioisotopes are used in medicine to provide radiation for radiation treatment. Radioactive isotopes of various chemicals are used to check how organs function or if they are diseased: for example, radioisotopes of iodine are used to investigate thyroid activity

radiologist [reɪdi'ɒlədʒɪst] *noun* doctor who specializes in radiology

radiology [reɪdi'ɒlədʒi] *noun* use of radiation to diagnose disorders (as in the use of X-rays or radioactive tracers) or to treat diseases such as cancer

radionuclide [reɪdəu'njuːklaɪd] *noun* element which gives out radiation; **radionuclide scan** = scan (especially of the brain) where radionuclides are put in compounds which are concentrated in certain parts of the body

radio-opaque [reɪdiəuəu'peɪk] *adjective* (substance) which absorbs all or most of a radiation

COMMENT: radio-opaque substances appear dark on X-rays and are used to make it easier to have clear radiographs of certain organs

radiopharmaceutical [reɪdiəufɑːmə'suːtɪkl] *noun* radioisotope used in medical diagnosis or treatment

radio pill ['reɪdɪəu 'pɪl] *noun* tablet with a tiny radio transmitter

COMMENT: the patient swallows the pill and as it passes through the body it gives off information about the digestive system

radioscopy [reɪdɪ'ɒskəpi] *noun* examining an X-ray photograph on a fluorescent screen

radiosensitive [reɪdɪəu'sensətɪv] *adjective* (cancer cell) which is sensitive to radiation and can be treated by radiotherapy

radiosensitivity [reɪdɪəusensɪ'tɪvəti] *noun* sensitivity of a cell to radiation

radiotherapy [reɪdɪəu'θerəpi] *noun* treating a disease by exposing the affected part to radioactive rays such as X-rays or gamma rays

COMMENT: many forms of cancer can be treated by directing radiation at the diseased part of the body

radium ['reɪdɪəm] *noun* radioactive metallic element (NOTE: chemical symbol is **Ra**)

radius ['reɪdɪəs] *noun* the shorter and outer of the two bones in the forearm between the elbow and the wrist (the other bone is the ulna); *see illustrations at* HAND, SKELETON (NOTE: the plural is **radii**)

radix ['reɪdɪks] *noun* root; (i) point from which a part of the body grows; (ii) part of a tooth which is connected to a socket in the jaw

radon ['reɪdɒn] *noun* radioactive gas, formed from the radioactive decay of radium, and used in capsules (known as radon seeds) to treat cancers inside the body (NOTE: chemical symbol is **Rn**)

COMMENT: radon occurs naturally in soil, in construction materials and even in ground water. It can seep into houses and causes radiation sickness

raise [reɪz] *verb* (a) to lift; *lie with your legs raised above the level of your head* (b) to increase; *anaemia causes a raised level of white blood cells in the body*

rale [rɑːl] = CREPITATION

Ramstedt's operation ['rɑːmstets ɒpə'reɪʃn] = PYLOROTOMY

ramus ['reɪməs] *noun* (a) branch of a nerve, artery or vein (b) the ascending part on each side of the mandible (NOTE: the plural is **rami**)

randomized ['rændəmaɪzd] *adjective* which has been selected or carried out at random; **double-blind randomized controlled trial (RCT)** = trial in which patients are randomly placed in the treatment or control group without either the patient or doctor knowing which, used to test new treatments

range [reɪndʒ] *noun* (i) series of different but similar things; (ii) difference between lowest and highest values in a series of data; *the drug offers protection against a wide range of diseases*; *doctors have a range of drugs which can be used to treat arthritis*

ranula ['rænjʊlə] *noun* small cyst under the tongue, on the floor of the mouth, which forms when a salivary duct is blocked

Ranvier [rɑːnvɪ'eɪ] *see* NODE

raphe ['reɪfi] *noun* long thin fold which looks like a seam, along a midline such as on the dorsal face of the tongue

rapid ['ræpɪd] *adjective* fast; **rapid eye movement (REM) sleep** = phase of normal sleep with fast movements of the eyeballs which occur at intervals

COMMENT: During REM sleep, a person dreams, breathes lightly and has a raised blood pressure and an increased rate of heartbeat. The eyes may be half-open, and the sleeper may make facial movements

rapid-acting ['ræpɪd'æktɪŋ] *adjective* (drug or treatment) which has an effect very quickly

rare [reə] *adjective* not common, (disease) of which there are very few cases; *he is suffering from a rare blood disorder*; *AO is not a rare blood group*

rarefaction [reərɪ'fækʃn] *noun* condition where bone tissue becomes more porous and less dense because of lack of calcium

rarefy ['reərɪfaɪ] *verb (of bones)* to become less dense

rash [ræʃ] *noun* mass of small spots which stays on the skin for a period of time, and then disappears; **to break out in a rash** = to have a rash which starts suddenly; *she had a high temperature and then broke out in a rash*; **nappy rash,** *US* **diaper rash** = sore red skin on a baby's buttocks and groin, caused by long contact with ammonia in a wet nappy

COMMENT: many common diseases such as chickenpox and measles have a special rash as their main symptom. Rashes can be very irritating, but the itching can be relieved by applying calamine lotion

raspatory ['ræspətəri] *noun* surgical instrument like a file, which is used to scrape the surface of a bone

ratbite fever *or* **disease** ['rætbaɪt 'fiːvə or dɪ'ziːz] *noun* fever caused by either of two bacteria *Spirillum minor* or *Streptobacillus moniliformis* and transmitted to humans by rats

rate [reɪt] *noun* (a) amount or proportion of something compared to something else; **birth rate** = number of children born per 1000 of population; **fertility rate** = number of births per year calculated per 1000 females aged between 15 and 44 (b) number of times something happens; *the heart was beating at a rate of only 59 per minute*; **heart rate** = number of times the heart beats per minute; **pulse rate** = number of times the pulse beats per minute

COMMENT: pulse rate is the heart rate felt at various parts of the body

ratio ['reɪʃiəu] *noun* number which shows a proportion or which is the result of one number divided by another; *an IQ is the ratio of the person's mental age to his chronological age*

Rauwolfia [rɔː'wulfiə] *noun* tranquillizing drug extracted from a plant *Rauwolfia serpentina* sometimes used to treat high blood pressure; *see also* RESERPINE

raw [rɔː] *adjective* (a) not cooked (b) (i) sensitive (skin); (ii) (skin) scraped or partly removed; *the scab came off leaving the raw wound exposed to the air*

ray [reɪ] *noun* line of light, radiation or heat; **infrared rays** = long invisible rays, below the visible red end of the spectrum, used to warm body tissue; **ultraviolet rays (UV rays)** = short invisible rays beyond the violet end of the spectrum, which form the element in sunlight which tans the skin; *see also* X-RAY

Raynaud's diseas [reɪ'nəuz dɪ'ziːz] *noun* condition where the fingers and toes become cold, white and numb at temperatures that would not affect a normal person, commonly called 'dead man's fingers'

RBC ['ɑː 'biː 'siː] = RED BLOOD CELL

RCGP ['ɑː 'siː 'dʒiː 'piː] = ROYAL COLLEGE OF GENERAL PRACTITIONERS

RCN ['ɑː 'siː 'en] = ROYAL COLLEGE OF NURSING

RCOG ['ɑː 'siː 'əu 'dʒiː] = ROYAL COLLEGE OF OBSTETRICIANS AND GYNAECOLOGISTS

RCP ['ɑː 'siː 'piː] = ROYAL COLLEGE OF PHYSICIANS

RCPsych = ROYAL COLLEGE OF PSYCHIATRISTS

RCS ['ɑː 'siː 'es] = ROYAL COLLEGE OF SURGEONS

RCT ['ɑː 'siː 'tiː]= RANDOMIZED CONTROLLED TRIAL

reabsorb [riːəb'sɔːb] *verb* to absorb again; *glucose is reabsorbed by the tubules in the kidney*

reabsorption [riːəb'sɔːpʃn] *noun* process of being reabsorbed; *some substances which are filtered into the tubules of the kidney, then pass into the bloodstream by tubular reabsorption*

reach [riːtʃ] 1 *noun* distance which one can stretch a hand; distance which one can travel easily; *medicines should be kept out of the reach of children*; *the hospital is in easy reach of the railway station* 2 *verb* to arrive at a point; *infection has reached the lungs*

react [ri'ækt] *verb* (a) to react to something = to act because of something else, to act in response to something; *the tissues reacted to the cortisone injection*; *the patient reacted badly to the penicillin*; *she reacted positively to the Widal test* (b) *(of a chemical substance)* to react with something = to change because of the presence of another substance

reaction [ri'ækʃn] *noun* (a) (i) action which takes place because of something which has happened earlier; (ii) effect produced by a stimulus; *a rash appeared as a reaction to the penicillin injection*; *the patient suffers from an allergic reaction to oranges*; **immune reaction** = reaction of a body to an antigen (b) particular response of a patient to a test; **Wassermann reaction** = reaction to a blood test for syphilis

reactivate [ri'æktɪveɪt] *verb* to make active again; *his general physical weakness has reactivated the dormant virus*

reactive *or* **reactionary** [ri'æktɪv or ri'ækʃnəri] *adjective* which takes place because of a reaction; **reactionary haemorrhage** = bleeding which follows an operation; **reactive hyperaemia** = congestion of blood vessels after an occlusion has been removed

reading ['ri:dɪŋ] *noun* note taken of figures, especially of degrees on a scale; *the sphygmomanometer gave a diastolic reading of 70*

reagent [rɪ'eɪdʒnt] *noun* chemical substance which reacts with another substance (especially when used to detect the presence of the second substance)

reagin ['rɪədʒɪn] *noun* antibody which reacts against an allergen

reappear [ri:ə'pɪə] *verb* to appear again

reappearance [ri:ə'pɪərns] *noun* appearing again; *the reappearance of the symptoms after a period of several months*

reason ['ri:zn] *noun* **(a)** thing which explains why something happens; *what was the reason for the sudden drop in the patient's pulse rate?* **(b)** being mentally stable; *her reason was beginning to fail*

reassurance [ri:ə'ʃʊərns] *noun* act of reassuring

reassure [ri:ə'ʃʊə] *verb* to make someone sure, to give someone hope; *the doctor reassured her that the drug had no unpleasant side-effects; he reassured the old lady that she should be able to walk again in a few weeks*

Reaven's Syndrome ['ri:vənz 'sɪndrəʊm] *noun* clinical syndrome characterized by Type 2 diabetes, abdominal obesity, hypertension and dyslipidaemia, insulin resistance may be a key factor

rebore ['ri:bɔ:] *noun* (*informal*) endarterectomy, the surgical removal of the lining of a blocked artery

rebuild [ri:'bɪld] *verb* to reconstruct a defective or damaged part of the body; *after the accident, she had several operations to rebuild her pelvis*

recalcitrant [rɪ'kælsɪtrnt] *adjective* (condition) which does not respond to treatment

recall [rɪ'kɔ:l] **1** *noun* act of remembering something from the past; **total recall** = being able to remember something in complete detail **2** *verb* to remember something which happened in the past

receive [rɪ'si:v] *verb* to get something (especially a transplanted organ); *she received six pints of blood in a transfusion; he received a new kidney from his brother*

receptaculum [ri:sep'tækjʊləm] *noun* part of a tube which is expanded to form a sac

receptor [rɪ'septə] *noun* nerve ending which senses a change (such as cold or heat) in the surrounding environment or in the body and reacts to it by sending an impulse to the central nervous system; *see also* ADRENERGIC, CHEMORECEPTOR, EXTEROCEPTOR, INTEROCEPTOR, THERMORECEPTOR, VISCERORECEPTOR

recess [rɪ'ses] *noun* hollow part in an organ

recessive [rɪ'sesɪv] *adjective & noun* (trait) which is weaker than and hidden by a dominant gene

COMMENT: since each physical characteristic is governed by two genes, if one is dominant and the other recessive, the resulting trait will be that of the dominant gene. Traits governed by recessive genes will appear if both genes are recessive

recipient [rɪ'sɪpiənt] *noun* person who receives something, such as a transplant or a blood transfusion from a donor

bone marrow from donors has to be carefully matched with the recipient or graft-versus-host disease will ensue

Hospital Update

Recklinghausen ['reklɪŋhaʊzən] *see* VON RECKLINGHAUSEN

recognize ['rekəgnaɪz] *verb* **(a)** to sense something (as to see a person or to taste a food) and remember it from an earlier sensing; *she did not recognize her mother* **(b)** to approve of something officially; *the diploma is recognized by the Department of Health*

recommend [rekə'mend] *verb* to suggest that it would be a good thing if someone did something; *the doctor recommended that she should stay in bed; I would recommend following a diet to try to lose some weight*

reconstruct [rɪkən'strʌkt] *verb* to rebuild a defective or damaged part of the body

reconstruction [rɪkən'strʌkʃn] *noun* rebuilding a defective or damaged part of the body

reconstructive surgery [ri:kən'strʌktɪv 'sɜ:dʒəri] *noun* plastic surgery, surgery which rebuilds a defective or damaged part of the body

reconvert [ri:kən'vɜ:t] *verb* to convert back into an earlier form; *the liver reconverts some of its stored glycogen into glucose*

record 1 [rɪ'kɔːd] *verb* to note information; *the chart records the variations in the patient's blood pressure; you must take the patient's temperature every hour and record it in this book* **2** ['rekɔːd] *noun* piece of information about something; **medical records** = information about a patient's medical history

COMMENT: patients have a legal right to access to their medical records

recover [rɪ'kʌvə] *verb* **(a)** to get better after an illness, operation or accident; *she recovered from her concussion in a few days; it will take him weeks to recover from the accident* (NOTE: you recover **from** an illness) **(b)** to get back something which has been lost; *will he ever recover the use of his legs?; she recovered her eyesight after all the doctors thought she would be permanently blind*

recovery [rɪ'kʌvəri] *noun* getting better after an illness, accident or operation; **he is well on the way to recovery** = he is getting better; **she made only a partial recovery** = she is better, but will never be completely well; **she has made a complete** *or* **splendid recovery** = she is completely well; **recovery room** = room in a hospital where a patient who has had an operation is placed until the effects of the anaesthetic have worn off and he can be moved into an ordinary ward

recovery position [rɪ'kʌvəri pə'zɪʃn] *noun* lying face downwards, with one knee and one arm bent forwards and the face turned to one side

COMMENT: called the recovery position because it is recommended for accident victims or for people who are suddenly ill, while waiting for an ambulance to arrive. The position prevents the patient from swallowing and choking on blood or vomit

recrudescence [riːkruː'desns] *noun* reappearance of symptoms (of a disease which seemed to have got better)

recrudescent [riːkruː'desnt] *adjective* (symptom) which has reappeared

recruit [rɪ'kruːt] *verb* to get people to join the staff or a group; *we are trying to recruit more nursing staff*

patients presenting with symptoms of urinary tract infection were recruited in a general practice surgery
Journal of the Royal College of General Practitioners

rect- *or* **recto-** ['rekt *or* 'rektəu] *prefix* referring to the rectum

rectal ['rektl] *adjective* referring to the rectum; **rectal fissure** = crack in the wall of the anal canal; **rectal prolapse** = condition where part of the rectum moves downwards and passes through the anus; **rectal temperature** = temperature in the rectum, taken with a rectal thermometer; **rectal thermometer** = thermometer which is inserted into the patient's rectum to take the temperature; **rectal triangle** = the anal triangle, the posterior part of the perineum

rectally ['rektli] *adverb* through the rectum; *the temperature was taken rectally*

rectocele ['rektəusiːl] *noun* proctocele, condition associated with prolapse of the uterus, where the rectum protrudes into the vagina

rectopexy ['rektəupeksi] *noun* surgical operation to attach a rectum which has prolapsed

rectoscope ['rektəskəup] *noun* instrument for looking into the rectum

rectosigmoidectomy [rektəusɪgmɔɪ'dektəmi] *noun* surgical removal of the sigmoid colon and the rectum

rectovaginal examination [rektəu'vædʒɪnl ɪgzæmɪ'neɪʃn] *noun* examination of the rectum and vagina

rectovesical [rektəu'vesɪkl] *adjective* referring to the rectum and the bladder

rectum ['rektəm] *noun* end part of the large intestine leading from the sigmoid colon to the anus; *see illustrations at* DIGESTIVE SYSTEM, UROGENITAL TRACT (NOTE: for terms referring to the rectum, see words beginning with **procto-**)

rectus ['rektəs] *noun* straight muscle; **rectus abdominis** = long straight muscle which runs down the front of the abdomen; **rectus femoris** = flexor muscle in the front of the thigh, one of the four parts of the quadriceps femoris; *see also* MEDIAL (NOTE: the plural is **recti**)

there are four recti muscles and two oblique muscles in each eye, which coordinate the movement of the eyes and enable them to work as a pair

Nursing Times

recumbent [rɪˈkʌmbənt] *adjective* lying down

recuperate [rɪˈkjuːpəreɪt] *verb* to recover, to get better after an illness or accident; *he is recuperating after an attack of flu*; *she is going to stay with her mother while she recuperates*

recuperation [rɪkjuːpəˈreɪʃn] *noun* getting better after an illness; *his recuperation will take several months*

recur [rɪˈkɜː] *verb* to return; *the headaches recurred frequently, but usually after the patient had eaten chocolate*

recurrence [rɪˈkʌrəns] *noun* act of returning; *he had a recurrence of a fever which he had caught in the tropics*

recurrent [rɪˈkʌrənt] *adjective* **(a)** which occurs again; **recurrent abortion** = condition where a woman has miscarriages with one pregnancy after another; **recurrent fever** = fever (like malaria) which returns at regular intervals **(b)** (vein, artery or nerve) which forms a loop; **radial recurrent** = artery in the arm which forms a loop beside the brachial artery

red [red] *adjective & noun* (of) a colour like the colour of blood; *blood in an artery is bright red, but venous blood is darker*; **red blood cell (RBC)** = erythrocyte, a blood cell which contains haemoglobin and carries oxygen; **red eye** = PINK EYE

Red Crescent [ˈred ˈkrezənt] *noun* organization similar to the Red Cross, working in Muslim countries

Red Cross [ˈred ˈkrɒs] *noun* **International Committee of the Red Cross (ICRC)** = international organization which provides mainly emergency medical help, but also relief to victims of earthquakes, floods, etc., or to prisoners of war; *Red Cross officials or officials of the Red Cross arrived in the disaster area this morning*

redness [ˈrednəs] *noun* being red; red colour; *the redness showed where the skin had reacted to the injection*

reduce [rɪˈdjuːs] *verb* **(a)** to make something smaller or lower; *they used ice packs to try to reduce the patient's temperature* **(b)** to put (a dislocated or a fractured bone, a displaced organ or part, a

hernia) back into its proper position so that it can heal

blood pressure control reduces the incidence of first stroke and aspirin appears to reduce the risk of stroke after transient ischaemic attacks by some 15%

British Journal of Hospital Medicine

reducible [rɪˈdjuːsəbl] *adjective* (hernia) where the organ can be pushed back into place without an operation

reduction [rɪˈdʌkʃn] *noun* **(a)** making less, becoming less; *they noted a reduction in body temperature* **(b)** putting (a hernia, dislocated joint or a broken bone) back into the correct position

re-emerge [riːɪˈmɜːdʒ] *verb* to come out again

re-emergence [riːɪˈmɜːdʒəns] *noun* coming out again

refer [rɪˈfɜː] *verb* **(a)** to mention or to talk about something; *the doctor referred to the patient's history of sinus problems* **(b)** to suggest that someone should consult something; *for method of use, please refer to the manufacturer's instructions*; *the user is referred to the page giving the results of the tests* **(c)** to pass on information about a patient to someone else; *she was referred to a gynaecologist*; *the GP referred the patient to a consultant* = he passed details about the patient's case to the consultant so that the consultant could examine him **(d)** to send to another place; **referred pain** = SYNALGIA

27 adult patients admitted to hospital with acute abdominal pains were referred for study because their attending clinicians were uncertain whether to advise an urgent laparotomy

Lancet

many patients from outside districts were referred to London hospitals by their GPs

Nursing Times

referral [rɪˈfɜːrəl] *noun* sending a patient to a specialist; *she asked for a referral to a gynaecologist*

he subsequently developed colicky abdominal pain and

tenderness which caused his referral

British Journal of Hospital Medicine

reflex ['ri:fleks] *noun* automatic reaction to something (such as a knee jerk); **accommodation reflex** = reaction of the pupil when the eye focuses on an object which is close; **corneal reflex** = reflex from touching or hitting the cornea which makes the eyelid close; **light reflex** *or* **pupillary reflex to light** = reaction of the pupil of the eye which changes size according to the amount of light going into the eye; **reflex action** = automatic reaction to a stimulus (such as a sneeze); **reflex arc** = basic system of a reflex action, where a receptor is linked to a motor neurone which in turn is linked to an effector muscle; *see also* PATELLAR, PLANTAR, RADIAL

reflexologist [ri:flək'sɒlədʒɪst] *noun* person specializing in reflexology

reflexology [ri:flek'sɒlədʒi] *noun* treatment to relieve tension by massaging the soles of the feet and thereby stimulating the nerves and increasing the blood supply

reflux ['ri:flʌks] *noun* flowing backwards (of a liquid) in the opposite direction to normal flow; *the valves in the veins prevent blood reflux*; **reflux oesophagitis** = inflammation of the oesophagus caused by regurgitation of acid juices from the stomach; *see also* VESICOURETERIC

refract [rɪ'frækt] *verb* to make light rays change direction as they go from one medium (such as air) to another (such as water) at an angle; *the refracting media in the eye are the cornea, the aqueous humour, the vitreous humour and the lens*

refraction [rɪ'frækʃn] *noun* (i) change of direction of light rays as they enter a medium (such as the eye); (ii) measuring the angle at which the light rays bend, as a test to see if someone needs to wear glasses

refractometer [ri:fræk'tɒmɪtə] *noun* optometer, instrument which measures the refraction of the eye

refractory [rɪ'fræktəri] *adjective* which it is difficult or impossible to treat, (condition) which does not respond to treatment; **refractory period** = short space of time after the ventricles of the heart have contracted, when they cannot contract again

refrigerate [rɪ'frɪdʒəreɪt] *verb* to make something cold; *the serum should be kept refrigerated*

refrigeration [rɪfrɪdʒə'reɪʃn] *noun* (i) making something cold; (ii) making part of the body very cold, to give the effect of an anaesthetic

refrigerator [rɪ'frɪdʒəreɪtə] *noun* machine which keeps things cold

regain [rɪ'geɪn] *verb* to get back something which was lost; *he has regained the use of his left arm*; *she went into a coma and never regained consciousness*

regenerate [rɪ'dʒenəreɪt] *verb* to grow again

regeneration [rɪdʒenə'reɪʃn] *noun* growing again of tissue which has been destroyed

regimen ['redʒɪmen] *noun* fixed course of treatment (such as a course of drugs or a special diet)

region ['ri:dʒn] *noun* area or part which is around something; *she experienced itching in the anal region*; *the rash started in the region of the upper thigh*; *the plantar region is very sensitive*

regional ['ri:dʒənl] *adjective* in a particular region, referring to a particular region; **Regional Health Authority (RHA)** = administrative unit in the National Health Service which is responsible for the planning of health services in a large part of the country; **regional ileitis** *or* **regional enteritis** = *see* ILEITIS

register ['redʒɪstə] **1** *noun* official list; **the Medical Register** = list of doctors approved by the General Medical Council; *the committee ordered his name to be struck off the register* **2** *verb* to write a name on an official list, especially to put your name on the official list of patients treated by a GP or dentist, or on the list of patients suffering from a certain disease; *she registered with her local GP*; *he is a registered heroin addict*; *they went to register the birth with the Registrar of Births, Marriages and Deaths*; *before registering with the GP, she asked if she could visit him*; *all practising doctors are registered with the General Medical Council*; **registered midwife** = qualified midwife who is registered to practise; **Registered Nurse (RN)** *or* **Registered General Nurse (RGN)** *or* **Registered Theatre Nurse (RTN)** = nurses who have been registered by the UKCC; *see also note at* NURSE

registrar [redʒɪ'strɑ:] *noun* **(a)** qualified doctor or surgeon in a hospital who supervises house officers **(b)** person who registers something officially; **Registrar of Births, Marriages and Deaths** = official who keeps the records of people who have been born, married or who have died in a certain area

registration [redʒɪ'streɪʃn] *noun* act of registering; *a doctor cannot practise without registration by the General Medical Council*

regress [rɪ'gres] *verb* to return to an earlier stage or condition

regression [rɪ'greʃn] *noun* **(a)** stage where symptoms of a disease are disappearing and the patient is getting better **(b)** *(in psychiatry)* returning to a mental state which existed when the patient was younger

regular ['regjʊlə] *adjective* which takes place again and again after the same period of time; which happens at the same time each day; *he was advised to make regular visits to the dentist*; *she had her regular six-monthly checkup*

regularly ['regjʊləli] *adverb* happening repeatedly after the same period of time; *the tablets must be taken regularly every evening*; *you should go to the dentist regularly*

regulate ['regjuleɪt] *verb* to make something work (in a regular way); *the heartbeat is regulated by the sinoatrial node*

regulation [regju'leɪʃn] *noun* act of regulating; *the regulation of the body's temperature*

regurgitate [rɪ'gɜːdʒɪteɪt] *verb* to bring into the mouth food which has been partly digested in the stomach

regurgitation [rɪgɜːdʒɪ'teɪʃn] *noun* flowing back in the opposite direction to the normal flow, especially bringing up partly digested food from the stomach into the mouth; **aortic regurgitation** = flow of blood backwards, caused by a defective heart valve

rehabilitate [riːhə'bɪlɪteɪt] *verb* to make someone fit to work or to lead a normal life

rehabilitation [riːhəbɪlɪ'teɪʃn] *noun* making a patient fit to work or to lead a normal life again

rehydration [riːhaɪ'dreɪʃn] *noun* giving water or liquid to a patient suffering from dehydration

reinfect [riːɪn'fekt] *verb* to infect again

Reiter's syndrome *or* **Reiter's disease** ['raɪtəz 'sɪndrəʊm *or* dɪ'ziːz] *noun* illness which may be venereal, with arthritis, urethritis and conjunctivitis at the same time, affecting mainly men

reject [rɪ'dʒekt] *verb* not to accept; *the new heart was rejected by the body*; *they gave the patient drugs to prevent the transplant being rejected*

rejection [rɪ'dʒekʃn] *noun* act of rejecting tissue; *the patient was given drugs to reduce the possibility of tissue rejection*

relapse [rɪ'læps] **1** *noun (of patient or disease)* becoming worse, reappearing (after seeming to be getting better) **2** *verb* to become worse, to return; *he relapsed into a coma*; **relapsing fever** = disease caused by a bacterium, where attacks of fever recur at regular intervals; **relapsing pancreatitis** = form of pancreatitis where the symptoms recur, but in a milder form

relate [rɪ'leɪt] *verb* to connect to; *the disease is related to the weakness of the heart muscles*

-related [rɪ'leɪtɪd] *suffix* connected to; *drug-related diseases*

relationship [rɪ'leɪʃənʃɪp] *noun* way in which someone or something is connected to another; *the incidence of the disease has a close relationship to the environment*; *he became withdrawn and broke off all relationships with his family*

relax [rɪ'læks] *verb* to become less tense or less strained; *he was given a drug to relax the muscles*; *after a hard day in the clinic the nurses like to relax by playing tennis*; *the muscle should be fully relaxed*

relaxant [rɪ'læksənt] *adjective* (substance) which relieves strain; **muscle relaxant** = drug (such as baclofen) which reduces contractions in muscles

relaxation [riːlæk'seɪʃn] *noun* (i) reducing strain in a muscle; (ii) reducing stress in a person; **relaxation therapy** = treatment of a patient where he is encouraged to relax his muscles to reduce stress

relaxative [rɪ'læksətɪv] *noun US* drug which reduces stress

relaxin [rɪ'læksɪn] *noun* hormone which may be secreted by the placenta to make the cervix relax and open fully in the final stages of pregnancy before childbirth

release [rɪ'liːs] **1** *noun* allowing something to go out; *the slow release of the drug into* *the bloodstream* **2** *verb* to let something out, to let something go free; *hormones are released into the body by glands*; **releasing hormones** = hormones secreted by the hypothalamus which make the pituitary gland release certain hormones

relief [rɪ'liːf] *noun* making better or easier; *the drug provides rapid relief for patients with bronchial spasms*

> complete relief of angina is experienced by 85% of patients subjected to coronary artery bypass surgery
>
> *British Journal of Hospital Medicine*

relieve [rɪ'liːv] *verb* to make better, to make easier; *nasal congestion can be relieved by antihistamines*; *the patient was given an injection of morphine to relieve the pain*; *the condition is relieved by applying cold compresses*

> replacement of the metacarpophalangeal joint is mainly undertaken to relieve pain, deformity and immobility due to rheumatoid arthritis
>
> *Nursing Times*

REM [rem] = RAPID EYE MOVEMENT

remedial [rɪ'miːdiəl] *adjective* which cures

remedy ['remədi] *noun* cure, drug which will cure; *honey and glycerine is an old remedy for sore throats*

remember [rɪ'membə] *verb* to bring back into the mind something which has been seen or heard before; *he remembers nothing* or *he can't remember anything about the accident*

remission [rɪ'mɪʃn] *noun* period when an illness or fever is less severe

re. mist. ['riː 'mɪst] *abbreviation for the Latin phrase* 'repetatur mistura': repeat the same mixture (written on a prescription)

remittent fever [rɪ'mɪtənt 'fiːvə] *noun* fever which goes down for a period each day, like typhoid fever

removal [rɪ'muːvl] *noun* action of removing; *an appendicectomy is the surgical removal of an appendix*

remove [rɪ'muːv] *verb* to take away; *he will have an operation to remove an ingrowing toenail*

ren- *or* **reni-** *or* **reno-** [ren *or* 'reni *or* 'riːnəʊ] *prefix* referring to the kidneys

renal ['riːnl] *adjective* referring to the kidneys; **renal arteries** = pair of arteries running from the abdominal aorta to the kidneys; **renal calculus** = stone in the kidney; **renal capsule** = fibrous tissue surrounding a kidney; **renal colic** = sudden pain caused by kidney stone or stones in the ureter; **renal corpuscle** = part of a nephron in the cortex of a kidney; **renal cortex** = outer covering of the kidney, immediately beneath the capsule; **renal hypertension** = high blood pressure linked to kidney disease; **renal pelvis** = upper and wider part of the ureter leading from the kidney where urine is collected before passing down the ureter into the bladder; **renal rickets** = form of rickets caused by kidneys which do not function properly; **renal sinus** = cavity in which the renal pelvis and other tubes leading into the kidney fit; **renal transplant** = kidney transplant; **renal tubule** = uriniferous tubule, tiny tube which is part of a nephron

renew [rɪ'njuː] *verb* **to renew a prescription** = to get a new prescription for the same drug as before

renin ['riːnɪn] *noun* enzyme secreted by the kidney to prevent loss of sodium, and which also affects blood pressure

rennin ['renɪn] *noun* enzyme which makes milk coagulate in the stomach, so as to slow down the passage of the milk through the digestive system

renography [riː'nɒgrəfi] *noun* examination of a kidney after injection of a radioactive substance, using a gamma camera

reovirus ['riːəʊvaɪrəs] *noun* virus which affects both the intestine and the respiratory system, but does not cause serious illness; *compare* ECHOVIRUS

rep [rep] *abbreviation of the Latin word* 'repetatur': repeat (a prescription)

repair [rɪ'peə] *verb* to mend, to make something good again; *surgeons operated to repair a hernia* or *defective heart valve*

repeat [rɪ'piːt] *verb* to say or do something again; *the course of treatment was repeated after two months*; **repeat prescription** = prescription which is exactly the same as the previous one, and is often given without examination of the patient by the doctor and may sometimes be requested by telephone

repel [rɪ'pel] *verb* to make something go away; *if you spread this cream on your skin it will repel insects*

repetitive strain injury or **repetitive stress injury (RSI)** [rɪˈpetɪtɪv ˈstreɪn ˈɪndʒəri or ˈstres ˈɪndʒəri] noun pain in the arm felt by someone who performs the same movement many times over a certain period, as when operating a computer terminal or playing a musical instrument

replace [rɪˈpleɪs] verb (i) to put back; (ii) to exchange one part for another; *an operation to replace a prolapsed uterus*; *the surgeons replaced the diseased hip with a metal one*

replacement [rɪˈpleɪsmənt] noun operation to replace part of the body with an artificial part; **replacement transfusion** = exchange transfusion, treatment for leukaemia or erythroblastosis where almost all the abnormal blood is removed from the body and replaced by normal blood; **hip replacement** = surgical operation to replace a defective or arthritic hip with an artificial one; **total hip replacement** = replacing both the head of the femur and the acetabulum with an artificial joint

replicate [ˈreplɪkeɪt] verb (of a cell) to make a copy of itself

replication [replɪˈkeɪʃn] noun process in the division of a cell, where the DNA makes copies of itself

report [rɪˈpɔːt] **1** noun official note stating what action has been taken, what treatment given, what results have come from a test, etc.; *the patient's report card has to be filled in by the nurse*; *the inspector's report on the hospital kitchens is good* **2** verb to make an official report about something; *the patient reported her doctor for misconduct*; *occupational diseases or serious accidents at work must be reported to the local officials*; **reportable diseases** = diseases (such as asbestosis, hepatitis or anthrax) which may be caused by working conditions or may infect other workers and must be reported to the District Health Authority

repositor [rɪˈpɒzɪtə] noun surgical instrument used to push a prolapsed organ back into its normal position

repress [rɪˈpres] verb (in psychiatry) to hide in the back of the mind feelings or thoughts which may be unpleasant or painful

repression [rɪˈpreʃn] noun (in psychiatry) hiding feelings or thoughts which might be unpleasant

reproduce [riːprəˈdjuːs] verb **(a)** to produce children; (of bacteria, etc.) to produce new cells **(b)** to do a test again in exactly the same way

reproduction [riːprəˈdʌkʃn] noun process of making children, derived cells, etc; **organs of reproduction** = REPRODUCTIVE ORGANS

reproductive [riːprəˈdʌktɪv] adjective referring to reproduction; **reproductive organs** = parts of the bodies of men and women which are involved in the conception and development of a fetus; **reproductive system** = arrangement of organs and ducts in the bodies of men and women which produces spermatozoa and ova; **reproductive tract** = series of tubes and ducts which carry spermatozoa and ova from one part of the body to another

COMMENT: in the human male, the testes produce the spermatozoa which pass through the vasa efferentia and the vasa deferentia where they receive liquid from the seminal vesicles, then out of the body through the urethra and penis on ejaculation. In the female, an ovum, produced by one of the two ovaries, passes through the Fallopian tube where it is fertilized by a spermatozoon from the male. The fertilized ovum moves down into the uterus where it develops into an embryo

require [rɪˈkwaɪə] verb to need; *his condition may require surgery*; *is it a condition which requires immediate treatment?*; **required effect** = effect which a drug is expected to have; *if the drug does not produce the required effect, the dose should be increased*

requirement [rɪˈkwaɪəmənt] noun something which is necessary; *one of the requirements of the position is a qualification in pharmacy*

RES [ˈɑː ˈiː ˈes] = RETICULOENDOTHELIAL SYSTEM

research [rɪˈsɜːtʃ] **1** noun scientific study which investigates something new; *he is the director of a medical research unit*; *she is doing research into finding a cure for leprosy*; *research workers or research teams are trying to find a vaccine against AIDS*; **research and development (R&D)** = the process by which pharmaceutical companies find new drugs and test their suitability; **the Medical Research Council (MRC)** = government body which organizes and pays for medical research **2** verb to carry out scientific study; *he is researching the origins of cancer*

resect [rɪ'sekt] *verb* to remove part of the body by surgery

resection [rɪ'sekʃn] *noun* surgical removal of part of an organ; **submucous resection** = removal of bent cartilage from the nasal septum; **transurethral resection (TUR)** *or* **resection of the prostate** = surgical removal of the prostate gland through the urethra

resectoscope [rɪ'sektəskəup] *noun* surgical instrument used to carry out a transurethral resection

reset [riːˈset] *verb* to break a badly set bone and set it again correctly; *his arm had to be reset*

residency ['rezɪdənsi] *noun US* period when a doctor is receiving specialist training in a hospital

resident ['rezɪdnt] *noun & adjective* **(a)** (person) who lives in a place; *all the residents of the old people's home were tested for food poisoning*; **resident doctor** *or* **nurse** = doctor or nurse who lives in a certain building (such as an old people's home) **(b)** *US* qualified doctor who is employed by a hospital and sometimes lives in the hospital; *compare* INTERN

residential [rezɪ'denʃl] *adjective* living in a hospital; living at home; **residential care** = care of patients either in a hospital or at home (but not as outpatients)

residual [rɪ'zɪdjuəl] *adjective* remaining, which is left behind; **residual urine** = urine left in the bladder after a person has passed as much water as possible; **residual air** *or* **residual volume** = air left in the lungs after a person has breathed out as much air as possible

resin ['rezɪn] *noun* sticky juice which comes from some types of tree

resist [rɪ'zɪst] *verb* to be strong enough to fight against a disease, to avoid being killed or attacked by a disease; *a healthy body can resist some infections*

resistance [rɪ'zɪstəns] *noun* **(a)** (i) ability of a person not to get a disease; (ii) ability of a microbe not to be affected by antibiotics; *the bacteria have developed a resistance to certain antibiotics*; *after living in the tropics his resistance to colds was low*; **penicillin resistance** = ability of bacteria to resist penicillin **(b)** opposition to force; **peripheral resistance** = ability of the peripheral blood vessels to slow down the flow of blood inside them

resistant [rɪ'zɪstənt] *adjective* able not to be affected by something; *the bacteria are resistant to some antibiotics*; **resistant strain** = strain of bacterium which is not affected by antibiotics

resolution [rezə'luːʃn] *noun* (i) amount of detail which can be seen in a microscope or on a computer monitor; (ii) point in the development of a disease where the inflammation begins to disappear

resolve [rɪ'zɒlv] *verb (of inflammation)* to begin to disappear

> valve fluttering disappears as
> the pneumothorax resolves.
> Always confirm resolution with
> a physical examination and
> X-ray
>
> *American Journal of Nursing*

resonance ['rezənəns] *noun* sound made by a hollow part of the body when hit; *see also* MAGNETIC

resorption [rɪ'sɔːpʃn] *noun* absorbing again of a substance already produced back into the body

respiration [respə'reɪʃn] *noun* action of breathing; **artificial respiration** = way of reviving someone who has stopped breathing (as by mouth-to-mouth resuscitation); **assisted respiration** = breathing with the help of a machine; **controlled respiration** = control of a patient's breathing by an anaesthetist during an operation, if normal breathing has stopped; **external respiration** = part of respiration concerned with oxygen in the air being exchanged in the lungs for carbon dioxide from the blood; **internal respiration** = part of respiration concerned with the passage of oxygen from the blood to the tissues, and the passage of carbon dioxide from the tissues to the blood; **respiration rate** = number of times a person breathes per minute

COMMENT: respiration includes two stages: breathing in (inhalation) and breathing out (exhalation). Air is taken into the respiratory system through the nose or mouth, and goes down into the lungs through the pharynx, larynx, and windpipe. In the lungs, the bronchi take the air to the alveoli (air sacs) where oxygen in the air is passed to the bloodstream in exchange for waste carbon dioxide which is then breathed out

respirator ['respəreɪtə] *noun* **(a)** machine which gives artificial respiration; **cuirass respirator** = type of iron lung, where the patient's limbs are not enclosed; **Drinker respirator** = iron lung, machine which encloses all a patient's body, except the head, and in which air pressure is increased and decreased in turn, so forcing the patient to breathe; **positive pressure respirator** = machine which forces air into a patient's lungs through a tube inserted in the mouth or in the trachea (after a tracheostomy), and then let out by releasing pressure; **the patient was put on a respirator** = the patient was attached to a machine which forced him to breathe **(b)** mask worn to prevent someone breathing harmful gas or fumes

respiratory [rɪ'spɪrətəri] *adjective* referring to breathing; **respiratory bronchiole** = end part of a bronchiole in the lung, which joins the alveoli; **respiratory centre** = nerve centre in the brain which regulates the breathing; **respiratory distress syndrome** = hyaline membrane disease, a condition of newborn babies, where the lungs do not expand properly, due to lack of surfactant (the condition is common among premature babies); **respiratory failure** = failure of the lungs to oxygenate the blood correctly; **respiratory illness** = illness which affects the patient's breathing; **upper respiratory infection** = infection in the upper part of the respiratory system; **respiratory pigment** = blood pigment which can carry oxygen collected in the lungs and release it in tissues; **respiratory quotient (RQ)** = ratio of the amount of carbon dioxide taken into the alveoli of the lungs from the blood to the amount the oxygen which the alveoli take from the air; **respiratory syncytial virus (RSV)** = virus which causes infections of the nose and throat in adults but serious bronchiolitis in children; **respiratory system** *or* **respiratory tract** = series of organs and passages which take air into the lungs, and exchange oxygen for carbon dioxide

respond [rɪ'spɒnd] *verb* to react to something, to begin to get better because of a treatment; *the cancer is not responding to drugs*; *she is responding to treatment*

> many severely confused
> patients, particularly those
> in advanced stages of
> Alzheimer's disease, do not
> respond to verbal
> communication
>
> *Nursing Times*

response [rɪ'spɒns] *noun* reaction by an organ, tissue or a person to an external stimulus; **immune response** = (i) reaction of a body to an antigen; (ii) reaction of a body which rejects a transplant

> anaemia may be due to
> insufficient erythrocyte
> production, in which case the
> reticulocyte count will be low,
> or to haemolysis or
> haemorrhage, in which cases
> there should be a reticulocyte
> response
>
> *Southern Medical Journal*

responsible [rɪ'spɒnsəbl] *adjective* which is the cause of something; *the allergen which is responsible for the patient's reaction*; *this is one of several factors which can be responsible for high blood pressure*

responsiveness [rɪ'spɒnsɪvnəs] *noun* being able to respond to other people or to sensations

rest [rest] **1** *noun* lying down, being calm; *what you need is a good night's rest*; *I had a few minutes' rest and then I started work again*; *the doctor prescribed a month's total rest* **2** *verb* to lie down, to be calm; *don't disturb your mother - she's resting*

restless ['restləs] *adjective* not still, not calm; *the children are restless in the heat*; *she had a few hours' restless sleep*

restore [rɪ'stɔː] *verb* to give back; *she needs vitamins to restore her strength*; *the physiotherapy should restore the strength of the muscles*; *a salpingostomy was performed to restore the patency of the Fallopian tube*

restrict [rɪ'strɪkt] *verb* (i) to make less or smaller; (ii) to set limits to something; *the blood supply is restricted by the tight bandage*; *the doctor suggested she should restrict her intake of alcohol*

restrictive [rɪ'strɪktɪv] *adjective* which restricts, which makes smaller

result [rɪ'zʌlt] **1** *noun* figures at the end of a calculation, at the end of a test; *what was the result of the test?*; *the doctor told the patient the result of the pregnancy test*; *the result of the operation will not be known for some weeks* **2** *verb* to happen because of something; *the cancer resulted from exposure to radiation at work*; *his illness resulted in his being away from work for several weeks*

resuscitate [rɪˈsʌsɪteɪt] *verb* to make someone who appears to be dead start breathing again, and to restart the circulation of blood

resuscitation [rɪsʌsɪˈteɪʃn] *noun* reviving someone who seems to be dead, by making him breathe again and restarting the heart; **cardiopulmonary resuscitation (CPR)** = method of reviving someone where stimulation is applied to both heart and lungs

COMMENT: the commonest methods of resuscitation are artificial respiration and cardiac massage

retain [rɪˈteɪn] *verb* to keep or to hold; *he was incontinent and unable to retain urine in his bladder*; *see also* RETENTION

retard [rɪˈtɑːd] *verb* to make something slower, to slow down the action of a drug; *the drug will retard the onset of the fever*; *the injections retard the effect of the anaesthetic*

retardation [riːtɑːˈdeɪʃn] *noun* making slower; **mental retardation** = condition where a person's mind has not developed as fully as normal, so that he is not as advanced mentally as others of the same age; **psychomotor retardation** = slowing of movement and speech, caused by depression

retarded [rɪˈtɑːdɪd] *adjective* (person) who has not developed mentally as far as others of the same age; *a school for retarded children*; *by the age of four, he was showing signs of being mentally retarded*

retch [retʃ] *verb* to try to vomit without bringing any food up from the stomach

retching [ˈretʃɪŋ] *noun* attempting to vomit without being able to do so

rete [ˈriːtiː] *noun* structure, formed like a net, made up of tissue fibres, nerve fibres or blood vessels; **rete testis** = network of channels in the testis which take the sperm to the epididymis; *see also* RETICULAR (NOTE: the plural is **retia**)

retention [rɪˈtenʃn] *noun* holding back (such as holding back urine in the bladder); **retention cyst** = cyst which is formed when a duct from a gland is blocked; **retention of urine** = condition where passing urine is difficult or impossible because the urethra is blocked or because the prostate gland is enlarged

reticular [rɪˈtɪkjʊlə] *adjective* made like a net, (fibres) which criss-cross or branch; **reticular fibres** *or* **reticular tissue** = fibres

in connective tissue which support organs, blood vessels, etc.

reticulin [rɪˈtɪkjʊliːn] *noun* fibrous protein which is one of the most important components of reticular fibres

reticulocyte [rɪˈtɪkjʊləʊsaɪt] *noun* red blood cell which has not yet fully developed

reticulocytosis [rɪtɪkjʊləʊsaɪˈtəʊsɪs] *noun* condition where the number of reticulocytes in the blood increases abnormally

reticuloendothelial system (RES) [rɪtɪkjʊləʊendəʊˈθiːliəl ˈsɪstəm] *noun* series of phagocytic cells in the body (found especially in bone marrow, lymph nodes, liver and spleen) which attack and destroy bacteria and form antibodies; **reticuloendothelial cell** = phagocytic cell in the RES

reticuloendotheliosis [rɪtɪkjʊləʊendəʊθiːliˈəʊsɪs] *noun* condition where cells in the RES grow large and form swellings in bone marrow or destroy bones

reticulosis [rɪtɪkjʊˈləʊsɪs] *noun* any of several conditions where cells in the reticuloendothelial system grow large and form usually malignant tumours

reticulum [rɪˈtɪkjʊləm] *noun* series of small fibres or tubes forming a network; **endoplasmic reticulum (ER)** = network in the cytoplasm of a cell; **sarcoplasmic reticulum** = network in the cytoplasm of striated muscle fibres

retina [ˈretɪnə] *noun* inside layer of the eye which is sensitive to light; **detached retina** = RETINAL DETACHMENT; *see illustration at* EYE

COMMENT: light enters the eye through the pupil and strikes the retina. Light-sensitive cells in the retina (cones and rods) convert the light to nervous impulses; the optic nerve sends these impulses to the brain which interprets them as images. The point where the optic nerve joins the retina has no light-sensitive cells, and is known as the blind spot

retinaculum [retɪˈnækjʊləm] *noun* band of tissue which holds a structure in place, as found in the wrist and ankle over the flexor tendons

retinal [ˈretɪnəl] *adjective* referring to the retina; **retinal artery** = sole artery of the retina (it accompanies the optic nerve); **retinal detachment** = condition where the retina is partly detached from the choroid

retinitis [reti'naitis] *noun* inflammation of the retina; **retinitis pigmentosa** = hereditary condition where inflammation of the retina can result in blindness

retinoblastoma [retinəʊblæ'stəʊmə] *noun* rare tumour in the retina, affecting infants

retinol ['retinɒl] *noun* vitamin A, vitamin (found in liver, vegetables, eggs and cod liver oil) which is essential for good vision

retinopathy [reti'nɒpəθi] *noun* any disease of the retina; **diabetic retinopathy** = defect in vision linked to diabetes; **solar retinopathy** = irreparable damage (blurred vision, reading difficulties, etc.) to the most sensitive part of the retina (the macula) caused by looking at the sun with no protection or inadequate protection, as when looking at an eclipse of the sun

retinoscope ['retinəskəʊp] *noun* instrument with various lenses, used to measure the refraction of the eye

retire [ri'taiə] *verb* to stop work at a certain age; *most men retire at 65, but women only go on working until they are 60*; *although she has retired, she still does voluntary work at the clinic*

retirement [ri'taiəmənt] *noun* act of retiring; being retired; *the retirement age for men is 65*

retraction [ri'trækʃn] *noun* moving backwards, becoming shorter; *there is retraction of the overlying skin*; **retraction ring** = groove round the uterus, separating the upper and lower parts of the uterus, which, in obstructed labour, prevents the baby from moving forward normally into the cervical canal (NOTE: also called **Bandl's ring**)

retractor [ri'træktə] *noun* surgical instrument which pulls and holds back the edge of the incision in an operation

retro- ['retrəʊ] *prefix* meaning at the back, behind

retrobulbar neuritis [retrəʊ'bʌlbə nju:'raitis] *noun* optic neuritis, inflammation of the optic nerve which makes objects appear blurred

retroflexion [retrəʊ'flekʃn] *noun* being bent backwards; **uterine retroflexion** *or* **retroflexion of the uterus** = condition where the uterus bends backwards away from its normal position

retrograde ['retrəʊgreid] *adjective* going backwards; **retrograde pyelography** = X-ray examination of the kidney where a catheter is passed into the kidney through the ureter, and the opaque liquid is injected directly into it

retrogression [retrəʊ'greʃn] *noun* returning to an earlier state

retrolental fibroplasia [retrəʊ'lentl faibrəʊ'pleiziə] *noun* condition where fibrous tissue develops behind the lens of the eye, resulting in blindness

COMMENT: the condition is likely in premature babies if they are treated with large amounts of oxygen immediately after birth

retro-ocular [retrəʊ'ɒkjʊlə] *adjective* at the back of the eye

retroperitoneal [retrəʊperitəʊ'ni:əl] *adjective* at the back of the peritoneum

retropharyngeal [retrəʊfærin'dʒi:əl] *adjective* at the back of the pharynx

retropubic [retrəʊ'pju:bik] *adjective* at the back of the pubis; **retropubic prostatectomy** = removal of the prostate gland which is carried out through a suprapubic incision and by cutting the membrane which surrounds the gland

retrospection [retrəʊ'spekʃn] *noun* recalling what happened in the past

retrospective [retrəʊ'spektiv] *adjective* (study) applying to the past, tracing what has happened already to selected patients; *compare* PROSPECTIVE

retroversion [retrəʊ'vɜ:ʃn] *noun* sloping backwards; **uterine retroversion** *or* **retroversion of the uterus** = condition where the uterus slopes backwards away from its normal position

retroverted uterus ['retrəʊvɜ:tid 'ju:tərəs] *noun* condition where the uterus slopes backwards away from its normal position

retrovirus ['retrəʊvairəs] *noun* virus whose genetic material contains RNA from which DNA is synthesized

COMMENT: the AIDS virus and many carcinogenic viruses are retroviruses

reveal [ri'vi:l] *verb* to show; *digital palpation revealed a growth in the breast*

reversal [ri'vɜ:səl] *noun* the procedure to change back; *reversal of sterilization*

revision [ri'viʒn] *noun* subsequent examination of a surgical operation; *a revision of a radical mastoidectomy*

revive [rɪ'vaɪv] *verb* to bring back to life, to consciousness; *they tried to revive him with artificial respiration*; *she collapsed on the floor and had to be revived by the nurse*

Reye's syndrome ['raɪz 'sɪndrəʊm] *noun* encephalopathy affecting young children possibly due to viral infection, and a suspected link with aspirin

RGN ['ɑː 'dʒiː 'en] = REGISTERED GENERAL NURSE

Rh *abbreviation for* rhesus

RHA ['ɑː 'eɪtʃ 'eɪ] = REGIONAL HEALTH AUTHORITY

rhabdovirus ['ræbdəvaɪrəs] *noun* any of a group of viruses containing RNA, one of which causes rabies

rhachio- ['reɪkɪəʊ] *suffix* referring to the spine

rhagades ['rægədiːz] *noun* fissures, long thin scars in the skin round the nose, mouth or anus, seen in syphilis

rhesus factor *or* **Rh factor** ['riːsəs 'fæktə *or* 'ɑː 'eɪtʃ 'fæktə] *noun* antigen in red blood cells, which is an element in blood grouping; **rhesus baby** = baby with erythroblastosis fetalis; **Rh-negative** = (person) who does not have the rhesus factor in his blood; **Rh-positive** = (person) who has the rhesus factor in his blood; **rhesus factor disease** *or* **Rh disease** = disease which occurs when the blood of a fetus is incompatible with that of the mother

COMMENT: the rhesus factor is important in blood grouping, because, although most people are Rh-positive, a Rh-negative patient should not receive a Rh-positive blood transfusion as this will cause the formation of permanent antibodies. If a Rh-negative mother has a child by a Rh-positive father, the baby will inherit Rh-positive blood, which may then pass into the mother's circulation at childbirth and cause antibodies to form. This can be prevented by an injection of anti D immunoglobulin immediately after the birth of the first Rh-positive child and any subsequent Rh-positive children. If a Rh-negative mother has formed antibodies to Rh-positive blood in the past, these antibodies will affect the blood of the fetus and may cause erythroblastosis fetalis

rheumatic [ruː'mætɪk] *adjective* referring to rheumatism; **rheumatic fever** *or* **acute rheumatism** = collagen disease of young people and children, caused by haemolytic streptococci, where the joints and also the valves and lining of the heart become inflamed

COMMENT: rheumatic fever often follows another streptococcal infection such as a strep throat or tonsillitis. Symptoms are high fever, pains in the joints, which become red, formation of nodules on the ends of bones, and difficulty in breathing. Although recovery can be complete, rheumatic fever can recur and damage the heart permanently

rheumatism ['ruːmətɪzm] *noun* general term for pains and stiffness in the joints and muscles; *she has rheumatism in her hips*; *he has a history of rheumatism*; *she complained of rheumatism in her knees*; **muscular rheumatism** = pains in muscles or joints, usually caused by fibrositis, inflammation of the muscles or osteoarthritis; *see also* RHEUMATOID ARTHRITIS, RHEUMATIC FEVER, OSTEOARTHRITIS

rheumatoid ['ruːmətɔɪd] *adjective* similar to rheumatism; **rheumatoid arthritis** = general painful disabling collagen disease affecting any joint, but especially the hands, feet and hips, making them swollen and inflamed; **rheumatoid erosion** = erosion of bone and cartilage in the joints caused by rheumatoid arthritis

rheumatoid arthritis is a chronic inflammatory disease which can affect many systems of the body, but mainly the joints. 70% of sufferers develop the condition in the metacarpophalangeal joints
Nursing Times

rheumatologist [ruːmə'tɒlədʒɪst] *noun* doctor who specializes in rheumatology

rheumatology [ruːmə'tɒlədʒi] *noun* branch of medicine dealing with rheumatic disease of muscles and joints

Rh factor ['ɑː 'eɪtʃ 'fæktə] *see* RHESUS FACTOR

rhin- *or* **rhino-** [raɪn *or* 'raɪnəʊ] *prefix* referring to the nose

rhinitis [raɪ'naɪtɪs] *noun* inflammation of the mucous membrane in the nose, which makes the nose run, caused by a virus infection (cold), an allergic reaction to dust or flowers, etc.; **acute rhinitis** = common cold, a virus infection which causes inflammation of the mucous membrane in the nose and throat; **allergic rhinitis** = HAY FEVER; **chronic**

catarrhal rhinitis = chronic form of inflammation of the nose where excess mucus is secreted by the mucous membrane

rhinology [raɪˈnɒlədʒi] *noun* branch of medicine dealing with diseases of the nose and the nasal passage

rhinomycosis [raɪnəʊmaɪˈkəʊsɪs] *noun* infection of the nasal passages by a fungus

rhinophyma [raɪnəʊˈfaɪmə] *noun* condition caused by rosacea, where the nose becomes permanently red and swollen

rhinoplasty [ˈraɪnəʊplæsti] *noun* plastic surgery to correct the appearance of the nose

rhinorrhoea [raɪnəʊˈrɪə] *noun* watery discharge from the nose

rhinoscope [ˈraɪnəskəʊp] *noun* instrument for examining the inside of the nose

rhinoscopy [raɪˈnɒskəpi] *noun* examination of the inside of the nose

rhinosporidiosis [raɪnəʊspɒrɪdiˈəʊsɪs] *noun* infection of the nose, eyes, larynx and genital organs by a fungus *Rhinosporidium seeberi*

rhinovirus [raɪnəʊˈvaɪrəs] *noun* group of viruses containing RNA, which cause infection of the nose, including the virus which causes the common cold

rhiz- *or* **rhizo-** [raɪz *or* ˈraɪzəʊ] *prefix* referring to a root

rhizotomy [raɪˈzɒtəmi] *noun* surgical operation to cut or divide the roots of a nerve to relieve severe pain

rhodopsin [rəʊˈdɒpsɪn] *noun* visual purple, light-sensitive purple pigment in the rods of the retina, which makes it possible to see in dim light

rhombencephalon [rɒmbenˈsefələn] *noun* the hindbrain, the part of the brain which contains the cerebellum, the medulla oblongata and the pons

rhomboid [ˈrɒmbɔɪd] *noun* one of two muscles in the top part of the back which move the shoulder blades

rhonchus [ˈrɒŋkəs] *noun* abnormal sound in the chest, heard through a stethoscope, caused by a partial blockage in the bronchi (NOTE: the plural is **rhonchi**)

rhythm [ˈrɪðəm] *noun* regular movement or beat; *see also* CIRCADIAN; **rhythm method** = method of birth control where sexual intercourse should take place only during the safe periods, when conception is least likely to occur, that is at the beginning and at the end of the menstrual cycle

COMMENT: this method is not as safe as other methods of contraception because the time when ovulation takes place cannot be accurately calculated if a woman does not have regular periods

rhythmic [ˈrɪðmɪk] *adjective* regular, with a repeated rhythm

rib [rɪb] *noun* one of twenty-four curved bones which protect the chest; **cervical rib** = extra rib sometimes found attached to the cervical vertebrae and which may cause thoracic inlet syndrome; **false ribs** = bottom five ribs on each side which are not directly attached to the breastbone; **floating ribs** = two lowest false ribs on each side, which are not attached to the breastbone; **true ribs** = top seven pairs of ribs

rib cage [ˈrɪb ˈkeɪdʒ] *noun* the ribs and the space enclosed by them (NOTE: for other terms referring to the ribs, see words beginning with **cost-**)

COMMENT: the rib cage is formed of twelve pairs of curved bones. The top seven pairs (the true ribs) are joined to the breastbone in front by costal cartilage; the other five pairs of ribs (the false ribs) are not attached to the breastbone, though the 8th, 9th and 10th pairs are each attached to the rib above. The bottom two pairs, which are not attached to the breastbone at all, are called the floating ribs

riboflavine *US* **riboflavin** [raɪbəʊˈfleɪvɪn] = VITAMIN B_2

ribonuclease [raɪbəʊˈnjuːklieɪz] *noun* enzyme which breaks down RNA

ribonucleic acid (RNA) [raɪbəʊnjuˈkliːɪk ˈæsɪd] *noun* one of the nucleic acids in the nucleus of all living cells, which takes coded information from DNA and translates it into specific enzymes and proteins; *see also* DNA

ribose [ˈraɪbəʊs] *noun* type of sugar found in RNA

ribosomal [raɪbəˈsəʊml] *adjective* referring to ribosomes

ribosome [ˈraɪbəsəʊm] *noun* tiny particle in a cell, containing RNA and protein, where protein is synthesized

rice [raɪs] *noun* common food plant, grown in hot countries, of which the whitish grains are eaten

ricewater stools ['raɪswɔːtə 'stuːlz] *noun* typical watery stools, passed by patients suffering from cholera

rich [rɪtʃ] *adjective* **(a) rich in** = having a lot of something; *green vegetables are rich in minerals*; *the doctor has prescribed a diet which is rich in protein or a protein-rich diet* **(b)** (food) which has high calorific value

> the sublingual region has a rich blood supply derived from the carotid artery
> *Nursing Times*

ricin ['raɪsɪn] *noun* highly toxic albumin found in the seeds of the castor oil plant

rickets ['rɪkɪts] *noun* rachitis, a disease of children, where the bones are soft and do not develop properly because of lack of vitamin D; **renal rickets** = form of rickets caused by poor kidney function

> COMMENT: initial treatment for rickets in children is a vitamin-rich diet, together with exposure to sunshine which causes vitamin D to form in the skin

Rickettsia [rɪ'ketsɪə] *noun* genus of microorganisms which causes several diseases including Q fever and typhus

rickettsial [rɪ'ketsɪəl] *adjective* referring to Rickettsia; **rickettsial pox** = disease found in North America, caused by *Rickettsia akari* passed to humans by bites from mites which live on mice

rid [rɪd] *verb* **to get rid of something** = to make something go away; **to be rid of something** = not to have something unpleasant any more; *he can't get rid of his cold - he's had it for weeks*; *I'm very glad to be rid of my flu*

ridge [rɪdʒ] *noun* long raised part on the surface of a bone or organ

right [raɪt] **1** *adjective & adverb & noun* not left, referring to the side of the body which usually has the stronger hand (which most people use to write with); *my right arm is stronger than my left*; *he writes with his right hand* **2** *noun* what the law says a person is bound to have; *the patient has no right to inspect his medical records*; *you always have the right to ask for a second opinion*

right-hand [raɪt'hænd] *adjective* on the right side; *the stethoscope is in the right-hand drawer of the desk*

right-handed [raɪt'hændɪd] *adjective* using the right hand more often than the left; *he's right-handed*; *most people are right-handed*

rigid ['rɪdʒɪd] *adjective* stiff, not moving

rigidity [rɪ'dʒɪdəti] *noun* being rigid, bent or not able to be moved; *see also* SPASTICITY

rigor ['rɪɡə] *noun* attack of shivering, often with fever; **rigor mortis** = condition where the muscles of a dead body become stiff a few hours after death and then become relaxed again

> COMMENT: rigor mortis starts about eight hours after death, and begins to disappear several hours later; environment and temperature play a large part in the timing

rima ['raɪmə] *noun* narrow crack or cleft; **rima glottidis** = space between the vocal cords

ring [rɪŋ] *noun* circle of tissue; tissue or muscle shaped like a circle; **ring finger** = the third finger, the finger between the little finger and the middle finger

ringing in the ear ['rɪŋɪŋ ɪn ði 'ɪə] *see* TINNITUS

ringworm ['rɪŋwɜːm] *noun* any of various infections of the skin by a fungus, in which the infection spreads out in a circle from a central point (ringworm is very contagious and difficult to get rid of); *see also* TINEA

Rinne's test ['rɪnɪz 'test] *noun* hearing test

> COMMENT: a tuning fork is hit and its handle placed near the ear (to test for air conduction) and then on the mastoid process (to test for bone conduction). It is then possible to determine the type of lesion which exists by finding if the sound is heard for a longer period by air or by bone conduction

rinse out ['rɪns 'aʊt] *verb* to wash the inside of something to make it clean; *she rinsed out the measuring jar*; *rinse your mouth out with mouthwash*

ripple bed ['rɪpl 'bed] *noun* type of bed with an air-filled mattress divided into sections, in which the pressure is continuously being changed so that the patient's body can be massaged and bedsores can be avoided

rise [raɪz] *verb* to go up; *his temperature rose sharply* (NOTE: **rising - rose - has risen**)

risk [rɪsk] **1** *noun* **(a)** possible harm, possibility of something happening; *there is a risk of a cholera epidemic*; *there is no risk of the disease spreading to other members of* the family; businessmen are particularly at risk of having a heart attack; **children at risk** = children who are more likely to be harmed or to catch a disease; **attributable risk (AR)** = measure of the excess risk of disease due to exposure to a particular risk: the excess risk of bacteriuria in oral contraceptive users attributable to the use of oral contraceptives is 1,566 per 100,000; **relative risk (RR)** = measure of the association between an exposure and a disease, it indicates the likelihood of developing the disease in the exposed group relative to the non-exposed: the relative risk of myocardial infarction for oral contraceptive users is 1.6 times that of non-users; **risk factor** = characteristic that increases a person's likelihood of getting a particular disease; *smoking is a risk factor for lung cancer, obesity is a risk factor for diabetes*; *see also* HIGH-RISK, LOW-RISK **2** *verb* to do something which may possibly harm or have bad results; *if the patient is not moved to an isolation ward, all the patients and staff in the hospital risk catching* the disease

---

adenomatous polyps are a risk factor for carcinoma of the stomach

Nursing Times

---

three quarters of patients aged 35 - 64 on GPs' lists have at least one major risk factor: high cholesterol, high blood pressure or addiction to tobacco

Health Services Journal

---

risus sardonicus ['raɪsəs sɑː'dɒnɪkəs] *noun* twisted smile which is a symptom of tetanus

river blindness ['rɪvə 'blaɪndnəs] *noun* blindness caused by larvae getting into the eye in cases of onchocerciasis

RM ['ɑː 'em] = REGISTERED MIDWIFE

RMN ['ɑː 'em 'en] = REGISTERED MENTAL NURSE

Rn *chemical symbol for* radon

RN ['ɑː 'en] = REGISTERED NURSE

RNA ['ɑː 'en 'eɪ] = RIBONUCLEIC ACID; **messenger RNA** = type of RNA which transmits information from DNA to form enzymes and proteins

RNMH ['ɑː 'en 'em 'eɪtʃ] = REGISTERED NURSE FOR THE MENTALLY HANDICAPPED

Rocky Mountain spotted fever ['rɒki 'maʊntɪn 'spɒtɪd 'fiːvə] *noun* type of typhus caused by *Rickettsia rickettsii,* transmitted to humans by ticks

rod [rɒd] *noun* **(a)** long thin round stick; *some bacteria are shaped like rods or are rod-shaped* **(b)** one of two types of light-sensitive cell in the retina of the eye; *see also* CONE

COMMENT: rods are sensitive to poor light. They contain rhodopsin or visual purple, which produces the nervous impulse which the rod transmits to the optic nerve

---

rodent ulcer ['rəʊdənt 'ʌlsə] *noun* basal cell carcinoma, a malignant tumour on the face

---

COMMENT: rodent ulcers are different from some other types of cancer in that they do not spread to other parts of the body and do not metastasize, but remain on the face, usually near the mouth or eyes. Rodent ulcer is rare before middle age

---

roentgen ['rɒntgən] *noun* unit which measures the amount of exposure to X-rays or gamma rays (NOTE: with figures usually written **R**); **roentgen rays** = X-rays or gamma rays which can pass through tissue and leave an image on a photographic film

roentgenogram ['rɒntgenəgræm] *noun* X-ray photograph

roentgenology [rɒntgə'nɒlədʒi] *noun* study of X-rays and their use in medicine

rolled bandage *or* **roller bandage** ['rəʊld or 'rəʊlə 'bændɪdʒ] *noun* bandage in the form of a long strip of cloth which is rolled up from one or both ends

Romberg's sign ['rɒmbɜːgz 'saɪn] *noun* symptom of a sensory disorder in the position sense

---

COMMENT: if a patient cannot stand upright when his eyes are closed, this shows that nerves in the lower limbs which transmit position sense to the brain are damaged

---

rongeur [rɒn'gɜːr] *noun* strong surgical instrument like a pair of pliers, used for cutting bone

roof [ruːf] *noun* top part of the mouth or other cavity

root [ruːt] *noun* radix; (i) origin, point from which a part of the body grows; (ii) part of a tooth which is connected to a socket in the jaw; *root of hair or hair root*; *root of nerve or nerve root*; **root canal** = canal in the root of a tooth through which the nerves and blood vessels pass; *see illustration at* TOOTH

Rorschach test ['rɔːʃɑːk 'test] *noun* the ink blot test, used in psychological diagnosis, where the patient is shown a series of blots of ink on paper, and is asked to say what each blot reminds him of. The answers give information about the patient's psychological state

rosacea [rəʊ'zeɪʃə] *noun* common skin disease affecting the face, and especially the nose, which becomes red because of enlarged blood vessels; the cause is not known

rosea ['rəʊziə] *see* PITYRIASIS

roseola [rəʊ'ziːələ] *noun* any disease with a light red rash; **roseola infantum** = sudden infection of small children, with fever, swelling of the lymph glands and a rash (NOTE: also called **exanthem subitum**)

rostral ['rɒstrl] *adjective* like the beak of a bird

rostrum ['rɒstrəm] *noun* projecting part of a bone, structure shaped like a beak (NOTE: the plural is **rostra**)

rot [rɒt] *verb* to decay, to become putrefied; *the flesh was rotting round the wound as gangrene set in*; *the fingers can rot away in leprosy*

rota ['rəʊtə] *noun* **duty rota** = list of duties which have to be done and the names of the people who will do them

rotate [rəʊ'teɪt] *verb* to move in a circle

rotation [rəʊ'teɪʃn] *noun* moving in a circle; **lateral and medial rotation** = turning part of the body to the side, towards the midline

rotator [rəʊ'teɪtə] *noun* muscle which makes a limb rotate

rotavirus ['rəʊtəvaɪrəs] *noun* any of a group of viruses associated with gastroenteritis in children

rotavirus is now widely accepted as an important cause of childhood diarrhoea in many different parts of the world
East African Medical Journal

Rothera's test ['rɒðərəz 'test] *noun* test to see if acetone is present in urine, a sign of ketosis which is a complication of diabetes mellitus

Roth spot ['rəʊt 'spɒt] *noun* pale spot which sometimes occurs on the retina of a person suffering from leukaemia or some other diseases

rotunda [rəʊ'tʌndə] *see* FENESTRA

rough [rʌf] *adjective* not smooth; *she put cream on her hands which were rough from heavy work*

roughage ['rʌfɪdʒ] *noun* dietary fibre, fibrous matter in food, which cannot be digested

COMMENT: roughage is found in cereals, nuts, fruit and some green vegetables. It is believed to be necessary to help digestion and avoid developing constipation, obesity and appendicitis

rouleau [ruː'ləʊ] *noun* roll of red blood cells which have stuck together like a column of coins (NOTE: the plural is **rouleaux**)

round [raʊnd] **1** *adjective* shaped like a circle; **round ligament** = band of ligament which stretches from the uterus to the labia; **round window** = round opening between the middle ear and the inner ear (NOTE: also called **fenestra rotunda**) **2** *noun* regular visit; **to do the rounds of the wards** = to visit various wards in a hospital and talk to the nurses and check on patients' progress or condition; **a health visitor's rounds** = regular series of visits made by a health visitor

roundworm ['raʊndwɜːm] *noun* any of several common types of parasitic worms with round bodies, such as hookworms (as opposed to flatworms)

Rovsing's sign ['rɒvsɪŋs 'saɪn] *noun* pain in the right iliac fossa when the left iliac fossa is pressed

COMMENT: a sign of acute appendicitis

Royal College of Nursing ['rɔɪəl 'kɒlɪdʒ əv 'nɜːsɪŋ] *noun* professional association which represents nurses

RQ ['ɑː 'kjuː] = RESPIRATORY QUOTIENT

RR ['ɑː 'ɑː] = RECOVERY ROOM

-rrhage *or* **-rrhagia** [rɪdʒ *or* 'reɪdʒə] *suffix* referring to abnormal flow or discharge of blood

-rrhaphy ['rəfi] *suffix* referring to surgical sewing or suturing

-rrhexis ['reksɪs] *suffix* referring to splitting or rupture

-rrhoea ['rɪə] *suffix* referring to an abnormal flow or discharge of fluid from an organ

RSCN ['ɑː 'es 'siː 'en] = REGISTERED SICK CHILDREN'S NURSE

RSI ['ɑː 'es 'aɪ] = REPETITIVE STRAIN INJURY

RSV ['ɑː 'es 'viː] = RESPIRATORY SYNCYTIAL VIRUS

RTN ['ɑː 'tiː 'en] = REGISTERED THEATRE NURSE

rub [rʌb] **1** *noun* lotion used to rub on the skin; *the ointment is used as a rub* **2** *verb* **(a)** to move something (especially the hands) backwards and forwards over a surface; *she rubbed her leg after she knocked it against the table*; *he rubbed his hands to make the circulation return* **(b) rub into** = to make an ointment go into the skin by rubbing; *rub the liniment gently into the skin*

rubber ['rʌbə] *noun* **(a)** material which can be stretched and compressed, made from the thick white liquid (latex) from a tropical tree; **rubber sheet** = waterproof sheet put on hospital beds or on the bed of a child who suffers from bedwetting, to protect the mattress **(b)** *(informal)* condom

rubbing alcohol ['rʌbɪŋ 'ælkəhɒl] *noun* US ethyl alcohol, used as a disinfectant or for rubbing on the skin (NOTE: British English is **surgical spirit**)

rubefacient [ruːbiˈfeɪʃnt] *adjective & noun* (substance) which makes the skin warm, and pink or red

rubella [ruˈbelə] = GERMAN MEASLES

rubeola [ruˈbiːələ] = MEASLES

Rubin's test ['ruːbɪnz 'test] *noun* test to see if the Fallopian tubes are free from obstruction

rubor ['ruːbə] *noun* redness (of the skin or tissue)

rubra ['ruːbrə] *see PITYRIASIS*

rudimentary [ruːdɪˈmentəri] *adjective* which exists in a small form, which has not developed fully; *the child was born with rudimentary arms*

Ruffini corpuscles *or* **Ruffini nerve endings** [ruˈfiːni 'kɔːpʌslz or 'nɜːv 'endɪŋz] *see CORPUSCLE*

ruga ['ruːgə] *noun* fold or ridge (especially in mucous membrane such as the lining of the stomach) (NOTE: the plural is **rugae**)

rule out ['ruːl 'aut] *verb* to state a patient does not have a certain disease; *we can rule out shingles*

rumbling ['rʌmblɪŋ] *noun* borborygmus, noise in the abdomen, caused by gas in the intestine

run [rʌn] *verb (of the nose)* to drip with liquid secreted from the mucous membrane in the nasal passage; *his nose is running*; *if your nose is running, blow it on a handkerchief*; *one of the symptoms of a cold is a running nose*

R-unit ['ɑːˈjuːnɪt] = ROENTGEN UNIT

runny nose ['rʌni 'nəuz] *noun* nose which is dripping with liquid from the mucous membrane

rupture ['rʌptʃə] **1** *noun* **(a)** breaking or tearing (of an organ such as the appendix) **(b)** hernia, condition where the muscles or wall round an organ become weak and the organ bulges through the wall **2** *verb* to break or tear; **ruptured spleen** = spleen which has been torn by piercing or by a blow

Russell traction ['rʌsl 'trækʃn] *noun* type of traction with weights and slings used to straighten a femur which has been fractured

Ryle's tube ['raɪlz 'tjuːb] *noun* thin tube which is passed into a patient's stomach through either the nose or mouth, used to pump out the contents of the stomach or to introduce a barium meal in the stomach

Ss

S *chemical symbol for* sulphur

Sabin vaccine ['seɪbɪn 'væksiːn] *noun* vaccine against poliomyelitis; *compare* SALK

COMMENT: the Sabin vaccine is given orally and consists of weak live polio virus

sac [sæk] *noun* part of the body shaped like a bag; **amniotic sac** = thin sac which covers an unborn baby in the uterus, containing the amniotic fluid; **hernial sac** = membranous sac of peritoneum where an organ has pushed through a cavity in the body; **pericardial sac** = the serous pericardium

sacchar- *or* **saccharo-** ['sækə or 'sækərəʊ] *prefix* referring to sugar

saccharide ['sækəraɪd] *noun* form of carbohydrate

saccharin ['sækərɪn] *noun* sweet substance, used in place of sugar because although it is nearly 500 times sweeter than sugar it contains no carbohydrates

saccule *or* **sacculus** ['sækjuːl or 'sækjuləs] *noun* smaller of two sacs in the vestibule of the inner ear which is part of the mechanism which relates information about the position of the head in space

sacral ['seɪkrl] *adjective* referring to the sacrum; **sacral foramina** = openings or holes in the sacrum through which pass the sacral nerves; *see illustration at* PELVIS; **sacral nerves** = nerves which branch from the spinal cord in the sacrum; **sacral plexus** = plexus, a group of nerves inside the pelvis near the sacrum, which supply nerves in the buttocks, back of the thigh and lower leg, foot and the urogenital area; **sacral vertebrae** = five vertebrae in the lower part of the spine which are fused together to form the sacrum

sacralization [sækrəlaɪˈzeɪʃn] *noun* abnormal condition where the lowest lumbar vertebra fuses with the sacrum

sacro- ['seɪkrəʊ] *prefix* referring to the sacrum

sacrococcygeal [seɪkrəʊkɒkˈsiːdʒɪəl] *adjective* referring to the sacrum and the coccyx

sacroiliac [seɪkrəʊˈɪliæk] *adjective* referring to the sacrum and the ilium; **sacroiliac joint** = joint where the sacrum joins the ilium

sacroiliitis [seɪkrəʊɪliˈaɪtɪs] *noun* inflammation of the sacroiliac joint

sacrotuberous ligament [seɪkrəʊˈtjuːbərəs 'lɪgəmənt] *noun* large ligament between the iliac spine, the sacrum, the coccyx and the ischial tuberosity

sacro-uterine ligament ['seɪkrəʊˈjuːtəraɪn 'lɪgəmənt] *noun* ligament which goes from the neck of the uterus to the sacrum, passing on each side of the rectum

sacrum ['seɪkrəm] *noun* flat triangular bone, between the lumbar vertebrae and the coccyx with which it articulates, formed of five sacral vertebrae fused together; it also articulates with the hip bones; *see illustrations at* PELVIS, VERTEBRAL COLUMN

SAD ['es 'eɪ 'diː] = SEASONAL AFFECTIVE DISORDER

saddle joint ['sædl 'dʒɔɪnt] *noun* synovial joint where one element is concave and the other convex, like the joint between the thumb and the wrist

saddle-nose ['sædl'nəʊz] *noun* deep bridge of the nose, normally a sign of injury but sometimes a sign of tertiary syphilis

sadism ['seɪdɪzm] *noun* abnormal sexual condition, where a person finds sexual pleasure in hurting others

sadist ['seɪdɪst] *noun* person whose sexual urge is linked to sadism

sadistic [səˈdɪstɪk] *adjective* referring to sadism; *compare* MASOCHISM

safe [seif] *adjective* not likely to hurt or cause damage; *medicines should be kept in a place which is safe from children*; *this antibiotic is safe to be used on very small babies*; *it is a safe painkiller, with no harmful side-effects*; *it is not safe to take the drug and also drink alcohol*; **safe dose** = amount of a drug which can be taken without causing harm to the patient; **safe period** = time during the menstrual cycle, when conception is not likely to occur, and sexual intercourse can take place (used as a method of contraception); **safe sex** = measures to reduce the possibility of catching a sexually transmitted disease, such as using a contraceptive sheath and having only one sexual partner (NOTE: **safe - safer - safest**)

> a good collateral blood supply makes occlusion of a single branch of the coeliac axis safe
> *British Medical Journal*

safely ['seifli] *adverb* without danger, without being hurt; *you can safely take six tablets a day without any risk of side-effects*

safety ['seifti] *noun* being safe, without danger; **to take safety precautions** = to do certain things which make your actions or condition safe; **safety belt** = belt which is worn in a car or a plane to help to stop a passenger being hurt if there is an accident; **safety pin** = special type of bent pin with a guard which covers the point, used for attaching nappies or bandages, etc.

sagittal ['sædʒɪtl] *adjective* which goes from the front of the body to the back, dividing it into right and left; **sagittal plane** = median plane, the division of the body along the midline, at right angles to the coronal plane, dividing the body into right and left parts; **sagittal section** = any section or cut through the body, going from the front to the back along the length of the body; **sagittal suture** = joint along the top of the head where the two parietal bones are fused

salicylate [sə'lɪsɪleɪt] *noun* one of various pain-killing substances, derived from salicylic acid, such as aspirin

salicylic acid [sælɪ'sɪlɪk 'æsɪd] *noun* white antiseptic substance, which destroys bacteria and fungi and which is used in ointments to treat corns, warts and other skin disorders

saline ['seɪlaɪn] **1** *adjective* referring to salt; *the patient was given a saline transfusion*; *she is on a saline drip*; **saline drip** = drip containing a saline solution; **saline solution** = salt solution, made of distilled water and sodium chloride, which is introduced into the body intravenously through a drip **2** *noun* saline solution

saliva [sə'laɪvə] *noun* fluid in the mouth, secreted by the salivary glands, which starts the process of digesting food (NOTE: for terms referring to saliva, see words beginning with **ptyal-**, **sial-**)

COMMENT: saliva is a mixture of a large quantity of water and a small amount of mucus, secreted by the salivary glands. Saliva acts to keep the mouth and throat moist, allowing food to be swallowed easily. It also contains the enzyme ptyalin, which begins the digestive process of converting starch into sugar while food is still in the mouth. Because of this association with food, the salivary glands produce saliva automatically when food is seen, smelt or even simply talked about. The salivary glands are situated under the tongue (the sublingual glands), beneath the lower jaw (the submandibular glands) and in the neck at the back of the lower jaw joint (the parotid glands)

salivary ['sælɪvəri or sə'laɪvəri] *adjective* referring to saliva; **salivary calculus** = stone which forms in a salivary gland; **salivary gland** = gland which secretes saliva

salivate ['sælɪveɪt] *verb* to produce saliva

salivation [sælɪ'veɪʃn] *noun* production of saliva

Salk vaccine ['sɑːlk 'væksiːn] *noun* vaccine against poliomyelitis; *compare* SABIN

COMMENT: the Salk vaccine consists of dead polio virus and is given by injection

Salmonella [sælmə'nelə] *noun* genus of bacteria which are in the intestines, which are pathogenic, are usually acquired by eating contaminated food, and cause typhoid or paratyphoid fever, gastroenteritis or food poisoning; *five people were taken to hospital with Salmonella poisoning* (NOTE: plural is **Salmonellae**)

salmonellosis [sælmənə'ləusɪs] *noun* food poisoning caused by *Salmonella* in the digestive system

salping- *or* **salpingo-** ['sælpɪndʒ or sæl'pɪŋgəu] *prefix* referring to a tube (i) the Fallopian tubes; (ii) the auditory meatus

salpingectomy [sælpɪn'dʒektəmi] *noun* surgical operation to remove or cut a Fallopian tube (used as a method of contraception)

salpingitis [sælpɪn'dʒaɪtɪs] *noun* inflammation, usually of a Fallopian tube

salpingography [sælpɪŋ'gɒgrəfi] *noun* X-ray examination of the Fallopian tubes

salpingo-oophoritis *or* **salpingo-oothecitis** [sælpɪŋɡəʊəʊɒfə'raɪtɪs *or* sælpɪŋɡəʊəʊɒnθɪ'saɪtɪs] *noun* inflammation of a Fallopian tube and the ovary connected to it

salpingo-oophorocele *or* **salpingo-oothecocele** [sælpɪŋɡəʊəʊ'ɒfərəʊsiːl *or* sælpɪŋɡəʊəʊɒn'θiːkəʊsiːl] *noun* hernia where a Fallopian tube and its ovary pass through a weak point in surrounding tissue

salpingostomy [sælpɪŋ'gɒstəmi] *noun* surgical operation to open up a blocked Fallopian tube

salpinx ['sælpɪŋks] = FALLOPIAN TUBE

salt [sɔːlt] **1** *noun* **(a) common salt** = sodium chloride, white crystals used to make food, especially meat, fish and vegetables, taste better; **salt depletion** = loss of salt from the body, by sweating or vomiting, which causes cramp and other problems; *a patient with heart failure is put on a salt-restricted diet*; *he should reduce his intake of salt* **(b)** chemical compound formed from an acid and a metal; **bile salts** = alkaline salts in the bile; **Epsom salts** = magnesium sulphate ($MgSO_47H_2O$, white powder which when diluted in water is used as a laxative **2** *adjective* tasting of salt; *sea water is salt*; *sweat tastes salt*

> COMMENT: salt forms a necessary part of diet, as it replaces salt lost in sweating and helps to control the water balance in the body. It also improves the working of the muscles and nerves. Most diets contain more salt than each person actually needs, and it is generally wise to cut down on salt consumption. Salt is one of the four tastes, the others being sweet, sour and bitter

salt-free diet ['sɒlt'friː 'daɪət] *noun* diet in which no salt is allowed

salve [sælv] *noun* ointment; **lip salve** = ointment, usually sold as a soft stick, used to rub on lips to prevent them cracking

sample ['sɑːmpl] *noun* small quantity of something used for testing; *blood samples were taken from all the staff in the hospital*; *the doctor asked her to provide a urine sample*

sanatorium [sænə'tɔːrɪəm] *noun* institution (like a hospital) which treats certain types of disorder, such as tuberculosis, or offers special treatment such as hot baths, massage, etc. (NOTE: plural is **sanatoria, sanatoriums**)

sandflea ['sændfliː] *noun* the jigger, tropical insect which enters the skin between the toes and digs under the skin, causing intense irritation

sandfly fever ['sændflaɪ 'fiːvə] *noun* virus infection like influenza, which is transmitted by the bite of the sandfly *Phlebotomus papatasii* and is common in the Middle East

sanguineous [sæŋ'gwɪnɪəs] *adjective* referring to blood, containing blood

sanies ['seɪnɪiːz] *noun* discharge from a sore or wound which has an unpleasant smell

sanitary ['sænətri] *adjective* (i) clean; (ii) referring to hygiene or to health; **sanitary napkin** *or* **sanitary towel** = wad of absorbent cotton placed over the vulva to absorb the menstrual flow

sanitation [sænɪ'teɪʃn] *noun* being hygienic (especially referring to public hygiene); *poor sanitation in crowded conditions can result in the spread of disease*

SA node *or* **S - A node** ['es 'eɪ 'nəʊd] = SINOATRIAL NODE

saphenous nerve [sə'fiːnəs 'nɜːv] *noun* branch of the femoral nerve which connects with the sensory nerves in the skin of the lower leg; **saphenous opening** = hole in the fascia of the thigh through which the saphenous vein passes; **saphenous vein** *or* **saphena** = one of two veins which take blood from the foot up the leg

> COMMENT: the long (internal) saphenous vein, the longest vein in the body, runs from the foot up the inside of the leg and joins the femoral vein. The short (posterior) saphenous vein runs up the back of the lower leg and joins the popliteal vein

sapraemia [sæ'priːmɪə] *noun* blood poisoning by saprophytes

saprophyte ['sæprəfaɪt] *noun* microorganism which lives on dead or decaying tissue

saprophytic [sæprəʊ'fɪtɪk] *adjective* (organism) which lives on dead or decaying tissue

sarc- *or* **sarco-** ['sɑːk *or* 'sɑːkəʊ] *prefix* referring to (i) flesh; (ii) muscle

sarcoid ['sɑːkɔɪd] *noun* & *adjective* (tumour) which is like a sarcoma

sarcoidosis [sɑːkɔɪ'dəʊsɪs] *noun* disease causing enlargement of the lymph nodes, where small nodules or granulomas form in certain tissues, especially in the lungs or liver and other parts of the body (NOTE: also called **Boeck's disease** or **Boeck's sarcoid**)

COMMENT: the Kveim test confirms the presence of sarcoidosis

sarcolemma [sɑːkəʊˈlemə] *noun* membrane surrounding a muscle fibre

sarcoma [sɑːˈkəʊmə] *noun* cancer of connective tissue, such as bone, muscle or cartilage

sarcomatosis [sɑːkəʊməˈtəʊsɪs] *noun* condition where a sarcoma has spread through the bloodstream to many parts of the body

sarcomatous [sɑːˈkɒmətəs] *adjective* referring to a sarcoma

sarcomere [ˈsɑːkəmɪə] *noun* filament in myofibril

sarcoplasm [ˈsɑːkəplæzm] *noun* myoplasm, semi-liquid cytoplasm in muscle membrane

sarcoplasmic [sɑːkəʊˈplæzmɪk] *adjective* referring to sarcoplasm; **sarcoplasmic reticulum** = network in the cytoplasm of striated muscle fibres

sarcoptes [sɑːˈkɒptiːz] *noun* type of mite which causes scabies

sardonicus [sɑːˈdɒnɪkəs] *see* RISUS

sartorius [sɑːˈtɔːrɪəs] *noun* very long muscle (the longest muscle) which runs from the anterior iliac spine, across the thigh down to the tibia

saturated fat [ˈsætʃəreɪtɪd ˈfæt] *noun* fat which has the largest amount of hydrogen possible

COMMENT: animal fats such as butter and fat meat are saturated fatty acids. It is known that increasing the amount of unsaturated and polyunsaturated fats (mainly vegetable fats and oils, and fish oil), and reducing saturated fats in the food intake helps reduce the level of cholesterol in the blood, and so lessens the risk of atherosclerosis

saturnism [ˈsætənɪzm] *noun* lead poisoning

satyriasis [sætəˈraɪəsɪs] *noun* abnormal sexual urge in a man (NOTE: in a woman, called **nymphomania**)

save [seɪv] *verb* to rescue someone, to stop someone from being hurt or killed; to stop

something from being damaged; *the doctors saved the little boy from dying of cancer*; *the surgeons were unable to save the sight of their patient*; **the surgeons saved her life** = they stopped the patient from dying

saw [sɔː] **1** *noun* tool with a long metal blade with teeth along its edge, used for cutting **2** *verb* to cut with a saw (NOTE: **sawing - sawed - has sawn**)

Sayre's jacket [ˈseɪəz ˈdʒækɪt] *noun* plaster cast which supports the spine when vertebrae have been deformed by tuberculosis or spinal disease

s.c. [ˈes ˈsiː] = SUB CUTANEOUS

scab [skæb] *noun* crust of dry blood which forms over a wound and protects it

scabicide [ˈskeɪbəsaɪd] *noun & adjective* (solution) which kills mites

scabies [ˈskeɪbiːz] *noun* very irritating infection of the skin caused by a mite which lives under the skin

scala [ˈskɑːlə] *noun* spiral canal in the cochlea

COMMENT: the cochlea is formed of three spiral canals: the scala vestibuli which is filled with perilymph and connects with the oval window; the scala media which is filled with endolymph and transmits vibrations from the scala vestibuli through the basilar membrane to the scala tympani, which in turn transmits the sound vibrations to the round window

scald [skɔːld] **1** *noun* injury to the skin caused by touching a very hot liquid or steam **2** *verb* to injure the skin with a very hot liquid or steam

scalding [ˈskɔːldɪŋ] *adjective* (i) very hot (liquid); (ii) (urine) which gives a burning sensation when passed

scale [skeɪl] **1** *noun* **(a)** flake of dead tissue (as dead skin in dandruff) **(b) scales** = machine for weighing; *the nurses weighed the baby on the scales* **2** *verb* to scrape teeth to remove plaque

scalenus or **scalene** [skeɪˈliːnəs or ˈskeɪliːn] *noun* one of a group of muscles in the neck which bend the neck forwards and sideways, and also help expand the lungs in deep breathing; **scalenus syndrome** = thoracic outlet syndrome, pain in an arm, caused by the scalenus anterior muscle pressing the subclavian artery and the brachial plexus against the vertebrae

scale off [ˈskeɪl ˈɒf] *verb* to fall off in scales

scaler ['skeɪlə] *noun* surgical instrument for scaling teeth

scalp [skælp] *noun* thick skin and muscle (with the hair) which covers the skull; **scalp wound** = wound in the scalp

scalpel ['skælpəl] *noun* small sharp pointed knife used in surgery

scaly ['skeɪli] *adjective* covered in scales; *the pustules harden and become scaly*

scan [skæn] **1** *noun* (i) examination of part of the body using computer-interpreted X-rays to create a picture of the part on a screen; (ii) picture of part of the body created on a screen using computer-interpreted X-rays; **brain scan** = examining the inside of the brain by passing X-rays through the head using a scanner, and reconstituting the images on a computer monitor; **CAT scan** *or* **CT scan** = scan where a narrow X-ray beam, guided by a computer, photographs a thin section of the body or an organ from different angles; the results are fed into the computer which analyses them and produces a picture of a slice of the body or organ **2** *verb* to examine part of the body, using computer-interpreted X-rays, and create a picture of the part on a screen

scanner ['skænə] *noun* **(a)** machine which scans a part of the body; **brain scanner, body scanner** = machines which scan only the brain, or all the body **(b)** (i) person who examines a test slide; (ii) person who operates a scanning machine

scanning speech ['skænɪŋ 'spiːtʃ] *noun* defect in speaking, where each sound is spoken separately and given equal stress

scaphocephalic [skæfəusə'fælɪk] *adjective* having a long narrow skull

scaphocephaly [skæfəu'sefəli *or* skæfəu'kefəli] *noun* condition where the skull is abnormally long and narrow

scaphoid (bone) ['skæfɔɪd 'bəun] *noun* one of the carpal bones in the wrist

scaphoiditis [skæfəu'daɪtɪs] *noun* degeneration of the navicular bone in children

scapula ['skæpjulə] *noun* shoulder blade, one of two large flat bones covering the top part of the back (NOTE: plural is **scapulae**)

scapular ['skæpjulə] *adjective* referring to the shoulder blade

scapulohumeral [skæpjuləu'hjuːmərl] *adjective* referring to the scapula and humerus; **scapulohumeral arthritis** = PERIARTHRITIS

scar [skɑː] **1** *noun* cicatrix, the mark left on the skin after a wound or surgical incision has healed; *he still has the scar of his appendicectomy*; **scar tissue** = fibrous tissue which forms a scar **2** *verb* to leave a scar on the skin; *the burns have scarred him for life*; *plastic surgeons have tried to repair the scarred arm*; *patients were given special clothes to reduce hypertrophic scarring*

scarification [skærɪfɪ'keɪʃn] *noun* scratching, making minute cuts on the surface of the skin (as for smallpox vaccination)

scarificator ['skærɪfəkeɪtə] *noun* instrument used for scarification

scarlatina *or* **scarlet fever** [skɑːlə'tiːnə *or* 'skɑːlət 'fiːvə] *noun* infectious disease with a fever, sore throat and red rash, caused by a haemolytic streptococcus

COMMENT: scarlet fever can sometimes have serious complications if the kidneys are infected

Scarpa's triangle ['skɑːpɑːz 'traɪæŋgl] *noun* femoral triangle, slight hollow in the groin; it contains the femoral vessels and nerve

scat- *or* **scato-** [skæt *or* 'skætəu] *prefix* referring to the faeces

scatole ['skætəul] *noun* substance in faeces, formed in the intestine, which causes a strong smell

SCD ['es 'siː 'diː] = SICKLE-CELL DISEASE

even children with the milder forms of SCD have an increased frequency of pneumococcal infection

Lancet

scent [sent] *noun* (i) pleasant smell; (ii) cosmetic substance which has a pleasant smell; (iii) smell given off by a substance which stimulates the sense of smell; *the scent of flowers makes me sneeze*

scented ['sentɪd] *adjective* with a strong pleasant smell; *he is allergic to scented soap*

schema ['skiːmə] *see* BODY SCHEMA

Scheuermann's disease ['ʃɔɪəmənz dɪ'ziːz] *noun* inflammation of the bones and cartilage in the spine, usually affecting adolescents

Schick test ['ʃɪk 'test] *noun* test to see if a person is immune to diphtheria

COMMENT: in this test, a small amount of diphtheria toxin is injected, and if the point of injection becomes inflamed it shows the patient is not immune to the disease (= positive reaction)

Schilling test ['ʃɪlɪŋ 'test] *noun* test to see if a patient can absorb vitamin B_{12} through the intestines, to determine cases of pernicious anaemia

-schisis ['skaɪsɪs] *suffix* referring to a fissure or split

schisto- *or* **schizo-** ['sɪstəʊ or 'skɪtsəʊ] *prefix* referring to something which is split

Schistosoma *or* **schistosome** [ʃɪstə'səʊmə or 'ʃɪstəsəʊm] = BILHARZIA

schistosomiasis [ʃɪstəsəʊ'maɪəsɪs] = BILHARZIASIS

schiz- *or* **schizo-** ['skɪts or 'skɪtsəʊ] *prefix* referring to something which is split

schizoid ['skɪtsɔɪd] **1** *adjective* referring to schizophrenia; **schizoid personality** = split personality, a disorder where the patient is cold towards other people, thinks mainly about himself and behaves in an odd way **2** *noun* person suffering from a less severe form of schizophrenia

schizophrenia [skɪtsə'friːniə] *noun* mental disorder where the patient withdraws from contact with other people, has delusions and seems to lose contact with the real world; **catatonic schizophrenia;** *see* CATATONIC

schizophrenic [skɪtsə'frenɪk] *noun & adjective* (person) suffering from schizophrenia

schizotypal [skɪtsəʊ'taɪpəl] *adjective* **schizotypal personality disorder** = schizoid personality type disorder

Schlatter's disease ['ʃlætəz dɪ'ziːz] *noun* inflammation in the bones and cartilage at the top of the tibia

Schlemm's canal ['ʃlemz kə'næl] *noun* circular canal in the sclera of the eye, which drains the aqueous humour

Schönlein's purpura ['ʃɜːnlaɪnz 'pɜːpərə] *see* PURPURA

school [skuːl] *noun* **(a)** place where children are taught; **school health service** = special service, part of the Local Health Authority, which looks after the health of children in school **(b)** specialized section of a university; **medical school** = section of a university which teaches medicine; *he is at medical school; she is taking a course at the School of Dentistry*

Schwann cells ['ʃvɒn selz] *noun* cells which form the myelin sheath round a nerve fibre; *see illustration at* NEURONE

schwannoma [ʃvɒ'nəʊmə] *noun* neurofibroma, benign tumour of a peripheral nerve

Schwartze's operation ['ʃvɔːtsɪz ɒpə'reɪʃn] *noun* the original surgical operation to drain fluid and remove infected tissue from the mastoid process

sciatic [saɪ'ætɪk] *adjective* referring to (i) the hip; (ii) the sciatic nerve; **sciatic nerve** = one of two main nerves which run from the sacral plexus into the thighs, dividing into a series of nerves in the lower legs and feet; it is the largest nerve in the body

sciatica [saɪ'ætɪkə] *noun* pain along the sciatic nerve, usually at the back of the thighs and legs

COMMENT: sciatica can be caused by a slipped disc which presses on a spinal nerve, or can simply be caused by straining a muscle in the back

science ['saɪəns] *noun* study based on looking at and noting facts, especially facts arranged into a system

scientific [saɪən'tɪfɪk] *adjective* referring to science; *he carried out scientific experiments*

scientist ['saɪəntɪst] *noun* person who specializes in scientific studies

scintigram ['sɪntɪgræm] *noun* recording radiation from radioactive isotopes injected into the body

scintillascope [sɪn'tɪləskəʊp] *noun* instrument which produces a scintigram

scintillator ['sɪntɪleɪtə] *noun* substance which produces a flash of light when struck by radiation

scintiscan ['sɪntɪskæn] *noun* scintigram which shows the variations in radiation from one part of the body to another

scirrhous ['sɪrəs] *adjective* hard (tumour)

scirrhus ['sɪrəs] *noun* hard malignant tumour (especially in the breast)

scissors ['sɪzəz] *plural noun* instrument for cutting, made of two blades and two handles; **scissor legs** = deformed legs, where one leg is permanently crossed over in front of the other

(NOTE: say 'a pair of scissors' when referring to one instrument)

scler- or **sclero-** [sklɪə or 'sklɪərəʊ] *prefix* (i) meaning hard, thick; referring to; (ii) sclera; (iii) sclerosis

sclera or **sclerotic (coat)** ['sklɪərə or sklə'rɒtɪk 'kəʊt] *noun* hard white outer covering of the eyeball; *see illustration at* EYE

COMMENT: the front part of the sclera is the transparent cornea, through which the light enters the eye. The conjunctiva, or inner skin of the eyelids, connects with the sclera and covers the front of the eyeball

scleral ['sklɪərl] *adjective* referring to the sclera; **scleral lens** = large contact lens which covers most of the front of the eye

scleritis [sklə'raɪtɪs] *noun* inflammation of the sclera

scleroderma [sklɪərə'dɜːmə] *noun* collagen disease which thickens connective tissue and produces a hard thick skin

scleroma [sklə'rəʊmə] *noun* patch of hard skin or hard mucous membrane

scleromalacia (perforans) [sklɪərəʊmə'leɪʃiə pə'fɔːrəns] *noun* condition of the sclera in which holes appear

sclerosant or **sclerosing** [sklə'rəʊzənt or sklə'rəʊsɪŋ] *adjective* which becomes hard, which makes tissue hard; **sclerosant agent** or **sclerosing agent** or **sclerosing solution** = irritating liquid injected into tissue to harden it

sclerosis [sklə'rəʊsɪs] *noun* hardening of tissue; **multiple sclerosis** or **disseminated sclerosis** = nervous disease which gets progressively worse, where patches of the fibres of the central nervous system lose their myelin, causing numbness in the limbs and progressive weakness and paralysis; *see also* ARTERIOSCLEROSIS, ATHEROSCLEROSIS, GEHRIG'S DISEASE

sclerotherapy [sklɪərəʊ'θerəpi] *noun* treatment of a varicose vein by injecting a sclerosing agent into the vein, and so encouraging the blood in the vein to clot

sclerotic [sklə'rɒtɪk] **1** *adjective* referring to sclerosis; suffering from sclerosis **2** *noun* hard white covering of the eyeball

sclerotome ['sklɪərətəʊm] *noun* sharp knife used in sclerotomy

sclerotomy [sklə'rɒtəmi] *noun* surgical operation to cut into the sclera

scolex ['skəʊleks] *noun* head of a tapeworm, with hooks which attach it to the wall of the intestine

scoliosis [skəʊli'əʊsɪs] *noun* condition where the spine curves sideways

scoliotic [skəʊli'ɒtɪk] *adjective* (spine) which curves sideways

scoop stretcher ['skuːp 'stretʃə] *noun* type of stretcher formed of two jointed sections which can slide under a patient and lock together

-scope [skəʊp] *suffix* referring to an instrument for examining by sight

scorbutic [skɔː'bjuːtɪk] *adjective* referring to scurvy; *see note at* SCURVY

scorbutus [skɔː'bjuːtəs] *noun* scurvy, disease caused by lack of vitamin C or ascorbic acid which is found in fruit and vegetables

scoto- ['skəʊtə] *prefix* meaning dark

scotoma [skɒ'təʊmə] *noun* small area in the field of vision where the patient cannot see

scotometer [skəʊ'tɒmɪtə] *noun* instrument used to measure areas of defective vision

scotopia [skəʊ'təʊpiə] *noun* the power of the eye to adapt to poor lighting conditions and darkness

scotopic [skəʊ'tɒpɪk] *adjective* referring to scotopia; **scotopic vision** = vision in the dark and in dim light (the rods of the retina are used instead of the cones which are used for photopic vision); *see* DARK ADAPTATION

scrape [skreɪp] *verb* to remove the surface of something by moving a sharp knife across it

scratch [skrætʃ] **1** *noun* slight wound on the skin made when a sharp point is pulled across it; *she had scratches on her legs and arms*; *wash the dirt out of that scratch in case it gets infected* **2** *verb* to harm the skin by moving a sharp point across it; *the cat scratched the girl's face*; *be careful not to scratch yourself on the wire*

scream [skriːm] **1** *noun* loud sharp cry; *you could hear the screams of the people in the burning building* **2** *verb* to make a loud sharp cry; *she screamed when a man suddenly opened the door*

screen [skriːn] **1** *noun* **(a)** light wall, sometimes with a curtain, which can be moved about and put round a bed to shield the patient **(b)** = SCREENING 2 *verb* to examine large numbers of people to test them for a disease; *the population of the village was screened for meningitis*

> in the UK the main screen is carried out by health visitors at 6 - 10 months. With adequately staffed and trained community services, this method of screening can be extremely effective
>
> *Lancet*

screening ['skriːnɪŋ] *noun* testing large numbers of people to see if any has a certain type of disease; *see also* GENETIC

> GPs are increasingly requesting blood screening for patients concerned about HIV
>
> *Journal of the Royal College of General Practitioners*

scrofula ['skrɒfjʊlə] *noun* form of tuberculosis in the lymph nodes in the neck, formerly caused by unpasteurized milk, but now rare

scrofuloderma [skrɒfjʊləʊ'dɜːmə] *noun* form of tuberculosis of the skin, forming ulcers, and secondary to tuberculous infection of an underlying lymph gland or structure

scrofulous ['skrɒfjʊləs] *adjective* suffering from scrofula

scrotal ['skrəʊtl] *adjective* referring to the scrotum

scrotum ['skrəʊtəm] *noun* bag of skin hanging from behind the penis, containing the testes, epididymides and part of the spermatic cord; *see illustration at* UROGENITAL SYSTEM (male)

scrub nurse ['skrʌb 'nɜːs] *noun* nurse who cleans the operation site on a patient's body before an operation

scrub typhus ['skrʌb 'taɪfəs] *noun* tsutsugamushi disease, severe form of typhus caused by Rickettsia bacteria, passed to humans by mites, found in South-East Asia

scrub up ['skrʌb 'ʌp] *verb (of surgeon or theatre nurse)* to wash the hands and arms carefully before an operation

scurf [skɜːf] *noun* dandruff or pityriasis capitis, pieces of dead skin which form on the scalp and fall out when the hair is combed

scurvy ['skɜːvi] *noun* scorbutus, disease caused by lack of vitamin C or ascorbic acid which is found in fruit and vegetables

> COMMENT: scurvy causes general weakness and anaemia, with bleeding from the gums, joints, and under the skin. In severe cases, the teeth drop out. Treatment consists of vitamin C tablets and a change of diet to include more fruit and vegetables

scybalum ['sɪbələm] *noun* very hard faeces

Se *chemical symbol for* selenium

sea [siː] *noun* area of salt water which covers a large part of the earth; *when the sea is rough he is often sick*

seasick ['siːsɪk] *adjective* feeling sick because of the movement of a ship; *as soon as the ferry started to move she felt seasick*

seasickness ['siːsɪknəs] *noun* travel sickness or motion sickness, illness, with nausea, vomiting and sometimes headache, caused by the movement of a ship; *take some seasickness tablets if you are going on a long journey*

seasonal affective disorder (SAD) ['siːzənl ə'fektɪv dɪ'sɔːdə] *noun* condition in which the patient becomes depressed and anxious during the winter when there are fewer hours of daylight: the precise cause is not known, but it is thought that the shortage of daylight may provoke a reaction between various hormones and neurotransmitters in the brain

sebaceous [sə'beɪʃəs] *adjective* (i) referring to sebum; (ii) which produces oil; **sebaceous cyst** = cyst which forms when a sebaceous gland is blocked; **sebaceous gland** = gland in the skin which secretes sebum at the base of each hair follicle; *see illustration at* SKIN & SENSORY RECEPTORS

seborrhoea [sebə'riːə] *noun* excessive secretion of sebum by the sebaceous glands, common in young people at puberty, and sometimes linked to seborrhoeic dermatitis

seborrhoeic [sebə'riːɪk] *adjective* (i) caused by seborrhoea; (ii) with an oily secretion; **seborrhoeic dermatitis** *or* **seborrhoeic eczema** = type of eczema where scales form on the skin; **seborrhoeic rash** = rash where the skin surface is oily

sebum ['siːbəm] *noun* oily substance secreted by a sebaceous gland, which makes the skin smooth; it also protects the skin against bacteria and the body against rapid evaporation of water

second ['sekənd] **1** *noun* unit of time equal to 1/60 of a minute **2** *adjective* coming after the first; **second intention** = healing of an infected wound or ulcer, which takes place slowly and leaves a prominent scar; **second molars** = molars at the back of the jaw, before the wisdom teeth, erupting at about 12 years of age; **second opinion** = a diagnosis or opinion on treatment from a second doctor, often a hospital specialist; **to ask for a second opinion** = to ask another doctor or consultant to examine a patient and give his opinion on diagnosis or treatment

secondary ['sekəndri] **1** *adjective* (i) which comes after the first; (ii) (condition) which develops from another condition (the primary condition); *he was showing symptoms of secondary syphilis*; **secondary amenorrhoea** = *see* AMENORRHOEA; **secondary bronchi** = air passages supplying a lobe of a lung; **secondary growth** = metastasis, the spreading of a malignant disease from one part of the body to another through the bloodstream or the lymph system; **secondary haemorrhage** = haemorrhage which occurs some time after an injury, usually due to infection of the wound; **secondary medical care** = specialized treatment provided by a hospital; **secondary prevention** = ways (such as screening tests) of avoiding a serious disease by detecting it early; **secondary sexual characteristics** = sexual characteristics (such as pubic hair or breasts) which develop after puberty **2** *noun* malignant tumour which metastasized from another malignant tumour; *see also* PRIMARY

secrete [sɪ'kriːt] *verb; (of a gland)* to produce a substance (such as hormone, oil or enzyme)

secretin [sɪ'kriːtɪn] *noun* hormone secreted by the duodenum, which encourages the production of pancreatic juice

secretion [sɪ'kriːʃn] *noun* **(a)** process by which a substance is produced by a gland; *the pituitary gland stimulates the secretion of hormones by the adrenal gland* **(b)** substance produced by a gland; *sex hormones are bodily secretions*

secretor [sɪ'kriːtə] *noun* person who secretes ABO blood group substances into mucous fluids in the body (such as the semen, the saliva)

secretory [sɪ'kriːtəri] *adjective* referring to, accompanied by or producing a secretion

section ['sekʃn] *noun* **(a)** part of something; *the middle section of the aorta* **(b)** (i) action of cutting tissue; (ii) cut made in tissue; **Caesarean section** = surgical operation to deliver a baby by cutting through the abdominal wall into the uterus **(c)** slice of tissue cut for examination under a microscope **(d)** part of a document, such as an Act of Parliament; *she was admitted under section 5 of the Mental Health Act*

sedate [sɪ'deɪt] *verb* to calm (a patient) by giving a drug which acts on the nervous system and relieves stress or pain, and in larger doses makes a patient sleep; *elderly or confused patients may need to be sedated to prevent them wandering*

sedation [sɪ'deɪʃn] *noun* calming a patient with a sedative; **under sedation** = having been given a sedative; *he was still under sedation, and could not be seen by the police*

sedative ['sedətɪv] *noun & adjective* old term for an anxiolytic or hypnotic drug such as benzodiazepine, which acts on the nervous system to help a patient sleep or to relieve stress; *she was prescribed sedatives by the doctor*

sedentary ['sedntri] *adjective* sitting; **sedentary occupations** = jobs where the workers sit down for most of the time

changes in lifestyle factors have been related to the decline in mortality from ischaemic heart disease. In many studies a sedentary lifestyle has been reported as a risk factor for ischaemic heart disease
Journal of the American Medical Association

sediment ['sedɪmənt] *noun* solid particles, usually insoluble, which fall to the bottom of a liquid

sedimentation [sedɪmen'teɪʃn] *noun* action of solid particles falling to the bottom of a liquid; **erythrocyte sedimentation rate (ESR)** = test to show how fast erythrocytes settle in a sample of blood plasma, used as a diagnostic of various blood conditions

segment ['segmənt] *noun* part of an organ or piece of tissue which is clearly separate from other parts

segmental [seg'mentl] *adjective* formed of segments; **segmental ablation** = surgical removal of part of a nail, as treatment for an ingrowing toenail; *see also* BRONCHI

segmentation [segmen'teɪʃn] *noun* movement of separate segments of the wall of the intestine to mix digestive juice with the food before it is passed along by the action of peristalsis

segmented [seg'mentɪd] *adjective* formed of segments

seizure ['siːʒə] *noun* fit, convulsion or sudden contraction of the muscles, especially in a heart attack or stroke or epileptic fit

select [sɪ'lekt] *verb* to make a choice, to choose some things, but not others; *the committee is meeting to select the company which will supply kitchen equipment for the hospital service*; *she was selected to go on a midwifery course*

selection [sɪ'lekʃn] *noun* act of choosing some things, but not others; *the candidates for the post have to go through a selection process*; *the selection of suitable donor for a bone marrow transplant*; **genetic selection** = choosing only the best examples of a genus for reproduction

selective [sɪ'lektɪv] *adjective* which choose only certain things, and not others; **selective oestrogen receptor modulator** = drug (such as raloxifene hydrochloride) which acts on specific oestrogen receptors to prevent bone loss without affecting other oestrogen receptors; **selective serotonin re-uptake inhibitor (SSRI)** = drug (such as fluoxetine) which inhibits the reuptake of serotonin causing a selective accumulation of the neurotransmitter in the CNS, used in the treatment of depression

COMMENT: the drug should not be started immediately after stopping an MAOI and should be withdrawn slowly

selenium [sɪ'liːniəm] *noun* non-metallic trace element (NOTE: chemical symbol is **Se**)

self- ['self] *prefix* referring to oneself

self-admitted ['selfəd'mɪtɪd] *adjective* (patient) who has admitted himself to hospital without being sent by a doctor

self-care ['self'keə] *noun* looking after yourself properly, so that you remain healthy

self-defence ['selfdɪ'fens] *noun* defending yourself when someone is attacking you

self-governing hospital ['self'ɡʌvənɪŋ 'hɒspɪtl] *noun* NHS hospital trust, a hospital which earns its revenue from services provided to the District Health Authorities and family doctors

sella turcica ['selə 'tɜːsɪkə] *noun* pituitary fossa, a hollow in the upper surface of the sphenoid bone in which the pituitary gland sits

semeiology [siːmaɪ'ɒlədʒi] = SYMPTOMATOLOGY

semen ['siːmen] *noun* thick pale fluid containing spermatozoa, produced by the testes and seminal vesicles, and ejaculated from the penis

semi- ['semi] *prefix* meaning half

semicircular [semi'sɜːkjʊlə] *adjective* shaped like half a circle; **semicircular canals** = three canals in the inner ear filled with fluid and which regulate the sense of balance; *see illustration at* EAR; **semicircular ducts** = ducts inside the canals in the inner ear

COMMENT: the three semicircular canals are on different planes. When a person's head moves (as when he bends down), the fluid in the canals moves and this movement is communicated to the brain through the vestibular section of the auditory nerve

semi-conscious ['semi'kɒnʃəs] *adjective* half conscious, only partly aware of what is going on; *she was semi-conscious for most of the operation*

semi-liquid ['semi'lɪkwɪd] *adjective* half liquid and half solid

semilunar [semi'luːnə] *adjective* shaped like half a moon; **semilunar cartilage** = one of two pads of cartilage (lateral meniscus and medial meniscus) between the femur and the tibia in the knee; **semilunar valve** = one of two valves in the heart, either the pulmonary or the aortic valve, through which blood flows out of the ventricles

seminal ['semɪnl] *adjective* referring to semen; **seminal fluid** = fluid part of semen, formed in the epididymis and seminal vesicles; **seminal vesicles** = two glands near the prostate gland which secrete fluid into the vas deferens; *see illustration at* UROGENITAL SYSTEM (male)

seminiferous tubule [semi'nɪfərəs 'tjuːbjuːl] *noun* tubule in the testis which carries semen

seminoma [semi'nəumə] *noun* malignant tumour in the testis

semipermeable membrane
[semi'pɜːmiəbl 'membreɪn] *noun* membrane which allows some substances in liquid solution to pass through, but not others

semiprone [semi'prəʊn] *adjective* (position) where the patient lies face downwards, with one knee and one arm bent forwards and the face turned to one side

semi-solid ['semi'sɒlɪd] *adjective* half solid and half liquid

SEN ['es 'iː 'en] = STATE ENROLLED NURSE

senescence [sɪ'nesəns] *noun* the ageing process

senescent [sɪ'nesənt] *adjective* becoming old

Sengstaken tube ['seŋzteɪkən 'tjuːb] *noun* tube with a balloon, which is passed through the mouth into the oesophagus to stop oesophageal bleeding

senile ['siːnaɪl] *adjective* (i) referring to old age or to the infirmities of old age; (ii) (person) whose mental faculties have become weak because of age; **senile cataract** = cataract which occurs in an elderly person; **senile dementia** = old term for a form of mental degeneration sometimes affecting old people; *see also* PRESENILE

senilis [sə'naɪlɪs] *see* ARCUS

senility [sə'nɪləti] *noun* weakening of the mental and physical faculties in an old person

senior ['siːniə] *adjective & noun* (person) who has a more important position than others; *he is the senior anaesthetist in the hospital; senior members of staff are allowed to consult the staff records*

senna ['senə] *noun* laxative made from the dried fruit and leaves of a tropical tree

sensation [sen'seɪʃn] *noun* feeling or information about something which has been sensed by a sensory nerve and is passed to the brain; **burning sensation** = sensation similar to that of being hurt by fire

sense [sens] **1** *noun* one of the five faculties by which a person notices things in the outside world (sight, hearing, smell, taste and touch); *when he had a cold, he lost his sense of smell; blind people develop an acute sense of touch*; **sense organ** = organ (such as the nose, the skin) in which there are various sensory nerves and which can detect environmental stimuli (such as scent, heat and pain) and transmit information about them to the central nervous system **2** *verb* to notice something; *teeth can sense changes in temperature*

sensibility [sensə'bɪləti] *noun* being able to detect and interpret sensations

sensible ['sensəbl] *adjective* which can be detected by the senses; **sensible perspiration** = drops of sweat which can be seen on the skin

sensitive ['sensətɪv] *adjective* able to detect and respond to an outside stimulus

sensitivity [sensə'tɪvəti] *noun* (i) being able to detect and respond to an outside stimulus; (ii) rate of positive responses in a test from persons with a specific disease (a high rate of sensitivity means a low rate of false negatives) (NOTE: compare with **specificity**)

sensitization [sensətaɪ'zeɪʃn] *noun* (i) making a person sensitive; (ii) abnormal reaction to an allergen or to a drug, caused by the presence of antibodies which were created when the patient was exposed to the drug or allergen in the past

sensitize ['sensətaɪz] *verb* to make someone sensitive to a drug or allergen; **sensitized person** = person who is allergic to a drug, who reacts badly to a drug; **sensitizing agent** = substance which, by acting as an antigen, makes the body form antibodies

sensorineural deafness [sensərɪ'njuːrəl 'defnəs] *noun* perceptive deafness or hearing loss, deafness caused by a disorder in the auditory nerves or the brain centres which receive impulses from the nerves

sensory ['sensəri] *noun* referring to the detection of sensations by nerve cells; **sensory cortex** = term which was formerly used to refer to the area of the cerebral cortex which receives information from nerves in all parts of the body; **sensory deprivation** = condition where a person becomes confused because of lacking sensations; **sensory nerve** = afferent nerve which transmits impulses relating to a sensation (such as a taste or a smell) to the brain; **sensory neurone** = nerve cell which transmits impulses relating to sensations from the receptor to the central nervous system; **sensory receptor** = nerve ending, special cell which senses a change in the surrounding environment (such as cold or pressure) and reacts to it by sending out an impulse through the nervous system; *see illustration at* SKIN & SENSORY RECEPTORS

separate ['separeɪt] *verb* to move two things apart, to divide; *the surgeons believe it may be possible to separate the Siamese twins; the retina has become separated from the back of the eye*

separation [sepə'reɪʃn] *noun* act of separating or dividing

sepsis ['sepsɪs] *noun* presence of bacteria and their toxins in the body (usually following the infection of a wound), which kill tissue and produce pus

sept- *or* **septi-** ['sept *or* 'septɪ] *prefix* referring to sepsis

septa- ['septə] *prefix* referring to a septum

septal ['septl] *adjective* referring to a septum; **(atrial** *or* **ventricular) septal defect** = congenital defect where a hole exists in the wall between the two atria or the two ventricles of the heart which allows blood to flow abnormally through the heart and lungs

septate ['septeɪt] *adjective* divided by a septum

septic ['septɪk] *adjective* referring to or produced by sepsis

septicaemia [septɪ'siːmiə] *noun* blood poisoning, condition where bacteria or their toxins are present in the blood, multiply rapidly and destroy tissue

septicaemic [septɪ'siːmɪk] *adjective* caused by septicaemia, associated with septicaemia; *see also* PLAGUE

septo- ['septəu] *prefix* referring to a septum

septoplasty [septəu'plæsti] *noun* operation to straighten the cartilage in the septum

septum ['septəm] *noun* wall between two parts of an organ (as between two parts of the heart, between the two sides of the nose); *see illustration at* HEART; **deviated (nasal) septum** = abnormal position of the septum of the nose which may block the nose and cause nosebleeds; **interatrial septum** = membrane between the right and left atria in the heart; **interventricular septum** = membrane between the right and left ventricles in the heart; **nasal septum** = wall of cartilage between the two nostrils and the two parts of the nasal cavity; **septum defect** = condition where a hole exists in a septum (usually the septum of the heart) (NOTE: the plural is **septa**)

sequelae [sɪ'kwiːliː] *plural noun* disease or conditions which follow on from an earlier disease; *Kaposi's sarcoma can be a sequela of AIDS*; **biochemical and hormonal sequelae of the eating disorders** (NOTE: the singular is **sequela, sequel**)

sequence ['siːkwəns] **1** *noun* series of things, numbers, etc., which follow each other in order **2** *verb* to put in order; **to sequence amino acids** = to show how amino acids are linked together in chains to form protein

sequestrectomy [siːkwe'strektəmi] *noun* surgical removal of a sequestrum

sequestrum [sɪ'kwestrəm] *noun* piece of dead bone which is separated from whole bone

ser- *or* **sero-** [ser *or* 'sɪərəu] *prefix* referring to (i) blood serum; (ii) serous membrane

sera ['sɪərə] *see* SERUM

serine ['serɪn] *noun* an amino acid in protein

serious ['sɪəriəs] *adjective* very bad; *he's had a serious illness; there was a serious accident on the motorway; there is a serious shortage of plasma*

seriously ['sɪəriəsli] *adverb* in a serious way; *she is seriously ill*

serological [sɪərəu'lɒdʒɪkl] *adjective* referring to serology; **serological diagnosis** = diagnosis which comes from testing serum; **serological type** = SEROTYPE

serology [sɪ'rɒlədʒi] *noun* scientific study of serum and antibodies contained in it

seronegative [sɪərəu'negətɪv] *adjective* (person) who gives a negative reaction to a serological test

seropositive [sɪərəu'pɒzətɪv] *adjective* (person) who gives a positive reaction to a serological test

seropositivity [sɪərəupɒzɪtɪvəti] *noun* giving a positive reaction to a serological test

seropus [sɪərəu'pʌs] *noun* mixture of serum and pus

serosa [sɪ'rəusə] *noun* serous membrane, the membrane which lines an internal cavity which has no contact with air (such as the peritoneum)

serositis [sɪərəu'saɪtɪs] *noun* inflammation of serous membrane

serotherapy [sɪərəu'θerəpi] *noun* treatment of a disease using serum from immune individuals or immunized animals

serotonin [sɪərəu'təunɪn] *noun* compound (5-hydroxytryptamine) which exists mainly in blood platelets and is released after tissue is injured; it is a neurotransmitter important in sleep, mood and vasoconstriction

serotype _or_ **serological type** ['sɪərəʊtaɪp _or_ sɪərəʊ'lɒdʒɪkl 'taɪp] **1** _noun_ (i) category of microorganisms or bacteria that have some antigens in common; (ii) series of common antigens which exists in microorganisms and bacteria **2** _verb_ to group microorganisms and bacteria according to their antigens

serous ['sɪərəs] _adjective_ referring to serum, producing serum, like serum; **serous membrane** _or_ **serosa** = membrane which lines an internal cavity which has no contact with air (such as the peritoneum and pleura) and covers the organs in the cavity (such as the heart and lungs)

serpens ['sɜːpens] _see_ ERYTHEMA

serpiginous [sə'pɪdʒɪnəs] _adjective_ (i) (ulcer or eruption) which creeps across the skin; (ii) (wound or ulcer) with a wavy edge

serrated [sə'reɪtɪd] _adjective_ (wound) with a zigzag or saw-like edge

serration [sə'reɪʃn] _noun_ one of the points in a zigzag or serrated edge

Sertoli cells [sə'təʊli 'selz] _noun_ cells which support the seminiferous tubules in the testis

serum ['sɪərəm] _noun_ **(a) blood serum =** yellowish watery liquid which separates from (whole) blood when the blood clots; **serum albumin** = major protein in blood serum; **serum globulin** = major protein in blood serum which is an antibody **(b) antitoxic serum** = immunizing agent formed of serum taken from an animal which has developed antibodies to a disease and used to protect a patient from that disease; **snake bite serum** = ANTIVENENE; **serum hepatitis** = HEPATITIS B; **serum sickness** = anaphylactic shock, an allergic reaction to a serum injection; _see also_ ANTISERUM (NOTE: the plural is **sera, serums**)

COMMENT: blood serum is plasma without the clotting agents. It contains salt and small quantities of albumin, globulin, amino acids, fats and sugars; its main component is water. Serum used in serum therapy is taken from specially treated animals; in rare cases this can cause an allergic reaction in a patient

service ['sɜːvɪs] _noun_ group of people working together; **the National Health Service** = British medical system, including all doctors, nurses, dentists, hospitals, clinics, etc., which provide free or cheap treatment to patients

sesamoid bone ['sesəmɔɪd 'bəʊn] _noun_ any small bony nodule in a tendon, the largest being the kneecap

sessile ['sesaɪl] _adjective_ anything which has no stem (often applied to a tumour) (NOTE: the opposite is **pedunculate**)

session ['seʃn] _noun_ visit of a patient to a therapist for treatment; _she has two sessions a week of physiotherapy_; _the evening session had to be cancelled because the therapist was ill_

set [set] _verb_ **(a)** to put the parts of a broken bone back into their proper places and keep the bone fixed until it has mended; _the doctor set his broken arm_ **(b)** _(of a broken bone)_ to mend, to form a solid bone again; _his arm has set very quickly_; _her broken wrist is setting very well_; _see also_ RESET

settle ['setl] _verb (of a sediment)_ to fall to the bottom of a liquid; _(of a parasite)_ to attach itself, to stay in a part of the body; _the fluke settles in the liver_

sever ['sevə] _verb_ to cut off; _his hand was severed at the wrist_; _surgeons tried to sew the severed finger back onto the patient's hand_

severe [sɪ'vɪə] _adjective_ very bad; _the patient is suffering from severe bleeding_; _a severe outbreak of whooping cough occurred during the winter_; _she is suffering from severe vitamin D deficiency_

severely [sɪ'vɪəli] _adverb_ very badly; _severely handicapped children need special care_; _her breathing was severely affected_

many severely confused patients, particularly those in advanced stages of Alzheimer's disease, do not respond to verbal communication

Nursing Times

severity [sɪ'verəti] _noun_ degree to which something is bad; _treatment depends on the severity of the attack_

sex [seks] _noun_ **(a)** one of two groups (male and female) into which animals and plants can be divided; _the sex of a baby can be identified before birth_; _the relative numbers of the two sexes in the population are not equal, more males being born than females;_ **sex act** = act of sexual intercourse; **sex chromatin** = Barr body, chromatin found only in female cells, which can be used to identify the sex of a baby before birth; **sex determination** = way in which the sex of an individual organism is fixed by the number of chromosomes which make up its cell structure; **sex organs** = organs which are associated with reproduction and sexual intercourse (such as the testes and penis in men, and the ovaries, Fallopian tubes, vagina and vulva in women) **(b)** sexual intercourse; **safe sex** = measures to reduce the possibility of catching a sexually transmitted disease, such as using a contraceptive sheath and having only one sexual partner

sex chromosome ['seks 'krəuməusəum] *noun* chromosome which determines if a person is male or female

COMMENT: out of the twenty-three pairs of chromosomes in each human cell, two are sex chromosomes which are known as X and Y. Females have a pair of X chromosomes and males have a pair consisting of one X and one Y chromosome. The sex of a baby is determined by the father's sperm. While the mother's ovum only carries X chromosomes, the father's sperm can carry either an X or a Y chromosome. If the ovum is fertilized by a sperm carrying an X chromosome, the embryo will contain the XX pair and so be female

sex hormone ['seks 'hɔːməun] *noun* hormone secreted by the testis or ovaries, which regulates sexual development and reproductive functions

COMMENT: the male sex hormones are androgens (testosterone and androsterone), and the female hormones are oestrogen and progesterone

sex-linkage ['seks'lɪŋkɪdʒ] *noun* existence of characteristics which are transmitted through the X chromosomes

sex-linked ['seks'lɪŋkt] *adjective* (i) (genes) which are linked to X chromosomes; (ii) (characteristics, such as colour-blindness) which are transmitted through the X chromosomes

sexology [seks'ɒlədʒi] *noun* study of sex and sexual behaviour

sextuplet ['sekstjuplət] *noun* one of six babies born to a mother at the same time; *see also* QUADRUPLET, QUINTUPLET, TRIPLET, TWIN

sexual ['sekʃul] *adjective* referring to sex; **sexual act** *or* **sexual intercourse** = action of inserting the man's erect penis into the woman's vagina, and releasing spermatozoa from the penis by ejaculation, which may fertilize ova from the woman's ovaries; **sexual reproduction** = reproduction in which gametes from two individuals fuse together

sexually transmitted disease (STD) ['sekʃuli træns'mɪtɪd dɪ'ziːz] *noun* any of several diseases which are transmitted from an infected person to another person during sexual intercourse

COMMENT: among the commonest STDs are non-specific urethritis, genital herpes, hepatitis B and gonorrhoea; AIDS is also a sexually transmitted disease

shaft [ʃɑːft] *noun* (i) long central section of a long bone; (ii) main central section of the erect penis

shake [ʃeɪk] *verb* to move or make something move with short quick movements

sharp [ʃɑːp] **1** *adjective* **(a)** which cuts easily; *a surgeon's knife has to be kept sharp* **(b)** acute (pain) (as opposed to dull pain); *she felt a sharp pain in her shoulder* **2** *noun* (*informal*) **sharps** = objects with points, such as syringes

sharply ['ʃɑːpli] *adverb* suddenly; *his condition deteriorated sharply during the night*

shave [ʃeɪv] **1** *noun* cutting off hair level with the skin with a razor **2** *verb* to cut off hair level with the skin with a razor; *he cut himself while shaving*; *the nurse shaved the area where the surgeon was going to make the incision*

sheath [ʃiːθ] *noun* **(a)** layer of tissue which surrounds a muscle or a bundle of nerve fibres **(b)** **(contraceptive) sheath** = condom, rubber covering put over the penis before sexual intercourse as a protection against infection and also as a contraceptive

shed [ʃed] *verb* to lose (blood or tissue); *the lining of the uterus is shed at each menstrual period*; *he was given a transfusion because he had shed a lot of blood* (NOTE: **shedding - shed - has shed**)

sheet [ʃiːt] *noun* large piece of cloth which is put on a bed; *the sheets must be changed each day*; *the soiled sheets were sent to the hospital laundry*; *see also* DRAW-SHEET

shelf operation ['ʃelf ɒpə'reɪʃn] *noun* surgical operation to treat congenital dislocation of the hip in children, where bone tissue is grafted onto the acetabulum

sheltered accommodation or **sheltered housing** ['ʃeltəd əkɒmə'deɪʃn or 'hauzɪŋ] *noun* rooms or small flats provided for elderly people, with a resident supervisor or nurse

shift [ʃɪft] *noun* (a) way of working, where one group of workers work for a period and are then replaced by another group; period of time worked by a group of workers; *she is working on the night shift*; *the day shift comes on duty at 6.30 in the morning* (b) movement; **Purkinje shift** = change in colour sensitivity which takes place in the eye in low light when the eye starts using the rods in the retina because the light is too weak to stimulate the cones

Shigella [ʃɪ'gelə] *noun* genus of bacteria which causes dysentery

shigellosis [ʃɪge'ləʊsɪs] *noun* infestation of the digestive tract with *Shigella*, causing bacillary dysentery

shin [ʃɪn] *noun* front part of the lower leg; **shin splints** = extremely sharp pains in the front of the lower leg, felt by athletes

shinbone ['ʃɪnbəʊn] *noun* the tibia

shingles ['ʃɪŋgəlz] = HERPES ZOSTER

Shirodkar's operation or **Shirodkar pursestring** [ʃɪ'rɒdkɑːz ɒpə'reɪʃn or ʃɪ'rɒdkɑː 'pɜːsstrɪŋ] *noun* pursestring operation, a surgical operation to narrow the cervix of the uterus in a woman who suffers from habitual abortion, to prevent another miscarriage, the suture being removed before labour starts

shiver ['ʃɪvə] *verb* to tremble or shake all over the body because of cold or a fever, caused by the involuntary rapid contraction and relaxation of the muscles

shivering ['ʃɪvərɪŋ] *noun* trembling or shaking all over the body because of cold or a fever, caused by the involuntary rapid contraction and relaxation of the muscles

shock [ʃɒk] **1** *noun* (a) weakness caused by illness or injury, which suddenly reduces the blood pressure; *the patient went into shock*; *several of the passengers were treated for shock*; *a patient in shock should be kept warm and lying down, until plasma or blood transfusions can be* given; **neurogenic shock** = state of shock caused by bad news or an unpleasant surprise; **traumatic shock** = state of shock caused by an injury which leads to loss of blood; **shock syndrome** = group of symptoms (pale face, cold skin, low blood pressure, rapid and irregular pulse) which show that a patient is in a state of shock; *see also* ANAPHYLACTIC (NOTE: you say that someone is **in shock, in a state of shock** or **went into shock**) (b) **electric shock** = sudden pain caused by the passage of an electric current through the body; **shock therapy** or **shock treatment** = method of treating some mental disorders by giving the patient an electric shock to induce convulsions **2** *verb* to give someone an unpleasant surprise, and so put him in a state of shock; *she was still shocked several hours after the accident*

shoe [ʃuː] *noun* piece of clothing made of leather or hard material which is worn on the foot; **surgical shoe** = specially made shoe to support or correct a deformed foot

short [ʃɔːt] *adjective* lacking, with not enough of something; **short of breath** = unable to breathe quickly enough to supply the oxygen needed; *after running up the stairs he was short of breath*

shortness of breath ['ʃɔːtnəs əv 'breθ] *noun* panting, being unable to breathe quickly enough to supply the oxygen needed

shortsighted [ʃɔːt'saɪtɪd] = MYOPIC

shortsightedness [ʃɔːt'saɪtɪdnəs] = MYOPIA

shot [ʃɒt] *noun* (*informal*) injection; *the doctor gave him a tetanus shot*; *he needed a shot of morphine to relieve the pain*

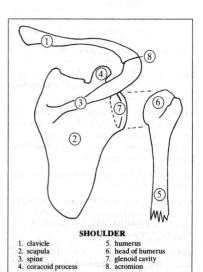

SHOULDER

1. clavicle	5. humerus
2. scapula	6. head of humerus
3. spine	7. glenoid cavity
4. coracoid process	8. acromion

shoulder ['ʃəʊldə] *noun* joint where the top of the arm joins the main part of the body; *he dislocated his shoulder*; *she was complaining of pains in her shoulder or of shoulder pains*; **shoulder blade** = scapula, one of two large triangular flat bones covering the top part of the back; **shoulder girdle** = pectoral girdle, the shoulder bones (scapulae and clavicles) to which the arm bones are attached; **shoulder joint** = ball and socket joint which allows the arm to rotate and move in any direction; **shoulder lift** = way of carrying a heavy patient where the upper part of his body rests on the shoulders of two carriers; **frozen shoulder** = stiffness and pain in the shoulder, after injury or after the shoulder has been immobile for some time, when it may be caused by inflammation of the membranes of the shoulder joint with deposits forming in the tendons

show [ʃəʊ] *noun* first discharge of blood at the beginning of childbirth

shrivel ['ʃrɪvl] *verb* to become dry and wrinkled

shuffling walk *or* **shuffling gait** ['ʃʌflɪŋ 'wɔːk *or* 'geɪt] *noun* way of walking (as in Parkinson's disease) where the feet are not lifted off the ground

shunt [ʃʌnt] **1** *noun* (i) passing of fluid through a channel which is not the usual one; (ii) channel which links two different blood vessels and carries blood from one to the other; **portocaval shunt** = artificial passage made between the portal vein and the inferior vena cava to relieve pressure on the liver; **right-left shunt** = defect in the heart, allowing blood to flow from the pulmonary artery to the aorta; **ventriculo-peritoneal shunt** = artificial drain used in hydrocephalus to drain CSF from the ventricles **2** *verb (of blood)* to pass through a channel which is not the normal one; *as much as 5% of venous blood can be shunted unoxygenated back to the arteries*

shunting ['ʃʌntɪŋ] *noun* condition where some of the deoxygenated blood in the lungs does not come into contact with air, and full gas exchange does not take place

Si *chemical symbol for* silicon

SI ['es 'aɪ] *abbreviation for* Système International, the international system of metric measurements; **SI units** = international system of units for measuring physical properties (such as weight, speed, light, etc.)

sial- *or* **sialo-** ['saɪəl *or* 'saɪələʊ] *prefix* meaning (i) saliva; (ii) a salivary gland

sialadenitis *or* **sialodenitis** *or* **sialitis** [saɪəlædɪ'naɪtɪs *or* saɪələʊædɪ'naɪtɪs *or* saɪə'laɪtɪs] *noun* inflammation of a salivary gland

sialagogue *or* **sialogogue** [saɪ'æləgɒg] *noun* substance which increases the production of saliva

sialography [saɪə'lɒgrəfi] *noun* ptyalography, X-ray examination of a salivary gland

sialolith [saɪ'æləʊlɪθ] *noun* ptyalith, stone in a salivary gland

sialorrhoea [saɪələʊ'riːə] *noun* production of an excessive amount of saliva

Siamese twins ['saɪəmiːz 'twɪnz] *noun* conjoined twins, twins who are joined together at birth

COMMENT: Siamese twins are always identical twins, and can be joined at the head, chest or hip. In some cases Siamese twins can be separated by surgery, but this is not possible if they share a single important organ, such as the heart

sib [sɪb] = SIBLING

sibilant ['sɪbɪlənt] *adjective (applied to a rale)* whistling (sound)

sibling ['sɪblɪŋ] *noun* brother or sister

Sichuan flu ['sɪtʃwɑːn 'fluː] *noun (informal)* virulent type of flu

COMMENT: the virus was first discovered in 1987 in Sichuan, a southwestern province of China; the symptoms are the same as those of ordinary flu (fever, sore throat, aching muscles, etc.) but more pronounced

sick [sɪk] *adjective* **(a)** ill, not well; *he was sick for two weeks*; *she's off sick from work*; **to report sick** = to say officially that you are ill and cannot work **(b)** wanting to vomit, having a condition where food is brought up from the stomach into the mouth; *the patient got up this morning and felt sick*; *he was given something to make him sick*; *the little boy ate too much and was sick all over the floor*; *she had a sick feeling or she felt sick* = she felt that she wanted to vomit

sickbay ['sɪkbeɪ] *noun* room where patients can visit a doctor for treatment in a factory or on a ship

sickbed ['sɪkbed] *noun* bed where a person is lying sick; *she sat for hours beside her daughter's sickbed*

sick building syndrome ['sɪk 'bɪldɪŋ 'sɪndrəʊm] *noun* condition where many people working in a building feel ill or have headaches, caused by blocked air-conditioning ducts in which stale air is recycled round the building, often carrying allergenic substances or bacteria

sicken for ['sɪkən 'fɔ:] *verb (informal)* to begin to have an illness, to feel the first symptoms of an illness; *she's looking pale - she must be sickening for something*

sickle cell ['sɪkl 'sel] *noun* drepanocyte, an abnormal red blood cell shaped like a sickle, due to an abnormal haemoglobin (HbS), which can cause blockage of capillaries; **sickle-cell disease (SCD)** = disease caused by sickle cells in the blood; **sickle-cell anaemia** = drepanocytosis, hereditary condition where the patient develops sickle cells which block the circulation, causing anaemia and pains in the joints and abdomen; **sickle-cell chest syndrome** = common complication of sickle-cell disease, with chest pain, fever and leucocytosis

COMMENT: sickle-cell anaemia is a hereditary condition which is mainly found in Africa and the West Indies

children with sickle-cell anaemia are susceptible to severe bacterial infection. Even children with the milder forms of sickle-cell disease have an increased frequency of pneumococcal infection
Lancet

sicklist ['sɪklɪst] *noun* list of people (children in a school or workers in a factory) who are sick; *we have five members of staff on the sicklist*

sickly ['sɪkli] *adjective (usually of children)* always slightly ill, never completely well; weak, subject to frequent sickness; *he was a sickly child, but now is a strong and healthy man*

sickness ['sɪknəs] *noun* **(a)** illness, not being well; *there is a lot of sickness in the winter months*; *many children are staying away from school because of sickness*; *see also* SEASICKNESS, TRAVEL SICKNESS **(b)** feeling of wanting to vomit

sickroom ['sɪkru:m] *noun* bedroom where someone is ill; *visitors are not allowed into the sickroom*

side [saɪd] *noun* (i) part of the body between the hips and the shoulder; (ii) part of an object which is not the front, back, top or bottom; *she was lying on her side*; *the nurse wheeled the trolley to the side of the bed*; **side rails** = rails at the side of a bed which can be lifted to prevent a patient falling out; *see also* BEDSIDE

side-effect ['saɪdɪ'fekt] *noun* effect produced by a drug or treatment which is not the main effect intended; *one of the side-effects of chemotherapy is that the patient's hair falls out*; *doctors do not recommend using the drug for long periods because of the unpleasant side-effects*; *the drug is being withdrawn because of its side-effects*

the treatment is not without possible side-effects, some of which can be particularly serious. The side-effects may include middle ear discomfort, claustrophobia, increased risk of epilepsy
New Zealand Medical Journal

sidero- ['saɪdərəʊ] *prefix* referring to iron

sideropenia [saɪdərəʊ'pi:niə] *noun* lack of iron in the blood probably caused by insufficient iron in diet

siderophilin [saɪdə'rɒfəlɪn] *noun* transferrin, substance found in the blood, which carries iron in the bloodstream

siderosis [saɪdə'rəʊsɪs] *noun* (i) condition where iron deposits form in tissue; (ii) inflammation of the lungs caused by inhaling dust containing iron

SIDS ['es 'aɪ 'di: 'es] = SUDDEN INFANT DEATH SYNDROME

sight [saɪt] *noun* one of the five senses, the ability to see; *his sight is beginning to fail*; *surgeons are fighting to save her sight*; **he lost his sight** = he became blind

sighted ['saɪtɪd] *adjective* (person) who can see; **the sighted** = people who can see; *he is partially sighted and uses a white stick*

sigmoid *or* **sigmoid colon** *or* **sigmoid flexure** ['sɪgmɔɪd *or* 'sɪgmɔɪd 'kəʊlən *or* 'sɪgmɔɪd 'flekʃə] *noun* fourth section of the colon which joins the rectum; *see illustration at* DIGESTIVE SYSTEM

sigmoidectomy [sɪgmɔɪ'dektəmi] *noun* surgical operation to remove the sigmoid colon

sigmoidoscope [sɪg'mɔɪdəskəup] *noun* surgical instrument with a light at the end which can be passed into the rectum so that the sigmoid colon can be examined

sigmoidostomy [sɪgmɔɪ'dɒstəmi] *noun* surgical operation to bring the sigmoid colon out through a hole in the abdominal wall

sign [saɪn] **1** *noun* **(a)** movement, mark, colouring or change which has a meaning and can be recognized by a doctor as indicating a condition (NOTE: a change in function which is also noticed by the patient is a **symptom**) **(b) sign language** = signs made with the fingers and hands, used to indicate words when talking to a deaf and dumb person, or when such a person wants to communicate **2** *verb* to write one's name on a form, cheque, etc., or at the end of a letter; *the doctor signed the death certificate*

signature ['sɪgnətʃə] *noun* name which someone writes when he signs; *the chemist could not read the doctor's signature*; *her signature is easy to recognize*

significant [sɪg'nɪfɪkənt] *adjective* important, worth noting; *no significant inflammatory responses were observed*

significantly [sɪg'nɪfɪkəntli] *adverb* in an important manner, in a manner worth noting; *he was not significantly better on the following day* = he was not much better

silence ['saɪləns] *noun* lack of noise, lack of speaking; *the crowd waited in silence*

silent ['saɪlənt] *adjective* **(a)** not making any noise, not talking **(b)** not visible, showing no symptoms; *genital herpes may be silent in women*; *graft occlusion is often silent with 80% of patients*

silica ['sɪlɪkə] *noun* silicon dioxide, mineral which forms quartz and sand

silicon ['sɪlɪkən] *noun* non-metallic chemical element; **silicon dioxide** = SILICA (NOTE: chemical symbol is **Si**)

silicosis [sɪlɪ'kəusɪs] *noun* form of pneumoconiosis, disease of the lungs caused by inhaling silica dust from mining or stone-crushing operations

COMMENT: this is a serious disease which makes breathing difficult and can lead to emphysema and bronchitis

silver ['sɪlvə] *noun* white-coloured metallic element (chemical symbol is **Ag**)

silver nitrate (AgNO₃) ['sɪlvə 'naɪtreɪt] *noun* salt of silver, mixed with a cream or solution, used to disinfect burns, to kill warts, etc.

Silvester method [sɪl'vestə 'meθəd] *noun* method of giving artificial respiration where the patient lies on his back and the first-aider brings the patient's hands together on his chest and then moves them above the patient's head; *see also* HOLGER-NIELSEN METHOD

Simmonds' disease ['sɪməndz dɪ'ziːz] *noun* condition of women where there is lack of activity in the pituitary gland, resulting in wasting of tissue, brittle bones and premature senility, due to postpartum haemorrhage

simple ['sɪmpl] *adjective* ordinary, not very complicated; **simple epithelium** = epithelium formed of a single layer of cells; **simple fracture** = fracture where the skin surface around the damaged bone has not been broken and the broken ends of the bone are close together; *see also* TACHYCARDIA

simplex ['sɪmpleks] *see* HERPES

sinew ['sɪnjuː] *noun* ligament, the tissue which holds together the bones at a joint; tendon or tissue which attaches a muscle to a bone

singultus [sɪŋ'gʌltəs] = HICCUP 1

sino- *or* **sinu-** ['saɪnəu *or* 'saɪnə] *prefix* referring to a sinus

sinoatrial node (SA node) [saɪnəu'eɪtriəl 'nəud] *noun* node in the heart at the junction of the superior vena cava and the right atrium, which regulates the heartbeat

sinogram ['saɪnəugræm] *noun* X-ray photograph of a sinus

sinography [saɪ'nɒgrəfi] *noun* examining a sinus by taking an X-ray photograph

sinuatrial node [saɪnə'eɪtriəl 'nəud] = SINOATRIAL NODE

sinus ['saɪnəs] *noun* (i) cavity inside the body, including the cavities inside the head behind the cheekbone, forehead and nose; (ii) tract or passage which develops between an infected place where pus has gathered and the surface of the skin; (iii) wide venous blood space; *he has had sinus trouble during the winter*; *the doctor diagnosed a sinus infection*; **carotid sinus** = expanded part attached to the carotid artery which monitors and regulates blood pressure and oxygen content; **cavernous sinus** = one of two cavities in the skull behind the eyes, which form part of the venous drainage system; **coronary sinus** = vein which takes most of the venous blood from the heart muscles to the right atrium; **ethmoidal sinuses** = air cells inside the ethmoid bone; **frontal sinus** = one of two sinuses in the front of the face above the eyes and near the nose; **maxillary sinus** = one of two sinuses behind the cheekbones in the upper jaw; **paranasal sinus** = one of the four pairs of sinuses in the skull near the nose (the frontal, maxillary, ethmoidal and sphenoidal); **renal sinus** = cavity in which the tubes leading into a kidney go; **sphenoidal sinus** = one of two sinuses behind the nasal passage; **sinus nerve** = nerve which branches from the glossopharyngeal nerve; *see also* TACHYCARDIA

sinusitis *or* **sinus trouble** [saɪnəˈsaɪtɪs or ˈsaɪnəs ˈtrʌbl] *noun* inflammation of the mucous membrane in the sinuses, especially the maxillary sinuses; **she has sinus trouble** = she has an inflammation of the sinuses

sinusoid [ˈsaɪnəsɔɪd] *noun* specially shaped small blood vessel in the liver, adrenal glands and other organs

sinus venosus [ˈsaɪnəs vəˈnəʊsəs] *noun* cavity in the heart of an embryo, part of which develops into the coronary sinus, and part of which is absorbed into the right atrium

siphonage [ˈsaɪfənɪdʒ] *noun* removing liquid from one place to another, with a tube, as used to empty the stomach of its contents

Sippy diet [ˈsɪpi ˈdaɪət] *noun US* alkaline diet of milk and dry biscuits as a treatment for peptic ulcers

sister [ˈsɪstə] *noun* (a) female who has the same father and mother as another child; *he has three sisters*; *her sister works in a children's clinic* (b) senior nurse; **sister in charge** *or* **ward sister** = senior nurse in charge of a hospital ward; **nursing sister** = sister with certain administrative duties (NOTE: sister can be used with names: **Sister Jones**)

site [saɪt] **1** *noun* position of something, place where something happened; place where an incision is to be made in an operation; *the X-ray showed the site of the infection* **2** *verb* to put something in a certain place; to be in a particular place; *the infection is sited in the right lung*

arterial thrombi have a characteristic structure: platelets adhere at sites of endothelial damage and attract other platelets to form a dense aggregate

British Journal of Hospital Medicine

the sublingual site is probably the most acceptable and convenient for taking temperature

Nursing Times

with the anaesthetist's permission, the scrub nurse and surgeon began the process of cleaning up the skin round the operation site

NATNews

situ [ˈsaɪtuː] *see* CARCINOMA-IN-SITU

situated [ˈsɪtjueɪtɪd] *adjective* in a place; *the tumour is situated in the bowel*; *the atlas bone is situated above the axis*

sit up [ˈsɪt ˈʌp] *verb* (a) to sit with your back straight; *the patient is sitting up in bed* (b) to move from a lying to a sitting position; *he finds it difficult to sit up* (NOTE: **sitting - sat - has sat**)

situs inversus viscerum [ˈsaɪtəs ɪnˈvɜːsəs ˈvɪsərəm] *noun* abnormal congenital condition, where the organs are not on the normal side of the body (i.e. where the heart is on the right side and not the left)

sitz bath [ˈsɪts ˈbɑːθ] *noun* small low bath where a patient can sit, but not lie down

Sjögren's syndrome [ˈʃɜːgrenz ˈsɪndrəʊm] *noun* chronic autoimmune disease where the lacrimal and salivary glands become infiltrated with lymphocytes and plasma cells, and the mouth and eyes become dry

skatole *or* **scatole** [ˈskætəʊl] *noun* substance in faeces which causes a strong foul smell

skeletal [ˈskelɪtl] *adjective* referring to a skeleton; **skeletal muscle** = voluntary muscle, muscle which is attached to a bone, which makes a limb move

skeleton [ˈskelɪtən] *noun* all the bones which make up a body; **appendicular skeleton** = part of the skeleton, formed of the pelvic girdle, pectoral girdle and the bones of the arms and legs; **axial skeleton** = trunk, the main part of the skeleton, formed of the spine, skull, ribs and breastbone

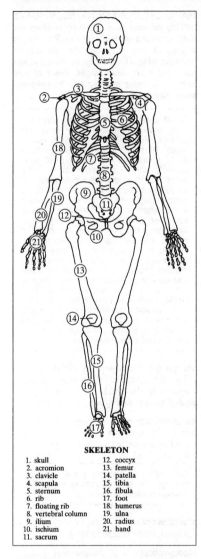

SKELETON

1. skull	12. coccyx
2. acromion	13. femur
3. clavicle	14. patella
4. scapula	15. tibia
5. sternum	16. fibula
6. rib	17. foot
7. floating rib	18. humerus
8. vertebral column	19. ulna
9. ilium	20. radius
10. ischium	21. hand
11. sacrum	

Skene's glands [ˈskiːnz ˈglændz] *noun* small mucous glands in the urethra in women

skia- [ˈskaɪə] *prefix* meaning shadow

skiagram [ˈskaɪəgræm] *noun* old term for X-ray photograph

skill [skɪl] *noun* ability to do difficult work, which is acquired by training; *you need special skills to become a doctor*

skilled [skɪld] *adjective* having acquired a particular skill by training; *he's a skilled plastic surgeon*

skin [skɪn] *noun* tissue (the epidermis and dermis) which forms the outside surface of the body; *his skin turned brown in the sun*; *after the operation she had to have a skin graft*; *skin problems in adolescents may be caused by diet*; *she went to see a specialist about her skin trouble*; **skin graft** = layer of skin transplanted from one part of the body to cover an area where the skin has been destroyed (NOTE: for other terms referring to skin, see words beginning with **cut-** or **derm-**)

COMMENT: the skin is the largest organ in the human body. It is formed of two layers: the epidermis is the outer layer, and includes the top layer of particles of dead skin which are continuously flaking off. Beneath the epidermis is the dermis, which is the main layer of living skin. Hairs and nails are produced by the skin, and pores in the skin secrete sweat from the sweat glands underneath the dermis. The skin is sensitive to touch and heat and cold, which are sensed by the nerve endings in the skin. The skin is a major source of vitamin D which it produces when exposed to sunlight

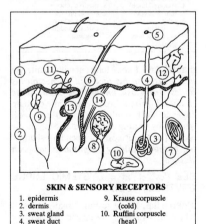

SKIN & SENSORY RECEPTORS

1. epidermis	9. Krause corpuscle
2. dermis	(cold)
3. sweat gland	10. Ruffini corpuscle
4. sweat duct	(heat)
5. pore	11. Merkel's discs
6. hair	(touch)
7. Pacinian corpuscle	12. free nerve endings
(pressure)	(pain)
8. Meissner's corpuscle	13. sebaceous gland
(touch)	14. arrector pili

skinny [ˈskɪni] *adjective (informal)* very thin

skull [skʌl] *noun* bones which are fused or connected together to form the head; **skull fracture** *or* **fracture of the skull** = condition where one of the bones in the skull has been fractured; *see also* VAULT (NOTE: for other terms referring to the skull, see words beginning with **crani-**)

COMMENT: the skull is formed of eight cranial bones which make up the head, and fourteen facial bones which form the face

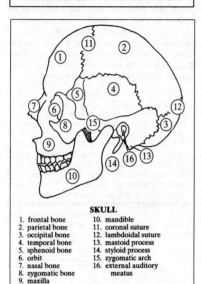

SKULL

1. frontal bone
2. parietal bone
3. occipital bone
4. temporal bone
5. sphenoid bone
6. orbit
7. nasal bone
8. zygomatic bone
9. maxilla
10. mandible
11. coronal suture
12. lambdoidal suture
13. mastoid process
14. styloid process
15. zygomatic arch
16. external auditory meatus

slash [slæʃ] **1** *noun* long cut with a knife, *he had bruises on his face and slashes on his hands*; *the slash on her leg needs three stitches* **2** *verb* **(a)** to cut with a knife or sharp edge; **to slash one's wrists** = to try to kill oneself by cutting the blood vessels in the wrists **(b)** to cut costs or spending sharply; *the hospital building programme has been slashed*

SLE ['es 'el 'iː] = SYSTEMIC LUPUS ERYTHEMATOSUS

sleep [sliːp] **1** *noun* resting (usually at night) when the eyes are closed and you are not conscious of what is happening; *most people need eight hours' sleep each night*; *you need to get a good night's sleep if you have a lot of work to do tomorrow*; *he had a short sleep in the middle of the afternoon*; **to get to sleep** *or* **go to sleep** = to start sleeping; *don't make a noise, the baby is trying to go to sleep*; **sleep apnoea** = condition relating to heavy snoring, with prolonged respiratory pauses leading to cerebral hypoxia and subsequent daytime drowsiness; *see also*

RAPID EYE MOVEMENT, SLOW-WAVE (NOTE: for other terms referring to sleep see words beginning with **hypn-**, **narco-**) **2** *verb* to be asleep, to rest with the eyes closed not knowing what is happening; *he always sleeps for eight hours each night*; *don't disturb him - he's trying to sleep* (NOTE: **sleeping - slept - has slept**)

COMMENT: sleep is a period when the body rests and rebuilds tissue, especially protein. Most adults need eight hours' sleep each night. Children require more (10 to 12 hours) but old people need less, possibly only four to six hours. Sleep forms a regular pattern of stages: during the first stage the person is still conscious of his surroundings, and will wake if he hears a noise; afterwards the sleeper goes into very deep sleep (slow-wave sleep), where the eyes are tightly closed, the pulse is regular and the sleeper breathes deeply. During this stage the pituitary gland produces the growth hormone somatotrophin. It is difficult to wake someone from deep sleep. This stage is followed by rapid eye movement sleep (REM sleep), where the sleeper's eyes are half open and move about, he makes facial movements, his blood pressure rises and he has dreams. After this stage he relapses into the first sleep stage again

sleeping pill *or* **sleeping tablet** ['sliːpɪŋ 'pɪl or 'sliːpɪŋ 'tæblət] *noun* drug (usually a barbiturate) which makes a person sleep; *she died of an overdose of sleeping tablets*

sleeping sickness ['sliːpɪŋ 'sɪknəs] *noun* African trypanosomiasis, an African disease, spread by the tsetse fly, where trypanosomes infest the blood

COMMENT: symptoms are headaches, lethargy and long periods of sleep. The disease is fatal if not treated

sleeplessness ['sliːpləsnəs] *noun* insomnia, being unable to sleep

sleepwalker ['sliːpwɔːkə] = SOMNAMBULIST

sleepwalking ['sliːpwɔːkɪŋ] = SOMNAMBULISM

sleepy ['sliːpi] *adjective* feeling ready to go to sleep; *the children are very sleepy by 10 o'clock*; **sleepy sickness** = encephalitis lethargica, virus infection, a form of encephalitis which occurred in epidemics in the 1920s (NOTE: **sleepy - sleepier - sleepiest**)

slice [slaɪs] *noun* thin flat piece of tissue which has been cut off; *he examined the slice of brain tissue under the microscope*

slide [slaɪd] **1** *noun* piece of glass, on which a tissue sample is placed, to be examined under a microscope **2** *verb* to move along smoothly; *the plunger slides up and down the syringe*; **sliding traction** = traction for a fracture of a femur, where weights are attached to pull the leg

slight [slaɪt] *adjective* not very serious; *he has a slight fever*; *she had a slight accident* (NOTE: **slight - slighter - slightest**)

slim [slɪm] **1** *adjective* pleasantly thin; *she has become slim again after being pregnant* **2** *verb* to try to become thinner, to weight less; *he stopped eating bread when he was slimming*; *she is trying to slim before she goes on holiday*; **slimming diet** *or* **slimming food** = special diet or special food which is low in calories and which is supposed to stop a person getting fat

sling [slɪŋ] *noun* triangular bandage attached round the neck, used to support an injured arm and prevent it from moving; *she had her left arm in a sling*; **elevation sling** = sling tied round the neck, used to hold an injured hand or arm in a high position to prevent bleeding

slipped disc ['slɪpt 'dɪsk] *noun* condition where a disc of cartilage separating two bones in the spine becomes displaced, where the soft centre of a disc passes through the hard cartilage outside and presses on a nerve

slough [slʌf] **1** *noun* dead tissue (especially dead skin) which has separated from healthy tissue **2** *verb* to lose dead skin which falls off

slow-release ['sləʊrɪ'liːs] *noun* **slow-release vitamin tablets** = vitamin tablets which will dissolve slowly in the body and to give a longer and more constant effect

slow-wave sleep ['sləʊ'weɪv 'sliːp] *noun* period of sleep when the sleeper sleeps deeply and the eyes do not move

COMMENT: during slow-wave sleep, the pituitary gland secretes the hormone somatotrophin

small [smɔːl] *adjective* **(a)** not large; *his chest was covered with small red spots*; *she has a small cyst on her neck;* **small intestine** = section of the intestine from the stomach to the caecum, consisting of the duodenum, jejunum and ileum; **small stomach** = stomach which is reduced in size after an operation, making the patient unable to eat large meals **(b)** young; *he had chickenpox when he was small*; **small children** = young children (between about 1 and 14 years of age)

small of the back ['smɔːl əv ðə 'bæk] *noun* middle part of the back between and below the shoulder blades

smallpox ['smɔːlpɒks] *noun* variola, formerly a very serious, usually fatal, contagious disease, caused by the poxvirus, with a severe rash, leaving masses of small scars on the skin

COMMENT: vaccination has proved effective in eradicating smallpox

In 1996 it will be the 200th anniversary of Jenner's first smallpox vaccine and smallpox is now clinically extinct

Guardian

smear [smɪə] *noun* sample of soft tissue (such as blood or mucus) taken from a patient and spread over a glass slide to be examined under a microscope; **cervical smear** = test for cervical cancer, where cells taken from the mucus in the cervix of the uterus are examined; **smear test** = PAP TEST

smegma ['smegmə] *noun* oily secretion with an unpleasant smell, which collects on and under the foreskin of the penis

smell [smel] **1** *noun* one of the five senses, the sense which is felt through the nose; *dogs have a good sense of smell*; *the smell of flowers makes him sneeze* **2** *verb* **(a)** to notice the smell of something through the nose; *I can smell smoke*; *he can't smell anything because he's got a cold* **(b)** to produce a smell; *it smells of gas in here* (NOTE: **smelling - smelled** *or* **smelt - has smelled** *or* **has smelt**)

COMMENT: the senses of smell and taste are closely connected, and together give the real taste of food. Smells are sensed by receptors in the nasal cavity which transmit impulses to the brain. When food is eaten, the smell is sensed at the same time as the taste is sensed by the taste buds, and most of what we think of as taste is in fact smell, which explains why food loses its taste when you have a cold and a blocked nose

smelling salts ['smelɪŋ 'sɔːlts] *noun* crystals of an ammonia compound, which give off a strong smell and can revive someone who has fainted

Smith-Petersen nail [ˈsmɪθ'piːtəsən 'neɪl] *noun* metal nail used to attach the fractured neck of a femur

smog [smɒg] *noun* pollution of the atmosphere in towns, caused by warm damp air combining with smoke and exhaust fumes from cars

smoke [sməʊk] **1** *noun* white, grey or black product made of small particles, given off by something which is burning; *the room was full of cigarette smoke*; *several people died from inhaling toxic smoke* **2** *verb* to breathe in smoke from a cigarette, cigar, pipe, etc., which is held in the lips; *she was smoking a cigarette*; *he only smokes a pipe*; *doctors are trying to persuade people to stop smoking*

COMMENT: the connection between smoking tobacco, especially cigarettes, and lung cancer has been proved to the satisfaction of the British government, which prints a health warning on all packets of cigarettes. Smoke from burning tobacco contains nicotine and other substances which stick in the lungs, and can in the long run cause cancer and heart disease

smokeless [ˈsməʊkləs] *adjective* where there is no smoke or where smoke is not allowed; **smokeless** *or* **smoke-free area** = part of a public place (restaurant, aircraft, etc.) where smoking is not allowed; **smokeless fuel** = special fuel which does not make smoke when it is burnt; **smokeless zone** = part of a town where open fires are not permitted

smoker [ˈsməʊkə] *noun* person who smokes cigarettes; **smoker's cough** = dry asthmatic cough, often found in people who smoke large numbers of cigarettes

smoking [ˈsməʊkɪŋ] *noun* action of smoking a cigarette, pipe, cigar, etc.; *smoking can injure your health*

three quarters of patients aged 35-64 on GPs' lists have at least one major risk factor: high cholesterol, high blood pressure or addiction to tobacco. Of the three risk factors, smoking causes a quarter of heart disease deaths

Health Services Journal

smooth [smuːð] **1** *adjective* flat, not rough; **smooth muscle** = involuntary muscle, muscle which moves without a person being

aware of it, such as the muscle in the walls of the intestine which makes the intestine contract; *compare* STRIATED, VOLUNTARY MUSCLE (NOTE: **smooth - smoother - smoothest**) **2** *verb* to make something smooth; *she smoothed down the sheets on the bed*

SMR [ˈes 'em 'ɑː] = SUBMUCOUS RESECTION

snake bite [ˈsneɪk 'baɪt] *noun* bite from a snake, especially a poisonous one

snare [sneə] *noun* surgical instrument made of a loop of wire, used to remove growths without the need of an incision; **diathermy snare** = snare which is heated by electrodes and burns away tissue

sneeze [sniːz] **1** *noun* reflex action to blow air suddenly out of the nose and mouth because of irritation in the nasal passages; *she gave a loud sneeze* **2** *verb* to blow air suddenly out of the nose and mouth because of irritation in the nasal passages; *the smell of flowers makes him sneeze*; *he was coughing and sneezing and decided to stay in bed*

COMMENT: a sneeze sends out a spray of droplets of liquid, which, if infectious, can then infect anyone who happens to inhale them

sneezing fit [ˈsniːzɪŋ fɪt] *noun* sudden attack when the patient sneezes many times

Snellen chart [ˈsnelən 'tʃɑːt] *noun* chart commonly used by opticians to test eyesight; **Snellen type** = different type sizes used on a Snellen chart

COMMENT: the Snellen chart has rows of letters, the top row being very large, and the bottom very small, with the result that the more rows a person can read, the better his eyesight

sniff [snɪf] **1** *noun* breathing in air or smelling through the nose; *they gave her a sniff of smelling salts to revive her* **2** *verb* to breathe in air or to smell through the nose; *he was sniffing because he had a cold*; *she sniffed and said that she could smell smoke*; *he is coughing and sniffing and should be in bed*

sniffle [ˈsnɪfl] *verb* to keep on sniffing, because you have a cold or are crying

sniffles [ˈsnɪflz] *noun (informal, used to children)* cold (when you sniff and sneeze); *don't go out into the cold when you have the sniffles*

snore [snɔː] **1** *noun* loud noise produced in the nose and throat when asleep **2** *verb* to make a loud noise in your nose and throat when you are asleep

COMMENT: a snore is produced by the vibration of the soft palate at the back of the mouth, and occurs when a sleeping person breathes through both mouth and nose

snoring ['snɔːrɪŋ] *noun* making a series of snores

snot [snɒt] *noun (informal)* mucus in the nose

snow [snəʊ] *noun* water which falls as white flakes in cold weather; **snow blindness** = temporary painful blindness caused by bright sunlight shining on snow; **carbon dioxide snow** = carbon dioxide which has been solidified at a very low temperature and is used in treating skin growths such as warts, or to preserve tissue samples

snuffles ['snʌflz] *noun (informal, used of small children)* breathing noisily through a nose which is blocked with mucus, which can sometimes be a sign of congenital syphilis

soak [səʊk] *verb* to put something in liquid, so that it absorbs some of it; *use a compress made of cloth soaked in warm water*

social ['səʊʃl] *adjective* referring to society or to groups of people; *US* **social diseases** = sexually transmitted diseases; **social medicine** = medicine as applied to treatment of diseases which occur in certain social groups; **social security** = payments made by the government to people or families who need money; **social worker** = government official who works to improve living standards of groups (such as families)

socket ['sɒkɪt] *noun* hollow part in a bone, into which another bone or organ fits; *the tip of the femur fits into a socket in the pelvis*; **ball and socket joint** = *see* JOINT; *(of tooth)* **dry socket** = inflammation of the tooth socket after a tooth has been extracted; **eye socket** = orbit, the hollow bony depression in the front of the skull in which each eye is placed

soda ['səʊdə] *see* BICARBONATE

sodium ['səʊdiəm] *noun* chemical element which is the basic substance in salt; **sodium balance** = balance maintained in the body between salt lost in sweat and urine and salt taken in from food, the balance is regulated by aldosterone; **sodium bicarbonate** ($NaHCO_3$) = sodium salt used in cooking, also as a relief for indigestion and acidity; **sodium chloride (NaCl)** = common salt; **sodium pump** = cellular process where sodium is immediately excreted from any cell which it enters and potassium is brought in (NOTE: chemical symbol is **Na**)

COMMENT: salt is an essential mineral and exists in the extracellular fluid of the body. Sweat and tears also contain a high proportion of sodium chloride

sodokosis *or* **sodoku** [səʊdəʊ'kəʊsɪs or 'səʊdəʊkuː] *noun* form of rat-bite fever, but without swellings in the jaws

sodomy ['sɒdəmi] *noun* anal sexual intercourse between men

soft [sɒft] *adjective* not hard; **soft palate** = back part of the palate, leading to the uvula; **soft sore** *or* **soft chancre** = chancroid, a venereal sore with a soft base, situated in the groin or on the genitals and caused by the bacterium *Haemophilus ducreyi* (NOTE: **soft - softer - softest**)

soften ['sɒfn] *verb* to make or become soft

soil [sɔɪl] **1** *noun* earth in which plants grow **2** *verb* to make dirty; *he soiled his sheets*; *soiled bedclothes are sent to the hospital laundry*

solarium [sə'leəriəm] *noun* room where patients can lie under sun lamps or where patients can lie in the sun

solar plexus ['səʊlə 'pleksəs] *noun* nerve network situated at the back of the abdomen between the adrenal glands

sole [səʊl] *noun* part under the foot; *the soles of the feet are very sensitive*

soleus ['səʊliəs] *noun* flat muscle which goes down the calf of the leg

solid ['sɒlɪd] *adjective* hard, not liquid; *water turns solid when it freezes*; **solid food** *or* **solids** = food which is chewed and eaten, not drunk; *she is allowed some solid food or she is allowed to eat solids*

COMMENT: solid foods are introduced gradually to babies and to patients who have had intestinal operations

solidify [sə'lɪdɪfaɪ] *verb* to become solid; *carbon dioxide solidifies at low temperatures*

soln *abbreviation for* SOLUTION

soluble ['sɒljʊbl] *adjective* which can dissolve; *a tablet of soluble aspirin*; **soluble**

fibre = fibre in vegetables, fruit and pulses and porridge oats, which is partly digested in the intestine and reduces the absorption of fats and sugar into the body, so lowering the level of cholesterol

solute ['sɒljuːt] *noun* solid substance which is dissolved in a solvent to make a solution

solution [sə'luːʃn] *noun* mixture of a solid substance dissolved in a liquid; **barium solution** = liquid solution containing barium sulphate (BaSO₄) which a patient drinks to increase the contrast of an X-ray of the alimentary tract

solvent ['sɒlvənt] *noun* liquid in which a solid substance can be dissolved; **solvent inhalation** *or* **solvent abuse** = glue sniffing, type of drug abuse where the addict inhales the toxic fumes given off by certain types of volatile chemical

deaths among teenagers caused by solvent abuse have reached record levels

Health Visitor

soma ['səʊmə] *noun* the body (as opposed to the mind) (NOTE: the plural is **somata** or **somas**)

somat- *or* **somato-** ['səʊmət *or* 'səʊmətəʊ] *prefix* (i) referring to the body; (ii) meaning somatic

somatic [səʊ'mætɪk] *adjective* referring to the body (i) as opposed to the mind; (ii) as opposed to the intestines and inner organs; **somatic nerves** = sensory and motor nerves which control skeletal muscles; *see also* PSYCHOSOMATIC

somatotrophic hormone *or* **somatotrophin** *US* **somatotropin** [səʊmətə'trɒfik 'hɔːməʊn *or* səʊmətə'trəʊfin *or* -trəʊpin] *noun* growth hormone, secreted by the pituitary gland, which stimulates the growth of long bones

-some [səʊm] *suffix* referring to tiny cell bodies

somnambulism [sɒm'næmbjʊlɪzm] *noun* sleepwalking, condition affecting some people (especially children), where the person gets up and walks about while still asleep

somnambulist [sɒm'næmbjʊlɪst] *noun* sleepwalker, person who walks in his sleep

somnambulistic [sɒmnæmbjʊ'lɪstɪk] *adjective* referring to sleepwalking

somnolent ['sɒmnələnt] *adjective* sleepy

somnolism ['sɒmnəlɪzm] *noun* trance which is induced by hypnotism

-somy [səʊmi] *suffix* referring to the presence of chromosomes

son [sʌn] *noun* male child of a parent; *they have two sons and one daughter*

Sonne dysentery ['sɒnə 'dɪsəntri] *noun* common form of mild dysentery in the UK, caused by *Shigella sonnei*

sonogram ['səʊnəgræm] *noun* chart produced using ultrasound waves to find where something is situated in the body

sonoplacentography [səʊnəplæsən'tɒgrəfi] *noun* use of ultrasound waves to find how the placenta is placed in a pregnant woman

sonotopography [səʊnətə'pɒgrəfi] *noun* use of ultrasound waves to produce a sonogram

soothe [suːð] *verb* to relieve pain; *the calamine lotion will soothe the rash*

soothing ['suːðɪŋ] *adjective* which relieves pain or makes someone less tense; *they played soothing music in the dentist's waiting room*

soporific [sɒpə'rɪfik] *noun & adjective* (drug) which makes a person go to sleep

sordes ['sɔːdiːz] *noun* dry deposits round the lips of a patient suffering from fever

sore [sɔː] **1** *noun* small wound on any part of the skin, usually with a discharge of pus; **cold sore** = herpes simplex, a burning sore, usually on the lips; **running sore** = sore which is discharging pus; **soft sore** = soft chancre, venereal sore with a soft base, situated in the groin or on the genitals and caused by the bacterium *Haemophilus ducreyi; see also* BEDSORE **2** *adjective* rough and inflamed (skin); painful (muscle); **sore throat** = condition where the mucous membrane in the throat is inflamed (sometimes because the patient has been talking too much, but usually because of an infection)

s.o.s. ['es 'əʊ 'es] *abbreviation for the Latin phrase* 'si opus sit': if necessary (written on a prescription to show that the dose should be taken once)

souffle [suːfl] *noun* soft breathing sound, heard through a stethoscope

sound [saʊnd] **1** *noun* **(a)** something which can be heard; *the doctor listened to the sounds of the patient's lungs; his breathing* *made a whistling sound* **(b)** long rod, used to examine or to dilate the inside of a cavity in the body **2** *adjective* strong and healthy; *he has a sound constitution; her heart is sound, but her lungs are congested* **3** *verb* **(a)** to make a noise; *her lungs sound as if she had pneumonia* **(b)** to examine the inside of a cavity using a rod

sour ['sauə] *adjective* one of the basic tastes, not bitter, salt or sweet

source [sɔːs] *noun* substance which produces something; place where something comes from; *sugar is a source of energy; vegetables are important sources of vitamins; the source of the allergy has been identified; the medical team has isolated the source of the infection*

soya ['sɔɪə] *noun* plant which produces edible beans which have a high protein and fat content and very little starch

space [speɪs] *noun* place, empty area between things; *an abscess formed in the space between the bone and the cartilage; write your name in the space at the top of the form;* **dead space** = breath in the last part of the inspiration which does not get further than the bronchial tubes

spare [speə] **1** *adjective* extra, which is only used in emergencies; *we have no spare beds in the hospital at the moment; the doctor carries a spare set of instruments in his car;* **spare part surgery** = surgery where parts of the body (such as bones or joints) are replaced by artificial pieces **2** *verb* to be able to give or spend; *can you spare the time to see the next patient?; we have only one bed to spare at the moment*

sparganosis [spɑːgə'nəʊsɪs] *noun* condition caused by the larvae of the worm Sparganum under the skin (it is widespread in the Far East)

spasm ['spæzm] *noun* sudden, usually painful, involuntary contraction of a muscle (as in cramp); *the muscles in his leg went into spasm; she had painful spasms in her stomach;* **clonic spasms** = spasms which recur regularly; **muscle spasm** = sudden sharp contraction of a muscle; *(of a muscle)* **to go into spasm** = to begin to contract

spasmo- ['spæzməʊ] *prefix* referring to a spasm

spasmodic [spæz'mɒdɪk] *adjective* (i) which occurs in spasms; (ii) which happens from time to time

spasmolytic [spæzmə'lɪtɪk] *noun* drug which relieves muscle spasms

spasmus nutans ['spæzməs 'njuːtəns] *noun* condition where the patient nods his head and at the same time has spasms in the neck muscles and rapid movements of the eyes

spastic ['spæstɪk] **1** *adjective* (i) with spasms or sudden contractions of muscles; (ii) referring to cerebral palsy; **spastic colon** = MUCOUS COLITIS; **spastic diplegia** = Little's disease, congenital form of cerebral palsy which affects mainly the legs; **spastic gait** = way of walking where the legs are stiff and the feet not lifted off the ground; **spastic paralysis** = cerebral palsy, disorder of the brain affecting spastics, due to brain damage which has occurred before birth; **spastic paraplegia** = paralysis of one side of the body after a stroke **2** *noun* **a spastic** = patient suffering from cerebral palsy

spasticity [spæ'stɪsəti] *noun* condition where a limb resists passive movement; *see also* RIGIDITY

speak [spiːk] *verb* to say words, to talk; *he is learning to speak again after a laryngectomy* (NOTE: **speaking - spoke - has spoken**)

speak up ['spiːk 'ʌp] *verb* to speak louder; *speak up, please - I can't hear you!*

special ['speʃl] *adjective* which refers to one particular thing, which is not ordinary; *he has been given a special diet to cure his allergy; she wore special shoes to correct a defect in her ankles;* **special care baby unit** = unit in a hospital which deals with premature babies or babies with serious disorders; **special hospital** = hospital for dangerous mental patients; **special school** = school for children who are handicapped

specialism ['speʃəlɪzm] = SPECIALITY

specialist ['speʃəlɪst] *noun* doctor who specializes in a certain branch of medicine; *he is a heart specialist; she was referred to an ENT specialist*

speciality [speʃɪ'ælɪti] *noun* particular branch of medicine

specialization [speʃəlaɪ'zeɪʃn] *noun* (i) act of specializing in a certain branch of medicine; (ii) particular branch of medicine which a doctor specializes in

specialize in ['speʃəlaɪz 'ɪn] *verb* to study or to treat one particular disease or one particular type of patient; *he specializes in* *children with breathing problems*; *she decided to specialize in haematology*

specialty ['speʃəltɪ] *US* = SPECIALITY

species ['spiːʃiːz] *noun* division of a genus, group of living things which can interbreed

specific [spə'sɪfɪk] **1** *adjective* particular, (disease) caused by one microbe; **specific urethritis** = inflammation of the urethra caused by gonorrhoea; *see also* NON-SPECIFIC **2** *noun* drug which is used to treat a particular disease

specificity [spesɪ'fɪsətɪ] *noun* rate of negative responses in a test from persons free from a disease (a high specificity means a low rate of false positives); *compare with* SENSITIVITY

specimen ['spesəmɪn] *noun* (i) small quantity of something given for testing; (ii) one item out of a group; *he was asked to bring a urine specimen*; *we keep specimens of diseased organs for students to examine*

spectacles ['spektəkəlz] *plural noun* glasses which are worn in front of the eyes to help correct defects in vision; *the optician said he needed a new pair of spectacles*; *she was wearing a pair of spectacles with gold frames*

> COMMENT: spectacles can correct defects in the focusing of the eye, such as shortsightedness, longsightedness and astigmatism. Where different lenses are required for reading, an optician may prescribe two pairs of spectacles, one for normal use and the other reading glasses. Otherwise, spectacles can be fitted with a divided lens (bifocals)

spectrography [spek'trɒgrəfɪ] *noun* recording of a spectrum on photographic film

spectroscope ['spektrəskəʊp] *noun* instrument used to analyse a spectrum

spectrum ['spektrəm] *noun* (i) range of colours (from red to violet) into which white light can be split (different substances in solution have different spectra); (ii) range of diseases which an antibiotic can be used to treat; **broad-spectrum antibiotic** = antibiotic used to control many types of bacteria (NOTE: the plural is **spectra**)

narrow-spectrum compounds have a significant advantage over broad-spectrum ones in that they do not upset the body's normal flora to the same extent
British Journal of Hospital Medicine

speculum ['spekjʊləm] *noun* surgical instrument which is inserted into an opening in the body (such as a nostril or the vagina) to keep it open, and allow a doctor to examine the inside (NOTE: the plural is **specula, speculums**)

speech [spiːtʃ] *noun* making intelligible sounds with the vocal cords; **speech block** = temporary inability to speak, caused by the effect of nervous stress on the mental processes; **speech impediment** = condition where a person cannot speak properly because of a deformed mouth or tongue; **speech therapist** = qualified person who practises speech therapy; **speech therapy** = treatment to cure a speech disorder such as stammering, or following a stroke

spell [spel] *noun* short period; *she has dizzy spells*; *he had two spells in hospital during the winter*

sperm [spɜːm] *noun* spermatozoon, a male sex cell; **sperm bank** = place where sperm can be stored for use in artificial insemination; **sperm count** = calculation of the number of sperm in a quantity of semen; **sperm duct** = the vas deferens, the tube along which sperm pass from the epididymis to the prostate gland (NOTE: no plural for **sperm: there are millions of sperm in each ejaculation)**

sperm- *or* **spermi(o)-** *or* **spermo-** ['spɜːm *or* 'spɜːmiəʊ *or* 'spɜːməʊ] *prefix* referring to sperm and semen

spermat- *or* **spermato-** ['spɜːmət *or* 'spɜːmətəʊ] *prefix* referring to (i) sperm; (ii) the male reproductive system

spermatic [spɜː'mætɪk] *adjective* referring to sperm; **spermatic artery** = artery which leads into the testes; **spermatic cord** = cord running from the testis to the abdomen carrying the vas deferens, the blood vessels, nerves and lymphatics of the testis

spermatid ['spɜːmətɪd] *noun* immature cell, formed from a spermatocyte, which becomes a spermatozoon

spermatocele ['spɜːmətəsiːl] *noun* cyst which forms in the scrotum

spermatocyte ['spɜːmətəsaɪt] *noun* early stage in the development of a spermatozoon

spermatogenesis [spɜːmətə'dʒenəsɪs] *noun* formation and development of spermatozoa in the testes

spermatogonium [spɜːmətə'gəʊnɪəm] *noun* cell which forms a spermatocyte

spermatorrhoea [spɜːmətəˈriːə] *noun* discharge of a large amount of semen frequently and without an orgasm

spermatozoon [spɜːmətəˈzəʊɒn] *noun* sperm, a mature male sex cell, which is ejaculated from the penis and is capable of fertilizing an ovum (NOTE: the plural is **spermatozoa**)

COMMENT: a human spermatozoon is very small and is formed of a head, neck and very long tail. A spermatozoon can swim by moving its tail from side to side. The sperm are formed in the testes and ejaculated through the penis. Each ejaculation may contain millions of sperm. Once a sperm has entered the female uterus, it remains viable for about three days

spermaturia [spɜːməˈtjʊəriə] *noun* sperm in the urine

spermicidal [spɜːmɪˈsaɪdl] *adjective* which can kill sperm; **spermicidal jelly** = jelly-like product which acts as a contraceptive

spermicide [ˈspɜːmɪsaɪd] *noun* substance which kills sperm

spheno- [ˈsfiːnəʊ] *prefix* referring to the sphenoid bone

sphenoid bone [ˈsfiːnɔɪd ˈbəʊn] *noun* one of two bones in the skull which form the side of the socket of the eye; **sphenoid sinus** *or* **sphenoidal sinus** = one of the sinuses in the skull behind the nasal passage

sphenopalatine ganglion [sfiːnəʊˈpælətaɪn ˈɡænɡliɒn] *noun* ganglion in the pterygopalatine fossa associated with maxillary sinus

spherocyte [ˈsfɪərəʊsaɪt] *noun* abnormal round red blood cell

spherocytosis [sfɪərəʊsaɪˈtəʊsɪs] *noun* condition where a patient has spherocytes in his blood, causing anaemia, enlarged spleen and gallstones, as in acholuric jaundice

sphincter [ˈsfɪŋktə] *noun* **sphincter** *or* **sphincter muscle** = ring of muscle at the opening of a passage in the body, which can contract to close the passage; **anal sphincter** = ring of muscle which closes the anus; **pyloric sphincter** = muscle which surrounds the pylorus, makes it contract and separates it from the duodenum; **sphincter pupillae muscle** = annular muscle in the iris which constricts the pupil

sphincterectomy [sfɪŋktəˈrektəmi] *noun* surgical operation to remove (i) a sphincter; (ii) part of the edge of the iris in the eye

sphincteroplasty [ˈsfɪŋktərəplæsti] *noun* surgery to relieve a tightened sphincter

sphincterotomy [sfɪŋktəˈrɒtəmi] *noun* surgical operation to make an incision into a sphincter

sphyg [sfɪɡ] *noun* (*informal*) = SPHYGMOMANOMETER

sphygmo- [ˈsfɪɡməʊ] *prefix* referring to the pulse

sphygmocardiograph [sfɪɡməˈkɑːdiəʊɡrɑːf] *noun* device which records heartbeats and pulse rate

sphygmograph [ˈsfɪɡməɡrɑːf] *noun* device which records the pulse

sphygmomanometer [sfɪɡməʊməˈnɒmɪtə] *noun* instrument which measures blood pressure in the arteries

COMMENT: the sphygmomanometer is a rubber sleeve connected to a scale with a column of mercury, allowing the nurse to take a reading; the rubber sleeve is usually wrapped round the arm and inflated until the blood flow is stopped; the blood pressure is determined by listening to the pulse with a stethoscope placed over an artery as the pressure in the rubber sleeve is slowly reduced, and by the reading on the scale

spica [ˈspaɪkə] *noun* way of bandaging a joint where the bandage crisscrosses over itself like the figure 8 on the inside of the bend of the joint (NOTE: the plural is **spicae** or **spicas**)

spicule [ˈspɪkjuːl] *noun* small splinter of bone

spina bifida [ˈspaɪnə ˈbɪfɪdə] *noun* rachischisis, serious condition where part of the spinal cord protrudes through the spinal column

COMMENT: spina bifida takes two forms: a mild form, spina bifida occulta, where only the bone is affected, and there are no visible signs of the condition; and the serious spina bifida cystica where part of the meninges or spinal cord passes through the gap; it may result in paralysis of the legs, and mental retardation is often present where the condition is associated with hydrocephalus

spinal [ˈspaɪnl] *adjective* referring to the spine; *he has spinal problems*; *she suffered spinal injuries in the crash*; **spinal accessory nerve** = eleventh cranial nerve which supplies the muscles in the neck and shoulders; **spinal anaesthesia** = local anaesthesia (subarachnoid or epidural) in which an anaesthetic is injected into the cerebrospinal fluid; **spinal block** = analgesia produced by injecting an analgesic solution into the space between the vertebral canal and the dura mater; **spinal canal** = the vertebral canal, the hollow running down through the vertebrae, containing the spinal cord; **spinal column** = backbone, spine or vertebral column; **spinal cord** = part of the central nervous system running from the medulla oblongata to the filum terminale, in the vertebral canal of the spine; **spinal curvature** *or* **curvature of the spine** = abnormal bending of the spine; **spinal fusion** = surgical operation to join two vertebrae together to make the spine more rigid; **spinal nerves** = 31 pairs of nerves which lead from the spinal cord; **spinal puncture** *or* **lumbar puncture,** *US* **spinal tap** = surgical operation to remove a sample of cerebrospinal fluid by inserting a hollow needle into the lower part of the spinal canal (NOTE: for terms referring to the spinal cord, see words beginning with **myel-, myelo-, rachi-, rachio-**)

spindle ['spɪndl] *noun* long thin structure; **spindle fibre** = one of the elements visible during cell division; **muscle spindles** = sensory receptors which lie along striated muscle fibres

spine [spaɪn] *noun* (i) backbone, the series of bones (the vertebrae) linked together to form a flexible supporting column running from the pelvis to the skull; (ii) any sharp projecting part of a bone; *she injured her spine or she had spine injuries in the crash*; **spine of the scapula** = ridge on the posterior face of the scapula; *see illustration at* SHOULDER

COMMENT: the spine is made up of twenty-four ring-shaped vertebrae, with the sacrum and coccyx, separated by discs of cartilage. The hollow canal of the spine (the spinal canal) contains the spinal cord. See also note at VERTEBRA

spino- ['spaɪnəʊ] *prefix* referring to (i) the spine; (ii) the spinal cord

spinocerebellar tracts [spaɪnəʊserə'belə 'trækts] *noun* nerve fibres in the spinal cord, taking impulses to the cerebellum

spinous process ['spaɪnəs 'prəʊses] *noun* projection on a vertebra or a bone, that looks like a spine; *see illustration at* VERTEBRAL COLUMN

spiral ['spaɪrəl] *adjective* which runs in a continuous circle upwards; **spiral bandage** = bandage which is wrapped round a limb, each turn overlapping the one before; **spiral ganglion** = ganglion in the eighth cranial nerve which supplies the organ of Corti; **spiral organ** = ORGAN OF CORTI

Spirillum [spɪ'rɪləm] *noun* one of the bacteria which cause rat-bite fever

spirit ['spɪrɪt] *noun* strong mixture of alcohol and water; **methylated spirit(s)** = almost pure alcohol, with wood alcohol and colouring added; **surgical spirit** = ethyl alcohol with an additive giving it an unpleasant taste, used as a disinfectant or for cleansing the skin

spiro- ['spaɪrəʊ] *prefix* referring to (i) a spiral; (ii) the respiration

spirochaetaemia [spaɪrəʊkɪ'tiːmiə] *noun* presence of spirochaetes in the blood

spirochaete *US* **spirochete** ['spaɪrəʊkiːt] *noun* bacterium with a spiral shape, such as that which causes syphilis

spirogram ['spaɪrəʊgræm] *noun* record of a patient's breathing made by a spirograph

spirograph ['spaɪrəʊgrɑːf] *noun* device which records depth and rapidity of breathing

spirography [spaɪ'rɒgrəfi] *noun* recording of a patient's breathing by use of a spirograph

spirometer [spaɪ'rɒmɪtə] *noun* instrument which measures how much air a person inhales or exhales

spirometry [spaɪ'rɒmətri] *noun* measurement of the vital capacity of the lungs by use of a spirometer

spit [spɪt] **1** *noun* saliva which is sent out of the mouth **2** *verb* to send liquid out of the mouth; *rinse your mouth out and spit into the cup provided*; *he spat out the medicine* (NOTE: **spitting - spat - has spat**)

Spitz-Holter valve ['spɪts'hɒltə 'vælv] *noun* valve with a one-way system, surgically placed in the skull, and used to drain excess fluid from the brain in hydrocephalus

splanchnic ['splæŋknɪk] *adjective* referring to viscera; **splanchnic nerve** = any sympathetic nerve which supplies organs in the abdomen

splanchnology [splæŋk'nɒlədʒi] *noun* special study of the organs in the abdominal cavity

spleen [spliːn] *noun* organ in the top part of the abdominal cavity behind the stomach and below the diaphragm; *see illustration at* DIGESTIVE SYSTEM

> COMMENT: the spleen, which is the largest endocrine (ductless) gland, appears to act to remove dead blood cells and fight infection, but its functions are not fully understood and an adult can live normally after his spleen has been removed

splen- *or* **spleno-** [splən or 'spliːnəʊ] *prefix* referring to the spleen

splenectomy [sple'nektəmi] *noun* surgical operation to remove the spleen

splenic ['splenɪk] *adjective* referring to the spleen; **splenic anaemia** = type of anaemia where the patient has portal hypertension, an enlarged spleen and haemorrhages, caused by cirrhosis of the liver (NOTE: also called **Banti's syndrome** *or* **Banti's disease**); **splenic flexure** = bend in the colon, where the transverse colon joins the descending colon

splenitis [splə'naɪtɪs] *noun* inflammation of the spleen

splenomegaly [spliːnəʊ'megəli] *noun* condition where the spleen is abnormally large, associated with several disorders including malaria and some cancers

splenorenal anastomosis [spliːnəʊ'riːnl ənæstə'məʊsɪs] *noun* surgical operation to join the splenic vein to a renal vein, as a treatment for portal hypertension

splenovenography [spliːnəʊvə'nɒgrəfi] *noun* X-ray examination of the spleen and the veins which are connected to it

splint [splɪnt] *noun* **(a)** stiff support attached to a limb to prevent a broken bone from moving; *he had to keep his arm in a splint for several weeks*; *see also* BRAUN'S SPLINT, DENIS BROWNE SPLINT, FAIRBANKS' SPLINT, THOMAS'S SPLINT **(b)** shin splints = *see* SHIN

splinter ['splɪntə] *noun* tiny thin piece of wood or metal which gets under the skin and can be irritating and cause infection

split [splɪt] *verb* to divide

split-skin graft ['splɪt'skɪn 'grɑːft] *noun* Thiersch graft, a type of skin graft where thin layers of skin are grafted over a wound

spondyl ['spɒndɪl] *noun* a vertebra

spondyl- *or* **spondylo-** ['spɒndɪl or 'spɒndɪləʊ] *prefix* referring to the vertebrae

spondylitis [spɒndɪ'laɪtɪs] *noun* inflammation of the vertebrae; **ankylosing spondylitis** = condition with higher incidence in young men, where the vertebrae and sacroiliac joints are inflamed and become stiff

spondylolisthesis [spɒndɪləʊ'lɪsθəsɪs] *noun* condition where one of the lumbar vertebrae moves forward over the one beneath

spondylosis [spɒndɪ'ləʊsɪs] *noun* stiffness in the spine and degenerative changes in the intervertebral discs, with osteoarthritis (it is common in older people); **cervical spondylosis** = degenerative change in the neck bones

sponge ['spʌnʒ] *noun* piece of light absorbent material, either natural or synthetic, used in bathing, cleaning, etc.; **contraceptive sponge** = piece of synthetic sponge impregnated with spermicide, which is inserted into the vagina before intercourse

sponge bath ['spʌnʒ 'bɑːθ] *noun* washing a patient in bed, using a sponge or damp cloth; *the nurse gave the old lady a sponge bath*

spongioblastoma [spʌnʒiəʊblæ'stəʊmə] = GLIOBLASTOMA

spongiosum [spʌnʒɪ'əʊsəm] *see* CORPUS

spongy ['spʌnʒi] *adjective* soft and full of holes like a sponge; **spongy bone** = cancellous bone, light spongy bone tissue which forms the inner core of a bone and also the ends of long bones; *see illustration at* BONE STRUCTURE

spontaneous [spɒn'teɪnɪəs] *adjective* which happens without any particular outside cause; **spontaneous abortion** = MISCARRIAGE

spoon [spuːn] *noun* instrument with a long handle at one end and a small bowl at the other, used for taking liquid medicine; *a 5 ml spoon*

spoonful ['spuːnfʊl] *noun* quantity which a spoon can hold; *take two 5 ml spoonfuls of the medicine twice a day*

sporadic [spə'rædɪk] *adjective* (disease) where outbreaks occur as separate cases, not in epidemics

spore [spɔː] *noun* reproductive body of certain bacteria and fungi which can survive in extremely hot or cold conditions for a long time

sporicidal [spɔːrɪ'saɪdl] *adjective* which kills spores

sporicide ['spɔ:rɪsaɪd] *noun* substance which kills bacterial spores

sporotrichosis [spɔ:rəʊtraɪ'kəʊsɪs] *noun* fungus infection of the skin which causes abscesses

Sporozoa [spɔ:rə'zəʊə] *noun* type of parasitic Protozoa which includes Plasmodium, the cause of malaria

sport [spɔ:t] *noun* playing of games; **sports injuries** = injuries commonly occurring when playing sports (injuries to the neck in Rugby, ligament injuries in football, etc.); **sports medicine** = study of the treatment of sports injuries

spot [spɒt] *noun* small round mark or pimple; *the disease is marked by red spots on the chest; he suddenly came out in spots on his chest;* **black spots (in front of the eyes)** = moving black dots seen when looking at something, more noticeable when a person is tired or run-down, more common in shortsighted people; **to break out in spots** *or* **to come out in spots** = to have a sudden rash; *see also* KOPLIK

spotted fever ['spɒtɪd 'fi:və] *noun* meningococcal meningitis, the commonest epidemic form of meningitis, caused by a bacterial infection, where the meninges become inflamed causing headaches and fever; *see also* ROCKY MOUNTAIN

spotty ['spɒti] *adjective* covered with pimples

sprain [spreɪn] **1** *noun* condition where the ligaments in a joint are stretched or torn because of a sudden movement **2** *verb* to tear the ligaments in a joint with a sudden movement; *she sprained her wrist when she fell*

spray [spreɪ] **1** *noun* **(a)** mass of tiny drops; *an aerosol sends out a liquid in a fine spray* **(b)** special liquid for spraying onto an infection; *throat spray or nasal spray* **2** *verb* to send out a liquid in fine drops; *they sprayed the room with disinfectant*

spread [spred] *verb* to go out over a large area; *the infection spread right through the adult population; sneezing in a crowded bus can spread infection* (NOTE: **spreading - spread - has spread**)

> spreading infection may give rise to cellulitis of the abdominal wall and abscess formation
>
> *Nursing Times*

Sprengel's deformity *or* **Sprengel's shoulder** ['spreŋgəlz dɪ'fɔ:məti *or* 'spreŋgəlz 'ʃəʊldə] *noun* congenitally deformed shoulder, where one scapula is smaller and higher than the other

sprue [spru:] = PSILOSIS

spud [spʌd] *noun* needle used to get a piece of dust or other foreign body out of the eye

spur [spɜ:] *noun* sharp projecting part of a bone

sputum ['spju:təm] *noun* phlegm, mucus which is formed in the inflamed nose, throat or lungs and is coughed up; *she was coughing up bloodstained sputum*

squama ['skweɪmə] *noun* thin piece of hard tissue, such as a thin flake of bone or scale on the skin (NOTE: the plural is **squamae**)

squamous ['skweɪməs] *adjective* thin and hard like a scale; **squamous bone** = part of the temporal bone which forms the side of the skull; **squamous epithelium** = epithelium with flat cells like scales which forms the lining of the pericardium, the peritoneum and the pleura (NOTE: also called **pavement epithelium**)

squint [skwɪnt] **1** *noun* strabismus, a condition where the eyes focus on different points; **convergent squint** = condition where one or both eyes look towards the nose; **divergent squint** = condition where one or both eyes look away from the nose **2** *verb* to have one eye or both eyes looking towards the nose; *babies often appear to squint, but it is corrected as they grow older*

Sr *chemical symbol for* strontium

SRN ['es 'ɑ: 'en] = STATE REGISTERED NURSE

SSRI ['es 'es 'ɑ: 'aɪ] = SELECTIVE SEROTONIN RE-UPTAKE INHIBITOR

stab [stæb] **1** *noun* **(a)** **stab wound** = deep wound made by the point of a knife **(b)** sharp pain; *he had a stab of pain in his right eye* **2** *verb* to cut by pushing the point of a knife into the flesh; *he was stabbed in the chest*

stabbing ['stæbɪŋ] *adjective* (pain) in a series of short sharp stabs; *he had stabbing pains in his chest*

stabilize ['steɪbəlaɪz] *verb* to make a condition stable; *we have succeeded in stabilizing his blood sugar level*

stable ['steɪbl] *adjective* not changing; *his condition is stable*; **stable angina** = angina which has not changed for a long time

staccato speech [stə'kɑːtəʊ 'spiːtʃ] *noun* abnormal way of speaking, with short pauses between each word

Stacke's operation ['stækɪz ɒpə'reɪʃn] *noun* surgical operation to remove the posterior and superior wall of the auditory meatus

stadium invasioni ['steɪdiəm ɪnveɪʃi'əʊni] *noun* incubation period, the period between catching an infectious disease and the appearance of the first symptoms of the disease

staff [stɑːf] *noun* people who work in a hospital, clinic, doctor's surgery, etc.; *we have 25 full-time medical staff; the hospital is trying to recruit more nursing staff; the clinic has a staff of 100*; **staff midwife** = midwife who is on the permanent staff of a hospital; **staff nurse** = senior nurse who is employed full-time (NOTE: when used as a subject, **staff** takes a plural verb: **a staff of 25** but **the ancillary staff work very hard**)

stage [steɪdʒ] *noun* point in the development of a disease, which allows a decision to be taken about the treatment which should be given; *the disease has reached a critical stage; this is a symptom of the second stage of syphilis*

memory changes are associated with early stages of the disease; in later stages, the patient is frequently incontinent, immobile and unable to communicate
Nursing Times

stagger ['stægə] *verb* to move from side to side while walking, to walk unsteadily

stagnant loop syndrome ['stægnənt 'luːp 'sɪndrəʊm] *see* LOOP

stain [steɪn] **1** *noun* dye, substance used to give colour to tissues which are going to be examined under the microscope; *see also* COUNTERSTAIN **2** *verb* to treat a piece of tissue with a dye to increase contrast before it is examined under the microscope

COMMENT: some stains are designed to have an affinity only with those chemical, cellular or bacterial elements in a specimen that are of interest to a microbiologist; thus the concentration or uptake of a stain, as well as giving the overall picture, can be diagnostic

staining ['steɪnɪŋ] *noun* colouring of tissue, bacterial samples, etc., to make it possible to examine them and to identify them under the microscope; **immunological staining** = checking if cancer is likely to return after the patient has been declared free of the disease, by staining cells

stalk [stɔːk] *noun* stem, piece of tissue which attaches a growth to the main tissue

stammer ['stæmə] **1** *noun* speech defect, where the patient repeats parts of a word or the whole word several times or stops to try to pronounce a word; *he has a bad stammer; she is taking therapy to try to correct her stammer* **2** *verb* to speak with a stammer

stammerer ['stæmərə] *noun* person who stammers

stammering ['stæmərɪŋ] *noun* dysphemia, difficulty in speaking, where the person repeats parts of a word or the whole word several times or stops to try to pronounce a word; *see also* STUTTER

stamp out ['stæmp 'aʊt] *verb* to remove completely; *international organizations have succeeded in stamping out smallpox; the government is trying to stamp out waste in the hospital service*

standard ['stændəd] **1** *adjective* normal; *it is standard practice to take the patient's temperature twice a day* **2** *noun* something which has been agreed upon and is used to measure other things by; *the standard of care in hospitals has increased over the last years; the report criticized the standards of hygiene in the clinic*; **gold standard** = the best measure of a disease against which screening tests, diagnostic methods, etc., are compared

stand up ['stænd 'ʌp] *verb* **(a)** to get up from being on a seat; *he tried to stand up, but did not have the strength* **(b)** to hold yourself upright; *she still stands up straight at the age of ninety-two*

stapedectomy [steɪpi'dektəmi] *noun* surgical operation to remove the stapes

stapediolysis *or* **stapedial mobilization** [stəpi:di'ɒləsɪs *or* stə'piːdiəl məʊbɪlaɪ'zeɪʃn] *noun* surgical operation to relieve deafness by detaching an immobile stapes from the fenestra ovalis

stapes ['steɪpiːz] *noun* one of the three ossicles in the middle ear, shaped like a stirrup; **mobilization of the stapes** = STAPEDIOLYSIS; *see illustration at* EAR

COMMENT: the stapes fills the fenestra ovalis, and is articulated with the incus, which in turn articulates with the malleus

staphylectomy [stæfɪ'lektəmi] *noun* surgical operation to remove the uvula

staphylococcal [stæfɪlə'kɒkl] *adjective* referring to Staphylococci; **staphylococcal poisoning** = poisoning by Staphylococci which have spread in food

Staphylococcus [stæfɪlə'kɒkəs] *noun* bacterium which grows in a bunch like a bunch of grapes, and causes boils and food poisoning (NOTE: the plural is **Staphylococci**)

staphyloma [stæfɪ'ləʊmə] *noun* swelling of the cornea or the white of the eye

staphylorrhaphy [stæfɪ'lɔːrəfi] = PALATORRHAPHY

staple ['steɪpl] **1** *noun* small piece of bent metal, used to attach tissues together **2** *verb* to attach tissues with staples

stapler ['steɪplə] *noun* device used in surgery to attach tissues with staples, instead of suturing

starch [staːtʃ] *noun* usual form in which carbohydrates exist in food, especially in bread, rice and potatoes

COMMENT: starch is present in common foods, and is broken down by the digestive process into forms of sugar

starchy ['staːtʃi] *adjective* (food) which contains a lot of starch; *he eats too much starchy food*

Starling's Law ['staːlɪŋz 'lɔː] *noun* law that the contraction of the ventricles is in proportion to the length of the ventricular muscle fibres at end of diastole

starvation [staː'veɪʃn] *noun* having had very little or no food; **starvation diet** = diet which contains little nourishment, and is not enough to keep a person healthy

starve [staːv] *verb* to have little or no food or nourishment; *the parents let the baby starve to death*

-stasis ['steɪsɪs] *suffix* referring to stoppage in the flow of a liquid

stasis ['steɪsɪs] *noun* stoppage or slowing in the flow of a liquid (such as blood in veins, food in the intestine)

A decreased blood flow in the extremities has been associated with venous stasis which may precipitate vascular complications

British Journal of Nursing

stat. *abbreviation for the Latin word* 'statim': immediately (written on prescriptions)

state [steɪt] *noun* **(a)** the condition of something or of a person; *his state of health is getting worse*; *the disease is in an advanced state* **(b)** *(formerly in Britain)* **State Registered Nurse** = nurse qualified to carry out all nursing services

statin ['stætɪn] *noun* a lipid-lowering drug which inhibits an enzyme in cholesterol synthesis, used to treat patients with, or at high risk of developing coronary heart disease

-statin ['stætɪn] *suffix* used in generic names of lipid-lowering drugs; *pravastatin*

statistics [stə'tɪstɪks] *plural noun* study of facts in the form of official figures; *population statistics show that the birth rate is slowing down*

status ['steɪtəs] *Latin for* 'state'; **status asthmaticus** = attack of bronchial asthma which lasts for a long time and results in exhaustion and collapse; **status epilepticus** = repeated and prolonged epileptic seizures without recovery of consciousness between them; **status lymphaticus** = condition where the glands in the lymphatic system are enlarged

the main indications being inadequate fluid and volume status and need for evaluation of patients with a history of severe heart disease
Southern Medical Journal

the standard pulmonary artery catheters have four lumens from which to obtain information about the patient's haemodynamic status
RN Magazine

stay [steɪ] **1** *noun* time which someone spends in a place; *the patient is only in hospital for a short stay*; **long stay patient** = patient who will stay in hospital for a long time; **long stay ward** = ward for patients who will stay in hospital for a long time **2** *verb* to stop in a place for some time; *she stayed in hospital for two weeks*; *he's ill with flu and has to stay in bed*

STD ['es 'tiː 'diː] = SEXUALLY TRANSMITTED DISEASE

steapsin [stiˈæpsɪn] *noun* enzyme produced by the pancreas, which breaks down fats in the intestine

stearic acid [stiˈærɪk ˈæsɪd] *noun* one of the fatty acids

steat- *or* **steato-** [ˈstiːət *or* ˈstiːətəʊ] *prefix* referring to fat

steatoma [stiːəˈtəʊmə] *noun* sebaceous cyst, a cyst in a blocked sebaceous gland

steatorrhoea [stiːətəˈriːə] *noun* condition where fat is passed in the faeces

Stein-Leventhal syndrome [ˈstaɪnˈlevəntɑːl ˈsɪndrəʊm] *noun* condition in young women, where menstruation becomes rare, or never takes place, together with growth of body hair, usually due to cysts in the ovaries

Steinmann's pin [ˈstaɪnmænz ˈpɪn] *noun* pin for attaching traction wires to a fractured bone

stellate [ˈsteleɪt] *adjective* shaped like a star; **stellate fracture** = fracture of the kneecap, shaped like a star; **stellate ganglion** = inferior cervical ganglion, group of nerve cells in the neck

Stellwag's sign [ˈstelvɑːgz ˈsaɪn] *noun* symptom of exophthalmic goitre, where the patient does not blink often, because the eyeball is protruding

stem [stem] *noun* thin piece of tissue which attaches an organ or growth to the main tissue; **brain stem** = lower part of the brain which connects the brain to the spinal cord

steno- [ˈstenəʊ] *prefix* meaning (i) narrow; (ii) constricted

stenose [steˈnəʊz] *verb* to make narrow; **stenosed valve** = valve which has become narrow or constricted; **stenosing condition** = condition which makes a passage narrow

stenosis [steˈnəʊsɪs] *noun* condition where a passage becomes narrow; **aortic stenosis** = condition where the aortic valve is narrow; **mitral stenosis** = condition where the opening in the mitral valve becomes smaller because the cusps have fused (almost always the result of rheumatic endocarditis); **pulmonary stenosis** = condition where the opening to the pulmonary artery in the right ventricle becomes narrow

stenostomia *or* **stenostomy** [stenəʊˈstəʊmiə *or* steˈnɒstəmi] *noun* abnormal narrowing of an opening

Stensen's duct [ˈstensənz ˈdʌkt] *noun* duct which carries saliva from the parotid gland

stent [stent] *noun* support of artificial material, often inserted in a tube or vessel which has been sutured, or in an artery which has been cleared

step [step] *noun* movement of the foot and the leg as in walking; *he took two steps forward*; *the baby is taking his first steps*

step up [ˈstep ˈʌp] *verb* (*informal*) to increase; *the doctor has stepped up the dosage*

sterco- [ˈstɜːkəʊ] *prefix* referring to faeces

stercobilin [stɜːkəˈbaɪlɪn] *noun* brown pigment which colours the faeces

stercobilinogen [stɜːkəbaɪˈlɪnədʒen] *noun* substance which is broken down from bilirubin and produces stercobilin

stercolith [ˈstɜːkəlɪθ] *noun* hard ball of dried faeces in the bowel

stercoraceous [stɜːkəˈreɪʃəs] *adjective* made of faeces; similar to faeces; containing faeces

stereognosis [steriɒgˈnəʊsɪs] *noun* being able to tell the shape of an object in three dimensions by means of touch

stereoscopic vision [steriəˈskɒpɪk ˈvɪʒn] *noun* being able to judge the distance and depth of an object by binocular vision

stereotaxy *or* **stereotaxic surgery** [steriəʊˈtæksi *or* steriəʊˈtæksɪk ˈsɜːdʒəri] *noun* surgical procedure to identify a point in the interior of the brain, before an operation can begin, to locate exactly the area to be operated on

stereotypy [ˈsteriəʊtaɪpi] *noun* repeating the same action or word again and again

sterile [ˈsteraɪl] *adjective* (a) with no microbes or infectious organisms; *she put a sterile dressing on the wound*; *he opened a pack of sterile dressings* (b) infertile, not able to produce children

sterility [stəˈrɪləti] *noun* (i) being free from microbes; (ii) infertility, being unable to produce children

sterilization [sterɪlaɪˈzeɪʃn] *noun* (i) action of making instruments, etc., free from microbes; (ii) action of making a person sterile

COMMENT: sterilization of a woman can be done by removing the ovaries or cutting the Fallopian tubes; sterilization of a man is carried out by cutting the vas deferens (vasectomy)

sterilize ['sterəlaɪz] *verb* **(a)** to make something sterile (by killing microbes); *surgical instruments must be sterilized before use*; *not using sterilized needles can cause infection* **(b)** to make a person unable to have children

sterilizer ['sterəlaɪzə] *noun* machine for sterilizing surgical instruments by steam, boiling water, etc.

sternal ['stɜːnl] *adjective* referring to the breastbone; **sternal angle** = ridge of bone where the manubrium articulates with the body of the sternum; **sternal puncture** = surgical operation to remove a sample of bone marrow from the breastbone for testing

sternoclavicular angle [stɜːnəʊklə'vɪkjʊlə 'æŋgəl] *noun* angle between the sternum and the clavicle

sternocleidomastoid muscle [stɜːnəʊklaɪdəʊ'mæstɔɪd 'mʌsl] *noun* muscle in the neck, running from the breastbone to the mastoid process

sternocostal joint [stɜːnəʊ'kɒstl 'dʒɔɪnt] *noun* joint where the breastbone joins a rib

sternohyoid muscle [stɜːnəʊ'haɪɔɪd 'mʌsl] *noun* muscle in the neck which runs from the breastbone into the hyoid bone

sternomastoid [stɜːnəʊ'mæstɔɪd] *adjective* referring to the breastbone and the mastoid; **sternomastoid muscle = STERNOCLEIDOMASTOID MUSCLE; sternomastoid tumour** = benign tumour which appears in the sternomastoid muscle in newborn babies

sternotomy [stɜː'nɒtəmi] *noun* surgical operation to cut through the breastbone, so as to be able to operate on the heart

sternum ['stɜːnəm] *noun* the breastbone, bone in the centre of the front of the chest

COMMENT: the sternum runs from the neck to the bottom of the diaphragm. It is formed of the manubrium (the top section), the body of the sternum, and the xiphoid process. The upper seven pairs of ribs are attached to the sternum

sternutatory [stɜː'njuː'teɪtəri] *noun* substance which makes someone sneeze

steroid ['stɪərɔɪd] *noun* any of several chemical compounds with characteristic ring systems, including the sex hormones, which affect the body and its functions

COMMENT: the word steroid is usually used to refer to corticosteroids. Synthetic steroids are used in steroid therapy, to treat arthritis, asthma and some blood disorders. They are also used by some athletes to improve their physical strength, but these are banned by athletic organizations and can have serious side-effects

steroidal ['stɪərɔɪdəl] *adjective* containing steroids (NOTE: the opposite is **non-steroidal**)

sterol ['stiərɒl] *noun* insoluble substance which belongs to the steroid alcohols such as cholesterol

stertor ['stɜːtə] *noun* noisy breathing sounds in an unconscious patient

steth- *or* **stetho-** ['steθ *or* 'steθə] *prefix* referring to the chest

stethograph ['steθəgrɑːf] *noun* instrument which records breathing movements of the chest

stethography [ste'θɒgrəfi] *noun* recording movements of the chest

stethometer [ste'θɒmɪtə] *noun* instrument which records how far the chest expands when a person breathes in

stethoscope ['steθəskəʊp] *noun* surgical instrument with two earpieces connected to a tube and a metal disc, used by doctors to listen to sounds made inside the body (such as the sound of the heart or lungs); **electronic stethoscope** = stethoscope with an amplifier which makes sounds louder

Stevens-Johnson syndrome ['stiːvənz'dʒɒnsən 'sɪndrəʊm] *noun* severe form of erythema multiforme affecting the face and genitals, caused by an allergic reaction to drugs

stick [stɪk] *verb* to attach, to fix together (as with glue); *in bad cases of conjunctivitis the eyelids can stick together*

sticking plaster ['stɪkɪŋ 'plɑːstə] *noun* adhesive plaster or tape used to cover a small wound or to attach a pad of dressing to the skin

sticky ['stɪki] *adjective* which attached like glue; **sticky eye** = condition in babies where the eyes remain closed because of conjunctivitis

stiff [stɪf] *adjective* which cannot be bent or moved easily; *my knee is stiff after playing football*; **stiff neck** = condition where moving the neck is painful, usually caused by a strained muscle or by sitting in cold draughts (NOTE: **stiff - stiffer - stiffest**)

stiffly ['stɪfli] *adverb* in a stiff way; *he is walking stiffly because of the pain in his hip*

stiffness ['stɪfnəs] *noun* being stiff; *arthritis accompanied by stiffness in the joints*

stigma ['stɪgmə] *noun* visible symptom which shows that a patient has a certain disease (NOTE: the plural is **stigmas, stigmata**)

stilet *or* **stilette** [staɪ'let] *noun* thin wire inside a catheter to make it rigid

stillbirth ['stɪlbɜːθ] *noun* birth of a dead fetus, more than 28 weeks after conception

stillborn ['stɪlbɔːn] *adjective* (baby) born dead; *her first child was stillborn*

Still's disease ['stɪlz dɪ'ziːz] *noun* arthritis affecting children, similar to rheumatoid arthritis in adults

stimulant ['stɪmjʊlənt] *noun & adjective* (substance) which makes part of the body function faster; *caffeine is a stimulant*

COMMENT: natural stimulants include some hormones, and drugs such as digitalis which encourage a weak heart. Drinks such as tea and coffee contain stimulants

stimulate ['stɪmjʊleɪt] *verb* to make a person or organ react, respond or function; *the drug stimulates the heart*; *the therapy should stimulate the patient into attempting to walk unaided*

stimulation [stɪmjʊ'leɪʃn] *noun* action of stimulating

stimulus ['stɪmjʊləs] *noun* something (drug, impulse, etc.) which makes part of the body react (NOTE: the plural is **stimuli**)

sting [stɪŋ] **1** *noun* piercing of the skin by an insect which passes a toxic substance into the bloodstream **2** *verb* (of an insect) to make a hole in the skin and pass a toxic substance into the blood; *he was stung by a wasp*; **stinging sensation** = burning sensation as if after being stung by an insect (NOTE: **stinging - stung**)

COMMENT: stings by some insects, such as the tsetse fly can transmit a bacterial infection to a person. Other insects such as bees have toxic substances which they

pass into the bloodstream of the victim, causing irritating swellings. Some people are particularly allergic to insect stings

stirrup ['stɪrəp] *noun* stapes, one of the three ossicles in the middle ear

stitch [stɪtʃ] **1** *noun* **(a)** suture, a small loop of thread or gut, used to attach the sides of a wound or incision to help it to heal; *he had three stitches in his head*; *the doctor told her to come back in ten days' time to have the stitches taken out* **(b)** pain caused by cramp in the side of the body after running; *he had to stop running because he developed a stitch* **2** *verb* to attach with a suture; *they tried to stitch back the finger which had been cut off in an accident*

St John Ambulance Association and Brigade ['sənt 'dʒɒnz 'æmbjʊləns] *noun* voluntary organization which gives training in first aid and whose members provide first aid at public events such as football matches, demonstrations, etc.

St Louis encephalitis ['seɪnt 'luːɪs ensefə'laɪtɪs] *noun* sometimes fatal form of encephalitis, transmitted by the ordinary house mosquito, *Culex pipiens*

stock culture ['stɒk 'kʌltʃə] *noun* basic culture of bacteria, from which other cultures can be taken

Stokes-Adams syndrome ['stəʊks'ædəmz 'sɪndrəʊm] *noun* loss of consciousness due to the stopping of the action of the heart because of asystole or fibrillation

stocking ['stɒkɪŋ] *noun* close-fitting piece of clothing to cover the leg; **support stocking** = stocking worn to prevent postural hypotension and peripheral oedema; **thrombo-embolic deterrent stocking (TED)** = support stocking to prevent thrombus formation following surgery

stoma ['stəʊmə] *noun* (i) any opening into a cavity in the body; (ii) the mouth; (iii); *(informal)* colostomy (NOTE: the plural is **stomata**)

stomach ['stʌmək] *noun* **(a)** part of the body shaped like a bag, into which food passes after being swallowed and where the process of digestion continues; *she complained of pains in the stomach or of stomach pains*; *he has had stomach trouble for some time*; **acid stomach** = *see* ACIDITY; **stomach ache** = pain in the abdomen or stomach (caused by eating too much food or by an infection); **stomach cramp** = sharp spasm of the stomach muscles; **stomach pump** = instrument for sucking out the contents of a patient's stomach, especially if he has just swallowed a poisonous substance; **stomach tube** = tube passed into the stomach to wash it out or to take samples of the contents; **stomach upset** = slight infection of the stomach **(b)** region of the abdomen; *he had been kicked in the stomach* (NOTE: for other terms referring to the stomach, see words beginning with **gastr-**)

COMMENT: the stomach is situated in the top of the abdomen, and on the left side of the body between the oesophagus and the duodenum. Food is partly broken down by hydrochloric acid and other gastric juices secreted by the walls of the stomach and is mixed and squeezed by the action of the muscles of the stomach, before being passed on into the duodenum. The stomach continues the digestive process started in the mouth, but few substances (except alcohol and honey) are actually absorbed into the bloodstream in the stomach

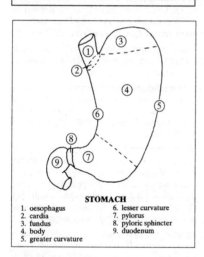

STOMACH

1. oesophagus	6. lesser curvature
2. cardia	7. pylorus
3. fundus	8. pyloric sphincter
4. body	9. duodenum
5. greater curvature	

stomachic [stə'mækɪk] *noun* substance which increases the appetite of a person by stimulating the secretion of gastric juice by the stomach

stomal ['stəʊml] *adjective* referring to a stoma; **stomal ulcer** = ulcer in the region of the jejunum

stomat- *or* **stomato-** ['stəʊmət *or* 'stəʊmətə] *prefix* referring to the mouth

stomatitis [stəʊmə'taɪtɪs] *noun* inflammation of the inside of the mouth

stomatology [stəʊmə'tɒlədʒi] *noun* branch of medicine which studies diseases of the mouth

-stomy [stəmi] *suffix* meaning an operation to make an opening

stone [stəʊn] *noun* **(a)** calculus, a hard mass of calcium like a little piece of stone which forms inside the body; *see also* GALLSTONE, KIDNEY STONE (NOTE: for other terms referring to stones, see words beginning or ending with **lith**) **(b)** measure of weight (= 14 pounds or 6.35 kilograms); *he tried to lose weight and lost three stone; she weighs eight stone ten (i.e. 8 stone 10 pounds)* (NOTE: no plural for in this meaning: '*she weighs ten stone*')

stone-deaf ['stəʊn'def] *adjective* totally deaf

stools [stuːlz] *plural noun* faeces, solid waste matter passed from the bowel through the anus (NOTE: can also be used in the singular: '*he passed an abnormal stool*')

stoop [stuːp] **1** *noun* position where especially the top of your back is bent forward; *he walks with a stoop* **2** *verb* to have a stoop; *he is seventy-five and stoops*

stop needle ['stɒp 'niːdl] *noun* needle with a ring round it, so that it can only be pushed a certain distance into the body

stoppage ['stɒpɪdʒ] *noun* act of stopping the function of an organ; **heart stoppage** = condition where the heart has stopped beating

storage disease ['stɔːrɪdʒ dɪ'ziːz] *noun* disease where abnormal amounts of a substance accumulate in a part of the body

stove-in chest ['stəʊv'ɪn 'tʃest] *noun* result of an accident, where several ribs are broken and pushed towards the inside

strabismal [strə'bɪzml] *adjective* cross-eyed

strabismus [strə'bɪzməs] *noun* squint, a condition where the eyes focus on different points; **convergent strabismus** = condition where one or both eyes look towards the nose; **divergent strabismus** = condition where one or both eyes look away from the nose

straight [streɪt] *adjective* (line) with no irregularities such as bends, curves or angles

straighten ['streɪtn] *verb* to make straight; *his arthritis is so bad that he cannot straighten his knees*

strain [streɪn] **1** *noun* **(a)** condition where a muscle has been stretched or torn by a strong or sudden movement; **back strain** = condition where the muscles or ligaments in the back have been stretched; *see also* EYESTRAIN **(b)** group of microorganisms which are different from others of the same type; *a new strain of influenza virus* **(c)** nervous tension and stress; *her work is causing her a lot of strain; he is suffering from nervous strain and needs to relax* **2** *verb* to stretch a muscle too far; *he strained his back lifting the table; she had to leave the game with a strained calf muscle; the effort of running upstairs strained his heart*

strand [strænd] *noun* thread; **DNA strand** = single thread of DNA

strangle ['stræŋgəl] *verb* to kill someone by squeezing his throat so that he cannot breathe or swallow

strangulated ['stræŋgjuleɪtɪd] *adjective* (part of the body) caught in an opening in such a way that the circulation of blood is stopped; **strangulated hernia** = condition where part of the intestine is squeezed in a hernia and the supply of blood to it is cut

strangulation [stræŋgju'leɪʃn] *noun* **(a)** squeezing a passage in the body **(b)** the act of strangling someone

strangury ['stræŋgjəri] *noun* condition where very little urine is passed, although the patient wants to pass water, caused by a bladder disorder or by a stone in the urethra

strap [stræp] *verb* **to strap (up)** = to wrap a bandage round a limb tightly, to attach tightly; *the nurses strapped up his stomach wound; the patient was strapped to the stretcher*

strapping ['stræpɪŋ] *noun* wide strong bandages or adhesive plaster used to bandage a large part of the body

stratified ['strætɪfaɪd] *adjective* made of several layers; **stratified epithelium** = epithelium formed of several layers of cells

stratum ['strɑːtəm] *noun* layer of tissue forming the epidermis (NOTE: the plural is **strata**)

> COMMENT: the main layers of the epidermis are: the **stratum germinativum** or **stratum basale**: this layer produces the cells that are pushed up to form the other layers; the **stratum granulosum**, a layer with granular cells under the **stratum lucidum**, a thin clear layer of dead and dying cells, and the surface layer, or **stratum corneum**, a layer of dead keratinized cells which progressively fall off

strawberry mark ['strɔːbəri mɑːk] *noun* naevus, a red birthmark in children, which will disappear in later life

streak [striːk] *noun* long thin line of a different colour

strength [streŋθ] *noun* being strong; *after her illness she had no strength in her limbs*; **full strength solution** = solution which has not been diluted

strengthen ['streŋθən] *verb* to make strong

strenuous ['strenjuəs] *adjective* (exercise) which involves using a lot of force; *avoid doing any strenuous exercise for some time while the wound heals*

strep throat ['strep 'θrəʊt] *noun; (informal)* infection of the throat by a streptococcus

strepto- ['streptə] *prefix* referring to organisms which grow in chains

streptobacillus [streptəbə'sɪləs] *noun* type of bacterium which forms a chain

streptococcal [streptə'kɒkl] *adjective* (infection) caused by a streptococcus

streptococcus [streptə'kɒkəs] *noun* genus of bacteria which grows in long chains, and causes fevers such as scarlet fever, tonsillitis and rheumatic fever (NOTE: the plural is **streptococci**)

streptodornase [streptə'dɔːneɪz] *noun* enzyme formed by streptococci which can make pus liquid

streptokinase [streptə'kaɪneɪz] *noun* enzyme formed by streptococci which can break down blood clots and is therefore used in the acute treatment of myocardial infarction

streptolysin [strep'tɒləsɪn] *noun* toxin produced by streptococci in rheumatic fever, which acts to destroy red blood cells

Streptomyces [streptə'maɪsiːz] *noun* genus of bacteria used to produce antibiotics

streptomycin [streptə'maɪsɪn] *noun see* DRUGS TABLE IN SUPPLEMENT

stress [stres] *noun* **(a)** physical pressure; **stress fracture** = fracture of a bone caused by excessive force, as in certain types of sport; **stress incontinence** = condition where the sufferer is not able to retain his urine when coughing **(b)** condition where an outside influence changes the working of the body, used especially of mental or emotional stress which can affect the hormone balance; **stress disorder** = disorder caused by stress; **stress reaction** = response to an outside stimulus which disturbs the normal physiological balance of the body; **stress-related illness** = illness which is due in part or completely to stress

stretch [stretʃ] *verb* to pull out, to make longer; **stretch reflex** = reflex reaction of a muscle which contracts after being stretched; **stretch mark** = mark on the skin of the abdomen of a pregnant woman or of a woman who has recently given birth; *see also* STRIAE GRAVIDARUM

stretcher ['stretʃə] *noun* folding bed, with handles, on which an injured person can be carried by two people; *she was carried out of the restaurant on a stretcher*; *some of the accident victims could walk to the ambulances, but there were several stretcher cases*; **stretcher bearer** = person who helps to carry a stretcher; **stretcher case** = person who is so ill that he has to be carried on a stretcher; **stretcher party** = group of people who carry a stretcher and look after the patient on it; **Furley stretcher** *or* **standard stretcher** = stretcher made of a folding frame with a canvas bed, with carrying poles at each side and small feet underneath; **paraguard stretcher** *or* **Neil Robertson stretcher** = type of strong stretcher to which the injured person is attached, so that he can be carried upright (used for rescuing people from mountains or from tall buildings); **pole and canvas stretcher** = simple stretcher made of a piece of canvas and two poles which slide into tubes at the side of the canvas; **scoop stretcher** = stretcher in two sections which slide under the patient and can lock together

stria ['straɪə] *noun* pale line on skin which is stretched (as in obese people); **striae gravidarum** = stretchmarks, lines on the skin of the abdomen of a pregnant woman or of a woman who has recently given birth (NOTE: the plural is **striae**)

striated [straɪ'eɪtɪd] *adjective* marked with pale lines; **striated muscle** = voluntary muscle which is attached to the bone which it moves; *compare* SMOOTH

strict [strɪkt] *adjective* severe, which must not be changed; *she has to follow a strict diet*; *the doctor was strict with the patients who wanted to drink alcohol in the hospital*

stricture ['strɪktʃə] *noun* narrowing of a passage in the body; **urethral stricture** = narrowing or blocking of the urethra by a growth

stridor *or* **stridulus** ['straɪdɔː or 'straɪdjuləs] *noun* sharp high sound made when air passes an obstruction in the larynx; *see also* LARYNGISMUS

strike-through ['straɪk'θruː] *noun* blood absorbed right through a dressing so as to be visible on the outside

---

If strike-through occurs, the wound dressing should be repadded, not removed
British Journal of Nursing

---

string sign ['strɪŋ 'saɪn] *noun* thin line which appears on the ileum, a sign of regional ileitis or Crohn's disease

strip [strɪp] **1** *noun* long thin piece of material or tissue; *the nurse bandaged the wound with strips of gauze*; *he grafted a strip of skin over the burn* **2** *verb* to take off (especially clothes); *the patients had to strip for the medical examination*; **to strip to the waist** = to take off the clothes on the top part of the body

stripper ['strɪpə] *noun* instrument (a flexible wire with an olive-shaped end) used for stripping varicose veins

stripping ['strɪpɪŋ] *noun* surgical operation to remove varicose veins

stroke [strəuk] **1** *noun* **(a)** sudden loss of consciousness caused by a cerebral haemorrhage or a blood clot in the brain; *he had a stroke and died*; *she was paralysed after a stroke*; **stroke patient** = person who has suffered a stroke; *see also* HEAT STROKE, SUNSTROKE **(b)** **stroke volume** = amount of blood pumped out the ventricle at each heartbeat **2** *verb* to touch softly with the fingers

---

COMMENT: there are two causes of stroke: cerebral haemorrhage (haemorrhagic stroke), when an artery bursts and blood leaks into the brain, and cerebral thrombosis (occlusive stroke), where a blood clot blocks an artery

---

stroke is the third most frequent cause of death in developed countries after ischaemic heart disease and cancer

British Journal of Hospital Medicine

raised blood pressure may account for as many as 70% of all strokes. The risk of stroke rises with both systolic and diastolic blood pressure

British Journal of Hospital Medicine

stroma ['strəumə] *noun* tissue which supports an organ, as opposed to parenchyma or functioning tissues in the organ

Strongyloides [strɒndʒi'lɔidiːz] *noun* parasitic worm which infests the intestines

strongyloidiasis [strɒndʒilɔi'daiəsis] *noun* being infested with *Strongyloides* which enters the skin and then travels to the lungs and the intestines

strontium ['strɒntiəm] *noun* metallic element; **strontium-90** = isotope of strontium which is formed in nuclear reactions and, because it is part of the fallout of nuclear explosions, can enter the food chain, attacking in particular the bones of humans and animals (NOTE: chemical symbol is **Sr**)

structure ['strʌktʃə] *noun* way in which an organ or muscle is formed

struma ['struːmə] *noun* goitre

strychnine ['strikniːn] *noun* poisonous alkaloid drug, made from the seeds of a tropical tree, and formerly used in small dose as a tonic

student ['stjuːdənt] *noun* person who is studying at a college or university; *all the medical students have to spend some time in hospital*; **student nurse** = person who is studying to become a nurse

study ['stʌdi] **1** *noun* examining something to learn about it; *he's making a study of diseases of small children*; *they have finished their study of the effects of the drug on pregnant women*; **blind study** = an investigation to test an intervention (often a drug) in which the patient does not know if he or she has taken the active medicine or the placebo; **case control study** = an investigation in which a group of patients with a disease (cases) are compared with a group without the disease in order to study possible causes; **cohort study** = an investigation in which a group of people (a cohort) without the disease are classified according to their exposure to a certain risk and are studied over a period of time to see if they develop the disease, in order to study links between risk and disease; **double blind study** = an investigation to test an intervention in which neither the doctor nor the patient knows if he or she has taken the active medicine or the placebo **2** *verb* to examine something to learn about it; *he's studying pharmacy*; *doctors are studying the results of the screening programme*

stuffy *or* **stuffed up** ['stʌfi *or* 'stʌft 'ʌp] *adjective* (nose) which is blocked with inflamed mucous membrane and mucus

stump [stʌmp] *noun* short piece of a limb which is left after the rest has been amputated

stun [stʌn] *verb* to concuss, to knock out by a blow to the head

stunt [stʌnt] *verb* to stop something growing; *the children's development was stunted by disease*

stupe [stjuːp] *noun* wet medicated dressing used as a compress

stupor ['stjuːpə] *noun* state of being semi-conscious; *after the party several people were found lying on the floor in a stupor*

Sturge-Weber syndrome ['stɜːdʒ'webə 'sindrəum] *noun* dark red mark on the skin above the eye, together with similar marks inside the brain, possibly causing epileptic fits

stutter ['stʌtə] **1** *noun* speech defect where the patient repeats the sound at the beginning of a word several times; *he is taking therapy to try to cure his stutter* **2** *verb* to speak with a stutter

stuttering ['stʌtəriŋ] *noun* dysphemia, difficulty in speaking where the person repeats parts of words or stops to try to pronounce words

St Vitus' dance [sənt 'vaitəs 'dɑːns] *noun* old name for Sydenham's chorea

stye [stai] *noun* hordeolum, inflammation of the gland at the base of an eyelash

stylo- ['stailəu] *prefix* referring to the styloid process

styloglossus [stailəu'glɒsəs] *noun* muscle which links the tongue to the styloid process

styloid ['stailɔid] *adjective* pointed; **styloid process** = piece of bone which projects from the bottom of the temporal bone; *see illustration at* SKULL

stylus ['staɪləs] *noun* long thin instrument used for applying antiseptics or ointments onto the skin

styptic ['stɪptɪk] *adjective & noun* (substance) which stops bleeding; **styptic pencil** = stick of alum, used to stop bleeding from small cuts

sub- [sʌb] *prefix* meaning underneath or below

subacute [sʌbə'kjuːt] *adjective* (condition) which is not acute but may become chronic; **subacute bacterial endocarditis** *or* **subacute infective endocarditis** = infection of the endocardium (the membrane covering the inner surfaces of the heart) by bacteria; **subacute combined degeneration (of the spinal cord)** = condition (caused by vitamin B_{12} deficiency) where the sensory and motor nerves in the spinal cord become damaged and the patient has difficulty in moving

subarachnoid [sʌbə'ræknɔɪd] *adjective* beneath the arachnoid membrane; **subarachnoid haemorrhage** = bleeding into the cerebrospinal fluid of the subarachnoid space; **subarachnoid space** = space between the arachnoid membrane and the pia mater in the brain, containing cerebrospinal fluid

subclavian [sʌb'kleɪvɪən] *adjective* underneath the clavicle; **subclavian artery** = one of two arteries branching from the aorta on the left, and from the innominate artery on the right, continuing into the brachial arteries and supplying blood to each arm; **subclavian veins** = veins which continue the axillary veins into the brachiocephalic vein

subclinical [sʌb'klɪnɪkl] *adjective* (disease) which is present in the body, but which has not yet developed any symptoms

subconscious [sʌb'kɒnʃəs] *adjective & noun* (referring to) mental processes (such as the memory) of which people are not aware all the time, but which can affect their actions

subcortical [sʌb'kɔːtɪkl] *adjective* beneath a cortex

subcostal [sʌb'kɒstl] *adjective* below the ribs; **subcostal plane** = imaginary horizontal line drawn across the front of the abdomen below the ribs

subculture ['sʌbkʌltʃə] *noun* culture of bacteria which is taken from a stock culture

subculturing [sʌb'kʌltʃərɪŋ] *noun* taking of a bacterial culture from a stock culture

subcutaneous [sʌbkjuː'teɪnɪəs] *adjective* under the skin; **subcutaneous injection** = injection made just under the skin (as to administer pain-killing drugs); **subcutaneous oedema** = fluid collecting under the skin, usually at the ankles; **subcutaneous tissue** = fatty tissue under the skin

subdural [sʌb'djʊərl] *adjective* between the dura mater and the arachnoid

subinvolution [sʌbɪnvə'luːʃn] *noun* condition where a part of the body does not go back to its former size and shape after having swollen or stretched (as in the case of the uterus after childbirth)

subject ['sʌbdʒekt] *noun* **(a)** patient, person suffering from a certain disease; *the hospital has developed a new treatment for arthritic subjects* **(b)** thing which is being studied or written about; *the subject of the article is 'Rh-negative babies'*

subjective [səb'dʒektɪv] *adjective* (*of views, account, etc.*) referring to the person concerned and not impartial; *the psychiatrist gave a subjective opinion on the patient's problem*

subject to ['sʌbdʒekt tʊ] *adverb* likely to suffer from; *the patient is subject to fits*; *after returning from the tropics he was subject to attacks of malaria*

sublimate 1 ['sʌblɪmət] *noun* deposit left when a vapour condenses **2** ['sʌblɪmeɪt] *verb* to convert violent emotion into a certain action which is not antisocial

sublimation [sʌblɪ'meɪʃn] *noun* doing a certain action as an unconscious way of showing violent emotions which would otherwise be expressed in antisocial behaviour

subliminal [sʌb'lɪmɪnl] *adjective* (stimulus) which is too slight to be noticed by the senses

sublingual [sʌb'lɪŋgwl] *adjective* under the tongue; **sublingual gland** = salivary gland under the tongue; *see illustration at* THROAT

> the sublingual region has a rich blood supply derived from the carotid artery and indicates changes in central body temperature more rapidly than the rectum
>
> *Nursing Times*

subluxation [sʌblʌk'seɪʃn] *noun* condition where a joint is partially dislocated

submandibular gland or **submaxillary gland** [sʌbˈmænˈdɪbjʊlə ˈglænd or sʌbmækˈsɪləri ˈglænd] noun salivary gland on each side of the lower jaw; see illustration at THROAT

submental [sʌbˈmentl] adjective under the chin

submucosa [sʌbmjuˈkəʊsə] noun tissue under mucous membrane

submucous [sʌbˈmjuːkəs] adjective under mucous membrane; **submucous resection (SMR)** = removal of a bent cartilage from the septum in the nose

subnormal [sʌbˈnɔːml] adjective (patient) with a mind which has not developed fully; **severely subnormal** = (patient) whose mind has not developed and is incapable of looking after himself

subnormality [sʌbnɔːˈmæləti] noun condition where a patient's mind has not developed fully

suboccipital [sʌbɒkˈsɪpɪtl] adjective beneath the back of the head

subphrenic [sʌbˈfrenɪk] adjective under the diaphragm; **subphrenic abscess** = abscess which forms between the diaphragm and the liver

subside [səbˈsaɪd] verb to go down or to become less violent; after being given the antibiotics, his fever subsided

substance [ˈsʌbstəns] noun chemical material; toxic substances released into the bloodstream; he became addicted to certain substances; **substance P** = neurotransmitter involved in pain pathways

substitution [sʌbstɪˈtjuːʃn] noun replacing one thing with another; **substitution therapy** = treating a condition by using a different drug from the one used before

substrate [ˈsʌbstreɪt] noun substance which is acted on by an enzyme

insulin is a protein hormone and the body's major anabolic hormone, regulating the metabolism of all body fuels and substrates

Nursing 87

subsultus [sʌbˈsʌltəs] noun twitching of the muscles and tendons, caused by fever

subtertian fever [sʌbˈtɜːʃn ˈfiːvə] noun type of malaria, where the fever is present most of the time

subtotal [sʌbˈtəʊtl] adjective (operation) to remove most of an organ; **subtotal gastrectomy** = surgical removal of most of the stomach; **subtotal hysterectomy** = removal of the uterus, but not the cervix; **subtotal thyroidectomy** = removal of most of the thyroid gland

subungual [sʌbˈʌŋgwəl] adjective under a nail

succeed [səkˈsiːd] verb to do well, to do what one was trying to do; scientists have succeeded in identifying the new influenza virus; they succeeded in stopping the flow of blood

success [səkˈses] noun **(a)** doing something well, doing what one was trying to do; they tried to isolate the virus but without success **(b)** something which does well; the operation was a complete success

successful [səkˈsesfʊl] adjective which works well; the operation was completely successful

succession [səkˈseʃn] noun line of things, one after the other; she had a succession of miscarriages

successive [səkˈsesɪv] adjective (things) which follow one after the other; she had a miscarriage with each successive pregnancy

succus [ˈsʌkəs] noun juice secreted by an organ; **succus entericus** = juice formed of enzymes, produced in the intestine to help the digestive process

succussion [səˈkʌʃn] noun splashing sound made when there is a large amount of liquid inside a cavity in the body (as in the stomach)

suck [sʌk] verb to pull liquid or air into the mouth or into a tube; they applied the stomach pump to suck out the contents of the patient's stomach; the baby is sucking its thumb

suckle [ˈsʌkl] verb to breastfeed a baby

sucrase [ˈsuːkreɪz] noun enzyme in the intestine which breaks down sucrose into glucose and fructose

sucrose [ˈsuːkrəʊz] noun sugar found in plants, especially in sugar cane, beet and maple syrup (sucrose is formed of glucose and fructose)

suction [ˈsʌkʃn] noun action of sucking; the dentist hooked a suction tube into the patient's mouth

sudamen [sʊˈdeɪmən] noun little blister caused by sweat (NOTE: the plural is **sudamina**)

sudden ['sʌdən] *adjective* which happens quickly; **sudden death** = death without identifiable cause, not preceded by an illness; **sudden infant death syndrome (SIDS)** = sudden death of a baby in bed, without any identifiable cause

COMMENT: occurs in very young children, up to the age of about 12 months; the causes are still being investigated

Sudeck's atrophy ['suːdeks 'ætrəfi] *noun* osteoporosis in the hand or foot

sudor ['suːdɔː] *noun* sweat

sudorific [suːdə'rɪfɪk] *noun* drug which makes a patient sweat

suffer ['sʌfə] *verb* **(a)** to have an illness for a long period of time; *she suffers from headaches*; *he suffers from not being able to distinguish certain colours* **(b)** to feel pain; *did she suffer much in her last illness?*; *he did not suffer at all and was conscious until he died* **(c)** to receive (an injury); *he suffered multiple injuries in the accident*

sufferer ['sʌfərə] *noun* person who has a certain disease; *a drug to help asthma sufferers or sufferers from asthma*

suffering ['sʌfərɪŋ] *noun* feeling pain over a long period of time; *the doctor gave him a morphine injection to relieve his suffering*

suffocate ['sʌfəkeɪt] *verb* to make someone stop breathing by cutting off the supply of air to his nose and mouth

suffocation [sʌfə'keɪʃn] *noun* making someone become unconscious by cutting off his supply of air

suffuse [sə'fjuːz] *verb* to spread over or through something

suffusion [sə'fjuːʒn] *noun* spreading (of a red flush) over the skin

sugar ['ʃʊgə] *noun* any of several sweet carbohydrates; **blood sugar level** = amount of glucose in the blood; **sugar content** = percentage of sugar in a substance or food; **sugar intolerance** = diarrhoea caused by sugar which has not been absorbed (NOTE: for other terms referring to sugar, see words beginning with **glyc-**)

COMMENT: there are several natural forms of sugar: sucrose (in plants), lactose (in milk), fructose (in fruit), glucose and dextrose (in fruit and in body tissue). Edible sugar used in the home is a form of refined sucrose. All sugars are useful sources of energy, though excessive amounts of sugar can increase weight and cause tooth decay. Diabetes mellitus is a condition where the body is incapable of absorbing sugar from food

suggest [sə'dʒest] *verb* to mention an idea; *the doctor suggested that she should stop smoking*

suggestion [sə'dʒestʃn] *noun* **(a)** idea which has been mentioned; *the doctor didn't agree with the suggestion that the disease had been caught in the hospital* **(b)** *(in psychiatry)* making a person's ideas change, by suggesting different ideas which the patient can accept, such as that he is in fact cured

suicidal [suːɪ'saɪdl] *adjective* (person) who wants to kill himself; *he has suicidal tendencies*

suicide ['suːɪsaɪd] *noun* act of killing oneself; **to commit suicide** = to kill yourself; *after his wife died he committed suicide*; **attempted suicide** = trying to kill yourself, but not succeeding

sulcus ['sʌlkəs] *noun* groove or fold (especially between the gyri in the brain); **Harrison's sulcus** = hollow on either side of the chest which develops in children with rickets and who breathe in with difficultry; **lateral sulcus and central sulcus** = two grooves which divide a cerebral hemisphere into lobes (NOTE: the plural is **sulci**)

sulphate *US* **sulfate** ['sʌlfeɪt] *noun* salt of sulphuric acid; **barium sulphate (BaSO₄)** = salt of barium not soluble in water and which shows as opaque in X-ray photographs; *see also* **MAGNESIUM**

sulphonamide *or* **sulpha drug** *or* **sulpha compound** [sʌl'fɒnəmaɪd *or* 'sʌlfə 'drʌg *or* 'sʌlfə 'kɒmpaʊnd] *noun* bacteriostatic drug (such as trimethoprim) used to treat bacterial infection, especially in the intestine and urinary system, but now less important due to increasing bacterial resistance

sulphur *US* **sulfur** ['sʌlfə] *noun* yellow non-metallic chemical element which is contained in some amino acids and is used in creams to treat some skin disorders (NOTE: chemical symbol is **S**. Note also that words beginning **sulph-** are spelt **sulf-** in American English)

sun [sʌn] *noun* very hot star round which the earth travels and which gives light and heat

sunbarrier ['sʌnbæriə] *noun* cream used on the skin to protect it against the effects of the sun

sunbathing ['sʌnbeɪðɪŋ] *noun* lying in the sun to absorb sunlight

sun blindness ['sʌn 'blaɪndnəs] = PHOTORETINITIS

sunburn ['sʌnbɜːn] *noun* damage to the skin by excessive exposure to sunlight

sunburnt ['sʌnbɜːnt] *adjective* (skin) made brown or red by exposure to sunlight

sunglasses ['sʌnglɑːsɪz] *plural noun* dark glasses which are worn to protect the eyes from the sun

sunlight ['sʌnlaɪt] *noun* light from the sun; *he is allergic to strong sunlight*

COMMENT: sunlight is essential to give the body vitamin D, but excessive exposure to sunlight will not simply turn the skin brown, but also may burn the surface of the skin so badly that it dies and pus forms beneath. Constant exposure to the sun can cause cancer of the skin

sunscreen ['sʌnskriːn] *noun* = SUNBARRIER

sunstroke ['sʌnstrəʊk] *noun* serious condition caused by excessive exposure to the sun or to hot conditions, where the patient becomes dizzy and has a high body temperature but does not perspire

super- ['suːpə] *prefix* meaning (i) above; (ii) extremely

superciliary [suːpə'sɪliəri] *adjective* referring to the eyebrows

superego [suːpər'iːgəʊ] *noun* (in psychology) part of the mind which is the conscience, which is concerned with right and wrong

superfecundation [suːpəfiːkən'deɪʃn] *noun* condition where two or more ova produced at the same time are fertilized by different males

superfetation [suːpəfiː'teɪʃn] *noun* condition where an ovum is fertilized in a woman who is already pregnant

superficial [suːpə'fɪʃl] *adjective* on the surface, close to the surface or on the skin; **superficial burn** = burn on the skin surface; **superficial fascia** = membranous layers of connective tissue found just under the skin; **superficial vein** = vein near the surface of the skin (as opposed to deep vein)

superinfection [suːpərɪn'fekʃn] *noun* second infection which affects the treatment of the first infection, because it is resistant to the drug used to treat the first

superior [suː'pɪəriə] *adjective (of part of the body)* higher up than another part; **superior aspect** = view of the body from above; **superior vena cava** = branch of the large vein into the heart, carrying blood from the head and the top part of the body

superiority [suːpɪəri'ɒrəti] *noun* being better than something or someone else; **superiority complex** = condition where a person feels he is better in some way than others and pays little attention to them (NOTE: the opposite is **inferior, inferiority**)

supernumerary [suːpə'njuːmərəri] *adjective* extra; *(of teeth, etc.)* one (or more than one) more than the usual number

allocation of supernumerary students to clinical areas is for their educational needs and not for service requirements
Nursing Times

supervise ['suːpəvaɪz] *verb* to manage or to organize something; *the administration of drugs has to be supervised by a qualified person*; *she has been appointed to supervise the transfer of patients to the new ward*

supervision [suːpə'vɪʒn] *noun* management or organization; *elderly patients need constant supervision*; *the sheltered housing is under the supervision of a full-time nurse*

supervisor ['suːpəvaɪzə] *noun* person who supervises; *the supervisor of hospital catering services*

supinate ['suːpɪneɪt] *verb* to turn (the hand) so that the palm is upwards

supination [suːpɪ'neɪʃn] *noun* turning the hand so that palm faces upwards (NOTE: the opposite is **pronation**)

supinator ['suːpɪneɪtə] *noun* muscle which turns the hand so that the palm faces upwards

supine ['suːpaɪn] *adjective* (i) lying on the back; (ii) with the palm of the hand facing upwards (NOTE: the opposite is **prone**)

the patient was to remain in the supine position, therefore a pad was placed under the Achilles tendon to raise the legs
NATNews

supply [sə'plaɪ] **1** *noun* something which is provided; *the arteries provide a continuous supply of oxygenated blood to the tissues*; *the hospital service needs a constant supply of blood for transfusion*; *the government sent medical supplies to the disaster area* **2** *verb* to provide or to give something which is needed; *a balanced diet will supply the body with all the vitamins and trace elements it needs*; *the brachial artery supplies the arm and hand*

support [sə'pɔːt] **1** *noun* **(a)** help to keep something in place; *the bandage provides some support for the knee*; *he was so weak that he had to hold onto a chair for support* **(b)** handle, metal rail which a person can hold; *there are supports at the side of the bed*; *the bath is provided with metal supports* **2** *verb* to hold something, to keep something in place; *he wore a truss to support a hernia*

supportive [sə'pɔːtɪv] *adjective* (person) who helps or comforts someone in trouble; *her family were very supportive when she was in hospital*; *the local health authority has been very supportive of the hospital management*

suppository [sə'pɒzɪtəri] *noun* piece of soluble material (such as glycerine jelly) containing a drug, which is placed in the rectum (to act as lubricant), or in the vagina (to treat disorders such as vaginitis) and is dissolved by the body's fluids

suppress [sə'pres] *verb* to remove (a symptom), to reduce the action of something completely, to stop (the release of a hormone); *a course of treatment which suppresses the painful irritation*; *the drug suppresses the body's natural instinct to reject the transplanted tissue*; *the release of adrenaline from the adrenal cortex is suppressed*

suppression [sə'preʃn] *noun* act of suppressing; *the suppression of allergic responses*; *the suppression of a hormone*

suppurate ['sʌpjureɪt] *verb* to form and discharge pus

suppurating ['sʌpjureɪtɪŋ] *adjective* purulent, containing or discharging pus

suppuration [sʌpju'reɪʃn] *noun* formation and discharge of pus

supra- ['suːprə] *prefix* meaning above or over

supraoptic nucleus [suːprə'ɒptɪk 'njuːkliəs] *noun* nucleus in the hypothalamus from which nerve fibres run to the posterior pituitary gland

supraorbital [suːprə'ɔːbɪtl] *adjective* above the orbit of the eye; **supraorbital ridge** = ridge of bone above the eye, covered by the eyebrow

suprapubic [suːprə'pjuːbɪk] *adjective* above the pubic bone or pubic area

suprarenal [suːprə'riːnl] *adjective* above the kidney; **suprarenal area** = the area of the body above the kidney; **suprarenal glands** *or* **suprarenals** = the adrenal glands, two endocrine glands at the top of the kidneys, which secrete adrenaline and other hormones

suprasternal [suːprə'stɜːnl] *adjective* above the sternum

surface ['sɜːfɪs] *noun* top layer of something; *the surfaces of the two membranes may rub together*

surfactant [sɜː'fæktnt] *noun* substance in the alveoli of the lungs which keeps the surfaces of the lungs wet and prevents lung collapse

surgeon ['sɜːdʒn] *noun* doctor who specializes in surgery; **eye surgeon** = surgeon who specializes in operations on eyes; **heart surgeon** = surgeon who specializes in operations on hearts; **plastic surgeon** = surgeon who repairs defective or deformed parts of the body *US*; **surgeon general** = government official responsible for all aspects of public health (NOTE: although surgeons are doctors, in the UK they are traditionally called 'Mr' and not 'Dr', so 'Dr Smith' may be a GP, but 'Mr Smith' is a surgeon)

surgery ['sɜːdʒəri] *noun* **(a)** treatment of a disease or disorder which requires an operation to cut into, to remove or to manipulate tissue, organs or parts; *the patient will need plastic surgery to remove the scars he received in the accident*; *the surgical ward is for patients waiting for surgery*; *two of our patients had to have surgery*; *she will have to undergo surgery*; **cosmetic surgery** = surgical operation carried out to improve the appearance of the patient; **exploratory surgery** = surgical operations in which the aim is to discover the cause of the patient's symptoms or the extent of the illness; **major surgery** = surgical operations involving important organs in the body; **plastic surgery** = surgery to repair defective or deformed parts of the body (NOTE: also called **reconstructive surgery**); **spare part surgery** = surgical operations where parts of the body (such as bones or joints) are replaced by artificial pieces; *see also* CRYOSURGERY, KEYHOLE, INVASIVE, MICROSURGERY **(b)** room where a doctor or dentist sees and examines patients; *there are ten patients waiting in the surgery*; *surgery hours are from 8.30 in the morning to 6.00 at night*

surgical ['sɜːdʒɪkl] *adjective* (i) referring to surgery; (ii) (disease) which can be treated by surgery; *all surgical instruments must be sterilized*; *we manage to carry out two surgical operations in an hour*; **surgical care** = looking after patients who have had surgery; **surgical emphysema** = air bubbles in tissue, not in the lungs; **surgical gloves** = thin plastic gloves worn by surgeons; **surgical neck** = narrow part at the top of the humerus, where the arm can easily be broken; **a surgical procedure** = a surgical operation; **surgical spirit** = ethyl alcohol with an additive which gives it an unpleasant taste, used as a disinfectant or for rubbing on the skin (NOTE: the American English is **rubbing alcohol**); **surgical stockings** = strong elastic stockings worn to support a weak joint in the knee or to hold varicose veins tightly; **surgical ward** = ward in a hospital for patients who have to have operations

surgically ['sɜːdʒɪkli] *adverb* using surgery; *the growth can be treated surgically*

surrogate ['sʌrəgət] *adjective* taking the place of; **surrogate mother** = (i) person who takes the place of a real mother; (ii) woman who has a child by artificial insemination for a couple where the wife cannot bear children, with the intention of handing the child over to them when it is born

surround [sə'raʊnd] *verb* to be all around something; *the wound is several millimetres deep and the surrounding flesh is inflamed*

surroundings [sə'raʊndɪŋz] *noun* area round something; *the cottage hospital is set in pleasant surroundings*

survival [sə'vaɪvl] *noun* continuing to live; *the survival rate of newborn babies has begun to fall*

survive [sə'vaɪv] *verb* to continue to live; *he survived two attacks of pneumonia*; *they survived a night on the mountain without food*; *the baby only survived for two hours*

survivor [sə'vaɪvə] *noun* person who survives

susceptibility [səseptə'bɪləti] *noun* lack of resistance to a disease

low birthweight has been associated with increased susceptibility to infection
East African Medical Journal

even children with the milder forms of sickle-cell disease have an increased frequency of pneumococcal infection. The reason for this susceptibility is a profound abnormality of the immune system
Lancet

susceptible [sə'septəbl] *adjective* likely to catch (a disease); *she is susceptible to colds or to throat infections*

suspect 1 ['sʌspekt] *noun* person who doctors believe may have a disease; *they are screening all typhoid suspects* **2** [səs'pekt] *verb* to think that someone may have a disease; *he is a suspected diphtheria carrier*; *several cases of suspected meningitis have been reported*

those affected are being nursed in five isolation wards and about forty suspected sufferers are being barrier nursed in other wards
Nursing Times

suspension [sə'spenʃn] *noun* liquid with solid particles in it

suspensory [sə'spensri] *adjective* which is hanging down; **suspensory bandage** = bandage to hold a part of the body which hangs; **suspensory ligament** = ligament which holds a part of the body in position

sustain [sə'steɪn] *verb* **(a)** to keep, to support, to maintain; *these bones can sustain quite heavy weights*; *he is not eating enough to sustain life* **(b)** to suffer (an injury); *he sustained a severe head injury*

sustentacular [sʌstən'tækjʊlə] *adjective* referring to sustentaculum

sustentaculum [sʌstən'tækjʊləm] *noun* part of the body which supports another part

suture ['suːtʃə] **1** *noun* **(a)** fixed joint where two bones are fused together, especially the bones in the skull; *see illustration at* SKULL; **coronal suture** = horizontal joint across the top of the skull between the parietal and frontal bones; **lambdoidal suture** = horizontal joint across the back of the skull between the parietal and occipital bones;

sagittal suture = joint along the top of the head between the two parietal bones **(b)** attaching the sides of an incision or wound with thread, so that healing can take place **(c)** thread used for attaching the sides of a wound so that they can heal **2** *verb* to attach the sides of a wound or incision together with thread so that healing can take place

COMMENT: wounds are usually stitched using thread or catgut which is removed after a week or so. Sutures are either absorbable (made of a substance which is eventually absorbed into the body) or non-absorbable, in which case they need to be removed after a certain time

swab [swɒb] *noun* **(a)** cotton wool pad, often attached to a small stick, used to clean a wound, to apply ointment, to take a specimen, etc. **(b)** specimen taken with a swab; *a cervical swab*

swallow ['swɒləʊ] *verb* to make liquid or food (and sometimes air) go down from the mouth to the stomach; *patients suffering from nosebleeds should try not to swallow the blood*

swallowing ['swɒləʊɪŋ] *noun* deglutition, action of passing food or liquids (sometimes also air) from the mouth into the oesophagus and down into the stomach; *see also* AEROPHAGY

sweat [swet] **1** *noun* sudor or perspiration, salt moisture produced by the sweat glands; *sweat was running off the end of his nose*; *her hands were covered with sweat*; **sweat duct** = thin tube connecting the sweat gland with the surface of the skin; **sweat gland** = gland which produces sweat, situated beneath the dermis and connected to the surface of the skin by a thin tube; **sweat pore** = hole in the skin through which the sweat comes out; *see illustration at* SKIN & SENSORY RECEPTORS **2** *verb* to perspire, to produce moisture through the sweat glands and onto the skin; *after working in the fields he was sweating*

COMMENT: sweat cools the body as the moisture evaporates from the skin. Sweat contains salt, and in hot countries it may be necessary to take salt tablets to replace the salt lost through the skin

sweet [swiːt] *adjective* one of the basic tastes, not bitter, sour or salt; *sugar is sweet, lemons are sour*

swell [swel] *verb* to become larger; *the disease affects the lymph glands, making*

them swell; *the doctor noticed that the patient had swollen glands in his neck*; *she finds her swollen ankles painful* (NOTE: swelling - swelled - has swollen)

swelling ['swelɪŋ] *noun* condition where fluid accumulates in tissue, making the tissue become large; *they applied a cold compress to try to reduce the swelling*

sycosis [saɪˈkəʊsɪs] *noun* bacterial infection of hair follicles; **sycosis barbae** = infection of hair follicles on the sides of the face and chin (NOTE: also called **barber's rash**)

Sydenham's chorea ['sɪdənhæmz kɔːˈrɪə] *see* CHOREA

Sylvius ['sɪlvɪəs] *see* AQUEDUCT

symbiosis [sɪmbɪˈəʊsɪs] *noun* condition where two organisms exist together and help each other to survive

symblepharon [sɪmˈblefərɒn] *noun* condition where the eyelid sticks to the eyeball

symbol ['sɪmbl] *noun* sign or letter which means something; **chemical symbol** = letters which indicate a chemical substance; *Na is the symbol for sodium*; *° is the symbol for degree*

Syme's amputation ['saɪmz æmpjuˈteɪʃən] *noun* surgical operation to amputate the foot above the ankle

sympathectomy [sɪmpəˈθektəmi] *noun* surgical operation to cut part of the sympathetic nervous system, as a treatment of high blood pressure

sympathetic nervous system [sɪmpəˈθetɪk ˈnɜːvəs ˈsɪstəm] *noun* part of the autonomic nervous system, which leaves the spinal cord from the thoracic and lumbar regions to various important organs, such as the heart, the lungs, the sweat glands, etc. , and which prepares the body for emergencies and vigorous muscular activity; *see also* PARASYMPATHETIC

sympatholytic [sɪmpəθəʊˈlɪtɪk] *noun* drug which stops the sympathetic nervous system working

sympathomimetic [sɪmpəθəʊmɪˈmetɪk] *adjective* (drug, such as dopamine hydrochloride) which stimulates the activity of the sympathetic nervous system, used in cardiac shock following myocardial infarction and in cardiac surgery

symphysiectomy [sɪmfɪzi'ektəmi] *noun* surgical operation to remove part of the pubic symphysis to make childbirth easier

symphysiotomy [sɪmfɪzi'ɒtəmi] *noun* surgical operation to make an incision in the pubic symphysis to make the passage for a fetus wider

symphysis ['sɪmfəsɪs] *noun* point where two bones are joined by cartilage which makes the joint rigid; **pubic symphysis** *or* **symphysis pubis** = interpubic joint, a piece of cartilage which joins the two sections of the pubic bone; **symphysis menti** = point in the front of the lower jaw where the two halves of the jaw are fused to form the chin

symptom ['sɪmtəm] *noun* change in the way the body works or change in the body's appearance, which shows that a disease or disorder is present and is noticed by the patient himself; *the symptoms of hay fever are running nose and watering eyes*; *a doctor must study the symptoms before making his diagnosis*; *the patient presented all the symptoms of rheumatic fever* (NOTE: if a symptom is noticed only by the doctor, it is a **sign**)

symptomatic [sɪmtə'mætɪk] *adjective* which is a symptom; *the rash is symptomatic of measles*

symptomatology [sɪmtəmə'tɒlədʒi] *noun* semeiology, branch of medicine concerned with the study of symptoms

syn- ['sɪn] *prefix* meaning joint, fused

synalgia [sɪ'nældʒə] *noun* referred pain, pain which is felt in one part of the body, but is caused by a condition in another part (such as pain in the groin which can be a symptom of kidney stone and pain in the right shoulder which can indicate gall bladder infection)

synapse ['saɪnæps] **1** *noun* point in the nervous system where the axons of neurones are in contact with the dendrites of other neurones **2** *verb* to link with a neurone

synaptic [sɪn'æptɪk] *adjective* referring to a synapse; **synaptic connection** = link between the dendrites of one neurone with another neurone

synarthrosis [sɪnɑː'θrəʊsɪs] *noun* joint (as in the skull) where the bones have fused together

synchondrosis [sɪŋkɒn'drəʊsɪs] *noun* joint, as in children, where the bones are linked by cartilage, before the cartilage has changed to bone

synchysis ['sɪŋkɪsɪs] *noun* condition where the vitreous humour in the eye becomes soft

syncope ['sɪŋkəpi] *noun* fainting fit, becoming unconscious for a short time because of reduced flow of blood to the brain

syncytium [sɪn'sɪʃiəm] *noun* continuous length of tissue in muscle fibres; **respiratory syncytial virus** = virus which causes infections of the nose and throat in children

syndactyly [sɪn'dæktɪli] *noun* condition where two toes or fingers are joined together with tissue

syndesm- *or* **syndesmo-** [sɪn'desm or sɪn'desməʊ] *prefix* referring to ligaments

syndesmology [sɪndes'mɒlədʒi] *noun* branch of medicine which studies joints

syndesmosis [sɪndes'məʊsɪs] *noun* joint where the bones are tightly linked by ligaments

syndrome ['sɪndrəʊm] *noun* group of symptoms and other changes in the body's functions which, when taken together, show that a particular disease is present

synechia [sɪ'nekiə] *noun* condition where the iris sticks to another part of the eye

syneresis [sɪ'nɪərəsɪs] *noun* releasing of fluid as in a blood clot when it becomes harder

synergism ['sɪnədʒɪzm] *noun* (*of two things*) acting together in such a way that both are more effective

synergist ['sɪnədʒɪst] *noun* muscle or drug which acts with another and increases the effectiveness of both

synergy ['sɪnədʒi] *noun* working together, so that the combination is twice as effective

syngraft ['sɪngrɑːft] *noun* isograft, graft of tissue from an identical twin

synoptophore [sɪ'nɒptəfɔː] *noun* instrument used to correct a squint

synostosed [sɪnɒ'stəʊzd] *adjective* (*of bones*) fused together with new bone tissue

synostosis [sɪnɒ'stəʊsɪs] *noun* fusing of two bones together by forming new bone tissue

synovectomy [saɪnəʊ'vektəmi] *noun* surgical operation to remove the synovial membrane of a joint

synovia [saɪ'nəʊviə] = SYNOVIAL FLUID

synovial [saɪ'nəʊviəl] *adjective* referring to the synovium; **synovial cavity** = space inside a synovial joint; **synovial fluid** = fluid secreted by a synovial membrane to lubricate a joint; **synovial joint** = diarthrosis, joint where two bones are covered with an articular capsule which allows them to move freely; **synovial membrane** *or* **synovium** = smooth membrane which forms the inner lining of the capsule covering a joint and secretes the fluid which lubricates the joint

synovioma [sɪnəuviˈəumə] *noun* tumour in a synovial membrane

synovitis [saɪnəˈvaɪtɪs] *noun* inflammation of the synovial membrane

synovium [sɪˈnəuviəm] = SYNOVIAL MEMBRANE; *see illustration at* JOINTS

70% of rheumatoid arthritis sufferers develop the condition in the metacarpophalangeal joints. The synovium produces an excess of synovial fluid which is abnormal and becomes thickened

Nursing Times

synthesize [ˈsɪnθəsaɪz] *verb* to make a chemical compound from its separate components; *essential amino acids cannot be synthesized; the body cannot synthesize essential fatty acids and has to absorb them from food*

synthetic [sɪnˈθetɪk] *adjective* made by man, made artificially

synthetically [sɪnˈθetɪkli] *adverb* made artificially; *synthetically produced hormones are used in hormone therapy*

syphilide [ˈsɪfɪlaɪd] *noun* rash or open sore which is a symptom of the second stage of syphilis

syphilis [ˈsɪfəlɪs] *noun* sexually transmitted disease caused by a spirochaete *Treponema pallidum;* **congenital syphilis** = syphilis which is passed on from a mother to her unborn child

COMMENT: syphilis is a serious sexually transmitted disease, but it is curable with penicillin injections if the treatment is started early. Syphilis has three stages: in the first (or primary) stage, a hard sore (chancre) appears on the genitals or sometimes on the mouth; in the second (or secondary) stage about two or three months later, a rash appears, with sores round the mouth and genitals. It is at this stage that the disease is particularly infectious. After this stage, symptoms disappear for a long time, sometimes many years. The disease reappears in the third (or tertiary) stage in many different forms: blindness, brain disorders, ruptured aorta, or general paralysis leading to insanity and death. The tests for syphilis are the Wassermann test and the less reliable Kahn test

syphilitic [sɪfəˈlɪtɪk] *noun & adjective* (person) suffering from syphilis

syring- *or* **syringo-** [ˈsɪrɪndʒ or sɪˈrɪŋgəu] *prefix* referring to tubes, especially the central canal of the spinal cord

syringe [sɪˈrɪndʒ] **1** *noun* surgical instrument made of a tube with a plunger which slides down inside it, forcing the contents out through a needle (as in an injection) or slides up the tube, allowing a liquid to be sucked into it **2** *verb* to wash out (the ears) using a syringe

syringobulbia [sɪrɪŋgəuˈbʌlbiə] *noun* syringomyelia in the brain stem

syringocystadenoma *or* **syringoma** [sɪrɪŋgəusɪstədɪˈnəumə or sɪrɪŋˈgəumə] *noun* benign tumour in sweat glands and ducts

syringomyelia [sɪrɪŋgəumaɪˈiːliə] *noun* disease which forms cavities in the neck section of the spinal cord, affecting the nerves so that the patient loses his sense of touch and pain

syringomyelocele [sɪrɪŋgəuˈmaɪələusiːl] *noun* severe form of spina bifida where the spinal cord pushes through a hole in the spine

syrinx [ˈsɪrɪŋks] = EUSTACHIAN TUBE

system [ˈsɪstəm] *noun* **(a)** the body as a whole; *amputation of a limb gives a serious shock to the system* **(b)** arrangement of certain parts of the body so that they work together; **the alimentary system** = system of organs and tracts which digest and break down food (including the alimentary canal, the salivary glands, the liver, etc.); **the cardiopulmonary system** = the functional unit of heart and lungs; **the cardiovascular system** = system of organs and blood vessels where the blood circulates round the body (including the heart, arteries and veins); **central nervous system** = the brain and spinal cord which link together all the nerves; **renovascular system** = the blood vessels associated with the kidney; **respiratory system** = series of organs and passages which take air into the lungs and exchange oxygen for carbon dioxide; **urinary system** = system of organs and ducts which separate waste liquids from blood and excrete them as urine (including the kidneys, bladder, ureters and urethra); *see also* AUTONOMIC, PARASYMPATHETIC, PERIPHERAL, SYMPATHETIC

Système International [sɪˈstem ænteənæsjɒˈnæl] *see* SI

systemic [sɪˈstiːmɪk] *adjective* referring to the whole body; *septicaemia is a systemic infection*; **systemic circulation** = circulation of blood around the whole body (except the lungs), starting with the aorta and returning through the venae cavae; **systemic lupus erythematosus (SLE)** = one of several collagen diseases, forms of lupus, where red patches form on the skin and spread throughout the body

systole [ˈsɪstəli] *noun* phase in the beating of the heart when it contracts as it pumps blood out; **the heart is in systole** = the heart is contracting and pumping (NOTE: often used without **the:** 'at systole the heart pumps blood into the arteries')

systolic [sɪˈstɒlɪk] *adjective* referring to the systole; **systolic pressure** = blood pressure taken at the systole, normally 160 mmHg; *compare* DIASTOLE, DIASTOLIC

COMMENT: systolic pressure is always higher than diastolic

Tt

T *symbol for* tera-

Ta *chemical symbol for* tantalum

TAB vaccine [ˈtiː ˈeɪ ˈbiː ˈvæksiːn] *noun* vaccine which immunizes against typhoid fever and paratyphoid A and B; *he was given a TAB injection*; *TAB injections give only temporary immunity against paratyphoid*

tabes [ˈteɪbiːz] *noun* wasting away; **tabes dorsalis** = locomotor ataxia, disease of the nervous system, caused by advanced syphilis, where the patient loses his sense of feeling, the control of his bladder, the ability to coordinate movements of the legs, and suffers severe pains; **tabes mesenterica** = wasting of glands in the abdomen

tabetic [təˈbetɪk] *adjective* which is wasting away or affected by tabes dorsalis

table [ˈteɪbl] *noun* piece of furniture with a flat top and legs, used to eat at or to work at; **operating table** = special flat table on which a patient lies while undergoing an operation

tablet [ˈtæblət] *noun* small flat round piece of dry drug which a patient swallows; *a bottle of aspirin tablets*; *the soluble tablets dissolve in water*; *take two tablets three times a day*

taboparesis [teɪbəʊpəˈriːsɪs] *noun* final stage of syphilis where the patient has locomotor ataxia and general paralysis of the insane

tachy- [ˈtæki] *prefix* meaning fast

tachycardia [tækiˈkɑːdiə] *noun* rapid beating of the heart; **nodal tachycardia** *or* **paroxysmal tachycardia** = sudden attack of rapid heartbeats; **sinus tachycardia** *or* **simple tachycardia** = rapid heartbeats caused by stimulation of the sinoatrial node

tachyphrasia [tækiˈfreɪziə] *noun* rapid speaking, as in some mentally disturbed patients

tachyphyl(l)axis [tækifiˈlæksɪs] *noun* effect of a drug or neurotransmitter which becomes less with repeated doses

tachypnoea [tækɪpˈniːə] *noun* very fast breathing

tactile [ˈtæktaɪl] *adjective* which can be sensed by touch; **tactile anaesthesia** = loss of sensation of touch

taenia [ˈtiːniə] *noun* **(a)** long ribbon-like part of the body; **taenia coli** = outer band of muscle running along the large intestine **(b)** **Taenia** = genus of tapeworm (NOTE: the plural is **taeniae, Taeniae**)

COMMENT: the various species of Taenia which affect humans are taken into the body from eating meat which has not been properly cooked. The most obvious symptom of tapeworm infestation is a sharply increased appetite, together with a loss of weight. The most serious infestation is with *Taenia solium*, found in pork, where the larvae develop in the body and can form hydatid cysts

taeniacide [ˈtiːniəsaɪd] *adjective* substance which kills tapeworms

taeniafuge [ˈtiːniəfjuːdʒ] *noun* substance which makes tapeworms leave the body

taeniasis [tiːˈnaɪəsɪs] *noun* infestation of the intestines with tapeworms

take [teɪk] **1** *noun* **on (the) take** = on duty (admitting patients to hospital) **2** *verb* **(a)** to swallow, to drink (a medicine); *she has to take her tablets three times a day*; *the medicine should be taken in a glass of water* **(b)** to do certain actions; *the dentist took an X-ray of his teeth*; *the patient has been allowed to take a bath* **(c)** *(of graft)* to be accepted by the body; *the skin graft hasn't taken*; *the kidney transplant took easily* (NOTE: **taking - took - has taken**)

take after [ˈteɪk ˈɑːftə] *verb* to be like (a parent); *he takes after his father*

take care of [ˈteɪk ˈkeə əv] *verb* to look after, to attend to (a patient); *the nurses will take care of the accident victims*

take off ['teɪk 'ɒf] *verb* to remove (especially clothes); *the doctor asked him to take his shirt off or to take off his shirt*

talc [tælk] *noun* soft white powder used to dust on irritated skin

talcum powder ['tælkəm 'paʊdə] *noun* scented talc

talipes ['tælɪpiːz] *noun* club foot, congenitally deformed foot

COMMENT: the most usual form (talipes equinovarus) is where the person walks on the toes because the foot is permanently bent forward; in other forms, the foot either turns towards the inside (talipes varus), towards the outside (talipes valgus), or upwards (talipes calcaneus) at the ankle, so that the patient cannot walk on the sole of the foot

tall [tɔːl] *adjective* high, usually higher than other people; *he's the tallest in the family - he's taller than all his brothers*; *how tall is he?*; *he's 5 foot 7 inches (5'7") tall or 1.25 metres tall* (NOTE: **tall - taller - tallest**)

talo- ['teɪləʊ] *prefix* referring to the ankle bone

talus ['teɪləs] *noun* ankle bone, the top bone in the tarsus which articulates with the tibia and fibula in the leg, and with the calcaneus in the heel; *see illustration at* FOOT

tampon ['tæmpɒn] *noun* (i) wad of absorbent material put into a wound to soak up blood during an operation; (ii) wad of absorbent material which is inserted into the vagina to absorb menstrual flow

tamponade [tæmpə'neɪd] *noun* (i) putting a tampon into a wound; (ii) abnormal pressure on part of the body; **cardiac tamponade** *or* **heart tamponade** = pressure on the heart when the pericardial cavity fills with blood

tan [tæn] *verb (of skin)* to become brown (in sunlight); *he tans easily*; *she is using a tanning lotion*

tannin *or* **tannic acid** ['tænɪn *or* 'tænɪk 'æsɪd] *noun* substance found in the bark of trees and in tea and other liquids, which stains brown

tantalum ['tæntələm] *noun* rare metal, used to repair damaged bones; **tantalum mesh** = type of net made of tantalum wire, used to repair cranial defects (NOTE: chemical symbol is **Ta**)

tantrum ['tæntrəm] *noun* violent attack of bad behaviour, usually in a child, where the child breaks things or lies on the floor and screams

tap [tæp] **1** *noun* pipe with a handle which can be turned to make a liquid or gas come out of a container **2** *verb* **(a)** to remove or drain liquid from part of the body; *see also* SPINAL **(b)** to hit lightly; *the doctor tapped his chest with his finger*

tape [teɪp] *noun* long thin flat piece of material; **adhesive tape** = dressing with a sticky substance on the back so that it can stick to the skin; **tape measure** *or* **measuring tape** = tape with marks on it showing centimetres or inches

tapeworm ['teɪpwɜːm] *noun* parasitic worm with a small head and long body like a ribbon

COMMENT: tapeworms enter the intestine when a person eats raw meat or fish. The worms attach themselves with hooks to the side of the intestine and grow longer by adding sections to their bodies. Tapeworm larvae do not develop in humans, with the exception of the pork tapeworm, *Taenia solium*

tapotement ['tɑːpəʊtmɒŋ *or* tə'pɒtmənt] *noun* type of massage where the therapist taps the patient with his hands

tapping ['tæpɪŋ] *noun* paracentesis, removing liquid from part of the body using a hollow needle

target ['tɑːgɪt] *noun* place which is to be hit by something; **target cell** *or* **target organ** = (i) cell or organ which receives the effect of a drug, by a hormone or by a disease; (ii) large red blood cell which shows a red spot in the middle when stained

the target cells for adult myeloid leukaemia are located in the bone marrow

British Medical Journal

tars(o)- ['tɑːsəʊ] *prefix* referring to (i) the ankle bones; (ii) the edge of an eyelid

tarsal ['tɑːsl] **1** *adjective* referring to the tarsus; **tarsal bones** = seven small bones in the ankle, including the talus (ankle bone) and calcaneus (heel bone); **tarsal gland** = MEIBOMIAN GLAND **2** *noun*; **the tarsals** = seven small bones which form the ankle

tarsalgia [tɑː'sældʒə] *noun* pain in the ankle

tarsectomy [tɑː'sektəmi] *noun* surgical operation to remove (i) one of the tarsal bones in the ankle; (ii) the tarsus of the eyelid

tarsitis [tɑːˈsaɪtɪs] *noun* inflammation of the edge of the eyelid

tarsorrhaphy [tɑːˈsɒrəfi] *noun* operation to join the two eyelids together to protect the eye after an operation

tarsotomy [tɑːˈsɒtəmi] *noun* incision of the tarsus (of the eyelid)

tarsus [ˈtɑːsəs] *noun* **(a)** the seven small bones of the ankle **(b)** connective tissue which supports an eyelid; *see illustration at* FOOT (NOTE: the plural is **tarsi**)

> COMMENT: the seven bones of the tarsus are: calcaneus, cuboid, the three cuneiforms, navicular and talus

tartar [ˈtɑːtə] *noun* hard deposit of calcium which forms on teeth, and has to be removed by scaling

tartrazine [ˈtɑːtrəziːn] *noun* yellow substance (E102) added to food to give it an attractive colour (although widely used, tartrazine provokes reactions in hypersensitive people and is banned in some countries)

taste [teɪst] **1** *noun* one of the five senses, where food or substances in the mouth are noticed through the tongue; *he doesn't like the taste of onions*; *he has a cold, so food seems to have lost all taste or seems to have no taste*; **taste bud** = tiny sensory receptor in the vallate and fungiform papillae of the tongue and in part of the back of the mouth **2** *verb* (i) to notice the taste of something with the tongue; (ii) to have a taste; *you can taste the salt in this butter*; *this cake tastes of chocolate*; *he has a cold so he can't taste anything*

> COMMENT: the taste buds can tell the difference between salt, sour, bitter and sweet tastes. The buds on the tip of the tongue identify salt and sweet tastes, those on the sides of the tongue identify sour, and those at the back of the mouth the bitter tastes. Note that most of what we think of as taste is in fact smell, and this is why when someone has a cold and a blocked nose, food seems to lose its taste. The impulses from the taste buds are received by the taste cortex in the temporal lobe of the cerebral hemisphere

taurine [ˈtɔːriːn] *noun* amino acid which forms bile salts

taxis [ˈtæksɪs] *noun* pushing or massaging dislocated bones or hernias to make them return to their normal position

-taxis [ˈtæksɪs] *suffix* meaning manipulation

Tay-Sachs disease [ˈteɪˈsæks dɪˈziːz] *noun* amaurotic familial idiocy, inherited form of mental abnormality, where the legs are paralysed and the child becomes blind and mentally retarded

TB [ˈtiː ˈbiː] *abbreviation for* TUBERCULOSIS; *he is suffering from TB*; *she has been admitted to a TB sanatorium*

T bandage [ˈtiː ˈbændɪdʒ] *noun* bandage shaped like the letter T, used for bandaging the area between the legs

TBI [ˈtiː ˈbiː ˈaɪ] = TOTAL BODY IRRADIATION

T-cell *or* **T-lymphocyte** [ˈtiːˈsel *or* ˈtiː ˈlɪmfəsaɪt] *noun* lymphocyte produced by the thymus gland

t.d.s. *or* **TDS** [ˈtiː ˈdiː ˈes] *abbreviation for* the Latin phrase 'ter in diem sumendus': three times a day (written on prescriptions)

tea [tiː] *noun* (i) dried leaves of a plant used to make a hot drink; (ii) hot drink made by pouring boiling water onto the dried leaves of a plant; **herb tea** = hot drink made from the leaves of a herb; *she drank a cup of peppermint tea*

teach [tiːtʃ] *verb* (i) to give lessons; (ii) to show someone how to do something; *Professor Smith teaches neurosurgery*; *she was taught first aid by her mother*; **teaching hospital** = hospital which is part of a medical school, where student doctors work and study as part of their training (NOTE: **teaching - taught - has taught**)

team [tiːm] *noun* group of people who work together; *the heart-lung transplant was carried out by a team of surgeons*

tear 1 *noun* **(a)** [tɪə]salty excretion which forms in the lacrimal gland when a person cries; *tears ran down her face*; **she burst into tears** = she suddenly started to cry; **tear duct** = lacrimal duct, the canal which takes tears from the lacrimal sac into the nose; **tear gland** = lacrimal gland, the gland which secretes tears (NOTE: for other terms referring to tears, see words beginning with **dacryo-**, **lacrim-**, **lacrym-**) **(b)** [teə]a hole or a split in a tissue often due to over-stretching; *an episiotomy was needed to avoid a tear in the perineal tissue* **2** [teə] *verb* to make a hole or a split in a tissue by pulling or stretching too much; *he tore a ligament in his ankle*; *they carried out an operation to repair a torn ligament* (NOTE: **tearing - tore - has torn**)

teat [ti:t] *noun* rubber nipple on the end of a baby's feeding bottle

technician [tek'nɪʃn] *noun* qualified person who does practical work in a laboratory or scientific institution; *he is a laboratory technician in a laboratory attached to a teaching hospital*; **dental technician** = qualified person who makes false teeth, plates, etc.

technique [tek'niːk] *noun* way of doing scientific or medical work; *a new technique for treating osteoarthritis*; *she is trying out a new laboratory technique*

> few parts of the body are inaccessible to modern catheter techniques, which are all performed under local anaesthesia
>
> *British Medical Journal*

> the technique used to treat aortic stenosis is similar to that for any cardiac catheterization
>
> *Journal of the American Medical Association*

> cardiac resuscitation techniques used by over half the nurses in a recent study were described as 'completely ineffective'
>
> *Nursing Times*

tectorial membrane [tek'tɔːrɪəl 'membreɪn] *noun* membrane in the inner ear which contains the hair cells which transmit impulses to the auditory nerve

tectospinal tract [tektəʊ'spaɪnl 'trækt] *noun* tract which takes nerve impulses from the mesencephalon to the spinal cord

TED = THROMBO-EMBOLIC DETERRENT STOCKING

teeth [ti:θ] *see* TOOTH

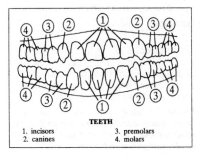

TEETH
1. incisors   3. premolars
2. canines   4. molars

teething ['ti:ðɪŋ] *noun* period when a baby's milk teeth are starting to erupt, and the baby is irritable; *he is awake at night because he is teething*; *she has teething trouble and won't eat*

teflon ['teflɒn] *noun* synthetic polymer injected into the joints of the larynx to increase movement and help hoarseness of voice

tegmen ['tegmən] *noun* covering for an organ (NOTE: the plural is **tegmina**)

tel- or **tele-** [tel or 'telɪ] *prefix* meaning done at a distance

telangiectasis *or* **telangiectasia** [telændʒi'ektəsɪs telændʒiek'teɪsɪə] *noun* small dark red spots on the skin, formed by swollen capillaries

teleceptor ['telɪseptə] *noun* sensory receptor which receives sensations from a distance

telencephalon [telen'kefəlɒn] *noun* cerebrum, the main part of the brain

> COMMENT: the telencephalon is the largest part of the brain, formed of two cerebral hemispheres. It controls the main mental processes, including the memory

teleradiography [telɪreɪdi'ɒgrəfi] *noun* radiography where the source of the X-rays is at a distance from the patient

teleradiotherapy [telɪreɪdiəʊ'θerəpi] *noun* radiotherapy, where the patient is some way away from the source of radiation

telo- ['teləʊ] *prefix* meaning end

telophase ['teləʊfeɪz] *noun* final stage of mitosis, the stage in cell division after anaphase

temper ['tempə] *noun* (usually bad) state of mind; **he's in a (bad) temper** = he is annoyed; **he lost his temper** = he became very angry; **temper tantrum** = violent attack of bad behaviour, usually in a child, where the child breaks things or lies on the floor and screams

temperature ['temprətʃə] *noun* **(a)** heat of the body or of the surrounding air, measured in degrees; *the doctor asked the nurse what the patient's temperature was*; *his temperature was slightly above normal*; *the thermometer showed a temperature of 99°F*; **to take a patient's temperature** = to insert a thermometer in a patient's body to see what his body temperature is; *they took his temperature every four hours*; *when her* temperature was taken this morning, it was normal; **central temperature** = temperature of the brain, thorax and abdomen, which is constant; **environmental temperature** = temperature of the air outside the body **(b)** sickness when the temperature of the body is higher than normal; *he's in bed with a temperature*; *her mother says she's got a temperature, and can't come to work*

COMMENT: the normal average body temperature is about 37º Celsius or 98º Fahrenheit. This temperature may vary during the day, and can rise if a person has taken a hot bath or had a hot drink. If the environmental temperature is high, the body has to sweat to reduce the heat gained from the air around it. If the outside temperature is low, the body shivers, because rapid movement of the muscles generates heat. A fever will cause the body temperature to rise sharply, to 40ºC (103ºF) or more. Hypothermia exists when the body temperature falls below about 35ºC (95ºF)

temple ['templ] *noun* flat part of the side of the head between the top of the ear and the eye

temporal ['temprəl] *adjective* referring to the temple; **temporal arteritis** = inflammation of the arteries in the temple; **temporal fossa** = depression at the side of the temporal bone, above the zygomatic arch; **temporal lobe** = lobe above the ear in each cerebral hemisphere; **temporal lobe epilepsy** = epilepsy due to a disorder of the temporal lobe and causing impaired memory, hallucinations and automatism

temporal bone ['temprəl 'bəʊn] *noun* one of the bones which form the sides and base of the cranium; *see illustrations at* SKULL, EAR

COMMENT: the temporal bone is in two parts: the petrous part forms the base of the skull and the inner and middle ears, while the squamous part forms the side of the skull. The lower back part of the temporal bone is the mastoid process, while the part between the ear and the cheek is the zygomatic arch

temporalis (muscle) [tempə'reɪlɪs 'mʌsl] *noun* flat muscle running down the side of the head from the temporal bone to the coronoid process, which makes the jaw move up

temporary ['temprəri] *adjective* which is not permanent, which is not final; *the dentist gave him a temporary filling*; *the accident team put a temporary bandage on the wound*

temporo- ['tempərə] *prefix* referring to (i) the temple; (ii) the temporal lobe

temporomandibular joint [tempərəmæn'dɪbjʊlə 'dʒɔɪnt] *noun* joint between the jaw and the skull, in front of the ear

tenaculum [tə'nækjʊləm] *noun* surgical instrument shaped like a hook, used to pick up small pieces of tissue during an operation

tend [tend] *verb* **to tend to do something** = to do something generally, as a normal process; *the prostate tends to enlarge as a man grows older*

tendency ['tendənsi] *noun* being likely to do something; **to have a tendency to something** = to be likely to have something; *there is a tendency to obesity in her family*; *the children of the area show a tendency to vitamin-deficiency diseases*

premature babies have been shown to have a higher tendency to develop a squint during childhood

Nursing Times

tender ['tendə] *adjective* (skin or flesh) which is painful when touched; *the bruise is still tender*; *her shoulders are still tender where she got sunburnt*; *a tender spot on the abdomen indicates that an organ is inflamed*

tenderness ['tendənəs] *noun* feeling painful when touched; *tenderness when pressure is applied is a sign of inflammation*

tendineae ['tendɪniː] *noun;* **chordae tendineae** = tiny fibrous ligaments in the heart which attach the edges of some of the valves to the walls of the ventricles

tendinitis [tendɪ'naɪtɪs] *noun* inflammation of a tendon, especially after playing sport, and often associated with tenosynovitis

tendinous ['tendɪnəs] *adjective* referring to a tendon

tendo calcaneus ['tendəʊ kæl'keɪnɪəs] *noun* Achilles tendon, the tendon at the back of the ankle which connects the calf muscles to the heel and which acts to pull up the heel when the calf muscle is contracted

tendon ['tendən] *noun* strip of connective tissue which attaches a muscle to a bone; **tendon sheath** = tube of membrane which covers and protects a tendon

tendovaginitis [tendəʊvædʒə'naɪtɪs] *noun* inflammation of a tendon sheath, especially in the thumb (NOTE: for other terms referring to a tendon, see also words beginning with **teno-**)

tenens ['tenəns] *see* LOCUM

tenesmus [tə'nezməs] *noun* condition where the patient feels he needs to pass faeces (or sometimes urine) but is unable to do so and experiences pain

tennis elbow ['tenɪs 'elbəʊ] *noun* lateral epicondylitis, inflammation of the tendons of the extensor muscles in the hand which are attached to the bone near the elbow

teno- ['tenəʊ] *prefix* referring to a tendon

Tenon's capsule [tə'nɒnz 'kæpsjuːl] *noun* tissue which lines the orbit of the eye

tenoplasty ['tenəplæsti] *noun* surgical operation to repair a torn tendon

tenorrhaphy [te'nɒrəfi] *noun* surgical operation to stitch pieces of a torn tendon together

tenosynovitis [tenəʊsaɪnəʊ'vaɪtɪs] *noun* peritendinitis, painful inflammation of the tendon sheath and the tendon inside

tenotomy [tə'nɒtəmi] *noun* surgical operation to cut through a tendon

tenovaginitis [tenəʊvædʒə'naɪtɪs] *noun* inflammation of the tendon sheath, especially in the thumb

tense [tens] *adjective* **(a)** *(of a muscle)* contracted **(b)** nervous and worried; *the patient was very tense while he waited for the report from the laboratory*

tension ['tenʃn] *noun* nervous stress; **tension headache** = headache all over the head, caused by worry and stress

tensor ['tensə] *noun* muscle which makes a joint stretch out; *compare* EXTENSOR, FLEXOR

tent [tent] *noun* small shelter put over and round a patient's bed so that gas or vapour can be passed inside; **oxygen tent** = type of cover put over a patient's bed so that he can inhale oxygen

tentorium cerebelli [ten'tɔːriəm serə'beli] *noun* part of the dura mater which separates the cerebellum from the cerebral hemispheres

tera- ['terə] *prefix* meaning 10^{12} (NOTE: the chemical symbol is **T**)

terat- *or* **terato-** ['terət *or* 'terətəʊ] *prefix* meaning congenitally abnormal

teratogen ['terətədʒen] *noun* substance (such as the German measles virus) which causes an abnormality to develop in an embryo

teratogenesis [terətə'dʒenəsɪs] *noun* development of abnormalities in an embryo and fetus

teratology [terə'tɒlədʒi] *noun* study of abnormal development of embryos and fetuses

teratoma [terə'təʊmə] *noun* tumour which is formed of abnormal tissue, usually developing in an ovary or testis

teres ['tɪəriːz] *noun* one of two shoulder muscles running from the shoulder blade to the top of the humerus

COMMENT: the larger of the two muscles, the teres major, makes the arm turn towards the inside, and the smaller, the teres minor, makes it turn towards the outside

term [tɜːm] *noun* **(a)** length of time, especially the period from conception to childbirth; **she was coming near the end of her term** = she was near the time when she would give birth **(b)** part of a college or school year; *the anatomy exams are at the beginning of the third term*

terminal ['tɜːmɪnl] **1** *adjective* (i) referring to the last stage of a fatal illness; (ii) referring to the end; being at the end of something; *the disease is in its terminal stages*; *he is suffering from terminal cancer*; **terminal branch** = end part of a neurone which is linked to a muscle; *see illustration at* NEURONE; **terminal illness** = illness from which the patient will soon die **2** *noun* ending, part at the end of an electrode or nerve

terminale [tɜːmɪ'neɪli] *see* FILUM

terminally ill ['tɜːmɪnəli 'ɪl] *adjective* very ill and about to die; *she was admitted to a hospice for terminally ill patients or for the terminally ill*

termination [tɜːmɪ'neɪʃn] *noun* ending; **termination (of pregnancy)** = abortion

-terol ['terɒl] *suffix* used in names of bronchodilators

tertian fever ['tɜːʃn 'fiːvə] *noun* type of malaria where the fever returns every two days; *see also* QUARTAN

tertiary ['tɜːʃəri] *adjective* third, coming after secondary and primary; **tertiary**

bronchi = air passages supplying a segment of a lung; *see also* SYPHILIS

test [test] **1** *noun* short examination to see if a sample is healthy or if part of the body is working well; *he had an eye test this morning*; *laboratory tests showed that she was a meningitis carrier*; *tests are being carried out on swabs taken from the operating theatre*; **blood test** = laboratory test of a blood sample to analyse its chemical composition; *the patient will have to have a blood test*; **laboratory test** = test carried out in a laboratory; **the urine test was positive** = the examination of the urine sample showed the presence of an infection or a diagnostic substance **2** *verb* to examine a sample of tissue to see if it is healthy or an organ to see if it is is working well; *they sent the urine sample away for testing*; *I must have my eyes tested*

testicle *or* **testis** ['testɪkl *or* 'testɪs] *noun* one of two male sex glands in the scrotum (NOTE: the plural of **testis** is **testes.** For other terms referring to the testes, see words beginning with **orchi-**); *see illustration at* UROGENITAL SYSTEM (male)

COMMENT: the testes produce both spermatozoa and the sex hormone, testosterone. Spermatozoa are formed in the testes, and passed into the epididymis to be stored. From the epididymis they pass along the vas deferens through the prostate gland which secretes the seminal fluid, and are ejaculated through the penis

testicular [te'stɪkjʊlə] *adjective* referring to the testes; *testicular cancer comprises only 1% of all malignant neoplasms in the male*; **testicular hormone** = testosterone

test meal ['test 'miːl] *noun* meal given to a patient to test the secretion of gastric juices

testosterone [te'stɒstərəʊn] *noun* male sex hormone, secreted by the Leydig cells in the testes, which causes physical changes (such as the development of body hair and deep voice) to take place in males as they become sexually mature

test tube ['test 'tjuːb] *noun* small glass tube open at the top and with a rounded bottom, used in laboratories to hold liquids and gas during experiments or analysis; **test-tube baby** = baby which develops after the mother's ova have been removed from the ovaries, fertilized with a man's spermatozoa in a laboratory, and returned to the mother's uterus to continue developing normally

COMMENT: this process of in vitro fertilization is carried out in cases where the mother is unable to conceive, though both she and the father are normally fertile

tetanic [te'tænɪk] *adjective* referring to tetanus

tetanus ['tetənəs] *noun* **(a)** continuous contraction of a muscle, under repeated stimuli from a motor nerve **(b)** lockjaw, an infection caused by *Clostridium tetani* in the soil, which affects the spinal cord and causes spasms in the muscles which occur first in the jaw

COMMENT: people who are liable to infection with tetanus, such as farm workers, should be immunized against it, though booster injections are needed from time to time

tetany ['tetəni] *noun* spasms of the muscles in the feet and hands, caused by a reduction in the level of calcium in the blood or by lack of carbon dioxide; *see* PARATHYROID HORMONE

tetracycline [tetrə'saɪkliːn] *noun* antibiotic used to treat a wide range of bacterial diseases such as chlamydia

COMMENT: because of its side-effects tetracycline should not be given to children. Many bacteria are now resistant to tetracycline

tetradactyly [tetrə'dæktɪli] *noun* congenital deformity where a child has only four fingers or toes

tetralogy of Fallot *or* **Fallot's tetralogy** [te'trælədʒi əv 'fæləʊ *or* 'fæləʊz te'trælədʒi] *noun* disorder of the heart which makes a child's skin blue; *see also* BLALOCK'S OPERATION, WATERSTON'S OPERATION

COMMENT: the condition is formed of four disorders occurring together: the artery leading to the lungs is narrow, the right ventricle is enlarged, there is a defect in the membrane between the ventricles, and the aorta is not correctly placed

tetraplegia [tetrə'pliːdʒə] = QUADRIPLEGIA

textbook ['teksbʊk] *noun* book which is used by students; *a haematology textbook or a textbook on haematology*; **textbook case** = case which shows symptoms which are exactly like those described in a textbook

thalam- *or* **thalamo-** ['θæləm or 'θæləməʊ] *prefix* referring to the thalamus

thalamencephalon [θæləmen'sefəlɒn] *noun* group of structures in the brain linked to the brain stem, formed of the epithalamus, hypothalamus, and thalamus

thalamic syndrome [θə'læmɪk 'sɪndrəʊm] *noun* condition where a patient is extremely sensitive to pain, caused by a disorder of the thalamus

thalamocortical tract [θæləməʊ'kɔːtɪkl 'trækt] *noun* tract containing nerve fibres, running from the thalamus to the sensory cortex

thalamotomy [θælə'mɒtəmi] *noun* surgical operation to make an incision into the thalamus to treat intractable pain

thalamus ['θæləməs] *noun* one of two masses of grey matter situated beneath the cerebrum where impulses from the sensory neurones are transmitted to the cerebral cortex; *see illustration at* BRAIN (NOTE: the plural is **thalami**)

thalassaemia [θælæ'siːmiə] *noun* Cooley's anaemia, hereditary type of anaemia, found in Mediterranean countries, due to a defect in the production of haemoglobin

thaw [θɔː] *verb* to bring something which is frozen back to normal temperature

theatre ['θɪətə] *noun* **(operating) theatre,** *US* **operating room** = special room in a hospital where surgeons carry out operations; **theatre gown** = gown worn by a patient, by a surgeon or nurse in an operating theatre; **theatre nurse** = nurse who is specially trained to assist in operations

---

> While waiting to go to theatre, parents should be encouraged to participate in play with their children
>
> *British Journal of Nursing*

---

theca ['θiːkə] *noun* tissue shaped like a sheath

thenar ['θiːnə] *adjective* (referring to) the palm of the hand; **thenar eminence** = the ball of the thumb, lump of flesh in the palm of the hand below the thumb; *compare* HYPOTHENAR

theory ['θɪəri] *noun* argument which explains a scientific fact

therapeutic [θerə'pjuːtɪk] *adjective* (treatment or drug) which is given in order to

cure a disorder or disease; **therapeutic abortion** = legal abortion carried out because the health of the mother is in danger

therapeutics [θerə'pjuːtɪks] *noun* study of various types of treatment and their effect on patients

therapist ['θerəpɪst] *noun* person specially trained to give therapy; *an occupational therapist*; *see also* PSYCHOTHERAPIST, THERAPY

therapy ['θerəpi] *noun* treatment of a patient to help cure a disease or disorder; **aversion therapy** = treatment where the patient is cured of a type of behaviour by making him develop a great dislike for it; **behaviour therapy** = psychiatric treatment where the patient learns to improve his condition; **group therapy** = type of treatment where a group of people with the same disorder meet together with a therapist to discuss their condition and try to help each other; **heat therapy** = thermotherapy, using heat (from infrared lamps, hot water, etc.) to treat certain conditions such as arthritis and bad circulation; **light therapy** = treatment of a disorder by exposing the patient to light (sunlight, UV light, etc); **occupational therapy** = light work or hobbies used as a means of treatment to promote independence, especially for handicapped or mentally ill patients and during the recovery period after an illness or operation; **shock therapy** = method of treating some mental disorders by giving the patient an electric shock to induce convulsions and loss of consciousness; **speech therapy** = treatment to cure a speech disorder such as stammering; *see also* PSYCHOTHERAPY, RADIOTHERAPY (NOTE: both therapy and therapist are used as suffixes: **psychotherapist, radiotherapy**)

thermal ['θɜːml] *adjective* referring to heat; **thermal anaesthesia** = loss of feeling of heat

thermo- ['θɜːməʊ] *prefix* referring to (i) heat; (ii) temperature

thermoanaesthesia [θɜːməʊænəs'θiːziə] *noun* condition where the patient cannot tell the difference between hot and cold

thermocautery [θɜːməʊ'kɔːtəri] *noun* removing dead tissue by heat

thermocoagulation [θɜːməʊkəʊægju'leɪʃn] *noun* removing tissue and coagulating blood by heat

thermogram ['θɜːməgræm] *noun* infrared photograph of part of the body

thermography [θɜːˈmɒgrəfi] *noun* technique of photographing part of the body using infrared rays, which record the heat given off by the skin, and show variations in the blood circulating beneath the skin, used especially in screening for breast cancer

thermolysis [θɜːˈmɒləsɪs] *noun* loss of body temperature (as by sweating)

thermometer [θəˈmɒmɪtə] *noun* instrument for measuring temperature; **clinical thermometer** = thermometer used in a hospital or by a doctor for taking a patient's body temperature; **oral thermometer** = thermometer which is put into the mouth to take a patient's temperature; **rectal thermometer** = thermometer which is inserted into the patient's rectum to take the temperature

thermophilic [θɜːməʊˈfɪlɪk] *adjective* (organism) which needs a high temperature to grow

thermoreceptor [θɜːməʊrɪˈseptə] *noun* sensory nerve which registers heat

thermotaxis [θɜːməʊˈtæksɪs] *noun* automatic regulation of the body's temperature

thermotherapy [θɜːməʊˈθerəpi] *noun* heat treatment, using heat (as from hot water or infrared lamps) to treat conditions such as arthritis and bad circulation

thiamine [ˈθaɪəmiːn] = VITAMIN B$_1$

thicken [ˈθɪkn] *verb* **(a)** to become wider or larger; *the walls of the arteries thicken under deposits of fat* **(b)** (of liquid) to become more dense and viscid and flow less easily; *the liquid thickens as its cools*

Thiersch graft [ˈtɪəʃ ˈgrɑːft] = SPLIT-SKIN GRAFT

thigh [θaɪ] *noun* top part of the leg from the knee to the groin

thighbone [ˈθaɪbəʊn] *noun* femur, the bone in the top part of the leg, which joins the acetabulum at the hip and the tibia at the knee (NOTE: for other terms referring to the thigh, see words beginning with **femor-**)

thin [θɪn] *adjective* **(a)** not fat; *his arms are very thin*; *she's getting too thin - she should eat more*; *he became quite thin after his illness* (NOTE: **thin - thinner - thinnest**) **(b)** not thick; *they cut a thin slice of tissue for examination under the microscope* **(c)** (blood) which is watery

thirst [θɜːst] *noun* feeling of wanting to drink; *he had a fever and a violent thirst*

thirsty [ˈθɜːsti] *adjective* wanting to drink; *if the patient is thirsty, give her a glass of water* (NOTE: **thirsty - thirstier - thirstiest**)

Thomas splint [ˈtɒməs ˈsplɪnt] *noun* type of splint used on a fractured femur, with a ring at the top round the thigh, and a bar under the foot at the lower end

thorac(o)- [ˈθɔːrəkəʊ] *prefix* referring to the chest

thoracectomy [θɔːrəˈsektəmi] *noun* surgical operation to remove one or more ribs

thoracentesis [θɔːrəsenˈtiːsɪs] *noun* operation where a hollow needle is inserted into the pleura to drain fluid

thoracic [θɔːˈræsɪk] *adjective* referring to the chest or thorax; **thoracic cavity** = chest cavity, containing the diaphragm, heart and lungs; **thoracic duct** = one of the main terminal ducts in the lymphatic system, running from the abdomen to the left side of the neck; **thoracic inlet** = small opening at the top of the thorax; **thoracic outlet** = large opening at the bottom of the thorax; **thoracic outlet syndrome** = pain in an arm, caused by the scalenus anterior muscle pressing the subclavian artery and the brachial plexus against the vertebrae (NOTE: also called **scalenus syndrome**); **thoracic vertebrae** = the twelve vertebrae in the spine behind the chest, to which the ribs are attached; *see illustration at* VERTEBRAL COLUMN

thoracocentesis [θɔːrəkəʊsenˈtiːsɪs] *noun* operation where a hollow needle is inserted into the pleura to drain fluid

thoracoplasty [ˈθɔːrəkəʊplæsti] *noun* surgical operation to cut through the ribs to allow the lungs to collapse, formerly a treatment for pulmonary tuberculosis

thoracoscope [ˈθɔːrəkəskəʊp] *noun* surgical instrument, like a tube with a light at the end, used to examine the inside of the chest

thoracoscopy [θɔːrəˈkɒskəpi] *noun* examination of the inside the chest, using a thoracoscope

thoracotomy [θɔːrəˈkɒtəmi] *noun* surgical operation to make a hole in the wall of the chest

thorax [ˈθɔːræks] *noun* chest, the cavity in the top part of the front of the body above the abdomen, containing the diaphragm, heart and lungs, and surrounded by the ribcage

thread [θred] **1** *noun* thin piece of cotton, suture, etc.; *the surgeon used strong thread* *to make the suture* **2** *verb* to insert a thin piece of cotton, suture, etc., through the eye of (a needle)

threadworm ['θredwɜ:m] *noun* pinworm, a thin parasitic worm, *Enterobius,* which infests the large intestine and causes itching round the anus

thready ['θredi] *adjective* (pulse) which is very weak and can hardly be felt

threonine ['θri:əni:n] *noun* essential amino acid

threshold ['θreʃhəʊld] *noun* (i) point below which a drug has no effect; (ii) point at which a sensation is strong enough to be sensed by the sensory nerves; *she has a low hearing threshold*; **pain threshold** = point at which a person cannot bear pain without crying

> if intracranial pressure rises above the treatment threshold, it is imperative first to validate the reading and then to eliminate any factors exacerbating the rise in pressure
>
> *British Journal of Hospital Medicine*

thrill [θrɪl] *noun* vibration which can be felt with the hands

thrive [θraɪv] *verb* to do well, to live and grow strongly; **failure to thrive** = wasting disease of small children who have difficulty in absorbing nutrients or who are suffering from malnutrition

throat [θrəʊt] *noun* (i) top part of the tube which goes down from the mouth to the stomach; (ii) front part of the neck below the chin; *if it is cold, wrap a scarf round your throat*; *a piece of meat got stuck in his throat*; **to clear the throat** = to give a little cough; **sore throat** = condition where the mucous membrane in the pharynx is inflamed (sometimes because the person has been talking too much, but usually because of an infection)

> COMMENT: the throat carries both food from the mouth and air from the nose and mouth. It divides into the oesophagus, which takes food to the stomach, and the trachea, which takes air into the lungs

throb [θrɒb] *verb* to have a regular beat, like the heart; *his head was throbbing with pain*

throbbing ['θrɒbɪŋ] *adjective* (pain) which comes again and again like a heart beat; *she has a throbbing pain in her finger*; *he has a throbbing headache*

thrombectomy [θrɒm'bektəmi] *noun* surgical operation to remove a blood clot

thrombin ['θrɒmbɪn] *noun* substance which converts fibrinogen to fibrin and so coagulates blood

thrombo- ['θrɒmbəʊ] *prefix* referring to (i) blood clot; (ii) thrombosis

thromboangiitis obliterans
[θrɒmbəʊændʒi'aɪtɪs əb'lɪtərəns] *noun* disease of the arteries, where the blood vessels in a limb (usually the leg) become narrow, causing gangrene (NOTE: also called **Buerger's disease**)

thromboarteritis [θrɒmbəʊɑːtə'raɪtɪs] *noun* inflammation of an artery caused by thrombosis

thrombocyte ['θrɒmbəʊsaɪt] *noun* platelet, a little blood cell which encourages the coagulation of blood

thrombocythaemia [θrɒmbəʊsi'θi:miə] *noun* disease where the patient has an abnormally high number of platelets in his blood

thrombocytopenia
[θrɒmbəʊsaɪtəʊ'pi:niə] *noun* condition where the patient has an abnormally low number of platelets in his blood

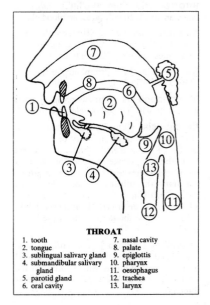

THROAT

1. tooth	7. nasal cavity
2. tongue	8. palate
3. sublingual salivary gland	9. epiglottis
4. submandibular salivary gland	10. pharynx
	11. oesophagus
5. parotid gland	12. trachea
6. oral cavity	13. larynx

thrombocytopenic
[θrɒmbəʊsaɪtəʊ'penɪk] *adjective* referring to thrombocytopenia

thrombocytosis [θrɒmbəʊsaɪ'təʊsɪs] *noun* increase in the number of platelets in a patient's blood

thrombo-embolic deterrent stocking (TED) [θrɒmbəʊem'bɒlɪk dɪ'terənt 'stɒkɪŋ] *noun* support stocking to prevent thrombus formation following surgery

thromboembolism [θrɒmbəʊ'embəlɪzm] *noun* condition where a blood clot forms in one part of the body and moves through the blood vessels to block another, usually narower, part

thromboendarterectomy [θrɒmbəʊendɑːtə'rektəmi] *noun* surgical operation to open an artery to remove a blood clot which is blocking it

thromboendarteritis [θrɒmbəʊendɑːtə'raɪtɪs] *noun* inflammation of the inside of an artery, caused by thrombosis

thrombokinase [θrɒmbəʊ'kaɪneɪz] *noun* thromboplastin, substance which converts prothrombin into thrombin, so starting the sequence for coagulation

thrombolysis [θrɒm'bɒləsɪs] *noun* breaking up of blood clots

thrombolytic [θrɒmbəʊ'lɪtɪk] *adjective* (substance) which will break up blood clots

thrombophlebitis [θrɒmbəʊflɪ'baɪtɪs] *noun* blocking of a vein by a blood clot, sometimes causing inflammation

thromboplastin [θrɒmbəʊ'plæstɪn] = THROMBOKINASE

thrombopoiesis [θrɒmbəʊpɔɪ'iːsɪs] *noun* process by which blood platelets are formed

thrombosis [θrɒm'bəʊsɪs] *noun* blood clotting, blocking of an artery or vein by a mass of coagulated blood; **cerebral thrombosis** = stroke, a condition where a blood clot enters and blocks a brain artery; **coronary thrombosis** = blood clot which blocks one of the coronary arteries, leading to a heart attack; **deep vein thrombosis (DVT)** = blood clot in the deep veins of the leg or pelvis

thrombus ['θrɒmbəs] *noun* soft mass of coagulated blood in a vein or artery; **mural thrombus** = thrombus which forms on the wall of a vein or artery (NOTE: the plural is **thrombi**)

throw up ['θrəʊ 'ʌp] *verb* to be sick, to vomit; *she threw up all over the bathroom floor*; *he threw up his dinner* (NOTE: throwing - threw - has thrown)

thrush [θrʌʃ] *noun* infection of the mouth (or sometimes the vagina) with the bacterium *Candida albicans*

thumb [θʌm] *noun* short thick finger, with only two phalanges, which is separated from the other four fingers on the hand; *he hit his thumb with the hammer*; *the baby was sucking its thumb*

thumb-sucking ['θʌmsʌkɪŋ] *noun* action of sucking a thumb; *thumb-sucking tends to push the teeth forward*

thym- ['θaɪm] *prefix* referring to the thymus gland

thymectomy [θaɪ'mektəmi] *noun* surgical operation to remove the thymus gland

-thymia ['θaɪmiə] *suffix* referring to a state of mind

thymic ['θaɪmɪk] *adjective* referring to the thymus gland

thymine ['θaɪmiːn] *noun* basic element in DNA

thymitis [θaɪ'maɪtɪs] *noun* inflammation of the thymus gland

thymocyte ['θaɪməʊsaɪt] *noun* lymphocyte formed in the thymus gland

thymoma [θaɪ'məʊmə] *noun* tumour in the thymus gland

thymus (gland) ['θaɪməs 'glænd] *noun* endocrine gland in the front part of the top of the thorax, behind the breastbone

COMMENT: the thymus gland produces lymphocytes and is responsible for developing the system of natural immunity in children. It grows less active as the person becomes an adult. Lymphocytes produced by the thymus are known as T-lymphocytes or T-cells

thyro- ['θaɪrəʊ] *prefix* referring to the thyroid gland

thyrocalcitonin [θaɪrəʊkælsi'təʊnɪn] *noun* hormone, produced by the thyroid gland, which is believed to regulate the level of calcium in the blood

thyrocele ['θaɪrəʊsiːl] *noun* swelling of the thyroid gland

thyroglobulin [θaɪrəʊ'glɒbjʊlɪn] *noun* protein stored in the thyroid gland which is broken down into thyroxine

thyroglossal [θaɪrəʊ'glɒsl] *adjective* referring to the thyroid gland and the throat; **thyroglossal cyst** = cyst in the front of the neck

thyroid ['θaɪrɔɪd] **1** *adjective* referring to the thyroid gland; **thyroid cartilage** = large cartilage in the larynx, part of which forms the Adam's apple; *see illustration at* LUNGS; **thyroid dysfunction** = abnormal functioning of the thyroid gland; **thyroid extract** = substance extracted from thyroid glands of animals and used to treat hypothyroidism; **thyroid hormone** = hormone produced by the thyroid gland **2** *noun;* **thyroid (gland)** = endocrine gland in the neck below the larynx

COMMENT: the thyroid gland is activated by the pituitary gland, and produces thyroxine, a hormone which regulates the body's metabolism. The thyroid gland needs a supply of iodine in order to produce thyroxine. If the thyroid gland malfunctions, it can result in hyperthyroidism (producing too much thyroxine) leading to goitre, or in hypothyroidism (producing too little thyroxine) which causes cretinism in children and myxoedema in adults. Hyperthyroidism can be treated with carbimazole

thyroidectomy [θaɪrɔɪ'dektəmi] *noun* surgical operation to remove all or part of the thyroid gland

thyroiditis [θaɪrɔɪ'daɪtɪs] *noun* inflammation of the thyroid gland

thyroid-stimulating hormone (TSH) or **thyrotrophin** *US* **thryotropin**
['θaɪrɔɪd'stɪmjuleɪtɪŋ 'hɔːməʊn or θaɪrəʊ'trəʊfɪn or θaɪrəʊ'trəʊpɪn] *noun* hormone secreted by the pituitary gland which stimulates the thyroid gland

thyrotomy [θaɪ'rɒtəmi] *noun* surgical opening made in the thyroid cartilage or the thyroid gland

thyrotoxic [θaɪrəʊ'tɒksɪk] *adjective* referring to severe hyperthyroidism; **thyrotoxic crisis** = sudden illness caused by hyperthyroidism; **thyrotoxic goitre** = goitre caused by thyrotoxicosis

thyrotoxicosis [θaɪrəʊtɒksɪ'kəʊsɪs] *noun* type of goitre, caused by hyperthyroidism, where the heart beats faster, the thyroid gland swells, the patient trembles and his eyes protrude (NOTE: also called **Graves' disease** or **exophthalmic goitre** or **Basedow's disease**)

thyrotrophin *US* **thyrotropin**
[θaɪrəʊ'trəʊfɪn *US* θaɪrəʊ'trəʊpɪn] *noun* thyroid-stimulating hormone, hormone secreted by the pituitary gland which stimulates the thyroid gland

thyrotrophin-releasing hormone (TRH) [θaɪrəʊ'trəʊfɪnrɪ'liːsɪŋ 'hɔːməʊn] *noun* hormone secreted by the hypothalamus, which makes the pituitary gland release thyrotrophin, which in turn stimulates the thyroid gland

thyroxine [θaɪ'rɒksiːn] *noun* hormone produced by the thyroid gland which regulates the body's metabolism and conversion of food into heat

COMMENT: synthetic thyroxine is used in treatment of hypothyroidism

Ti *chemical symbol for* titanium

TIA ['tiː 'aɪ 'eɪ] = TRANSIENT ISCHAEMIC ATTACK

blood pressure control reduces the incidence of first stroke and aspirin appears to reduce the risk of stroke after TIAs by some 15%
British Journal of Hospital Medicine

tibia ['tɪbiə] *noun* shinbone, the larger of the two long bones in the lower leg running from the knee to the ankle (the other, thinner, bone in the lower leg is the fibula)

tibial ['tɪbiəl] *adjective* referring to the tibia; **tibial arteries** = two arteries which run down the front and back of the lower leg

tibialis [tɪbi'eɪlɪs] *noun* one of two muscles in the lower leg running from the tibia to the foot

tibio- ['tɪbiəʊ] *prefix* referring to the tibia

tibiofibular [tɪbiəʊ'fɪbjʊlə] *adjective* referring to both the tibia and the fibula

tic [tɪk] *noun* involuntary twitching of the muscles (usually in the face); **tic douloureux** = pain in the trigeminal nerve which sends intense pains shooting across the face (NOTE: also called **trigeminal neuralgia**)

tick [tɪk] *noun* tiny parasite which sucks blood from the skin; **tick fever** = infectious disease transmitted by bites from ticks

t.i.d. *or* **TID** ['tiː 'aɪ 'diː] *abbreviation for the Latin phrase* 'ter in die': three times a day (written on prescriptions)

-tidine ['tɪdɪn] *suffix* used for antihistamines; *loratidine; cimetidine*

tie [taɪ] *verb* to attach a thread with a knot; *the surgeon quickly tied up the stitches*; *the nurse had tied the bandage too tight* (NOTE: tying - tied - has tied)

tight [taɪt] *adjective* which fits firmly, which is not loose; *make sure the bandage is not too tight*; *the splint must be kept tight, or the bone may move*; *tight-fitting clothes can affect the circulation* (NOTE: tight - tighter - tightest)

tightly ['taɪtli] *adverb* in a tight way; *she tied the bandage tightly round his arm*

time [taɪm] *noun* period of hours, minutes, seconds, etc.; **bleeding time =** test of clotting of a patient's blood, by timing the length of time it takes for the blood to congeal; **clotting time** *or* **coagulation time =** the time taken for blood to coagulate under normal conditions

tincture ['tɪŋktʃə] *noun* medicinal substance dissolved in alcohol; **tincture of iodine =** disinfectant made of iodine and alcohol

tinea ['tɪniə] *noun* ringworm, infection by a fungus, in which the infection spreads out in a circle from a central point; **tinea barbae =** ringworm in the beard; **tinea capitis =** ringworm on the scalp; **tinea pedis =** athlete's foot, fungal infection between the toes

tingle ['tɪŋgl] *verb* to give a feeling like a slight electric shock; *he had a tingling feeling in his fingers*

tinnitus [tɪ'naɪtəs] *noun* ringing sound in the ears

COMMENT: tinnitus can sound like bells, or buzzing, or a loud roaring sound. In some cases it is caused by wax blocking the auditory canal, but it is also associated with Ménière's disease, infections of the middle ear and acoustic nerve conditions

tipped womb ['tɪpt 'wuːm] *noun* US condition where the uterus slopes backwards away from its normal position (NOTE: the British English is **retroverted uterus**)

tired ['taɪəd] *adjective* feeling sleepy, feeling that a person needs to rest; *the patients are tired, and need to go to bed*; *there is something wrong with her - she's always tired*

tiredness ['taɪədnəs] *noun* being tired

tired out ['taɪəd 'aut] *adjective* feeling extremely tired, feeling in need of a rest; *she is tired out after the physiotherapy*

tissue ['tɪʃuː] *noun* material made of cells, of which the parts of the body are formed; *most of the body is made up of soft tissue, with the exception of the bones and cartilage*; *the main types of body tissue are connective, epithelial, muscular and nerve tissue*; **adipose tissue =** tissue where the cells contain fat; **connective tissue =** tissue which forms the main part of bones and cartilage, ligaments and tendons, in which a large amount of fibrous material surrounds the tissue cells; **elastic tissue =** connective tissue as in the walls of arteries, which contains elastic fibres; **epithelial tissue =** tissue which forms the skin; **fibrous tissue =** strong white tissue which makes tendons and ligaments and also scar tissue; **lymphoid tissue =** tissue in the lymph nodes, the tonsils and the spleen, which forms lymphocytes and antibodies; **muscle tissue** *or* **muscular tissue** **=** tissue which forms the muscles, and which can contract and expand; **nerve tissue =** tissue which forms nerves, and which is able to transmit nerve impulses; **tissue culture =** live tissue grown in a culture in a laboratory; **tissue plasminogen activator (TPA) =** agent given to cause fibrinolysis in blood clots; **tissue typing =** identifying various elements in tissue from a donor and comparing them to those of the recipient to see if a transplant is likely to be rejected (the two most important factors are the ABO blood grouping and the HLA antigen system) (NOTE: for other terms referring to tissue, see words beginning with **hist-, histo-**)

titanium [tɪ'teɪniəm] *noun* light metallic element which does not corrode (NOTE: chemical symbol is **Ti**)

titration [taɪ'treɪʃn] *noun* process of measuring the strength of a solution

titre ['taɪtə] *noun* measurement of the quantity of antibodies in a serum

tobacco [tə'bækəu] *noun* leaves of a plant which are dried and smoked, either in a pipe or as cigarettes or cigars

COMMENT: tobacco contains nicotine, which is an addictive stimulant. This is why it is difficult for a person who smokes a lot of cigarettes to give up the habit. Nicotine can enter the bloodstream and cause poisoning; tobacco smoking also causes cancer, especially of the lungs and throat, and heart disease

toco- ['tɔkəu] *prefix* referring to childbirth

tocography [tɒ'kɒgrəfi] *noun* recording of the contractions of the uterus during childbirth

Todd's paralysis *or* **Todd's palsy** ['tɒdz pə'ræləsɪs *or* 'tɒdz 'pɔ:lzi] *noun* temporary paralysis of part of the body which has been the starting point of focal epilepsy

toe [təʊ] *noun* one of the five separate parts at the end of the foot (each toe is formed of three bones or phalanges, except the big toe, which only has two); **big toe** *or* **great toe and little toe** = biggest and smallest of the five toes

toenail ['təʊneɪl] *noun* thin hard growth covering the end of a toe

toilet ['tɔɪlət] *noun* **(a)** cleaning of the body; *she was busy with her toilet* **(b)** lavatory, place or room where a person can pass urine or faeces

toilet paper ['tɔɪlət 'peɪpə] *noun* special paper for wiping oneself after defecating or urinating

toilet roll ['tɔɪlət 'rəʊl] *noun* roll of toilet paper

toilet training ['tɔɪlət 'treɪnɪŋ] *noun* teaching a small child to pass urine or faeces in a toilet, so that it no longer requires nappies

tolerance ['tɒlərəns] *noun* ability of the body to tolerate a substance or an action; *he has been taking the drug for so long that he has developed a tolerance to it*; **drug tolerance** = condition where a drug has been given to a patient for so long that his body no longer reacts to it, and the dosage has to be increased; **glucose tolerance test** = test for diabetes mellitus, where the patient eats glucose and his blood and urine are tested regularly

26 patients were selected from the outpatient department on grounds of disabling breathlessness, severely limiting exercise tolerance and the performance of activities of normal daily living

Lancet

tolerate ['tɒləreɪt] *verb* to accept, not to react to (a drug)

tomo- ['təʊməʊ] *prefix* meaning a cutting or section

tomogram ['təʊməgræm] *noun* picture of part of the body taken by tomography

tomography [tə'mɒgrəfi] *noun* scanning of a particular part of the body using X-rays or ultrasound; **computerized axial tomography (CAT** *or* **CT) =** system of scanning a patient's body, where a narrow X-ray beam, guided by a computer, can photograph a thin section of the body or of an organ from several angles, using the computer to build up an image of the section; **positron-emission tomography =** scanning of the brain for function using the emission of positrons; **single photon emission computed tomography =** scan to study brain blood flow in conditions such as Alzheimer's disease

tomotocia [təʊmə'təʊsiə] *noun* Caesarean section, the surgical operation to deliver a baby by cutting through the mother's abdominal wall into the uterus

-tomy [təmi] *suffix* referring to a surgical operation

tone [təʊn] *noun* tonus or tonicity, normal slightly tense state of a healthy muscle when it is not fully relaxed

tongue [tʌŋ] *noun* glossa, the long muscular organ inside the mouth which can move and is used for tasting, swallowing and speaking; *the doctor told him to stick out his tongue and say 'Ah'*; **furred tongue** *or* **coated tongue** = condition when the papillae of the tongue are covered with a whitish coating

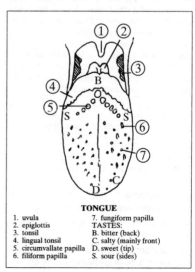

TONGUE

1. uvula
2. epiglottis
3. tonsil
4. lingual tonsil
5. circumvallate papilla
6. filiform papilla
7. fungiform papilla
TASTES:
B. bitter (back)
C. salty (mainly front)
D. sweet (tip)
S. sour (sides)

(NOTE: for other terms referring to the tongue, see **lingual** and words beginning with **gloss-**)

COMMENT: the top surface of the tongue is covered with papillae, some of which contain buds. The tongue is also necessary for speaking certain sounds such as 'l', 'd', 'n' and 'th'

tonic ['tɒnɪk] **1** *adjective* (muscle) which is contracted **2** *noun* substance which improves the patient's general health, which makes a tired person stronger; *he is taking a course of iron tonic tablets*; *she asked the doctor to prescribe a tonic for her anaemia*

tonicity [təʊ'nɪsəti] *noun* tonus or tone, normal state of a healthy muscle which is not fully relaxed

tono- ['təʊnəʊ] *prefix* referring to pressure

tonography [təʊ'nɒgrəfi] *noun* measurement of the pressure inside an eyeball

tonometer [təʊ'nɒmɪtə] *noun* instrument which measures the pressure inside an organ, especially the eye

tonometry [təʊ'nɒmɪtri] *noun* measurement of pressure inside an organ, especially the eye

tonsil *or* **palatine tonsil** ['tɒnsl *or* 'pælətaɪn 'tɒnsl] *noun* area of lymphoid tissue at the back of the throat in which lymph circulates and protects the body against germs entering through the mouth; *the doctor looked at her tonsils*; *they recommended that she should have her tonsils out*; *there are red spots on his tonsils*; **lingual tonsil** = lymphoid tissue on the top surface of the back of the tongue; **pharyngeal tonsil** *or* **adenoidal tissue** = lymphoid tissue at the back of the throat where the passages from the nose join the pharynx; *see illustration at* TONGUE

COMMENT: the tonsils are larger in children than in adults, and are more liable to infection. When infected, the tonsils become enlarged and can interfere with breathing

tonsillar ['tɒnsələ] *adjective* referring to the tonsils

tonsillectomy [tɒnsə'lektəmi] *noun* surgical operation to remove the tonsils

tonsillitis [tɒnsə'laɪtɪs] *noun* inflammation of the tonsils

tonsillotome [tɒn'sɪlətəʊm] *noun* surgical instrument used in operations on the tonsils

tonsillotomy [tɒnsɪ'lɒtəmi] *noun* surgical operation to make an incision into the tonsils

tonus ['təʊnəs] *noun* tone or tonicity, normal state of a healthy muscle which is not fully relaxed

tooth [tu:θ] *noun* one of a set of bones in the mouth which are used to chew food; *dental hygiene involves cleaning the teeth every day after breakfast*; *you will have to see the dentist if one of your teeth hurts*; *he had to have a tooth out* = he had to have a tooth taken out by the dentist; **impacted tooth** = tooth which is held against another tooth and so cannot grow normally; **milk teeth** *or* **deciduous teeth** = a child's first twenty teeth, which are gradually replaced by the permanent teeth; **permanent teeth** = adult's teeth, which replace a child's teeth during late childhood; *see also* HUTCHINSON'S TOOTH; *see illustration at* TOOTH, TEETH (NOTE: the plural is **teeth**. For terms referring to teeth, see words beginning with **dent-**, **odont-**)

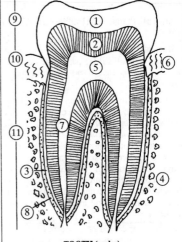

TOOTH (molar)

1. enamel	7. root canal
2. dentine	8. periodontal membrane
3. cementum	9. crown
4. bone	10. neck
5. pulp cavity	11. root
6. gingiva (gum)	

COMMENT: a tooth is formed of a soft core of pulp, covered with a layer of hard dentine. The top part of the tooth (the crown), which can be seen above the gum, is covered with hard shiny enamel which is very hard-wearing. The lower part of the tooth (the root), which attaches the tooth to the jaw, is covered with cement, also a hard substance, but which is slightly rough and holds the periodontal ligament which links the tooth to the jaw. The milk teeth in a child appear over the first two years of childhood and consist of incisors, canines and molars. The permanent teeth which replace them are formed of eight incisors, four canines, eight premolars and twelve molars, the last four molars (the third molars or wisdom teeth), are not always present, and do not appear much before the age of twenty. Permanent teeth start to appear about the age of 5 to 6. The order of eruption of the permanent teeth is: first molars, incisors, premolars, canines, second molars, wisdom teeth

toothache ['tu:θeɪk] *noun* pain in a tooth; *he went to the dentist because he had toothache*

toothbrush ['tu:θbrʌʃ] *noun* small brush which is used to clean the teeth

toothpaste ['tu:θpeɪst] *noun* soft cleaning material which is spread on a toothbrush and then used to brush the teeth; *he always brushes his teeth with fluoride toothpaste*

topagnosis [təʊpə'gnəʊsɪs] *noun* being unable to tell which part of your body has been touched, caused by a disorder of the brain

tophus ['təʊfəs] *noun* deposit of solid crystals in the skin, or in the joints, especially with gout (NOTE: the plural is **tophi**)

topical ['tɒpɪkl] *adjective* referring to one particular part of the body; **topical drug** = drug which is applied to one external part of the body only

one of the most common routes of neonatal poisoning is percutaneous absorption following topical administration

Southern Medical Journal

topically ['tɒpɪkli] *adverb* (applied) to one external part of the body only; *the drug is applied topically*

topographical [tɒpə'græfɪkl] *adjective* referring to topography

topography [tə'pɒgrəfi] *noun* description of each particular part of the body

tormina ['tɔ:mɪnə] *noun* colic, pain in the intestine

torpor ['tɔ:pə] *noun* condition where a patient seems sleepy or slow to react

torso ['tɔ:səʊ] *noun* main part of the body, not including the arms, legs and head

torticollis [tɔ:tɪ'kɒlɪs] *noun* wry neck, a deformity of the neck, where the head is twisted to one side by contraction of the sternocleidomastoid muscle

total ['təʊtl] *adjective* complete, covering the whole body; *he has total paralysis of the lower part of the body*; **total hip arthroplasty** *or* **replacement** = replacing both the head of the femur and the acetabulum with an artificial joint

totally ['təʊtəli] *adverb* completely; *she is totally paralysed*; *he will never totally regain the use of his left hand*

touch [tʌtʃ] *noun* one of the five senses, where sensations are felt by part of the skin, especially by the fingers and lips

COMMENT: touch is sensed by receptors in the skin which send impulses back to the brain. The touch receptors can tell the difference between hot and cold, hard and soft, wet and dry, and rough and smooth

tough [tʌf] *adjective* solid, which cannot break or tear easily; *the meninges are covered by a layer of tough tissue, the dura mater* (NOTE: **tough - tougher - toughest**)

Tourette's *or* **Tourette syndrome** [tu:'ret 'sɪndrəʊm] *noun (Gilles de la Tourette syndrome)* condition which includes involuntary movements, tics, use of foul language and respiratory disorders

tourniquet ['tɔ:nɪkeɪ] *noun* instrument or tight bandage wrapped round a limb to constrict an artery, so reducing the flow of blood and stopping bleeding from a wound

towel ['taʊəl] *noun* **(a)** piece of soft cloth which is used for drying **(b) sanitary towel** = wad of absorbent cotton placed over the vulva to absorb the menstrual flow

tox- *or* **toxo-** ['tɒks *or* 'tɒksəʊ] *prefix* meaning poison

toxaemia *US* **toxemia** [tɒk'si:miə] *noun* blood poisoning, presence of poisonous substances in the blood; **toxaemia of pregnancy** = condition which can affect pregnant women towards the end of pregnancy, where the patient develops high blood pressure and passes protein in the urine

toxic ['tɒksɪk] *adjective* poisonous; **toxic goitre** = thyrotoxicosis, type of goitre where the thyroid gland swells, the patient's limbs tremble and the eyes protrude

toxicity [tɒk'sɪsəti] *noun* degree to which a substance is poisonous or harmful; amount of poisonous or harmful material in a substance; *scientists are measuring the toxicity of car exhaust fumes*; **acute toxicity** = level of concentration of a toxic substance which makes people seriously ill or can cause death; **chronic toxicity** = short exposure to high exposure to harmful levels of a toxic substance over a period of time

toxico- ['tɒksɪkəʊ] *prefix* meaning poison

toxicologist [tɒksɪ'kɒlədʒɪst] *noun* scientist who specializes in the study of poisons

toxicology [tɒksɪ'kɒlədʒi] *noun* scientific study of poisons and their effects on the human body

toxicosis [tɒksɪ'kəʊsɪs] *noun* poisoning

toxin ['tɒksɪn] *noun* poisonous substance produced in the body by microorganisms, and which, if injected into an animal, stimulates the production of antitoxins

toxocariasis [tɒksəkə'raɪəsɪs] *noun* visceral larva migrans, the infestation of the intestine with worms from a dog or cat

toxoid ['tɒksɔɪd] *noun* toxin which has been treated and is no longer poisonous, but which can still provoke the formation of antibodies

COMMENT: toxoids are used as vaccines, and are injected into a patient to give immunity against a disease

toxoid-antitoxin ['tɒksɔɪdæntɪ'tɒksɪn] *noun* mixture of toxoid and antitoxin, used as a vaccine

toxoplasmosis [tɒksəʊplæz'məʊsɪs] *noun* disease caused by the parasite *Toxoplasma* which is carried by animals; **congenital toxoplasmosis** *or* **toxoplasma encephalitis** = condition of a baby which has been infected with toxoplasmosis by its mother while still in the uterus

COMMENT: toxoplasmosis can cause encephalitis or hydrocephalus and can be fatal

TPA ['ti: 'pi: 'eɪ] = **TISSUE PLASMINOGEN ACTIVATOR**

trabecula [trə'bekjʊlə] *noun* thin strip of stiff tissue which divides an organ or bone tissue into sections (NOTE: the plural is **trabeculae**)

trabeculectomy [trəbekjʊ'lektəmi] *noun* surgical operation to treat glaucoma by cutting a channel through trabeculae to link with Schlemm's canal

trace [treɪs] *noun* very small amount; *there are traces of the drug in the blood sample*; *the doctor found traces of alcohol in the patient's urine*; **trace element** = element which is essential to the human body, but only in very small quantities

COMMENT: the trace elements are cobalt, chromium, copper, magnesium, manganese, molybdenum, selenium and zinc

tracer ['treɪsə] *noun* substance (often radioactive) injected into a substance in the body, so that doctors can follow its passage round the body

trachea ['treɪkɪə] *noun* the windpipe, the main air passage which runs from the larynx to the lungs, where it divides into the two main bronchi; *see illustrations at* LUNGS, THROAT

COMMENT: the trachea is about 10 centimetre long, and is formed of rings of cartilage and connective tissue

tracheal ['treɪkɪəl] *adjective* referring to the trachea; **tracheal tugging** = feeling that something is pulling on the windpipe when the patient breathes in, a symptom of aneurysm

tracheitis [treɪki'aɪtɪs] *noun* inflammation of the trachea due to an infection

trachelorrhaphy [treɪki'lɒrəfi] *noun* surgical operation to repair tears in the cervix of the uterus

tracheobronchitis [treɪkiəʊbrɒŋ'kaɪtɪs] *noun* inflammation of both the trachea and the bronchi

tracheostomy *or* **tracheotomy** [treɪkɪ'ɒstəmi *or* treɪkɪ'ɒtəmi] *noun* surgical operation to make a hole through the throat into the windpipe, so as to allow air to get to the lungs in cases where the trachea is blocked, as in pneumonia, poliomyelitis or diphtheria

COMMENT: after the operation, a tube is inserted into the hole to keep it open. The tube may be permanent if it is to bypass an obstruction, but can be removed if the condition improves

trachoma [trə'kəʊmə] *noun* contagious viral inflammation of the eyelids, common in tropical countries, which can cause blindness if the conjunctiva becomes scarred

tract [trækt] *noun* (i) series of organs or tubes which allow something to pass from one part of the body to another; (ii) series or bundle of nerve fibres connecting two areas of the nervous system and transmitting nervous impulses in one or in both directions; **cerebrospinal tracts** = main motor pathways in the anterior and lateral white columns of the spinal cord; **olfactory tract** = nerve tract which takes the olfactory nerve from the nose to the brain; **pyramidal tract** = tract in the brain and spinal cord carrying motor neurone fibres from the cerebral cortex; *see also* DIGESTIVE TRACT

GI fistulae are frequently associated with infection because the effluent contains bowel organisms which initially contaminate the fistula tract

Nursing Times

traction ['trækʃn] *noun* pulling applied to straighten a broken or deformed limb; *the patient was in traction for two weeks*

COMMENT: a system of weights and pulleys is fixed over the patient's bed so that the limb can be pulled hard enough to counteract the tendency of the muscles to contract and pull it back to its original position. Traction can also be used for slipped discs and other dislocations. Other forms of traction include frames attached to the body

tractotomy [træk'tɒtəmi] *noun* surgical operation to cut the nerve pathway taking sensations of pain to the brain, as treatment for intractable pain

tragus ['treigəs] *noun* piece of cartilage in the outer ear which projects forward over the entrance to the auditory canal

training ['treiniŋ] *noun* educating by giving instruction and the opportunity to practise; *see also* TOILET

trait [trei or treit] *noun* characteristic which is particular to a person; **physical genetic trait** = characteristic of the body of a person (such as red hair or big feet) which is inherited

trance [trɑːns] *noun* condition where a person is in a dream, but not asleep, and seems not to be aware of what is happening round him; *he walked round the room in a trance*; *the hypnotist waved his hand and she went into or came out of a trance*

tranquillizer *or* **tranquillizing drug** ['træŋkwəlaizə or 'træŋkwəlaiziŋ 'drʌg] *noun* old term for an antipsychotic, anxiolytic or hypnotic drug which relieves a patient's anxiety and calms him or her down; *she's taking tranquillizers to calm her nerves*; *he's been on tranquillizers ever since he started his new job*

trans- [træns] *prefix* meaning through or across; **transdiaphragmatic approach** = operation carried out through the diaphragm

transaminase [træn'sæmineiz] *noun* enzyme involved in the transamination of amino acids

transamination [trænsæmi'neiʃn] *noun* process by which amino acids are metabolized in the liver

transdermal [trænz'dɜːməl] *adjective (as of drugs, etc., in a patch applied directly on the skin)* (released) through the skin

transdiaphragmatic [trænzdaiəfræg'mætik] *adjective* through a diaphragm; **transdiaphragmatic approach** = operation carried out through the diaphragm

transection [træn'sekʃn] noun (i) cutting across part of the body; (ii) sample of tissue which has been taken by cutting across a part of the body

transfer [træns'fɜː] *verb* to pass from one place to another; *the hospital records have been transferred to the computer*; *the patient was transferred to a special burns unit*

transference ['trænsfrəns] *noun (in psychiatry)* condition where the patient transfers to the psychoanalyst the characteristics belonging to a strong character from his past (such as a parent), and reacts to the analyst as if he were that person

transferrin [træns'fɜːrin] *noun* siderophilin, substance found in the blood, which carries iron in the bloodstream

transfusion [træns'fjuːʒn] *noun* transferring blood or saline fluids from a container into a patient's bloodstream; **blood transfusion** = transferring blood which has been given by another person into a patient's vein; **exchange transfusion** = method of treating leukaemia or erythroblastosis where almost all the abnormal blood is removed from the body and replaced by normal blood; *see also* AUTOLOGOUS

transient ['trænziənt] *adjective* which does not last long; **transient ischaemic attack**

(TIA) = mild stroke caused by a short stoppage of blood supply

transillumination [trænsiluːmɪˈneɪʃn] *noun* examination of an organ by shining a bright light through it

transitional [trænˈzɪʃnl] *adjective* which is in the process of developing into something; **transitional epithelium** = type of epithelium found in the urethra

translocation [trænsləʊˈkeɪʃn] *noun* moving of part of a chromosome to a different chromosome pair which causes abnormal development of the fetus

translumbar [trænsˈlʌmbə] *adjective* through the lumbar region

transmigration [trænzmaɪˈgreɪʃn] *noun* movement of a cell through a membrane

transmit [trænzˈmɪt] *verb* to pass (a message or a disease); *impulses are transmitted along the neural pathways*; *the disease is transmitted by lice*

transparent [trænsˈpærənt] *adjective* which you can see through; *the cornea is a transparent tissue on the front of the eye*

transplacental [trænspləˈsentl] *adjective* through the placenta

transplant 1 [ˈtrænsplɑːnt] *noun* (i) act of taking an organ (such as the heart or kidney) or tissue (such as skin) and grafting it into a patient to replace an organ or tissue which is diseased or not functioning properly; (ii) the organ or tissue which is grafted; *she had a heart-lung transplant; the kidney transplant was rejected* **2** [trænsˈplɑːnt] *verb* to graft an organ or tissue onto a patient to replace an organ or tissue which is diseased or not functioning correctly

transplantation [trænsplɑːnˈteɪʃn] *noun* transplant, the act of transplanting

> bone marrow transplantation has the added complication of graft-versus-host disease
>
> *Hospital Update*

transport [trænsˈpɔːt] *verb* to carry to another place; *arterial blood transports oxygen to the tissues*

> insulin's primary metabolic function is to transport glucose into muscle and fat cells, so that it can be used for energy
>
> *Nursing 87*

transposition [trænspəˈzɪʃn] *noun* congenital condition where the aorta and pulmonary artery are placed on the opposite side of the body to their normal position

transpyloric plane [trænspaɪˈlɒrɪk ˈpleɪn] *noun* plane at right angles to the sagittal plane, passing midway between the suprasternal notch and the symphysis pubis

transrectal [trænsˈrektl] *adjective* through the rectum

transsexual [trænˈsekʃul] *noun & adjective* (person) who feels a desire to be a member of the opposite sex; (behaviour) showing that a person wants to be a member of the opposite sex

transsexualism [trænˈsekʃulɪzm] *noun* sexual abnormality where a person wants to be a member of the opposite sex

transtubercular plane [trænstjuˈbɜːkjʊlə ˈpleɪn] *noun* plane at right angles to the sagittal plane, passing through the tubercles of the iliac crests

transudation [trænsjuˈdeɪʃn] *noun* passing of a fluid from the body's cells outside the body

transurethral [trænsjuˈriːθrl] *adjective* through the urethra; **transurethral prostatectomy** *or* **transurethral resection (TUR)** = surgical operation to remove the prostate gland, where the operation is carried out through the urethra

transverse [trænzˈvɜːs] *adjective* across, at right angles to an organ; **transverse arch** = arched structure across the sole of the foot; **transverse colon** = second section of the colon, which crosses the body below the stomach; *see illustration at* DIGESTIVE SYSTEM; **transverse fracture** = fracture where the bone is broken straight across; **transverse plane** = plane at right angles to the sagittal plane, running horizontally across the body; **transverse presentation** = position of the baby in the uterus, where the baby's side will appear first, normally requiring urgent manipulation or Caesarean section to prevent complications; **transverse process** = part of a vertebra which protrudes at the side

transvesical prostatectomy [trænsˈvesɪkl prɒstəˈtektəmi] *noun* operation to remove the prostate gland, where the operation is carried out through the bladder

transvestite [trænzˈvestaɪt] *noun* person who dresses in the clothes of the opposite sex, as an expression of transsexualism

trapezium [trə'piːziəm] *noun* one of the eight small carpal bones in the wrist; *see illustration at* HAND

trapezius [trə'piːziəs] *noun* triangular muscle in the upper part of the back and the neck, which moves the shoulder blade and pulls the head back

trapezoid (bone) ['træpɪzɔɪd 'bəʊn] *noun* one of the eight small carpal bones in the wrist; *see illustration at* HAND

trauma ['trɔːmə] *noun* (a) wound or injury; (b) mental shock caused by a sudden happening which was not expected to take place; *in trauma* = suffering the effects of great shock

traumatic [trɔː'mætɪk] *adjective* referring to trauma, caused by an injury; **traumatic fever** = fever caused by an injury; **traumatic shock** = state of general weakness caused by an injury and loss of blood

traumatology [trɔːmə'tɒlədʒi] *noun* branch of surgery which deals with injuries received in accidents

travel sickness ['trævl 'sɪknəs] *noun* motion sickness, illness and nausea felt when travelling

COMMENT: the movement of liquid inside the labyrinth of the middle ear causes motion sickness, which is particularly noticeable in vehicles which are closed, such as planes, coaches, hovercraft

tray [treɪ] *noun* (i) flat board for carrying plates of food for a patient to eat; (ii) flat metal plate for carrying equipment needed to a surgical intervention (such as a 'rectoscopy tray')

treat [triːt] *verb* to look after a sick or injured person, to try to cure a sick person; to try to cure a disease; *after the accident the passengers were treated in hospital for cuts*; *she has been treated with a new antibiotic*; *she's being treated by a specialist for heart disease*

treatment ['triːtmənt] *noun* way of looking after a sick or injured person; way of trying to cure a disease; *this is a new treatment for heart disease*; *he is receiving or undergoing treatment for a slipped disc*; *she's in hospital for treatment to her back*; *we are going to try some cortisone treatment*

trematode ['tremətəʊd] *noun* fluke, parasitic flatworm

tremble ['trembl] *verb* to shake or shiver slightly; *his hands are trembling with cold*; *her body trembled with fever*

trembling ['tremblɪŋ] *noun* making rapid small movements of a limb or muscles; *trembling of the hands is a symptom of Parkinson's disease*

tremens ['triːmenz] *see* DELIRIUM

tremor ['tremə] *noun* shaking, making slight movements of a limb or muscle; **coarse tremor** = severe trembling; **essential tremor** = involuntary slow trembling movement of the hands often seen in old people; **intention tremor** = trembling of the hands when a person suffering from certain brain disease makes a voluntary movement to try to touch something; **physiological tremor** = normal small movements of limbs which take place when a person tries to remain still

trench fever ['trenʃ 'fiːvə] *noun* fever caused by Rickettsia bacteria, similar to typhus but recurring every five days; **trench foot** = immersion foot, a condition, caused by exposure to cold and damp, where the skin of the foot becomes red and blistered and in severe cases turns black when gangrene sets in. (The condition was common among soldiers serving in the trenches during the First World War); **trench mouth** = *see* GINGIVITIS

Trendelenburg's position [tren'delənbɜːgz pə'zɪʃn] *noun* position where the patient lies on a sloping bed, with the head lower than the feet, and the knees bent (used in surgical operations to the pelvis); **Trendelenburg's operation** = operation to tie a saphenous vein in the groin before removing varicose veins; **Trendelenburg's sign** = symptom of congenital dislocation of the hip, where the patient's pelvis is lower on the opposite side to the dislocation

trepan [trɪ'pæn] *verb* (*formerly*) to cut a hole in the skull, as a treatment for some diseases of the head

trephination [trɪfɪ'neɪʃn] *noun* surgical operation which consists of removing a small part of the skull with a trephine in order to perform surgery on the brain

trephine [trɪ'fiːn] *noun* surgical instrument for making a round hole in the skull, or for removing a round piece of tissue

Treponema [trepə'niːmə] *noun* spirochaete which causes disease such as syphilis or yaws

treponematosis [trepəni:mə'təusɪs] *noun* yaws, an infection by the bacterium *Treponema pertenue*

TRH ['ti: 'ɑː 'eɪtʃ] = THYROTROPHIN-RELEASING HORMONE

triad ['traɪæd] *noun* three organs or symptoms which are linked together in a group

trial ['traɪəl] *noun* test; **clinical trial** = trial carried out in a medical laboratory on a patient or on tissue from a patient; **multicentric trial** = trial carried out in several centres at the same time

triangle ['traɪæŋgl] *noun* flat shape which has three sides; part of the body with three sides; **rectal triangle** *or* **anal triangle** = posterior part of the perineum; *see also* FEMORAL, SCARPA

triangular [traɪ'æŋgjʊlə] *adjective* with three sides; **triangular bandage** = bandage made of a triangle of cloth, used to make a sling for the arm; **triangular muscle** = muscle in the shape of a triangle

triceps ['traɪseps] *noun* muscle formed of three parts, which are joined to form one tendon; **triceps brachii** = muscle in the back part of the upper arm which makes the forearm stretch out

trichiasis [trɪ'kaɪəsɪs] *noun* painful condition where the eyelashes grow in towards the eye and scratch the eyeball

trichinosis *or* **trichiniasis** [trɪkɪ'nəusɪs *or* trɪkɪ'naɪəsɪs] *noun* disease caused by infestation of the intestine by larvae of roundworms or nematodes, which pass round the body in the bloodstream and settle in muscles

COMMENT: the larvae enter the body from eating meat, especially pork, which has not been properly cooked

trich(o)- ['trɪkə] *prefix* (i) referring to hair; (ii) like hair

Trichocephalus [trɪkə'sefləs] *noun* whipworm, thin round parasitic worm which infests the caecum

trichology [trɪ'kɒlədʒi] *noun* study of hair and the diseases which affect it

Trichomonas [trɪkəu'məunəs] *noun* species of long thin parasite which infests the intestines; **Trichomonas vaginalis** = parasite which infests the vagina and causes an irritating discharge

trichomoniasis [trɪkəumə'naɪəsɪs] *noun* infestation of the intestine or vagina with Trichomonas

trichomycosis [trɪkəumaɪ'kəusɪs] *noun* disease of the hair caused by a corynebacterium

Trichophyton [traɪ'kɒfɪtɒn] *noun* fungus which affects the skin, hair and nails

trichophytosis [trɪkəufaɪ'təusɪs] *noun* infection caused by Trichophyton

trichosis [traɪ'kəusɪs] *noun* abnormal condition of the hair

trichotillomania [trɪkəutɪləu'meɪniə] *noun* condition where a person pulls his hair out compulsively

trichromatic [traɪkrəu'mætɪk] *adjective* (vision) which is normal, where the person can tell the difference between the three primary colours; *compare* DICHROMATIC

trichrome stain ['traɪkrəum 'steɪn] *noun* stain in three colours used in histology

trichuriasis [trɪkju'raɪəsɪs] *noun* infestation of the intestine with whipworms

Trichuris [trɪ'kjʊərɪs] *noun* whipworm, thin round parasitic worm which infests the caecum

tricuspid valve [traɪ'kʌspɪd 'vælv] *noun* inlet valve with three cusps between the right atrium and the right ventricle in the heart; *see illustration at* HEART

tricyclic antidepressant drug [traɪ'saɪklɪk æntidɪ'presənt 'drʌg] *noun* drug (such as amitriptyline hydrochloride) used to treat depression and panic disorder

COMMENT: antimuscarinic and cardiac side-effects can occur; rapid withdrawal should be avoided

trifocal lenses *or* **trifocal glasses** *or* **trifocals** [traɪ'fəukl lenzɪz *or* 'glɑːsɪz *or* traɪ'fəuklz] *plural noun* type of glasses, where three lenses are combined in one piece of glass to give clear vision over different distances; *see also* BIFOCAL

trigeminal [traɪ'dʒemɪnl] *adjective* in three parts; **trigeminal nerve** = fifth cranial nerve (formed of the ophthalmic nerve, the maxillary nerve, and the mandibular nerve) which controls the sensory nerves in the forehead, face and chin, and the muscles in the jaw; **trigeminal neuralgia** = tic douloureux, pain in the trigeminal nerve, which sends intense pains shooting across the face

trigeminy [traɪ'dʒemɪnɪ] *noun* irregular heartbeat, where a normal beat is followed by two ectopic beats

trigger ['trɪgə] *verb* to start something happening; *it is not known what triggers the development of shingles*

the endocrine system releases hormones in response to a change in the concentration of trigger substances in the blood or other body fluids

Nursing 87

trigger finger ['trɪgə 'fɪŋgə] *noun* condition where a finger can bend but is difficult to straighten, probably because of a nodule on the flexor tendon

triglyceride [traɪ'glɪsəraɪd] *noun* substance (such as fat) which contains three fatty acids

trigone ['traɪgəun] *noun* triangular piece of the wall of the bladder, between the openings for the urethra and the two ureters

trigonitis [trɪgə'naɪtɪs] *noun* inflammation of the bottom part of the wall of the bladder

trigonocephalic [traɪgɒnəsə'fælɪk] *adjective* (skull) which shows signs of trigonocephaly

trigonocephaly [traɪgɒnə'sefli] *noun* condition where the skull is deformed in the shape of a triangle, with points on either side of the face in front of the ears

triiodothyronine [traɪaɪəudəu'θaɪrəniːn] *noun* hormone synthesized in the body from thyroxine secreted by the thyroid gland

trimester [traɪ'mestə] *noun* one of the three 3-month periods of a pregnancy

trip [trɪp] **1** *noun* **(a)** journey; *he finds it too difficult to make the trip to the outpatients department twice a week* **(b)** trance induced by drugs; **bad trip** = trance induced by drugs, producing a very bad reaction **2** *verb* **(a)** to fall down because of knocking the foot on something; *he tripped over the piece of wood*; *she tripped up and fell down* **(b)** to experience a trance induced by drugs (NOTE: **tripping - tripped**)

triphosphate [traɪ'fɒsfeɪt] *see* ADENOSINE TRIPHOSPHATE (ATP)

triplet ['trɪplət] *noun* one of three babies born to a mother at the same time; *she gave birth to triplets*; *see also* QUADRUPLET, QUINTUPLET, SEXTUPLET, TWIN

triploid ['trɪplɔɪd] *noun & adjective* (cell, organ, etc.) having 3N chromosomes, three times the haploid number

triquetral (bone) *or* **triquetrum** [traɪ'kwetrəl 'bəun or traɪ'kwetrəm] *noun* one of the eight small carpal bones in the wrist; *see illustration at* HAND

trismus ['trɪzməs] *noun* lockjaw, spasm in the lower jaw, which makes it difficult to open the mouth, a symptom of tetanus

trisomic [traɪ'səumɪk] *adjective* referring to Down's syndrome

trisomy ['traɪsəumi] *noun* condition where a patient has three chromosomes instead of a pair; **trisomy 21** = DOWN'S SYNDROME

tritanopia [traɪtə'nəupiə] *noun* rare form of colour blindness, a defect in vision where the patient cannot see blue; *compare* DALTONISM, DEUTERANOPIA

trocar ['trəukɑː] *noun* surgical instrument or pointed rod which slides inside a cannula to make a hole in tissue to drain off fluid

trochanter [trə'kæntə] *noun* two bony lumps on either side of the top end of the femur where muscles are attached

COMMENT: the lump on the outer side is the greater trochanter, and that on the inner side is the lesser trochanter

trochlea ['trɒkliə] *noun* any part of the body shaped like a pulley, especially (i) part of the lower end of the humerus, which articulates with the ulna; (ii) curved bone in the frontal bone through which one of the eye muscles passes (NOTE: the plural is **trochleae**)

trochlear ['trɒkliə] *adjective* referring to a ring in a bone; **trochlear nerve** = fourth cranial nerve, which controls the muscles of the eyeball

trochoid joint ['trəukɔɪd 'dʒɔɪnt] *noun* pivot joint, joint where a bone can rotate freely about a central axis as in the neck, where the atlas articulates with the axis

trolley ['trɒli] *noun* wheeled table or cupboard, which can be pushed from place to place; *she takes newspapers and books round the wards on a trolley*; *the patient was placed on a trolley to be taken to the operating theatre* (NOTE: the American English is **cart**)

troph(o)- ['trɒfəu] *prefix* referring to food or nutrition

trophoblast ['trɒfəublæst] *noun* tissue which forms the wall of a blastocyst

-trophy [trəfi] *suffix* meaning (i) nourishment; (ii) development of an organ

-tropic ['trɒpɪk] *suffix* meaning (i) turning towards; (ii) which influences

tropical ['trɒpɪkl] *adjective* referring to the tropics; *the disease is carried by a tropical insect*; **tropical countries** = the tropics, countries near the equator; *disease which is endemic in tropical countries*; **tropical disease** = disease which is found in tropical countries, such as malaria, dengue, Lassa fever; **tropical medicine** = branch of medicine which deals with tropical diseases; **tropical ulcer** = Naga sore, large area of infection which forms round a wound, especially in tropical countries

tropics ['trɒpɪks] *plural noun* hot areas of the world, countries near the equator; *he lives in the tropics*; *disease which is endemic in the tropics*

trouble ['trʌbl] *noun* any type of illness or disorder; *he has had stomach trouble for the last few months*; *she is undergoing treatment for back trouble*; *his bladder is giving him some trouble*; **what seems to be the trouble?** = what are your symptoms? what are you suffering from?

Trousseau's sign [tru'səuz 'saɪn] *noun* spasm in the muscles in the forearm, causing the index and middle fingers to extend, when a tourniquet is applied to the upper arm, a sign of latent tetany, showing that the blood contains too little calcium

true [tru:] *adjective* correct or right; **true ribs** = top seven pairs of ribs which are attached to the breastbone

truncus ['trʌŋkəs] *noun* main blood vessel in a fetus, which develops into the aorta and pulmonary artery

trunk [trʌŋk] *noun* main part of the body, without the head, arms and legs; *see also* BRONCHOMEDIASTINAL, COELIAC

truss [trʌs] *noun* belt worn round the waist, with pads to hold a hernia in place

trust [trʌst] *noun* **trust status** = position of a hospital which is a self-governing trust; **hospital trust** = self-governing hospital, a hospital which earns its revenue from services provided to the District Health Authorities and PCGs

trypanocide [trɪ'pænəusaɪd] *noun* drug which kills trypanosomes

Trypanosoma *or* **trypanosome** [trɪpənəu'səumə *or* 'trɪpənəusəum *or* trɪ'pænəsəum] *noun* genus of parasite which causes sleeping sickness and Chagas' disease

trypanosomiasis [trɪpənəusəu'maɪəsɪs] *noun* disease, spread by insect bites, where trypanosomes infest the blood

COMMENT: symptoms are pains in the head, general lethargy and long periods of sleep. In Africa, sleeping sickness, and in South America, Chagas' disease, are both caused by trypanosomes

trypsin ['trɪpsɪn] *noun* enzyme converted from trypsinogen by the duodenum and secreted into the digestive system where it absorbs protein

trypsinogen [trɪp'sɪnədʒn] *noun* enzyme secreted by the pancreas into the duodenum

tryptophan ['trɪptəfæn] *noun* essential amino acid

tsetse fly ['tetsi 'flaɪ] *noun* African insect which passes trypanosomes into the human bloodstream, causing sleeping sickness

TSH ['ti: 'es 'eɪtʃ] = THYROID-STIMULATING HORMONE

tsutsugamushi disease [tsu:tsəgə'mu:ʃi dɪ'zi:z] *noun* scrub typhus, a form of typhus caused by the Rickettsia bacteria, passed to humans by mites (found in South East Asia)

tubal ['tju:bl] *adjective* referring to a tube; **tubal ligation** = surgical operation to tie up the Fallopian tubes as a sterilization procedure; **tubal pregnancy** = the most common form of ectopic pregnancy, where the fetus develops in a Fallopian tube instead of the uterus

tube [tju:b] *noun* **(a)** long hollow passage in the body, like a pipe; *see also* EUSTACHIAN, FALLOPIAN **(b)** soft flexible pipe for carrying liquid or gas; *the tube leading to the colostomy bag had become detached* **(c)** soft plastic or metal pipe, sealed at one end and with a lid at the other, used to dispense a paste or gel; *a tube of eye ointment*; *an empty tube of toothpaste*

tuber ['tju:bə] *noun* swollen or raised area; **tuber cinereum** = part of the brain to which the stalk of the pituitary gland is connected

tubercle ['tju:bəkl] *noun* **(a)** small bony projection (as on a rib) **(b)** small infected lump characteristic of tuberculosis, where tissue is destroyed and pus forms; **primary tubercle** = first infected spot where tuberculosis starts to infect a lung

tubercular [tju'bɜ:kjʊlə] *adjective* (i) which causes or refers to tuberculosis; (ii) (patient) suffering from tuberculosis; (iii) with small lumps, though not always due to tuberculosis

tuberculid(e) [tju'bɜ:bjʊlɪd] *noun* skin wound caused by tuberculosis

tuberculin [tjʊ'bɜ:kjʊlɪn] *noun* substance which is derived from the culture of the tuberculosis bacillus and is used to test patients for the presence of tuberculosis; **tuberculin test** = Mantoux test, test to see if someone has tuberculosis, where the patient is given an intracutaneous injection of tuberculin and the reaction of the skin is noted; *see also* PATCH TEST

tuberculosis (TB) [tjubɜ:kju'ləʊsɪs] *noun* infectious disease caused by the tuberculosis bacillus, where infected lumps form in the tissue; **miliary tuberculosis** = form of tuberculosis which occurs as little nodes in many parts of the body, including the meninges of the brain and spinal cord; **post-primary tuberculosis** = reappearance of tuberculosis in a patient who has been infected before; **primary tuberculosis** = infection with tuberculosis for the first time; **pulmonary tuberculosis** = tuberculosis in the lungs, which makes the patient lose weight, cough blood and have a fever

COMMENT: tuberculosis can take many forms: the commonest form is infection of the lungs (pulmonary tuberculosis), but it can also attack the bones (Pott's disease), the skin (lupus), or the lymph nodes (scrofula). Tuberculosis is caught by breathing in bacillus or by eating contaminated food, especially unpasteurized milk; it can be passed from one person to another, and the carrier sometimes shows no signs of the disease. Tuberculosis can be cured by treatment with antibiotics, and can be prevented by inoculation with BCG vaccine. The tests for the presence of TB are the Mantoux test and patch test; it can also be detected by X-ray screening

tuberculous [tju'bɜ:kjʊləs] *adjective* referring to tuberculosis

tuberose ['tju:bərəʊz] *adjective* with lumps or nodules; **tuberose sclerosis** = epiloia, a hereditary disease of the brain, where a child is mentally retarded, suffers from epilepsy and many little tumours appear on the skin and on the brain

tuberosity [tju:bə'rɒsəti] *noun* large lump on a bone; **deltoid tuberosity** = raised part

of the humerus to which the deltoid muscle is attached

tuberous ['tju:brəs] *adjective* with lumps or nodules

tubo- ['tju:bəʊ] *prefix* referring to a Fallopian tube or the auditory meatus

tuboabdominal [tju:bəʊæb'dɒmɪnl] *adjective* referring to a Fallopian tube and the abdomen

tubo-ovarian [tju:bəʊəʊ'veəriən] *adjective* referring to a Fallopian tube and an ovary

tubotympanal [tju:bəʊ'tɪmpənl] *adjective* referring to the Eustachian tube and the tympanum

tubular ['tju:bjʊlə] *adjective* (i) shaped like a tube; (ii) referring to a tubule; **tubular bandage** = bandage made of a tube of elastic cloth; **tubular reabsorption** = process where some substances filtered into the kidney are reabsorbed into the bloodstream; **tubular secretion** = secretion of substances by the tubules of a kidney into the urine

tubule ['tju:bju:l] *noun* small tube in the body; **renal tubule** = small tube in the kidney, part of the nephron

tuft [tʌft] *noun* small group of hairs, of blood vessels; **glomerular tuft** = group of blood vessels in the kidney which filters the blood

tugging ['tʌgɪŋ] *see* TRACHEAL

tularaemia US **tularemia** [tu:lə'ri:miə] *noun* rabbit fever, a disease of rabbits, caused by the bacterium *Pasteurella* or *Brucella tularensis*, which can be passed to humans

COMMENT: in humans, the symptoms are headaches, fever and swollen lymph nodes

tulle gras ['tju:l 'grɑ:] *noun* dressing made of open gauze covered with soft paraffin wax which prevents sticking

tumefaction [tju:mɪ'fækʃn] *noun* oedema, swelling of tissue caused by liquid which accumulates underneath

tumescence [tju:'mesns] *noun* oedema, swollen tissue where liquid has accumulated underneath

tumid ['tju:mɪd] *adjective* swollen

tummy ['tʌmi] *noun (informal)* child's word for stomach or abdomen; **tummy ache** = child's expression for stomach pain; *see also* GIPPY

tumoral *or* **tumorous** ['tju:mərəl *or* 'tju:mərəs] *adjective* referring to a tumour

tumour *US* **tumor** ['tjuːmə] *noun* abnormal swelling or growth of new cells; *the X-ray showed a tumour in the breast*; *she died of a brain tumour*; *the doctors diagnosed a tumour in the liver*; **benign tumour** = tumour which is not cancerous, and which will not grow again or spread to other parts of the body if is is removed surgically; **malignant tumour** = tumour which is cancerous and can grow again or spread into other parts of the body, even if removed surgically (NOTE: for other terms referring to tumours, see words beginning with **onco-**)

tunable dye laser ['tjuːnəbl 'daɪ 'leɪzə] *noun* laser which coagulates fine blood vessels, used to blanch portwine stains

tunica ['tjuːnɪkə] *noun* layer of tissue which covers an organ; **tunica albuginea testis** = white fibrous membrane covering the testes and the ovaries; **tunica vaginalis** = membrane covering the testes and epididymis

COMMENT: the wall of a blood vessel is made up of several layers: the outer layer (tunica adventitia); the inner layer (tunica intima); and in between the central layer (tunica media)

tuning fork ['tjuːnɪŋ 'fɔːk] *noun* special metal fork which, if hit, gives out a perfect note, used in hearing tests, such as Rinne's test

tunnel vision ['tʌnl 'vɪʒn] *noun* field of vision which is restricted to the area directly in front of the eye

TUR ['tiː 'juː 'ɑː] = TRANSURETHRAL RESECTION

turbinal bones *or* **turbinate bones** ['tɜːbɪnl *or* 'tɜːbɪnət bəʊnz] *plural noun* three little bones which form the sides of the nasal cavity (NOTE: also called the **nasal conchae**)

turbinectomy [tɜːbɪ'nektəmi] *noun* surgical operation to remove a turbinate bone

turbulent flow ['tɜːbjʊlənt 'fləʊ] *noun* rushing or uneven flow of blood in a vessel, usually caused by a partial obstruction

turcica ['tɜːsɪkə] *see* SELLA

turgescence [tɜː'dʒesns] *noun* swelling of tissue, when fluid accumulates underneath

turgid ['tɜːdʒɪd] *adjective* swollen with blood

turgor ['tɜːgə] *noun* being swollen

turn [tɜːn] **1** *noun (informal)* slight illness, attack of dizziness; *she had one of her turns on the bus*; *he had a bad turn at the office and had to be taken to hospital* **2** *verb* **(a)** to move the head or body to face in another direction; *he turned to look at the camera*; *she has difficulty in turning her head* **(b)** to change into something different; *the solution is turned blue by the reagent*; *his hair has turned grey*

turn away ['tɜːn ə'weɪ] *verb* to send people away; *the casualty ward is closed, so we have had to turn the accident victims away*

Turner's syndrome ['tɜːnəz 'sɪndrəʊm] *noun* congenital condition of females, where sexual development is retarded and no ovaries develop

COMMENT: the condition is caused by the absence of one of the pair of X chromosomes

turricephaly [tʌrɪ'sefəli] = OXYCEPHALY

tussis ['tʌsɪs] *noun* coughing

tutor ['tjuːtə] *noun* teacher, person who teaches small groups of students; **nurse tutor** = experienced nurse who teaches student nurses

tweezers ['twiːzəz] *noun* instrument shaped like small scissors, with ends which pinch, and do not cut, used to pull out or pick up small objects; *she pulled out the splinter with her tweezers*; *he removed the swab with a pair of tweezers*

twenty-twenty vision ['twenti'twenti 'vɪʒn] *noun* perfect normal vision

twice [twaɪs] *adverb* two times; **twice daily** = two times a day; **twice daily dose** = dose to be taken two times a day

twilight ['twaɪlaɪt] *noun* time of day when the light is changing from daylight to night; **twilight myopia** = condition of the eyes, where the patient has difficulty in seeing in dim light; **twilight state** = condition (of epileptics and alcoholics) where the patient can do certain automatic actions, but is not conscious of what he is doing; **twilight sleep** = type of anaesthetic sleep, where the patient is semi-conscious but cannot feel any pain

COMMENT: twilight state is induced at childbirth, by introducing anaesthetics into the rectum

twin [twɪn] *noun* one of two babies born to a mother at the same time; **fraternal** *or*

dizygotic twins = twins who are not identical because they come from two different ova fertilized at the same time; **identical** *or* **monozygotic twins** = twins who are exactly the same in appearance because they developed from the same ovum; *see also* QUADRUPLET, QUINTUPLET, SEXTUPLET, SIAMESE, TRIPLET

COMMENT: twins are relatively frequent (about one birth in eighty) and are often found in the same family, where the tendency to have twins is passed through females

twinge [twɪnʒ] *noun* sudden feeling of sharp pain; *he sometimes has a twinge in his right shoulder*; *she complained of having twinges in the knee*

twist [twɪst] *verb* to turn or bend a joint in a wrong way; **he twisted his ankle** = he hurt it by bending it in an odd direction

twitch [twɪtʃ] **1** *noun* small movement of a muscle in the face or hands **2** *verb* to make small movements of the muscles; *the side of his face was twitching*

twitching ['twɪtʃɪŋ] *noun* small movements of the muscles in the face or hands

tylosis [taɪ'ləʊsɪs] *noun* development of a callus

tympan(o)- ['tɪmpənəʊ] *prefix* referring to the eardrum

tympanic [tɪm'pænɪk] *adjective* referring to the eardrum; **tympanic cavity** = middle ear, the section of the ear between the eardrum and the inner ear, containing the three ossicles; **tympanic membrane** *or* **tympanum** = the eardrum, the membrane at the inner end of the external auditory meatus which vibrates with sound and passes the vibrations on to the ossicles in the middle ear

tympanites [tɪmpə'naɪtiːz] *noun* meteorism, the expansion of the stomach with gas

tympanitis [tɪmpə'naɪtɪs] *noun* otitis, middle ear infection

tympanoplasty ['tɪmpənəʊplæsti] *noun* myringoplasty, surgical operation to correct a defect in the eardrum

tympanotomy [tɪmpə'nɒtəmi] *noun* myringotomy, surgical operation to make an opening in the eardrum to allow fluid to escape

tympanum ['tɪmpənəm] *noun* **(a)** eardrum, the membrane at the inner end of the external auditory meatus leading from the outer ear, which vibrates with sound and passes the vibrations on to the ossicles in the middle ear; *see illustration at* EAR **(b)** the tympanic cavity, the section of the ear between the eardrum and the inner ear, containing the three ossicles

typhlitis [tɪ'flaɪtɪs] *noun* inflammation of the caecum (large intestine)

typhoid fever ['taɪfɔɪd 'fiːvə] *noun* infection of the intestine caused by *Salmonella typhi* in food and water

COMMENT: typhoid fever gives a fever, diarrhoea and the patient may pass blood in the faeces. It can be fatal if not treated; patients who have had the disease may become carriers, and the Widal test is used to detect the presence of typhoid fever in the blood

typhus ['taɪfəs] *noun* one of several fevers caused by the Rickettsia bacterium, transmitted by fleas and lice; **endemic typhus** = fever transmitted by fleas from rats; **epidemic typhus** = fever with headaches, mental disturbance and a rash, caused by lice which come from other humans; *see also* SCRUB TYPHUS

COMMENT: typhus victims have a fever, feel extremely weak and develop a dark rash on the skin. The test for typhus is Weil-Felix reaction

typical ['tɪpɪkl] *adjective* showing the usual symptoms of a condition; *his gait was typical of a patient suffering from Parkinson's disease*

typically ['tɪpɪkli] *adverb* in a typical way; *the anorexia patient is typically an adolescent or young woman, who is suffering from stress*

tyramine ['taɪrəmiːn] *noun* enzyme found in cheese, beans, tinned fish, red wine and yeast extract, which can cause high blood pressure if found in excessive quantities in the brain; *see also* MONOAMINE OXIDASE

tyrosine ['taɪrəsiːn] *noun* amino acid in protein which is a component of thyroxine, and is a precursor to the catecholamines dopamine, noradrenaline and adrenaline

tyrosinosis [taɪrəʊsɪ'nəʊsɪs] *noun* condition caused by abnormal metabolism of tyrosine

Uu

UKCC ['ju: 'keɪ 'si: 'si:] = UNITED KINGDOM CENTRAL COUNCIL

ulcer ['ʌlsə] *noun* open sore in the skin or in mucous membrane, which is inflamed and difficult to heal; *he is on a special diet because of his stomach ulcers*; **aphthous ulcer** = little ulcer in the mouth; **decubitus ulcer** = bedsore, an inflamed patch of skin on a bony part of the body (usually found on the shoulder blades, buttocks, base of the back or heels), which develops into an ulcer, caused by pressure of the part of the body against the mattress; **dendritic ulcer** = branching ulcer on the cornea, caused by herpesvirus; **duodenal ulcer** = ulcer in the duodenum; **gastric ulcer** = ulcer in the stomach; **peptic ulcer** = benign ulcer in the stomach or duodenum; **trophic ulcer** = ulcer caused by lack of blood (such as a bedsore); **varicose ulcer** = ulcer in the leg as a result of bad circulation and varicose veins; *see also* RODENT

ulcerated ['ʌlsəreɪtɪd] *adjective* covered with ulcers

ulcerating ['ʌlsereɪtɪŋ] *adjective* which is developing into an ulcer

ulceration [ʌlsə'reɪʃn] *noun* (i) condition where ulcers develop; (ii) the development of an ulcer

ulcerative ['ʌlsrətɪv] *adjective* referring to ulcers, characterized by ulcers; **ulcerative colitis** = severe pain in the colon, with diarrhoea and ulcers in the rectum, possibly with a psychosomatic cause

ulceromembranous gingivitis [ʌlsərəʊ'membrənəs dʒɪndʒɪ'vaɪtɪs] *noun* inflammation of the gums, which can also affect the mucous membrane in the mouth

ulcerous ['ʌlsrəs] *adjective* (i) referring to an ulcer; (ii) like an ulcer

ulitis [ju'laɪtɪs] *noun* inflammation of the gums

ulna ['ʌlnə] *noun* the longer and inner of the two bones in the forearm between the elbow and the wrist (the other, outer bone, is the radius); *see illustration at* HAND

ulnar ['ʌlnə] *adjective* referring to the ulna; **ulnar artery** = artery which branches from the brachial artery at the elbow and runs down the inside of the forearm to join the radial artery in the palm of the hand; **ulnar nerve** = nerve which runs from the neck to the elbow and controls the muscles in the forearm and some of the fingers (and passes near the surface of the skin at the elbow, where it can easily be hit, giving the effect of the 'funny bone'); **ulnar pulse** = secondary pulse in the wrist, taken near the inner edge of the forearm

> the whole joint becomes disorganised, causing ulnar deviation of the fingers resulting in the typical deformity of the rheumatoid arthritic hand
>
> *Nursing Times*

ultra- ['ʌltrə] *prefix* meaning (i) further than; (ii) extremely

ultrafiltration [ʌltrəfɪl'treɪʃn] *noun* filtering of the blood where tiny particles are removed, as when the blood is filtered by the kidney

ultramicroscopic [ʌltrəmaɪkrə'skɒpɪk] *adjective* so small that it cannot be seen using a normal microscope

ultrasonic [ʌltrə'sɒnɪk] *adjective* referring to ultrasound

ultrasonics [ʌltrə'sɒnɪks] *noun* study of ultrasound and its use in medical treatments

ultrasonograph [ʌltrə'sɒnəgrɑːf] *noun* machine which takes pictures of internal organs, using ultrasound

ultrasonography [ʌltrəsə'nɒgrəfi] *noun* passing ultrasound waves through the body and recording echoes which show details of internal organs

ultrasonotomography

[ʌltrəsɒnətə'mɒɡrəfi] *noun* making pictures of organs which are placed at different depths inside the body, using ultrasound

ultrasound *or* ultrasonic waves

['ʌltrəsaund *or* ʌltrə'sɒnɪk 'weɪvz] *noun* very high frequency sound wave; *the nature of the tissue may be made clear on ultrasound examination*; *ultrasound scanning provides a picture of the ovary and the eggs inside it*; **ultrasound treatment** = treatment of soft tissue inflammation using ultrasound waves (NOTE: no plural for **ultrasound**)

> COMMENT: the very high frequency waves of ultrasound can be used to detect and record organs or growths inside the body (in a similar way to the use of X-rays), by recording the differences in echoes sent back from different tissues. Ultrasound is used routinely to monitor growth of the foetus in the uterus, and to treat some conditions such as internal bruising; it can also destroy bacteria and calculi

ultraviolet radiation (UVR) [ʌltrə'vaɪələt reɪdi'eɪʃn] *noun* invisible rays of light, which have very short wavelengths and are beyond the violet end of the spectrum, and form the tanning and burning element in sunlight; **ultraviolet lamp** = lamp which gives off ultraviolet rays which tan the skin, help the skin produce Vitamin D, and kill bacteria

umbilical [ʌm'bɪlɪkl] *adjective* referring to the navel; **umbilical circulation** = circulation of blood from the mother's bloodstream through the umbilical cord into the fetus; **umbilical hernia** = exomphalos, a hernia which bulges at the navel, mainly in young children; **umbilical region** = central part of the abdomen, lower than the epigastrium

umbilical cord [ʌm'bɪlɪkl 'kɔːd] *noun* cord containing two arteries and one vein which links the fetus inside the uterus to the placenta

> COMMENT: the arteries carry the blood and nutrients from the placenta to the fetus and the vein carries the waste from the fetus back to the placenta. When the baby is born, the umbilical cord is cut and the end tied in a knot. After a few days, this drops off, leaving the navel marking the place where the cord was originally attached

umbilicated [ʌm'bɪlɪkeɪtɪd] *adjective* with a small depression, like a navel, in the centre

umbilicus [ʌm'bɪlɪkəs] *noun* navel or omphalus, the scar with a depression in the middle of the abdomen where the umbilical cord was attached to the fetus

umbo ['ʌmbəʊ] *noun* projecting part in the middle of the outer side of the eardrum

un- [ʌn] *prefix* meaning not

unaided [ʌn'eɪdɪd] *adjective* without any help; *two days after the operation, he was able to walk unaided across the ward*

unblock [ʌn'blɒk] *verb* to remove something which is blocking; *an operation to unblock an artery*; *if you swallow it will unblock your ears*

unboiled [ʌn'bɔɪld] *adjective* which has not been boiled; *in some areas, it is dangerous to drink unboiled water*

unborn [ʌn'bɔːn] *adjective* not yet born; *a pregnant woman and her unborn child*

unciform bone ['ʌnsɪfɔːm 'bəʊn] *noun* hamate bone, one of the eight small carpal bones in the wrist, shaped like a hook; *see illustration at* HAND

uncinate ['ʌnsɪnət] *adjective* shaped like a hook; **uncinate epilepsy** = type of temporal lobe epilepsy, where the patient has hallucinations of smell and taste

unconscious [ʌn'kɒnʃəs] **1** *adjective* not conscious, not aware of what is happening; *he was found unconscious in the street*; *the nurses tried to revive the unconscious accident victims*; *she was unconscious for two days after the accident*; *she became unconscious and did not revive* **2** *noun (in psychology)* **the unconscious** = the part of the mind which stores feelings, memories or desires, which the patient cannot consciously call up, but which influence his actions; *see also* SEMI-CONSCIOUS, SUBCONSCIOUS

unconsciousness [ʌn'kɒnʃəsnəs] *noun* being unconscious (it may be the result of lack of oxygen or some other external cause such as a blow on the head); *he relapsed into unconsciousness, and never became conscious again*

uncontrollable [ʌnkən'trəʊləbl] *adjective* which cannot be controlled; *she has an uncontrollable desire to drink alcohol*; *the uncontrollable spread of the disease through the population*

uncoordinated [ʌnkəʊˈɔːdɪneɪtɪd] *adjective* not working together; *his finger movements are completely uncoordinated; the symptoms are uncoordinated movements of the arms and legs*

uncus [ˈʌŋkəs] *noun* projecting part of the cerebral hemisphere, shaped like a hook

under- [ˈʌndə] *prefix* meaning less than, not as strong as; **underactivity** = less activity than usual; **underhydration** = having too little water in the body; **undernourished** = having too little food; **underproduction** = producing less than normal

undergo [ʌndəˈgəʊ] *verb* **to undergo surgery** = to have an operation; *he underwent an appendicectomy; she will probably have to undergo another operation*

undertake [ʌndəˈteɪk] *verb* to carry out (a surgical operation); *replacement of the joint is mainly undertaken to relieve pain*

underweight [ʌndəˈweɪt] *adjective* too thin, not heavy enough; *he is several pounds underweight for his age*

undescended testis [ʌndɪˈsendɪd ˈtestɪs] *noun* condition where a testis has not descended into the scrotum

undigested [ʌndɪˈdʒestɪd] *adjective* (food) which is not digested in the body

undine [ˈʌndiːn] *noun* glass container for a solution to bathe the eyes

undress [ʌnˈdres] *verb* to take off all or most of your clothes; *the doctor asked the patient to undress or to get undressed*

undulant fever [ˈʌndjʊlənt ˈfiːvə] = BRUCELLOSIS

unfertilized [ʌnˈfɜːtəlaɪzd] *adjective* which has not been fertilized; *unfertilized ova are produced in the ovaries and can be fertilized by spermatozoa*

unfit [ʌnˈfɪt] *adjective* not fit, not healthy; *she used to play a lot of tennis, but she became unfit during the winter*

ungual [ˈʌŋgwəl] *adjective* referring to the fingernails or toenails

unguent [ˈʌŋgwənt] *noun* ointment, smooth oily medicinal substance which can be spread on the skin to soothe irritations

unguentum [ʌnˈgwentəm] *noun* (in pharmacy) ointment

unguis [ˈʌŋgwɪs] = NAIL

unhealthy [ʌnˈhelθi] *adjective* not healthy; which does not make someone healthy; *the children have a very unhealthy diet; not taking any exercise is an unhealthy way of living; the office is an unhealthy place, and everyone always feels ill there*

unhygienic [ʌnhaɪˈdʒiːnɪk] *adjective* which is not hygienic; *the conditions in the hospital laundry have been criticized as unhygienic*

uni- [ˈjuːni] *prefix* meaning one

unicellular [juːniˈseljʊlə] *adjective* (organism) formed of one cell

uniform [ˈjuːnɪfɔːm] **1** *noun* special clothes worn by a group of people, such as the nurses in a hospital; *the nurses' uniform does not include a cap; he was wearing the uniform of the St John Ambulance Brigade* **2** *adjective* the same or similar; *healthy red blood cells are of a uniform shape and size*

unigravida [juniˈɡrævɪdə] = PRIMIGRAVIDA

unilateral [juːniˈlætərəl] *adjective* affecting one side of the body only; **unilateral oophorectomy** = surgical removal of one ovary

union [ˈjuːniən] *noun* joining together of two parts of a fractured bone; *see also* MALUNION (NOTE: opposite is **non-union**)

uniovular twins [juːniˈɒvjʊlə ˈtwɪnz] *noun* monozygotic twins, twins who are identical in appearance because they developed from a single ovum

unipara [juˈnɪpərə] = PRIMIPARA

unipolar [juːniˈpəʊlə] *adjective* (neurone) with a single process; *compare with* BIPOLAR, MULTIPOLAR

unit [ˈjuːnɪt] *noun* **(a)** single part (as of a series of numbers); **SI units** = international system of measurement for physical properties; *lumen is the SI unit of illumination* **(b)** specialized section of a hospital; *she is in the maternity unit; he was rushed to the intensive care unit; the burns unit was full after the plane accident*

> the blood loss caused his haemoglobin to drop dangerously low, necessitating two units of RBCs and one unit of fresh frozen plasma
>
> *RN Magazine*

United Kingdom Central Council (for Nursing, Midwifery and Health Visiting) (UKCC) [juˈnaɪtɪd ˈkɪŋdəm ˈsentrl ˈkaʊnsɪl] *noun* official body which regulates and registers nurses, midwives and health visitors

univalent [ˌjuːniˈveɪlənt] *adjective* = MONOVALENT

universal [ˌjuːniˈvɜːsəl] *adjective* **universal donor** = subject with blood group O, whose blood may, in theory, be given to anyone; **universal recipient** = subject with blood group AB, who can receive blood from all the other groups

unmedicated dressing [ʌnˈmedɪkeɪtɪd ˈdresɪŋ] *noun* sterile dressing with no antiseptic or other medication on it

unpasteurized [ʌnˈpæstʃəraɪzd] *adjective* which has not been pasteurized; *unpasteurized milk can carry bacilli*

unprofessional conduct [ʌnprəˈfeʃənl ˈkɒndʌkt] *noun* action by a professional person (a doctor, nurse, etc.) which is considered wrong by the body which regulates the profession

refusing to care for someone with HIV-related disease may well result in disciplinary procedure for unprofessional conduct

Nursing Times

unqualified [ʌnˈkwɒlɪfaɪd] *adjective* (person) who has no qualifications, who has no licence to practise; *the hospital is employing unqualified nursing staff*

unsaturated fat [ʌnˈsætʃəreɪtɪd ˈfæt] *noun* fat which does not have a large amount of hydrogen, and so can be broken down more easily; *see also* FAT, SATURATED

unstable [ʌnˈsteɪbl] *adjective* not stable, which may change easily; *the patient was showing signs of an unstable mental condition*; **unstable angina** = angina which has suddenly become worse

unsteady [ʌnˈstedi] *adjective* likely to fall down when walking; *he is still very unsteady on his legs*

unsterilized [ʌnˈsterəlaɪzd] *adjective* which has not been sterilized; *he had to carry out the operation using unsterilized equipment*

unsuitable [ʌnˈsuːtəbl] *adjective* not suitable; *radiotherapy is unsuitable in this case*

untreated [ʌnˈtriːtɪd] *adjective* which has not been treated; *the disease is fatal if left untreated*

unwanted [ʌnˈwɒntɪd] *adjective* which is not wanted; *a cream to remove unwanted facial hair*

unwashed [ʌnˈwɒʃt] *adjective* which has not been washed; *dysentery can be caused by eating unwashed fruit*

unwell [ʌnˈwel] *adjective* sick, not well; *she felt unwell and had to go home* (NOTE: not used before a noun: **a sick woman** but **the woman was unwell**)

upper [ˈʌpə] *adjective* at the top, higher; **the upper limbs** = the arms; **upper arm** = part of the arm from the shoulder to the elbow; *he had a rash on his right upper arm*; **upper respiratory infection** = infection of the upper part of the respiratory system; *see also* NEURONE (NOTE: the opposite is **lower**)

upright [ˈʌpraɪt] *adjective & adverb* in a vertical position or standing; *he became dizzy as soon as he stood upright*

upset 1 [ˈʌpset] *noun* slight illness; **stomach upset** = slight infection of the stomach; *she is in bed with a stomach upset* **2** [ʌpˈset] *adjective* slightly ill; *she is in bed with an upset stomach*

upside down [ˈʌpsaɪd ˈdaun] *adverb* with the top turned to the bottom; *US* **upside-down stomach** = DIAPHRAGMATIC HERNIA

uraemia *US* **uremia** [juˈriːmiə] *noun* disorder caused by kidney failure, where urea is retained in the blood, and the patient develops nausea, convulsions and in severe cases goes into a coma

uraemic *US* **uremic** [juˈriːmɪk] *adjective* referring to and suffering from uraemia

uran- [ˈjuərən] *prefix* referring to the palate

uraniscorrhaphy [juərənɪˈskɒrəfi] = PALATORRHAPHY

urataemia [juərəˈtiːmiə] *noun* condition where urates are present in the blood, as in gout

urate [ˈjuəreɪt] *noun* salt of uric acid found in urine

uraturia [juərəˈtjuəriə] *noun* presence of excessive amounts of urates in the urine, as in gout

urea [juˈriːə] *noun* substance produced in the liver from excess amino acids, and excreted by the kidneys into the urine

urease [ˈjuərieɪz] *noun* enzyme which converts urea into ammonia and carbon dioxide

urecchysis [juˈrekɪsɪs] *noun* condition where uric acid leaves the blood and enters connective tissue

uresis [juˈriːsɪs] *noun* passing urine

ureter [ˈjuərɪtə] *noun* one of two tubes which take urine from the kidneys to the urinary bladder; *see illustration at* KIDNEY

ureter- *or* **uretero-** [juˈriːtə *or* juˈriːtərəu] *prefix* referring to the ureters

ureteral *or* **ureteric** [juˈriːtərl *or* juərɪˈterɪk] *adjective* referring to the ureters; **ureteric calculus** = kidney stone in the ureter; **ureteric catheter** = catheter passed through the ureter to the kidney, to inject an opaque solution into the kidney before taking an X-ray; *see also* IMPACTED

ureterectomy [juərɪtəˈrektəmi] *noun* surgical removal of a ureter

ureteritis [juərətəˈraɪtɪs] *noun* inflammation of a ureter

ureterocele [juˈriːtərəusiːl] *noun* swelling in a ureter caused by narrowing of the opening where the ureter enters the bladder

ureterocolostomy [juriːtərəukɒˈlɒstəmi] *noun* surgical operation to implant the ureter into the sigmoid colon, so as to bypass the bladder

ureteroenterostomy [juriːtərəuentəˈrɒstəmi] *noun* artificially formed passage between the ureter and the intestine

ureterolith [juˈriːtərəulɪθ] *noun* calculus, stone in a ureter

ureterolithotomy [juriːtərəulɪˈθɒtəmi] *noun* surgical removal of a stone from the ureter

ureteronephrectomy [juriːtərəunɪˈfrektəmi] *noun* nephroureterectomy, surgical removal of a kidney and the ureter attached to it

ureteroplasty [juˈriːtərəuplæsti] *noun* surgical operation to repair a ureter

ureteropyelonephritis [juriːtərəupaɪləunɪˈfraɪtɪs] *noun* inflammation of the ureter and the pelvis of the kidney to which it is attached

ureterosigmoidostomy [juriːtərəusɪgmɔɪˈdɒstəmi] = URETEROCOLOSTOMY

ureterostomy [juərɪtəˈrɒstəmi] *noun* surgical operation to make an artificial opening for the ureter into the abdominal wall, so that urine can be passed directly out of the body

ureterotomy [juərɪtəˈrɒtəmi] *noun* surgical operation to make an incision into the ureter mainly to remove a stone

ureterovaginal [juriːtərəuvæˈdʒaɪnl] *adjective* referring to the ureter and the vagina

urethr- *or* **urethro-** [juˈriːθr *or* juˈriːθrəu] *prefix* referring to the urethra

urethra [juˈriːθrə] *noun* tube which takes urine from the bladder to be passed out of the body; *see illustration at* UROGENITAL SYSTEM; **penile urethra** = channel in the penis through which both urine and semen pass; **prostatic urethra** = section of the urethra which passes through the prostate

COMMENT: in males, the urethra serves two purposes: the discharge of both urine and semen. The male urethra is about 20cm long; in women it is shorter, about 3cm and this relative shortness is one of the reasons for the predominance of bladder infection and inflammation (cystitis) in women. The urethra has sphincter muscles at either end which help control the flow of urine

urethral [juˈriːθrl] *adjective* referring to the urethra; **urethral catheter** = catheter passed up the urethra to allow urine to flow out of the bladder, used to empty the bladder before an abdominal operation; **urethral stricture** = URETHROSTENOSIS

urethritis [juərəˈθraɪtɪs] *noun* inflammation of the urethra; **specific urethritis** = inflammation of the urethra caused by gonorrhoea; *see also* NON-SPECIFIC URETHRITIS

urethrocele [juˈriːθrəsiːl] *noun* (i) swelling formed in a weak part of the wall of the urethra; (ii) prolapse of the urethra in a woman

urethrogram [juˈriːθrəgræm] *noun* X-ray photograph of the urethra

urethrography [juərɪˈθrɒgrəfi] *noun* X-ray examination of the urethra after an opaque substance has been introduced into it

urethroplasty [juˈriːθrəplæsti] *noun* surgical operation to repair a urethra

urethrorrhaphy [juərɪˈθrɒrəfi] *noun* surgical operation to repair a torn urethra

urethrorrhoea [juriːθrəˈriːə] *noun* discharge of fluid from the urethra, usually associated with urethritis

urethroscope [juˈriːθrəskəup] *noun* surgical instrument, used to examine the interior of a man's urethra

urethroscopy [juərɪˈθrɒskəpi] *noun* examination of the inside of a man's urethra with a urethroscope

urethrostenosis *or* **urethral stricture** [juriːθrəstəˈnəusɪs *or* juˈriːθrl ˈstrɪktʃə] *noun* narrowing, blocking of the urethra by a growth

urethrostomy [juərɪˈθrɒstəmi] *noun* surgical operation to make an opening for a man's urethra between the scrotum and the anus

urethrotomy [juərɪˈθrɒtəmi] *noun* surgical operation to open a blocked or narrowed urethra

urge [ɜːdʒ] *noun* strong need to do something; *he was given drugs to reduce his sexual urge*

urgent [ˈɜːdʒənt] *adjective* which has to be done quickly; *he had an urgent message to go to the hospital; urgent cases are referred to the accident unit; she had an urgent operation for strangulated hernia*

urgently [ˈɜːdʒəntli] *adverb* immediately; *the relief team urgently requires more medical supplies*

-uria [ˈjuəriə] *suffix* meaning (i) a condition of the urine; (ii) a disease characterized by a condition of the urine

uric acid [ˈjuərɪk ˈæsɪd] *noun* chemical compound which is formed from nitrogen in waste products from the body and which also forms crystals in the joints of patients suffering from gout; *see also* LITHAEMIA

uricosuric (drug) [juərɪkəˈsjuərɪk ˈdrʌg] *noun* drug which increases the amount of uric acid excreted in the urine

uridrosis [juərɪˈdrəusɪs] *noun* condition where excessive urea forms in the sweat

urin- *or* **urino-** [ˈjuərɪn *or* ˈjuərɪnəu] *prefix* referring to urine

urinalysis [juərɪˈnæləsɪs] *noun* analysis of a patient's urine, to detect diseases such as diabetes mellitus

urinary [ˈjuərɪnəri] *adjective* referring to urine; **urinary bladder** = sac where the urine collects from the kidneys through the ureters, before being passed out of the body through the urethra; *see illustration at* KIDNEY, UROGENITAL SYSTEM; **urinary catheter** = catheter passed up the urethra to allow urine to flow out of the bladder, used to empty the bladder before an abdominal operation; **urinary duct** = ureter, one of two tubes which take urine from the kidneys to the bladder; **urinary obstruction** = blockage of the urethra which prevents urine being passed; **urinary retention** = inability to pass urine, usually because the urethra is blocked or the prostate gland is enlarged; **urinary system** = system of organs and ducts which separates waste liquids from the blood and excretes them as urine (including the kidneys, urinary bladder, ureters and urethra); **urinary tract** = tubes down which the urine passes from the kidneys to the bladder and from the bladder out of the body; **urinary trouble** = disorder of the urinary tract

urinate [ˈjuərɪneɪt] *verb* to pass urine from the body; *the patient has difficulty in urinating; he urinated twice this morning*

urination [juərɪˈneɪʃn] *noun* micturition, passing of urine out of the body

urine [ˈjuərɪn] *noun* yellowish liquid, containing water and waste products (mainly salt and urea), which is excreted by the kidneys and passed out of the body through the ureters, bladder and urethra

uriniferous [juərɪˈnɪfərəs] *adjective* which carries urine; **uriniferous tubule** = renal tubule, tiny tube which is part of a nephron

urinogenital *or* **urogenital** [juərɪnəˈdʒenɪtl *or* juərəˈdʒenɪtl] *adjective* referring to the urinary and genital systems

urinometer [juərɪˈnɒmɪtə] *noun* instrument which measures the specific gravity of urine

urobilin [juərəˈbaɪlɪn] *noun* yellow pigment formed when urobilinogen comes into contact with air

urobilinogen [juərəbaɪˈlɪnədʒən] *noun* colourless pigment formed when bilirubin is reduced to stercobilinogen in the intestines

urocele [ˈjuərəsiːl] *noun* swelling in the scrotum which contains urine

urochesia *US* **urochezia** [juərəˈkiːziə] *noun* passing of urine through the rectum, due to injury of the urinary system

urochrome [ˈjuərəkrəum] *adjective* pigment which colours the urine yellow

urogenital [juərəˈdʒenɪtl] *adjective* referring to the urinary and genital systems; **urogenital diaphragm** = layer of fibrous tissue beneath the prostate gland, through which the urethra passes; **urogenital system**

= the whole of the urinary tract and reproductive system

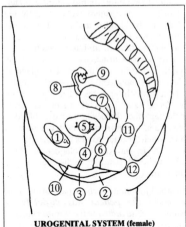

UROGENITAL SYSTEM (female)

1. pubic bone	7. uterus
2. labia majora	8. Fallopian tube
3. labia minora	9. ovary
4. urethra	10. clitoris
5. urinary bladder	11. rectum
6. vagina	12. anus

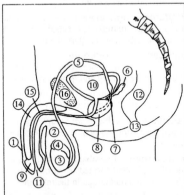

UROGENITAL SYSTEM (male)

1. penis	10. urinary bladder
2. scrotum	11. urethra
3. testis	12. rectum
4. epididymis	13. anus
5. ductus deferens	14. corpus cavernosum
6. seminal vesicle	15. corpus
7. ejaculatory duct	spongiosum
8. prostate gland	16. pubic bone
9. glans	

urography [juˈrɒgrəfi] *noun* X-ray examination of part of the urinary system after injection of radio-opaque dye

urokinase [jυərə'kaɪneɪz] *noun* enzyme formed in the kidneys, which begins the process of breaking down blood clots

urolith ['jυərəlɪθ] *noun* stone in the urinary system

urological [jυərə'lɒdʒɪkl] *adjective* referring to urology

urologist [juˈrɒlədʒɪst] *noun* doctor who specializes in urology

urology [juˈrɒlədʒi] *noun* scientific study of the urinary system and its diseases

urticaria [ɜːtɪ'keəriə] *noun* allergic reaction (to injections or to certain foods) where the skin forms irritating reddish patches (also called 'hives' or 'nettlerash')

USP ['juː 'es 'piː] = UNITED STATES PHARMACOPEIA; *see* PHARMACOPOEIA

uter- *or* **utero-** ['juːtə *or* 'juːtərəυ] *prefix* referring to the uterus

uterine ['juːtəraɪn] *adjective* referring to the uterus; *the fertilized ovum becomes implanted in the uterine wall*; **uterine cavity** = the inside of the uterus; **uterine fibroma** *or* **fibroid** = benign tumour in the muscle fibres of the uterus; **uterine subinvolution** = condition where the uterus does not go back to its normal size after childbirth; **uterine tube** = FALLOPIAN TUBE; *see also* INTRAUTERINE; **uterine procidentia** *or* **uterine prolapse** = condition where part of the uterus has passed through the vagina (usually after childbirth)

COMMENT: uterine prolapse has three stages of severity: in the first the cervix descends into the vagina, in the second the cervix is outside the vagina, but part of the uterus is still inside, and in the third stage, the whole uterus passes outside the vagina

uterocele ['juːtərəsiːl] *noun* hysterocele, hernia of the uterus

uterogestation [juːtərədʒe'steɪʃn] *noun* normal pregnancy, where the fetus develops in the uterus

uterography [juːtə'rɒgrəfi] *noun* X-ray examination of the uterus

utero-ovarian [juːtərəυəυ'veəriən] *adjective* referring to the uterus and the ovaries

uterosalpingography [juːtərəsælpɪŋ'gɒgrəfi] = HYSTEROSALPINGOGRAPHY

uterovesical [juːtərə'vesɪkl] *adjective* referring to the uterus and the bladder

uterus ['juːtərəs] *noun* womb, the hollow organ in a woman's pelvic cavity, behind the bladder and in front of the rectum; *see illustration at* UROGENITAL SYSTEM (female); **double uterus** = condition where the uterus is divided into two sections by a membrane; *see also* DIMETRIA (NOTE: for other terms referring to the uterus, see words beginning with **hyster-, metr-**)

COMMENT: the top of the uterus is joined to the Fallopian tubes which link it to the ovaries, and the lower end (cervix uteri or neck of the uterus) opens into the vagina. When an ovum is fertilized it becomes implanted in the wall of the uterus and develops into an embryo inside it. If fertilization and pregnancy do not take place, the lining of the uterus (endometrium) is shed during menstruation. At childbirth, strong contractions of the wall of the uterus (myometrium) help push the baby out through the vagina

utricle *or* **utriculus**   ['juːtrɪkl   or juˈtrɪkjʊləs] *noun* **(a)** large sac inside the vestibule of the ear, which relates information about the upright position of the head to the brain **(b) prostatic utricle** = sac branching off the urethra as it passes through the prostate gland

UV ['juː 'viː] = ULTRAVIOLET

UV-absorbing ['juː 'viː əbˈzɔːbɪŋ] *noun* UV-absorbing lens = lens specially devised to absorb UVR in order to protect the eyes against the sun

uvea ['juːvɪə] *noun* layer of organs in the eye beneath the sclera, formed of the iris, the ciliary body and the choroid

uveal ['juːvɪəl] *adjective* referring to the uvea; **uveal tract** = layer of organs in the eye beneath the sclera, containing the iris, the ciliary body and choroid

uveitis [juːviˈaɪtɪs] *noun* inflammation of any part of the uvea

uveoparotid fever *or* **syndrome** [juːvɪəˈpærətɪd 'fiːvə or 'sɪndrəʊm] *noun* inflammation of the uvea and of the parotid gland

UVR ['juː 'viː 'ɑː] = ULTRAVIOLET RADIATION

uvula ['juːvjʊlə] *noun* piece of soft tissue which hangs down from the back of the the soft palate

uvular ['juːvjʊlə] *adjective* referring to the uvula

uvulectomy [juːvjʊˈlektəmi] *noun* surgical removal of the uvula

uvulitis [juːvjʊˈlaɪtɪs] *noun* inflammation of the uvula; *see illustration at* TONGUE

Vv

vaccinate ['væksɪneɪt] *verb* to use a vaccine to give a person immunization against a specific disease; *she was vaccinated against smallpox as a child*; *see also* IMMUNIZE (NOTE: you vaccinate someone **against** a disease)

vaccination [væksɪ'neɪʃn] *noun* action of vaccinating; *see also* IMMUNIZATION (NOTE: Originally the words **vaccination** and **vaccine** applied only to smallpox immunization, but they are now used for immunization against any disease)

vaccine ['væksiːn] *noun* substance which contains the germs of a disease, used to inoculate or vaccinate; *the hospital is waiting for a new batch of vaccine to come from the laboratory*; *new vaccines are being developed all the time*; *MMR vaccine is given to control measles, mumps and rubella*; *there is, as yet, no vaccine for meningococcal meningitis*

COMMENT: a vaccine contains the germs of the disease, sometimes alive and sometimes dead, and this is injected into the patient so that his body will develop immunity to the disease. The vaccine contains antigens, and these provoke the body to produce antibodies, some of which remain in the bloodstream for a very long time and react against the same antigens if they enter the body naturally at a later date when the patient is exposed to the disease. Vaccination is mainly given against cholera, diphtheria, rabies, smallpox, tuberculosis, and typhoid

vaccinia [væk'sɪnɪə] = COWPOX

vaccinotherapy [væksɪnəʊ'θerəpi] *noun* treatment of a disease with a vaccine

vacuole ['vækjuəʊl] *noun* space in a fold of a cell membrane

vacuum ['vækjuəm] *noun* space which is completely empty of all matter, including air; **vacuum extraction** = method used to help deliver a baby using a vacuum extractor

vacuum extractor ['vækjuəm ɪk'stræktə] *noun* surgical instrument formed of a rubber suction cup applied to the head of the baby, which is used in vacuum extraction, by pulling on the head of the baby during childbirth

vagal ['veɪgl] *adjective* referring to the vagus nerve; **vagal tone** = action of the vagus nerve to slow the beat of the SA node

vagin- [və'dʒaɪn] *prefix* referring to the vagina

vagina [və'dʒaɪnə] *noun* passage in a woman's reproductive tract between the entrance to the uterus (the cervix) and the vulva, able to stretch enough to allow a baby to pass through during childbirth

vaginal [və'dʒaɪnl] *adjective* referring to the vagina; **vaginal bleeding** = bleeding from the vagina; **vaginal diaphragm** = contraceptive device, inserted into the woman's vagina and placed over the neck of the uterus; **vaginal discharge** = flow of liquid from the vagina; **vaginal douche** = (i) washing out of the vagina; (ii) the device used to wash out the vagina; *see also* DOUCHE; **vaginal examination** = checking the vagina for signs of disease or growth; **vaginal orifice** = opening leading from the vulva to the uterus; *see illustration at* UROGENITAL SYSTEM (female) (NOTE: for other terms referring to the vagina, see words beginning with **colp-**)

vaginalis [vædʒɪ'neɪlɪs] *see* TRICHOMONAS, TUNICA

vaginectomy [vædʒɪ'nektəmi] *noun* surgical operation to remove the vagina or part of it

vaginismus [vædʒɪ'nɪzməs] *noun* painful contraction of the vagina which prevents sexual intercourse

vaginitis [vædʒɪ'naɪtɪs] *noun* inflammation of the vagina which is mainly caused by the bacterium *Trichomonas vaginalis* or by a fungus *Candida albicans*

vaginography [væd͡ʒɪˈnɒgrəfi] *noun* X-ray examination of the vagina

vaginoplasty [vəˈd͡ʒaɪnəplæsti] *noun* surgical operation to graft tissue on to the vagina

vaginoscope [ˈvæd͡ʒɪnəʊskəʊp] *noun* colposcope, surgical instrument inserted into the vagina to inspect the inside of it

vago- [ˈveɪgɒ] *prefix* referring to the vagus nerve

vagotomy [veɪˈgɒtəmi] *noun* surgical operation to cut through the vagus nerve which controls the nerves in the stomach, as a treatment for peptic ulcers

vagus nerve [ˈveɪgəs ˈnɜːv] *noun* tenth cranial nerve, which controls swallowing and the nerve fibres in the heart, stomach and lungs

valency *or* **valence** [ˈveɪləns *or* ˈveɪlənsi] *noun* number of atoms with which any single atom will combine chemically

valgus [ˈvælgəs] *noun* type of deformity where the foot or hand bends away from the centre of the body; **genu valgum** = knock knee, state where the knees touch and the feet are apart when a person is standing straight; **hallux valgus** = condition of the foot, where the big toe turns towards the other toes and a bunion is formed; *compare* VARUS

validity [vəˈlɪdəti] *adjective (of a study)* characteristic of good design in order to exclude alternative explanations of a result

valine [ˈveɪliːn] *noun* essential amino acid

vallate papillae [ˈvæleɪt pəˈpiliː] *noun* large papillae which form a line towards the back of the tongue and contain taste buds; *see illustration at* TONGUE

vallecula [vəˈlekjʊlə] *noun* natural depression or fissure in an organ as between the hemispheres of the brain (NOTE: the plural is **valleculae**)

value [ˈvæljuː] *noun* quantity shown as a number; **calorific value** = number of calories which a certain amount of a certain food contains; **energy value** = amount of energy produced by a certain amount of a certain food

valve [vælv] *noun* flap, mainly in the heart, blood vessels or lymphatic vessels but also in other organs, which opens and closes to allow liquid to pass in one direction only; **aortic valve** = valve with three flaps at the opening into the aorta; **bicuspid (mitral) valve** = valve in the heart which allows blood to flow from the left atrium to the left ventricle but not in the opposite direction; **ileocaecal valve** = valve at the end of the ileum, which allows food to pass from the ileum into the caecum; **pulmonary valve** = valve at the opening of the pulmonary artery; **semilunar valve** = one of two valves in the heart, either the aortic valve or pulmonary valve; **tricuspid valve** = inlet valve with three cusps between the right atrium and the right ventricle in the heart

valvotomy *or* **valvulotomy** [vælˈvɒtəmi *or* vælvjuˈlɒtəmi] *noun* surgical operation to cut into a valve to make it open wider; **mitral valvotomy** = surgical operation to separate the cusps of the mitral valve in mitral stenosis

valvula [ˈvælvjʊlə] *noun* small valve (NOTE: the plural is **valvulae**)

valvular [ˈvælvjʊlə] *adjective* referring to a valve; **valvular disease of the heart (VDH)** = inflammation of the membrane which lines the valves of the heart

valvulitis [vælvjuˈlaɪtɪs] *noun* inflammation of a valve in the heart

valvuloplasty [ˈvælvjʊləʊplæsti] *noun* surgery to repair valves in the heart without opening the heart

> in percutaneous balloon valvuloplasty a catheter introduced through the femoral vein is placed across the aortic valve and into the left ventricle; the catheter is removed and a valve-dilating catheter bearing a 15mm balloon is placed across the valve
> *Journal of the American Medical Association*

van den Bergh test [ˈvæn den ˈbɜːg ˈtest] *noun* test of blood serum to see if a case of jaundice is caused by an obstruction in the liver or by haemolysis of red blood cells

vaporize [ˈveɪpəraɪz] *verb* to turn a liquid into a vapour

vaporizer [ˈveɪpəraɪzə] *noun* device which warms a liquid to which medicinal oil has been added, so that it provides a vapour which a patient can inhale

vapour *US* **vapor** [ˈveɪpə] *noun* substance in the form of gas; medicinal oil in steam

Vaquez-Osler disease [væ'keɪ'əuslə dɪ'ziːz] = POLYCYTHAEMIA VERA

vara ['veərə] *see* VARUS

variation [veərɪ'eɪʃn] *noun* change from one level to another; *there is a noticeable variation in his pulse rate; the chart shows the variations in the patient's temperature over a twenty-four hour period*

varicectomy [værɪ'sektəmi] *noun* surgical operation to remove a vein or part of a vein

varicella [værɪ'selə] = CHICKENPOX

varices ['værɪsiːz] *see* VARIX

varicocele ['værɪkəusiːl] *noun* swelling of a vein in the spermatic cord and which can be corrected by surgery

varicose veins ['værɪkəus 'veɪnz] *plural noun* veins, usually in the legs, which become twisted and swollen; *she wears special stockings to support her varicose veins*; **varicose eczema** = form of eczema which develops on the legs, caused by bad circulation; **varicose ulcer** = ulcer in the leg as a result of varicose veins

varicosity [værɪ'kɒsəti] *noun (of veins)* being swollen and twisted

varicotomy [værɪ'kɒtəmi] *noun* surgical operation to make a cut into a varicose vein

variola [və'raɪələ] = SMALLPOX

varioloid ['veərɪəlɔɪd] *noun* type of mild smallpox which affects patients who have already had smallpox or have been vaccinated against it

varix ['veərɪks] *noun* swollen blood vessel, especially a swollen vein in the leg (NOTE: the plural is **varices**)

Varolii [və'rəuliː] *see* PONS (b)

varus ['veərəs] *noun* deformity where the foot or hand bends in towards the centre of the body; **coxa vara** = deformity of the hip bone, making the legs bow; **genu varum** = bow legs, state where the ankles touch and the knees are apart when a person is standing straight; *compare* VALGUS

vary ['veəri] *verb* to change, to try different actions; *the dosage varies according to the age of the patient; the patient was recommended to change to a more varied diet*

vas- [væs] *prefix* referring to (i) a blood vessel; (ii) the vas deferens

vas [væs] *noun* tube in the body; **vasa vasorum** = tiny blood vessels in the walls of larger blood vessels (NOTE: the plural is vasa)

vascular ['væskjʊlə] *adjective* referring to blood vessels; **vascular dementia** = dementia caused by oxygen starvation to the brain due to disease of the blood vessels; **peripheral vascular disease** = disease affecting the blood vessels which supply the arms and legs; **vascular lesion** = damage to a blood vessel; **vascular system** = series of vessels such as veins, arteries and capillaries, carrying blood around the body

vascularization [væskjʊləraɪ'zeɪʃn] *noun* development of new blood vessels

vasculitis [væskju'laɪtɪs] *noun* inflammation of a blood vessel

vas deferens ['væs 'defərenz] *noun* one of two tubes along which sperm passes from the epididymis to the prostate gland for ejaculation (NOTE: also called **ductus deferens** *or* **sperm duct**. Note also the plural is **vasa deferentia**); *see illustration at* UROGENITAL SYSTEM (male)

vasectomy [væ'sektəmi] *noun* surgical operation to cut a vas deferens, to prevent sperm travelling from the epididymis up the duct; **bilateral vasectomy** = surgical operation to cut both vasa deferentia and so make the patient sterile

COMMENT: bilateral vasectomy is a safe method of male contraception

vas efferens ['væs 'efərenz] *noun* one of many tiny tubes which take the spermatozoa from the testis to the epididymis (NOTE: the plural is **vasa efferentia**)

vaso- ['veɪzə] *prefix* referring to (i) a blood vessel; (ii) the vas deferens

vasoactive [veɪzəʊ'æktɪv] *adjective* (agent) which has an effect on the blood vessels (especially one which constricts the arteries)

vasoconstriction [veɪzəkən'strɪkʃn] *noun* contraction of blood vessels which makes them narrower

vasoconstrictor [veɪzəkən'strɪktə] *noun* chemical substance (such as ephedrine hydrochloride) which makes blood vessels become narrower, so that blood pressure rises

vasodilatation [veɪzədaɪle'teɪʃn] *noun* relaxation of blood vessels which makes them wider

vasodilator [veɪzədaɪˈleɪtə] *noun* chemical substance (such as hydralazine hydrochloride) which makes blood vessels become wider, so that blood flows more easily and blood pressure falls; **peripheral vasodilator** = chemical substance (such as nifedipine) which acts to widen the blood vessels in the arms and legs, and so helps bad circulation as in Raynaud's disease

Volatile anaesthetic agents are potent vasodilators and facilitate blood flow to the skin

British Journal of Nursing

vasoligation [veɪzəlaɪˈgeɪʃn] *noun* surgical operation to tie the vasa deferentia to prevent infection entering the epididymis from the urinary system

vasomotion [veɪzəˈməʊʃn] *noun* vasoconstriction or vasodilatation

vasomotor [veɪzəˈməʊtə] *adjective* which makes blood vessels narrower or wider; **vasomotor centre** = nerve centre in the brain which changes the rate of heartbeat and the diameter of blood vessels and so regulates blood pressure; **vasomotor nerve** = nerve in the wall of a blood vessel which affects the diameter of the vessel

vasopressin [veɪzəˈpresɪn] *noun* antidiuretic hormone (ADH), a hormone secreted by the posterior pituitary gland which acts on the kidneys to regulate the quantity of salt in body fluids and the amount of urine excreted by the kidneys

vasopressor [veɪzəˈpresə] *noun* substance which increases blood pressure by narrowing the blood vessels

vasospasm [ˈveɪzəspæzm] *noun* Raynaud's disease, a condition where the fingers become cold, white and numb

vasovagal [veɪzəˈveɪgl] *adjective* referring to the vagus nerve and its effect on the heartbeat and blood circulation; **vasovagal attack** = fainting fit (following a slowing down of the heartbeats caused by the vagus nerve)

vasovasostomy [veɪzəvəˈsɒstəmi] *noun* surgical operation to reverse a vasectomy

vasovesiculitis [veɪzəvesɪkjuˈlaɪtɪs] *noun* inflammation of the seminal vesicles and a vas deferens

vastus intermedius *or* **vastus medialis** *or* **vastus lateralis** [ˈvæstəs ɪntəˈmiːdiəs *or* miːdiˈeɪlɪs *or* lætəˈreɪlɪs] *noun* three of the four parts of the quadriceps femoris, the muscle of the thigh

vault [vɒlt] *noun* **vault of the skull** = part of the skull which includes the frontal bone, the temporal bones and the occipital bone

VD [ˈviː ˈdiː] = VENEREAL DISEASE; **VD clinic** = clinic specializing in the diagnosis and treatment of venereal diseases; *he is attending a VD clinic*; *the treatment for VD takes several weeks*

VDH [ˈviː ˈdiː ˈeɪtʃ] = VALVULAR DISEASE OF THE HEART

vectis [ˈvektɪs] *noun* curved surgical instrument used in childbirth

vector [ˈvektə] *noun* insect, an animal which carries a disease and can pass it to humans; *the tsetse fly is a vector of sleeping sickness*

vegan [ˈviːgn] *noun & adjective* strict vegetarian, (person) who does not eat meat, dairy produce, eggs or fish and eats only vegetables and fruit; *compare* LACTOVEGETARIAN, VEGETARIAN

vegetable [ˈvedʒtəbl] *noun* plant grown for food, not usually sweet; *green vegetables are a source of dietary fibre*

vegetarian [vedʒəˈteəriən] *noun & adjective* (person) who does not eat meat, but eats mainly vegetables and fruit and sometimes dairy produce, eggs or fish; *he is on a vegetarian diet*; *she is a vegetarian*; *compare* LACTOVEGETARIAN, VEGAN

vegetation [vedʒəˈteɪʃn] *noun* growth on a membrane (as on the cusps of valves in the heart)

vegetative [ˈvedʒətətɪv] *adjective* (i) referring to growth of tissue or organs; (ii) (state) after brain damage, where a person is alive and breathing but shows no responses; **persistent vegetative state (PVS)** = condition where a patient is alive and breathes, but shows no brain activity, and will never recover consciousness

vehicle [ˈviːɪkl] *noun* liquid in which a dose of a drug is put

vein [veɪn] *noun* blood vessel which takes deoxygenated blood containing waste carbon dioxide from the tissues back to the heart; **azygos vein** = vein which brings blood back into the vena cava from the abdomen; **basilic vein** = large vein running along the inside of the arm; **deep vein** = vein which is deep in tissue, near the bones; **hepatic vein** = vein which carries blood from the liver to the vena cava; **lingual vein** = vein which takes blood away from the tongue; **portal vein** = vein which takes blood from the stomach, pancreas, intestines and spleen to the liver; **pulmonary vein** = vein which carries oxygenated blood from the lungs back to the left atrium of the heart (it is the only vein - one of two for each lung - which carries oxygenated blood); **superficial vein** = vein which is near the surface of the skin (NOTE: for other terms referring to the veins, see words beginning with **phleb-**)

vena cava ['viːnə 'keɪvə] *noun* one of two large veins which take deoxygenated blood from all the other veins into the right atrium of the heart; *see illustrations at* HEART, KIDNEY (NOTE: the plural is **venae cavae**)

> COMMENT: the superior vena cava brings blood from the head and the top part of the body, while the inferior vena cava brings blood from the abdomen and legs

vene- *or* **veno-** ['venɪ or 'viːnəʊ] *prefix* referring to veins

venene [və'niːn] *noun* mixture of different venoms, used to produce antivenene

venepuncture *or* **venipuncture** ['venɪpʌŋktʃə] *noun* puncturing a vein either to inject a drug or to take a blood sample

venereal disease (VD) [və'nɪərɪəl dɪ'ziːz] *noun* disease which is passed from one person to another during sexual intercourse (NOTE: now usually called **sexually transmitted diseases (STDs)**)

> COMMENT: the main types of venereal disease are syphilis, gonorrhoea, AIDS, non-specific urethritis, genital herpes and chancroid. The spread of sexually transmitted diseases can be limited by use of condoms. Other forms of contraceptive offer no protection against the spread of disease

venereologist [vənɪərɪ'ɒlədʒɪst] *noun* doctor who specializes in the study of venereal diseases

venereology [vənɪərɪ'ɒlədʒi] *noun* scientific study of venereal diseases

venereum [və'nɪərɪəm] *see* LYMPHOGRANULOMA

veneris ['venərɪs] *see* MONS

venesection [venɪ'sekʃn] *noun* operation where a vein is cut so that blood can be removed (as when taking blood from a donor)

venoclysis [və'nɒkləsɪs] *noun* introducing slowly a saline or other solution into a vein

venogram ['viːnəgræm] = PHLEBOGRAM

venography [vɪ'nɒgrəfi] = PHLEBOGRAPHY

venom ['venəm] *noun* poison in the bite of a snake or insect

> COMMENT: depending on the source of the bite, venom can have a wide range of effects, from a light irritating spot after a mosquito sting, to death from a scorpion. Antivenene will counteract the effects of venom, but is only effective if the animal which gave the bite can be correctly identified

venomous ['venəməs] *adjective* (animal) which has poison in its bite; *the cobra is a venomous snake*; *he was bitten by a venomous spider*

venosus [vɪ'nəʊsəs] *see* DUCTUS

venous ['viːnəs] *adjective* referring to the veins; **venous bleeding** = bleeding from a vein; **venous blood** = deoxygenated blood, from which most of the oxygen has been removed by the tissues and is darker than oxygenated arterial blood (it is carried by all the veins except for the pulmonary veins which carry oxygenated blood); **venous system** = system of veins which bring blood back to the heart from the tissues; **venous thrombosis** = blocking of a vein by a blood clot; **venous ulcer** = ulcer in the leg, caused by varicose veins or by a blood clot; **central venous pressure** = blood pressure in the right atrium, which can be measured by means of a catheter

> venous air embolism is a potentially fatal complication of percutaneous venous catheterization
>
> *Southern Medical Journal*

> a pad was placed under the Achilles tendon to raise the legs, thus aiding venous return and preventing deep vein thrombosis
>
> *NATNews*

ventilation [ventɪ'leɪʃn] *noun* breathing air in or out of the lungs, so removing waste products from the blood in exchange for oxygen; *see also* DEAD SPACE; **artificial ventilation** = breathing which is assisted or controlled by a machine; **mouth-to-mouth**

ventilation = making a patient start to breathe again by blowing air through his mouth into his lungs

ventilator ['ventɪleɪtə] *noun* respirator, a machine which pumps air into and out of the lungs of a patient who has difficulty in breathing; *the newborn baby was put on a ventilator*

ventilatory failure ['ventɪleɪtri 'feɪljə] *noun* failure of the lungs to oxygenate the blood correctly

ventral ['ventrl] *adjective* referring to (i) the abdomen; (ii) the front of the body (NOTE: the opposite is **dorsal**)

ventricle ['ventrɪkl] *noun* cavity in an organ, especially in the heart or brain; *see illustration at* HEART

COMMENT: there are two ventricles in the heart: the left ventricle takes oxygenated blood from the pulmonary veins through the left atrium, and pumps it into the aorta to circulate round the body; the right ventricle takes blood from the veins through the right atrium, and pumps it into the pulmonary artery to be passed to the lungs to be oxygenated. There are four ventricles in the brain, each containing cerebrospinal fluid. The two lateral ventricles in the cerebral hemispheres contain the choroid processes which produce cerebrospinal fluid. The third ventricle lies in the midline between the two thalami. The fourth ventricle is part of the central canal of the hindbrain

ventricul- [ven'trɪkjʊl] *prefix* referring to a ventricle in the brain or heart

ventricular [ven'trɪkjʊlə] *adjective* referring to the ventricles; **ventricular fibrillation (VF)** = serious heart condition where the ventricular muscles flutter and the heart no longer beats; **ventricular folds** = the vocal cords, two folds in the larynx which can be brought together to make sounds as air passes between them

ventriculitis [ventrɪkju'laɪtɪs] *noun* inflammation of the brain ventricles

ventriculoatriostomy [ventrɪkjʊləveɪtri'ɒstəmi] *noun* operation to relieve pressure caused by excessive quantities of cerebrospinal fluid in the brain ventricles

ventriculogram [ven'trɪkjʊləgræm] *noun* X-ray picture of the brain ventricles

ventriculography [ventrɪkju'lɒgrəfi] *noun* method of taking X-ray pictures of the ventricles of the brain after air has been introduced to replace the cerebrospinal fluid

ventriculoscopy [ventrɪkju'lɒskəpi] *noun* examination of the brain using an endoscope

ventriculostomy [ventrɪkju'lɒstəmi] *noun* surgical operation to pass a hollow needle into a brain ventricle so as to reduce pressure, take a sample of fluid, or enlarge the ventricular opening to prevent the need for a shunt

ventro- ['ventrəʊ] *prefix* (i) meaning ventral; (ii) referring to the abdomen

ventrofixation [ventrəʊfik'seɪʃn] *noun* surgical operation to treat retroversion of the uterus by attaching the uterus to the wall of the abdomen

ventrosuspension [ventrəʊsə'spenʃn] *noun* surgical operation to treat retroversion of the uterus

venule ['venjuːl] *noun* small vein or vessel leading from tissue to a larger vein

vera ['vɪərə] *see* DECIDUA

verbigeration [vɜːbɪdʒə'reɪʃn] *noun* condition seen in mental patients, where the patient keeps saying the same words over and over again

vermicide ['vɜːmɪsaɪd] *noun* substance which kills worms in the intestine

vermiform ['vɜːmɪfɔːm] *adjective* shaped like a worm; **vermiform appendix** = small tube attached to the caecum which serves no function, but can become infected, causing appendicitis

vermifuge ['vɜːmɪfjuːdʒ] *noun & adjective* (substance) which removes worms from the intestine

vermil(l)ion border [və'mɪliən 'bɔːdə] *noun* external red parts of the lips

vermis ['vɜːmɪs] *noun* central part of the cerebellum, which forms the top of the fourth ventricle

vermix ['vɜːmɪks] *noun* vermiform appendix

vernix caseosa ['vɜːnɪks keɪsi'əʊsə] *noun* oily substance which covers a baby's skin at birth

verruca [və'ruːkə] *noun* wart, small hard benign growth on the skin, caused by a virus (NOTE: the plural is **verrucae**)

version ['vɜːʃn] *noun* turning the fetus in a uterus so as to put it in a better position for birth; **cephalic version** = turning a wrongly positioned fetus round in the uterus, so that the head will appear first at birth; **pelvic version** = version performed by moving the buttocks of the fetus; **podalic version** = turning a fetus in the uterus so that the baby will be born feet first; **spontaneous version** = movement of a fetus to take up another position in the uterus, caused by the contractions of the uterus during childbirth or by movements of the baby itself before birth

VERTEBRAL COLUMN (lateral view)

1. sacrum	7. atlas
2. coccyx	8. axis
3. cervical vertebrae	9. intervertebral foramen
4. thoracic vertebrae	10. spinous process
5. lumbar vertebrae	11. vertebra
6. intervertebral disc	

vertebra ['vɜːtɪbrə] *noun* one of twenty-four ring-shaped bones which link together to form the backbone (NOTE: the plural is **vertebrae**)

COMMENT: the top vertebra (the atlas) supports the skull; the first seven vertebrae in the neck are the cervical vertebrae; then follow the twelve thoracic or dorsal vertebrae which are behind the chest and five lumbar vertebrae in the lower part of the back. The sacrum and coccyx are formed of five sacral vertebrae and four coccygeal vertebrae which have fused together

vertebral ['vɜːtɪbrl] *adjective* referring to the vertebrae; **vertebral arteries** = two arteries which go up the back of the neck into the brain; **vertebral canal** = channel formed of the holes in the centre of each vertebra, through which the spinal cord passes; **vertebral column** = backbone, series of bones and discs linked together to form a flexible column running from the base of the skull to the pelvis; **vertebral disc** = thick piece of cartilage which lies between two vertebrae and acts as a cushion (NOTE: also called **intervertebral disc**); **vertebral foramen** = hole in the centre of a vertebra which links with others to form the vertebral canal (NOTE: the vertebrae are referred to by numbers and letters: **C6** = the sixth cervical vertebra; **T11** = the eleventh thoracic vertebra, and so on)

vertebro-basilar insufficiency ['vɜːtɪbrəʊ'bæzɪlə ɪnsə'fɪʃənsi] *noun* brainstem ischaemia due to temporary occlusion of the arteries

vertex ['vɜːteks] *noun* top of the skull; **vertex delivery** = normal birth of a baby, where the head appears first

vertigo ['vɜːtɪgəʊ] *noun* (a) dizziness or giddiness, loss of balance where the patient feels that everything is rushing round him, caused by a malfunction of the sense of balance (b) fear of heights, sensation of dizziness which is felt when high up (especially on a tall building); *he won't sit near the window - he suffers from vertigo*

vesical ['vesɪkl] *adjective* referring to the bladder

vesicant ['vesɪkənt] *noun* epispastic, a substance which makes the skin blister

vesicle ['vesɪkl] *noun* (a) small blister on the skin (such as those caused by eczema) (b) sac which contains liquid; **seminal vesicles** =

two organs near the prostate gland which secrete seminal fluid into the vas deferens; *see illustration at* UROGENITAL SYSTEM (male)

vesico- ['vesɪkəʊ] *prefix* referring to the urinary bladder

vesicofixation [vesɪkəʊfik'seɪʃn] *noun* cystopexy, surgical operation to fix the urinary bladder in a different position

vesicostomy [vesɪ'kɒstəmi] = CYSTOSTOMY

vesicotomy [vesɪ'kɒtəmi] = CYSTOTOMY

vesicoureteric reflux [vesɪkəʊjʊərə'terɪk 'riːflʌks] *noun* flowing of urine back from the bladder up the ureters, which may carry infection from the bladder to the kidneys

vesicovaginal [vesɪkəʊ'vædʒɪnl] *adjective* referring to the bladder and the vagina; **vesicovaginal fistula** = abnormal opening which connects the bladder to the vagina

vesicular [və'sɪkjʊlə] *adjective* referring to a vesicle; **vesicular breathing sound** = faint breathing sound as the air enters the alveoli of the lung

vesiculation [vəsɪkju'leɪʃn] *noun* formation of blisters on the skin

vesiculectomy [vəsɪkju'lektəmi] *noun* surgical operation to remove a seminal vesicle

vesiculitis [vəsɪkju'laɪtɪs] *noun* inflammation of the seminal vesicles

vesiculography [vəsɪkju'lɒgrəfi] *noun* X-ray examination of the seminal vesicles

vesiculopapular [vəsɪkjʊləʊ'pæpjʊlə] *adjective* (skin disorder) which has both blisters and papules

vesiculopustular [vəsɪkjʊləʊ'pʌstjʊlə] *adjective* (skin disorder) which has both blisters and pustules

vessel ['vesəl] *noun* tube in the body along which liquid flows, especially a blood vessel; **afferent vessel** = tube which brings lymph to a gland; **blood vessel** = any tube (artery, vein or capillary) which carries blood round the body; **efferent vessel** = tube which drains lymph from a gland; **lymphatic vessel** = tube which carries lymph round the body (NOTE: for other terms referring to vessels, see words beginning with **vasc-, vaso-**)

vestibular [ve'stɪbjʊlə] *adjective* referring to a vestibule, especially the vestibule of the

inner ear; **vestibular folds** = folds in the larynx, above the vocal cords; *see also* VOCAL CORDS; **vestibular glands** = glands at the point where the vagina and vulva join, which secrete a lubricating substance; **greater vestibular gland** = Bartholin's gland, the more posterior of the vestibular glands; **lesser vestibular gland** = the more anterior of the vestibular glands; **vestibular nerve** = part of the auditory nerve which carries information about balance to the brain

vestibule ['vestɪbjuːl] *noun* cavity in the body at the entrance to an organ, especially (i) the first cavity in the inner ear; (ii) the space in the larynx above the vocal cords; (iii) a nostril

vestibuli [ve'stɪbjʊlaɪ] *see* FENESTRA

vestibulocochlear nerve [vestɪbjʊləʊ'kɒkliə 'nɜːv] *noun* eighth cranial nerve which governs hearing and balance (NOTE: also called the **acoustic nerve** *or* **auditory nerve**)

vestigial [ves'tɪdʒiəl] *adjective* which exists in a rudimentary form; *the coccyx is a vestigial tail*

VF ['viː 'ef] = VENTRICULAR FIBRILLATION; **in VF** = (patient) whose heart is no longer able to beat

viability [vaɪə'bɪləti] *noun* being viable; *the viability of the fetus before the 22nd week is doubtful*

viable ['vaɪəbl] *adjective* (fetus) which can survive if born; *a fetus is viable by about the 28th week of pregnancy*

vial ['vaɪəl] = PHIAL

vibrate [vaɪ'breɪt] *verb* to move rapidly and continuously

vibration [vaɪ'breɪʃn] *noun* rapid and continuous movement; *speech is formed by the vibrations of the vocal cords; sounds make the eardrum vibrate and the vibrations are sent to the brain as nervous impulses*; **vibration white finger** = condition caused by using a chain saw or pneumatic drill, which affects the circulation in the fingers

vibrator [vaɪ'breɪtə] *noun* device to produce vibrations, which may be used for massages

Vibrio ['vɪbriəʊ] *noun* genus of Gram-negative bacteria which are found in water and cause cholera

vibrissae [vaɪ'brɪsiː] *plural noun* hairs in the nostrils or ears

vicarious [vɪ'keərɪəs] *adjective* (done by one organ or agent) in place of another; **vicarious menstruation** = discharge of blood other than by the vagina during menstrual periods

victim ['vɪktɪm] *noun* person who is injured in an accident, who has caught a disease; *the victims of the rail crash were taken to the local hospital*; *half the people eating at the restaurant fell victim to salmonella poisoning*; *the health authority is planning a special hospital for AIDS victims*

vigour *US* **vigor** ['vɪgə] *see* HYBRID

villous ['vɪləs] *adjective* shaped like a villus; formed of villi

villus ['vɪləs] *noun* tiny projection like a finger on the surface of mucous membrane; **arachnoid villi** = villi in the arachnoid membrane which absorb cerebrospinal fluid; **chorionic villi** = tiny folds in the membrane covering the fertilized ovum; **intestinal villi** = projections on the walls of the intestine which help in the digestion of food (NOTE: the plural is **villi**)

Vincent's angina ['vɪnsents æn'dʒaɪnə] = ULCERATIVE GINGIVITIS

vinculum ['vɪŋkjuləm] *noun* thin connecting band of tissue (NOTE: the plural is **vincula**)

violent ['vaɪələnt] *adjective* very strong, very severe; *he had a violent headache*; *her reaction to the injection was violent*

violently ['vaɪələntli] *adverb* in a strong way; *he reacted violently to the antihistamine*

violet ['vaɪələt] *noun* dark, purplish blue colour at the end of the visible spectrum; *see also* CRYSTAL, GENTIAN

viraemia *US* **viremia** [vaɪ'riːmɪə] *noun* virus in the blood

viral ['vaɪrəl] *adjective* caused by a virus, referring to a virus; *he caught viral pneumonia on a plane*; **viral infection** = infection caused by a virus; *see also* HEPATITIS

virgin ['vɜːdʒɪn] *noun* female who has not experienced sexual intercourse

virginity [və'dʒɪnəti] *noun* condition of a female who has not experienced sexual intercourse

virile ['vɪraɪl] *adjective* like a man, with strong male characteristics

virilism ['vɪrɪlɪzm] *noun* male characteristics (such as body hair, deep voice) in a woman

virilization [vɪrɪlaɪ'zeɪʃn] *noun* development of male characteristics in a woman, caused by a hormone defect or therapy

virology [vaɪ'rɒlədʒi] *noun* scientific study of viruses

virulence ['vɪruləns] *noun* (i) ability of a microbe to cause a disease; (ii) violent effect (of a disease)

virulent ['vɪrulənt] *adjective* (i) (microbe) which can cause a disease; (ii) (disease) which has violent effects and develops rapidly

virus ['vaɪrəs] *noun* tiny germ cell which can only develop in other cells, and often destroys them; *scientists have isolated a new flu virus*; *shingles is caused by the same virus as chickenpox*; **infectious virus hepatitis** = hepatitis transmitted by a carrier through food or drink; **virus pneumonia** = inflammation of the lungs caused by a virus

COMMENT: many common diseases such as measles or the common cold are caused by viruses; viral diseases cannot be treated with antibiotics

viscera ['vɪsərə] *plural noun* internal organs (such as the heart, lungs, stomach, intestines); **abdominal viscera** = the organs inside the abdomen (NOTE: the singular (rarely used) is **viscus**)

visceral ['vɪsərəl] *adjective* referring to the internal organs; **viscera larva migrans** = toxocariasis, infestation of the intestine with worms from a dog or cat; **visceral muscle** = smooth muscle in the wall of the intestine which makes the intestine contract; **visceral pericardium** = inner layer of serous pericardium attached to the wall of the heart; **visceral peritoneum** = part of the peritoneum which covers the organs in the abdominal cavity; **visceral pleura** = inner pleura, membrane attached to the surface of a lung; **visceral pouch** = PHARYNGEAL POUCH

visceromotor [vɪsərə'məutə] *adjective* (reflex, etc.) which controls the movement of viscera

visceroptosis [vɪsərə'təusɪs] *noun* movement of an internal organ downwards from its usual position

visceroreceptor [vɪsərərɪ'septə] *noun* receptor cell which reacts to stimuli from organs such as the stomach, heart and lungs

viscid ['vɪsɪd] *adjective* sticky, slow-moving (liquid)

viscosity [vɪ'skɒsəti] *noun* state of a liquid which moves slowly

viscous ['vɪskəs] *adjective* thick, slow-moving (liquid)

viscus ['vɪskəs] *see* VISCERA

visible ['vɪzəbl] *adjective* which can be seen; *there were no visible symptoms of the disease*

vision ['vɪʒn] *noun* ability to see, eyesight; *after the age of 50, many people's vision begins to fail*; **binocular vision** = ability to see with both eyes at the same time, which gives a stereoscopic effect and allows a person to judge distances; **blurred vision** = condition where the patient does not see objects clearly; **field of vision** = area which can be seen without moving the eye; **impaired vision** = eyesight which is not fully clear; **monocular vision** = seeing with one eye only, so that the sense of distance is impaired; **partial vision** = being able to see only part of the total field of vision; **stereoscopic vision** = being able to judge how far something is from you, because of seeing it with both eyes at the same time; **tunnel vision** = field of vision which is restricted to the area immediately in front of the eye; **twenty-twenty vision** *or* **20/20 vision** = perfect normal vision

visit ['vɪzɪt] **1** *noun* **(a)** short stay with someone (especially to comfort a patient); *the patient is too weak to have any visits*; *he is allowed visits of ten minutes only* **(b)** short stay with a professional person; *they had a visit from the district nurse*; *she paid a visit to the chiropodist*; *on the patient's last visit to the physiotherapy unit, nurses noticed a great improvement in her walking* **2** *verb* to stay a short time with someone; *I am going to visit my brother in hospital*; *she was visited by the health visitor*; **visiting times** *or* **hours** = times of day when friends are allowed into a hospital to visit patients

visitor ['vɪzɪtə] *noun* person who visits; *visitors are allowed into the hospital on Sunday afternoons*; *how many visitors did you have this week?*; **health visitor** = registered nurse with qualifications in midwifery or obstetrics and preventive medicine, who visits mothers and babies, and sick people in their homes and advises on treatment

visual ['vɪʒuəl] *adjective* referring to sight or vision; **visual acuity** = being able to see objects clearly; **visual axis** = the line between the object on which the eye focuses, and the fovea; **visual cortex** = part of the cerebral cortex which receives information about sight; **visual field** = field of vision, the area which can be seen without moving the eye; **visual purple** = rhodopsin, purple pigment in the rods of the retina which makes it possible to see in bad light

vitae ['vaɪtiː] *see* ARBOR

vital ['vaɪtl] *adjective* most important for life; *if circulation is stopped, vital nerve cells begin to die in a few minutes*; *oxygen is vital to the human system*; **vital capacity** = largest amount of air which a person can exhale; **vital centre** = group of nerve cells in the brain which govern a particular function of the body (such as the five senses); **vital organs** = the most important organs in the body, without which a human being cannot live (such as the heart, lungs, brain); **vital signs** = measurement of pulse, breathing and temperature; **vital statistics** = official statistics relating to the population of a place (such as the percentage of live births per thousand, the incidence of a certain disease, the numbers of births and deaths)

vitamin ['vɪtəmɪn] *noun* essential substance not synthesized in the body, but found in most foods, and needed for good health; **vitamin deficiency** = lack of necessary vitamins; *he is suffering from Vitamin A deficiency*; *Vitamin C deficiency causes scurvy*

vitelline sac [vɪ'telaɪn 'sæk] *noun* sac attached to an embryo, where the blood cells first form

vitellus [vɪ'teləs] *noun* yolk of an egg (ovum)

vitiligo [vɪtɪ'laɪgəʊ] *noun* leucoderma, condition where white patches appear on the skin

vitreous body *or* **vitreous humour** ['vɪtriəs 'bɒdi *or* 'hjuːmə] *noun* transparent jelly which fills the main cavity behind the lens in the eye

vitro ['viːtrəʊ] *see* IN VITRO

Vitus ['vaɪtəs] *see* ST VITUS

viviparous [vɪ'vɪpərəs] *adjective* (animal) which bears live young (such as humans, as opposed to birds and reptiles which lay eggs)

vivisection [vɪvɪˈsekʃn] *noun* dissecting a living animal as an experiment

vocal [ˈvəʊkl] *adjective* referring to the voice; **true vocal cords** = cords in the larynx which can be brought together to make sounds as air passes between them; *see also* FOLD, VESTIBULAR CORDS; **vocal fremitus** = vibration of the chest as a patient speaks or coughs; **vocal ligament** = ligament in the centre of the vocal cords; **vocal resonance** = sound heard by a doctor when he listens through a stethoscope while a patient is speaking

voice [vɔɪs] *noun* sound made when a person speaks or sings; *the doctor has a quiet and comforting voice*; *I didn't recognize your voice over the phone*; **to lose your voice** = not to be able to speak because of a throat infection; **his voice has broken** = his voice has become deeper and adult, with the onset of puberty

voice box [ˈvɔɪs ˈbɒks] *noun* larynx, the organ at the back of the throat which produces sounds

COMMENT: the voice box is a hollow organ containing the vocal cords, situated behind the Adam's apple

volar [ˈvəʊlə] *adjective* referring to the palm of the hand or sole of the foot

volatile [ˈvɒlətaɪl] *adjective* (liquid) which turns into gas at normal room temperature; **volatile oils** = concentrated oils from plants used in cosmetics and as antiseptics

volitantes [vɒlɪˈtæntiːz] *see* MUSCAE

volition [vəˈlɪʃn] *noun* ability to use the will

Volkmann's canal [ˈfɒlkmɑːnz kəˈnæl] *noun* canal running horizontally through compact bone, carrying blood to the Haversian systems

Volkmann's contracture [ˈfɒlkmɑːnz kənˈtræktʃə] *see* CONTRACTURE

volsella *or* **vulsella** [vɒlˈselə *or* vʌlˈselə] *noun* type of forceps with hooks at the end of each arm

volume [ˈvɒljuːm] *noun* amount of a substance; **blood volume** = total amount of blood in the body; **stroke volume** = amount of blood pumped out of a ventricle at each heartbeat

voluntary [ˈvɒləntəri] *adjective* not forced, (action) done because one wishes to do it; **voluntary admission** = admitting a patient into a psychiatric hospital with the consent of the patient; **voluntary movement** = movement (such as walking or speaking) directed by the person's willpower, using voluntary muscles; **voluntary muscles** = muscles which are moved by the willpower of the person acting through the brain

COMMENT: voluntary muscles work in pairs, where one contracts and pulls, while the other relaxes to allow the bone to move

volunteer [vɒlənˈtɪə] **1** *noun* person who offers to do something freely, without being paid; *the hospital relies on volunteers to help with sports for handicapped children*; *they are asking for volunteers to test the new cold cure* **2** *verb* to offer to do something freely; *the research team volunteered to test the new drug on themselves*

volvulus [ˈvɒlvjʊləs] *noun* condition where a loop of intestine is twisted and blocked, so cutting off its blood supply

vomer [ˈvəʊmə] *noun* thin flat vertical bone in the septum of the nose

vomica [ˈvɒmɪkə] *noun* **(a)** cavity in the lungs containing pus **(b)** action of vomiting pus from the throat or lungs

vomit [ˈvɒmɪt] **1** *noun* vomitus, partly digested food which has been brought up into the mouth from the stomach; *his bed was covered with vomit*; *she died after choking on her own vomit* **2** *verb* to bring up partly digested food from the stomach into the mouth; *he had a fever, and then started to vomit*; *she vomited her breakfast*

vomiting [ˈvɒmɪtɪŋ] *noun* emesis, being sick, bringing up vomit into the mouth

vomitus [ˈvɒmɪtəs] *noun* vomit

von Hippel-Lindau syndrome [vɒn ˈhɪpəlˈlɪndaʊ ˈsɪndrəʊm] *noun* disease in which angiomas of the brain are related to angiomas and cysts in other parts of the body

von Recklinghausen's disease [vɒn ˈreklɪŋhauzənz dɪˈziːz] *noun* **(a)** = NEUROFIBROMATOSIS **(b)** osteitis fibrosa, weakness of the bones caused by excessive activity of the thyroid gland

von Willebrand's disease [vɒn ˈvɪlɪbrændz dɪˈziːz] *noun* hereditary blood disease (occurring in both sexes) where the mucous membrane starts to bleed without any apparent reason (involving a deficiency of a clotting factor in the blood, called 'von Willebrand's factor')

voyeurism ['vwaɪɜːrɪzm] *noun* condition where a person experiences sexual pleasure by watching others having intercourse

vu [vuː] *see* DEJA VU

vulgaris [vʌlˈgeərɪs] *see* ACNE, LUPUS

vulnerable ['vʌlnərəbl] *adjective* likely to catch (a disease) because of being in a weakened state; *premature babies are especially vulnerable to infection*

vulsella [vʌlˈselə] = VOLSELLA

vulv- ['vʌlv] *prefix* referring to the vulva

vulva ['vʌlvə] *noun* a woman's external sexual organs, at the opening leading to the vagina; *see also* KRAUROSIS

COMMENT: the vulva is formed of folds (the labia), surrounding the clitoris and the entrance to the vagina

vulvectomy [vʌlˈvektəmi] *noun* surgical operation to remove the vulva

vulvitis [vʌlˈvaɪtɪs] *noun* inflammation of the vulva, causing intense irritation

vulvovaginitis [vʌlvəuvædʒɪˈnaɪtɪs] *noun* inflammation of the vulva and vagina (NOTE: for other terms referring to the vulva, see words beginning with **episio-**)

Ww

wad [wɒd] *noun* pad of material used to put on a wound, etc.; *the nurse put a wad of absorbent cotton over the sore*

wadding ['wɒdɪŋ] *noun* material used to make a wad; *put a layer of cotton wadding over the eye*

waist [weɪst] *noun* narrow part of the body below the chest and above the buttocks; *he measures 85 centimetres around the waist*

wait [weɪt] *verb* to stay somewhere until something happens or someone arrives; *he has been waiting for his operation for six months*; *there are ten patients waiting to see Dr Smith*; **waiting list** = list of patients waiting for admission to hospital usually for treatment of non-urgent disorders; *the length of waiting lists for non-emergency surgery varies enormously from one region to another*; *it is hoped that hospital waiting lists will get shorter*; **waiting room** = room at a doctor's or dentist's surgery where patients wait; *please sit in the waiting room - the doctor will see you in ten minutes*; **waiting time** = period between the time when the name of a patient has been put on the waiting list and his admission into hospital

wake [weɪk] *verb* (i) to interrupt someone's sleep; (ii) to stop sleeping; *the nurse woke the patient or the patients was woken by the nurse*; *the patient had to be woken to have his injection* (NOTE: **waking - woke - has woken**)

wakeful ['weɪkfʊl] *adjective* being wide awake, not wanting to sleep

wakefulness ['weɪkfʊlnəs] *noun* being wide awake

wake up ['weɪk 'ʌp] *verb* to stop sleeping; *the old man woke up in the middle of the night and started calling for the nurse*

Waldeyer's ring ['vɑːldaɪəz 'rɪŋ] *noun* ring of lymphoid tissue made by the tonsils

walk [wɔːk] *verb* to go on foot; *the baby is learning to walk*; *he walked when he was only eleven months old*; *she can walk a few steps with a Zimmer*

walking frame *or* **walker** ['wɔːkɪŋ 'freɪm or 'wɔːkə] *noun* metal frame which is used to support someone who has difficulty in walking

wall [wɔːl] *noun* side part of an organ or a passage in the body; *an ulcer formed in the wall of the duodenum*; *the doctor made an incision in the abdominal wall*; *they removed a fibroma from the wall of the uterus or from the uterine wall*

wall eye *or* **walleye** ['wɔːl 'aɪ] *noun* eye which is very pale, eye which is squinting so strongly that only the white sclera is visible

Wangensteen tube ['wæŋɡənstiːn 'tjuːb] *noun* tube which is passed into the stomach to remove the stomach's contents by suction

ward [wɔːd] *noun* room or set of rooms in a hospital, with beds for the patients; *he is in Ward 8B*; *the children's ward is at the end of the corridor*; **ward sister** = senior nurse in charge of a ward; **accident ward** *or* **casualty ward** = ward for urgent accident victims; **emergency ward** = ward for patients who require urgent attention; **geriatric ward** = ward for the treatment of geriatric patients; **isolation ward** = special ward where patients suffering from dangerous infectious diseases can be kept isolated from other patients; **medical ward** = ward for patients who are not undergoing surgery; **surgical ward** = ward for patients who have undergone surgery

warm [wɔːm] *adjective* quite hot, pleasantly hot; *the patients need to be kept warm in cold weather* (NOTE: **warm - warmer - warmest)**

warn [wɔːn] *verb* to tell someone that a danger is possible; *the children were warned about the dangers of solvent abuse*; *the doctors warned her that her husband would not live more than a few weeks*

warning ['wɔːnɪŋ] *noun* telling someone about a danger; *there's a warning on the bottle of medicine, saying that it should be kept away from children*; *each packet of cigarettes has a government health warning printed on it*; *the health department has given out warnings about the danger of hypothermia*

wart [wɔːt] *noun* verruca, a small hard benign growth on the skin; **common wart** = wart which appears mainly on the hands; **plantar wart** = wart on the sole of the foot; **venereal wart** = wart on the genitals or in the urogenital area

> COMMENT: warts are caused by a virus, and usually occur on the hands, feet or face

washbasin ['wɒʃbeɪsɪn] *noun* bowl in a kitchen or bathroom where you can wash your hands

washout ['wɒʃaʊt] *noun* thorough cleaning with a liquid, especially water; **stomach washout** = gastric lavage or lavage of the stomach to remove poison

Wassermann reaction (WR) *or* **Wassermann test** ['wæsəmæn rɪˈækʃn or 'wæsəmæn 'test] *noun* blood serum test to see if a patient has syphilis

waste [weɪst] **1** *adjective* (material or matter) which is useless, which has no use; *the veins take blood containing waste carbon dioxide back into the lungs*; *waste matter is excreted in the faeces or urine*; **waste product** = substance which is not needed in the body (and is excreted in urine or faeces) **2** *verb* to use more than is needed; *the hospital kitchens waste a lot of food*

waste away ['weɪst əˈweɪ] *verb* to become thinner, to lose flesh; *when he caught the disease he simply wasted away*

wasting ['weɪstɪŋ] *noun* condition where a person or a limb loses weight and becomes thin; **wasting disease** = disease which causes severe loss of weight or reduction in size (of an organ)

water ['wɔːtə] **1** *noun* **(a)** common liquid which forms rain, rivers, the sea, etc., and which makes up a large part of the body; *can I have a glass of water please?*; *they suffered dehydration from lack of water*; **water balance** = state where the water lost by the body (in urine, perspiration, etc.) is balanced by water absorbed from food and drink; **water on the knee** = fluid in the knee joint under the kneecap, caused by a blow on the knee **(b)** urine; *he passed a lot of water during the night*; *she noticed blood streaks in her water*; *the nurse asked him to give a sample of his water* **(c)** **the waters** = amniotic fluid, the fluid in the amnion in which a fetus float; **breaking of the waters** = rupture of the amniotic membrane releasing the amniotic fluid, before a baby is born; *see also* BAG **2** *verb* to fill with tears or saliva; *onions made his eyes water*; *her mouth watered when she saw the ice cream*; **watering eye** = eye which fills with tears because of an irritation (NOTE: for other terms referring to water, see words beginning with **hydr-**)

> COMMENT: since the body is formed of about 50% water, a normal adult needs to drink about 2.5 litres (5 pints) of fluid each day. Water taken into the body is passed out again as urine or sweat

water bed ['wɔːtə 'bed] *noun* mattress made of a large sack filled with water, used to prevent bedsores

waterbrash ['wɔːtəbræʃ] *noun* condition caused by dyspepsia, where there is a burning feeling in the stomach and the mouth suddenly fills with acid saliva

Waterhouse-Friderichsen syndrome ['wɔːtəhaʊs'friːdərɪksən 'sɪndrəʊm] *noun* condition caused by blood poisoning with meningococci, where the tissues of the adrenal glands die and haemorrhage

waterproof ['wɔːtəpruːf] *adjective* which will not let water through; *put a waterproof sheet on the baby's bed*

water sac *or* **bag of waters** ['wɔːtə 'sæk or 'bæg əv 'wɔːtəz] = AMNION

Waterston's operation ['wɔːtəstənz ɒpəˈreɪʃn] *noun* surgical operation to treat Fallot's tetralogy, where the right pulmonary artery is joined to the ascending aorta

waterworks ['wɔːtəwɜːks] *noun (informal)* the urinary system; *there's nothing wrong with his waterworks*

watery ['wɔːtəri] *adjective* liquid, like water; *he passed some watery stools*

Watson knife ['wɒtsən 'naɪf] *noun* type of very sharp surgical knife for skin transplants

wax [wæks] *noun* **(a)** soft yellow substance produced by bees, also made from petroleum; **hot wax treatment** = treatment for arthritis in which the joints are painted with hot liquid wax **(b)** **ear wax** = cerumen, wax which forms in the ear

WBC ['dʌbəljuː 'biː 'siː] = WHITE BLOOD CELL

weak [wiːk] *adjective* not strong; *after his illness he was very weak*; *she is too weak to dress herself*; *he is allowed to drink weak tea or coffee*; **weak pulse** = pulse which is not strong, which is not easy to feel (NOTE: **weak - weaker - weakest**)

weaken ['wiːkən] *verb* to make something or someone weak; to become weak; *he was weakened by the disease and could not resist further infection*; *the swelling is caused by a weakening of the wall of the artery*

weakness ['wiːknəs] *noun* not being strong; *the doctor noticed the weakness of the patient's pulse*

weal *or* **wheal** [wiːl] *noun* small area of skin which swells because of a sharp blow or an insect bite

wean [wiːn] *verb* (i) to make a baby start to eat solid food after having only had liquids to drink; (ii) to make a baby start to drink from a bottle and start eating solid food after having been only breastfed; *the baby was breastfed for two months and then was gradually weaned onto the bottle*

wear [weə] *verb* to become damaged through being used; *the cartilage of the knee was worn from too much exercise* (NOTE: **wearing - wore - has worn**)

wear and tear ['weə ən 'teə] *noun* normal use which affects an organ; *a heart has to stand a lot of wear and tear*; *the wear and tear of a strenuous job has begun to affect his heart*

wear off ['weə 'ɒf] *verb* to disappear gradually; *the effect of the painkiller will wear off after a few hours*; *he started to open his eyes, as the anaesthetic wore off*

Weber-Christian disease ['veɪbə'krɪstʃən dɪ'ziːz] *noun* type of panniculitis where the liver and spleen become enlarged

Weber's test ['veɪbəz 'test] *noun* test to see if both ears hear correctly, where a tuning fork is struck and the end placed on the head

Wegener's granulomatosis ['vegənəz grænjʊləʊmə'təʊsɪs] *noun* disease of connective tissue, where the nasal passages, lungs and kidneys are inflamed and ulcerated, with formation of granulomas; it is usually fatal

weigh [weɪ] *verb* (i) to measure how heavy something is; (ii) to have a certain weight; *the nurse weighed the baby on the scales*; *she weighed seven pounds (3.5 kilos) at birth*; *a woman weighs less than a man of similar height*; *the doctor asked him how much he weighed*; *I weigh 120 pounds or I weigh 54 kilos*

weight [weɪt] *noun* **(a)** how heavy a person is; *what's the patient's weight?*; **her weight is only 105 pounds** = she weighs only 105 pounds; **to lose weight** = to get thinner; *she's trying to lose weight before she goes on holiday*; **to put on weight** = to become fatter; *he's put on a lot of weight in the last few months*; **weight gain** *or* **gain in weight** = becoming fatter or heavier; **weight loss** = action of losing weight or of becoming thinner; *weight loss can be a symptom of certain types of cancer* **(b)** something which is heavy; *don't lift heavy weights, you may hurt your back*

weightlessness ['weɪtləsnəs] *noun* state where the body seems to weigh nothing (as experienced by astronauts)

Weil-Felix reaction *or* **Weil-Felix test** ['vaɪl'feɪlɪks rɪ'ækʃn *or* 'vaɪl'feɪlɪks 'test] *noun* test to see if the patient has typhus, where the patient's serum is tested for antibodies against *Proteus vulgaris*

Weil's disease ['vaɪlz dɪ'ziːz] = LEPTOSPIROSIS

welder's flash ['weldəz 'flæʃ] *noun* condition where the eye is badly damaged by very bright light

welfare ['welfeə] *noun* **(a)** good health, good living conditions; *they look after the welfare of the old people in the town* **(b)** money paid by the government to people who need it; *he exists on welfare payments*

well [wel] *adjective* healthy; *he's not a well man*; *you're looking very well after your holiday*; *he's quite well again after his flu*; *he's not very well, and has had to stay in bed*; **well-woman clinic** = clinic which specializes in preventive medicine for women (such as breast screening and cervical smear tests) and gives advice on pregnancy, contraception, the menopause, etc.

wellbeing ['welbiːɪŋ] *noun* being in good health, in good living conditions; *she is responsible for the wellbeing of the patients under her care*

wen [wen] *noun* cyst which forms in a sebaceous gland

Wernicke's encephalopathy ['vɜːnɪkəz ensefə'lɒpəθi] *noun* condition caused by lack of vitamin B (often in alcoholics), where the patient is delirious, moves his eyes about rapidly (nystagmus), walks unsteadily and is subject to constant vomiting

Wertheim's operation [ˈvɜːthaɪmz ɒpəˈreɪʃn] *noun* type of hysterectomy, surgical operation to remove the uterus, the lymph nodes which are next to it, and most of the vagina, the ovaries and the tubes, as treatment for cancer of the uterus

wet [wet] **1** *adjective* not dry, covered in liquid; *he got wet waiting for the bus in the rain and caught a cold*; *the baby has nappy rash from wearing a wet nappy*; **wet burn** = scald, an injury to the skin caused by touching a very hot liquid or steam; **wet dream** = NOCTURNAL EMISSION (NOTE: **wet - wetter - wettest**) **2** *verb* to urinate (in bed); *he is eight years old and he still wets his bed every night*; *see also* BEDWETTING

wet dressing [ˈwet ˈdresɪŋ] *noun see* COMPRESS

Wharton's duct [ˈwɔːtənz ˈdʌkt] *noun* duct which takes saliva into the mouth from the salivary glands under the lower jaw, the submandibular salivary glands

Wharton's jelly [ˈwɔːtənz ˈdʒeli] *noun* jelly-like tissue in the umbilical cord

wheal [wiːl] = WEAL

wheel [wiːl] *verb* to push along something which has wheels; *the orderly wheeled the trolley into the operating theatre*

wheelchair [ˈwiːltʃeə] *noun* chair with wheels in which an invalid can sit and move around; *he manages to get around in a wheelchair*; *she has been confined to a wheelchair since her accident*

Wheelhouse's operation [ˈwiːlhaʊsɪz ɒpəˈreɪʃn] *noun* urethrotomy, surgical operation to relieve blockage of the urethra by making an incision into the urethra

wheeze [wiːz] **1** *noun* whistling noise in the bronchi; *the doctor listened to his wheezes* **2** *verb* to make a whistling sound when breathing; *when she has an attack of asthma, she wheezes and has difficulty in breathing*

wheezing [ˈwiːzɪŋ] *noun* whistling noise in the bronchi when breathing

COMMENT: wheezing is often found in asthmatic patients and is also associated with bronchitis and heart disease

wheezy [ˈwiːzi] *adjective* making a whistling sound when breathing; *he was quite wheezy when he stopped running*

whiplash injury [ˈwɪplæʃ ˈɪndʒəri] *noun* injury to the vertebrae in the neck, caused when the head jerks backwards, often occurring in a car that is struck from behind

Whipple's disease [ˈwɪpəlz dɪˈziːz] *noun* disease where the patient has difficulty in absorbing nutrients and passes fat in the faeces, where the joints are inflamed and the lymph glands enlarged

Whipple's operation [ˈwɪpəlz ɒpəˈreɪʃn] = PANCREATECTOMY

whipworm [ˈwɪpwɜːm] *noun Trichuris,* thin round parasitic worm which infests the caecum

whisper [ˈwɪspə] **1** *noun* speaking very quietly; *she has a sore throat and can only speak in a whisper* **2** *verb* to speak in a very quiet voice; *he whispered to the nurse that he wanted something to drink*

white [waɪt] **1** *adjective & noun* of a colour like snow or milk; *white patches developed on his skin*; *her hair has turned quite white*; **white blood cell (WBC)** = leucocyte, a blood cell which contains a nucleus, is formed in bone marrow, and creates antibodies; **white commissure** = part of the white matter in the spinal cord near the central canal; **white leg** = acute oedema of the leg, a condition which affects women after childbirth, where a leg becomes pale and inflamed as a result of lymphatic obstruction (NOTE: also called **milk leg** or **phlegmasia alba dolens**); **white matter** = nerve tissue in the central nervous system which contains more myelin than grey matter (NOTE: **white - whiter - whitest**) **2** *noun* main part of the eye which is white; *the whites of his eyes turned yellow when he developed jaundice*; *see also* LEUCORRHOEA

whitlow [ˈwɪtləʊ] *noun* felon, an inflammation caused by infection, near the nail in the fleshy part of the tip of a finger; *see also* PARONYCHIA

WHO [ˈdʌbəlju: ˈeɪtʃ ˈəʊ] = WORLD HEALTH ORGANIZATION

whoop [wuːp or huːp] *noun* loud noise made when inhaling by a person suffering from whooping cough

whooping cough [ˈhuːpɪŋ ˈkɒf] *noun* pertussis, an infectious disease caused by *Bordetella pertussis* affecting the bronchial tubes, common in children, and sometimes very serious

COMMENT: the patient coughs very badly and makes a characteristic 'whoop' when he breathes in after a coughing fit. Whooping cough can lead to pneumonia, and is treated with antibiotics. Vaccination against whooping cough is given to infants

Widal reaction or **Widal test** [viːˈdɑːl rɪˈækʃn or viːˈdɑːl ˈtest] *noun* test to detect typhoid fever

COMMENT: a sample of the patient's blood is put into a solution containing typhoid bacilli or anti-typhoid serum is added to a sample of bacilli from the patient's faeces. If the bacilli agglutinate (i.e. form into groups) this indicates that the patient is suffering from typhoid fever

widen [ˈwaɪdən] *verb* to make wider; *an operation to widen the blood vessels near the heart*

widespread [ˈwaɪdspred] *adjective* affecting a large area or a large number of people; *the government advised widespread immunization*; *glaucoma is widespread in the northern part of the country*

will [wɪl] *noun* power of the mind to decide to do something

Willis [ˈwɪlɪs] *see* CIRCLE OF WILLIS

willpower [ˈwɪlpaʊə] *noun* having a strong will; *the patient showed the willpower to start walking again unaided*

Wilms' tumour [ˈvɪlmz ˈtjuːmə] = NEPHROBLASTOMA

Wilson's disease [ˈwɪlsənz dɪˈziːz] *noun* hepatolenticular degeneration, hereditary disease where copper deposits accumulate in the liver and the brain, causing cirrhosis

wind [wɪnd] *noun* (i) flatus, gas which forms in the digestive system; (ii) flatulence, accumulation of gas in the digestive system; *the baby is suffering from wind*; *he has pains in the stomach caused by wind*; *to* **break wind** = to let gas escape from the anus

windchill factor [ˈwɪndtʃɪl ˈfæktə] *noun* way of calculating the risk of exposure in cold weather by adding the speed of the wind to the number of degrees of temperature below zero

window [ˈwɪndəʊ] *noun* small opening in the ear; **oval window** = fenestra ovalis, oval-shaped opening between the middle ear and the inner ear, closed by a membrane and covered by the base of the stapes; **round window** = fenestra rotunda, round opening

closed by a membrane, between the middle ear and the cochlea; *see illustration at* EAR

windpipe [ˈwɪndpaɪp] *noun* the trachea, the main air passage from the nose and mouth to the lungs

wink [wɪŋk] *verb* to close one eye and open it again rapidly

wisdom tooth [ˈwɪzdəm ˈtuːθ] *noun* third molar, one of the four teeth in the back of the jaw, which only appears at about the age of 20 and sometimes does not appear at all; *see illustration at* TEETH

witch hazel [ˈwɪtʃ ˈheɪzl] *noun* hamamelis, lotion made from the bark of a tree, used to check bleeding and harden inflamed tissue and bruises

withdraw [wɪðˈdrɔː] *verb* (a) to stop being interested in the world, to become isolated; *the patient withdrew into himself and refused to eat* (b) to remove (a drug), to stop (a treatment); *the doctor decided to withdraw the drug from the patient* (NOTE: **withdrawing - withdrew - has withdrawn**)

withdrawal [wɪðˈdrɔːl] *noun* (a) removing of interest, becoming isolated (b) removal of a drug or treatment; **withdrawal symptom** = unpleasant physical condition (vomiting, headaches or fever) which occurs when a patient stops taking an addictive drug

she was in the early stages of physical withdrawal from heroin and showed classic symptoms: sweating, fever, sleeplessness and anxiety

Nursing Times

woman [ˈwʊmən] *noun* female adult person; *it is a common disease of women of 45 to 60 years of age*; *on average, women live longer than men*; **women's ward** or **women's hospital** = ward or hospital for female patients; *see also* WELL-WOMAN CLINIC (NOTE: plural is **women**. For other terms referring to women, see words beginning with **gyn-**)

womb [wuːm] *noun* uterus, hollow organ in a woman's pelvic cavity in which a fertilized ovum develops into a fetus (NOTE: for other terms referring to the womb, see words beginning with **hyster-, hystero-, metr-, metro-, utero-**)

wood [wʊd] *noun* material that comes from trees; **wood alcohol** = methyl alcohol, a poisonous alcohol used as fuel

Wood's lamp [ˈwʊdz ˈlæmp] *noun* lamp which allows a doctor to see fluorescence in the hair of a patient suffering from fungal infection

woolsorter's disease ['wʊlsɔːtəz dɪ'ziːz] *noun* form of anthrax which affects the lungs

word [wɜːd] *noun* separate part of language, either written or spoken; *there are seven words in this sentence*

word blindness ['wɜːd 'blaɪndnəs] *see* ALEXIA

World Health Organization (WHO) ['wɜːld 'helθ ɔːgənaɪ'zeɪʃn] *noun* organization (part of the United Nations Organization) which aims to improve health in the world by teaching or publishing information, etc.

worm [wɜːm] *noun* long thin animal with no legs or backbone, which can infest the human body, especially the intestines; *compare* RINGWORM; *see also* FLATWORM, HOOKWORM, ROUNDWORM, TAPEWORM, WHIPWORM

worn out ['wɔːn 'aʊt] *adjective* very tired; *he came home worn out after working all day in the hospital*; *she was worn out by looking after the children*; *see also* WEAR

wound [wuːnd] **1** *noun* damage to external tissue which allows blood to escape; *he had a knife wound in his leg*; *the doctors sutured the wound in his chest*; **contused wound** = wound caused by a blow, where the skin is bruised, torn and bleeding; **gunshot wound** = wound caused by a pellet or bullet from a gun; **incised wound** = wound with clear edges, caused by a sharp knife or razor; **lacerated wound** = wound where the skin is torn; **puncture wound** = wound made by a sharp point which makes a hole in the flesh; **surgical wound** = incision

made during a surgical operation **2** *verb* to harm someone by making a hole in the tissue of the body; *he was wounded three times in the head*

WR ['dʌbəljuː 'ɑː] = WASSERMANN REACTION

wrinkle ['rɪŋkl] *noun* fold in the skin; *old people have wrinkles on the neck*; *she had a face lift to remove wrinkles*

wrinkled ['rɪŋkld] *adjective* covered with wrinkles

wrist [rɪst] *noun* joint between the hand and forearm; *he sprained his wrist and can't play tennis tomorrow*; **wrist drop** = paralysis of the wrist muscles, where the hand hangs limp, caused by damage to the radial nerve in the upper arm (NOTE: for other terms referring to the wrist, see words beginning with **carp-**); *see illustration at* HAND

COMMENT: the wrist is formed of eight small bones in the hand which articulate with the bones in the forearm. The joint allows the hand to rotate and move downwards and sideways. The joint is easily fractured or sprained

writer's cramp ['raɪtəz 'kræmp] *noun* painful spasm of the muscles in the forearm and hand which comes from writing too much

writhe [raɪð] *verb* **to writhe in pain** = to twist and turn because the pain is very severe

wry neck *or* **wryneck** ['raɪ 'nek] *noun* torticollis, deformity of the neck, where the head is twisted to one side by contraction of the sternocleidomastoid muscle

Wuchereria [vʊkə'rɪəriə] *noun* type of tiny nematode worm which infests the lymph system, causing elephantiasis

Xx Yy Zz

xanth- *or* **xantho-** [ˈzænθ *or* ˈzænθəʊ] *prefix* meaning yellow

xanthaemia *US* **xanthemia** [zænˈθiːmiə] = CAROTENAEMIA

xanthelasma [zænθəˈlæzmə] *noun* formation of little yellow fatty tumours on the eyelids

xanthochromia [zænθəˈkrəʊmiə] *noun* yellow colour of the skin as in jaundice

xanthoma [zænˈθəʊmə] *noun* yellow fatty mass (often on the eyelids and hands), found in patients with a high level of cholesterol in the blood (NOTE: the plural is **xanthomata**)

xanthomatosis [zænθəməˈtəʊsɪs] *noun* condition where several small masses of yellow fatty substance appear in the skin or some internal organs, caused by an excess of fat in the body

xanthopsia [zænˈθɒpsiə] *noun* disorder of the eyes, making everything appear yellow

xanthosis [zænˈθəʊsɪs] *noun* yellow colouring of the skin, caused by eating too much food containing carotene

X chromosome [ˈeks ˈkrəʊməsəʊm] *noun* sex chromosome

COMMENT: every person has a series of pairs of chromosomes, one of which is always an X chromosome; a normal female has one pair of XX chromosomes, while a male has one XY pair. Defective chromosomes affect sexual development: a person with an XO chromosome pair (i.e. one X chromosome alone) has Turner's syndrome; a person with an extra X chromosome (making an XXY set) has Klinefelter's syndrome. Haemophilia is a disorder linked to the X chromosome

xeno- [ˈzenəʊ] *prefix* meaning different

xenograft [ˈzenəɡrɑːft] *noun* heterograft, tissue taken from an individual of one species and grafted on an individual of another species (NOTE: the opposite is **homograft** *or* **allograft**)

xero- [ˈzɪərəʊ] *prefix* meaning dry

xeroderma [zɪərəˈdɜːmə] *noun* skin disorder where dry scales form on the skin

xerophthalmia [zɪərɒfˈθælmiə] *noun* condition of the eye, where the cornea and conjunctiva become thick and dry, a symptom of lack of Vitamin A

xeroradiography [zɪərəʊreɪdiˈɒɡrəfi] *noun* X-ray technique used in producing mammograms on selenium plates

xerosis [zɪˈrəʊsɪs] *noun* dry eye, abnormally dry condition of the eye

xerostomia [zɪərəˈstəʊmiə] *noun* dryness of the mouth, caused by lack of saliva

xiphisternal plane [zɪfiˈstɜːnl ˈpleɪn] *noun* imaginary horizontal line across the middle of the chest at the· point where the xiphoid process starts

xiphisternum *or* **xiphoid process** *or* **xiphoid cartilage** [zɪfiˈstɜːnəm *or* ˈzɪfɔɪd ˈprəʊses *or* ˈzɪfɔɪd ˈkɑːtɪlɪdʒ] *noun* bottom part of the breastbone or sternum, which in young people is formed of cartilage and becomes bone only by middle age

X-ray [ˈeksreɪ] **1** *noun* **(a)** ray with a very short wavelength, which is invisible, but can go through soft tissue and register as a photograph on a film; *the X-ray examination showed the presence of a tumour in the colon*; *the X-ray department is closed for lunch* **(b)** photograph taken using X-rays; *the dentist took some X-rays of the patient's teeth*; *he pinned the X-rays to the light screen*; *all the staff had to have chest X-rays* **2** *verb* to take an X-ray photograph of a patient; *there are six patients waiting to be X-rayed*

COMMENT: because X-rays go through soft tissue, it is sometimes necessary to make internal organs opaque so that they will show up on the film. In the case of stomach X-rays, patients take a barium meal before being photographed (contrast radiography); in other cases, such as kidney X-rays, radioactive substances are injected into the bloodstream or into the organ itself. X-rays are used not only in radiography for diagnosis but as a treatment in radiotherapy as rapidly dividing cells such as cancer cells are most affected. Excessive exposure to X-rays, either as a patient being treated, or as a radiographer, can cause radiation sickness

xylose ['zaɪləʊz] *noun* pentose which has not been metabolized

yawn [jɔːn] **1** *noun* reflex action when tired or sleepy, where the mouth is opened wide and after a deep intake of air, the breath exhaled slowly; *his yawns made everyone feel sleepy* **2** *verb* to open the mouth wide and breathe in deeply and then breathe out slowly

COMMENT: yawning can be caused by tiredness as the body prepares for sleep, but it can have other causes, such as a hot room, or even can be started by unconsciously imitating someone who is yawning near you

yaws [jɔːz] *noun* framboesia or pian, a tropical disease caused by the spirochaete *Treponema pertenue*

COMMENT: symptoms include fever with raspberry-like swellings on the skin, followed in later stages by bone deformation

Y chromosome ['waɪ 'krəʊməsəʊm] *noun* male chromosome

COMMENT: the Y chromosome has male characteristics and does not form part of the female genetic structure. A normal male has an XY pair of chromosomes. See also the note at X CHROMOSOME

yeast [jiːst] *noun* fungus which is used in the fermentation of alcohol and in making bread

COMMENT: yeast is a good source of Vitamin B and can be taken in dried form in tablets

yellow ['jeləʊ] *adjective & noun* of a colour like that of the sun or of gold; *his skin turned yellow when he had hepatitis*; *the whites of the eyes become yellow as a symptom of jaundice*; **yellow atrophy** = old name for

severe damage to the liver; **yellow fibres** = elastic fibres, fibres made of elastin, which can expand easily and are found in the skin and in the walls of arteries or the lungs; **yellow spot** = macula lutea, yellow patch on the retina of the eye around the fovea

yellow fever ['jeləʊ 'fiːvə] *noun* infectious disease, found especially in Africa and South America, caused by an arbovirus carried by the mosquito *Aedes aegypti*

COMMENT: the fever affects the liver and causes jaundice. There is no known cure for yellow fever and it can be fatal, but vaccination can prevent it

Yersinia pestis [jɜːˈsɪniə ˈpestɪs] *noun* bacterium which causes plague

yolk sac ['jəʊk 'sæk] = VITELLINE SAC

yuppie flu ['jʌpi 'fluː] *noun (informal)* = MYALGIC ENCEPHALOMYELITIS

Zadik's operation ['zeɪdɪks ɒpəˈreɪʃn] *noun* surgical operation to remove the whole of an ingrowing toenail

zidovudine [zɪˈdəʊvjudiːn] *noun* azidothymidine or AZT, a drug used in the treatment of AIDS; it helps to slow the progress of the disease

Zimmer (frame) ['zɪmə 'freɪm] *noun* trade mark for a metal frame used by patients who have difficulty in walking; *she managed to walk some steps with a Zimmer*

zinc [zɪŋk] *noun* white metallic trace element (NOTE: chemical symbol is **Zn**)

zinc ointment ['zɪŋk 'ɔɪntmənt] *noun* soothing ointment made of zinc oxide and oil

zinc oxide (ZnO) ['zɪŋk 'ɒksaɪd] *noun* compound of zinc and oxygen, which forms a soft white soothing powder used in creams and lotions

Z line ['zed laɪn] *noun* part of the pattern of muscle tissue, a dark line seen in the light I band

Zn *chemical symbol for* zinc

Zollinger-Ellison syndrome ['zɒlɪndʒərˈelɪsən 'sɪndrəʊm] *noun* condition where tumours are formed in the islet cells of the pancreas together with peptic ulcers

zona ['zəʊnə] *noun* **(a)** = HERPES ZOSTER **(b)** zone or area; **zona pellucida** = membrane which forms around an ovum

zone [zəʊn] *noun* area of the body; **erogenous zone** = part of the body which, if stimulated, produces sexual arousal (such as the penis, clitoris or nipples)

zonula or **zonule** ['zɒnjʊlə or 'zɒnjuːl] *noun* small area of the body; **zonule of Zinn** = suspensory ligament of the lens of the eye

zonulolysis [zɒnjuˈlɒləsɪs] *noun* removal of a zonule by dissolving it

zoonosis [zəʊɒˈnəʊsɪs] *noun* disease which a human can catch from an animal (NOTE: the plural is **zoonoses**)

zoster ['zɒstə] *see* HERPES ZOSTER

zygoma [zaɪˈgəʊmə] *noun* (i) zygomatic arch; (ii) zygomatic bone or cheekbone (NOTE: the plural is **zygomata**)

zygomatic [zaɪgəˈmætɪk] *adjective* referring to the zygoma; **zygomatic arch** or **zygoma** = ridge of bone across the temporal bone, running between the ear and the bottom of the eye socket; **zygomatic bone** = cheekbone or malar bone, bone which forms the prominent part of the cheek and the lower part of the eye socket; **zygomatic process** = one of the bony projections which form the zygomatic arch; *see illustration at* SKULL

zygomycosis [zaɪgəmaɪˈkəʊsɪs] *noun* disease caused by a fungus which infests the blood vessels in the lungs

zygote ['zaɪgəʊt] *noun* fertilized ovum, the first stage of development of an embryo

zym- ['zaɪm] *prefix* meaning (i) enzymes; (ii) fermentation

zymogen ['zaɪmədʒen] = PROENZYME

zymosis [zaɪˈməʊsɪs] *noun* fermentation, the process where carbohydrates are broken down by enzymes and produce alcohol

zymotic [zaɪˈmɒtɪk] *adjective* referring to zymosis

SUPPLEMENT

ANATOMICAL TERMS

The body is always described as if standing upright with the palms of the hands facing forward. There is only one central vertical plane, termed the *median* or *sagittal* plane, and this passes through the body from front to back. Planes parallel to this on either side are *parasagittal* or *paramedian* planes. Vertical planes at right angles to the median are called *coronal* planes. The term *horizontal* (or *transverse) plane* speaks for itself. Two specific horizontal planes are (a) the *transpyloric,* midway between the suprasternal notch and the symphysis pubis, and (b) the *irons tubercular* or *intra-tubercutar* plane, which passes through the tubercles of the iliac crests. Many other planes are named from the structures they pass through.

Views of the body from some different points are shown on the diagram; a view of the body from above is called the *superior aspect,* and that from below is the *inferior aspect. Cephalic* means toward the head; *caudal* refers to positions (or in a direction) towards the tail. *Proximal* and *distal* refer to positions respectively closer to and further from the centre of the body in any direction, while *lateral* and *medial* relate more specifically to relative sideways positions, and also refer to movements. *Ventral* refers to the abdomen, front or anterior, while *dorsal* relates to the back of a part or organ. The hand has a *dorsal* and a *palmar* surface, and the foot a *dorsal* and a *plantar* surface.

Note that *flexion of the thigh* moves it forward while *flexion of the leg* moves it backwards; the movements of *extension* are similarly reversed. Movement and rotation of limbs can be *medial,* which is with the front moving towards the centre line, or *lateral,* which is in the opposite direction. Specific terms for limb movements are *adduction,* towards the centre line, and *abduction,* which is away from the centre line. Other specific terms are *supination* and *pronation* for the hand, and *inversion* and *eversion* for the foot.

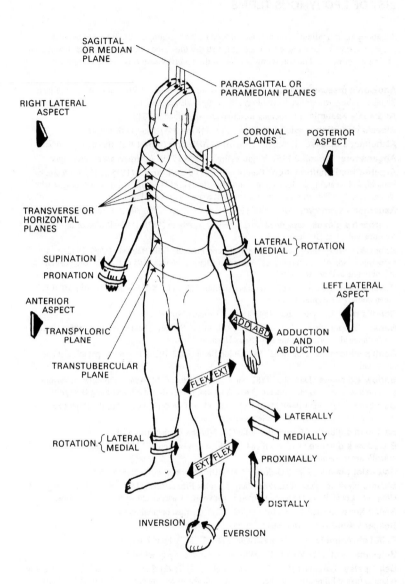

LIST OF EPONYMOUS TERMS

An eponym, in medicine, is a disease, procedure or anatomical structure that bears a person's name or the name of a place. It is usually the name of the person who discovered or first described it. The following is a list of the *eponymous* terms in this dictionary.

Addison's disease described 1849. Thomas Addison (1793-1860), from Northumberland, founder of the science of endocrinology. His name is also applied to

Addison's anaemia (pernicious anaemia) also described in 1849.

Albee's operation Frederick Houdlett Albee (1876-1945), New York surgeon.

Alzheimer's disease Described 1906. Alois Alzheimer (1864-1915), Bavarian physician.

Apgar score Described 1952. Virginia Apgar (1909-1974), American anaesthesiologist.

Arnold-Chiari malformation Described 1894. Julius A. Arnold (1835-1915), Professor of Pathological Anatomy at Heidelberg. Hans von Chiari (1851-1916), Viennese pathologist who was Professor of Pathological Anatomy at Strasbourg and later at Prague.

Asperger's syndrome Described 1944. Hans Asperger (1906-80), Austrian psychiatrist.

Auerbach's plexus Described 1862. Leopold Auerbach (1828-1897), Professor of Neuropathology at Breslau.

Babinski reflex, test Described 1896. Joseph François Felix Babinski (1857-1932), French-born son of Polish refugees. A pupil of Charcot, he was head of the Neurological clinic at Hôpital de la Pitié, 1890-1927.

Baker's cyst Described 1877. William Morrant Baker (1838-1896), member of staff at St Bartholomew's Hospital, London.

Bandl's ring Ludwig Bandl (1842-1892), German obstetrician.

Bankart's operation First performed 1923. Arthur Sydney Blundell Bankart (1879-1951), first orthopaedic surgeon at the Middlesex Hospital, London.

Banti's syndrome Described 1882. Guido Banti (1852-1925), Florentine pathologist and physician.

Barlow's disease Described 1882. Sir Thomas Barlow (1845-1945), physician at various London hospitals; also physician to Queen Victoria, King Edward VII and King George V.

Barr body Described 1949. Murray Llewellyn Barr (1908-1995), head of the Department of Anatomy at the University of Western Ontario, Canada.

Bartholin's glands Caspar Bartholin (1655-1748), Danish anatomist.

Basedow's disease Described 1840. Carl Adolph Basedow (1799-1854), general practitioner in Mersburg, Germany.

Batchelor plaster J.S. Bachelor (b. 1905), British orthopaedic surgeon

Bazin's disease Described 1861. Pierre Antoine Ernest Bazin (1807-1878), dermatologist at Hôpital St Louis, Paris. He was an expert in parasitology associated with skin conditions.

Beer's knife George Joseph Beer (1763-1821), German ophthalmologist.

Behçet's syndrome Described 1937. Halushi Behçet (1889-1948), Turkish dermatologist.

Bellocq's cannula Jean Jacques Bellocq (1732-1807), French surgeon.

Bell's mania Luther Vose Bell (1806-1862), American physiologist.

Bell's palsy Described 1821. Sir Charles Bell (1774-1842), Scottish surgeon. He ran anatomy schools, first in Edinburgh and then in London. Professor of Anatomy at the Royal Academy.

Bence Jones protein Described 1848. Henry Bence Jones (1814-1873), physician at St George's Hospital, London.

Benedict's test Described 1915. Stanley Rossiter Benedict (1884-1936), physiological chemist at Cornell University, New York.

Bennett's fracture   Described 1886. Edward Halloran Bennett (1837-1907), Irish anatomist, later Professor of Surgery at Trinity College, Dublin.

Besnier's prurigo   Ernest Besnier (1831-1909), French dermatologist.

Billroth's operations   Described 1881. Christian Albert Theodore Billroth (1829-1894), Prussian surgeon; studied at Greifswald, Göttingen and Berlin.

Binet's test   Originally described 1905 but later modified at Stanford University, California. Alfred Binet (1857-1911), French psychologist and physiologist.

Bitot's spots   Described 1863. Pierre A. Bitot (1822-1888), Bordeaux physician.

Blalock's operation   Described 1945. Alfred Blalock (1899-1964), Professor of Surgery at Johns Hopkins University, Baltimore.

Boeck's sarcoid   Described 1899. Caesar Peter Moeller Boeck (1845-1913), Professor of Dermatology at Oslo.

Bonney's blue   William Francis Victor Bonney (1872-1953), London gynaecologist.

Bowman's capsule   Described 1842. Sir William Paget Bowman (1816-1892), surgeon in Birmingham and later in London. A pioneer in work on the kidney and also in ophthalmology.

Bradford's frame   Edward Hickling Bradford (1848-1926), American orthopaedic surgeon.

Braille   Introduced 1829-1830. Louis Braille (1809-1852), blind Frenchman and teacher of the blind; he introduced the system which had originally been proposed by Charles Barbier in 1820.

Braun's splint, frame   Heinrich Friedrich Wilhelm Braun (1862-1934), German surgeon.

Braxton-Hicks contractions   Dr Braxton-Hicks, 19th century London physician.

Bright's disease   Described 1836. Richard Bright (1789-1858), physician at Guy's Hospital, London

Broadbent's sign   Sir William Henry Broadbent (1835-1907), English physician.

Broca's area   Described 1861. Pierre Henri Paul Broca (1824-1880), Paris surgeon and anthropologist. A pioneer of neurosurgery, he also invented various instruments, described muscular dystrophy before Duchenne, and recognized rickets as a nutritional disorder before Virchow.

Brodie's abscess   Described 1832. Sir Benjamin Collins Brodie (1783-1862), English surgeon.

Brown-Séquard syndrome   Described 1851. Charles Edouard Brown-Séquard (1817-1894), French physiologist.

Brunner's glands   Described 1687. Johann Konrad Brunner (1653-1727), Swiss anatomist at Heidelberg, then at Strasbourg.

Budd-Chiari syndrome   Described 1845. George Budd (1808-1882), Professor of Medicine at King's College Hospital, London. Hans von Chiari (1851-1916), Viennese pathologist who was Professor of Pathological Anatomy at Strasbourg and later at Prague.

Buerger's disease   Described 1908. Leo Buerger (1879-1943), New York physician of Viennese origins.

Burkitt's lymphoma   Described 1957. Denis Parsons Burkitt (1911-1993), formerly Senior Surgeon, Kampala, Uganda; later a member of the Medical Research Council (UK).

Caldwell-Luc operation   Described 1893. George Walter Caldwell (1834-1918), American physician; Henri Luc (1855-1925), French laryngologist.

Calmette-Guérin (bacille)   A. Calmette (1863-1933) and C. Guérin (1872-1961), French bacteriologists.

Celsius   Described 1742. Anders Celsius (1701-1744), Swedish astronomer and scientist.

Chagas' disease   Described 1909. Carlos Chagas (1879-1934), Brazilian scientist and physician.

Charcot's joints   Described 1868. Jean-Martin Charcot (1825-1893), French neurologist.

Cheyne-Stokes respiration   Described 1818 by Cheyne and 1854 by Stokes. John Cheyne (1777-1836), Scottish physician; William Stokes (1804-1878), Irish physician.

Christmas disease Named after Mr Christmas, the patient in whom the disease was first studied in detail.

Clutton's joints Described 1886. Henry Hugh Clutton (1850-1909), surgeon at St Thomas's Hospital, London.

Colles' fracture Abraham Colles (1773-1843), Irish surgeon.

Cooley's anaemia Described 1927. Thomas Benton Cooley (1871-1945), Professor of Paediatrics at Wayne College of Medicine, Detroit.

Coombs' test Described 1945. Robin Royston Amos Coombs (1921-), Quick Professor of Biology, and Fellow of Corpus Christi College, Cambridge.

Corti (organ of) Described 1851. Marquis Alfonso Corti (1822-1888), Italian anatomist and histologist.

Cowper's glands Described 1700. William Cowper (1666-1709), English surgeon.

Coxsackie virus Named after Coxsackie, New York, where the virus was first identified.

Credé's method Described 1860. Karl Sigmund Franz Credé (1819-1892), German gynaecologist.

Creutzfeldt-Jakob disease Described 1920 by Creutzfeldt; 1921 by Jakob. H.G. Creutzfeldt (1885-1964), A.M. Jakob (1884-1931), German psychiatrists

Crohn's disease Described 1932. Burrill Bernard Crohn (1884-1983), New York physician.

Cushing's disease Described 1932. Harvey Williams Cushing (1869-1939), Boston, USA, surgeon.

da Costa's syndrome Described 1871. Jacob Mendes da Costa (1833-1900), Philadelphia surgeon, who described this condition in soldiers in the American Civil War.

Daltonism Described 1794. John Dalton (1766-1844), English chemist and physician. Founder of the atomic theory, he himself was colour-blind.

Denis Browne splint Described 1934. Sir Denis John Wolko Browne (1892-1967), Australian orthopaedic and general surgeon working in Britain.

Dercum's disease Described 1888. François Xavier Dercum (1856-1931), Professor of Neurology at Jefferson Medical College, Philadelphia.

Descemet's membrane Described 1785. Jean Descemet (1732-1810), French physician; Professor of Anatomy and Surgery in Paris.

Devic's disease Described 1894. Devic was a French physician who died in 1930.

Dick test Described 1924. George Frederick Dick (1881-1967), American physician who, in 1923 with Gladys Rowena Dick (1881-1963), identified streptococci as the cause of scarlet fever.

Dietl's crisis Joseph Dietl (1804-1878), Polish physician.

Döderlein's bacillus Albert Siegmund Gustav Döderlein (1860-1941), German obstetrician and gynaecologist.

Down's syndrome Described 1866. John Langdon Haydon Down (1828-1896), English physician at Normansfield Hospital, Teddington.

Duchenne muscular dystrophy Described 1849. Guillaume Benjamin Arnaud Duchenne (1806-1875), French neurologist.

Ducrey's bacillus Described 1889. Augusto Ducrey (1860-1940), Professor of Dermatology in Pisa, then Rome.

Dupuytren's contracture Described 1831. Baron Guillaume Dupuytren (1775-1835), French surgeon.

Eisenmenger complex Described 1897. Victor Eisenmenger (1864-1932), German physician.

Epstein-Barr virus Isolated and described 1964. Michael Anthony Epstein (b. 1921), Bristol pathologist; Murray Llewellyn Barr (1908-1995), Canadian anatomist and cytologist, head of the Department of Anatomy at the University of Western Ontario, Canada.

Erb's palsy Described 1874. Wilhelm Erb (1840-1921), professor of Medicine at Leipzig and later at Heidelberg.

Esmarch's bandage Described 1869. Johann Friedrich August von Esmarch (1823-1908), Professor of Surgery at Kiel.

Eustachian tube Described 1562, but actually named after Eustachio by Valsalva a century later. Bartolomeo Eustachio (1520-1574), physician to the Pope and Professor of Anatomy in Rome.

Ewing's tumour Described 1922. James Ewing (1866-1943), Professor of Pathology at Cornell University, New York.

Fallopian tube described 1561. Gabriele Fallopio (1523-1563), Italian man of medicine. He was Professor of Surgery and Anatomy at Padua, where he was also Professor of Botany.

Fallot's tetralogy Described 1888. Etienne-Louis Arthur Fallot (1850-1911), Professor of Hygiene and Legal medicine at Marseilles.

Fanconi syndrome Described 1927. Guido Fanconi (b.1892), Professor of Paediatrics at the University of Zürich.

Fehling's solution Described 1848. Hermann Christian von Fehling (1812-1885), Professor of Chemistry at Stuttgart.

Felty's syndrome Described 1924. Augustus Roi Felty (1895-1963), physician at Hartford Hospital, Connecticut.

Fothergill's operation W.E. Fothergill (1865-1926), English gynaecologist.

Frei test Described 1925. Wilhelm Siegmund Frei (1885-1943), Professor of Dermatology at Berlin; he settled in New York.

Freiberg's disease Described 1914. Albert Henry Freiberg (1869-1940), Cincinnati surgeon.

Friedländer's bacillus Described 1882. (Now known as *Klebsiella pneumoniae*). Carl Friedländer (1847-1887), pathologist at the Friedrichshain Hospital, Berlin.

Friedman's test Maurice H. Friedman (b. 1903), American physician.

Friedreich's ataxia Described 1863. Nicholaus Friedreich (1825-1882), Professor of Pathological Anatomy at Würzburg, later Professor of Pathology and Therapy at Heidelberg.

Fröhlich's syndrome Described 1901. Alfred Fröhlich (1871-1953), Professor of Pharmacology at the University of Vienna.

Gallie's operation Described 1921. William Edward Gallie (1882-1959), Professor of Surgery at the University of Toronto, Canada.

Ganser's state Sigbert Joseph Maria Ganser (1853-1931), psychiatrist at Dresden and Munich.

Gasserian ganglion Johann Laurentius Gasser (1723-1765), Professor of Anatomy at Vienna. He left no writings, and the ganglion was given his name by Anton Hirsch, one of his students, in his thesis of 1765.

Gaucher's disease Described 1882. Philippe Charles Ernest Gaucher (1854-1918), French physician and dermatologist.

Geiger counter Described 1908. Hans Geiger (1882-1945), German physicist who worked with Rutherford at Manchester University.

Ghon's focus Described 1912. Anton Ghon (1866-1936), Professor of Pathological Anatomy at Prague.

Gilliam's operation David Tod Gilliam (1844-1923), Columbus, Ohio, physician.

Girdlestone's operation Gathorne Robert Girdlestone (1881-1950), Nuffield Professor of Orthopaedics at Oxford.

Glisson's capsule Francis Glisson (1597-1677), philosopher, physician and anatomist at Cambridge and London.

Golgi apparatus Described 1898. Camillo Golgi (1843-1926), Professor of Histology and later Rector of the University of Pavia. In 1906 he shared the Nobel Prize with Santiago Ramón y Cajal for work on the nervous sytem.

Goodpasture's syndrome Described 1919. Ernest William Goodpasture (1886-1960), American pathologist.

Graafian follicle Reijnier de Graaf (1641-1673), Dutch physician.

Graefe's knife Friedrich Wilhelm Ernst Albrecht von Graefe (1828-1870), Professor of Ophthalmology in Berlin.

Gram's stain Described 1884. Hans Christian Joachim Gram (1853-1938), Professor of Medicine in Copenhagen. He discovered the stain by accident as a student in Berlin.

Graves' disease Described 1835. Robert James Graves (1796-1853), Irish physician at the Meath Hospital, Dublin, where he was responsible for introducing clinical ward work for medical students.

Grawitz tumour Described 1883. Paul Albert Grawitz (1850-1932), Professor of Pathology at Griefswald.

Guillain-Barré syndrome Described 1916. Georges Guillain (1876-1961), Professor of Neurology at Paris; Jean Alexandre Barré (1880-1967), Professor of Neurology at Strasbourg.

Guthrie test R. Guthrie (b. 1916), American paediatrician.

Hand-Schüller-Christian disease First described 1893. (Described 1915 by Schüller and 1920 by Christian). Alfred Hand Jr. (1868-1949), Phildelphia paediatrician; Artur Schüller (1874-1958), Vienna neurologist; Henry Asbury Christian (1876-1951), Professor of Medicine at Harvard.

Hansen's bacillus (*Mycobacterium leprae*) Discovered 1873. Gerhard Henrik Armauer Hansen (1841-1912), Norwegian physician.

Harris's operation S.H. Harris (1880-1936), Australian surgeon.

Harrison's sulcus Edward Harrison (1766-1838), Lincolnshire general practitioner. Also ascribed to Edwin Harrison (1779-1874), London physician.

Hartmann's solution Described 1932. Alexis Frank Hartmann (1898-1964), St Louis, Missouri, paediatrician.

Hartnup disease Name of the family in which this hereditary disease was first recorded.

Hashimoto's disease Described 1912. Hakuru Hashimoto (1881-1934), Japanese surgeon.

Haversian canals Described 1689. Clopton Havers (1657-1702), English surgeon.

Heberden's nodes Described 1802. William Heberden (1767-1845), London physician, specialist in rheumatic diseases.

Hegar's sign Alfred Hegar (1830-1914), Professor of Obstetrics and Gynaecology at Freiburg.

Heller's operation E. Heller (1877-1964), German surgeon.

Heller's test Johann Florenz Heller (1813-1871), Austrian physician.

Henle's loop Described 1862. Friedrich Gustav Jakob Henle (1809-1885), Professor of Anatomy at Göttingen.

Henoch-Schönlein purpura Described 1832 by Schönlein and 1865 by Henoch. Eduard Heinrich Henoch (1820-1910), Professor of Paedriatrics at Berlin; Johannes Lukas Schönlein (1793-1864), physician and pathologist at Würzburg, Zürich and Berlin.

Hering-Breuer reflex Karl Ewald Konstantin Hering (1834-1918), physiologist in Vienna and Leipzig; Josef Breuer (1842-1925), Vienna psychiatrist.

Higginson's syringe Alfred Higginson (1808-1884), Liverpool surgeon.

Highmore (antrum of) Described 1651. Nathaniel Highmore (1613-1685), Dorset physician.

Hirschsprung's disease Described 1888. Harald Hirschsprung (1830-1916), Professor of Paediatrics in Copenhagen.

His (bundle of) Described 1893. Ludwig His (1863-1934), Professor of Anatomy successively at Leipzig, Basle, Göttingen and Berlin.

Hodgkin's disease Described 1832. Thomas Hodgkin (1798-1866), London physician.

Homans' sign Described 1941. John Homans (1877-1954), Professor of Clinical Surgery at Harvard.

Horner's syndrome Described 1869. Johann Friedrich Horner (1831-1886), Professor of Ophthalmology at Zürich.

Horton's headache, syndrome Bayard Taylor Horton (b. 1895), Minnesota physician.

Huhner's test Max Huhner (1873-1947), New York urologist.

Huntington's chorea Described 1872. George Sumner Huntington (1850-1916), New York physician.

Hurler's syndrome Described 1920. Gertrud Hurler, Munich paediatrician.

Hutchinson's tooth Sir Jonathan Hutchinson (1828-1913), English surgeon.

Jacksonian epilepsy Described 1863. John Hughlings Jackson (1835-1911), English neurologist.

Jacquemier's sign Jean Marie Jacquemier (1806-1879), French obstetrician.

Kahn test Described 1922. Reuben Leon Kahn, Lithuanian-born serologist who worked in the USA.

Kaposi's sarcoma Described 1872. Moritz Kohn Karposi (1837-1902), Professor of Dermatology at Vienna.

Kayser-Fleischer rings Described 1902 by Kayser, 1903 by Fleischer. Bernard Kayser (1869-1954), German ophthalmologist; Bruno Richard Fleischer (1848-1904), German physician.

Keller's operation Described 1904. William Lordan Keller (1874-1959), American surgeon.

Kernig's sign Described 1882. Vladimir Mikhailovich Kernig (1840-1917), St Petersburg neurologist.

Killian's operation Gustav Killian (1860-1921), Berlin laryngologist.

Kimmelstiel-Wilson disease Described 1936. Paul Kimmelstiel (1900-1970), Boston pathologist; Clifford Wilson (1906-1998), Professor of Medicine, London University.

Kirschner wire Described 1909. Martin Kirschner (1879-1942), Professor of Surgery at Heidelberg.

Klebs-Leoffler bacillus (*Borynebacterium diphtheriae*) Theodor Albrecht Klebs (1834-1913), bacteriologist in Zürich and Chicago; Friedrich August Loeffler (1852-1915), Berlin bacteriologist.

Klinefelter's syndrome Described 1942. Harry Fitch Klinefelter Jr. (b. 1912), Associate Professor of Medicine, John Hopkins Medical School, Baltimore.

Klumpke's paralysis Described 1885. Augusta Klumpke (Madame Déjerine-Klumpke) (1859-1937), Paris neurologist, one of the first women to qualify there in 1888.

Koch's bacillus (*Mycobacterium tuberculosis*) Described 1882. Robert Koch (1843-1910), Professor of Hygiene in Berlin, later Director of the Institute for Infectious Diseases. (Nobel Prize 1905).

Köhler's disease Described 1908 and 1926. Alban Köhler (1874-1947), German radiologist.

Koplik's spots Described 1896. Henry Koplik (1858-1927), American paediatrician.

Korsakoff's syndrome, psychosis Described 1887. Sergei Sergeyevich Korsakoff (1854-1900), Russian psychiatrist.

Krause corpuscles Described 1860. Wilhelm Johann Friedrich Krause (1833-1910), Göttingen and Berlin anatomist.

Krebs cycle Described 1937. Sir Hans Adolf Krebs (1900-1981), German biochemist who emigrated to England in 1934. Shared the Nobel prize for Medicine 1953 with F.A. Lipmann.

Krukenberg tumour Friedrich Krukenberg (1871-1946), Bonn gynaecologist.

Kuntscher nail Described 1940. Gerhard Kuntscher (1900-1972), Kiel surgeon.

Kupffer's cells Described 1876. Karl Wilhelm von Kupffer (1829-1902), German anatomist.

Kveim test Morten Ansgar Kveim (b. 1892), Oslo physician.

Laennec's cirrhosis Described 1819. René Théophile Hyacinthe Laennec (1781-1826), Professor of medicine at the Collège de France, and inventor of the stethoscope.

Landry's paralysis Jean-Baptiste Octave Landry (1826-1865), Paris physician.

Lange test Described 1912. Carl Friedrich August Lange (b. 1883), German physician.

Langerhans (islets of) Described 1869. Paul Langerhans (1847-1888), Professor of Pathological Anatomy at Freiburg.

Lassa fever named after a village in northern Nigeria where the fever was first reported.

Lassar's paste Oskar Lassar (1849-1907), Berlin dermatologist.

Legg-Calvé-Perthes disease Described 1910 separately by all three workers. Arthur Thornton Legg (1874-1939), American orthopaedic surgeon; Jacques Calvé (1875-1954), French orthopaedic surgeon; Georg Clemens Perthes (1869-1927), Leipzig surgeon.

Lembert's suture Described 1826. Antoine Lembert (1802-1851), Paris surgeon.

Leydig's cells Described 1850. Franz von Leydig (1821-1908), Professor of Histology at Würzburg, Tübingen and then Bonn.

Lieberkuhn's glands Described 1745. Johann Nathaniel Lieberkuhn (1711-1756), Berlin anatomist and physician.

Little's disease Described 1843. William John Little (1810-1894), physician at the London Hospital.

Ludwig's angina Described 1836. Wilhelm Friedrich von Ludwig (1790-1865), Professor of Surgery and Midwifery at Tübingen, and Court Physician to King Frederick II.

Magendie (foramen of) Described 1828. François Magendie (1783-1855), Paris physician and physiologist.

Mallory-Weiss tears Described 1929. G. Kenneth Mallory (b. 1900), Professor of Pathology, Boston University.

Malpighian body Described 1666. Marcello Malpighi (1628-1694), anatomist and physiologist in Rome and Bologna.

Mantoux test Described 1908. Charles Mantoux (1877-1947), Paris physician.

Marfan's syndrome Described 1896. Bernard Jean Antonin Marfan (1858-1942), Paris paediatrician.

McBurney's point Described 1899. Charles McBurney (1845-1913), New York surgeon.

Meckel's diveticulum Described 1809. Johann Friedrich Meckel II (1781-1833), Halle surgeon and anatomist.

Meissner's plexus Described 1853. Georg Meissner (1829-1905), German anatomist and physiologist.

Mendel's laws Described 1865. Gregor Johann Mendel (1822-1884), Austrian Augustinian monk and naturalist of Brno, whose work was rediscovered by de Vries in 1900.

Mendelson's syndrome Described 1946. Curtis L. Mendelson (b. 1913), American obstetrician and gynaecologist.

Ménière's disease Described 1861. Prosper Ménière (1799-1862) and his son, Emile Antoine Ménière (1839-1905), Paris physicians.

Merkel's disc Friedrich Siegmund Merkel (1845-1919), German anatomist.

Michel's clips Gaston Michel (1874-1937), Professor of Clinical Surgery at Nancy.

Milroy's disease Described 1892. William Forsyth Milroy (1855-1942), Professor of Clinical medicine in Nebraska.

Mönckeberg's arteriosclerosis Described 1903. Johann Georg Mönckeberg (1877-1925), Bonn physician and pathologist.

Montgomery's glands William Fetherstone Montgomery (1797-1859), Dublin gynaecologist.

Mooren's ulcer Albert Mooren (1828-1899), ophthalmologist in Düsseldorf.

Moro reflex Ernst Moro (1874-1951), paediatrician in Heidelberg.

Müllerian duct Described 1825. Johannes Peter Müller (1801-1858), Professor of Anatomy at Bonn, later Professor of Anatomy and Physiology at Berlin.

Munchhausen's syndrome Described by Richard Asher in 1951, and named after Baron von Munchhausen, a 16th century traveller and inveterate liar.

Murphy's sign Described 1912. John Benjamin Murphy (1857-1916), Chicago surgeon.

Negri bodies Described 1903. Adelchi Negri (1876-1912), Professor of Bacteriology at Pavia.

Nissl bodies Described 1894. Franz Nissl (1860-1919), Heidelberg psychiatrist.

Ortolani's sign Described 1937. Marius Ortolani, contemporary Italian orthopaedic surgeon.

Osler's nodes Described 1885. Sir William Osler (1849-1919), Professor of Medicine in Montreal, Philadelphia, Baltimore and then Oxford.

Pacinian corpuscles Described 1835. Filippo Pacini (1812-1883), anatomist and physiologist in Pisa and Florence.

Paget's disease Described 1877. Sir James Paget (1814-1899), London surgeon.

Papanicolaou test Described 1933. George Nicholas Papanicolaou (1883-1962), Greek anatomist and physician who worked in the USA.

Parkinson's disease Described 1817. James Parkinson (1755-1824), English physician.

Paschen body Enrique Paschen (1860-1936), Hamburg pathologist.

Pasteurization Louis Pasteur (1822-1895), Paris chemist and bacteriologist.

Paul-Bunnell reaction Described 1932. John Rodman Paul (b. 1893), New Haven physician; Walls Willard Bunnell (1902-1966), Connecticut physician.

Paul's tube Described 1891. Frank Thomas Paul (1851-1941), English surgeon.

Pel-Ebstein fever Described 1885. Pieter Klaases Pel (1852-1919), Professor of Medicine in Amsterdam; Wilhelm Ebstein (1836-1912), Professor of Medicine at Göttingen.

Pelligrini-Stieda disease Described 1905. Augusto Pelligrini, surgeon in Florence; Alfred Stieda (1869-1945), Professor of Surgery at Königsberg.

Peyer's patches Described 1677. Johann Conrad Peyer (1653-1712), Swiss anatomist.

Peyronie's disease Described 1743. François de la Peyronie (1678-1747), Surgeon to Louis XV in Paris.

Placido's disc A. Placido, Portuguese oculist.

Plummer-Vinson syndrome Described 1912 by Plummer, 1919 by Vinson (also described in 1919 by Patterson and Brown Kelly, whose names are frequently associated with the syndrome). Henry Stanley Plummer (1874-1937), Minnesota physician; Porter Paisley Vinson (1890-1959), physician at the Mayo Clinic, Minnesota.

Politzer's bag Described 1863. Adam Politzer (1835-1920), Professor of Otology in Vienna.

Pott's disease Described 1779.

Pott's fracture Described 1765. Sir Percivall Pott (1714-1788), London surgeon.

Poupart's ligament Described 1705. François Poupart (1616-1708), Paris surgeon and anatomist.

Purkinje cells described 1837.

Purkinje fibres Described 1839. Johannes Evangelista Purkinje (1787-1869), Professor of Physiology at Breslau and then Prague.

Queckenstedt test Described 1916. Hans Heinrich George Queckenstedt (1876-1918), German physician.

Quick test Described 1932. Armand James Quick (1894-1978), Professor of Biochemistry, Marquette University.

Ramstedt's operation Described 1912. Wilhelm Conrad Ramstedt (1867-1963), Münster surgeon.

Raynaud's disease Described 1862. Maurice Raynaud (1834-1881), Paris physician.

Reaven's syndrome Described 1988. Gerald Reaven, Californian physician.

Reiter's syndrome Described 1916. Hans Conrad Reiter (1881-1969), German bacteriologist and hygienist.

Rinne's test Described 1855. Friedrich Heinrich Rinne (1819-1868), otologist at Göttingen.

Roentgen Named after Wilhelm Konrad von Röntgen (1845-1923), physicist at Strasbourg, Geissen. Würzburg and Munich, and then Director of the physics laboratory at Würzburg where he discovered X-rays in 1895. Nobel prize for Physics 1901.

Romberg's sign Described 1846. Moritz Heinrich Romberg (1795-1873), Berlin physician and pioneer neurologist.

Rorschach test Described 1921. Hermann Rorschach (1884-1922), German-born psychiatrist who worked in Bern, Switzerland.

Roth spots Moritz Roth (1839-1915), Basle pathologist and physician.

Rothera's test Arthur Cecil Hamel Rothera (1880-1915), biochemist in Melbourne, Australia.

Rovsing's sign Described 1907. Nils Thorkild Rovsing (1862-1927), Professor of Surgery at Copenhagen.

Rubin's test Isador Clinton Rubin (b. 1883), New York gynaecologist.

Ruffini corpuscles Described 1893. Angelo Ruffini (1864-1929), histologist at Bologna.

Russell traction (Hamilton Russell traction) Described 1924. R. Hamilton Russell (1860-1933), Melbourne surgeon.

Ryle's tube Described 1921. John Alfred Ryle (1882-1950), physician at London, Cambridge and Oxford.

Sabin vaccine Developed 1955. Albert Bruce Sabin (1906-1993), Russian-born New York bacteriologist.

Salk vaccine Developed 1954. Jonas Edward Salk (1914-1995), virologist in Pittsburgh.

Sayre's jacket Lewis Albert Sayre (1820-1901), New York surgeon.

Scarpa's triangle Antonio Scarpa (1747-1832), Italian anatomist and surgeon.

Scheuermann's disease Described 1920. Holger Werfel Scheuermann (1877-1960), Danish orthopaedic surgeon and radiologist.

Schick test Described 1908. Bela Schick (1877-1967), paediatrician in Vienna and New York.

Schilling test Robert Frederick Schilling (b. 1919), Wisconsin physician.

Schlatter's disease Described 1903. Carl Schlatter (1864-1934), Professor of Surgery at Zürich.

Schlemm's canal Described 1830. Friedrich Schlemm (1795-1858), Professor of Anatomy in Berlin.

Schönlein-Henoch purpura *see* HENOCH-SCHONLEIN PURPURA.

Schwann cell Described 1839. Friedrich Theodor Schwann (1810-1882), German anatomist.

Schwartze's operation Hermann Schwartze (1837-1910), Halle otologist.

Sengstaken tube Robert William Sengstaken (b. 1923), New Jersey surgeon.

Sertoli cells Described 1865. Enrico Sertoli (1842-1910), Italian histologist, Professor of Experimental Physiology at Milan.

Shirodkar's operation N. V. Shirodkar (1900-1971), Indian obstetrician.

Simmonds' disease Described 1914. Morris Simmonds (1855-1925), German physician and pathologist.

Sippy diet Bertram Welton Sippy (1866-1924), physician in Chicago.

Skene's glands Described 1880. Alexander Johnston Chalmers Skene (1838-1900), Scottish-born New York gynaecologist.

Smith-Petersen nail Described 1931. Marius Nygaard Smith-Petersen (1886-1953), Norwegian-born Boston orthopaedic surgeon.

Snellen chart Described 1862. Hermann Snellen (1834-1908), Utrecht ophthalmologist.

Sonne dysentry Described 1915. Carl Olaf Sonne (1882-1948), Danish bacteriologist and physician.

Sprengel's deformity Described 1891. Otto Gerhard Karl Sprengel (1852-1915), German surgeon.

Stacke's operation Ludwig Stacke (1859-1918), German otologist.

Stein-Leventhal syndrome Described 1935. Irving F. Stein (b. 1887), American gynaecologist; Michael Leo Leventhal (1901-1971), American obstetrician and gynaecologist.

Steinmann's pin Described 1907. Fritz Steinmann (1872-1932), Berne surgeon.

Stellwag's sign Carl Stellwag von Carion (1823-1904), ophthalmologist in Vienna.

Stensen's duct described 1661. Niels Stensen (1638-1686), Danish physician and priest, anatomist, physiologist and theologian.

Stevens-Johnson syndrome Described 1922. Albert Mason Stevens (1884-1945), Frank Chambliss Johnson (1894-1934), physicians in New York.

Still's disease Described 1896. Sir George Frederic Still (1868-1941), London paediatrician and physician to the King.

St Louis encephalitis From St Louis, Missouri, where it was first diagnosed.

Stokes-Adams syndrome William Stokes (1804-1878), Irish physician; Robert Adams (1791-1875), Irish surgeon.

Sudeck's atrophy Described 1900. Paul Hermann Martin Sudeck (1866-1938), Hamburg surgeon.

Sydenham's chorea Described 1686. Thomas Sydenham (1624-1689), English physician.

Syme's amputation Described 1842. James Syme (1799-1870), Edinburgh surgeon and teacher; one of the first to adopt antisepsis (Joseph Lister was his son-in-law), and also among the early users of anaesthesia.

Tay-Sachs disease Described 1881. Warren Tay (1843-1927), London ophthalmologist; Bernard Sachs (1858-1944), New York neurologist.

Tenon's capsule Jacques René Tenon (1724-1816), Paris surgeon.

Thiersch's graft Described 1874. Karl Thiersch (1822-1895), German surgeon.

Thomas's Splint Described 1875. Hugh Owen Thomas (1834-1891), Liverpool surgeon and bonesetter.

Trendelburg operation (position, sign) Friedrich Trendelburg (1844-1924), Leipzig surgeon.

Trousseau's sign Armand Trousseau (1801-1867), Paris physician.

Turner's syndrome Described 1938. Henry Hubert Turner (b. 1892), American endocrinologist, Clinical professor of Medicine, Oklahoma University.

van den Bergh test A.A. Hijmans van den Bergh (1869-1943), Dutch physician.

Vaquez-Osler disease Henri Vaquez (1860-1936), Paris physician, Sir William Osler (1849-1919), Professor of Medicine in Montreal, Philadelphia, Baltimore and then Oxford.

Varolii (pons) Constanzo Varolius (1543-1575), Italian physician and anatomist, doctor to Pope Gregory XIII.

Vincent's angina Described 1898. Jean Hyacinthe Vincent (1862-1950), physician and bacteriologist in Paris.

Volkmann's canal, contracture Richard von Volkmann (1830-1889), German surgeon.

von Recklinghausen's disease Described 1882. Friedrich Daniel von Recklinghausen (1833-1910), Professor of Pathology at Strasbourg.

von Willebrand's disease Described 1926. E. A. von Willebrand (1870-1949), Finnish physician.

Waldeyer's ring Described 1884. Heinrich Wilhelm Gottfried Waldeyer-Hartz (1836-1921), Berlin anatomist.

Wangensteen tube Described 1832. Owen Harding Wangensteen (1898-1980), Minneapolis surgeon.

Wassermann reaction, test Described 1906. August Paul von Wassermann (1866-1925), Berlin bacteriologist.

Waterhouse-Friderichsen syndrome Described 1911 by Rupert Waterhouse (1873-1958), physician at Bath; described 1918 by Carl Friderichsen (b. 1886), Copenhagen physician.

Waterston's anastomosis David James Waterston (1910-1985), paediatric surgeon in London.

Weber-Christian disease Frederick Parkes Weber (1863-1962), London physician; Henry Asbury Christian (1876-1951), Boston physician.

Weber's test Friedrich Eugen Weber-Liel (1832-1891), German otologist.

Weil-Felix test, reaction Described 1916. Edmund Weil (1880-1922) Viennese physician and bacteriologist; Arthur Felix (1887-1956), London bacteriologist.

Weil's disease Described 1886. Adolf Weil (1848-1916), physician in Estonia who also practised in Wiesbaden.

Wernicke's encephalopathy Described 1875. Karl Wernicke (1848-1905), Breslau psychiatrist and neurologist.

Wertheim's operation Described 1900. Ernst Wertheim (1864-1920), Vienna gynaecologist.

Wharton's duct, jelly Thomas Wharton (1614-1673), English physician and anatomist at St Thomas's Hospital, London.

Wheelhouse's operation Claudius Galen Wheelhouse (1826-1909), Leeds surgeon.

Whipple's disease Described 1907. George Hoyt Whipple (1878-1976), American pathologist. Nobel prize for Pathology and Medicine 1934.

Widal reaction Described 1896. Georges Fernand Isidore Widal (1862-1929), Paris physician and teacher.

Willis (circle of) Described 1664. Thomas Willis (1621-1675), English physician and anatomist.

Wilms' tumour Described 1899. Max Wilms (1867-1918), Professor of Surgery at Leipzig, Basle and Heidelberg.

Wilson's disease Described 1912. Samuel Alexander Kinnier Wilson (1878-1937), London neurologist.

Wood's lamp Robert Williams Wood (1868-1955), Baltimore physicist.

Zollinger-Ellison syndrome Described 1955. Robert Milton Zollinger (b. 1903), Professor of Surgery at Ohio State University; Edwin H. Ellison (1918-1970), Associate Professor of Surgery at Ohio State University.

DRUGS

drug	type	use
acarbose	oral antidiabetic	type 2 diabetes
aciclovir	antiviral	herpes, varicella
alfuzosin hydrochloride	alpha-blocker	relax smooth muscle in urinary retention
Algicon®	antacid	gastro-intestinal disease
allopurinol	reduces uric acid	gout
amantadine hydrochloride	dopamine agonist	parkinsonism
amiloride hydrochloride	potassium-sparing diuretic	hypertension, oedema
aminophylline	theophylline bronchodilator	asthma
amiodarone hydrochloride	anti-arrhythmic	cardiac arrhythmias
amitriptyline	tricyclic antidepressant	depression
amlodipine besylate	calcium-channel blocker	hypertension, angina
amoxycillin	penicillin antibacterial	see ampicillin
amphotericin	antifungal	Candida, oral infection
ampicillin	penicillin antibacterial	sinusitis, gonorrhoea, urinary tract infection
Asilone® (aluminium hydroxide)	antacid	dyspepsia
aspirin (acetylsalicylic acid)	analgesic, antiplatelet oral anticoagulant	pyrexia, analgesia, prophylaxis of thrombus
atenolol	beta-blocker	hypertension, angina, arrhythmia
azathioprine	cytotoxic immunosuppressant	suppression of transplant organ rejection, inflammatory disease
azithromycin	macrolide antibacterial	respiratory tract infection, chlamydia, otitis media
baclofen	skeletal muscle relaxant	spasticity from trauma & multiple sclerosis
beclomethasone dipropionate	corticosteroid	anti-inflammatory, asthma
bendrofluazide	diuretic	hypertension, oedema
benzhexol hydrochloride	muscarinic antagonist	parkinsonism
benzylpenicillin	penicillin antibacterial	throat infections, otitis media, meningococcal meningitis
betamethasone	corticosteroid	inflammation
bezafibrate	lipid-lowering	hyperlipidaemia
biphasic insulin	insulin antidiabetic	diabetes
bisacodyl	stimulant laxative	constipation
budesonide	corticosteroid	anti-inflammatory, asthma
bumetanide	diuretic	hypertension, oedema
bupivacaine hydrochloride	local anaesthetic	spinal block in surgery & labour
captopril	angiotensin-converting enzyme (ACE) inhibitor	hypertension, heart failure

carbamazepine	antiepileptic	epilepsy, neuropathy, neuralgia
carbimazole	antithyroid	hyperthyroidism
cefaclor	cephalosporin antibacterial	septicaemia, meningitis, pneumonia, urinary tract infection
cefuroxime	cephalosporin antibacterial	sinusitis, gonorrhoea, urinary tract infection
cephradine	cephalosporin antibacterial	sinusitis, gonorrhoea, urinary tract infection
certoparin	parenteral anticoagulant	venous thrombosis, pulmonary embolism
cetirizine	antihistamine	allergy
chloramphenicol	antibacterial	eye infection
chlormethiazole	hypnotic	insomnia, restlessness
chloroquine	antimalarial	prophylaxis & treatment of malaria
chlorpheniramine maleate	antihistamine	allergy, anaphylaxis
chlorpromazine hydrochloride	antipsychotic	schizophrenia, psychosis, mania
cimetidine	H_2-receptor antagonist	gastric and duodenal ulcers
ciprofloxacin	4-quinolone antibacterial	gram-negative infection such as salmonella, eye infection
cisapride	gut motility stimulant	oesphageal reflux, non-ulcer dyspepsia
citalopram	selective serotonin re-uptake inhibitor (SSRI)	depression
clarithromycin	macrolide antibacterial	respiratory tract infection, skin infection
co-amoxiclav	penicillin antibacterial	see ampicillin
co-beneldopa	dopamine precursor & enzyme inhibitor	parkinsonism
co-careldopa	dopamine precursor & enzyme inhibitor	parkinsonism
codeine phosphate	opioid analgesic	analgesia, antidiarrhoeal, cough suppressant
co-fluampicil	penicillin antibacterial	mixed infection
colchicine	anti-inflammatory	gout
cyclizine	antihistamine	nausea, vomiting
cyclosporin	corticosteroid	prevention of tissue & organ transplant rejection
cyproterone acetate	anti-androgen	prostate cancer
danazol	inhibitor of pituitary gonadotrophins	endometriosis, menstrual disorders
dexamethasone	corticosteroid	inflammation, allergy, tumour suppression
diamorphine hydrochloride	opioid analgesic	severe pain
diazepam	benzodiazepine anxiolytic	anxiety, insomnia
diclofenac sodium	non-steroidal anti-inflammatory drug (NSAID)	rheumatic disease, gout
digoxin	cardiac glycoside	atrial fibrillation
dihydrocodeine tartrate	opioid analgesic	severe pain

diltiazem hydrochloride	calcium-channel blocker	hypertension, angina
dipyridamole	antiplatelet oral anticoagulant	prophylaxis of thrombus
disodium etidronate	biphosphonate drug for bone metabolism	osteoporosis, Paget's disease
disopyramide	anti-arrhythmic	cardiac arrhythmia
domperidone	anti-nausea	nausea, vomiting
dopamine hydrochloride	inotropic sympathomimetic	cardiac shock
dorzolamide	carbonic anhydrase inhibitor	glaucoma
dothiepin hydrochloride	tricyclic antidepressant	depression
doxazosin	alpha-blocker	hypertension
doxycycline	tetracycline antibacterial	chlamydia, acne
enalapril maleate	angiotensin-converting enzyme (ACE) inhibitor	hypertension, heart failure
ergometrine maleate	obstetric drug	haemorrhage, labour
erythromycin	macrolide antibacterial	alternative to penicillin in sensitive patients
famciclovir	antiviral	herpes
ferrous sulphate	oral iron salt	iron deficiency anaemia
flucloxacillin	penicillin antibacterial	staphylococcal infection
fluconazole	triazole	antifungal Candida
fludrocortisone acetate	corticosteroid	replacement in adrenocortical insufficiency
fluoxetine	selective serotonin re-uptake inhibitor (SSRI)	depression
flupenthixol decanoate	thioxanthene antipsychotic	schizophrenia, psychosis, depression
flutamide	anti-androgen	prostate cancer
fluticasone propionate	corticosteroid	anti-inflammatory, asthma
folic acid	nutrient	anaemia, prevention of foetal neural tube defect
frusemide	diuretic	hypertension, oedema, heart failure
gaviscon®	antacid	dyspepsia
gemfibrozil	lipid-lowering	hyperlipidaemia
gentamicin	aminoglycoside antibacterial	septicaemia, pneumonia, meningitis
glibenclamide	sulphonylurea oral antidiabetic	type 2 diabetes
gliclazide	sulphonylurea oral antidiabetic	type 2 diabetes
glucagon	pancreatic hormone	hypoglycaemia
glyceryl trinitrate	nitrate	angina
goserelin	anti-endocrine drug	endometriosis, breast & prostate cancer
haloperidol	butyrophenone antipsychotic	schizophrenia, psychosis, mania
halothane	inhalation anaesthetic	induction of general anaesthesia
heparin	parenteral anticoagulant	venous thrombosis, pulmonary embolism
hydralazine hydrochloride	vasodilator anti-hypertensive	hypertension
hydrocortisone	corticosteroid	inflammation
hydroxocobalamin	parenteral form of vitamin B_{12}	anaemia
hydroxyzine hydrochloride	antihistamine	anxiety, pruritus

hypromellose	artificial tears	tear deficiency
ibuprofen	non-steroidal anti-inflammatory drug (NSAID)	rheumatic disease, dysmenorrhoea, fever & pain in children
indapamide	diuretic	hypertension, oedema
indomethacin	non-steroidal anti-inflammatory drug (NSAID)	rheumatic disease, gout, dysmenorrhoea
indoramin	alpha-blocker	hypertension
insulin lispro	insulin antidiabetic	diabetes
ipratropium bromide	antimuscarinic bronchodilator	asthma, chronic obstructive pulmonary disease
isophane insulin	insulin antidiabetic	diabetes
isosorbide mononitrate	nitrate	angina
ketoconazole	antifungal	systemic mycosis
labetalol hydrochloride	beta-blocker	hypertension
lacidipine	calcium-channel blocker	hypertension, angina
lactulose	osmotic laxative	constipation
lamotrigine	antiepileptic	epilepsy
lansoprazole	proton pump inhibitor	oesophagitis, peptic ulceration
levodopa	dopamine precursor	parkinsonism
levonorgestrel	sex hormones	contraception
lignocaine hydrochloride	anti-arrhythmic	cardiac arrhythmia
lignocaine hydrochloride	local anaesthetic	surface use, nerve block
lisinopril	angiotensin-converting enzyme (ACE) inhibitor	hypertension, heart failure
lithium carbonate	antipsychotic	psychosis, depression
lofepramine	tricyclic antidepressant	depression
loperamide hydrochloride	antimotility	anti-diarrhoeal
loratadine	antihistamine	allergy
lorazepam	benzodiazepine anxiolytic	anxiety, insomnia
losartan potassium	angiotensin-II receptor antagonist	hypertension
magnesium trisilicate	antacid	dyspepsia
mannitol	osmotic diuretic	cerebral oedema
mebendazole	anthelmintic	threadworm, roundworm, hookworm
mebeverine hydrochloride	antimuscarinic antispasmodic	irritable bowel syndrome, diverticular disease
mefenamic acid	non-steroidal anti-inflammatory drug (NSAID)	rheumatic disease, osteoarthrosis, dysmenorrhoea
mefloquine	antimalarial	prophylaxis & treatment of malaria
mesalazine	aminosalicylate	ulcerative colitis, Crohn's disease
metformin hydrochloride	oral antidiabetic	type 2 diabetes
methyl phenidate	stimulant	attention-deficit hyperactivity disorder
metoclopramide hydrochloride	anti-nausea	nausea, vomiting
metolazone	diuretic	hypertension, oedema, heart failure
metronidazole	antimicrobial	anaerobic infection, protozoal infection

minocycline	tetracycline antibacterial	chlamydia, acne, meningococcal prophylaxis
morphine salts	opioid analgesic	severe pain
naproxen	non-steroidal anti-inflammatory drug (NSAID)	rheumatic disease, gout, dysmenorrhoea
neomycin sulphate	antibacterial	ear and skin infections
nicardipine hydrochloride	calcium-channel blocker	hypertension, angina
nicorandil	potassium-channel activator	angina
nifedipine	calcium-channel blocker	hypertension, angina
nitrazepam	benzodiazepine hypnotic	insomnia
nitrofurantoin	4-quinolone antibacterial	urinary tract infection
nitrous oxide	inhalation anaesthetic	analgesia in obstetrics, maintenance of anaesthesia
norethisterone	sex hormones	contraception, hormone replacement therapy
nystatin	antifungal	Candida
ofloxacin	4-quinolone antibacterial	urinary & respiratory tract infections, skin
omeprazole	proton pump inhibitor	oesophagitis, peptic ulceration
orphenadrine hydrochloride	antimuscarinic	parkinsonism
oxazepam	benzodiazepine anxiolytic	anxiety
oxybutynin hydrochloride	antimuscarinic	urinary frequency
oxytetracycline	tetracycline antibacterial	chlamydia, acne, respiratory infection
paracetamol	non-opioid analgesic	analgesia, pyrexia
paroxetine	selective serotonin re-uptake inhibitor (SSRI)	depression
perindopril	angiotensin-converting enzyme (ACE) inhibitor	hypertension, heart failure
pethidine hydrochloride	opioid analgesic	obstetric analgesia, severe pain
phenelzine	monoamine-oxidase inhibitor (MAOI)	depression
phenindione	oral anticoagulant	venous thrombosis, pulmonary embolism
phenoxymethylpenicillin	penicillin antibacterial	otitis media, tonsillitis, pneumococcal infection
phenytoin	antiepileptic	epilepsy
pholcodine	opioid analgesic	cough suppressant
pilocarpine	miotic muscarinic agonist	glaucoma
piperazine	anthelmintic	threadworm, roundworm
piroxicam	non-steroidal anti-inflammatory drug (NSAID)	rheumatic disease, gout
pizotifen	antihistamine, serotonin agonist	migraine prophylaxis
polymyxin sulphate	antibacterial	eye infection
pravastatin	statin	hyperlipidaemia, coronary heart disease
prednisolone	corticosteroid	inflammation, allergy

prochlorperazine	antinausea	nausea, vomiting
procyclidine hydrochloride	antimuscarinic	parkinsonism
progesterone	sex hormone	endometriosis, contraception, hormone replacement therapy
proguanil hydrochloride	antimalarial	prophylaxis of malaria
propranolol hydrochloride	beta-blocker	hypertension, angina, arrhythmia, migraine prophylaxis
propylthiouracil	antithyroid	hyperthyroidism
raloxifene hydrochloride	oestrogen modulator	osteoporosis
ranitidine	H_2-receptor antagonist	gastric and duodenal ulcers
risperidone	antipsychotic	psychosis
salbutamol	beta$_2$-adrenoceptor agonist bronchodilator	asthma
salmeterol	beta$_2$-adrenoceptor agonist bronchodilator	asthma
senna	stimulant laxative	constipation
sertraline	selective serotonin re-uptake inhibitor (SSRI)	depression
simvastatin	statin	hyperlipidaemia, coronary heart disease
sodium cromoglycate	cromoglycate	asthma, allergy
sodium valproate	antiepileptic	epilepsy
soluble insulin	insulin antidiabetic	diabetes
spironolactone	aldosterone antagonist diuretic	hypertension, oedema
streptokinase	fibrinolytic	venous thrombosis, pulmonary embolism, myocardial infarction
streptomycin	antibacterial	tuberculosis
sulphasalazine	aminosalicylate	ulcerative colitis, Crohn's disease
sumatriptan	serotonin-1-agonist	migraine
tamoxifen	oestrogen receptor antagonist	breast cancer, infertility
tamsulosin hydrochloride	alpha-blocker	relax smooth muscle in urinary retention
temazepam	benzodiazepine hypnotic	insomnia
terbinafine	antifungal	ringworm, nail infection
terbutaline sulphate	beta$_2$-adrenoceptor agonist bronchodilator	asthma
testosterone	sex hormone	hypogonadism, hypopituitarism
tetracycline	tetracycline antibacterial	chlamydia, acne, respiratory infection
thiopentone sodium	intravenous anaesthetic	induction of general anaesthesia
thioridazine	antipsychotic	schizophrenia, psychosis, mania
thyroxine sodium	thyroid hormone	hypothyroidism
timolol maleate	beta-blocker	glaucoma
tramadol hydrochloride	opioid analgesic	severe pain
trandolapril	angiotensin-converting enzyme (ACE) inhibitor	hypertension, heart failure
tranexamic acid	antifibrinolytic	stop haemorrhage
tranylcypromine	monoamine-oxidase inhibitor	depression

	(MAOI)	
trazodone hydrochloride	antidepressant	depression
trifluoperazine	antipsychotic	schizophrenia, psychosis
trimethoprim	sulphonamide antibacterial	urinary tract infection, bronchitis
venlafaxine	mixed antidepressant	depression
verapamil	calcium-channel blocker	cardiac arrhythmia
vigabatrin	antiepileptic	epilepsy
warfarin sodium	oral anticoagulant	venous thrombosis, pulmonary embolism
zopiclone	benzodiazepine hypnotic	insomnia

Request for further information

Use this form to request information about our range of dictionaries. Send to:
Peter Collin Publishing, 1 Cambridge Road, Teddington, TW11 8DT, UK
fax: +44 20 8943 1673   tel: +44 20 8943 3386   email: info@petercollin.com

Visit our web site: **www.petercollin.com** for more information, resources and
software versions of the dictionaries.

Title	ISBN	Send Details
English Dictionaries		
Accounting	0-948549-27-0	❏
Aeronautical Terms	1-901659-10-0	❏
Agriculture, 2nd ed	0-948549-78-5	❏
American Business, 2nd ed	1-901659-22-4	❏
Automobile Engineering	0-948549-66-1	❏
Banking & Finance, 2nd ed	1-901659-30-5	❏
Business, 2nd ed	0-948549-51-3	❏
Computing, 3rd ed	1-901659-04-6	❏
Ecology & Environment, 3rd ed	0-948549-74-2	❏
English Dictionary for Students	1-901659-06-2	❏
Government & Politics, 2nd ed	0-948549-89-0	❏
Hotels, Tourism, Catering Management	0-948549-40-8	❏
Human Resources & Personnel, 2nd ed	0-948549-79-3	❏
Information Technology, 2nd ed	0-948549-88-2	❏
Law, 3rd ed	1-901659-43-7	❏
Library and Information Management	0-948549-68-8	❏
Marketing, 2nd ed	0-948549-73-4	❏
Medicine, 3rd ed	1-901659-45-3	❏
Military Terms	1-901659-24-0	❏
Printing and Publishing, 2nd ed	0-948549-99-8	❏
Vocabulary Workbooks		
Banking and Finance	0-948549-96-3	❏
Business, 2nd ed	0-948549-72-6	❏
Computing, 2nd ed	1-901659-28-3	❏
Colloquial English	0-948549-97-1	❏
English for Students	1-901659-11-9	❏
Hotels, Tourism, Catering	0-948549-75-0	❏
Law, 2nd ed	1-901659-21-6	
Marketing	1-901659-48-8	❏
Medicine, 2nd ed	1-901659-47-X	❏
Bilingual Dictionaries		
Chinese-English		❏
French-English		❏
German-English		❏
Spanish-English		❏

Name: ....

Dept: ....

Address: ....

....

....Postcode: ....Country: ....